6th edition

comprehensive pharmacy review

EDITORS

Leon Shargel, PhD, RPh
Alan H. Mutnick, PharmD, FASHP, RPh
Paul F. Souney, MS, RPh
Larry N. Swanson, PharmD, FASHP, RPh

 Wolters Kluwer | Lippincott Williams & Wilkins
Health

Philadelphia • Baltimore • New York • London
Buenos Aires • Hong Kong • Sydney • Tokyo

Acquisitions Editor: David B. Troy
Managing Editor: Meredith L. Brittain
Marketing Manager: Marisa A. O'Brien
Production Editor: Paula C. Williams
Designer: Holly Reid McLaughlin
Compositor: Maryland Composition, Inc.
Printer: Data Reproductions Corporation

351 West Camden Street
Baltimore, MD 21201

530 Walnut Street
Philadelphia, PA 19106

Fourth Edition, 2001
Fifth Edition, 2004

Library of Congress Cataloging-in-Publication Data

Comprehensive pharmacy review / editors, Leon Shargel ... [et al.].—6th ed.
    p. ; cm.
  Includes index.
  ISBN-13: 978-0-7817-6561-9 (alk. paper)
  ISBN-10: 0-7817-6561-7 (alk. paper)
  1. Pharmacy—Examinations, questions, etc. I. Shargel, Leon, 1941-
  [DNLM: 1. Pharmacy—Examination Questions. QV 18.2 C737 2007]
  RS97.P49 2007
  615'.1076—dc22

               2006034922

To purchase additional copies of this book, call our customer service department at **(800) 638-3030** or fax orders to **(301) 223-2320.** International customers should call **(301) 223-2300.**

Visit Lippincott Williams & Wilkins on the Internet: http://www.LWW.com. Lippincott Williams & Wilkins customer service representatives are available from 8:30 am to 6:00 pm, EST.

07 08 09 10
3 4 5 6 7 8 9 10

6th edition

comprehensive pharmacy review

Preface

As with the previous editions, this 6th edition of *Comprehensive Pharmacy Review* reflects the continuing evolution of pharmacy practice and educational requirements. The main objective of the book is to provide a comprehensive study guide for pharmacy students and other candidates who are preparing for the North American Pharmacist Licensure Examination (NAPLEX). This volume represents the contributions of more than two dozen specialists, each delivering a current summary of his or her field to a review guide that is not only accurate and up to date but also comprehensible to students, teachers, and practitioners alike. This review publication, along with the separate booklet of simulated NAPLEX exams (*Comprehensive Pharmacy Review Practice Exams*, 6th edition) and the CD-ROM that supplements this review (*Comprehensive Pharmacy Review NAPLEX Preparation,* 6th Edition CD-ROM), provides both guidance and test practice for NAPLEX candidates.

Pharmaceutical education, including pharmaceutical science and practice, must prepare pharmacy practitioners for the future. The current pharmaceutical education provides greater career opportunities for pharmacists than ever before. Pharmacists now work in academic pharmacy, community pharmacy, long-term care, and consulting pharmacy, including hospice and home care, pharmaceutical and healthcare distributors, pharmaceutical industry, professional trade organizations, uniformed (public health) services, federal and state governments, hospital and institutional practice settings, and managed care pharmacy. Pharmacists are taking a more active role in healthcare, such as in counseling and medication therapy, disease-state management, and screening programs (diabetes and high cholesterol) as well as the more traditional role of dispensing medication and educating patients. A pharmaceutical education combined with a business (MBA), research (PhD), or law (JD) degree provides opportunities to relate pharmacy practice with other challenging fields.

Although the *Comprehensive Pharmacy Review* is principally written for NAPLEX candidates, the book is also intended for a broader audience of pharmacy undergraduates and health professionals who seek detailed summaries of pharmacy subjects. A wide range of topics central to the study of pharmacy—chemistry, pharmaceutics, pharmacology, pharmacy practice, drug therapy—is organized to parallel the pharmacy curriculum and presented in outline form for easy use. The *Comprehensive Pharmacy Review* may be used as a quick review (or preview) of essential topics by a diverse group of readers, including

- **Matriculating pharmacy students.** The organization and topical coverage of *Comprehensive Pharmacy Review* are such that many pharmacy students will want to purchase it in their first professional year and use it throughout their pharmacy education to prepare for course examinations.
- **Instructors and preceptors.** *Comprehensive Pharmacy Review* also functions as an instructor's manual and a reference for teachers and tutors in pharmacy schools. Chapter outlines can be used to organize courses and to plan specific lectures.
- **Professional pharmacists.** *Comprehensive Pharmacy Review* offers practitioners a convenient handbook of pharmacy facts. It can be used as a course refresher and as a source of recent information on pharmacy practice. The appendices include prescription dispensing information, common prescription drugs, and general pharmacy references.

What's New in This Edition

The continuing evolution of pharmacy practice is reflected by the licensure examinations developed by the National Association of Boards of Pharmacy (NABP) to assess the competence of pharmacy candidates. For this reason, we have requested and have been given permission by NABP to reproduce the competency statements for the NABP examination (NAPLEX) in the frontmatter of this edition of *Comprehensive Pharmacy Review.*

Furthermore, this edition has been extensively revised to reflect the current educational and competency requirements for a successful career in pharmacy. For example, the chapter on drug–drug and drug–nutrient interactions (Chapter 18) has been revised to reflect the greater use of nutraceuticals. A new chapter on medication errors (Chapter 23) has been added to reflect public health concerns by patients receiving drug therapy. Also, a new chapter on bowel disorders (Chapter 53), targeting irritable bowel disease and inflammatory bowel disease, was added because of the significant advances in drug therapy since the publication of the last edition.

Organizational Philosophy and Chapter Structure

The organization of the 6th edition has been revised to reflect the current changes in the undergraduate pharmacy curriculum. Part I, Pharmaceutical Sciences (Chapters 1–19), contains subject matter pertaining to the basic science of pharmacy. Part II, Pharmacy Practice (Chapters 20–61), contains subject matter for the practice of pharmacy with emphasis on pharmaceutical care. Each chapter of the book contains topic outlines and practice questions according to the pharmacy school curriculum.

At the front of the book you'll find guidelines for taking a test and an introduction to the NAPLEX exam, including the actual NAPLEX blueprint. The appendices of the book are compilations of handy reference tables.

Contributors

Loyd V. Allen Jr., PhD
Editor in Chief
International Journal of Pharmaceutical
  Compounding
Edmond, Oklahoma

Anton H. Amann, PhD, RPh
Vice President, Generic Development
Endo Pharmaceuticals
Westbury, New York

Rebekah Arthur, PharmD, BCPS
Assistant Professor
Department of Pharmacy Practice
Campbell University School of Pharmacy
Buies Creek, North Carolina
Clinical Pharmacist in Medicine/Psychiatry
Duke University Medical Center
Durham, North Carolina

Connie Lee Barnes, PharmD
Associate Professor
Director, Drug Information
Department of Pharmacy Practice
Campbell University School of Pharmacy
Buies Creek, North Carolina

Lawrence H. Block, PhD, RPh
Professor of Pharmaceutics
Division of Pharmaceutical Sciences
Mylan School of Pharmacy
Duquesne University
Pittsburgh, Pennsylvania

Riccardo L. Boni, PhD
Assistant Professor of Pharmaceutics
Division of Pharmaceutical Sciences
Mylan School of Pharmacy
Duquesne University
Pittsburgh, Pennsylvania

Donald F. Brophy, PharmD, MS, FCCP, BCPS
Associate Professor
Departments of Pharmacy and Internal
  Medicine
School of Pharmacy
Virginia Commonwealth University
Richmond, Virginia

Todd A. Brown, MHP, RPh
Associate Clinical Specialist and Vice Chair
Department of Pharmacy Practice
Northeastern University
Boston, Massachusetts

Marcia L. Buck, PharmD, FCCP
Clinical Pharmacy Specialist
Department of Pharmacy Services
University of Virginia Health System
Clinical Associate Professor
Department of Pediatrics
University of Virginia
Charlottesville, Virginia

Judy Chase, PharmD, FASHP
Director, Clinical Pharmacy Services
The University of Texas
M.D. Anderson Cancer Center
Division of Pharmacy
Houston, Texas

Robert Cisneros, MS, MBA, PhD
Assistant Professor
Department of Pharmacy Practice
Campbell University School of Pharmacy
Buies Creek, North Carolina

Eric Coldiron, PharmD
Medical Scientific Manager
Field Medical Affairs
Berlex Laboratories Affiliate of Schering AG
Omaha, Nebraska

Ron J. DeBellis, PharmD
Chair and Associate Professor
Department of Pharmacy Practice
Massachusetts College of Pharmacy and
    Health Sciences
Worcester, Massachusetts

Stephen C. Dragotakes, RPh, BCNP
PET Nuclear Pharmacist
Division of Nuclear Medicine, Department
    of Radiology
Massachusetts General Hospital
Boston, Massachusetts
Adjunct Instructor
Department of Pharmacy Practice
Massachusetts College of Pharmacy and
    Allied Health Science
Boston, Massachusetts

Alice C. Engelbrecht, PharmD
Clinical Coordinator for Pharmacy Clinical
    Services
OU Medical Center
Oklahoma City, Oklahoma
Adjunct Professor
Department of Pharmacy Practice
College of Pharmacy, University of
    Oklahoma
Oklahoma City, Oklahoma

Maria Evasovich, MD
Assistant Professor
Department of Surgery
Medical School
University of Minnesota
Minneapolis, Minnesota

John Fanikos, RPh, MBA
Clinical Assistant Professor
Department of Pharmacy Practice
Northeastern University
Massachusetts College of Pharmacy
Boston, Massachusetts
Assistant Director of Pharmacy
Brigham and Women's Hospital
Boston, Massachusetts

Godwin W. Fong, PhD
Senior Consultant, Research and
    Development
Pharmaceutical Development Consulting
Westborough, Massachusetts

Gail Goodman-Snitkoff, PhD
Associate Professor
Department of Basic and Pharmaceutical
    Sciences
Albany College of Pharmacy
Albany, New York

James B. Groce III, PharmD, CACP
Professor
Department of Pharmacy Practice
Campbell University School of Pharmacy
Buies Creek, North Carolina
Clinical Pharmacy
    Specialist—Anticoagulation
Department of Pharmacy
The Moses H. Cone Memorial Hospital
Greensboro, North Carolina

Marc W. Harrold, PhD
Professor of Medicinal Chemistry
Department of Pharmaceutical Sciences
Duquesne University School of Pharmacy
Pittsburgh, Pennsylvania

John E. Janosik, PharmD, RPh
Regional Manager, Primary Care
Scientific Field Operations, Medical Affairs
Roche
Nutley, New Jersey

Alan F. Kaul, PharmD, MS, MBA, FCCP
President
Medical Outcomes Management, Inc.
Foxborough, Massachusetts
Adjunct Professor of Pharmacy
Department of Pharmacy Practice
University of Rhode Island College of
    Pharmacy
Kingston, Rhode Island
Adjunct Professor of Pharmacy Practice
School of Pharmacy
Massachusetts College of Pharmacy and
    Health Sciences
Boston, Massachusetts

Kevin P. Keating, MD
Director, Surgical Critical Care
Department of Surgery
Hartford Hospital
Hartford, Connecticut
Assistant Professor of Surgery
Department of Surgery
University of Connecticut School of
Medicine
Farmington, Connecticut

Julie L. Kelsey, PharmD
Clinical Pharmacy Specialist
Department of Pharmacy Services
University of Virginia Health System
Charlottesville, Virginia

Teresa Klepser, PharmD, BCPS
Associate Professor
Department of Pharmacy Practice
Ferris State University College of
Pharmacy
Big Rapids, Michigan
ProMed Physicians-Family Practice
Portage, Michigan

Charles Lee, MS
Director, Regulatory Affairs
Roche-Regulatory Affairs
Nutley, NJ

Pui-Kai Li, PhD
Associate Professor of Medicinal
Chemistry
Medicinal Chemistry Division Chair
College of Pharmacy
Ohio State University
Columbus, Ohio

Scott F. Long, RPh, PhD
Associate Professor
Department of Pharmaceutical Sciences
Southwestern Oklahoma State University
College of Pharmacy
Weatherford, Oklahoma

D. Byron May, PharmD, BCPS
Associate Professor
Department of Pharmacy Practice
Campbell University School of Pharmacy
Buies Creek, North Carolina
Clinical Specialist—Adult Internal
Medicine
Duke University Medical Center
Durham, North Carolina

David I. Min, PharmD, MS, FCCP
Associate Professor
Department of Pharmacy Practice and
Administration
College of Pharmacy
Western University of Health Sciences
Pomona, California

J. Edward Moreton, PhD
Professor of Pharmacology and Toxicology
Department of Pharmaceutical Sciences
University of Maryland School of Pharmacy
Baltimore, Maryland

**Alan H. Mutnick, PharmD, FASHP,
RPh**
Assistant Director/ Clinical Pharmacy
Services
Department of Pharmacy
University of Virginia Health System
Charlottesville, Virginia
Associate Clinical Professor
Department of Pharmacy Practice
Medical College of Virginia College of
Pharmacy
Richmond, Virginia

**Jeffrey P Norenberg, PharmD, BCNP,
FASHP, FAPhA**
Associate Professor
College of Pharmacy
University of New Mexico Health Sciences
Center
Albuquerque, NM

Laura K. Williford Owens, PharmD
Assistant Professor
Department of Pharmacy Practice
Campbell University School of Pharmacy
Buies Creek, North Carolina
Chief of Pharmacy Services
Carolina Family Health Centers, Inc.
Wilson, North Carolina

Robert C. Pavlan Jr., BS Pharm, JD
Assistant Professor
Department of Pharmacy Practice
Loma Linda University School of Pharmacy
San Bernardino, California

Roy A. Pleasants, PharmD, BCPS
Associate Professor
Department of Pharmacy Practice
Campbell University School of Pharmacy
Buies Creek, North Carolina
Clinical Specialist—Pulmonary
Division of Pulmonary Medicine
Duke University
Durham, NC

John J. Ponzillo, PharmD
Critical Care Pharmacist
Department of Pharmacy
St. John's Mercy Medical Center
St. Louis, Missouri
Adjunct Assistant Professor
Department of Internal Medicine
Division of Pulmonary, Critical Care and
    Sleep Medicine
Saint Louis University
St. Louis, Missouri

Robert A. Quercia, MS, RPh
Clinical Manager
Director, Drug Information Center
Department of Pharmacy
Hartford Hospital
Hartford, Connecticut
Adjunct Associate Professor
University of Connecticut
School of Pharmacy
Storrs, Connecticut

Azita Razzaghi, RPh, PharmD
Manager, Pharmacovigilance
Genzyme Corporation
Cambridge, Massachusetts

Gerald Schumacher, PharmD, MS, PhD
Professor of Pharmacy
Department of Pharmacy Practice
Northeastern University
Boston, Massachusetts

Jamie Shapiro, PharmD
Oncology Pharmacy Practice Resident
The University of Texas
M.D. Anderson Cancer Center
Division of Pharmacy
Houston, Texas

Leon Shargel, PhD, RPh
Applied Biopharmaceutics
Raleigh, North Carolina
Adjunct Associate Professor
Department of Pharmaceutical Sciences
University of Maryland School of
    Pharmacy
Baltimore, Maryland

**Jennifer D. Smith, PharmD, CPP,
    BC-ADM, CDE**
Assistant Professor
Department of Pharmacy Practice
Campbell University School of Pharmacy
Buies Creek, North Carolina
Pharmacist Clinician
Wilson Community Health Center
Wilson, North Carolina

Paul F. Souney, RPh, MS
National Director, Field Medical Affairs
Berlex Laboratories Affiliate of Schering
    AG
Wayne, New Jersey

Linda M. Spooner, PharmD, BCPS
Assistant Professor
Department of Pharmacy Practice
Massachusetts College of Pharmacy and
    Health Sciences
Worcester, Massachusetts

**Larry N. Swanson, PharmD, FASHP,
    RPh**
Professor and Chairman
Department of Pharmacy Practice
Campbell University School of Pharmacy
Buies Creek, North Carolina

Barbara Szymusiak-Mutnick, RPh, MHP
Lake Monticello, Virginia

Tina Harrison Thornhill, PharmD, FASCP, CGP
Associate Professor
Department of Pharmacy Practice
Campbell University School of Pharmacy
Buies Creek, North Carolina

Ashiwel S. Undie, PhD
Associate Professor
Neuroscience, Pharmacology, and
  Molecular Medicine
Department of Pharmaceutical Sciences
University of Maryland School of
  Pharmacy
Baltimore, Maryland

Jenny A. Van Amburgh, BPharm, PharmD, CDE
Assistant Clinical Specialist
Department of Pharmacy Practice
Northeastern University
Boston, Massachusetts

Habiba O. U. Vongtau, PhD
Neuropharmacology Fellow
Department of Pharmaceutical Sciences
University of Maryland School of
  Pharmacy
Baltimore, Maryland

Jennifer L. Whetstone, PhD
Adjunct Assistant Professor of Medicinal
  Chemistry
College of Pharmacy
Ohio State University
Columbus, Ohio

Andrew L. Wilson, PharmD
Chief Pharmacy Officer
National Institutes of Health Clinical
  Center
Bethesda, Maryland

Peter K. Wong, PhD, MS, MBA, RPh
Vice President, Quality & Clinical
  Effectiveness
Department of Clinical Integration
Mercy Health Partners, Southwest Region,
  Ohio
Cincinnati, Ohio
Assistant Clinical Professor
Center for Global Health Systems
  Management and Policy
Boonshoft School of Medicine
Wright State University
Dayton, Ohio

Peggy C. Yarborough, PharmD, MS, BC-ADM, CDE, CPP
Diabetes Clinician and Clinical Pharmacist
  Practitioner
Diabetes Care and Risk Reduction
  Program
Urban Ministries Open Door Clinic
Raleigh, North Carolina
Professor (retired)
Department of Pharmacy Practice
Campbell University School of Pharmacy
Buies Creek, North Carolina

Nelson Shu-Sang Yee, MD, PhD, RPh
Assistant Professor
Division of Hematology, Oncology,
  Blood & Marrow Transplantation
Department of Internal Medicir e
University of Iowa
Carver College of Medicine
Iowa City, Iowa
Attending Physician
University of Iowa Hospitals and Clinics
Iowa City, Iowa

Anthony E. Zimmerman, PharmD, RPh
Associate Professor
Department of Pharmacy Practice
Massachusetts College of Pharmacy
Worcester, Massachusetts
Critical Care Specialist
Mercy Medical Center
Department of Pharmacy
Springfield, Massachusetts

Contents

NAPLEX Blueprint
PART I: Pharmaceutical Sciences

Taking a Test

One of the least attractive aspects of pursuing an education is the necessity of being examined on the material that has been presented. Instructors do not like to prepare tests, and students do not like to take them.

However, students are required to take many examinations during their learning careers, and little if any time is spent acquainting them with the positive aspects of tests and with systematic and successful methods for approaching them. Students perceive tests as punitive and sometimes feel as if they were merely opportunities for the instructor to discover what the student has forgotten or has never learned. Students need to view tests as opportunities to display their knowledge and to use them as tools for developing prescriptions for further study and learning.

While preparing for any exam, class and board exams as well as practice exams, it is important that students learn as much as they can about the subject they will be tested and are prepared to discover just how much they may not know. Students should study to acquire knowledge, not just to prepare for tests. For the well-prepared student, the chances of passing far exceed the chances of failing.

Materials Needed for Test Preparation

In preparing for a test, most students collect far too much study material, only to find that they simply do not have time to go through all of it. They are defeated before they begin because either they cannot get through all the material, leaving areas unstudied, or they race through the material so quickly that they cannot benefit from the activity.

It is generally more efficient for the student to use materials already at hand—that is, class notes, one good outline to cover and strengthen all areas and to quickly review the whole topic, and one good text as a reference for complex material that requires further explanation.

Also, many students attempt to memorize far too much information, rather than learning and understanding less material and then relying on that learned information to determine the answers to questions at the time of the examination. Relying too heavily on memorized material causes anxiety, and the more anxious students become during a test, the less learned knowledge they are likely to use.

Attitude and Approach

A positive attitude and a realistic approach are essential to successful test taking. If the student concentrates on the negative aspects of tests or on the potential for failure, anxiety increases and performance decreases. A negative attitude generally develops if the student concentrates on "I must pass" rather than on "I can pass." "What if I fail?" becomes the major factor motivating the student to run from failure rather than toward success. This results from placing too much emphasis on scores. The score received is only one aspect of test performance. Test performance also indicates the student's ability to use differential reasoning.

In each question with five alternatives, of which one is correct, there are four alternatives that are incorrect. If deductive reasoning is used, the choices can be viewed as having possibilities of being correct. The elimination of wrong choices increases the odds that a student will be able to recognize the correct choice. Even if the correct choice does not become evident, the probability of guessing correctly increases. Eliminating incorrect choices on a test can result in choosing the correct answer.

Answering questions based on what is incorrect is difficult for many students because they have had nearly 20 years of experience taking tests with the implied assertion that knowledge can be displayed only by knowing what is correct. It must be remembered, however, that students can display knowledge by knowing something is wrong, just as they can display it by knowing something is right.

Preparing for the Examination

1. **Study for yourself.** Although some of the material may seem irrelevant, the more you learn now, the less you will have to learn later. Also, do not let the fear of the test rob you of an important part of your education. If you study to learn, the task is less distasteful than studying solely to pass a test.
2. **Review all areas.** You should not be selective by studying perceived weak areas and ignoring perceived strong areas. Cover all of the material, putting added emphasis on weak areas.
3. **Attempt to understand, not just to memorize, the material.** Ask yourself: To whom does the material apply? When does it apply? Where does it apply? How does it apply? Understanding the connections among these points allows for longer retention and aids in those situations when guessing strategies may be needed.

4. **Try to anticipate questions that might appear on the test.** Ask yourself how you might construct a question on a specific topic.
5. **Give yourself a couple days of rest before the test.** Studying up to the last moment will increase your anxiety and cause potential confusion.

Taking the Examination

1. Be sure to pace yourself to use the test time optimally. You should use all of your allotted time; if you finish too early, you probably did so by moving too quickly through the test.
2. Read each question and all the alternatives carefully before you begin to make decisions. Remember, the questions contain clues, as do the answer choices.
3. Read the directions for each question set carefully. You would be amazed at how many students make mistakes in tests simply because they have not paid close attention to the directions.
4. It is not advisable to leave blanks with the intention of coming back to answer questions later. If you feel that you must come back to a question, mark the best choice and place a note in the margin. Generally speaking, it is best not to change answers once you have made a decision. Your considered reaction and first response are correct more often than are changes made out of frustration or anxiety.
5. Do not let anxiety destroy your confidence. If you have prepared conscientiously, you know enough to pass. Use all that you have learned.
6. Do not try to determine how well you are doing as you proceed. You will not be able to make an objective assessment, and your anxiety will increase.
7. Do not become frustrated or angry about what appear to be bad or difficult questions. You simply do not know the answers; you cannot know everything.

Specific Test-Taking Strategies

Read the entire question carefully, regardless of format. Test questions have multiple parts. Concentrate on picking out the pertinent key words that will help you problem-solve. Words such as *always, all, never, mostly, primarily,* and so forth play significant roles. In all types of questions, distractors with terms such as *always* or *never* most often are incorrect. Adjectives and adverbs can completely change the meaning of questions—pay close attention to them. The knowledge and application of grammar often are key to dissecting questions.

Multiple-Choice Questions

Read the question and the choices carefully to become familiar with the data provided. Remember, in multiple-choice questions there is one correct answer and there are four distractors, or incorrect answers. (Distractors are plausible and possibly correct, or they would not be called distractors.) They are generally correct for part of the question but not for the entire question. Dissecting the question into parts helps eliminate distractors.

Many students think that they must always start at option A and make a decision before they move to B, thus forcing decisions they are not ready to make. Your first decisions should be made on those choices you feel the most confident about.

Compare the choices with each part of the question. To be wrong, a choice needs to be incorrect for only part of the question. To be correct, it must be totally correct. If you believe a choice is partially incorrect, tentatively eliminate that choice. Make notes next to the choices regarding tentative decisions. One method is to place a minus sign next to the choices you are certain are incorrect and a plus sign next to those that potentially are correct. Finally, place a zero next to any choice you do not understand or need to come back to for further inspection. Do not feel that you must make final decisions until you have examined all choices carefully.

When you have eliminated as many choices as you can, decide which of those that remain has the highest probability of being correct. Above all, be honest with yourself. If you do not know the answer, eliminate as many choices as possible and choose reasonably.

Multiple True-False Questions

Multiple true–false questions are not as difficult as some students make them. These are the questions for which you must select from the following choices:

A if **only I** is correct
B if **only III** is correct
C if **I and II** are correct
D if **II and III** are correct
E if **I, II, and III** are correct

Remember that the name for this type of question is *multiple true–false,* and then use this concept. Become familiar with each choice, and make notes. Then concentrate on the one choice you feel is definitely incorrect. If you can find one incorrect alternative, you can eliminate three choices immediately and be down to a 50-50 probability of guessing the correct answer. If choice A is incorrect, so are C and E; if choice B is incorrect, so are choices D and E. Therefore, you are down to a 50-50 probability of guessing the correct answer.

After eliminating the choices you are sure are incorrect, concentrate on the choice that will make your final decision. For instance, if you discard choice I, you have eliminated alternatives A, C, and E. This leaves B (III) and D (II and III). Concentrate on choice II, and decide if it is true or false. (Take the path of least resistance and concentrate on the smallest possible number of items while making a decision.) Obviously, if none of the choices is found to be incorrect, the answer is E (I, II, III).

Guessing

Nothing takes the place of a firm knowledge base, but having little information to work with, you may find it necessary to guess at the correct answer. A few simple rules can help increase your guessing accuracy. Always guess consistently if you have no idea what is correct—that is, after eliminating all that you can, make the choice that agrees with your intuition or choose the option closest to the top of the list that has not been eliminated as a potential answer.

When guessing at questions that present with choices in numeric form, you will often find the choices listed in an ascending or descending order. It is generally not wise to guess the first or last alternative because these are usually extreme values and are most likely incorrect.

Using a Practice Exam to Learn

All too often, students do not take full advantage of practice exams. There is a tendency to complete the exam, score it, look up the correct answer to those questions missed, and then forget the entire thing.

In fact, great educational benefits could be derived if students would spend more time using practice tests as learning tools. As mentioned previously, incorrect choices in test questions are plausible and partially correct, or they would not fulfill their purpose as distractors. This means that it is just as beneficial to look up the incorrect choices as the correct choices to discover specifically why they are incorrect. In this way, it is possible to learn better test-taking skills as the subtlety of question construction is uncovered.

In addition, it is advisable to go back and attempt to restructure each question to see if all the choices can be made correct by modifying the question. By doing this, you will learn four times as much. By all means, look up the right answer and explanation. Then, focus on each of the other choices, and ask yourself under what conditions, if any, they might be correct.

Summary

Ideally, examinations are designed to determine how much material students have learned and how that material is used in the successful completion of the examination. Students will be successful if these suggestions are followed:
- Develop a positive attitude, and maintain that attitude.
- Be realistic in determining the amount of material you attempt to master and in the score you hope to attain.
- Read the directions for each type of question and the questions themselves closely, and follow the directions carefully.
- Bring differential reasoning to each question in the examination.
- Guess intelligently and consistently when guessing strategies must be used.
- Use the test as an opportunity to display your knowledge and as a tool for developing prescriptions for further study and learning.

Board examinations are not easy. They may be almost impossible for those who have unrealistic expectations or for those who allow misinformation concerning the exams to produce anxiety out of proportion to the task at hand. Examinations are manageable if they are approached with a positive attitude and with consistent use of all of the information the student has learned.

Michael J. O'Donnell

Introduction to the NAPLEX

After graduation from an accredited pharmacy program, the prospective pharmacist must demonstrate the competency to practice pharmacy. The standards of competence for the practice of pharmacy are set by each state board of pharmacy. NAPLEX—The North American Pharmacist Licensure Examination—is the principal instrument used by the state board of pharmacy to assess the knowledge and proficiency necessary for a candidate to practice pharmacy. The National Association of Boards of Pharmacy (NABP) is an independent, international, and impartial association that assists member boards and jurisdictions in developing, implementing and enforcing uniform standards for the purpose of protecting the public health. NABP develops examinations that enable boards of pharmacy to assess the competence of candidates seeking licensure to practice pharmacy. Each state board of pharmacy may impose additional examinations. The two major examinations developed by NABP are

- The North American Pharmacist Licensure Examination (NAPLEX)
- Multistate Pharmacy Jurisprudence Examination (MPJE)

Registration information and a description of these computerized examinations may be found on the NABP Web site: www.nabp.net. Before submitting registration materials, the pharmacy candidate should contact the board of pharmacy for additional information regarding procedures, deadline dates, and required documentation.

The NAPLEX is a computer-adaptive test that measures a candidate's knowledge and ability by assessing the answers before presenting the next test question. If the answer is correct, the computer will select a more difficult question from the test item pool in an appropriate content area; if the answer is incorrect, an easier question will be selected by the computer. The NAPLEX score is based on the difficulty level of the questions answered correctly.

NAPLEX consists of 185 multiple-choice test questions. Of these, 150 questions are used to calculate the test score. The remaining 35 items serve as pretest questions and do not affect the NAPLEX score. Pretest questions are administered to evaluate the item's difficulty level for possible inclusion as a scored question in future exams. These pretest questions are dispersed throughout the exam and cannot be identified by the candidate.

A majority of the questions on the NAPLEX are asked in a scenario-based format (i.e., patient profiles with accompanying test questions). To properly analyze and answer the questions presented, the candidate must refer to the information provided in the patient profile. Some questions appear in a stand-alone format and should be answered solely from the information provided in the question.

All NAPLEX questions are based on competency statements that are reviewed and revised periodically. The NAPLEX Competency Statements describe the knowledge, judgment, and skills that the candidate is expected to demonstrate as an entry-level pharmacist. A complete description of the NAPLEX Competency Statements is published on the NABP Web site and is reproduced, with permission of NABP, in this edition (p. xxiii). The NAPLEX examines three general areas of competence:

- Ensure safe and effective pharmacotherapy and optimize therapeutic outcomes
- Ensure safe and accurate preparation and dispensing of medications
- Provide healthcare information and promote public health

The NAPLEX *Candidates' Review Guide* is no longer available. NABP offers candidates who are preparing for the NAPLEX the Pre-NAPLEX, which is similar to the actual NAPLEX and allows candidates to gain experience in answering questions before examination day. The Pre-NAPLEX can be accessed via the Internet at the following URL: www.nabp.net/prenaplex/.

NAPLEX Blueprint

The NAPLEX Competency Statements

The NAPLEX Competency Statements provide a blueprint of the topics covered on the examination. They offer important information about the knowledge, judgment, and skills you are expected to demonstrate as an entry-level pharmacist. A strong understanding of the Competency Statements will aid in your preparation to take the examination.

Area 1: Assure safe and effective pharmacotherapy and optimize therapeutic outcomes (approximately 54% of test)

1.1.0 Obtain, interpret and evaluate patient information to determine the presence of a disease or medical condition, assess the need for treatment and/or referral, and identify patient-specific factors that affect health, pharmacotherapy, and/or disease management.

1.1.1 Identify and assess patient information including medication, laboratory and disease state histories.

1.1.2 Identify and/or use instruments and techniques related to patient assessment and diagnosis.

1.1.3 Identify and define the terminology, signs, and symptoms associated with diseases and medical conditions.

1.1.4 Identify and evaluate patient factors, genetic factors, biosocial factors, and concurrent drug therapy that are relevant to the maintenance of wellness and the prevention or treatment of a disease or medical condition.

1.2.0 Identify, evaluate, and communicate to the patient or health-care provider, the appropriateness of the patient's specific pharmacotherapeutic agents, dosing regimens, dosage forms, routes of administration, and delivery systems.

1.2.1 Identify specific uses and indications for drug products.

1.2.2 Identify the known or postulated sites and mechanisms of action of pharmacotherapeutic agents.

1.2.3 Evaluate drug therapy for the presence of pharmacotherapeutic duplications and interactions with other drugs, food, diagnostic tests, and monitoring procedures.

1.2.4 Identify contraindications, warnings and precautions associated with a drug product's active and inactive ingredients.

1.2.5 Identify physicochemical properties of drug substances that affect their solubility, pharmacodynamic and pharmacokinetic properties, pharmacologic actions, and stability.

1.2.6 Interpret and apply pharmacodynamic and pharmacokinetic principles to calculate and determine appropriate drug dosing regimens.

1.2.7 Interpret and apply biopharmaceutic principles and the pharmaceutical characteristics of drug dosage forms and delivery systems, to assure bioavailability and enhance patient compliance.

1.3.0 Manage the drug regimen by monitoring and assessing the patient and/or patient information, collaborating with other health care professionals, and providing patient education.

1.3.1 Identify pharmacotherapeutic outcomes and endpoints.

1.3.2 Evaluate patient signs and symptoms, and the results of monitoring tests and procedures to determine the safety and effectiveness of pharmacotherapy.

1.3.3 Identify, describe the mechanism of, and remedy adverse reactions, allergies, side effects and iatrogenic or drug-induced illness.

1.3.4 Prevent, recognize, and remedy medication non-adherence, misuse or abuse.

1.3.5 Recommend pharmacotherapeutic alternatives.

Area 2: Assure safe and accurate preparation and dispensing of medications (approximately 35% of test)

2.1.0 Perform calculations required to compound, dispense, and administer medication.

2.1.1 Calculate the quantity of medication to be compounded or dispensed; reduce and enlarge formulation quantities and calculate the quantity of ingredients needed to compound the proper amount of the preparation.

2.1.2 Calculate nutritional needs and the caloric content of nutrient sources.

2.1.3 Calculate the rate of drug administration.

2.1.4 Calculate or convert drug concentrations, ratio strengths, and/or extent of ionization.

2.2.0 Select and dispense medications in a manner that promotes safe and effective use.

2.2.1 Identify drug products by their generic, brand, and/or common names.

2.2.2 Determine whether a particular drug dosage strength or dosage form is commercially available, and whether it is available on a nonprescription basis.

2.2.3 Identify commercially available drug products by their characteristic physical attributes.

2.2.4 Interpret and apply pharmacokinetic parameters and quality assurance data to determine equivalence among manufactured drug products, and identify products for which documented evidence of inequivalence exists.

2.2.5 Identify and communicate appropriate information regarding packaging, storage, handling, administration, and disposal of medications.

2.2.6 Identify and describe the use of equipment and apparatus required to administer medications.

2.3.0 Prepare and compound extemporaneous preparations and sterile products.

2.3.1 Identify and describe techniques and procedures related to drug preparation, compounding, and quality assurance.

2.3.2 Identify and use equipment necessary to prepare and extemporaneously compound medications.

2.3.3 Identify the important physicochemical properties of a preparation's active and inactive ingredients; describe the mechanism of, and the characteristic evidence of incompatibility or degradation; and identify methods for achieving stabilization of the preparation.

Area 3 Provide health care information and promote public health (approximately 11% of test)

3.1.0 Access, evaluate, and apply information to promote optimal health care.

3.1.1 Identify the typical content and organization of specific sources of drug and health information for both health-care providers and consumers.

3.1.2 Evaluate the suitability, accuracy, and reliability of information from reference sources by explaining and evaluating the adequacy of experimental design and by applying and evaluating statistical tests and parameters.

3.2.0 Educate the public and health-care professionals regarding medical conditions, wellness, dietary supplements, and medical devices.

3.2.1 Provide health care information regarding the prevention and treatment of diseases and medical conditions, including emergency patient care.

3.2.2 Provide health care information regarding nutrition, lifestyle, and other non-drug measures that are effective in promoting health or preventing or minimizing the progression of a disease or medical condition.

3.2.3 Provide information regarding the documented uses, adverse effects and toxicities of dietary supplements.

3.2.4 Provide information regarding the selection, use and care of medical/surgical appliances and devices, self-care products, and durable medical equipment, as well as products and techniques for self-monitoring of health status and medical conditions.

1

Drug Product Development in the Pharmaceutical Industry

Anton H. Amann

Leon Shargel

I. INTRODUCTION

A. Active pharmaceutical ingredient (API)

1. A **drug substance** is the API or component that produces pharmacological activity.

2. The API may be **produced by** chemical synthesis, recovery from a natural product, enzymatic reaction, recombinant DNA technology, fermentation, or a combination of these processes. Further purification of the API may be needed before it can be used in a drug product.

3. A **new chemical entity (NCE)** is a drug substance with unknown clinical, toxicologic, physical, and chemical properties. In addition, the U.S. Food and Drug Administration (FDA) considers an NCE as an API that has not been approved for marketing in the United States.

4. The **identity, strength, quality,** and **purity** of a drug substance depend on proper control of the manufacturing and synthetic process.

B. Drug product

1. A drug product is the **finished dosage form** (e.g., capsule, tablet, ointment) that contains the API, generally in association with other excipients, or inert ingredients.

2. The excipients in the drug product may affect the functionality and performance of the drug product, including modification of the rate of drug substance release, improving drug stability, and masking the drug taste.

3. Different **approaches** are generally used to produce drug products that contain NCEs, product line extensions, generic drug products, and specialty drug products.

C. Drug products containing new chemical entities. The following phases of product development proceed sequentially.

1. **Preclinical stage.** Animal pharmacology and toxicology data are obtained to determine the safety and efficacy of the drug. An **investigational new drug (IND) application** for human testing is submitted to the FDA. Because little is known about the human and the therapeutic/toxicologic potential, many drug products will not reach the marketplace. No attempt is made to develop a final formulation during the preclinical stage. **Nonclinical** studies are nonhuman studies that may continue at any stage of research to obtain additional information concerning the pharmacology and toxicology of the drug.

2. **Phase I**
   a. Clinical testing takes place after the IND application is submitted.
   b. Healthy volunteers are used in phase I clinical studies to determine drug tolerance and toxicity.

      c. For oral drug administration, a simple hard gelatin capsule formulation containing the API is usually used for IND studies.

      d. Toxicologic studies—including acute, chronic, subchronic, and mutagenicity—and other such studies in various animal species are planned during this phase.

3. Phase II

  a. A limited number of patients with the disease or condition for which the drug was developed are treated under close supervision.

  b. Dose–response studies and pharmacokinetics are performed to determine the optimum dosage regimen for treating the disease.

  c. Safety is measured by attempting to determine the **therapeutic index** (ratio of toxic dose to effective dose).

  d. A final drug formulation is developed. This formulation is bioequivalent to the dosage form used in the initial clinical studies.

  e. Chronic toxicity studies are started in two species; such studies normally last more than 2 years' duration.

4. Phase III

  a. Large-scale, **multicenter clinical studies** are performed with the final dosage form developed in phase II. These studies are done to determine the safety and efficacy of the drug product in a large patient population who have the disease or condition for which the drug was developed.

  b. **Side effects** are monitored. In a large population, new toxic effects may occur that were not evident in previous clinical trials.

5. Submission of a **new drug application (NDA).** An NDA is submitted to the FDA for review and approval after the completion of clinical trials that show to the satisfaction of the medical community that the drug product is effective by all parameters and is reasonably safe as demonstrated by animal and human studies.

6. Phase IV

  a. After the NDA is submitted and before approval to market the product is obtained from the FDA, manufacturing **scale-up** activities occur. Scaleup is the increase in the batch size from the clinical batch, submission batch, or both to the full-scale production batch size, using the finished, marketed product.

  b. The **drug formulation** may be modified slightly as a result of data obtained during the manufacturing scaleup and validation processes.

  c. Changes in **drug formulation** should always be within the scaleup and postapproval change (SUPAC) guidelines.

7. Phase V

  a. After the FDA grants market approval of the drug, product development may continue.

  b. The drug product may be improved as a result of equipment, regulatory, supply, or market demands.

  c. Additional clinical studies may be performed in special populations, such as the elderly, pediatric, and renal-impaired, to obtain information on the efficacy of the drug in these subjects.

  d. Additional clinical studies may be performed to determine if the drug can be used for a new indication.

D. Product line extensions are dosage forms in which the physical form or strength, but not the use or indication, of the product changes. Product line extension is usually performed during phase III, IV, or V.

  1. Developing a **transdermal patch** when only tablets have been available; for example:
- Progesterone
- Nicotine
- Estradiol
- Nitroglycerin

  2. Additional strengths as long as these strengths are within the total daily dose; for example:
- Ibuprofen

  3. Controlled-release or modified-release dosage forms when only an immediate-release dosage form is available. This is an ongoing project for all brand companies; almost every NCE has or will eventually have a modified-release dosage form of the immediate-release product.

E. Biologic products

1. A biologic product is any virus, serum, toxin, antitoxin, vaccine, blood, blood component or derivative, allergenic product, or analogous product applicable to the prevention, treatment, or cure of diseases or injuries.

2. Biologic products are a **subset** of drug products, distinguished by their manufacturing processes (biologic vs. chemical). In general, the term *drugs* includes biologic products.

3. **Biologic license application (BLA).** Biologic products are approved for marketing under the provisions of the Public Health Service (PHS) Act.

F. Generic drug products

1. After **patent expiration** of the brand drug product, a generic drug product may be marketed. A generic drug product is **therapeutically equivalent to the brand name drug product** and contains the same amount of the drug in the same type of dosage form (e.g., tablet, liquid, injectable).

2. A generic drug product must be **bioequivalent** (i.e., have the same rate and extent of drug absorption) to the brand drug product. Therefore, a generic drug product is expected to give the same clinical response (see Chapter 7). These studies are normally performed with healthy human volunteers.

3. Some generic products are not absorbed; for some others bioequivalence is not a good marker. Under those conditions, **comparative clinical trials** or studies with **pharmacodynamic end points** are considered to measure the equivalence of two products. Inhalation products and nonabsorbed drug products fall into this category.

4. The generic drug product may differ from the brand product in **physical appearance** (i.e., size, color, shape) or in the amount and type of excipients only for tablets.

5. A generic drug product may not differ in both the qualitative and the quantitative compositions for liquids, injectables, semisolids, transdermal patches, inhalation products, and ophthalmic products, unless adequate safety studies have been performed.

6. Before a drug product is marketed, the manufacturer must submit an **abbreviated new drug application (ANDA)** to the FDA for approval. Because preclinical safety and efficacy studies have already been performed for the NDA-approved brand product, human bioequivalence studies, instead of clinical trials, are generally required for the ANDA. The chemistry, manufacturing, and controls requirements for the generic drug product are similar to those for the brand name drug product.

G. Specialty drug products are existing products developed as a new delivery system or for a new therapeutic indication. The safety and efficacy of the drug product were established in the initial NDA-approved dosage form. For example, the nitroglycerin transdermal delivery system (patch) was developed after experience with nitroglycerin sublingual tablets.

II. PRODUCT DEVELOPMENT.
For each drug, various activities and information are required to develop a safe, effective, and stable dosage form.

A. New chemical entities

1. **Preformulation** is the characterization of the physical and chemical properties of the active drug substance and dosage form. The therapeutic indication of the drug and the route of administration dictate the type of drug product or drug delivery system (e.g., immediate release, controlled release, suppository, parenteral, transdermal) that needs to be developed.
   a. **Preformulation** activities are usually performed during the preclinical stage. However, these activities may continue into phases I and II.
   b. The following information is obtained during preformulation.
      (1) **General characteristics,** including particle size and shape, crystalline features, polymorphism, density, surface area, hygroscopicity (ability to take up and retain moisture), and powder flow

(2) **Solubility characteristics,** including intrinsic dissolution, pH solubility profile, and general solubility characteristics in various solvents

(3) **Chemical characteristics,** including surface energy, pH stability profile, pK_a, temperature stability (dry or under various humidity conditions), and excipient interactions

(4) **Analytical methods development,** including development of a stability indicating method (measures both the API and the degradation products), cleaning methods, and identification of impurities

2. **Formulation development** is a continuing process. Initial drug formulations are developed for early clinical studies. When the submission of an NDA is considered, the manufacturer attempts to develop the final (marketed) dosage form. The dose of the drug and the route of administration are important in determining the modifications needed.

   a. **Injectable drug product**
      (1) A final injectable drug product is usually developed in the preclinical phase.
      (2) Major concerns include the stability of the drug in solution and the sterility of the product.
      (3) Because few excipients are allowed in injectable products, the formulator must choose a final product early in the development process.
      (4) If the formulation is changed, bioavailability studies are not required for intravenous injections because the product is injected directly into the body.
      (5) Formulation changes may require acute toxicity studies.

   b. **Topical drug products for local application** include antibacterials, antifungals, corticosteroids, and local anesthetics.
      (1) The final dosage form for a topical drug product is usually developed during phase I because any major formulation changes may require further clinical trials.
      (2) The release of the drug from the matrix is measured in vitro with various diffusion cell models.
      (3) Significant problems encountered with locally acting topical drug products include local irritation and systemic drug absorption.

   c. **Topical drug products for systemic drug absorption** include drug delivery through the skin (transdermal), mucous membranes (intranasal), and rectal mucosa.
      (1) A prototype formulation is developed for phase I.
      (2) A final topical drug product is developed during phase III after the available technology and desired systemic levels are considered.

   d. **Oral drug products**
      (1) Prototype dosage forms are often developed during the **preclinical phase** to ensure that the drug is optimally available and that the product dissolves in the gastrointestinal tract.
      (2) In the early stages of product development, **hard gelatin** capsule dosage forms are often developed for **phase I** clinical trials. If the drug shows efficacy, the same drug formulation may be used in phase II studies.
      (3) Final product development begins when the drug proceeds during phase II and before initiating phase III clinical studies.

3. **Final drug product.** Considerations in the development of a final dosage form include the following:
   a. Color, shape, size, taste, viscosity, sensitivity, skin feel, and physical appearance of the dosage form
   b. Size and shape of the package or container
   c. Production equipment
   d. Production site
   e. Country of origin in which the drug is to be manufactured
   f. Country in which the drug will be marketed

B. **Product line extensions** are generally defined as drug products containing an NDA-approved drug in a different dosage strength or in a different dosage form (e.g., modified release, oral liquid).

1. **Solid oral product line extensions**
   a. The simplest dosage form to develop is a different dosage strength of a drug in a tablet or capsule. Only bioequivalence studies are needed.
   b. A **modified-release** dosage form is more difficult to develop when only an instant-release dosage form exists. Clinical trials are normally required.

    c. **Considerations** in developing these dosage forms are similar to those for the final drug product (see II.A.3).

    d. **Marketing** has a role in the choice of the dosage form.

    e. Because the original brand drug product information contributes to the body of knowledge about the drug, no preformulation is needed. All other factors considered for the original product are similar. If the relation between **in vitro** dissolution and **in vivo** bioavailability is known, the innovator can progress to a finished dosage form relatively quickly.

    f. **Regulatory approval** is based on the following:

      (1) Stability information

      (2) Analytical and manufacturing controls

      (3) Bioequivalence studies

      (4) Clinical trials (in the case of modified-release dosage forms)

    g. A new therapeutic indication for a drug requires new **efficacy studies** and a new NDA.

  2. **Liquid product line extensions**

    a. If the current marketed product is a liquid preparation, then the same factors as for the solid oral dosage forms are considered (see II.B.1.a–g).

    b. If the marketed product is a solid oral dosage form and the product line extension is a liquid, product development must proceed with caution because the rate and extent of absorption for liquid and solid dosage forms may not be the same.

    c. **Regulatory approval** requires

      (1) Bioequivalence studies

      (2) Stability information

      (3) Analytical and manufacturing controls

      (4) Safety studies (e.g., depending on the drug substance, local irritation)

      (5) Clinical trials, if the rate and extent of drug absorption are drastically altered from the original dosage form

C. **Combination products** are made up of two or more regulated components (e.g., drug/device, biologic/device, drug/biologic, or drug/device/biologic) that are physically, chemically, or otherwise combined or mixed and produced as a single entity.

  1. These may be two or more separate products packaged together in a single package or as a unit and may be composed of drug and device products, device and biologic products, or biologic and drug products.

  2. An **example** is an inhalation steroid (e.g., beclomethasone inhalation aerosol) in which the device component is important for delivery of the steroid.

III. PREAPPROVAL INSPECTIONS (PAIs)

A. The **manufacturing facility** is inspected by the FDA after an NDA, abbreviated antibiotic drug application (AADA), or ANDA is submitted and before the application is approved.

B. A PAI may be initiated if a **major change** is reported in a supplemental application to an NDA, AADA, or ANDA.

C. During the PAI, the FDA investigator:

  1. **Performs** a general current good manufacturing practice (cGMP) inspection relating specifically to the drug product intended for the market

  2. **Reviews** the development report to verify that the drug product has enough supporting documentation to ensure a validated product and a rationale for the manufacturing directions

  3. **Consults** the chemistry, manufacturing, and control (CMC) section of the NDA, AADA, or ANDA and determines the capability of the manufacturer to produce the drug product as described

  4. **Verifies** the traceability of the information submitted in the CMC section to the original laboratory notebooks, electronic information, and batch records

5. **Verifies and ensures** that all the quality systems are in place to manufacture the product so it retains the identity, strength, quality, and purity of the drug product that were approved by the center.

6. **Recommends** whether to approve the manufacture of the drug product after the PAI

IV. SCALEUP AND POSTAPPROVAL CHANGES (SUPACs)

A. **Purpose.** These guidelines are intended to reduce the number of manufacturing changes that require preapproval by the FDA. The guidelines are published by the FDA on the Internet (www.fda.gov/cder/guidance/index.htm).

B. **Function.** These guidelines provide recommendations to sponsors of NDAs, AADAs, and ANDAs during the postapproval period when

1. Making slight changes in the amount of the **excipient** to aid in the processing of the product during scaleup

2. Changing the **site** of manufacture

3. **Scaling up** (increasing) or **scaling down** (decreasing) the batch size of the formulation

4. Changing the manufacturing **process** or **equipment**

C. The FDA must be notified about a proposed change to a drug product through different **regulatory documentation,** depending on the type of change proposed.

1. **Annual report.** Changes that are unlikely to have any detectable effect on formulation quality and performance can be instituted without approval by the FDA and reported annually. Examples of these changes include
   a. **Compliance** with an official compendium
   b. **Label description** of the drug product or how it is supplied (not involving dosage strength or dosage form)
   c. Deletion of an **ingredient** that affects only the color of the product
   d. Extension of the expiration date based on full shelf-life data obtained from a protocol approved in the application
   e. **Container** and **closure system** for the drug product (except a change in container size for nonsolid dosage forms) based on equivalency to the approved system under a protocol approved in the application or published in an official compendium
   f. Addition or deletion of an **alternate analytical method**

2. **Changes being effected (CBE) supplement.** Changes that probably would not have any detectable effect but require some validation efforts require specific documentation, depending on the change. A supplement is submitted, and the change can be implemented without previous approval (CBE-0) by the FDA or, in some cases, the FDA has 30 days to review the change **(CBE-30).** FDA may reject this supplement. Examples of reasons for submitting a supplement include
   a. Addition of a **new specification** or test method or changes in methods, facilities, or controls
   b. **Label change** to add or strengthen a contraindication, warning, precaution, or adverse reaction
   c. Use of a **different facility** to manufacture the drug substance and drug product (the manufacturing process in the new facility does not differ materially from that in the former facility, and the new facility has received a satisfactory cGMP inspection within the previous 2 years covering that manufacturing process)

3. **Preapproval supplement.** Changes that could have a significant effect on formulation quality and performance require specific documentation. This supplement must be approved before the proposed change is initiated. Appropriate examples for preapproval supplement are
   a. Addition or deletion of an **ingredient**
   b. Relaxation of the limits for a **specification**
   c. Establishment of a new **regulatory analytical method**
   d. Deletion of a **specification** or regulatory analytical method

    e. Change in the method of **manufacture** of the drug product, including changing or relaxing an in-process control

    f. Extension of the **expiration date** of the drug product based on data obtained under a new or revised stability testing protocol that was been approved in the application

D. When any change to a drug product is proposed, the manufacturer must show that the resultant drug product is **bioequivalent** and **therapeutically equivalent** to the original approved drug product (see Chapter 7).

    1. A **minor change** is a change that has minimal potential to have an adverse effect on the identity, strength, quality, purity, or potency of the product as they may relate to the safety or effectiveness of the product. If the proposed change is considered **minor** by the FDA, bioequivalence may be demonstrated by comparative dissolution profiles for the original and new formulations.

    2. A **major change** is one that has substantial potential to have an adverse effect on the identity, strength, quality, purity, or potency of a product as they may relate to the safety or effectiveness of the product. If the proposed change is considered **major** by the FDA, bioequivalence must be demonstrated by an in vivo bioequivalence study comparing the original and new formulations.

V. GOOD MANUFACTURING PRACTICES (GMPs) are regulations developed by the FDA. GMPs are minimum requirements that the industry must meet when manufacturing, processing, packing, or holding human and veterinary drugs. These regulations, also known as **cGMPs,** establish criteria for personnel, facilities, and manufacturing processes to ensure that the finished drug product has the correct identity, strength, quality, and purity characteristics.

A. Good Manufacturing Practices are described in the Code of Federal Regulations (CFR), title 21, sections 210 and 211.

B. **Quality control (QC)** is the group within the manufacturer that is responsible for establishing process and product specifications.

    1. **Specifications** are the criteria to which a drug product should conform to be considered having acceptable quality for its intended use.

    2. The QC unit **tests** the product and verifies that the specifications are met. QC testing includes the **acceptance** or **rejection** of the incoming raw materials, packaging components, drug products, water system, and environmental conditions (e.g., heating, ventilation, air-conditioning, air quality, microbial load) that exist during the manufacturing process.

C. **Quality assurance (QA)** is the group within the manufacturer that determines that the systems and facilities are adequate and that the written procedures are followed to ensure that the finished drug product meets the applicable specifications for quality.

STUDY QUESTIONS

Directions: Each statement in this section can be correctly completed by **one or more** of the suggested phrases. Choose the **correct** answer, A–E:

A   if **I** only is correct
B   if **III** only is correct
C   if **I and II** are correct
D   if **II and III** are correct
E   if **I, II, and III** are correct

1. Healthy human volunteers are used in drug development for

   I. phase I testing after the submission of an investigational new drug (IND) application.
   II. generic drug development for an abbreviated new drug application (ANDA) submission.
   III. phase III testing just before the submission of a new drug application (NDA).

2. The required information contained in a new drug application (NDA) that is *not* included in the abbreviated new drug application (ANDA) consists of

   I. preclinical animal toxicity studies.
   II. clinical efficacy studies.
   III. human safety and tolerance studies.

3. A product line extension contains the new drug application (NDA) approved drug in a new

   I. dosage form.
   II. dosage strength.
   III. therapeutic indication.

Directions: Each statement in this section can be correctly completed by **one** of the suggested phrases. Choose the **best** answer.

4. The regulations developed by the U.S. Food and Drug Administration (FDA) for the pharmaceutical industry for meeting the minimum requirements in the manufacturing, processing, packing, or holding of human and veterinary drugs are known as

   (A) good manufacturing practices (GMPs).
   (B) quality assurance (QA).
   (C) quality control (QC).
   (D) preapproval inspection (PAI).
   (E) scaleup and postapproval changes (SUPACs).

5. The unit within the pharmaceutical manufacturer that ensures that the finished dosage form has met all the specifications for its intended use is the

   (A) analytical methods unit.
   (B) marketing and sales unit.
   (C) preapproval inspection (PAI) unit.
   (D) quality assurance (QA) unit.
   (E) quality control (QC) unit.

6. Manufacturers may make a change in the formulation after market approval. If the change in the formulation is considered a minor change, the manufacturer needs to report the change to the FDA only in the

   (A) annual report.
   (B) preapproval supplement.
   (C) investigational new drug (IND) submission.
   (D) changes being effected supplement, 30 days (CBE-30).
   (E) No report is required for a minor change.

ANSWERS AND EXPLANATIONS

1. The answer is C (I, II) *[see I.C.2.b; I.F.2]*.
Phase I testing is the first set of human studies performed during new drug development. Phase I studies establish the tolerance and toxicity of the drug in humans. Bioequivalence studies for generic drug development are most often performed in healthy human volunteers. These studies establish the bioequivalence of the generic drug product against the brand drug product. Phase III testing entails large-scale, multicenter clinical studies performed in patients with the disease or condition to be treated. Phase III studies determine the safety and efficacy of the drug in a large patient population.

2. The answer is E (I, II, and III) *[see I.C.5; I.F.6]*.
The development of a new drug requires extensive toxicity and efficacy testing in animals and humans. The NDA documents all studies performed on the drug. The ANDA is used for generic drug product submissions. The generic drug product is similar to the original brand drug product that has already been marketed. Because the efficacy, safety, and toxicity of this drug product have been studied and documented, further studies of this nature are unnecessary.

3. The answer is C (I, II) *[see I.D]*.
Product line extensions are developed after further studies with the original NDA-approved drug product. From these studies, the manufacturer may develop a new dosage form (e.g., controlled-release product) or a new dosage strength. A new therapeutic indication requires an NDA.

4. The answer is A *[see V]*.
Quality control and quality assurance follow GMP regulations to ensure that the finished product meets all applicable specifications for quality. The FDA may inspect a manufacturing site (PAI) before the drug application is approved. In addition, the FDA must be notified about any proposed changes to an approved drug product.

5. The answer is E *[see V.B]*.
The QC unit performs the appropriate tests on the dosage form. PAI is performed by FDA compliance inspectors, who examine the pharmaceutical manufacturer and review the procedures and records for manufacturing the finished dosage form before the administration grants market approval. The analytical development unit develops the analytical methods used in testing the drug product.

6. The answer is A *[see IV.C.1]*.
All changes in the formulation must be reported to the FDA. A **minor change** is a change that has minimal potential to have an adverse effect on the identity, strength, quality, purity, or potency of the product as they may relate to the product's safety or effectiveness. Changes that are unlikely to have any detectable effect on formulation quality and performance can be instituted without approval by the FDA and need only to be reported annually in the annual report.

2
Pharmaceutical Calculations and Statistics

Riccardo L. Boni

I. FUNDAMENTALS OF MEASUREMENT AND CALCULATION. The pharmacist is often required to perform or evaluate a variety of calculations in his or her practice. Many of these calculations involve the use of direct or inverse proportions. **Dimensional** (or **unit**) **analysis** and **approximation** can be useful in solving these problems. In dimensional analysis, dimensions (or units) are included with each number used in the calculation. Units common to the numerator and denominator may be canceled and the remaining units provide the units for the final answer. In approximation, each number used in the calculation is rounded to a single significant digit. Factors common to the numerator and denominator may be canceled and the answer to this approximation should be reasonably close to the final exact answer.

A. Ratio and proportion

1. **Ratio.** The relative magnitude of two like quantities is a ratio, which is expressed as a fraction. Certain basic principles apply to the ratio, as they do to all fractions.
   a. When the two terms of a ratio are multiplied or divided by the same number, the value of the ratio is unchanged.

   $$\frac{1}{3} \times \frac{2}{2} = \frac{2}{6} = \frac{1}{3}$$

   b. Two ratios with the same value are equivalent. Equivalent ratios have equal cross products and equal reciprocals. For example:

   $$\frac{1}{3} = \frac{2}{6}$$

   and

   $$1 \times 6 = 3 \times 2 = 6$$

   If two ratios are equal, then their reciprocals are equal:

   $$\text{if } \frac{1}{3} = \frac{2}{6}, \text{ then } \frac{3}{1} = \frac{6}{2}$$

2. **Proportion.** The expression of the equality of two ratios is a proportion. The product of the extremes is equal to the product of the means for any proportion. Furthermore, the numerator of the one fraction equals the product of its denominator and the other fraction (i.e., one missing term can always be found given the other three terms). Most pharmaceutical calculations can be performed by use of proportion.
   a. **Proper ratios.** Some pharmacists use proper ratios (in which similar units are used in the numerator and denominator of each ratio) in their proportion calculations. Several examples follow.
      (1) If 240 mL of a cough syrup contains 480 mg of dextromethorphan hydrobromide, then what mass of drug is contained in a child's dose, 1 teaspoonful (5 mL) of syrup?

      $$\frac{240 \text{ mL}}{5 \text{ mL}} = \frac{480 \text{ mg}}{x \text{ mg}}$$

      $$x = \frac{480 \times 5}{240} = 10 \text{ mg}$$

(2) If a child's dose (5 mL) of a cough syrup contains 10 mg of dextromethorphan hydrobromide, what mass of drug is contained in 240 mL?

$$\frac{240 \text{ mL}}{5 \text{ mL}} = \frac{x \text{ mg}}{10 \text{ mg}}$$

$$x = \frac{240 \times 10}{5} = 480 \text{ mg}$$

(3) If the amount of dextromethorphan hydrobromide in 240 mL of cough syrup is 480 mg, what would be the volume required for a child's dose of 10 mg?

$$\frac{x \text{ mL}}{240 \text{ mL}} = \frac{10 \text{ mg}}{480 \text{ mg}}$$

$$x = \frac{10 \times 240}{480} = 5 \text{ mL}$$

(4) How many milligrams of dextromethorphan base (molecular weight = 271.4) are equivalent to 10 mg of dextromethorphan hydrobromide (molecular weight = 352.3)?

$$\frac{x \text{ mg}}{10 \text{ mg}} = \frac{271.4}{352.3}$$

$$x = 10 \times \frac{271.4}{352.3} = 7.7 \text{ mg}$$

b. Mixed ratios. Some pharmacists use mixed ratios (in which dissimilar units are used in the numerator and denominator of each ratio) in their proportion calculations. Such computations generally give correct answers, providing the conditions in which mixed ratios cannot be used are known. A later example shows mixed ratios leading to failure in the case of dilution, when inverse proportions are required. For **inverse proportions,** similar units must be used in the numerator and denominator of each ratio. Following is an example of a mixed ratio calculation using the previous problem.

$$\frac{x \text{ mL}}{10 \text{ mL}} = \frac{240 \text{ mg}}{480 \text{ mg}}$$

$$x = 240 \times \frac{10}{480} = 5 \text{ mL}$$

The **same answer** is obtained in this example whether we use proper ratios, with similar units in numerator and denominator, or mixed ratios. This is not the case when dealing with inverse proportions.

3. Inverse proportion. The most common example of the need for inverse proportion for the pharmacist is the case of **dilution.** Whereas in the previous examples of proportion the relationships involved direct proportion, the case of dilution calls for an inverse proportion (i.e., as volume increases, concentration decreases). The necessity of using inverse proportions for dilution problems is shown in this example.

If 120 mL of a 10% stock solution is diluted to 240 mL, what is the final concentration? Using inverse proportion,

$$\frac{120 \text{ mL}}{240 \text{ mL}} = \frac{x\%}{10\%}$$

$$120 \times \frac{10}{240} = 5\%$$

As expected, the final concentration is one half the original concentration because the volume is doubled. However, if the pharmacist attempts to use direct proportion and neglects to estimate an appropriate answer, the resulting calculation would provide an answer of 20%, which is twice the actual concentration.

$$\frac{120 \text{ mL}}{240 \text{ mL}} = \frac{10\%}{x\%}$$

$$240 \times \frac{10}{120} = 20\% \text{ (incorrect answer)}$$

Likewise, the pharmacist using mixed ratios fails in this case.

$$\frac{120 \text{ mL}}{10\%} = \frac{240 \text{ mL}}{x\%}$$

and

$$10 \times \frac{240}{120} = 20\% \text{ (again, incorrect answer)}$$

B. Aliquot. A pharmacist requires the aliquot method of measurement when the **sensitivity** (the smallest quantity that can be measured with the required accuracy and precision) of the measuring device is not great enough for the required measurement. Aliquot calculations can be used for measurement of solids or liquids, allowing the pharmacist to realize the required precision through a process of measuring a multiple of the desired amount followed by dilution and finally selection and measurement of an aliquot part that contains the desired amount of material. This example problem involves weighing by the aliquot method, using a prescription balance.

A prescription balance has a sensitivity requirement of 6 mg. How would you weigh 10 mg of drug with an accuracy of ± 5%, using a suitable diluent?

1. First, calculate the least weighable quantity for the balance with a sensitivity requirement of 6 mg, assuming ± 5% accuracy is required.

$$\frac{6 \text{ mg}}{x \text{ mg}} = \frac{5}{100}; \ x = 120 \text{ mg (least weighable quantity for our balance)}$$

2. Now it is obvious that an aliquot calculation is required because 10 mg of drug is required, whereas the least weighable quantity is 120 mg to achieve the required percentage of error. Using the least weighable quantity method of aliquot measurement, use the smallest quantity weighable on the balance at each step to preserve materials.
   a. Weigh 12 × 10 mg = 120 mg of drug.
   b. Dilute the 120 mg of drug (from step **a**) with a suitable diluent by geometrical dilution to achieve a mixture that will provide 10 mg of drug in each 120-mg aliquot. The amount of diluent to be used can be determined through **proportion.**

$$\frac{120 \text{ mg drug}}{10 \text{ mg drug}} = \frac{x \text{ mg total mixture}}{120 \text{ mg aliquot mixture}}$$

$$x = 1440 \text{ mg total mixture}$$
$$1440 \text{ mg total } - 120 \text{ mg drug} = 1320 \text{ mg diluent}$$

   c. Weigh 120 mg (1/12) of the total mixture, which will contain the required 10 mg of drug.

II. SYSTEMS OF MEASURE. The pharmacist must be familiar with **three systems** of measure: the **metric system** and two common systems of measure (the **avoirdupois** and **apothecaries'** systems). The primary system of measure in pharmacy and medicine is the metric system. Most students find it easiest to convert measurements in the common systems to metric units. A table of conversion equivalents is provided and should be memorized by the pharmacist (see Appendix A). The metric system, because of its universal acceptance and broad use, will not be reviewed here.

A. Apothecaries' system of fluid measure. The apothecaries' system of fluid measure is summarized in Appendix A.

B. Apothecaries' system for measuring weight. The apothecaries' system for measuring weight includes units of grains, scruples, drams, ounces, and pounds (see Appendix A).

C. Avoirdupois system of measuring weight. The avoirdupois (AV) system of measuring weight includes the grain, ounce, and pound. The grain is a unit common with the apothecaries' system and allows for easy conversion between the systems. The avoirdupois pound, however, is 16 AV ounces in contrast to the apothecaries' pound, which is 12 apothecaries' ounces (see Appendix A).

D. Conversion equivalents. See Appendix A.

III. REDUCING AND ENLARGING FORMULAS.
The pharmacist is often required to reduce or enlarge a recipe. Problems of this type are solved through proportion, or by multiplication or division by the appropriate factor to obtain the required amount of each ingredient that will give the desired total mass or volume of the formula. Formulas can be provided in amounts or in parts.

A. Formulas that indicate parts. When dealing with formulas that specify parts, parts by weight will require the determination of weights of ingredients, whereas parts by volume warrant the calculation of volumes of ingredients. Always find the total number of parts indicated in the formula, and equate that total with the total mass or volume of the desired formula in order to set up a proportion. Such a proportion will allow calculation of the mass or volume of each ingredient in units common to the total mass or volume.

What quantities should be used to prepare 100 g of camphorated parachlorophenol?

R_x	parachlorophenol	7 parts
	camphor	13 parts

$$7 \text{ parts} + 13 \text{ parts} = 20 \text{ parts total}$$

$$\frac{7 \text{ parts}}{20 \text{ parts}} = \frac{x \text{ g}}{100 \text{ g}}; \; x = 35 \text{ g of parachlorophenol}$$

$$\frac{13 \text{ parts}}{20 \text{ parts}} = \frac{x \text{ g}}{100 \text{ g}}; \; x = 65 \text{ g of camphor}$$

B. Formulas that indicate quantities. The previous prescription for cold cream provides a 100 g quantity.

What mass of each ingredient is required to provide 1 pound (AV) of cream?

R_x	white wax	12.5 g
	mineral oil	60.0 g
	lanolin	2.5 g
	sodium borate	1.0 g
	rose water	24.0 g

$$1 \text{ lb} = 454 \text{ g}$$

$$\frac{454}{100} = 4.54 \text{ (factor to use in calculating the quantities of each ingredient)}$$

$$12.5 \text{ g} \times 4.54 = 56.8 \text{ g of white wax}$$
$$60.0 \text{ g} \times 4.54 = 272 \text{ g of mineral oil}$$
$$2.5 \text{ g} \times 4.54 = 11.4 \text{ g of lanolin}$$
$$1.0 \text{ g} \times 4.54 = 4.54 \text{ of sodium borate}$$
$$24.0 \text{ g} \times 4.54 = 109 \text{ g of rose water}$$

IV. CALCULATING DOSES.
Calculation of doses generally can be performed with dimensional analysis. **Problems** encountered in the pharmacy include calculation of the number of doses, quantities in a dose or total mass/volume, amount of active or inactive ingredients, and size of dose. Calculation of **children's doses** is commonly performed by the pharmacist. Dosage is optimally calculated by using the child's body weight or mass and the appropriate dose in milligrams per kilogram (mg/kg). Without these data, the following formulas based on an adult dose can be used.

A. Fried's rule for infants

$$\frac{\text{age (in months)} \times \text{adult dose}}{150} = \text{dose for infant}$$

B. Clark's rule

$$\frac{\text{weight (lb)} \times \text{adult dose}}{150 \text{ lb (avg wt of adult)}} = \text{dose for child}$$

C. Child's dosage based on body surface area (BSA)

$$\frac{\text{BSA of child (m}^2) \times \text{adult dose}}{1.73 \text{ m}^2 \text{ (avg adult BSA)}} = \text{approximate dose for child}$$

D. Young's rule for children $\geq$ 2 years old

$$\frac{\text{age (in years)}}{\text{age (in years)} + 12} \times \text{adult dose} = \text{dose for child}$$

E. Constant rate intravenous infusions. Some drugs are administered intravenously at a constant (zero-order) rate by using a continuous-drip infusion set or a constant-rate infusion pump. The flow rate (volume per unit time) required can be calculated from the volume to be administered and the duration of the infusion. The rate of drug administration can be calculated from the concentration of drug in the infused solution and the flow rate of the infusion set or pump. Conversion factors may be required to obtain the final answer in the correct units (drops per minute or milliliters per hour).

A vancomycin solution containing 1000 mg of vancomycin hydrochloride diluted to 250 mL with D5W is to be infused at a constant rate with a continuous-drip intravenous infusion set that delivers 25 drops/mL. **What flow rate (drops/min) should be used to infuse all 250 mL of the vancomycin hydrochloride solution in 2 hr?**

$$\frac{250 \text{ mL}}{2 \text{ hr}} \times \frac{1 \text{ hr}}{60 \text{ min}} \times \frac{25 \text{ drops}}{1 \text{ mL}} = 52 \text{ drops/min}$$

V. PERCENTAGE, RATIO STRENGTH, AND OTHER CONCENTRATION EXPRESSIONS

A. Percentage weight in volume (w/v)

1. **Definition.** Percentage, indicating parts per hundred, is an important means of expressing concentration in pharmacy practice. Percentage w/v indicates the number of grams of a constituent per 100 mL of solution or liquid formulation. The pharmacist may be required to perform **three types** of calculations: determine the **weight** of active ingredient in a certain volume when given the percentage strength, determine the **percentage w/v** when the weight of substance and volume of liquid formulation are known, and determine the **volume** of liquid mixture when the percentage strength and amount of substance are known.

2. **Tolu balsam syrup.** Tolu balsam tincture contains 20% w/v tolu balsam.

   What is the percentage concentration of tolu balsam in the syrup?

tolu balsam tincture	50 mL
magnesium carbonate	10 g
sucrose	820 g
purified water, qs ad	1000 mL

   a. First, determine what the amount of tolu balsam is in the 50 mL quantity of tincture used for the syrup. Then, by proportion, calculate the concentration of tolu balsam in the syrup.

   $$\text{tolu balsam tincture} = 50 \text{ mL} \times \frac{20 \text{ g}}{100 \text{ mL}} = 10 \text{ g tolu balsam}$$

   $$\frac{10 \text{ g}}{1000 \text{ mL}} = \frac{x \text{ g}}{100 \text{ mL}}; x = \frac{1 \text{ g}}{100 \text{ mL}} = 1\% \text{ tolu balsam in the syrup}$$

   In answering this one question, the first two types of problems listed above have been solved, while exhibiting two methods of solving percentage problems—namely, by **dimensional analysis** and **proportion.**

   b. For an example of the **third type** of percentage w/v problem, determine what volume of syrup could be prepared if we had only 8 g of magnesium carbonate. Use proportion to find the total volume of syrup that can be made using only 8 g of magnesium carbonate. If we have 8 g of magnesium carbonate in 1000 mL of solution, then, according to the recipe, 800 mL of solution can be prepared using all 8 g of the drug.

$$\frac{10 \text{ g}}{1000 \text{ mL}} = \frac{8 \text{ g}}{x \text{ mL}}; x = 800 \text{ mL}$$

B. Percentage volume in volume (v/v). Percentage v/v indicates the number of milliliters of a constituent in 100 mL of liquid formulation. The percentage strength of mixtures of liquids in liquids is indicated by percent v/v, which indicates the parts by volume of a substance in 100 parts of the liquid preparation. The **three types** of problems that are encountered involve calculating **percentage strength,** calculating **volume of ingredient,** and calculating **volume of the liquid preparation.** Using the same tolu balsam syrup formula from earlier, we'll now work a percent v/v problem.

What is the percentage strength v/v of the tolu balsam tincture in the syrup preparation? By proportion, we can solve the problem in one step.

$$\frac{50 \text{ mL tolu balsam tincture}}{x \text{ mL tolu balsam tincture}} = \frac{1000 \text{ mL syrup}}{100 \text{ mL syrup}}; x = 5\%$$

C. Percentage weight in weight (w/w). Percentage w/w indicates the number of grams of a constituent per 100 g of formulation (solid or liquid). Solution of problems involving percentage w/w is straightforward when the total mass of the mixture is available or when the total mass can be determined from the available data. In calculations similar to those for percentage w/v and v/v, the pharmacist might need to solve several types of problems, including determination of the weight of a constituent, the total weight of a mixture, or the percentage w/w.

1. **How many grams of drug substance should be used to prepare 240 g of a 5% w/w solution in water?**
   a. The first step in any percentage w/w problem is to attempt identification of the total mass of the mixture. In this problem, the total mass is, obviously, provided (240 g).
   b. The problem can be easily solved through **dimensional analysis.**

$$240 \text{ g mixture} \times \frac{5.0 \text{ g drug}}{100 \text{ g drug}} = 12 \text{ g}$$

2. When the total mass of the mixture is unavailable or cannot be determined, an **extra step** is required in the calculations. Because it is usually impossible to know how much volume is displaced by a solid material, the pharmacist is unable to prepare a specified volume of a solution given the percentage w/w.

   How much drug should be added to 30 mL of water to make a 10% w/w solution? The volume of water that is displaced by the drug is unknown, so the final volume is unknown. Likewise, even though the mass of solvent is known (30 mL $\times$ 1 g/mL = 30 g), it is not known how much drug is needed, so the total mass is unknown. The water represents 100% $-$ 10% = 90% of the total mixture. Then, by proportion, the mass of drug to be used can be identified.

$$\frac{30 \text{ g of mixture (water)}}{x \text{ g of mixture (drug)}} = \frac{90\%}{10\%}; x = 3.33 \text{ g of drug required to make a solution}$$

   The **common error** that many students make in solving problems of this type is to assume that 30 g is the total mass of the mixture. Solving the problem with that assumption gives the following incorrect answer.

$$\frac{x \text{ g drug}}{10 \text{ g drug}} = \frac{30 \text{ g mixture}}{100 \text{ g mixture}}; x = 3 \text{ g of drug (incorrect answer)}$$

D. Ratio strength. Solid or liquid formulations that contain low concentrations of active ingredients will often have concentration expressed in **ratio strength.** Ratio strength, as the name implies, is the expression of concentration by means of a ratio. The numerator and denominator of the ratio indicate grams (g) or milliliters (mL) of a solid or liquid constituent in the total mass (g) or volume (mL) of a solid or liquid preparation. Because **percentage strength** is essentially a ratio of parts per hundred, conversion between ratio strength and percentage strength is easily accomplished by proportion.

1. Express 0.1% w/v as a ratio strength.

a. Ratio strengths are by convention expressed in reduced form, so in setting up our proportion to solve for ratio strength, use the numeral 1 in the numerator of the right-hand ratio as shown:

$$\frac{0.1 \text{ g}}{100 \text{ mL}} = \frac{1 \text{ part}}{x \text{ parts}}; \ x = 1000 \text{ parts, for a ratio strength of 1:1000}$$

b. Likewise, conversion from ratio strength to percentage strength by proportion is easy, as seen in the following example. Keep in mind the definition of percentage strength (parts per hundred) when setting up the proportion.

2. Express 1:2500 as a percentage strength.

$$\frac{1 \text{ part}}{2500 \text{ parts}} = \frac{x \text{ parts}}{100 \text{ parts}}; \ x = 0.04, \text{ indicating } 0.04\%$$

E. Other concentration expressions

1. Molarity (M) is the expression of the number of moles of solute dissolved per liter of solution. It is calculated by dividing the moles of solute by the volume of solution in liters.

$$M_A = \frac{n_A}{\text{solution (L)}}$$

2. Normality. A convenient way of dealing with acids, bases, and electrolytes involves the use of equivalents. One equivalent of an acid is the quantity of that acid that supplies or donates 1 mole of H^+ ions. One equivalent of a base is the quantity that furnishes 1 mole of OH^- ions. One equivalent of acid reacts with 1 equivalent of base. Equivalent weight can be calculated for atoms or molecules.

$$\text{Equivalent weight} = \frac{\text{atomic weight or molecular weight}}{\text{valence}}$$

The **normality** (N) of a solution is the number of gram-equivalent weights (equivalents) of solute per liter of solution. Normality is analogous to molarity; however, it is defined in terms of equivalents rather than moles.

$$\text{Normality} = \frac{\text{\# equivalents of solute}}{\text{\# liters of solution}}$$

3. Molality (m) is the moles of solute dissolved per kilogram of solvent. Molality is calculated by dividing the number of moles of solute by the number of kilograms of solvent. Molality offers an advantage over molarity because it is based on solvent weight and avoids problems associated with volume expansion or contraction owing to the addition of solutes.

$$m_A = \frac{n_A}{\text{mass}_{\text{solvent (kg)}}}$$

4. Mole fraction (X) is the ratio of the number of moles of one component to the total moles of a mixture or solution.

$$X_A = \frac{n_A}{n_A, \ n_B, \ n_C \ldots}, \text{ where } X_A + X_B + X_C + \ldots = 1$$

VI. DILUTION AND CONCENTRATION. If the amount of drug remains constant in a dilution or concentration, then any change in the mass or volume of a mixture is inversely proportional to the concentration.

A. Dilution and concentration problems can be solved by:

1. Inverse proportion (as mentioned earlier)

2. The equation quantity$_1$ × concentration$_1$ = quantity$_2$ × concentration$_2$

3. Determining the amount of active ingredient present in the initial mixture and, with the assumption that the initial quantity does not change, calculating of the final concentration of the new total mass or volume

4. **Alligation medial.** A method for calculating the average concentration of a mixture of two or more substances

5. **Alligation alternate.** A method for calculating the number of parts of two or more components of known concentration to be mixed when the final desired concentration is known

B. Dilution of alcohols and acids

1. **Dilution of alcohols.** When alcohol and water are mixed, a contraction of volume occurs. As a result, the final volume of solution cannot be determined accurately. Nor can the volume of water needed to dilute to a certain percentage v/v be identified. Accordingly, percentage w/w is often used for solutions of alcohol.

2. The **percentage strength** of concentrated acids is expressed as percentage w/w. The concentration of diluted acids is expressed as percentage w/v. Determining the volume of concentrated acid to be used in preparing a diluted acid requires the specific gravity of the concentrated acid.

C. Dilution and concentration of liquids and solids. Dilution and concentration problems are often easily solved by identifying the amount of drug involved followed by use of an appropriate proportion.

1. **How many milliliters of a 1:50 stock solution of ephedrine sulfate should be used in compounding the following prescription?**

R_x ephedrine sulfate   0.25%
rose water, ad   30 mL

$$\frac{0.25 \text{ g}}{100 \text{ mL}} \times 30 \text{ mL} = 0.075 \text{ g drug required}$$

$$\frac{50 \text{ mL}}{1 \text{ g}} = \frac{x \text{ mL}}{0.075 \text{ g}};$$

$x = 3.75$ mL of stock solution required for prescription

2. **How many milliliters of a 15% w/v concentrate of benzalkonium chloride should be used in preparing 300 mL of a stock solution such that 15 mL diluted to 1 L will yield a 1: 5000 solution?**

a. First, determine the amount of drug in 1 L of a 1:5000 solution.

$$\frac{5000 \text{ mL}}{1000 \text{ mL}} = \frac{1 \text{ g}}{x \text{ g}}; x = 0.2 \text{ g of benzalkonium chloride in the final solution}$$

b. Now, because 15 mL of the stock solution is being diluted to 1 L, a stock solution is needed in which 15 mL contain 0.2 g of drug. The amount of drug required to make 300 mL of the stock solution is found by proportion.

$$\frac{0.2 \text{ g}}{x \text{ g}} = \frac{15 \text{ mL}}{300 \text{ mL}}; x = 4 \text{ g of drug required to make 300 mL of solution}$$

c. Finally, to determine the amount of 15% concentrate required,

$$\frac{15 \text{ g}}{4 \text{ g}} \times \frac{100 \text{ mL}}{x \text{ mL}}; x = 26.7 \text{ mL of 15% solution required to}$$
obtain necessary drug

3. When the relative amount of components must be determined for preparation of a mixture of a desired concentration, the problem is most easily solved using alligation alternate.

How many grams of 2.5% hydrocortisone cream should be mixed with 360 g of 0.25% cream to make a 1% hydrocortisone cream?

2.5%	0.75 parts of 2.5% cream	= 1 part	0.75/2.25 = 1/3
0.25%	1.5 parts of 0.25% cream	= 2 parts	1.5/2.25 =2/3
	2.25 parts total	= 3 parts	

1%

The relative amounts of the 2.5% and 1% creams are 1 to 2, respectively. By proportion, the mass of 2.5% cream to use can be determined. **If 2 parts of 0.25% cream is represented by 360 g, then the total mass (3 parts) is represented by what mass?**

$$\frac{2 \text{ parts}}{3 \text{ parts}} = \frac{360 \text{ g}}{x \text{ g}}; x = 540 \text{ g total}$$

With the total mass known, the amount of 2.5% cream can be identified. If 3 parts represent the total mass of 540 g, then 1 part represents the mass of 2.5% cream (x g = 180 g).

$$\frac{1 \text{ part}}{3 \text{ parts}} = \frac{x \text{ g}}{540 \text{ g}}; \ x = 180 \text{ g of 2.5\% cream}$$

VII. ELECTROLYTE SOLUTIONS. Electrolyte solutions contain species (electrolytes) that dissociate into ions. The **milliequivalent** (mEq) is the unit used to express the concentration of electrolytes in solution. Table 2-1 exhibits some physiologically important ions and their properties.

A. Milliequivalents. The milliequivalent is the amount, in milligrams, of a solute equal to 1/1000 of its gram-equivalent weight. Conversion of concentrations in the form of milliequivalent to concentrations in percentage strength, milligrams per milliliters (mg/mL) or any other terms, begins with calculation of the number of milliequivalents of drug. The following examples demonstrate the computation of milliequivalents and manipulation of data from Table 2-1 to perform the required calculations for preparing electrolyte solutions.

What is the concentration, in percent w/v, of a solution containing 2 mEq of potassium chloride per milliliter?
Calculations involving milliequivalents are easily solved if the practitioner follows a predefined procedure to determine the milliequivalent weight. This involves three steps.

1. Find the molecular weight (mol wt).

$$\text{Atomic wt K} = 39$$
$$\text{Atomic wt Cl} = 35.5$$
$$39 + 35.5 = 74.5 \text{ g} = \text{mol wt of KCl}$$

2. Calculate the equivalent weight (Eq wt) of KCl.

$$\text{Eq wt} = \frac{\text{mol wt}}{\text{valence}} = \frac{74.5}{1} = 74.5 \text{ g}$$

3. Determine the milliequivalent weight, which is $^1/_{1000}$ of the equivalent weight.

$$\text{mEq wt} = 74.5 \text{ g} / 1000 = 0.745 \text{ g or } 74.5 \text{ mg}$$

Table 2-1. Valences, Atomic Weights, and Milliequivalent Weights of Selected Ions

Ion	Formula	Valence	Atomic/Formula Weight	Milliequivalent Weight (mg)
Aluminum	Al^{+++}	3	27	9
Ammonium	NH_4^+	1	18	18
Calcium	Ca^{++}	2	40	20
Ferric	Fe^{+++}	3	56	18.7
Ferrous	Fe^{++}	2	56	28
Lithium	Li^+	1	7	7
Magnesium	Mg^{++}	2	24	12
Bicarbonate	HCO_3^-	1	61	61
Carbonate	CO_3^-	1	60	30
Chloride	Cl^-	1	35.5	35.5
Citrate	$C_6H_5O_7^{---}$	3	189	63
Gluconate	$C_6H_{11}O_7^-$	1	195	195
Lactate	$C_3H_5O_3^-$	1	89	89
Phosphate	$H_2PO_4^-$	1	97	97
Sulfate	SO_4^{--}	2	96	48
Potassium	K^+	1	29	39
Sodium	Na^+	1	23	23
Acetate	$C_2H_3O_2^-$	1	59	59

Now that we know the milliequivalent weight, we can calculate by dimensional analysis and proportion the concentration in percentage in a fourth step.

4. 0.0745 g/mEq × 2 mEq = 0.149 g of drug

$$\frac{0.149 \text{ g drug}}{1 \text{ mL}} = \frac{x \text{ g drug}}{100 \text{ mL}}; x = 14.9\text{g/100 mL} = 14.9\%$$

How many milliequivalents of Na^+ would be contained in a 15-mL volume of the following buffer?

$Na_2HPO_4\cdot7H_2O$		180 g
$NaH_2PO_4\cdot H_2O$		480 g
Purified water	ad	1000 mL

For each salt, the mass (and milliequivalents) must be found in a 15-mL dose.

$$\text{mol wt } Na_2HPO_4\cdot7H_2O \text{ (disodium hydrogen phosphate)} = 268 \text{ g}$$
$$\text{Eq wt} = 268 / 2 = 134 \text{ g}$$
$$1 \text{ mEq} = 0.134 \text{ g or } 134 \text{ mg}$$

$$\frac{180 \text{ g}}{x \text{ g}} = \frac{1000 \text{ mL}}{15 \text{ mL}}; x = 2.7 \text{ g of disodium hydrogen phosphate in each 15 mL}$$

$$2.7 \text{ g} \times \frac{1 \text{ mEq}}{0.134 \text{ g}} = 20.1 \text{ mEq of disodium hydrogen phosphate}$$

$$\text{mol wt } Na_2HPO_4\cdot H_2O \text{ (sodium biphosphate)} = 138 \text{ g}$$
$$\text{Eq wt} = 138 \text{ g}$$
$$1 \text{ mEq} = 0.138 \text{ g}$$

$$\frac{480 \text{ g}}{x \text{ g}} = \frac{1000 \text{ mL}}{15 \text{ mL}}; x = 7.2 \text{ g of sodium biphosphate in each 15 mL}$$

$$7.2 \text{ g} \times \frac{1 \text{ mEq}}{0.138 \text{ g}} = 52.2 \text{ mEq of sodium biphosphate}$$

$$20.1 \text{ mEq} + 52.2 \text{ mEq} = 72.3 \text{ mEq of sodium in each 15 mL of solution}$$

B. Milliosmoles (mOsmol). Osmotic pressure is directly proportional to the total number of particles in solution. The milliosmole is the unit of measure for osmotic concentration. For nonelectrolytes, 1 millimole represents 1 milliosmole. However, for electrolytes, the total number of particles in solution is determined by the number of particles produced in solution and influenced by the degree of dissociation. Assuming complete dissociation, 1 millimole of KCl represents 2 milliosmoles of total particles, 1 millimole of $CaCl_2$ represents 3 milliosmoles of total particles, etc. The ideal osmolar concentration can be calculated with the following equation.

$$\text{mOsmol/L} = \frac{\text{wt of substance in g/L}}{\text{mol wt in g}} \times \text{number of species} \times 1000$$

The pharmacist should recognize the difference between **ideal** osmolar concentration and **actual** osmolarity. As the concentration of solute increases, interaction between dissolved particles increases, resulting in a reduction of the actual osmolar values.

C. Isotonic solutions. An **isotonic** solution is one that has the same osmotic pressure as body fluids. **Isosmotic** fluids are fluids with the same osmotic pressure. Solutions to be administered to patients should be isosmotic with body fluids. A **hypotonic** solution is one with a lower osmotic pressure than body fluids, whereas a **hypertonic** solution has an osmotic pressure that is greater than body fluids.

1. Preparation of isotonic solutions. Colligative properties, including freezing point depression, are representative of the number of particles in solution and considered in preparation of isotonic solutions.
   a. When 1 g mol wt of any nonelectrolyte is dissolved in 1000 g of water, the freezing point of the solution is depressed by 1.86°C. By proportion, the weight of any nonelectrolyte needed to make the solution isotonic with body fluid can be calculated.

b. Boric acid (H_3BO_3) has a mol wt of 61.8 g. Thus 61.8 g of H_3BO_3 in 1000 g of water should produce a freezing point of 1.86°C. Therefore, knowing that the freezing point depression of body fluids is −0.52°C,

$$\frac{-1.86°C}{-0.52°C} = \frac{61.8 \text{ g}}{x \text{ g}}; \ x = 17.3 \text{ g}$$

and 17.3 g of H_3BO_3 in 1000 g of water provides a solution that is **isotonic.**

c. The degree of dissociation of electrolytes must be taken into account in such calculations. For example, NaCl is approximately 80% dissociated in weak solutions, yielding 180 particles in solution for each 100 molecules of NaCl. Therefore,

$$\frac{-1.86°C \times 1.8}{-0.52°C} = \frac{58 \text{ g}}{x \text{ g}}; \ x = 9.09 \text{ g}$$

indicating that 9.09 g of NaCl in 1000 g of water (0.9% w/v) should make a solution isotonic. Lacking any information on the degree of dissociation of an electrolyte, the following **dissociation values** (*i*) may be used.

(1) Substances that dissociate into two ions: 1.8
(2) Substances that dissociate into three ions: 2.6
(3) Substances that dissociate into four ions: 3.4
(4) Substances that dissociate into five ions: 4.2

2. Sodium chloride equivalents. The pharmacist will often be required to prepare an isotonic solution by adding an appropriate amount of another substance (drug or inert electrolyte or nonelectrolyte). Considering that isotonic fluids contain the equivalent of 0.9% NaCl, the question arises, How much of the added ingredient is required to make the solution isotonic? A **common method** for computing the amount of added ingredient to use for reaching isotonicity involves the use of **sodium chloride equivalents.**

a. Definition. The sodium chloride equivalent represents the amount of NaCl that is equivalent to the amount of particular drug in question. For every substance, there is one quantity that should have a constant tonic effect when dissolved in 1000 g of water. This is 1 g mol wt of the substance divided by its dissociation value (*i*).

b. Examples

(1) Considering H_3BO_3, from the last section, 17.3 g of H_3BO_3 is equivalent to 0.52 g of NaCl in tonicity. Therefore, the relative quantity of NaCl that is equivalent to H_3BO_3 in tonicity effects is determined as follows:

$$\frac{\text{mol wt of NaCl}/i \text{ value}}{\text{mol wt of } H_3BO_3/i \text{ value}} = \frac{58.5/1.8}{61.8/1.0}$$

Applying this method to atropine sulfate, recall that the molecular weight of NaCl and the molecular weight of atropine sulfate are 58.5 and 695 g, respectively, and their *i* values are 1.8 and 2.6, respectively. Calculate the mass of NaCl represented by 1 g of atropine sulfate (Table 2-2).

$$\frac{695 \times 1.8}{58.5 \times 2.6} = \frac{1 \text{ g}}{x \text{ g}}; \ x = 0.12 \text{ g NaCl represented by 1 g of atropine sulfate}$$

Table 2-2. Sodium Chloride (NaCl) Equivalents

Substance	NaCl Equivalent
Atropine sulfate (H_2O)	0.12
Boric acid	0.52
Chlorobutanol	0.24
Dextrose (anhydrous)	0.18
Ephedrine hydrochloride	0.29
Phenacaine hydrochloride	0.20
Potassium chloride	0.78

(2) An example of the practical use of sodium chloride equivalents is seen in the following problem.

How many grams of boric acid should be used in compounding the following prescription?

R_x	phenacaine hydrochloride	1%
	chlorobutanol	0.5%
	boric acid	qs
	purified water, ad	60.0 mL
	make isotonic solution	

The prescription calls for 0.3 g of chlorobutanol and 0.6 g of phenacaine. How much boric acid is required to prepare this prescription? The question is best answered in four steps.

(a) Find the mass of sodium chloride represented by all ingredients.

$0.20 \times 0.6 = 0.120$ g of sodium chloride represented by phenacaine hydrochloride

$0.24 \times 0.3 = \underline{0.072}$ g of sodium chloride represented by chlorobutanol

0.192 g of sodium chloride represented by the two active ingredients

(b) Find the mass of sodium chloride required to prepare an equal volume of isotonic solution.

$$\frac{0.9 \text{ g NaCl}}{100 \text{ mL}} = \frac{X \text{ g NaCL}}{60 \text{ mL}}; \; x = 0.540 \text{ g of sodium chloride}$$

in 60 mL of an isotonic sodium chloride solution

(c) Calculate, by subtraction, the amount of NaCl required to make the solution isotonic.

0.540 g NaCl required for isotonicity
$\underline{0.192}$ g NaCl represented by ingredients
0.348 g NaCl required to make isotonic solution

(d) Because the prescription calls for boric acid to be used, one last step is required.

$\frac{0.348 \text{ g}}{0.52}$ (sodium chloride equivalent for boric acid) $= 0.669$ g of boric acid to be used

VIII. STATISTICS

A. Introduction. Statistics can be used to describe and compare data distributions. Such **frequency distributions** are constructed by classifying individual observations into categories corresponding to fixed numeric intervals and plotting the number of observations in each such category (i.e., **interval frequency**) versus the category descriptor (e.g., the interval mean or range). Because of random errors, repeated observations or measurements (of the same value) are not identical. These observations have a **normal distribution.** Normally distributed data are described by a **bell-shaped (Gaussian) curve** with a maximum, μ (**population mean**), corresponding to the central tendency of the population and a spread characterized by the **population standard deviation** (σ). Statistics derived from a **sample** or subset of a population can be used as estimates of the population parameters.

B. Frequency distribution

1. Estimates of population mean. The population mean, μ, is the best estimate of the true value.

    a. The sample mean. For a finite number of observations, the arithmetic average or mean ($\bar{X}$) is the best estimate of the true value, μ.

$$\bar{X} = \frac{\sum x_i}{n}$$

where $\sum x_i$ is the sum of all (n) observations.

   (1) **Accuracy** is the degree to which a measured value (X or $\bar{X}$) agrees with the "true" value (μ).

   (2) **Error** (or bias) is the difference between a measured value (X or $\bar{X}$) and the "true" value (μ).

   b. **Median.** The median is the midmost value of a data distribution. When all the values are arranged in increasing (or decreasing) order, the median is the middle value for an **odd** number of observations. For an **even** number of observations, the median is the arithmetic mean of the two middle values. For a **normal distribution, the median equals the mean.** The median is less affected by "outliers" or by a skewed distribution.

   c. **Mode.** The mode is the most frequently occurring value (or values) in a frequency distribution. The mode is useful for non-normal distributions, especially those that are **bimodal.**

2. **Estimates of variability.** For an **infinite** number of observations, the **population variance** (σ^2) can be used to describe the variability or "spread" of observations in a data distribution. For a **finite** number of observations, the **sample variance** (s^2) can be used to describe the variability or spread of observations in a data distribution.

   a. **Sample variance** (s^2) is estimated by

   $$s^2 = \frac{\sum(x_i - \bar{X})^2}{(n-1)}$$

   $$s^2 = \frac{\sum x_i^2 - \frac{(\sum x_i)^2}{n}}{(n-1)}$$

   where $\bar{X}$ is the mean and $(n-1)$ is the number of degrees of freedom (df).

   b. **Range.** For a very small number of observations, the **range** (w) can be used to describe the variability in the data set:

   $$w = |X_{largest} - X_{smallest}|$$

   c. The **standard deviation** (s or SD), one of the most commonly encountered estimates of variability, is equal to the square root of the variance.

   $$s = \sqrt{s^2} = \sqrt{\frac{\sum(x_i - \bar{X})^2}{(n-1)}}$$

   or

   $$s = \sqrt{s^2} = \sqrt{\frac{\sum x_i^2 - \frac{(\sum x_i)^2}{n}}{(n-1)}}$$

   d. **Precision** (reproducibility) is the degree to which replicate measurements "made in exactly the same way" agree with each other. **Precision** is often expressed as the **relative standard deviation** (RSD or %RSD):

   $$\%RSD = \left(\frac{s}{\bar{X}} \times 100\right)$$

3. The **standard deviation of the mean** (s_m), or standard error of the mean (SEM), is an estimate of the **variability** or **error in the mean** obtained from n observations. It is often used to establish confidence intervals for describing the mean of a data set or when comparing the means of two data sets.

   $$s_m = \frac{s}{\sqrt{n}}$$

STUDY QUESTIONS

Directions for questions 1–30: Each question, statement, or incomplete statement in this section can be correctly answered or completed by **one** of the suggested answers or phrases. Choose the **best** answer.

1. If a vitamin solution contains 0.5 mg of fluoride ion in each milliliter, then how many milligrams of fluoride ion would be provided by a dropper that delivers 0.6 mL?

   (A) 0.3 mg
   (B) 0.1 mg
   (C) 1 mg
   (D) 0.83 mg

2. How many chloramphenicol capsules, each containing 250 mg, are needed to provide 25 mg per kg per day for 7 days for a person weighing 200 lb?

   (A) 90 capsules
   (B) 64 capsules
   (C) 13 capsules
   (D) 25 capsules

3. If 3.17 kg of a drug is used to make 50,000 tablets, how many milligrams will 30 tablets contain?

   (A) 1.9 mg
   (B) 1900 mg
   (C) 0.0019 mg
   (D) 3.2 mg

4. A capsule contains $\frac{1}{8}$ gr of ephedrine sulfate, $\frac{1}{4}$ gr of theophylline, and $\frac{1}{16}$ gr of phenobarbital. What is the total mass of the active ingredients in milligrams?

   (A) 20 mg
   (B) 8 mg
   (C) 28 mg
   (D) 4 mg

5. If 1 fluid ounce of a cough syrup contains 10 gr of sodium citrate, how many milligrams are contained in 10 mL?

   (A) 650 mg
   (B) 65 mg
   (C) 217 mg
   (D) 20 mg

6. How many capsules, each containing $\frac{1}{4}$ gr of phenobarbital, can be manufactured if a bottle containing 2 avoirdupois ounces of phenobarbital is available?

   (A) 771 capsules
   (B) 350 capsules
   (C) 3500 capsules
   (D) 1250 capsules

7. Using the formula for calamine lotion, determine the amount of calamine (in grams) necessary to prepare 240 mL of lotion.

Calamine	80 g
Zinc oxide	80 g
Glycerin	20 mL
Bentonite magma	250 mL
Calcium hydroxide topical solution	sufficient quantity to make 1000 mL

   (A) 19.2 g
   (B) 140 g
   (C) 100 g
   (D) 24 g

8. From the following formula, calculate the amount of white wax required to make 1 lb of cold cream. Determine the mass in grams.

Cetyl esters wax	12.5 parts
White wax	12.0 parts
Mineral oil	56.0 parts
Sodium borate	0.5 parts
Purified water	19.0 parts

   (A) 56.75 g
   (B) 254.24 g
   (C) 54.48 g
   (D) 86.26 g

9. How many grams of aspirin should be used to prepare 1.255 kg of the powder?

ASA	6 parts
Phenacetin	3 parts
Caffeine	1 part

   (A) 125 g
   (B) 750 g
   (C) 175 g
   (D) 360 g

10. A solution contains 1.25 mg of a drug per milliliter. At what rate should the solution be infused (drops/min) if the drug is to be administered at a rate of 80 mg/hr? (1 mL = 30 drops)

(A) 64 drops/min
(B) 1.06 drops/min
(C) 32 drops/min
(D) 20 drops/min

11. The recommended maintenance dose of aminophylline for children is 1.0 mg/kg/hr by injection. If 10 mL of a 25-mg/mL solution of aminophylline is added to a 100-mL bottle for dextrose, what should be the rate of delivery in mL/hr for a 40-lb child?

(A) 2.30 mL/hr
(B) 8.00 mL/hr
(C) 18.9 mL/hr
(D) 18.2 mL/hr

12. For children, streptomycin is to be administered at a dose of 30 mg/kg of body weight daily in divided doses every 6–12 hr. The dry powder is dissolved by adding water for injection, USP in an amount to yield the desired concentration as indicated in the following table (for a 1-g vial).

Approximate Concentration (mg/mL)	Volume (mL)
200	4.2
250	3.2
400	1.8

Reconstituting at the lowest possible concentration, what volume (in mL) would be withdrawn to obtain one day's dose for a 50-lb child?

(A) 3.4 mL
(B) 22.73 mL
(C) 2.50 mL
(D) 2.27 mL

13. The atropine sulfate is available only in the form of 1/150 gr tablets. How many atropine sulfate tablets would you use to compound the following prescription?

Atropine sulfate	1/200 gr
Codeine phosphate	1/4 gr
Aspirin	5 gr
d.t.d.	#24 capsules
Sig:	1 capsule p.r.n.

(A) 3 tablets
(B) 6 tablets
(C) 12 tablets
(D) 18 tablets

14. In 25.0 mL of a solution for injection, there are 4.00 mg of the drug. If the dose to be administered to a patient is 200 μg, what quantity (in mL) of this solution should be used?

(A) 1.25 mL
(B) 125 mL
(C) 12.0 mL
(D) None of the above

15. How many milligrams of papaverine will the patient receive each day?

R_x	papaverine hydrochloride	1.0 g
	aqua	30.0 mL
	syrup tolu, qs ad	90.0 mL
	Sig:	1 teaspoon t.i.d.

(A) 56 mg
(B) 5.6 mg
(C) 166 mg
(D) 2.5 mg

16. Considering the following formula, how many grams of sodium bromide should be used in filling this prescription?

R_x	sodium bromide	1.2 g
	syrup tolu	2.0 mL
	syrup wild cherry, qs ad	5.0 mL
	d.t.d.	#24

(A) 1.2 g
(B) 1200 g
(C) 28.8 g
(D) 220 g

17. How many milliliters of a 7.5% stock solution of $KMnO_4$ should be used to obtain the KMnO needed?

KMnO4, qs
Distilled water, ad 1000
Sig: 2 teaspoons diluted to 500 mL yield a 1:5000 solution

(A) 267 mL
(B) 133 mL
(C) 26.7 mL
(D) 13.3 mL

18. The formula for Ringer's solution follows. How much sodium chloride is needed to make 120 mL?

R_x	sodium chloride	8.60 g
	potassium chloride	0.30 g
	calcium chloride	0.33 g
	water for injection, qs ad	1000 mL

(A) 120 g
(B) 1.03 g
(C) 0.12 g
(D) 103 g

19. How many grams of talc should be added to 1 lb of a powder containing 20 g of zinc undecylenate per 100 g to reduce the concentration of zinc undecylenate to 3%?

(A) 3026.7 g
(B) 2572.7 g
(C) 17 g
(D) 257 g

20. How many milliliters of a 0.9% aqueous solution can be made from 20.0 g of sodium chloride?

(A) 2222 mL
(B) 100 mL
(C) 222 mL
(D) 122 mL

21. The blood of a reckless driver contains 0.1% alcohol. Express the concentration of alcohol in parts per million.

(A) 100 ppm
(B) 1000 ppm
(C) 1 ppm
(D) 250 ppm

22. Syrup is an 85% w/v solution of sucrose in water. It has a density of 1.313 g/mL. How many milliliters of water should be used to make 125 mL of syrup?

(A) 106.25 mL
(B) 164.1 mL
(C) 57.9 mL
(D) 25.0 mL

23. How many grams of benzethonium chloride should be used in preparing 5 gal. of a 0.025% w/v solution?

(A) 189.25 g
(B) 18.9 g
(C) 4.73 g
(D) 35 g

24. How many grams of menthol should be used to prepare this prescription?

R_x	menthol	0.8%
	alcohol, qs ad	60.0 mL

(A) 0.48 g
(B) 0.8 g
(C) 4.8 g
(D) 1.48 g

25. How many milliliters of a 1:1500 solution can be made by dissolving 4.8 g of cetylpyridinium chloride in water?

(A) 7200 mL
(B) 7.2 mL
(C) 48 mL
(D) 4.8 mL

26. The manufacturer specifies that one Domeboro tablet dissolved in 1 pint of water makes a modified Burow's solution approximately equivalent to a 1:40 dilution. How many tablets should be used in preparing ½ gal of a 1:10 dilution?

(A) 16 tablets
(B) 189 tablets
(C) 12 tablets
(D) 45 tablets

27. How many milliosmoles of calcium chloride ($CaCl_2 \cdot 2H_2O$ – mol wt = 147) are represented in 147 mL of a 10% w/v calcium chloride solution?

(A) 100 mOsmol
(B) 200 mOsmol
(C) 300 mOsmol
(D) 3 mOsmol

28. How many grams of boric acid should be used in compounding the following prescription?

Phenacaine HCl 1.0% (NaCl eq = 0.17)
Chlorobutanol 0.5% (NaCl eq = 0.18)
Boric acid, qs (NaCl eq = 0.52)
Purified H_2O, ad 30 mL
Make isotonic solution
Sig: 1 drop in each eye

(A) 0.37 g
(B) 0.74 g
(C) 0.27 g
(D) 0.47 g

29. A pharmacist prepares 1 gal of KCl solution by mixing 565 g of KCl (valence = 1) in an appropriate vehicle. How many milliequivalents of K^+ are in 15 mL of this solution? (atomic weights: K = 30; Cl = 35.5)

(A) 7.5 mEq
(B) 10 mEq
(C) 20 mEq
(D) 30 mEq
(E) 40 mEq

30. A vancomycin solution containing 1000 mg of vancomycin hydrochloride diluted to 250 mL with D5W is to be infused at a constant rate with an infusion pump in 2 hr. What is the rate of drug administration?

(A) 2.08 mg/min
(B) 8.33 mg/min
(C) 4.17 mg/min
(D) 16.7 mg/min
(E) 5.21 mg/min

For questions 31–34: Five ibuprofen tablets were assayed for drug content, and the following results were obtained by high-pressure liquid chromatography (HPLC) analysis: 198.2 mg, 199.7 mg, 202.5 mg, 201.3 mg, 196.4 mg.

31. What is the mean ibuprofen content?

(A) 196.9 mg
(B) 200.2 mg
(C) 199.6 mg
(D) 249.5 mg
(E) 202.5 mg

32. What is the standard deviation of ibuprofen content in the analyzed tablets?

(A) 2.17 mg
(B) 3.35 mg
(C) 2.42 mg
(D) 3.00 mg
(E) −2.17 mg

33. What is the percent relative standard deviation (%RSD) for this ibuprofen tablet analysis?

(A) 1.69%
(B) 1.21%
(C) 8.25%
(D) 3.35%
(E) 1.50%

34. What is the standard deviation of the mean drug content of this sample?

(A) 0.480 mg
(B) 0.605 mg
(C) 1.21 mg
(D) 1.08 mg
(E) 0.825 mg

ANSWERS AND EXPLANATIONS

1. The answer is A *[see I.A.2].*

2. The answer is B *[see II].*

3. The answer is B *[see II].*

4. The answer is C *[see II].*

5. The answer is C *[see I.A.2].*

6. The answer is C *[see II].*

7. The answer is A *[see III].*

8. The answer is C *[see II; III.A].*
The formula tells the pharmacist that white wax (W.W.) represents 12 parts out of the total 100 parts in the prescription. What we wish to determine is the mass of white wax required to prepare 454 g (1 lb) of the recipe. This can be easily solved by proportion:

$$\frac{12 \text{ parts W.W.}}{100 \text{ parts total}} = \frac{x}{454 \text{ parts (grams)}}; \; x = 54.48 \text{ g}$$

9. The answer is B *[see III.A].*

10. The answer is C *[see IV.E].*

11. The answer is B *[see II; IV].*

12. The answer is A *[see IV].*

13. The answer is D *[see II; III.B].*

14. The answer is A *[see I.A.2; II].*
Dimensional analysis is often useful for calculating doses. Considering that 4 mg of the drug is present in each 25 mL of solution, we can easily calculate the number of milliliters to be used to give a dose of 0.200 mg (200 μg). Always include units in your calculations.

$$\frac{25 \text{ mL}}{4 \text{ mg}} \times 0.200 \text{ mg} = 1.25 \text{ mL}$$

15. The answer is C *[see III.B].*

16. The answer is C *[see III.B].*

17. The answer is B *[see V.A; VI].*
First, determine the mass of drug in the final diluted solution.

$$\frac{1 \text{ part}}{5000 \text{ parts}} = \frac{x \text{ g}}{500 \text{ g}}; \; x = 0.1 \text{ g}$$

Now, if 0.1 g of drug is present in 500 mL of 1:5000 solution, 2 teaspoonfuls (10 mL) of the prescription contains the same amount of drug (0.1 g) before dilution. From this, the amount of drug in 1000 mL (the total volume) of the prescription can be determined:

$$\frac{0.1 \text{ g}}{10 \text{ mL}} = \frac{x \text{ g}}{1000 \text{ mL}}; \; x = 10 \text{ g}$$

Finally, to obtain the correct amount of drug to formulate the prescription (10 g), we are to use a 7.5% stock solution. Recalling the definition of percentage strength w/v:

$$\frac{100 \text{ mL}}{7.5 \text{ g}} \times 10 \text{ g} = 133.3 \text{ mL or } 133 \text{ mL}$$

18. The answer is B *[see III.B].*

19. The answer is B *[see V.C; VI.C].*

20. The answer is A *[see I.A.2; V.A].*
Using dimensional analysis

$$\frac{20 \text{ g} \times 100 \text{ mL}}{0.9 \text{ g}} = 2222 \text{ mL}$$

21. The answer is B *[see V.D.1].*

22. The answer is C *[see I.A; V.A.1].*
Using the density, the weight of 125 mL of syrup can be calculated:

$$125 \text{ mL} \times 1.313 \text{g/mL} = 164.125 \text{ g}$$

Using proportion and the sucrose concentration in w/v, the weight of sucrose in 125 mL of syrup can be calculated:

$$\frac{100 \text{ mL}}{125 \text{ mL}} = \frac{85 \text{ g}}{x \text{ g}}; \ x = 106.25\text{g}$$

Finally, the weight of water in 125 mL of syrup can be calculated:

$$164.125 \text{ g} - 106.25 \text{ g} = 57.875 \text{ g}$$

which has a volume of 57.9 mL.

23. The answer is C *[see I; II; V].*

24. The answer is A *[see I; V].*

25. The answer is A *[see I; V].*
The problem is easily solved by proportion. The question to be answered is, If 1 g of drug is present in 1500 mL of solution, what volume can be made with 4.8 g of drug?

$$\frac{1 \text{ g}}{4.8 \text{ g}} = \frac{1500 \text{ mL}}{x \text{ mL}}; \ x = 7200 \text{ mL}$$

(the volume of 1 to 1500 solution that can be prepared from 4.8 g of drug)

26. The answer is A *[see I; V].*

27. The answer is C *[see VII.B].*
Recalling the expression for ideal osmolar concentration:

$$mOsmol/L = \frac{100 \text{ g/L}}{147 \text{ g/mol}} \times 3 \times 1000$$

$$= mOsmol/L \times 0.147 \text{ L}$$
$$= 300 \text{ mOsmol}$$

28. The answer is A *[see VII.C].*

29. The answer is D *[see VII.A].*

30. The answer is B *[see IV.E].*
Using dimensional anaylsis:

$$\frac{1000 \text{ mg}}{250 \text{ mL}} \times \frac{250 \text{ mL}}{2 \text{ hr}} \times \frac{1 \text{ hr}}{60 \text{ min}} = 8.33 \text{ mg/min}$$

31. The answer is C *[see VIII.B.1].*
The mean is calculated directly from the equation:

$$\overline{X} = \frac{\sum X_i}{n} = \frac{998.1}{5} = 199.6 \text{ mg}$$

32. The answer is C *[see VIII.B.3].*

The standard deviation can be calculated with the most commonly used equation:

x_i	x_i^2
198.2	39,283.24*
199.7	39,880.09
202.5	41,006.25
201.3	40,521.69
196.4	38,572.96
$\sum x_i = 998.1$	$\sum x_i^2 = 199,264.23$

$$\sqrt{s^2} = \sqrt{\frac{199,264.23 - \frac{(988.1)^2}{5}}{(5-1)}} = 2.42 \text{ mg}$$

Note: It is important to carry enough significant figures through the calculation to minimize round-off error.

33. The answer is B *[see VIII.B.4].*

$$\%RSD = \left(\frac{s}{\bar{X}}\right) \times 100 = \left(\frac{2.42}{199.6}\right) \times 100 = 1.21\%$$

34. The answer is D *[see VIII.C].*

$$s_m = \frac{s}{\sqrt{n}} = \frac{2.42}{\sqrt{5}} = 1.08 \text{ mg}$$

3
Pharmaceutical Principles and Drug Dosage Forms

Lawrence H. Block

I. INTRODUCTION. Pharmaceutical principles are the underlying physicochemical principles that allow a drug to be incorporated into a pharmaceutical **dosage form** (e.g., solution, capsule). These principles apply whether the drug is extemporaneously compounded by the pharmacist or manufactured for commercial distribution as a **drug product.**

A. The finished **dosage form** contains the active drug ingredient in association with nondrug (usually inert) ingredients (**excipients**) that make up the **vehicle,** or **formulation matrix.**

B. The **drug delivery system** concept, which has evolved since the 1960s, is a more holistic concept. It embraces not only the drug (or prodrug) and its formulation matrix, but also the dynamic interactions among the drug, its formulation matrix, its container, and the physiologic milieux of the patient. These dynamic interactions are the subject of **biopharmaceutics** (see Chapter 4).

II. INTERMOLECULAR FORCES OF ATTRACTION

A. Introduction. The application of pharmaceutical principles to drug dosage forms is illustrated when drug dosage forms are **categorized** according to their **physical state, degree of heterogeneity,** and **chemical composition.** The usual relevant states of matter are **gases, liquids,** and **solids.** Intermolecular forces of attraction are weakest in gases and strongest in solids. Conversions from one physical state to another can involve simply overcoming intermolecular forces of attraction by adding energy (heat). Chemical composition can have a dramatic effect on physicochemical properties and behavior. For this reason, it is necessary to distinguish between **polymers,** or **macromolecules,** and more conventional (i.e., smaller) molecules, or **micromolecules.**

B. Intermolecular forces of attraction. Because atoms vary in their electronegativity, electron sharing between different atoms is likely to be unequal. This asymmetric electron distribution causes a shift in the overall electron cloud in the molecule. As a result, the molecule tends to behave as a **dipole** (i.e., as if it had a positive and a negative pole). The dipole associated with each covalent bond has a corresponding **dipole moment** (μ) defined as the product of the distance of charge separation (d) and the charge (q):

$$\mu = q \times d$$

The molecular dipole moment may be viewed as the vector sum of the individual bond moments.

1. Nonpolar molecules that have **perfect symmetry** (e.g., carbon tetrachloride) have dipole moments of zero (Figure 3-1).

2. Polar molecules are **asymmetric** and have nonzero dipole moments.

3. When **dipolar** molecules approach one another close enough—"positive to positive" or "negative to negative"—so that their electron clouds interpenetrate, **intermolecular repulsive forces** arise. When these dipolar molecules approach one another so that the positive

Figure 3-1. The carbon tetrachloride molecule.

pole of one is close to the negative pole of the other, molecular **attraction** occurs (**dipole–dipole interaction**). When the identically charged poles of the two molecules are closer, **repulsion** occurs.

C. Types of intermolecular forces of attraction include the following:

1. Nonpolar molecules do not have permanent dipoles. However, the instantaneous electron distribution in a molecule can be asymmetric. The resultant transient dipole moment can induce a dipole in an adjacent molecule. This **induced dipole–induced dipole interaction (London dispersion force),** with a force of 0.5–1 kcal/mol, is sufficient to facilitate order in a molecular array. These relatively weak electrostatic forces are responsible for the liquefaction of nonpolar gases.

2. The transient dipole induced by a permanent dipole, or **dipole–induced dipole interaction (Debye induction force),** is a stronger interaction, with a force of 1–3 kcal/mol.

3. **Permanent dipole interactions (Keesom orientation forces),** with a force of 1–7 kcal/mol, together with Debye and London forces, constitute **van der Waals forces.** Collectively, they are responsible for the more substantive structure and molecular ordering found in liquids.

4. **Hydrogen bonds.** Because they are small and have a large electrostatic field, hydrogen atoms can approach highly electronegative atoms (e.g., fluorine, oxygen, nitrogen, chlorine, sulfur) and interact electrostatically to form a hydrogen bond. Depending on the electronegativity of the second atom and the molecular environment in which hydrogen bonding occurs, hydrogen bond energy varies from approximately 1 to 8 kcal/mol.

5. **Ion–ion, ion–dipole, and ion-induced dipole forces. Positive–negative ion interactions** in the solid state involve forces of 100–200 kcal/mol. Ionic interactions are reduced considerably in liquid systems in the presence of other electrolytes. **Ion–dipole** interaction, or **dipole induction by an ion,** can also affect molecular aggregation, or ordering, in a system.

III. STATES OF MATTER

A. Gases. Molecules in the gaseous state can be pictured as moving along straight paths, in all directions and at high velocities (e.g., mean velocity for H_2O vapor: 587 m/sec; for O_2: 440 m/sec), until they collide with other molecules. As a result of these random collisions, molecular velocities and paths change, and the molecules continue to collide with other molecules and with the boundaries of the system (e.g., the walls of a container holding the gas). This process, repeated incessantly, is responsible for the **pressure** exhibited within the confines of the system.

1. The interrelation among **volume (V), pressure (P),** and the **absolute temperature (T)** is given by the **ideal gas law,** which is the equation of state for an ideal gas:

$$PV = nRT$$
$$PV = (g/M)RT$$

where n is the number of moles of gas—equivalent to the number of grams (g) of gas divided by the molecular weight of the gas (M)—and R is the **molar gas constant** (0.08205 L atm/mole deg).

2. Pharmaceutical gases include the **anesthetic gases** (e.g., nitrous oxide, halothane). **Compressed gases** include oxygen (for therapy), nitrogen, and carbon dioxide. **Liquefiable gases,** including certain **halohydrocarbons** and **hydrocarbons,** are used as propellants in **aerosol products (pressurized packaging),** as are compressed gases, such as nitrous oxide, nitrogen, and carbon dioxide. Ethylene oxide is a gas used to sterilize or disinfect heat-labile objects.

3. In general, as the temperature of a substance increases, its **heat content,** or **enthalpy,** increases as well.
    a. Substances can undergo a change of state, or phase change, from the solid to the liquid state (**melting**) or from the liquid to the gaseous state (**vaporization**).
    b. **Volatile liquids** (e.g., ether, halothane, methoxyflurane) are used as inhalation anesthetics. Amyl nitrite is a volatile liquid that is inhaled for its vasodilating effect in acute angina.
    c. **Sublimation** occurs when a solid is heated directly to the gaseous, or vapor, state without passing through the liquid state (e.g., camphor, iodine). Ice sublimes at pressures below

3 torr. The process of **freeze-drying,** or **lyophilization,** is a form of vacuum drying in which water is removed by sublimation from the frozen product. It is an especially useful process for drying aqueous solutions or dispersions of heat- or oxygen-sensitive drugs and biologicals (e.g., proteins, peptides).

  d. The reverse process (i.e., direct transition from the vapor state to the solid state) is also referred to as sublimation, but the preferred term is **deposition.** Some forms of sulfur and colloidal silicon dioxide are prepared in this way.

 4. The intermolecular forces of attraction in gases are virtually nonexistent at room temperature. Gases display little or no ordering.

B. Liquids. The intermolecular forces of attraction in liquids (**van der Waals forces**) are sufficient to impose some ordering, or regular arrangement, among the molecules. **Hydrogen bonding** increases the likelihood of cohesion in liquids and further affects their physicochemical behavior. However, these forces are much weaker than **covalent** or **ionic** forces. Therefore, liquids tend to display short-range rather than long-range order. Hypothetically, although molecules of a liquid would tend to aggregate in localized clusters, no defined structuring would be evident.

 1. Surface and interfacial tension
  a. Molecules in the bulk phase of a liquid are surrounded by other molecules of the same kind (Figure 3-2A). Molecules at the surface of a liquid are not completely surrounded by like molecules (Figure 3-2B). As a result, molecules at or near the surface of a liquid experience a net inward pull from molecules in the interior of the liquid. Because of this net inward intermolecular attraction, the liquid surface tends to spontaneously contract. Thus liquids tend to assume a spherical shape (i.e., a volume with the minimum surface area). This configuration has the least free energy.
  b. Any expansion of the surface increases the free energy of the system. Thus **surface free energy** can be defined by the work required to increase the surface area A of the liquid by 1 area unit. This value is expressed as the number of milli-Newtons (mN) needed to expand a 1-m^2 surface by 1 unit:

$$\text{work} = \gamma \times \Delta A$$

  where ΔA is the increase in surface area and γ is the **surface tension,** or **surface free energy,** in mN m^{-1}—equivalent to centimeter-gram-second (CGS) units of dynes cm^{-1}. At 20°C. water has a surface tension of 72 mN m^{-1}, whereas n-octanol has a surface tension of 27 mN m^{-1}. Thus more work must be expended to expand the surface of water than to expand the surface of n-octanol (i.e., to proceed from a given volume of bulk liquid to the corresponding volume of small droplets).
  c. At the **boundary,** or **interface,** between two immiscible liquids that are in contact with one another, the corresponding **interfacial tension** (i.e., free energy, or work required to expand the interfacial area) reflects the extent of the intermolecular forces of attraction and repulsion at the interface. When the interface is between two liquids, substantial molecular interaction occurs across the interface between the two phases. This interaction

Figure 3-2. A. Molecules in the bulk phase. **B.** Molecules at the surface of a liquid.

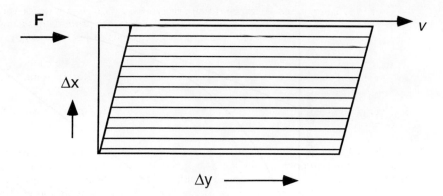

Figure 3-3. Liquid flow.

reduces the imbalance in forces of attraction within each phase. The interfacial tension between *n*-octanol and water is reduced to 8.5 mN m^{-1} from 72 mN m^{-1} (γ air/water). This reduction indicates, in part, the interfacial interaction between *n*-octanol and water.

2. The flow of a liquid across a solid surface can be examined in terms of the **velocity,** or rate of movement, of the liquid relative to the surface across which it flows. More insight can be gained by visualizing the flow of liquid as involving the movement of numerous parallel layers of liquid between an upper, movable plate and a lower, fixed plate (Figure 3-3). The application of a constant force (*F*) to the upper plate causes both this plate and the uppermost layer of liquid in contact with it to move with a velocity $\Delta y/\Delta x$. The interaction between the fixed bottom plate and the liquid layer closest to it prevents the movement of the bottom layer of liquid. The **velocity** (*v*) of the remaining layers of liquid between the two plates is proportional to their distance from the immovable plate (i.e., $\Delta y/\Delta x$). The **velocity gradient** leads to deformation of the liquid with time. This deformation is the **rate of shear,** d*v*/d*x*, or *D*. **Newton** defined flow in terms of the ratio of the force *F* applied to a plate of area *A*—**shear stress** (τ)—divided by the velocity gradient (*D*) induced by τ:

$$\frac{F}{A} = \eta \frac{dv}{dx}$$

or

$$\frac{\tau}{D} = \eta$$

The proportionality constant η is the coefficient of **viscosity.** It indicates the resistance to flow of adjacent layers of fluid. The reciprocal of η is **fluidity.** Units of viscosity in the CGS system are dynes cm^{-2}s^{-1}, or poise. In the SI system, the units are Newtons m^{-2}s^{-1}, which corresponds to 10 poise. The viscosity of water at 20°C is approximately 0.01 poise, or 1 centipoise (cps), which corresponds to 1 mN m^{-2}s^{-1}.

   a. Substances that flow in accordance with the equation in III.B.2 (Newton's law) are known as **Newtonian substances.** Liquids that consist of simple molecules and dilute dispersions tend to be **Newtonian.** For a Newtonian fluid, a plot of shear stress as a function of shear rate (a **flow curve** or **rheogram**) yields a straight line with a slope of η (Figure 3-4, *Curve 1*).
   b. **Non-Newtonian substances** do not obey Newton's equation of flow. These substances tend to exhibit **shear-dependent** or **time-dependent viscosity.** In either case, viscosity is more aptly termed **apparent viscosity** because Newton's law is not strictly obeyed. Heterogeneous liquids and solids are most likely non-Newtonian.
      (1) **Shear-dependent viscosity** involves either an *increase* in apparent viscosity (i.e., **shear thickening,** or **dilatancy**) (Figure 3-4, *Curve 3*) or a *decrease* in apparent viscosity (i.e., **shear thinning,** or **pseudo-plasticity**) (Figure 3-4, *Curve 2*) with an increase in the rate of shear. Shear thickening is displayed by suspensions that have a high solids content of small, deflocculated particles. Shear thinning is displayed by poly-

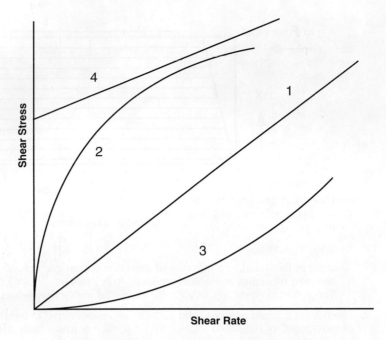

Figure 3-4. Non-Newtonian flow curves.

mer or macromolecule solutions. **Plastic,** or **Bingham body,** behavior (Figure 3-4, *Curve 4*) is exemplified by flocculated particles in concentrated suspensions that show no apparent response to low-level stress. Flow begins only after a limiting yield stress (**yield value**) is exceeded.

   (2) Time-dependent viscosity

    (a) The yield value of **plastic** systems may be time dependent (i.e., may depend on the time scale involved in the application of force). **Thixotropic** systems display shear-thinning behavior but do not immediately recover their higher apparent viscosity when the rate of shear is lowered. In a thixotropic system, structural recovery is relatively slow compared with structural breakdown.

    (b) Thixotropy occurs with heterogeneous systems that involve a three-dimensional structure or network. When such a system is at rest, it appears to have a relatively rigid consistency. Under shear, the structure breaks down and fluidity increases (i.e., **gel–sol** transformation).

    (c) Rheopexy (negative thixotropy, or antithixotropy) occurs when the apparent viscosity of the system continues to increase with continued application of shear up to some equilibrium value at a given shear rate. These systems display a **sol–gel** transformation. One explanation for antithixotropic behavior is that continued shear increases the frequency of particle or macromolecule interactions and leads to increased structure in the system.

C. Solids. Intermolecular forces of attraction are stronger in solids than in liquids or gases. Molecular arrangements in solids may be characterized as either crystalline or amorphous.

    1. Crystalline solids have the following attributes:

      a. Fixed **molecular order** (i.e., molecules occupy set positions in a specific array)

      b. A distinct melting point

      c. Anisotropicity (i.e., their properties are not the same in all directions), with the exception of cubic crystals

    2. Amorphous solids have the following attributes:

      a. Randomly arranged molecules with the short-range order typical of liquids

      b. No melting points

      c. Isotropicity (i.e., properties are the same in all directions)

> **d.** Less thermodynamic stability than the corresponding crystalline solid and therefore more apt to exhibit chemical and physical instability, increased dissolution rate, etc.

3. Polymorphism is the condition wherein substances can exist in more than one crystalline form. These **polymorphs** have different molecular arrangements or crystal lattice structures. As a result, the different polymorphs of a drug solid can have different properties. For example, the melting point, solubility, dissolution rate, density, and stability can differ considerably among the polymorphic forms of a drug. Many drugs exhibit polymorphic behavior. Fatty (triglyceride) excipients (e.g., theobroma oil, cocoa butter) are recognized for their polymorphic behavior.

4. The incorporation of solvent molecules into the crystal lattice of a solid results in a molecular adduct known as a **solvate** or **hydrate** (the latter term is used when water is the solvent). In general, solvates or hydrates exhibit different solubilities and dissolution rates than their unsolvated/anhydrous counterparts.

5. Melting point and heat of fusion. The melting point of a solid is the temperature at which the solid is transformed to a liquid. When 1 g of a solid is heated and melts, the heat absorbed in the process is referred to as the **latent heat of fusion.**

D. Phase diagrams and phase equilibria. A **phase diagram** represents the states of matter (i.e., solid, liquid, and gas) that exist as temperature and pressure are varied (Figure 3-5). The data

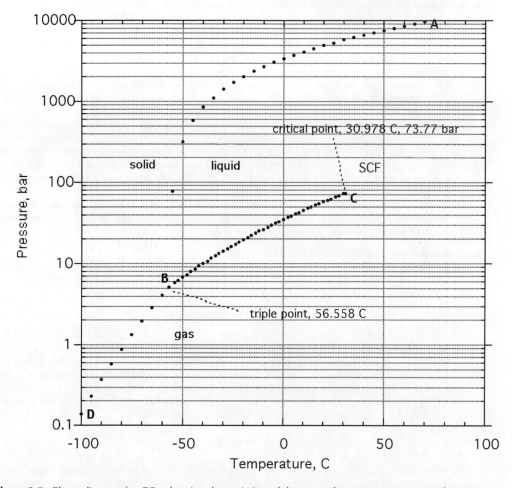

Figure 3-5. Phase diagram for CO_2 showing the variation of the state of matter as pressure and temperature are varied. The solid state exists in the region *ABD;* the liquid state, in the region *ABC;* and the gas state, in the region to the right of curve *CD.* *B* corresponds to the triple point, the pressure and temperature at which all three phases coexist. *C* corresponds to the critical point, the pressure and temperature above which the liquid and gas phases are indistinguishable.

arrays separating the phases in Figure 3-5 delineate the temperatures and pressures at which the phases can coexist. Thus gas (or vapor) and liquid coexist along "curve" *BC,* solid and liquid coexist along "curve" *AB,* and solid and gas (or vapor) coexist along "curve" *DB.* Depending on the change in temperature and pressure, **evaporation** or **condensation** occur along curve *BC,* **fusion** or **melting** along curve *AB,* and **sublimation** or **deposition** along curve *DB.* The three "curves" intersect at point *B.* Only at this unique temperature and pressure, known as the **triple point,** do all three phases exist in equilibrium. (The triple point for water is 0.01°C and 6.04 $\times$ 10^{-3} atm.) Continuing along curve *BC,* to higher temperatures and pressures, one ultimately reaches point *C,* known as the **critical point,** above which there is no distinction between the liquid and the gas phases. Substances that exist above this critical point are known as **supercritical fluids.** Supercritical fluids such as carbon dioxide (critical point, 30.98°C and 73.8 atm) often exhibit markedly altered physicochemical properties (e.g., density, diffusivity, or solubility characteristics) that render them useful as solvents and processing aids in the production of pharmaceuticals and drug delivery systems.

IV. PHYSICOCHEMICAL BEHAVIOR

A. Homogeneous systems

1. A **solution** is a homogeneous system in which a **solute** is molecularly dispersed, or dissolved, in a **solvent.** The solvent is the predominant species. **Saturated solutions** are solutions that, at a given temperature and pressure, contain the maximum amount of solute that can be accommodated by the solvent. If the saturation, or solubility, limit is exceeded, a fraction of the solute can separate from the solution and exist in equilibrium with it.
   a. **Solutes** can be gases, liquids, or solids, and nonelectrolytes or electrolytes.
      (1) **Nonelectrolytes** are substances that **do not form ions** when dissolved in water. Examples are estradiol, glycerin, urea, and sucrose. Their aqueous solutions do not conduct electric current.
      (2) **Electrolytes** are substances that **do form ions** in solution. Examples are sodium chloride, hydrochloric acid, and atropine. As a result, their aqueous solutions conduct electric current. Electrolytes are characterized as **strong** or **weak.** Strong electrolytes (e.g., sodium chloride, hydrochloric acid) are **completely ionized** in water at all concentrations. Weak electrolytes (e.g., aspirin, atropine) are **partially ionized** in water.
   b. The **colligative properties of a solution** depend on the total **number of ionic and nonionic solute molecules in the solution.** These properties depend on ionization but are **independent of other chemical properties of the solute.**

2. **Colligative properties** include the following:
   a. **Lowering of vapor pressure.** The **partial vapor pressure** of each volatile component in a solution is equal to the product of the mol fraction of the component in the solution and the vapor pressure of the pure component. This is **Raoult's law:**

$$P_A = P_A^0 \times x_A$$

   where p_A is the partial vapor pressure above a solution in which the mol fraction of the solute A is x_A and P_A^0 is the **vapor pressure** of the pure component A. The vapor pressure is the pressure at which an equilibrium is established between the molecules of A in the liquid state and the molecules of A in the gaseous (vapor) state in a closed, evacuated container. The vapor pressure is temperature dependent, but independent of the amount of liquid and vapor. Raoult's law holds for ideal solutions of nonelectrolytes. For a **binary solution** (i.e., a solution of component B in component A)

$$\frac{P_A^0 - P_A}{P_A^0} = (1 - x_A) = x_B$$

   The lowering of the vapor pressure of the solution relative to the vapor pressure of the pure solvent is proportional to the number of molecules of solute in the solution. The actual lowering of the vapor pressure by the solute, Δp_A, is given by

$$\Delta p_A = (P_A^0 - p_A) = x_B\, P_A^0$$

   b. **Elevation of the boiling point.** The **boiling point** is the temperature at which the vapor pressure of a liquid equals an external pressure of 760 mm Hg. A solution of a nonvolatile solute has a higher boiling point than a pure solvent because the solute lowers the vapor pressure of the solvent. The amount of elevation of the boiling point (ΔT_b) depends on the concentration of the solute:

$$\Delta T_b = \frac{RT_0^2 M_1 m}{1000 \times \Delta H_{vap}} = K_b m$$

where K_b is the molal boiling point elevation constant, R is the molar gas constant, T is absolute temperature (degrees K), M_1 is the molecular weight of the solute, m is the molality of the solution, and ΔH_{vap} is the molal enthalpy of vaporization of the solvent.

c. **Depression of the freezing point.** The **freezing point,** or melting point, of a pure compound is the temperature at which the solid and the liquid phases are in equilibrium under a pressure of 1 atmosphere (atm). The freezing point of a solution is the temperature at which the solid phase of the pure solvent and the liquid phase of the solution are in equilibrium under a pressure of 1 atm. The amount of depression of the freezing point (ΔT_f) depends on the molality of the solution:

$$\Delta T_f = \frac{RT_0^2 M_1 m}{1000 \times \Delta H_{fusion}} = K_f m$$

where K_f is the molal freezing point constant and ΔH_{fusion} is the molal heat of fusion.

d. **Osmotic pressure. Osmosis** is the process by which solvent molecules pass through a semipermeable membrane (a barrier through which only solvent molecules may pass) from a region of dilute solution to one of more concentrated solution. Solvent molecules transfer because of the inequality in chemical potential on the two sides of the membrane. Solvent molecules in a concentrated solution have a lower chemical potential than solvent molecules in a more dilute solution.
   (1) **Osmotic pressure** is the **pressure** that must be applied to the solution to prevent the flow of pure solvent into the concentrated solution.
   (2) Solvent molecules move from a region where their **escaping tendency is high** to one where their **escaping tendency is low.** The presence of dissolved solute lowers the escaping tendency of the solvent in proportion to the solute concentration.
   (3) The **van't Hoff equation** defines the osmotic pressure π as a function of the number of moles of solute n_2 in the solution of volume V:

$$\pi V = n_2 RT$$

3. **Electrolyte solutions and ionic equilibria**
   a. **Acid–base equilibria**
      (1) According to the **Arrhenius dissociation theory,** an **acid** is a substance that liberates H^+ in aqueous solution. A **base** is a substance that liberates hydroxyl ions (OH^-) in aqueous solution. This definition applies only under aqueous conditions.
      (2) The **Lowry-Brønsted theory** is a more powerful concept that applies to aqueous and nonaqueous systems. It is most commonly used for pharmaceutical and biologic systems because these systems are primarily aqueous.
         (a) According to this definition, an **acid** is a substance (charged or uncharged) that is capable of donating a proton. A **base** is a substance (charged or uncharged) that is capable of accepting a proton from an acid. The dissociation of an acid (HA) always produces a base (A^-) according to the following formula:

$$HA \leftrightarrow H^+ + A^-$$

         (b) HA and A^- are a **conjugate acid–base pair** (an acid and a base that exist in equilibrium and differ in structure by a proton). The proton of an acid does not exist free in solution, but combines with the solvent. In water, this **hydrated proton** is a **hydronium ion** (H_3O^+).
         (c) The relative **strengths** of acids and bases are determined by their ability to donate or accept protons. For example, in water, HCl donates a proton more readily than does acetic acid. Thus HCl is a stronger acid. Acid strength is also determined by the affinity of the solvent for protons. For example, HCl may dissociate completely in liquid ammonia, but only very slightly in glacial acetic acid. Thus HCl is a strong acid in liquid ammonia and a weak acid in glacial acetic acid.

(3) The **Lewis theory** extends the acid–base concept to reactions that do not involve protons. It defines an **acid** as a molecule or ion that accepts an electron pair from another atom and a **base** as a substance that donates an electron pair to be shared with another atom.

b. H^+ concentration values are very small. Therefore, they are expressed in **exponential notation as pH.** The pH is the logarithm of the reciprocal of the H^+ concentration

$$pH = \log\left(\frac{1}{[H^+]}\right)$$

where $[H^+]$ is the molar concentration of H^+. Because the logarithm of a reciprocal equals the **negative logarithm** of the number, this equation may be rewritten as:

$$pH = -\log[H^+]$$

or

$$[H^+] = 10^{-pH}$$

Thus the pH value may be defined as the negative logarithm of the $[H^+]$ value. For example, if the H^+ concentration of a solution is 5×10^{-6}, the pH value may be calculated as follows:

$$pH = -\log(5 \times 0^{-6})$$
$$\log 5 = 0.699$$
$$\log 10^{-6} = -6.0$$
$$pH = -(-6 + 0.699)$$
$$= -(-5.301)$$
$$= 5.301$$

c. As pH decreases, **H^+ concentration increases exponentially.** When the pH decreases from 6 to 5, the H^+ concentration increases from 10^{-6} to 10^{-5}, or 10 times its original value. When the pH falls from 5 to 4.7, the H^+ concentration increases from 1×10^{-5} to 2×10^{-5}, or double its initial value.

d. Dissociation constants. Ionization is the complete separation of the ions in a crystal lattice when the salt is dissolved. **Dissociation** is the separation of ions in solution when the ions are associated by interionic attraction.

(1) For **weak electrolytes,** dissociation is a reversible process. The equilibrium of this process can be expressed by the law of mass action. This law states that the rate of the chemical reaction is proportional to the product of the concentration of the reacting substances, each raised to a power of the number of moles of the substance in solution.

(2) For **weak acids,** dissociation in water is expressed as:

$$HA \leftrightarrow H^+ + A^-$$

The dynamic equilibrium between the simultaneous forward and reverse reactions is indicated by the arrows. By the law of mass action,

$$\text{rate of forward reaction} = K_1[HA]$$
$$\text{rate of reverse reaction} = K_2[H^+][A^-]$$

At equilibrium, the forward and reverse rates are equal. Therefore,

$$K_1[HA] = K_2[H^+][A^-]$$

Thus **the equilibrium expression for the dissociation of a weak acid** is written as:

$$K_a = \frac{K_1}{K_2} = \frac{[H^+][A^-]}{[HA]}$$

where K_a represents the acid dissociation constant. For a weak acid, the **acid dissociation constant** is conventionally expressed as **pK_a,** which is $-\log K_a$. For example, the K_a of acetic acid at 25°C is 1.75×10^{-5}. The pK_a is calculated as follows:

$$pKa = -\log(1.75 \times 10^{-5})$$
$$\log 1.75 = 0.243$$
$$\log 10^{-5} = -5$$
$$pH = -(-5 + 0.243)$$
$$= -(-4.757)$$
$$= 4.76$$

(3) For **weak bases,** dissociation may also be expressed with the K_a expression for the **conjugate acid of the base.** This acid is formed when a proton reacts with the base. For a base that does not contain a hydroxyl group,

$$BH^+ \leftrightarrow H^+ + B$$

The **dissociation constant** for this reaction is expressed as:

$$K_a = \frac{[H^+][B]}{[BH^+]}$$

However, a **base dissociation constant** is traditionally defined for a weak base with this expression:

$$B + H_2O \leftrightarrow OH^- + BH^+$$

$$K_b = \frac{[OH^-][BH^+]}{[B]}$$

where K_b represents the dissociation constant of a weak base. This **dissociation constant** can be expressed as **pK_b,** as follows:

$$pK_b = -\log K_b$$

(4) **Certain compounds** (acids or bases) can accept or donate more than one proton. Consequently, they have **more than one dissociation constant.**

e. **Henderson-Hasselbalch equations** describe the relation between the ionized and the unionized species of a weak electrolyte.

(1) For **weak acids,** the Henderson-Hasselbalch equation is obtained from the equilibrium relation described in IV.A.3d.(2):

$$pH = pK_a + \log \frac{[salt]}{[acid]}$$

(2) Similarly, the Henderson-Hasselbalch equation for **weak bases** is as follows:

$$pH = pK_a + \log \frac{[B]}{[BH^+]}$$

where B is the unionized weak base and BH^+ is the protonated base.

f. The **degree of ionization (α),** the fraction of a weak electrolyte that is ionized in solution, is calculated from the following equation:

$$\alpha = \frac{[I]}{[I] + [U]}$$

where [I] and [U] represent the concentrations of the ionized and unionized species, respectively. The degree of ionization depends solely on the pH of the solution and the pK_a of the weak electrolyte. **When pH = pK_a,** the Henderson-Hasselbalch equations are, for a weak acid and a weak base, respectively:

$$pH - pK_a = 0 = \log \frac{[A^-]}{[HA]}$$

thus

$$\frac{[A^-]}{[HA]} = 1$$

$$pH - pK_a = 0 = \log \frac{[B]}{[BH^+]}$$

thus

$$\frac{[B]}{[BH^+]} = 1$$

In effect, when the pH of the solution is numerically equivalent to the pK_a of the weak electrolyte, whether a weak base or a weak acid, $[I] = [U]$ and the degree of ionization $\alpha = 0.5$ (i.e., 50% of the solute is ionized).

g. **Solubility of a weak electrolyte** varies as a function of pH.
   (1) For a **weak acid,** the total solubility C_s is given by the expression:

$$C_s = [HA] + [A^-]$$

   where [HA] is the intrinsic solubility of the unionized weak acid and is denoted as C_0, whereas $[A^-]$ is the concentration of its anion. Because $[A^-]$ can be expressed in terms of C_0 and the dissociation constant K_a,

$$C_s = C_0 + \frac{K_a C_0}{[H^+]}$$

   Thus the **solubility of a weak acid increases with increasing pH** (i.e., with an increasing degree of ionization, as the anion is more polar and therefore more water soluble than the unionized weak acid).

   (2) Similarly, for **weak bases,**

$$C_s = C_0 + \frac{C_0[H^+]}{K_a}$$

   Thus the **solubility decreases with increasing pH** because more of the weak base is in the unprotonated form. This form is less polar and therefore less water soluble.

h. **Buffers and buffer capacity**
   (1) A **buffer** is a mixture of salt with acid or base that resists changes in pH when small quantities of acid or base are added. A buffer can be a **combination** of a weak acid and its conjugate base (salt) or a combination of a weak base and its conjugate acid (salt). However, buffer solutions are more **commonly prepared** from weak acids and their salts. They are not ordinarily prepared from weak bases and their salts because weak bases are often unstable and volatile.
      (a) For a **weak acid and its salt,** the following buffer equation is satisfactory for calculations with a pH of 4–10. It is important in the preparation of buffered pharmaceutical solutions:

$$pH = pK_a + \log \frac{[salt]}{[acid]}$$

      (b) For a **weak base and its salt,** the buffer equation is similar but also depends on the dissociation constant of water (pK_w). The equation becomes:

$$pH = pK_w - + pK_b \log \frac{[base]}{[salt]}$$

   (2) **Buffer action** is the resistance to a change in pH.
   (3) **Buffer capacity** is the ability of a buffer solution to resist changes in pH. The **smaller the pH change** caused by addition of a given amount of acid or base, the **greater the buffer capacity** of the solution.
      (a) Buffer capacity is the number of gram equivalents of an acid or base that changes the pH of 1 L of buffer solution by 1 unit.
      (b) Buffer capacity is affected by the concentration of the buffer constituents. A higher concentration provides a greater acid or base reserve. Buffer capacity (β) is related to total concentration (C) as follows:

$$\beta = \frac{2.3CK_a[H^+]}{(K_a + [H^+])^2}$$

where C represents the molar concentrations of the acid and the salt.
  (c) Thus buffer capacity depends on the value of the ratio of the salt to the acid form. It increases as the ratio approaches unity. Maximum buffer capacity occurs when $pH = pK_a$, and is represented by $\beta = 0.576C$.

B. Heterogeneous (disperse) systems

1. Introduction

  a. A **suspension** is a two-phase system that is composed of a solid material dispersed in an oily or aqueous liquid. The particle size of the dispersed solid is usually > 0.5 μm.
  b. An **emulsion** is a heterogeneous system that consists of at least one immiscible liquid that is intimately dispersed in another in the form of droplets. The droplet diameter usually exceeds 0.1 μm. Emulsions are **inherently unstable** because the droplets of the dispersed liquid tend to coalesce to form large droplets until all of the dispersed droplets have coalesced. The third component of the system is an **emulsifying agent.** This agent prevents coalescence and maintains the integrity of the individual droplets.

2. Dispersion stability.
In an **ideal dispersion,** the dispersed particles do not interact. The particles are uniform in size and undergo no change in position other than the random movement that results from Brownian motion. In contrast, in a **real dispersion,** the particles are not uniformly sized (i.e., they are not **monodisperse**). The particles are subject to particulate aggregation, or clumping, and the dispersion becomes more heterogeneous with time. The **rate of settling (separating, or creaming)** of the dispersed phase in the dispersion medium is a function of the particle size, dispersion phase viscosity, and difference in density between the dispersed phase and the dispersion medium, in accordance with **Stokes's law:**

$$\text{sedimentation rate} = \frac{d^2 g(\rho_1 - \rho_2)}{18\,\eta}$$

where d is the particle diameter, g is the acceleration owing to gravity, η is the viscosity of the dispersion medium, and $(\rho_1 - \rho_2)$ is the difference between the density of the particles (ρ_1) and the density of the dispersion medium (ρ_2). Although Stokes's law was derived to determine the settling, or sedimentation, of noninteracting spherical particles, it also provides guidance for determining the stabilization of dispersion:

  a. **Particle size** should be as **small** as possible. Smaller particles yield slower sedimentation, or flotation, rates.
  b. **High particulate (dispersed phase) concentrations** increase the rate of particle–particle collisions and interaction. As a result, particle aggregation occurs, and instability increases as the aggregates behave as larger particles. In the case of liquid–liquid dispersions, particle–particle collisions can lead to coalescence (i.e., larger particles) and decrease dispersion stability.
  c. **Avoidance of particle–particle interactions**
    (1) Aggregation can be prevented if the particles have a similar electrical charge. Particles in an aqueous system always have some electrical charge because of **ionization** of chemical groups on the particle surface or **adsorption** of charged molecules or ions at the interface. If the adsorbed species is an **ionic surfactant** (e.g., sodium lauryl sulfate), the charge associated with the surfactant ion (e.g., lauryl sulfate anion) will accumulate at the interface. However, if a relatively non-surface-active electrolyte is adsorbed, the sign of the charge of the adsorbed ion is less readily predicted.
    (2) The **magnitude of the charge** is the difference in electrical potential between the charged surface of the particle and the bulk of the dispersion medium. This magnitude is approximated by the **electrokinetic, or zeta, potential (ζ).** The zeta potential is measured from the fixed, avidly bound layers of ions and solvent molecules on the particle surface. When ζ is high (e.g., ≥ 25 mV), interparticulate **repulsive forces** exceed the attractive forces. As a result, the dispersion is **deflocculated** and relatively stable to collision and subsequent aggregation (**flocculation**). When ζ is so low that interparticulate **attractive forces** predominate, loose particle aggregates, or **flocs,** form (i.e., **flocculation** occurs).
  d. **Density** can be manipulated to decrease the rate of dispersion instability. The settling

rate decreases as $(\rho_1 - \rho_2)$ approaches zero. However, the density of the dispersion medium usually cannot be altered sufficiently to halt the settling (or flotation) process. In the dispersed phase, the density of solid particles is not readily altered; altering the density of liquid particles would require the addition of a miscible liquid of higher (or lower) density. Altering the composition of suspensions is also problematic because most solid particles are denser than the dispersion medium. Additives of higher (or lower) density might alter the biopharmaceutical characteristics of the formulation (e.g., rate of drug release, residence time at the site of administration, or absorption).

e. The **sedimentation, or flotation, rate** is inversely proportional to the **viscosity.** An **increase** in the **viscosity of the dispersion medium** decreases the rate of settling, or flotation. However, although the rate of destabilization can be slowed by an increase in viscosity, it cannot be halted.

3. **Emulsion stability. Coalescence** occurs in emulsion systems when the liquid particles of the dispersed phase merge to form larger particles. Coalescence is largely prevented by the **interfacial film** of surfactant around the droplets. This film prevents direct contact of the liquid phase of the droplets. Coalescence of droplets in oil in water (o/w) emulsions is also inhibited by the **electrostatic repulsion** of similarly charged particles. **Creaming** is the **reversible** separation of a layer of emulsified particles. Because mixing or shaking may be sufficient to reconstitute the emulsion system, creaming is not necessarily unacceptable. However, **cracking, or irreversible phase separation,** is never acceptable. **Phase inversion,** or emulsion-type reversal, involves the reversion of an emulsion from an o/w to a water in oil (w/o) form, or vice versa. Phase inversion can change the consistency or texture of the emulsion or cause further deterioration in its stability.

V. CHEMICAL KINETICS AND DRUG STABILITY

A. **Introduction.** The **stability** of the **active component** of a drug is a major criterion in the rational design and evaluation of drug dosage forms. Problems with **stability** can determine whether a given formulation is accepted or rejected.

1. Extensive chemical degradation of the active ingredient can cause **substantial loss** of active ingredient from the dosage form.

2. Chemical degradation can produce a **toxic product** that has undesirable side effects.

3. Instability of the drug product can cause **decreased bioavailability.** As a result, the therapeutic efficacy of the dosage form may be substantially reduced.

B. **Rates and orders of reactions**

1. The **rate of a reaction,** or degradation rate, is the velocity with which the reaction occurs. This rate is expressed as dC/dt (the change in concentration, or C, within a given time interval, or dt).

   a. Reaction rates depend on certain conditions (e.g., **reactant concentration, temperature, pH, presence of solvents or additives**). Radiation and catalytic agents (e.g., polyvalent cations) also have an effect.

   b. The effective study of reaction rates in the body requires application of **pharmacokinetic principles** (see Chapter 6).

2. The **order of a reaction** is the way in which the concentration of the drug or reactant in a chemical reaction affects the rate. The rate of a reaction, dC/dt, is proportional to the concentration to the nth power, where n is the order of the reaction—that is,

$$\frac{dC}{dt} \propto C^n$$

The study of reaction orders is a crucial aspect of pharmacokinetics (see Chapter 6). Usually, **pharmaceutical degradation** can be treated as a **zero-order, first-order,** or **higher-order reaction.** The first two are summarized as follows.

   a. In a **zero-order reaction,** the **rate is independent of the concentration of the reactants** (i.e., $dC/dt \propto C^0$) (see Chapter 6). Other factors, such as absorption of light in certain photochemical reactions, determine the rate.

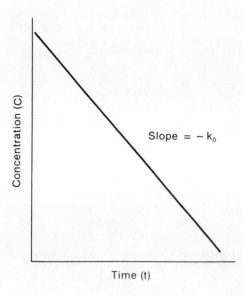

Figure 3-6. Concentration *(C)* versus time *(t)* for a zero-order reaction. The slope of the line equals $-k_0$. The slope of the line is not equal to the rate constant because it includes the minus sign.

(1) A **zero-order reaction** can be expressed as:

$$C = -k_0t + C_0$$

where C is the drug concentration, k_0 is the zero-order rate constant in units of concentration/time, t is the time, and C_0 is the initial concentration.

(2) When this equation is plotted with C on the vertical axis (ordinate) against t on the horizontal axis (abscissa), the **slope of the line is equal to $-k_0$** (Figure 3-6). The negative sign indicates that the slope is decreasing.

b. In a **first-order reaction, the rate depends on the first power of the concentration of a single reactant** (i.e., $dC/dt \propto C^1$).

(1) In a first-order reaction, **drug concentration decreases exponentially with time,** in accordance with the equation

$$C = C_0 e^{-k_1 t}$$

where C is the concentration of the reacting material, C_0 is the initial concentration, k_1 is the first-order rate constant in units of reciprocal time, and t is time. A plot of the logarithm of concentration against time produces a straight line with a slope of $-k/2.303$ (Figure 3-7).

(2) The **half-life** $(t_{1/2})$ of a reaction is the time required for the concentration of a drug to decrease by one half. For a first-order reaction, half-life is expressed by:

$$t_{1/2} = \frac{0.693}{k_1}$$

(3) The **time required for a drug to degrade** to 90% of its original concentration $(t_{90\%})$ is also important. This time represents a reasonable limit of degradation for the active ingredients. The $t_{90\%}$ can be calculated as:

$$t_{90\%} = \frac{2.303}{k_1} \log \frac{100}{90} = \frac{0.105}{k_1}$$

(a) Because

$$k_1 = 0.693 / t_{1/2}$$

(b) Then

$$t_{90\%} = \frac{0.105}{0.693/t_{1/2}} = 0.152 \times t_{1/2}$$

Figure 3-7. Logarithm of concentration (log C) versus time (t) for a first-order reaction. The slope of the line equals $-k/2.303$.

The graph shows:

Log of concentration (log C) on the vertical axis, Time (t) on the horizontal axis.

$$\text{Slope} = \frac{-k}{2.303}$$

    (4) Both $t_{1/2}$ and $t_{90\%}$ are **concentration independent.** Thus, for $t_{1/2}$, it takes the same amount of time to reduce the concentration of the drug from 100 mM to 50 mM as it does from 50 mM to 25 mM.

C. Factors that affect reaction rates. Factors other than concentration can affect the reaction rate and stability of a drug. These factors include temperature, the presence of a solvent, pH, and the presence of additives.

    1. Temperature. An **increase in temperature** causes an increase in reaction rate, as expressed in the equation first suggested by Arrhenius:

$$k = Ae^{-Ea/RT}$$

or

$$\log k = \log A - \left(\frac{Ea}{2.303} \times \frac{1}{RT} \right)$$

    where k is the specific reaction rate constant, A is a constant known as the frequency factor, Ea is the energy of activation, R is the molar gas constant (1.987 cal/degree $\times$ mole), and T is the absolute temperature.

    a. The **constants A and Ea** are obtained by determining k at several temperatures and then plotting log k against $1/T$. The slope of the resulting line equals $-Ea/(2.303 \times R)$. The intercept on the vertical axis equals log A.

    b. The activation energy (Ea) is the amount of energy required to put the molecules in an **activated state.** Molecules must be activated to react. As **temperature increases,** more molecules are activated, and the **reaction rate increases.**

    2. Presence of solvent. Many dosage forms require the incorporation of a water-miscible solvent—for example, low molecular weight alcohols, such as the polyethylene glycols (PEGs)—to stabilize the drug.

    a. A change in the solvent system **alters** the transition state and the **activity coefficients** of the reactant molecules. It can also cause simultaneous changes in physicochemical parameters, such as pK_a, surface tension, and viscosity. These changes **indirectly affect the reaction rate.**

    b. In some cases, **additional reaction pathways** are generated. For example, with an increasing concentration of ethanol in an aqueous solution, aspirin degrades by an extra route and forms the ethyl ester of acetylsalicylic acid. However, a **change in solvent can also stabilize the drug.**

3. **Change in pH.** The magnitude of the rate of a hydrolytic reaction catalyzed by H^+ and OH^- can vary considerably with pH.
   a. **H^+ catalysis** predominates at **lower pH,** whereas **OH^- catalysis** operates at **higher pH.** At **intermediate pH,** the rate may be **pH independent** or may be catalyzed by **both H^+ and OH^-**. Rate constants in the intermediate pH range are typically less than those at higher or lower pH.
   b. To determine the **effect of pH on degradation kinetics,** decomposition is measured at several H^+ concentrations. The **pH of optimum stability** can be determined by plotting the logarithm of the rate constant (k) as a function of pH (Figure 3-8). The **point of inflection** of the plot is the pH of optimum stability. This value is useful in the development of a stable drug formulation.

4. **Presence of additives**
   a. **Buffer salts** must be added to many drug solutions to maintain the formulation at optimum pH. These salts **can affect the rate of degradation,** primarily as a result of salt increasing the ionic strength.
      (1) Increasing salt concentrations, particularly from polyelectrolytes (e.g., citrate, phosphate), can **substantially affect the magnitude of pK_a**. In this way, they change the rate constant.
      (2) Buffer salts can also **promote drug degradation** through general acid or base catalysis.
   b. The **addition of surfactants** may accelerate or decelerate drug degradation.
      (1) **Acceleration of degradation** is common and is caused by micellar catalysis.
      (2) **Stabilization of a drug** through the addition of a surfactant is less common.
   c. **Complexing agents** can improve drug stability. Aromatic esters (e.g., benzocaine, procaine, tetracaine) **increase in half-life** in the presence of caffeine. This increased stability appears to result from the formation of a less reactive complex between the aromatic ester and the caffeine.

D. **Modes of pharmaceutical degradation.** The decomposition of active ingredients in a dosage form occurs through several pathways (e.g., hydrolysis, oxidation, photolysis; see Chapter 12, II.A).

1. **Hydrolysis** is the most common type of degradation because many medicinal compounds are esters, amides, or lactams.
   a. **H^+ and OH^-** are the most common catalysts of hydrolytic degradation in solution.
   b. **Esters** usually undergo hydrolytic reactions that cause drug instability. Because esters are rapidly degraded in aqueous solution, formulators are reluctant to incorporate drugs that have ester functional groups into liquid dosage forms.

Figure 3-8. Semilogarithmic plot of the rate constant (k) versus pH. This plot is used to determine the pH of optimum stability.

2. Oxidation is usually mediated through reaction with atmospheric oxygen under ambient conditions (auto-oxidation).

    a. Medicinal compounds that undergo auto-oxidation at room temperature are affected by **oxygen dissolved in the solvent** and in the head space of their packages. These compounds should be packed in an **inert atmosphere** (e.g., nitrogen) to exclude air from their containers.

    b. Most oxidation reactions involve a **free radical mechanism** and a **chain reaction.** Free radicals tend to take electrons from other compounds.

        (1) Antioxidants in the formulation react with the free radicals by providing electrons and easily available hydrogen atoms. In this way, they prevent the propagation of chain reactions.

        (2) Commonly used antioxidants include ascorbic acid, butylated hydroxyanisole (BHA), butylated hydroxytoluene (BHT), propyl gallate, sodium bisulfite, sodium sulfite, and the tocopherols.

3. Photolysis is the degradation of drug molecules by normal sunlight or room light.

    a. Molecules may absorb the proper wavelength of light and **acquire sufficient energy to undergo reaction.** Usually, photolytic degradation occurs on exposure to light of wavelengths < 400 nm.

    b. An **amber glass bottle** or an **opaque container** acts as a barrier to this light, thereby preventing or retarding photolysis. For example, sodium nitroprusside in aqueous solution has a shelf life of only 4 hr if exposed to normal room light. When protected from light, the solution is stable for at least 1 year.

E. Determination of shelf life. The shelf life of a drug preparation is the amount of time that the product can be stored before it becomes unfit for use, through either chemical decomposition or physical deterioration.

    1. Storage temperature affects shelf life. It is generally understood to be ambient temperature unless special storage conditions are specified.

    2. In general, a preparation is considered fit for use if it varies from the nominal concentration or dose by no more than 10%, provided that the decomposition products are not more toxic or harmful than the original material.

    3. Shelf-life testing aids in determining the standard shelf life of a formulation.

        a. Samples are stored at 3–5°C and at room temperature (20–25°C). The samples are then analyzed at various intervals to determine the **rate of decomposition.** Shelf life is calculated from this rate.

        b. Because storage time at these temperatures can result in an extended testing time, **accelerated testing** is conducted as well, with a range of higher temperatures. The **rate constants** obtained from these samples are used to predict shelf life at ambient or refrigeration temperatures. **Temperature-accelerated stability testing** is not useful if temperature changes are accompanied by changes in the reaction mechanism or by physical changes in the system (e.g., change from the solid to the liquid phase).

        c. Stability at room temperature can be predicted from accelerated testing data by the Arrhenius equation:

$$\log\left(\frac{k_{T_2}}{k_{T_1}}\right) = \frac{Ea(T_2 - T_1)}{2.303 \times R \times T_2 \times T_1}$$

        where k_{T_2} and k_{T_1} are the rate constants at the absolute temperatures T_2 and T_1, respectively; R is the molar gas constant; and Ea is the energy of activation.

        d. Alternatively, an expression of concentration can be plotted as a linear function of time. Rate constants (k) for degradation at several temperatures are obtained. The logarithm of the rate constant (log k) is plotted against the reciprocal of absolute temperature ($1/T$) to obtain, by extrapolation, the rate constant for degradation at room temperature (Figure 3-9).

        e. The **length of time that the drug will maintain its required potency** can also be predicted by calculation of the $t_{90\%}$ (see V.B.2.b.(3)). This method applies to chemical reactions with activation energies of 10–30 kcal/mol, the magnitude of the activation energy for many pharmaceutical degradations that occur in solution.

Figure 3-9. Semilogarithmic plot of the rate constant (k) versus the reciprocal of absolute temperature ($1/T$), showing the temperature dependency of degradation rates.

VI. DRUG DOSAGE FORMS AND DELIVERY SYSTEMS

A. Oral solutions. The *United States Pharmacopeia* (*USP*) 29/*National Formulary* (*NF*) 24 categorizes **oral solutions** as "liquid preparations, intended for oral administration, that contain one or more substances with or without flavoring, sweetening, or coloring agents dissolved in water or cosolvent-water mixtures." Oral solutions can contain certain polyols (e.g., sorbitol, glycerin) to inhibit crystallization and to modify solubility, taste, mouth feel, and other vehicle properties. They can be "formulated for direct oral administration to the patient or they may be dispensed in a more concentrated form that must be diluted prior to administration." **Drugs in solution** are more homogeneous and easier to swallow than drugs in solid form. For drugs that have a slow dissolution rate, onset of action and bioavailability are also improved. However, drugs in solution are bulkier dosage forms, degrade more rapidly, and are more likely to interact with constituents than those in solid form.

1. **Water** is the **most commonly used vehicle** for drug solutions. The *USP* recognizes seven types of water for the preparation of dosage forms:
    a. **Purified water** *USP* is water obtained by distillation, ion exchange, reverse osmosis, or other suitable treatment. It cannot contain more than 10 parts per million (ppm) of total solid and should have a pH between 5 and 7. Purified water is used in prescriptions and finished manufactured products except parenteral and ophthalmic products.
    b. **Water for injection** *USP* is water obtained by distillation or by reverse osmosis. It conforms to the standards of purified water but is also free of pyrogen. Water for injection is used as a solvent for the preparation of parenteral solutions.
    c. **Sterile water for injection** *USP* is water for injection that is sterilized and packaged in single-dose containers of type I and II glass. These containers do not exceed a capacity of 1 L. The limitations for total solids depend on the size of the container.
    d. **Bacteriostatic water for injection** *USP* is sterile water for injection that contains one or more suitable antimicrobial agents. It is also packaged in single- or multiple-dose containers of type I or II glass. These containers do not exceed the capacity of 30 mL.
    e. **Sterile water for inhalation** *USP* is water that is purified by distillation or by reverse osmosis (i.e., water for injection) and rendered sterile. It contains no antimicrobial agents, except when used in humidifiers or similar devices. This type of water should not be used for parenteral administration or for other sterile dosage forms.
    f. **Sterile water for irrigation** *USP* is water for injection that is sterilized and suitably packaged. It contains no antimicrobial agents or other added substance.

g. **Sterile purified water USP** is purified water sterilized and suitably packaged. It contains no antimicrobial agent. It is not intended for use in parenterals.

2. **Oral drug solutions** include **syrups** and **elixirs** as well as other less widely prescribed classic (**galenical**) formulations, such as **aromatic waters, tinctures, fluidextracts,** and **spirits.**

   a. **Syrups** are traditionally peroral solutions that contain high concentrations of sucrose or other sugars. Through common usage, the term *syrup* has also come to include any other liquid dosage form prepared in a sweet, viscous vehicle, including peroral suspensions.

      (1) **Syrup *NF* (simple syrup)** is a concentrated or nearly saturated aqueous solution of sugar (85%; 65% w/w).

      (2) Syrups have a **low solvent capacity for water-soluble drugs** because the hydrogen bonding between sucrose and water is very strong. For this reason, it can be difficult or impossible to dissolve a drug in a syrup. Often, the drug is best dissolved in a small quantity of water, and the flavoring syrup is added.

      (3) The **sucrose concentration** of syrup plays a crucial role in the control of microbial growth. Dilute sucrose solutions are excellent media for microorganisms. As the concentration of sucrose approaches saturation, the syrup becomes self-preserving (i.e., requires no additional preservative). However, a saturated solution is undesirable because temperature fluctuations may cause crystallization. **Syrup *NF*** is a self-preserved solution with a minimal tendency to undergo crystallization.

   b. **Elixirs** are traditionally peroral solutions that contain alcohol as a cosolvent. Many peroral solutions are not described as elixirs but contain alcohol.

      (1) To be considered an elixir, the solution **must contain alcohol.** Traditionally, the alcohol content of elixirs has varied from 5% to 40%. Most elixirs become turbid when moderately diluted by aqueous liquids. Elixirs are not the preferred vehicle for salts because alcohol accentuates saline taste. Salts also have limited solubility in alcohol. Therefore, the alcoholic content of salt-containing elixirs must be low.

      (2) **Aromatic elixir *NF,*** prepared in part from syrup, contains approximately 22% alcohol. The limited usefulness of this elixir as a solvent for drugs was offset by the development of **iso-alcoholic elixir.** It is a combination of **low-alcoholic elixir,** an elixir with low alcoholic content (8%–10% alcohol), and **high-alcoholic elixir,** an elixir with high alcoholic content (73%–78% alcohol). Mixing appropriate volumes of the two elixirs provides an alcoholic content sufficient to dissolve the drugs.

B. **Miscellaneous solutions**

1. **Aromatic waters** are clear, **saturated aqueous solutions of volatile oils** or other aromatic or volatile substances. Aromatic waters may be used as pleasantly flavored vehicles for a water-soluble drug or as an aqueous phase in an emulsion or suspension. If a large amount of water-soluble drug is added to an aromatic water, then an insoluble layer may form at the top. This **"salting out"** is a competitive process. The molecules of water-soluble drugs have more attraction for the solvent molecules of water than the "oil" molecules. The associated water molecules are pulled away from the oil molecules, which are no longer held in solution. Aromatic waters should be stored in tight, light-resistant bottles to reduce volatilization and degradation from sunlight. Aromatic waters are usually prepared by one of the following methods:

   a. **Distillation** is a universal method but is not practical or economical for most products. It is the only method, however, for preparing strong rose water and orange flower water.

   b. With the **solution method,** the volatile, or aromatic, substance is admixed with water, with or without the use of a dispersant (e.g., talc).

2. **Spirits,** or **essences,** are alcoholic or hydroalcoholic solutions of volatile substances, that contain 50%–90% alcohol. This **high alcoholic content** maintains the water-insoluble volatile oils in solution. If water is added to a spirit, the oils separate. Some spirits are **medicinal** (e.g., aromatic ammonia spirit). Many spirits (e.g., compound orange spirit, compound cardamom spirit) are used as flavoring agents. Spirits should be stored in tight containers to reduce loss by evaporation.

3. **Tinctures** are alcoholic or hydroalcoholic solutions of chemicals or soluble constituents of vegetable drugs. Although tinctures vary in drug concentration ($\leq$ 50%), those prepared from potent drugs are usually 10% in strength (i.e., 100 mL of the tincture has the activity of 10 g of the drug). Tinctures are usually considered stable. The alcohol content of the official tinctures varies from 17% to 21% for opium tincture *USP* and from 74% to 80% for compound benzoin tincture *USP.* Most tinctures are prepared by an **extraction process** of

maceration or percolation. The selection of a **solvent,** or menstruum, is based on the solubility of the active and inert constituents of the crude drugs. Aging can cause precipitation of the inactive constituents of tinctures. Glycerin may be added to the hydroalcoholic solvent to increase the solubility of the active constituent and reduce precipitation on storage. Tinctures must be tightly stoppered and kept from excessive temperatures. Because many of their constituents undergo a photochemical change when exposed to light, tinctures must be stored in light-resistant containers.

4. **Fluidextracts** are liquid extracts of vegetable drugs that contain alcohol as a solvent, preservative, or both. Fluidextracts are prepared by percolation so that each milliliter contains the therapeutic constituents of 1 g of the standard drug. Because of their high drug content, fluidextracts are sometimes referred to as "100% tinctures." Fluidextracts of potent drugs are usually 10 times as concentrated, or potent, as the corresponding tincture. For example, the usual dose of tincture belladonna is 0.6 mL; the equivalent dose of the more potent fluidextract is 0.06 mL. Many fluidextracts are considered too potent for self-administration by patients, so they are almost never prescribed. In addition, many fluidextracts are simply too bitter. Today, most fluidextracts are modified by either flavoring or sweetening agents.

5. **Nasal, ophthalmic, otic,** and **parenteral solutions** are classified separately because of their specific use and method of preparation.

6. **Mouthwashes** are solutions that are used to cleanse the mouth or treat diseases of the oral mucous membrane. They often contain alcohol or glycerin to aid in dissolving the volatile ingredients. Mouthwashes are more often used cosmetically than therapeutically.

7. **Astringents** are locally applied solutions that precipitate protein. They reduce cell permeability without causing injury. Astringents cause **constriction,** with wrinkling and blanching of the skin. Because astringents **reduce secretions,** they can be used as antiperspirants.
   a. **Aluminum acetate** and **aluminum subacetate solutions** are used as wet dressings in contact dermatitis. The precipitation is minimized by the addition of boric acid.
   b. **Calcium hydroxide solution** is a mild stringent that is used in lotions as a reactant and an alkalizer.

8. **Antibacterial topical solutions** (e.g., benzalkonium chloride, strong iodine, povidone–iodine) kill bacteria when applied to the skin or mucous membrane in the proper strength and under appropriate conditions.

C. Suspensions

1. **Lotions, magmas** (i.e., suspensions of finely divided material in a small amount of water), and **mixtures** are all suspensions that have had official formulas for some time (e.g., calamine lotion *USP,* kaolin mixture with pectin *NF*). Official formulas are given in the *USP/NF.*
   a. A **complete formula** and a **detailed method of preparation** are available for some official suspensions. For others, only the **concentration** of the active ingredients is given, and the manufacturer has considerable latitude in the formulation.
   b. Some drugs are packaged in a **dry form** to circumvent the instability of aqueous dispersions. Water is added at the time of dispensing to reconstitute the suspension.

2. **Purposes of suspension**
   a. **Sustaining effect.** For a sustained-release preparation, a suspension necessitates drug dissolution before absorption.
   b. **Stability.** Drug degradation in suspension or solid dosage forms occurs much more slowly than degradation in solution form.
   c. **Taste.** A drug with an unpleasant taste can be converted into an insoluble form and then prepared as a suspension.
   d. **Basic solubility.** When suitable solvents are not available, the suspension provides an alternative. For example, only water can be used as a solvent for ophthalmic preparations because of the possibility of corneal damage. Ophthalmic suspensions provide an alternative to ophthalmic solutions.

3. **Suspending agents** include hydrophilic colloids, clays, and a few other agents. Some are also used as **emulsifying agents** (see VI.D.3).
   a. **Hydrophilic colloids** (i.e., **hydrocolloids**) increase the viscosity of water by binding water molecules, thus limiting their mobility, or fluidity. Viscosity is proportional to the concentration of the hydrocolloid. These agents **support the growth of microorganisms** and require a preservative. They are mostly **anionic,** with the exception of methyl cellulose

(neutral) and chitosan (cationic). Thus the anionic hydrocolloids are incompatible with quaternary antibacterial agents and other positively charged drugs. Chitosan is incompatible with negatively charged drugs and excipients. Most hydrocolloids are **insoluble in alcoholic solutions.**

(1) **Acacia** is usually used as a 35% dispersion in water (mucilage). Its viscosity is greatest between pH 5 and pH 9. Acacia is susceptible to microbial decomposition.

(2) **Tragacanth** is usually used as a 6% dispersion in water (mucilage). One advantage of tragacanth over acacia is that less is needed. Also, tragacanth does not contain the oxidase that is present in acacia. This oxidase catalyzes the decomposition of organic chemicals. The viscosity of tragacanth is greatest at pH 5.

(3) **Methyl cellulose** is a polymer that is nonionic and stable to heat and light. It is available in several viscosity grades. Because it is soluble in cold water, but not in hot water, dispersions are prepared by adding methyl cellulose to boiling water and then cooling the preparation until the material dissolves.

(4) **Carboxymethylcellulose** is an anionic material that is soluble in water. Prolonged exposure to heat causes loss of viscosity.

b. **Clays** (e.g., bentonite, Veegum) are silicates that are anionic in aqueous dispersions. They are strongly hydrated and exhibit **thixotropy** (the property of forming a gel-like structure on standing and becoming fluid on agitation).

(1) The official form of **bentonite** is the 5% magma.

(2) **Veegum** is hydrated to a greater degree than bentonite. Thus it is more viscous at the same concentration.

c. **Other agents** include agar, chondrus (carrageenan), gelatin, pectin, and gelatinized starch. Their use is limited by their susceptibility to bacterial attack, their incompatibilities, and their cost. Xanthan gum is used in many modern suspension formulations because of its cosolvent compatibility, its stability, and its solution's high viscosity relative to concentration.

4. **Preparation**

a. **Solids are wetted initially** to separate individual particles and coat them with a layer of dispersion medium. Wetting is accomplished by **levigation** (i.e., addition of a suitable nonsolvent, or **levigating agent,** to the solid material, followed by blending to form a paste), using a glass mortar and pestle or an ointment slab. A **surfactant** can also be used.

b. **Suspending agents** are then added as dry powder along with the active ingredient. For best results, the suspending agent is added in the form of its **aqueous dispersion.**

(1) The aqueous dispersion is added to the solid (or the levigated solid) by **geometric dilution.**

(2) The preparation is brought to the desired volume by stirring in the appropriate vehicle.

D. **Emulsions**

1. **Purposes of emulsions**

a. **Increased drug solubility.** Many drugs have limited aqueous solubility but have maximum solubility in the oil phase of an emulsion. Drug partitioning from the oil phase to the water phase can maintain or enhance activity.

b. **Increased drug stability.** Many drugs are more stable when incorporated into an emulsion rather than an aqueous solution.

c. **Prolonged drug action.** Incorporation of a drug into an emulsion can prolong bioavailability, as with certain intramuscular injection preparations.

d. **Improved taste.** Drugs with an unpleasant taste are more palatable and thus more conveniently administered in emulsion form.

e. **Improved appearance.** Oily materials intended for topical application are more appealing in an emulsified form.

2. **Phases of emulsions.** Most emulsions are considered **two-phase systems.**

a. The **liquid droplet** is known as the **dispersed, internal,** or **discontinuous phase.** The other liquid is known as the **dispersion medium, external phase,** or **continuous phase.**

b. In pharmaceutical applications, one phase is usually an **aqueous solution.** The other phase is usually **lipid** or **oily.** The lipids range from vegetable or hydrocarbon oils to semisolid hydrocarbons and waxes. Emulsions are usually described in terms of water and oil. Oil is the lipid, or nonaqueous, phase, regardless of its composition.

      (1) If water is the **internal phase,** the emulsion is classified as **w/o.**

      (2) If water is the **external phase,** the emulsion is classified as **o/w.**

   c. The **type of emulsion** formed is primarily determined by the **relative phase volumes** and the **emulsifying agent** used.

      (1) For an ideal emulsion, the maximum concentration of internal phase is 74% (i.e., theoretically, an o/w emulsion can be prepared containing $\leq$ 74% oil).

      (2) The choice of an emulsifying agent is more important than the relative phase volumes in determining the final emulsion type. Most agents preferentially form one type of emulsion or the other if the phase volume permits.

3. Emulsifying agents. Any compound that lowers the interfacial tension and forms a film at the interface can potentially function as an emulsifying agent. The effectiveness of the emulsifying agent depends on its chemical structure, concentration, solubility, pH, physical properties, and electrostatic effect. **True emulsifying agents** (primary agents) can form and stabilize emulsions by themselves. **Stabilizers** (auxiliary agents) do not form acceptable emulsions when used alone, but assist primary agents in stabilizing the product (e.g., increase viscosity). Emulsifying agents are either **natural** or **synthetic.**

   a. Natural emulsifying agents:

      (1) Acacia forms a good, stable emulsion of low viscosity. It tends to cream easily, is acidic, and is stable at a pH range of 2–10. Like other gums, it is negatively charged, dehydrates easily, and usually requires a preservative. It is incompatible with Peruvian balsam, bismuth salts, and carbonates.

      (2) Tragacanth forms a stable emulsion that is coarser than acacia emulsion. It is anionic, is difficult to hydrate, and is used mainly for its effects on viscosity. Less than $^{1}/_{10}$ of the amount used for acacia is needed.

      (3) Agar is an anionic gum that is primarily used to increase viscosity. Its stability is affected by heating, dehydration, and destruction of charge. It is also susceptible to microbial degradation.

      (4) Pectin is a quasi-emulsifier that is used in the same proportion as tragacanth.

      (5) Gelatin provides good emulsion stabilization in a concentration of 0.5%–1.0%. It may be anionic or cationic, depending on its isoelectric point. Type A gelatin (+), prepared from an acid-treated precursor, is used in acidic media. Type B gelatin (−), prepared from an alkali-treated precursor, is used in basic media.

      (6) Methyl cellulose is nonionic and induces viscosity. It is used as a primary emulsifier with mineral oil and cod liver oil, and yields an o/w emulsion. It is usually used in 2% concentration.

      (7) Carboxymethylcellulose is anionic and is usually used to increase viscosity. It tolerates alcohol up to 40%, forms a basic solution, and precipitates in the presence of free acids.

   b. Synthetic emulsifying agents are anionic, cationic, or nonionic. Although these surfactants are amphiphilic molecules, their lipophilic and hydrophilic regions are seldom inverse equals of each other: Some surfactant molecules tend to be predominantly lipophilic, whereas others are predominantly hydrophilic. This imbalance is reflected in the hydrophilic–lipophilic balance (HLB) scale: The larger the HLB value, the more hydrophilic the molecule. Table 3-1 lists HLB values for surfactants and their corresponding uses.

Table 3-1. Hydrophilic–Lipophilic Balance (HLB)

HLB Value Range	Surfactant Application
0–3	Antifoaming agents
4–6	Water-in-oil emulsifying agents
7–9	Wetting agents
8–18	Oil-in-water emulsifying agents
13–15	Detergents
10–18	Solubilizing agents

    (1) Anionic synthetic agents include **sulfuric acid esters** (e.g., sodium lauryl sulfate), **sulfonic acid derivatives** (e.g., dioctyl sodium sulfosuccinate), and **soaps.** Soaps are for external use. They have a high pH and are, therefore, sensitive to the addition of acids and electrolytes.

    (a) Alkali soaps are hydrophilic and form an o/w emulsion.

    (b) Metallic soaps are water insoluble and form a w/o emulsion.

    (c) Monovalent soaps form an o/w emulsion.

    (d) Polyvalent soaps form a w/o emulsion.

    (2) Cationic synthetic agents (e.g., benzalkonium chloride) are used as surface-active agents in 1% concentration. They are incompatible with soaps.

    (3) Nonionic synthetic agents are resistant to the addition of acids and electrolytes (Table 3-1).

    (a) The **sorbitan esters** known as **Spans** are hydrophobic in nature and form w/o emulsions. They have low hydrophilic–lipophilic balance values (1–9) (Table 3-2).

    (b) The **polysorbates** known as **Tweens** are hydrophilic and tend to form o/w emulsions. They may form complexes with phenolic compounds. They have high hydrophilic–lipophilic balance values (11–20).

4. Preparation. Various methods are used to prepare emulsions, depending on the type of emulsifying agent.

    a. Classical, acacia-stabilized emulsions are prepared by one of the following four methods:

    (1) Wet gum (English) method. A primary emulsion of fixed oil, water, and acacia (in a 4:2:1 ratio) is prepared as follows:

    (a) Two parts of water are added all at once to one part of acacia. The mixture is triturated until a smooth mucilage is formed.

    (b) Oil is added in small increments (1–5 mL), with continuous trituration, until the primary emulsion is formed.

    (c) The mixture (an o/w emulsion) is triturated for another 5 min.

    (d) The o/w mixture can then be brought to volume with water and mixed to achieve homogeneity.

    (2) Dry gum (continental) method. A primary emulsion of the fixed oil, water, and acacia (in a 4:2:1 ratio) is prepared as follows:

Table 3-2. Commonly Used Surfactants and Their Hydrophilic–Lipophilic Balance (HLB) Values

Agent	HLB Value
Sorbitan trioleate (Span 85, Arlacel 85)	1.8
Sorbitan tristearate (Span 65)	2.1
Propylene glycol monostearate (pure)	3.4
Sorbitan sesquioleate (Arlacel C)	3.7
Sorbitan monooleate (Span 80y)	4.3
Sorbitan monostearate (Arlacel 60)	4.7
Sorbitan monopalmitate (Span 40, Arlacel 40)	6.7
Sorbitan monolaurate (Span 20, Arlacel 20)	8.6
Glyceryl monostearate (Aldo 28, Tegin)	5.5
Gelatin	9.8
Triethanolamine oleate (Trolamine)	12.0
Polyoxyethylene alkyl phenol (Igepal CA-630)	12.8
Tragacanth	13.2
Polyoxyethylene sorbitan monolaurate (Tween 21)	13.3
Polyoxyethylene castor oil (Atlas G-1794)	13.3
Polyoxyethylene sorbitan monooleate (Tween 80)	15.0
Polyoxyethylene sorbitan monopalmitate (Tween 40)	15.6
Polyoxyethylene sorbitan monolaurate (Tween 20)	16.7
Polyoxyethylene lauryl ether (Brij 35)	16.9
Sodium oleate	18
Sodium lauryl sulfate	40

    (a) Oil is added to the acacia, and the mixture is triturated until the powder is distributed uniformly throughout the oil. Water is added all at once, followed by rapid trituration to form the primary emulsion.

    (b) Any remaining water and other ingredients are added to finish the product.

        (i) Electrolytes in high concentration tend to crack an emulsion. They should be added last and in as dilute a form as possible.

        (ii) Alcoholic solutions tend to dehydrate and precipitate hydrocolloids. They should be added in as dilute a concentration as possible.

  (3) Bottle method (a variation of the dry gum method used for volatile oils). Oil is added to the acacia in a bottle. The ratio of oil, water, and acacia should be 3:2:1 or 2:1:1. The low viscosity of the volatile oil requires a higher proportion of acacia.

  (4) Nascent soap method. A soap is formed by mixing relatively equal volumes of an oil and an aqueous solution that contains a sufficient amount of alkali. The soap acts as an emulsifying agent.

    (a) This method is used to form an o/w or a w/o emulsion, depending on the soap formed. For example, olive oil, which contains oleic acid, is mixed with lime water during the preparation of calamine lotion to calcium oleate, an emulsifying agent.

    (b) A 50:50 ratio of oil to water ensures sufficient emulsion, provided that the oil contains an adequate amount of free fatty acid. Olive oil usually does. Cottonseed oil, peanut oil, and some other vegetable oils do not.

    (c) The addition of an acid destroys the emulsifying soap and causes the emulsion to separate.

 b. Emulsions stabilized by synthetic emulsifying agents are readily prepared by a two-phase procedure:

  (1) Oil-miscible ingredients and water-miscible ingredients are separately admixed, using heat if necessary to ensure liquefaction and ease of mixing of each phase.

    (a) High melting point oil-miscible ingredients (e.g., waxes) are melted before lower melting point ingredients (e.g., oils) are added.

  (2) The two phases are heated to 70°–80° and then combined with stirring until the resultant emulsion has cooled.

    (a) In general, heat-labile or volatile ingredients should not be incorporated in the separate phases but in the resultant emulsion after it has cooled to about 40°C. or less.

  (3) Further mechanical processing of the emulsion by a hand homogenizer, immersion blender, or other equipment may be warranted to improve the homogeneity and stability of the product.

5. Incorporation of medicinal agents. Medicinal agents can be incorporated into an emulsion either during or after its formation.

 a. Addition of a drug during emulsion formation. It is best to incorporate a drug into a vehicle during emulsion formation, when it can be incorporated in molecular form. Soluble drugs should be dissolved in the appropriate phase (e.g., drugs that are soluble in the external phase of the emulsion should be added as a solution to the primary emulsion).

 b. Addition of a drug to a preformed emulsion can present some difficulty, depending on the type of emulsion and the nature of the emulsifier (Table 3-3).

  (1) Addition of oleaginous materials to a w/o emulsion presents no problem because of the miscibility of the additive with the external phase. However, **addition of oleaginous materials to an o/w emulsion** can be difficult after emulsion formation.

    (a) Occasionally, a small amount of oily material is added if excess emulsifier was used in the original formation.

    (b) A small amount of an oil-soluble drug can be added if it is dissolved in a very small quantity of oil with geometric dilution techniques.

  (2) Addition of water or an aqueous material to a w/o emulsion is extremely difficult, unless enough emulsifier has been incorporated into the emulsion. However, **addition of aqueous materials to an o/w emulsion** usually presents no problems if the added material does not interact with the emulsifying agent. Potential interactions should be expected with cationic compounds and salts of weak bases.

  (3) Addition of small quantities of alcoholic solutions to an o/w emulsion is possible if the solute is compatible or dispersible in the aqueous phase of the emulsion. If

Table 3-3. Selected Commercial Emulsion Bases: Emulsion Type and Emulsifier Used

Commercial Base	Emulsion Type	Emulsifier Type
Allercreme skin lotion	o/w	Triethanolamine stearate
Almay emulsion base	o/w	Fatty acid glycol esters
Cetaphil	o/w	Sodium lauryl sulfate
Dermovan	o/w	Fatty acid amides
Eucerin	w/o	Wool wax alcohol
HEB base	o/w	Sodium lauryl sulfate
Keri lotion	o/w	Nonionic emulsifiers
Lubriderm	o/w	Triethanolamine stearate
Neobase	o/w	Polyhydric alcohol esters
Neutrogena lotion	o/w	Triethanolamine lactate
Nivea cream	w/o	Wool wax alcohols
pHorsix	o/w	Polyoxyethylene emulsifiers
Polysorb hydrate	w/o	Sodium sesquioleate
Velvachol	o/w	Sodium lauryl sulfate

o/w, oil in water; *w/o,* water in oil.

acacia or another gum is used as the emulsifying agent, the alcoholic solution should be diluted with water before it is added. Table 3-3 lists some commercial emulsion bases and their general composition.

(4) **Addition of crystalline drugs to a w/o emulsion** occurs more easily if the drugs are dissolved or dispersed in a small quantity of oil before they are added.

E. Ointments

1. **Introduction. Ointments** are **semisolid preparations intended for external use.** They are easily spread. Modifying the formulation controls their plastic viscosity. Ointments are typically used as:
   a. **Emollients** to make the skin more pliable
   b. **Protective barriers** to prevent harmful substances from coming in contact with the skin
   c. **Vehicles** in which to incorporate medication

2. **Ointment bases**
   a. **Oleaginous bases** are anhydrous and insoluble in water. They cannot absorb or contain water and are not washable in water.
      (1) **Petrolatum** is a good base for oil-insoluble ingredients. It forms an occlusive film on the skin, absorbs < 5% water under normal conditions, and does not become rancid. Wax can be incorporated to stiffen the base.
      (2) **Synthetic esters** are used as constituents of oleaginous bases. These esters include glyceryl monostearate, isopropyl myristate, isopropyl palmitate, butyl stearate, and butyl palmitate. Long-chain alcohols (e.g., cetyl alcohol, stearyl alcohol, PEG) can also be used.
      (3) **Lanolin derivatives** are often used in topical and cosmetic preparations. Examples are lanolin oil and hydrogenated lanolin.
   b. **Absorption bases** are anhydrous and water insoluble. Therefore, they are not washable in water, although they can absorb water. These bases permit water-soluble medicaments to be included through prior solution and uptake as the internal phase.
      (1) **Wool fat** (anhydrous lanolin) contains a high percentage of cholesterol as well as esters and alcohol that contain fatty acids. It absorbs twice its weight in water and melts between 36°C and 42°C.
      (2) **Hydrophilic petrolatum** is a white petrolatum combined with 8% beeswax, 3% stearyl alcohol, and 3% cholesterol. These components are added to a w/o emulsifier. Prepared forms include Aquaphor, which uses wool alcohol to render white petrolatum emulsifiable. Aquaphor is superior in its ability to absorb water.
   c. **Emulsion bases** may be w/o emulsions, which are water insoluble and are not washable in water. These emulsions can absorb water because of their aqueous internal phase. Emulsion bases may also be o/w emulsions, which are water insoluble but washable in water. They can absorb water in their aqueous external phase.

(1) Hydrous wool fat (lanolin) is a w/o emulsion that contains approximately 25% water. It acts as an emollient and occlusive film on the skin, effectively preventing epidermal water loss.

(2) Cold cream is a w/o emulsion that is prepared by melting white wax, spermaceti, and expressed almond oil together; adding a hot aqueous solution of sodium borate; and stirring until the mixture is cool.

    (a) The use of mineral oil rather than almond oil makes a more stable cold cream. However, cold cream prepared with almond oil makes a better emollient base.

    (b) This ointment should be freshly prepared.

(3) Hydrophilic ointment is an o/w emulsion that uses sodium lauryl sulfate as an emulsifying agent. It absorbs 30%–50% w/w without losing its consistency. It is readily miscible with water and is removed from the skin easily.

(4) Vanishing cream is an o/w emulsion that contains a large percentage of water as well as humectant (e.g., glycerin, propylene glycol) that retards moisture loss. An excess of stearic acid in the formula helps form a thin film when the water evaporates.

(5) Other emulsion bases include Dermovan, a hypoallergenic, greaseless emulsion base, and Unibase, a nongreasy emulsion base that absorbs approximately 30% of its weight in water and has a pH close to that of the skin.

d. Water-soluble bases may be anhydrous or may contain some water. They are washable in water and absorb water to the point of solubility.

(1) PEG ointment is a blend of water-soluble polyethylene glycols that form a semisolid base. This base can solubilize water-soluble drugs and some water-insoluble drugs. It is compatible with a wide range of drugs.

    (a) This base contains 40% PEG 3350 and 60% PEG 400. It is prepared by the fusion method (see VI.E.3.b).

    (b) Only a small amount of liquid ($< 5\%$) can be incorporated without loss of viscosity. This base can be made stiffer by increasing the amount of PEG 3350 to 60%.

    (c) If 6% to 25% of an aqueous solution is to be incorporated, 5 g of the 40 g of PEG 3350 can be replaced with an equal amount of stearyl alcohol.

(2) Propylene glycol and **propylene glycol–ethanol** form a clear gel when mixed with 2% hydroxypropyl cellulose. This base is a popular dermatologic vehicle.

3. Incorporation of medicinal agents. Medicinal substances may be incorporated into an ointment base by **levigation** or by the **fusion method.** Insoluble substances should be reduced to the finest possible form and levigated before incorporation with a small amount of compatible levigating agent or with the base itself.

a. Levigation. The substance is incorporated into the ointment by levigation on an ointment slab.

(1) A stainless-steel spatula with a long, broad, flexible blade should be used. If the substance may interact with a metal spatula (e.g., when incorporating iodine and mercuric salts), then a hard rubber spatula can be used.

(2) Insoluble substances should be powdered finely in a mortar and mixed with an equal quantity of base until a smooth, grit-free mixture is obtained. The rest of the base is added in increments.

(3) Levigation of powders into a small portion of base is facilitated by the use of a melted base or a small quantity of compatible levigation aid (e.g., mineral oil, glycerin).

(4) Water-soluble salts are incorporated by dissolving them in the smallest possible amount of water and incorporating the aqueous solution directly into a compatible base.

    (a) Usually, organic solvents (e.g., ether, chloroform, alcohol) are not used to dissolve the drug because the drug may crystallize as the solvent evaporates.

    (b) Solvents are used as levigating aids only if the solid will become a fine powder after the solvent evaporates.

b. Fusion method. This method is used when the base contains solids that have higher melting points (e.g., waxes, cetyl alcohol, glyceryl monostearate). This method is also useful for solid medicaments, which are readily soluble in the melted base.

(1) The oil phase should be melted separately, starting with materials that have the highest melting point. All other oil-soluble ingredients are added in decreasing order of melting point.

(2) The ingredients in the water phase are combined and heated separately to a temperature that is equal to or several degrees above that of the melted oil phase.

    (3) The two phases are combined. If a w/o system is desired, then the hot aqueous phase is incorporated into the hot oil phase with agitation. If an o/w system is preferred, then the hot oil phase is incorporated into the hot aqueous phase.

    (4) Volatile materials (e.g., menthol, camphor, iodine, alcohol, perfumes) are added after the melted mixture cools to 40°C or less.

F. Suppositories

1. Introduction. A suppository is a **solid or semisolid mass intended to be inserted into a body orifice** (i.e., rectum, vagina, urethra). After it is inserted, a suppository either melts at body temperature or dissolves (or disperses) into the aqueous secretions of the body cavity.

    a. Suppositories are often used for local effects (e.g., relief of hemorrhoids or infection).

    b. When used rectally, suppositories can provide systemic medication. The absorption of a drug from a suppository through the rectal mucosa into the circulation involves two steps:

        (1) The drug is released from a vehicle and partitions/diffuses through the mucosa.

        (2) The drug is transported through the veins or lymph vessels into systemic fluids or tissues. The first-pass effect is avoided because the rectal veins "bypass" the liver.

    c. Rectal suppositories are useful when oral administration is inappropriate, as with infants, debilitated or comatose patients, and patients who have nausea, vomiting, or gastrointestinal disturbances. Some drugs can cause disturbances of the gastrointestinal tract.

2. Types of suppositories

    a. Rectal suppositories are usually cylindrical and tapered to a point, forming a bullet-like shape. As the rectum contracts, a suppository of this shape moves inward rather than outward. Suppositories for adults weigh approximately 2 g. Suppositories for infants and children are smaller.

    b. Vaginal suppositories are oval and typically weigh approximately 5 g. Drugs administered by this route are intended to have a local effect, but systemic absorption can occur. Antiseptics, contraceptive agents, and drugs used to treat trichomonal, monilial, or bacterial infections are often formulated as vaginal suppositories.

    c. Urethral suppositories are typically long and tapered. They are approximately 60 mm long and 4–5 mm in diameter. They are administered for a local effect and are most often used for anti-infective agents. Alprostadil, or prostaglandin E_1 (PGE_1), when used to treat erectile dysfunction, is available for urethral insertion in the form of a micropellet, or microsuppository, that is only 3–6 mm long and 1.4 mm in diameter.

3. Suppository bases

    a. Criteria for satisfactory suppository bases. Suppository bases should

        (1) Remain firm at room temperature to allow insertion. The suppository should not soften < 30°C to avoid melting during storage.

        (2) Have a narrow, or sharp, melting range

        (3) Yield a clear melt just below body temperature or dissolve rapidly in the cavity fluid

        (4) Be inert and compatible with a variety of drugs

        (5) Be nonirritating and nonsensitizing

        (6) Have wetting and emulsifying properties

        (7) Have an acid value of < 0.2, a saponification value of 200–245, and an iodine value of < 7 if the base is fatty

    b. Selecting a suppository base. Lipid–water solubility must be considered because of its relation to the drug-release rate.

        (1) If an oil-soluble drug is incorporated into an oily base, then the rate of absorption is somewhat less than that achieved with a water-soluble base. The lipid-soluble drug tends to remain dissolved in the oily pool from the suppository. It is less likely to escape into the mucous secretions from which it is ultimately absorbed.

        (2) Conversely, a water-soluble drug tends to pass more rapidly from the oil phase to the aqueous phase. Therefore, if rapid onset of action is desired, the water-soluble drug should be incorporated into the oily base.

    c. Bases that melt include **cocoa butter,** other **combinations of fats and waxes, Witepsol bases,** and **Wecobee bases** (Table 3-4).

        (1) Cocoa butter (theobroma oil) is the most widely used suppository base. It is firm and solid up to a temperature of 32°C, at which point it begins to soften. At 34–35°C, it melts to produce a thin, bland, oily liquid.

Table 3-4. Composition, Melting Range, and Congealing Range of Selected Bases That Melt

Base	Composition	Melting Range (°C)	Congealing Range (°C)
Cocoa butter	Mixed triglycerides of oleic, palmitic, and stearic acids	34–35	28 or less
Cotmar	Partially hydrogenated cottonseed oil	34–75	—
Dehydag	Hydrogenated fatty alcohols		
Base I	and esters	33–36	32–33
Base II		37–39	36–37
Base III		9 ranges	9 ranges
Wecobee R	Glycerides of saturated fatty acids C_{12}–C_{18}	33–35	31–32
Wecobee SS	Triglycerides derived from coconut oil	40–43	33–35
Witepsol	Triglycerides of saturated fatty		
H-12	acids C_{12}–C_{18}, with varied	32–33	29–32
H-15	portions of the	33–35	32–34
H-85	corresponding partial glycerides	42–44	36–38

(a) Cocoa butter is a good base for a **rectal suppository,** but it is less than ideal for a vaginal or urethral suppository.

(b) A mixture of triglycerides, cocoa butter exhibits polymorphism. Depending on the fusion temperature, it can crystallize into any one of four crystal forms.

(c) **Major limitations of cocoa butter.** Because of the following limitations, many combinations of fats and waxes are used as substitutes (Table 3-4):

    (i) **An inability to absorb aqueous solutions.** The addition of nonionic surfactants to the base ameliorates this problem to some extent. However, the resultant suppositories have poor stability and may turn rancid rapidly.

    (ii) **The lowering of the melting point produced by certain drugs** (e.g., chloral hydrate)

(2) Witepsol bases contain natural saturated fatty acid chains between C_{12} and C_{18}. Lauric acid is the major component. All 12 bases of this series are colorless and almost odorless. The drug-release characteristics of Witepsol H15 are similar to those of cocoa butter.

    (a) Unlike cocoa butter, Witepsol bases do not exhibit polymorphism when heated and cooled.

    (b) The interval between softening and melting temperatures is very small. Because Witepsol bases solidify rapidly in the mold, lubrication of the mold is not necessary.

(3) Wecobee bases are derived from coconut oil. Their action is similar to that of Witepsol bases. Incorporation of glyceryl monostearate and propylene glycol monostearate makes these bases emulsifiable.

d. Bases that dissolve include **PEG** polymers with a molecular weight of 400–6000.

    (1) At room temperature, PEG 400 is a liquid, PEG 1000 is a semisolid, PEG 1500 and 1600 are fairly firm semisolids, and PEG 3350 and 6000 are firm wax-like solids.

    (2) These bases are water soluble, but the dissolution process is very slow. In the rectum and vagina, where the amount of fluid is very small, they dissolve very slowly, but they soften and spread.

    (3) PEGs complex with several drugs and affect drug release and absorption.

    (4) Mixtures of PEG polymers in varying proportions provide a base of different properties (Table 3-5).

4. Preparation. Suppositories are prepared by the following three methods:

    a. Hand-rolling involves molding the suppository with the fingers after a plastic mass is formed.

        (1) A finely powdered drug is mixed with the grated base in a mortar and pestle, using levigation and geometric dilution techniques. A small quantity of fixed oil may be added to facilitate preparation.

Table 3-5. Mixtures of Polyethylene Glycol (PEG) Bases Providing Satisfactory Room Temperature Stability and Dissolution Characteristics

Base	Comments	Components	Proportion (%)
1	Provides a good general-purpose, water-soluble suppository	PEG 6000	50
		PEG 1540	30
		PEG 400	20
2	Provides a good general-purpose base that is slightly softer than base 1 and dissolves more rapidly	PEG 4000	60
		PEG 1500	30
		PEG 400	10
3	Has a higher melting point than the other bases, which is usually sufficient to compensate for the melting-point lowering effect of such drugs as chloral hydrate and camphor	PEG 6000	30
		PEG 1540	70

    (2) The uniformly mixed semiplastic mass is kneaded further, rolled into a cylinder, and divided into the requisite number of suppositories. Each small cylinder is rolled by hand until a suppository shape is fashioned.

  b. Compression is generally used when cocoa butter is used as a base.

    (1) A uniform mixture of drug and base is prepared as for the hand-rolling method.

    (2) The mixture is placed into a suppository compression device. Pressure is applied, and the mixture is forced into lubricated compression mold cavities. The mold is then cooled and the suppositories ejected.

    (3) This procedure generally produces a 2-g suppository. However, a large volume of the active ingredients can affect the amount of cocoa butter required for an individual formula.

      (a) The amount of cocoa butter needed is determined by calculating the total amount of active ingredient to be used, dividing this number by the cocoa butter density factor (Table 3-6), and subtracting the resulting number from the total amount of cocoa butter required for the desired number of suppositories.

      (b) For example, suppose 12 suppositories, each containing 300 mg aspirin, are required. Each mold cavity has a 2-g capacity. For 13 suppositories (calculated to provide one extra), 3.9 g aspirin (13×0.3 g $= 3.9$ g) is required. This number is divided by the density factor of aspirin (1.1) (Table 3-6). Thus 3.9 g of aspirin replaces 3.55 g of cocoa butter. The total amount of cocoa butter needed for 13 suppositories of 2 g each equals 26 g. The amount of cocoa butter required is 26 g $-$ 3.55 g, or 22.45 g.

  c. The **fusion method** is the principal way that suppositories are made commercially. This method is used primarily for suppositories that contain cocoa butter, PEG, and glycerin–

Table 3-6. Cocoa Butter Density Factors of Drugs Commonly Used in Suppositories

Drug	Cocoa Butter Density Factor	Drug	Cocoa Butter Density Factor
Aloin	1.3	Dimenhydrinate	1.3
Aminophylline	1.1	Diphenhydramine hydrochloride	1.3
Aminopyrine	1.3	Gallic acid	2.0
Aspirin	1.1	Morphine hydrochloride	1.6
Barbital sodium	1.2	Pentobarbital	1.2
Belladonna extract	1.3	Phenobarbital sodium	1.2
Bismuth subgallate	2.7	Salicylic acid	1.3
Chloral hydrate	1.3	Secobarbital sodium	1.2
Codeine phosphate	1.1	Tannic acid	1.6
Digitalis leaf	1.6		

gelatin bases. Molds made of aluminum, brass, or nickel–copper alloys are used and can make 6–50 suppositories at one time.

(1) The **capacity of the molds** is determined by melting a sufficient quantity of base over a steam bath, pouring it into the molds, and allowing it to congeal. The "blank" suppositories are trimmed, removed, and weighed. Once the weight is known, the drug-containing suppositories are prepared.

    (a) To prepare suppositories, the drug is reduced to a fine powder. A small amount of grated cocoa butter is liquefied in a suitable container placed in a water bath at 33°C or less.

    (b) The finely powdered drug is mixed with melted cocoa butter with continuous stirring.

    (c) The remainder of the grated cocoa butter is added with stirring. The temperature is maintained at or below 33°C. The liquid should appear creamy rather than clear.

    (d) The mold is very lightly lubricated with mineral oil, and the creamy melt is poured into the mold at room temperature. The melt is poured continuously to avoid layering.

    (e) After the suppositories congeal, they are placed in a refrigerator to harden. After 30 min, they are removed from the refrigerator, trimmed, and unmolded.

(2) The fusion process should be used carefully with **thermolabile drugs** and **insoluble powders.**

    (a) Insoluble powders in the melt may settle or float during pouring, depending on their density. They may also collect at one end of the suppository before the melt congeals, and cause a nonuniform drug distribution.

    (b) Hard crystalline materials (e.g., iodine, merbromin) can be incorporated by dissolving the crystals in a minimum volume of suitable solvent before they are incorporated into the base.

    (c) Vegetable extracts can be incorporated by moistening with a few drops of alcohol and levigating with a small amount of melted cocoa butter.

G. Powders

1. Introduction. A pharmaceutical powder is a mixture of finely divided drugs or chemicals in dry form. The powder may be used internally or externally.

    a. Advantages of powders

        (1) Flexibility of compounding

        (2) Good chemical stability

        (3) Rapid dispersion of ingredients because of the small particle size

    b. Disadvantages of powders

        (1) Time-consuming preparation

        (2) Inaccuracy of dose

        (3) Unsuitability for many unpleasant-tasting, hygroscopic, and deliquescent drugs

    c. Milling is the mechanical process of reducing the particle size of solids (**comminution**) before mixing with other components, further processing, or incorporation into a final product (Tables 3-7 and 3-8). The particle size of a powder is related to the proportion of the powder that can pass through the opening of standard sieves of various dimensions in a specified amount of time. **Micromeritics** is the study of particles.

Table 3-7. *United States Pharmacopeia* Standards for Powders of Animal and Vegetable Drugs

Type of Powder	Sieve Size All Particles Pass Through	Sieve Size Percentage of Particles Pass Through
Very coarse (#8)	#20 sieve	20% through a #60 sieve
Coarse (#20)	#20 sieve	40% through a #60 sieve
Moderately coarse (#40)	#40 sieve	40% through a #80 sieve
Fine (#60)	#60 sieve	40% through a #100 sieve
Very fine (#80)	#80 sieve	No limit

Table 3-8. *United States Pharmacopeia* Standards for Powders of Chemicals

Type of Powder	Sieve Size All Particles Pass Through	Sieve Size Percentage of Particles Pass Through
Coarse (#20)	#20 sieve	60% through a #40 sieve
Moderately coarse (#40)	#40 sieve	60% through a #60 sieve
Fine (#80)	#80 sieve	No limit
Very fine (#120)	#120 sieve	No limit

    (1) Advantages of milling

        (a) Increases the surface area, which may increase the dissolution rate as well as bioavailability (e.g., griseofulvin)

        (b) Increases extraction, or leaching, from animal glands (e.g., liver, pancreas) and from crude vegetable extracts

        (c) Facilitates drying of wet masses by increasing the surface area and reducing the distance that moisture must travel to reach the outer surface. Micronization and subsequent drying, in turn, increase stability as occluded solvent is removed.

        (d) Improves mixing, or blending, of several solid ingredients if they are reduced to approximately the same size; also minimizes segregation and provides greater dose uniformity

        (e) Permits uniform distribution of coloring agents in artificially colored solid pharmaceuticals

        (f) Improves the function of lubricants used to coat the surface of the granulation or powder in compressed tablets and capsules

        (g) Improves the texture, appearance, and physical stability of ointments, creams, and pastes

    (2) Disadvantages of milling

        (a) Can change the polymorphic form of the active ingredient, rendering it less active

        (b) Can degrade the drug as a result of heat buildup, oxidation, or adsorption of unwanted moisture because of increased surface area

        (c) Decreases the bulk density of the active compound and excipients, causing flow problems and segregation.

        (d) Decreases the particle size of the raw materials and may create problems with static charge, which may cause particle aggregation and decrease the dissolution rate

        (e) Increases surface area, which may promote air adsorption and inhibit wettability

    (3) Comminution techniques. On a large scale, various mills and pulverizers (e.g., rotary cutter, hammer, roller, fluid energy mill) are used during manufacturing. On a small scale, the pharmacist usually uses one of the following comminution techniques:

        (a) Trituration. The substance is reduced to small particles by rubbing it in a mortar with a pestle. Trituration also describes the process by which fine powders are intimately mixed in a mortar.

        (b) Pulverization by intervention. Substances are reduced and subdivided with an additional material (i.e., solvent) that is easily removed after pulverization. This technique is often used with gummy substances that reagglomerate or resist grinding. For example, camphor is readily reduced after a small amount of alcohol or other volatile solvent is added. The solvent is then permitted to evaporate.

        (c) Levigation. The particle size of the substance is reduced by adding a suitable nonsolvent (levigating agent) to form a paste. The paste is then rubbed in a mortar and pestle or using an ointment slab and spatula. This method is often used to prevent a gritty feel when solids are incorporated into dermatologic or ophthalmic ointments and suspensions. Mineral oil is a common levigating agent.

  2. Mixing powders. Powders are mixed, or blended, by the following five methods:

    a. Spatulation. A spatula is used to blend small amounts of powders on a sheet of paper or a pill tile.

        (1) This method is not suitable for large quantities of powders or for powders that contain potent substances because homogeneous blending may not occur.

(2) This method is particularly useful for solid substances that liquefy or form **eutectic mixtures** (i.e., mixtures that melt at a lower temperature than any of their ingredients) when in close, prolonged contact with one another because little compression or compaction results.

    (a) These substances include phenol, camphor, menthol, thymol, aspirin, phenylsalicylate, and phenacetin.

    (b) To diminish contact, powders prepared from these substances are commonly mixed with an inert diluent (e.g., light magnesium oxide or magnesium carbonate, kaolin, starch, bentonite).

    (c) Silicic acid (approximately 20%) prevents eutexia with aspirin, phenylsalicylate, and other troublesome compounds.

  b. Trituration is used both to comminute and to mix powders.

    (1) If comminution is desired, a porcelain or ceramic mortar with a rough inner surface is preferred to a glass mortar with a smooth working surface.

    (2) A glass mortar is preferable for chemicals that stain a porcelain or ceramic surface as well as for simple admixture of substances without special need for comminution. A glass mortar cleans more readily after use.

  c. Geometric dilution is used when potent substances must be mixed with a large amount of diluent.

    (1) The potent drug and an approximately equal volume of diluent are placed in a mortar and thoroughly mixed by trituration.

    (2) A second portion of diluent, equal in volume to the powder mixture in the mortar, is added, and trituration is repeated. The process is continued; equal volumes of diluent are added to the powder mixture in the mortar until all of the diluent is incorporated.

  d. Sifting. Powders are mixed by passing them through sifters similar to those used to sift flour. This process results in a light, fluffy product. Usually, it is not acceptable for incorporating potent drugs into a diluent base.

  e. Tumbling is the process of mixing powders in a large container rotated by a motorized process. These blenders are widely used in industry, as are large-volume powder mixers that use motorized blades to blend the powder in a large mixing vessel.

3. Use and packaging of powders. Depending on their intended use, powders are packaged and dispensed by pharmacists as bulk powders or divided powders.

  a. Bulk powders are dispensed by the pharmacist in bulk containers. A **perforated,** or **sifter, can** is used for external dusting, and an **aerosol container** is used for spraying onto skin. A **wide-mouthed glass jar** permits easy removal of a spoonful of powder.

    (1) Powders commonly dispensed in bulk form

      (a) Antacid and laxative powders are used by mixing the directed amount of powder (usually approximately 1 teaspoon) in a portion of liquid, which the patient then drinks.

      (b) Douche powders are dissolved in warm water and applied vaginally.

      (c) Medicated and nonmedicated powders for external use are usually dispensed in a sifter for convenient application to the skin.

      (d) Dentifrices, or **dental cleansing powders,** are used for oral hygiene.

      (e) Powders for the **ear, nose, throat, tooth sockets,** or **vagina** are administered with an insufflator, or powder blower.

    (2) Nonpotent substances are usually dispensed in bulk powder form. Those intended for external use should be clearly labeled.

    (3) Hygroscopic, deliquescent, or **volatile** powders should be packed in glass jars rather than pasteboard containers. Amber or green glass should be used if needed to prevent decomposition of light-sensitive components. All powders should be stored in tightly closed containers.

  b. Divided powders are dispensed in individual doses, usually in folded **papers** (i.e., chartulae). They may also be dispensed in metal foil, small heat-sealed or resealable **plastic bags,** or other containers.

    (1) After the ingredients are weighed, comminuted, and mixed, the powders must be accurately **divided** into the prescribed number of doses.

    (2) Depending on the potency of the drug substance, the pharmacist decides whether to **weigh** each portion separately before packaging or to approximate portions by the **block-and-divide method.**

(3) Powder papers can be of any convenient size that fits the required dose. Four basic types are used:
  (a) Vegetable parchment is a thin, semiopaque, moisture-resistant paper.
  (b) White bond is an opaque paper that has no moisture-resistant properties.
  (c) Glassine is a glazed, transparent, moisture-resistant paper.
  (d) Waxed paper is a transparent waterproof paper.
(4) Hygroscopic and volatile drugs are best protected with waxed paper that is double wrapped and covered with a bond paper to improve the appearance. Parchment and glassine papers are of limited use for these drugs.

4. Special problems. Volatile substances, eutectic mixtures, liquids, and hygroscopic or deliquescent substances present problems when they are mixed into powders that require special treatment.
  a. Volatile substances (e.g., camphor, menthol, essential oils) can be lost by volatilization after they are incorporated into powders. This process is prevented or retarded by the use of heat-sealed plastic bags or by double wrapping with waxed or glassine paper inside white bond paper.
  b. Liquids are incorporated into divided powders in small amounts.
    (1) Magnesium carbonate, starch, or lactose can be added to increase the absorbability of the powders by increasing the surface area.
    (2) When the liquid is a solvent for a nonvolatile heat-stable compound, it is evaporated gently in a water bath. Some fluidextracts and tinctures are treated in this way.
  c. Hygroscopic and deliquescent substances that become moist because of an affinity for moisture in the air can be prepared as divided powders by adding inert diluents. Double wrapping is desirable for further protection.
  d. Eutectic mixtures

H. Capsules

1. Introduction. Capsules are solid dosage forms in which one or more medicinal or inert substances (as powder, compact, beads, or granulation) are enclosed within a small gelatin shell. Gelatin capsules may be hard or soft. Most capsules are intended to be swallowed whole, but occasionally, the contents are removed from the gelatin shell and used as a premeasured dose.

2. Hard gelatin capsules
  a. Preparation of filled hard capsules includes preparing the formulation, selecting the appropriate capsule, filling the capsule shells, and cleaning and polishing the filled capsules.
    (1) Empty hard capsule shells are manufactured from a mixture of gelatin, colorants, and sometimes an opacifying agent (e.g., titanium dioxide). The *USP* also permits the addition of 0.15% sulfur dioxide to prevent decomposition of gelatin during manufacture.
    (2) Gelatin *USP* is obtained by partial hydrolysis of collagen obtained from the skin, white connective tissue, and bones of animals. Types A and B are obtained by acid and alkali processing, respectively.
    (3) Capsule shells are cast by dipping cold metallic molds or pins into gelatin solutions that are maintained at a uniform temperature and an exact degree of fluidity.
      (a) Variation in the viscosity of the gelatin solution increases or decreases the thickness of the capsule wall.
      (b) After the pins are withdrawn from the gelatin solution, they are rotated while being dried in kilns. A strong blast of filtered air with controlled humidity is forced through the kilns. Each capsule is then mechanically stripped, trimmed, and joined.
  b. Storage. Hard capsules should be stored in tightly closed glass containers and protected from dust and extremes of humidity and temperature.
    (1) These capsules contain 12%–16% water, varying with storage conditions. When humidity is low, the capsules become brittle. When humidity is high, the capsules become flaccid and shapeless.
    (2) Storage at high temperatures also affects the quality of hard gelatin capsules.
  c. Sizes. Hard capsules are available in a variety of sizes.

(1) Empty capsules are **numbered** from 000, which is the largest size that can be swallowed, to 5, the smallest size. The approximate capacity of capsules ranges from 600 to 30 mg for capsules from 000 to 5, respectively. The capacity varies because of varying densities of powdered drug materials and the degree of pressure used to fill the capsules.

(2) Large capsules are available for **veterinary medicine.**

(3) Selecting capsules. Capsule size should be chosen carefully. A properly filled capsule should have its body filled with the drug mixture and its cap fully extended down the body. The cap is meant to enclose the powder, not to retain additional powder. Typically, hard gelatin capsules are used to encapsulate between 65 mg and 1 g of powdered material, including the drug and any diluents needed.

    (a) If the drug dose is inadequate to fill the capsule, a diluent (e.g., lactose) is added.

    (b) If the amount of drug needed for a usual dose is too large to place in a single capsule, two or more capsules may be required.

    (c) Lubricants such as magnesium stearate (frequently, 1%) are added to facilitate the flow of the powder when an automatic capsule-filling machine is used.

    (d) Wetting agents (e.g., sodium lauryl sulfate) may be added to capsule formulations to enhance drug dissolution.

d. Filling capsules. Whether on a large- or a small-production scale, the cap is first separated from the body of the capsule before filling the capsule body with the formulation and then reattaching the cap. Automated and semiautomated capsule-filling equipment fill the capsule bodies with the formulation by gravity fill, tamping, or a screw-feed (i.e., auger) mechanism. Extemporaneously compounded capsules are usually filled by the punch method.

(1) The powder is placed on paper and flattened with a spatula so that the layer of powder is no more than approximately one third the length of the capsule. The paper is held in the left hand. The body of the capsule is held in the right hand and repeatedly pressed into the powder until the capsule is filled. The cap is replaced and the capsule weighed.

(2) Granular material that does not lend itself well to the punch method can be poured into each capsule from the powder paper on which it was weighed.

(3) Crystalline materials, especially those that consist of a mass of filament-like crystals (e.g., quinine salts) will not fit into a capsule easily unless they are powdered.

(4) After they are filled, capsules must be cleaned and polished.

    (a) On a **small scale,** capsules are cleaned individually or in small numbers by rubbing them on a clean gauze or cloth.

    (b) On a **large scale,** many capsule-filling machines have a cleaning vacuum that removes any extraneous material as the capsules leave the machine.

3. Soft gelatin capsules

  a. Preparation

    (1) Soft gelatin capsules are prepared from gelatin shells. Glycerin or a polyhydric alcohol (e.g., sorbitol) is added to these shells to make them elastic or plastic-like.

    (2) These shells contain preservatives (e.g., methyl and propyl parabens, sorbic acid) to prevent the growth of fungi.

  b. Uses. Soft gelatin shells are oblong, elliptical, or spherical. They are used to contain liquids, suspensions, pastes, dry powders, or pellets.

    (1) Drugs that are commercially prepared in soft capsules include demeclocycline hydrochloride (Declomycin, Lederle), chloral hydrate, digoxin (Lanoxicaps, GlaxoSmithKline), vitamin A, and vitamin E.

    (2) Soft gelatin capsules are usually prepared by the plate process or by the rotary or reciprocating die process.

4. Uniformity and disintegration

  a. The **uniformity** of dosage forms can be demonstrated by either weight variation or content uniformity methods. The official compendia should be consulted for details of these procedures.

  b. Disintegration tests are not usually required for capsules unless they have been treated to resist solution in gastric fluid (enteric coated). In this case, they must meet the requirements for disintegration of enteric-coated tablets.

I. TABLETS

1. **Introduction**
   a. The **oral route** is the most important method for administering drugs for systemic effect. Oral drugs can be given as solids or liquids.
      (1) **Advantages of solid dosage forms**
         (a) Accurate dosage
         (b) Easy shipping and handling
         (c) Less shelf space needed per dose than for liquid
         (d) No preservation requirements
         (e) No taste-masking problem
         (f) Generally more stable than liquids, with longer expiration dates
      (2) **Advantages of liquid dosage forms**
         (a) For some drugs (e.g., adsorbents, antacids), greater effectiveness than solid form
         (b) Useful for patients who have trouble swallowing solid dosage forms
   b. **Tablets** are the **most commonly used solid dosage form.**
      (1) **Advantages**
         (a) Precision and low content variability of the unit dose
         (b) Low manufacturing cost
         (c) Easy to package and ship
         (d) Simple to identify
         (e) Easy to swallow
         (f) Appropriate for special-release forms
         (g) Best suited to large-scale production
         (h) Most stable of all oral dosage forms
            (i) Essentially tamperproof
      (2) **Disadvantages**
         (a) Some drugs resist compression into tablets.
         (b) Some drugs (i.e., those with poor wetting, slow dissolution properties, intermediate to large doses, optimum absorption high in the gastrointestinal tract, or any combination of these features) may be difficult to formulate to provide adequate bioavailability.
         (c) Some drugs (e.g., those with an objectionable taste or odor, those sensitive to oxygen or atmospheric moisture) require encapsulation or entrapment before compression. These drugs are more appropriate in capsule form.

2. **Tablet design and formulation**
   a. **Characteristics of ideal tablets**
      (1) Free of defects (e.g., chips, cracks, discoloration, contamination)
      (2) Strong enough to withstand the mechanical stresses of production
      (3) Chemically and physically stable over time
      (4) Capable of releasing medicinal agents in a predictable and reproducible manner
   b. **Tablet excipients.** Tablets are manufactured by **wet granulation, dry granulation,** or **direct compression.** Regardless of the method of manufacture, tablets for oral ingestion usually contain excipients, which are components added to the active ingredients that have special functions (Table 3-9).
      (1) **Diluents** are fillers designed to make up the required bulk of the tablet when the drug dosage amount is inadequate. Diluents may also improve cohesion, permit direct compression, or promote flow.
         (a) **Common diluents** include kaolin, lactose, mannitol, starch, microcrystalline cellulose, powdered sugar, and calcium phosphate.
         (b) **Selection of the diluent** is based on the experience of the manufacturer as well as on the cost of the diluent and its compatibility with the other tablet ingredients. For example, calcium salts cannot be used as fillers for tetracycline products because calcium interferes with the absorption of tetracycline from the gastrointestinal tract.
      (2) **Binders and adhesives** are added in either dry or liquid form to promote granulation or to promote cohesive compacts during direct compression.
         (a) **Common binding agents** include a 10%–20% aqueous preparation of cornstarch, a 25%–50% solution of glucose, molasses, various natural gums (e.g., acacia), cellulose derivatives (e.g., methylcellulose, carboxymethylcellulose, microcrys-

Table 3-9. Some Common Tablet Excipients

Diluents
Calcium phosphate dihydrate *NF* (dibasic)
Calcium sulfate dihydrate *NF*
Cellulose *NF* (microcrystalline)
Cellulose derivatives
Dextrose
Lactose *USP*
Lactose *USP* (anhydrous)
Lactose *USP* (spray dried)
Mannitol *USP*
Starches (directly compressible)
Starches (hydrolyzed)
Sorbitol
Sucrose *USP* (powder)
Sucrose-based materials

Binders and adhesives
Acacia
Cellulose derivatives
Gelatin
Glucose
PVP
Sodium alginate and alginate derivatives
Sorbitol
Starch (paste)
Starch (pregelatinized)
Tragacanth

Disintegrants
Alginates
Cellulose
Cellulose derivatives
Clays
PVP (cross-linked)
Starch
Starch derivatives

Lubricants
PEGs
Stearic acid
Stearic acid salts
Stearic acid derivatives
Surfactants
Talc
Waxes

Glidants
Cornstarch
Silica derivatives
Talc

Colors, flavors, and sweeteners
FD&C and D&C dyes and lakes
Flavors available in two forms (spray dried, oil)
Artificial sweetenersNatural sweetener

D&C, drugs and cosmetics; *FD&C,* food, drugs, and cosmetics; *NF, National Formulary; PEG,* polyethylene glycol; *PVP,* polyvinylpyrrolidone (more commonly, povidone); *USP, United States Pharmacopeia.*

talline cellulose), gelatins, and povidone. The natural gums are variable in composition and are usually contaminated with bacteria.

(b) If the drug substance is adversely affected by an aqueous binder, a **nonaqueous binder** can be used or the binder can be added dry. The binding action is usually more effective when the binder is mixed in liquid form.

(c) The **amount** of binder or adhesive used depends on the experience of the manufacturer as well as on the other tablet ingredients. Overwetting usually produces granules that are too hard to allow proper tableting. Underwetting usually produces tablets that are too soft and tend to crumble.

(3) **Disintegrants** are added to tablet formulations to facilitate disintegration when the tablet contacts water in the gastrointestinal tract. Disintegrants function by drawing water into the tablet, swelling, and causing the tablet to burst.

(a) Tablet disintegration may be critical to the subsequent dissolution of the drug and to satisfactory drug bioavailability.

(b) **Common disintegrants** include cornstarch and potato starch; starch derivatives (e.g., sodium starch glycolate); cellulose derivatives (e.g., sodium carboxymethylcellulose, croscarmellose sodium); clays (e.g., VEEGUM, bentonite); and cation exchange resins.

(c) The total **amount of disintegrant** is not always added to the drug–diluent mixture. A portion can be added, with the lubricant, to the prepared granulation of the drug. This approach causes double disintegration of the tablet. The portion of disintegrant that is added last causes the tablet to break into small pieces, or chunks. The portion that is added first breaks the pieces of tablet into fine particles.

(4) **Lubricants, antiadherents,** and **glidants** have overlapping function.

(a) **Lubricants** reduce the friction that occurs between the walls of the tablet and the walls of the die cavity when the tablet is ejected. Talc, magnesium stearate, and calcium stearate are commonly used.

(b) **Antiadherents** reduce sticking, or adhesion, of the tablet granulation or powder to the faces of the punches or the die walls.

(c) **Glidants** promote the flow of the tablet granulation or powder by reducing friction among particles.

(5) **Colors and dyes** disguise off-color drugs, provide product identification, and produce a more aesthetically appealing product. **Food, drug,** and **cosmetic dyes** are applied as solutions. **Lakes** are dyes that have been absorbed on a hydrous oxide. Lakes are typically used as dry powders.

(6) **Flavoring agents** are usually limited to chewable tablets or tablets that are intended to dissolve in the mouth.

(a) Water-soluble flavors usually have poor stability. For this reason, flavor oils or dry powders are typically used.

(b) Flavor oils may be added to tablet granulations in solvents, dispersed on clays and other adsorbents, or emulsified in aqueous granulating agents. Usually, the maximum amount of oil that can be added to a granulation without affecting its tablet characteristics is 0.5%–0.75%.

(7) **Artificial sweeteners,** like flavors, are typically used only with chewable tablets or tablets that are intended to dissolve in the mouth.

(a) Some **sweetness** may come from the diluent (e.g., mannitol, lactose). Other agents (e.g., saccharin, aspartame) may also be added.

(b) **Saccharin** has an unpleasant aftertaste.

(c) **Aspartame** is not stable in the presence of moisture and heat.

(8) **Adsorbents** (e.g., magnesium oxide, magnesium carbonate, bentonite, silicon dioxide) hold quantities of fluid in an apparently dry state.

3. Tablet types and classes. Tablets are classified according to their route of administration, drug delivery system, and form and method of manufacture (Table 3-10).

a. Tablets for oral ingestion are designed to be swallowed intact, with the exception of chewable tablets. Tablets may be coated for a number of reasons: to mask the taste, color, or odor of the drug; to control drug release; to protect the drug from the acid environment of the stomach; to incorporate another drug and provide sequential release or avoid incompatibility; or to improve appearance.

(1) **Compressed tablets** are formed by compression and have no special coating. They are made from powdered, crystalline, or granular materials, alone or in combination with excipients such as binders, disintegrants, diluents, and colorants.

(2) **Multiple compressed tablets** are layered or compression-coated.

(a) **Layered tablets** are prepared by compressing a tablet granulation around a previously compressed granulation. The operation is repeated to produce multiple layers.

(b) **Compression-coated, or dry-coated, tablets** are prepared by feeding previously compressed tablets into a special tableting machine. This machine compresses an outer shell around the tablets. This process applies a thinner, more uniform coating than sugar coating, and it can be used safely with drugs that are sensitive to moisture. This process can be used to separate incompatible materials, to

Table 3-10. Tablet Types and Classes

Tablets for oral ingestion	Tablets used in the oral cavity
Compressed	Buccal
Multiple compressed	Sublingual
Layered	Troches, lozenges, and dental
Compression coated	cones
Repeat-action	
Delayed action and enteric coated	**Tablets used to prepare solutions**
Sugar coated and chocolate coated	Effervescent
Film coated	Dispensing
Air suspension coated	Hypodermic
Chewable	Triturates

produce repeat-action or prolonged-action products or to produce tablets with a multilayered appearance.

(3) Repeat-action tablets are layered or compression-coated tablets in which the outer layer or shell rapidly disintegrates in the stomach (e.g., Repetabs, Schering; Extentabs, Wyeth). The components of the inner layer or inner tablet are insoluble in gastric media but soluble in intestinal media.

(4) Delayed-action and **enteric-coated tablets** delay the release of a drug from a dosage form. This delay is intended to prevent destruction of the drug by gastric juices, to prevent irritation of the stomach lining by the drug, or to promote absorption, which is better in the intestine than in the stomach.

    (a) Enteric-coated tablets are coated and remain intact in the stomach, but yield their ingredients in the intestines (e.g., Ecotrin, GlaxoSmithKline). Enteric-coated tablets are a form of delayed-action tablet. However, not all delayed-action tablets are enteric or are intended to produce an enteric effect.

    (b) Agents used to coat these tablets include fats, fatty acids, waxes, shellac, and cellulose acetate phthalate.

(5) Sugar-coated and **chocolate-coated tablets** are compressed tablets that are coated for various reasons. The coating may be added to protect the drug from air and humidity, to provide a barrier to a drug's objectionable taste or smell, or to improve the appearance of the tablet.

    (a) Tablets may be coated with a colored or an uncolored sugar. The process includes **seal coating** (waterproofing), **subcoating, syrup coating** (for smoothing and coloring), and **polishing.** These steps take place in a series of mechanically operated coating pans.

    (b) Disadvantages of sugar-coated tablets include the time and expertise required for the process and the increase in tablet size and weight. Sugar-coated tablets may be 50% larger and heavier than the original tablets.

    (c) Chocolate-coated tablets are rare today.

(6) Film-coated tablets are compressed tablets that are coated with a thin layer of a water-insoluble or water-soluble polymer (e.g., hydroxypropyl methylcellulose, ethylcellulose, povidone, PEG).

    (a) The film is usually colored. It is more durable, less bulky, and less time-consuming to apply than sugar coating. Although the film typically increases tablet weight by only 2%–3%, it increases formulation efficiency, resistance to chipping, and output.

    (b) Film-coating solutions usually contain a film former, an alloying substance, a plasticizer, a surfactant, opacifiers, sweeteners, flavors, colors, glossants, and a volatile solvent.

    (c) The volatile solvents used in these solutions are expensive and potentially toxic when released into the atmosphere. Specifically formulated **aqueous dispersion**s of polymers (e.g., ethylcellulose) are now available as alternatives to organic solvent–based coating solutions.

(7) Air suspension–coated tablets are fed into a vertical cylinder and supported by a column of air that enters from the bottom of the cylinder. As the coating solution enters the system, it is rapidly applied to the suspended, rotating solids (**Wurster process**). Rounding coats can be applied in < 1 hr when blasts of warm air are released in the chamber.

(8) Chewable tablets disintegrate smoothly and rapidly when chewed or allowed to dissolve in the mouth. These tablets contain specially colored and flavored mannitol and yield a creamy base.

    (a) Chewable tablets are especially useful in formulations for children.

    (b) They are commonly used for multivitamin tablets and are used for some antacids and antibiotics.

b. Tablets used in the oral cavity are allowed to dissolve in the mouth.

(1) Buccal and sublingual tablets allow absorption through the oral mucosa after they dissolve in the buccal pouch (buccal tablets) or below the tongue (sublingual tablets). These forms are useful for drugs that are destroyed by gastric juice or poorly absorbed from the intestinal tract. Examples include sublingual nitroglycerin tablets, which dissolve promptly to give rapid drug effects, and buccal progesterone tablets, which dissolve slowly.

(2) Troches, lozenges, and dental cones dissolve slowly in the mouth and provide primarily local effects.
    c. Tablets used to prepare solutions are dissolved in water before administration.
        (1) Effervescent tablets are prepared by compressing granular effervescent salts or other materials (e.g., citric acid, tartaric acid, sodium bicarbonate) that release carbon dioxide gas when they come into contact with water. Commercial alkalinizing analgesic tablets are often made to effervesce to encourage rapid dissolution and absorption (e.g., Alka-Seltzer, Bayer).
        (2) Other tablets used to prepare solutions include dispensing tablets, hypodermic tablets, and tablet triturates.

4. Processing problems
    a. Capping is the partial or complete separation of the top or bottom crown from the main body of the tablet. Lamination is separation of a tablet into two or more distinct layers. These problems are usually caused by entrapment of air during processing.
    b. Picking is removal of the surface material of a tablet by a punch. Sticking is adhesion of tablet material to a die wall. These problems are caused by excessive moisture or the inclusion of substances with low melting temperatures in the formulation.
    c. Mottling is unequal color distribution, with light or dark areas standing out on an otherwise uniform surface. This problem occurs when a drug has a different color than the tablet excipients or when a drug has colored degradation products. Colorants solve the problem but can create other problems.

5. Tablet evaluation and control
    a. The general appearance of tablets is an important factor in consumer acceptance. It also allows monitoring of lot-to-lot uniformity, tablet-to-tablet uniformity, and elements of the manufacturing process. The appearance of the tablet includes visual identity and overall appearance. The appearance of the tablet is controlled by measurement of attributes such as size, shape, color, odor, taste, surface, texture, physical flaws, consistency, and legibility of markings.
    b. Hardness and resistance to friability are necessary for tablets to withstand the mechanical shocks of manufacture, packaging, and shipping, and to ensure consumer acceptance. Hardness involves both tablet disintegration and drug dissolution. Certain tablets that are intended to dissolve slowly are made hard. Other tablets that are intended to dissolve rapidly are made soft. Friability is the tendency of the tablet to crumble.
        (1) Tablet hardness testers measure the degree of force required to break a tablet.
        (2) Friabilators determine friability by allowing the tablet to roll and fall within a rotating tumbling apparatus. The tablets are weighed before and after a specified number of rotations, and the weight loss is determined.
            (a) Resistance to weight loss indicates the ability of the tablet to withstand abrasion during handling, packaging, and shipping. Compressed tablets that lose < 0.5%–1% of their weight are usually considered acceptable.
            (b) Some chewable tablets and most effervescent tablets are highly friable and require special unit packaging.
    c. Tablets are routinely weighed to ensure that they contain the proper amount of drug.
        (1) The USP defines a weight variation standard to which tablets must conform.
        (2) These standards apply to tablets that contain 50 mg or more of drug substance when the drug substance is 50% or more (by weight) of the dosage form unit.
    d. Content uniformity is evaluated to ensure that each tablet contains the desired amount of drug substance, with little variation among contents within a batch. The USP defines content uniformity tests for tablets that contain 50 mg or less of drug substance.
    e. Disintegration is evaluated to ensure that the drug substance is fully available for dissolution and absorption from the gastrointestinal tract.
        (1) All USP tablets must pass an official disintegration test that is conducted in vitro with special equipment.
            (a) Disintegration times for uncoated USP tablets are as low as 2 min (nitroglycerin) to 5 min (aspirin). Most have a maximum disintegration time of less than 30 min.
            (b) Buccal tablets must disintegrate within 4 hr.
            (c) Enteric-coated tablets must show no evidence of disintegration after 1 hr in simulated gastric fluid. In simulated intestinal fluid, they should disintegrate in 2 hr plus the time specified.

(2) Dissolution requirements in the USP have replaced earlier disintegration requirements for many drugs.

    f. Dissolution characteristics are tested to determine drug absorption and physiologic availability.

        (1) The USP gives standards for tablet dissolution.

        (2) An increased emphasis on testing tablet dissolution and determining drug bioavailability has increased the use of sophisticated testing systems.

J. Aerosol products

    1. Introduction. Aerosol products, or aerosols, are pressurized dosage forms. They are designed to deliver drug systemically or topically with the aid of a liquefied or propelled gas (propellant). Aerosol products consist of a pressurizable container (tin-plated steel, aluminum, glass, or plastic); a valve that allows the pressurized product to be expelled from the container (either continuously or intermittently) when the actuator is pressed; and a dip tube that conveys the formulation from the bottom of the container to the valve assembly. Aerosols are prepared by special methods (cold filling, pressure filling) because of the gaseous components.

    2. Systemic or pulmonary drug delivery is provided by aerosol drug delivery systems, or metered dose inhalers (MDIs). These devices allow a drug to be inhaled as a fine mist of drug or drug-containing particles. MDIs use special metering valves to regulate the amount of formulation and drug that is dispensed with each dose (i.e., each actuation of the container). Aerosol products are used for topical drug delivery. The formulations range from solutions to dispersions. Metering valves may also be used with topical aerosol products to regulate the amount of drug applied per application.

    3. Propellants used in aerosol products

        a. Compressed gases include carbon dioxide, nitrogen, and nitrous oxide. Aerosol products that contain compressed gas tend to lose pressure over time as the product is dispensed. The drop in pressure reflects the expansion of the head space in the container (i.e., increase in the volume that the gas can occupy) as formulation is withdrawn for use. For this reason, higher initial pressures are typically used with compressed gas–based systems than with liquefiable gas–based formulations.

        b. Liquefiable gases include saturated hydrocarbons (n-butane, isobutane, propane); chlorofluorocarbons (CFCs), including tetrafluorodichloroethane (propellant 114), dichlorodifluoromethane (propellant 12), and trichlorofluoromethane (propellant 11); dimethyl ether; and hydrofluorocarbons, such as 1,1,1,2-fluoroethane (propellant 134a) and 1,1-difluoroethane (propellant 152a). The negative effect of older CFCs on atmospheric ozone and the potential for global warming led to the worldwide reduction in CFC production under the Montreal Protocol. This plan called for a general ban on CFC production in industrialized countries by January 1996. As a result, the use of CFCs in pharmaceutical products is being phased out. Temporary exemptions for CFCs in MDIs will eventually lapse (in 2008) as stable, safe, and effective alternative formulations are developed with more acceptable propellants (e.g., hydrofluorocarbons).

    4. Advantages of aerosol products include the convenience of push-button dispensing of medication and the stability afforded by a closed, pressurized container that minimizes the likelihood of tampering and protects the contents from light, moisture, air (oxygen), and microbial contamination. Aerosol formulations and packaging components (valves, actuators) permit a wide range of products to be dispensed as sprays, foams, or semisolids.

    5. The principal disadvantage of aerosol products is environmental (e.g., disposal of pressurized packages, venting of propellants to the atmosphere).

K. Controlled-release dosage forms

    1. Introduction. Controlled-release dosage forms are also known as delayed-release, sustained-action, prolonged-action, sustained-release, prolonged-release, timed-release, slow-release, extended-action, and extended-release forms. They are designed to release drug substance slowly to provide prolonged action in the body.

2. Advantages of controlled-release forms
  a. Fewer problems with patient compliance
  b. Use of less total drug
  c. Fewer local or systemic side effects
  d. Minimal drug accumulation with long-term dosage
  e. Fewer problems with potentiation or loss of drug activity with long-term use
  f. Improved treatment efficiency
  g. More rapid control of the patient's condition
  h. Less fluctuation in drug level
  i. Improved bioavailability for some drugs
  j. Improved ability to provide special effects (e.g., morning relief of arthritis by bedtime dosing)
  k. Reduced cost

3. Sustained-release forms can be grouped according to their pharmaceutical mechanism.
  a. Coated beads or granules (e.g., Spansules, GlaxoSmithKline; Sequels, Wyeth) produce a blood level profile similar to that obtained with multiple dosing.
    (1) A solution of the drug substance in a nonaqueous solvent (e.g., alcohol) is coated onto small, inert beads, or granules, made of a combination of sugar and starch. When the drug dose is large, the starting granules may be composed of the drug itself.
    (2) Some of the granules are left uncoated to provide immediate release of the drug.
    (3) Coats of a lipid material (e.g., beeswax) or a cellulosic material (e.g., ethylcellulose) are applied to the remaining granules. Some granules receive few coats, and some receive many. The various coating thicknesses produce a sustained-release effect.
  b. Microencapsulation is a process by which solids, liquids, or gases are encased in microscopic capsules. Thin coatings of a "wall" material are formed around the substance to be encapsulated.
    (1) Coacervation is the most common method of microencapsulation. It occurs when a hydrophilic substance is added to a colloidal drug dispersion and causes layering and the formation of microcapsules.
    (2) Film-forming substances that are used as the coating material include a variety of natural and synthetic polymers. These materials include shellacs, waxes, gelatin, starches, cellulose acetate phthalate, and ethylcellulose. After the coating material dissolves, all of the drug inside the microcapsule is immediately available for dissolution and absorption. The thickness of the wall can vary from 1 to 200 mm, depending on the amount of coating material used (3%–30% of total weight).
  c. Matrix tablets use insoluble plastics (e.g., polyethylene, polyvinyl acetate, polymethacrylate), hydrophilic polymers (e.g., methylcellulose, hydroxypropyl methylcellulose), or fatty compounds (e.g., various waxes, glyceryl tristearate). Examples include Gradumet (Abbott) and Dospan (Aventis).
    (1) The most common method of preparation is mixing of the drug with the matrix material followed by compression of the material into tablets.
    (2) The primary dose, or the portion of the drug to be released immediately, is placed on the tablet as a layer, or coat. The rest of the dose is released slowly from the matrix.
  d. Osmotic systems include the Oros system (Alza), which is an oral osmotic pump composed of a core tablet and a semipermeable coating that has a small hole (0.4 mm in diameter) for drug exit. The hole is produced by a laser beam. Examples include Glucotrol XL (glipizide extended-release tablets, Pfizer) and Procardia XL (nifedipine extended-release tablets, Pfizer).
    (1) This system requires only osmotic pressure to be effective. It is essentially independent of pH changes in the environment.
    (2) The drug-release rate can be changed by changing the tablet surface area, the nature of the membrane, or the diameter of the drug-release aperture.
  e. Ion-exchange resins can be complexed with drugs by passage of a cationic drug solution through a column that contains the resin. The drug is complexed to the resin by replacement of hydrogen atoms. Examples include Ionamin capsules (Celltech; resin complexes of phentermine) and the Pennkinetic system (Celltech), which incorporates a polymer barrier coating and bead technology in addition to the ion-exchange mechanism.

(1) After the components are complexed, the resin–drug complex is washed and tableted, encapsulated, or suspended in an aqueous vehicle.

(2) Release of drug from the complex depends on the ionic environment within the gastrointestinal tract and on the properties of the resin. Usually, release is greater in the highly acidic stomach than in the less acidic small intestine.

f. Complex formation is used for certain drug substances that combine chemically with other agents. For example, hydroxypropyl-β-cyclodextrin forms a chemical complex that can be only slowly soluble from body fluids, depending on the pH of the environment. Tannic acid (i.e., tannates) complexes with the amino groups of weak bases dissolve at a slow rate in the gastrointestinal tract, thereby providing for a prolonged release of drug. Examples of the latter include brompheniramine tannate (Brovex, Athlon) and chlorpheniramine/phenylephrine tannates (Rynatan, Wallace).

STUDY QUESTIONS

Directions for questions 1–28: Each of the questions, statements, or incomplete statements in this section can be correctly answered or completed by one of the suggested answers or phrases. Choose the best answer.

1. Which substance is classified as a weak electrolyte?

(A) glucose
(B) urea
(C) ephedrine
(D) sodium chloride
(E) sucrose

2. The pH value is calculated mathematically as the

(A) log of the hydroxyl ion (OH−) concentration.
(B) negative log of the OH^- concentration.
(C) log of the hydrogen ion (H^+) concentration.
(D) negative log of the H^+ concentration.
(E) ratio of H^+/OH^- concentration.

3. Which property is classified as colligative?

(A) solubility of a solute
(B) osmotic pressure
(C) hydrogen ion (H^+) concentration
(D) dissociation of a solute
(E) miscibility of the liquids

4. The colligative properties of a solution are related to the

(A) pH of the solution.
(B) number of ions in the solution.
(C) total number of solute particles in the solution.
(D) number of unionized molecules in the solution.
(E) pK_a of the solution.

5. The pH of a buffer system can be calculated with the

(A) Noyes-Whitney equation.
(B) Henderson-Hasselbalch equation.
(C) Michaelis-Menten equation.
(D) Young equation.
(E) Stokes equation.

6. Which mechanism is most often responsible for chemical degradation?

(A) racemization
(B) photolysis
(C) hydrolysis
(D) decarboxylation
(E) oxidation

7. Which equation is used to predict the stability of a drug product at room temperature from experiments at accelerated temperatures?

(A) Stokes equation
(B) Young equation
(C) Arrhenius equation
(D) Michaelis-Menten equation
(E) Hixson-Crowell equation

8. Based on the relation between the degree of ionization and the solubility of a weak acid, the drug aspirin (pK_a 3.49) will be most soluble at

(A) pH 1.0
(B) pH 2.0
(C) pH 3.0
(D) pH 4.0
(E) pH 6.0

9. Which solution is used as an astringent?

(A) strong iodine solution *USP*
(B) aluminum acetate topical solution *USP*
(C) acetic acid *NF*
(D) aromatic ammonia spirit *USP*
(E) benzalkonium chloride solution *NF*

10. The particle size of the dispersed solid in a suspension is usually greater than

(A) 0.5 μm
(B) 0.4 μm
(C) 0.3 μm
(D) 0.2 μm
(E) 0.1 μm

11. In the extemporaneous preparation of a suspension, levigation is used to

(A) reduce the zeta potential.
(B) avoid bacterial growth.
(C) reduce particle size.
(D) enhance viscosity.
(E) reduce viscosity.

12. Which compound is a natural emulsifying agent?

(A) acacia
(B) lactose
(C) polysorbate 20
(D) polysorbate 80
(E) sorbitan monopalmitate

13. Vanishing cream is an ointment that may be classified as

(A) a water-soluble base.
(B) an oleaginous base.
(C) an absorption base.
(D) an emulsion base.
(E) an oleic base.

14. Rectal suppositories intended for adult use usually weigh approximately

(A) 1 g.
(B) 2 g.
(C) 3 g.
(D) 4 g.
(E) 5 g.

15. In the fusion method of making cocoa butter suppositories, which substance is most likely to be used to lubricate the mold?

(A) mineral oil
(B) propylene glycol
(C) cetyl alcohol
(D) stearic acid
(E) magnesium silicate

16. A very fine powdered chemical is defined as one that

(A) completely passes through a #80 sieve.
(B) completely passes through a #120 sieve.
(C) completely passes through a #20 sieve.
(D) passes through a #60 sieve and not more than 40% through a #100 sieve.
(E) passes through a #40 sieve and not more than 60% through a #60 sieve.

17. Which technique is typically used to mill camphor?

(A) trituration
(B) levigation
(C) pulverization by intervention
(D) geometric dilution
(E) attrition

18. The dispensing pharmacist usually blends potent powders with a large amount of diluent by

(A) spatulation.
(B) sifting.
(C) trituration.
(D) geometric dilution.
(E) levigation.

19. Which type of paper best protects a divided hygroscopic powder?

(A) waxed paper
(B) glassine
(C) white bond
(D) blue bond
(E) vegetable parchment

20. Which capsule size has the smallest capacity?

(A) 5
(B) 4
(C) 1
(D) 0
(E) 000

21. The shells of soft gelatin capsules may be made elastic or plastic-like by the addition of

(A) sorbitol.
(B) povidone.
(C) polyethylene glycol (PEG).
(D) lactose.
(E) hydroxypropyl methylcellulose.

22. The *United States Pharmacopeia* (*USP*) content uniformity test for tablets is used to ensure which quality?

(A) bioequivalency
(B) dissolution
(C) potency
(D) purity
(E) toxicity

23. All of the following statements about chemical degradation are true *except*

(A) as temperature increases, degradation decreases.
(B) most drugs degrade by a first-order process.
(C) chemical degradation may produce a toxic product.
(D) chemical degradation may result in a loss of active ingredients.
(E) chemical degradation may affect the therapeutic activity of a drug.

24. All of the following statements concerning zero-order degradation are true *except*

(A) its rate is independent of the concentration.
(B) a plot of concentration versus time yields a straight line on rectilinear paper.
(C) its half-life is a changing parameter.
(D) its concentration remains unchanged with respect to time.
(E) the slope of a plot of concentration versus time yields a rate constant.

25. All of the following statements about first-order degradation are true *except*

(A) its rate is dependent on the concentration.
(B) its half-life is a changing parameter.
(C) a plot of the logarithm of concentration versus time yields a straight line.
(D) its $t_{90\%}$ is independent of the concentration.
(E) a plot of the logarithm of concentration versus time allows the rate constant to be determined.

26. A satisfactory suppository base must meet all of the following criteria *except*

(A) it should have a narrow melting range.
(B) it should be nonirritating and nonsensitizing.
(C) it should dissolve or disintegrate rapidly in the body cavity.
(D) it should melt $< 30°C$.
(E) it should be inert.

27. Cocoa butter (theobroma oil) exhibits all of the following properties *except*

(A) it melts at temperatures between 33°C and 35°C.
(B) it is a mixture of glycerides.
(C) it is a polymorph.
(D) it is useful in formulating rectal suppositories.
(E) it is soluble in water.

28. *United States Pharmacopeia* (*USP*) tests to ensure the quality of drug products in tablet form include all of the following *except*

(A) disintegration.
(B) dissolution.
(C) hardness and friability.
(D) content uniformity.
(E) weight variation.

Directions for questions 29–42: The questions and incomplete statements in this section can be correctly answered or completed by **one or more** of the suggested answers. Choose the answer, **A–E.**

A	if **I only** is correct
B	if **III only** is correct
C	if **I and II** are correct
D	if **II and III** are correct
E	if **I, II, and III** are correct

29. Forms of water that are suitable for use in parenteral preparations include

  I. purified water *USP.*
 II. water for injection *USP.*
III. sterile water for injection *USP.*

30. The particles in an ideal suspension should satisfy which of the following criteria?

  I. Their size should be uniform.
 II. They should be stationary or move randomly.
III. They should remain discrete.

31. The sedimentation of particles in a suspension can be minimized by

  I. adding sodium benzoate.
 II. increasing the viscosity of the suspension.
III. reducing the particle size of the active ingredient.

32. Ingredients that may be used as suspending agents include

  I. methylcellulose.
 II. acacia.
III. talc.

33. Mechanisms that are thought to provide stable emulsifications include the

  I. formation of interfacial film.
 II. lowering of interfacial tension.
III. presence of charge on the ions.

34. Nonionic surface-active agents used as synthetic emulsifiers include

  I. tragacanth.
 II. sodium lauryl sulfate.
III. sorbitan esters (Spans).

35. Advantages of systemic drug administration by rectal suppositories include

  I. avoidance of first-pass effects.
 II. suitability when the oral route is not feasible.
III. predictable drug release and absorption.

36. True statements about the milling of powders include

  I. a fine particle size is essential if the lubricant is to function properly.
 II. an increased surface area may enhance the dissolution rate.
III. milling may cause degradation of thermolabile drugs.

37. Substances used to insulate powder components that liquefy when mixed include

 I. talc.
 II. kaolin.
 III. light magnesium oxide.

38. A ceramic mortar may be preferable to a glass mortar when

 I. a volatile oil is added to a powder mixture.
 II. colored substances (dyes) are mixed into a powder.
 III. comminution is desired in addition to mixing.

39. Divided powders may be dispensed in

 I. individual-dose packets.
 II. a bulk container.
 III. a perforated, sifter-type container.

40. True statements about the function of excipients used in tablet formulations include

 I. binders promote granulation during the wet granulation process.
 II. glidants help promote the flow of the tablet granulation during manufacture.
 III. lubricants help the patient swallow the tablets.

41. Which manufacturing variables would be likely to affect the dissolution of a prednisone tablet in the body?

 I. the amount and type of binder added
 II. the amount and type of disintegrant added
 III. the force of compression used during tableting

42. Agents that may be used to coat enteric-coated tablets include

 I. hydroxypropyl methylcellulose.
 II. carboxymethylcellulose.
 III. cellulose acetate phthalate.

Directions for questions 43–46: Each of the following tablet-processing problems can be the result of one the following reasons. The processing problems may be used more than once or not at all. Choose the **best** answer, **A–E.**

 A   excessive moisture in the granulation
 B   entrapment of air
 C   tablet friability
 D   degraded drug
 E   tablet hardness

43. Picking

44. Mottling

45. Capping

46. Sticking

Directions for questions 47–49: Each of the following processes can be described by one of the following comminution procedures. The processes may be used more than once or not at all. Choose the **best** answer, **A–E.**

 A   trituration
 B   spatulation
 C   levigation
 D   pulverization by intervention
 E   tumbling

47. Rubbing or grinding a substance in a mortar that has a rough inner surface

48. Reducing and subdividing a substance by adding an easily removed solvent

49. Adding a suitable agent to form a paste and then rubbing or grinding the paste in a mortar

Directions for questions 50–53: Each of the following controlled-release dosage forms is represented by one of the following drug products. The dosage forms may be used more than once or not at all. Choose the **best** answer, **A–E.**

    A   matrix formulations
    B   ion-exchange resin complex
    C   drug complexes
    D   osmotic system
    E   coated beads or granules

50. Ionamin capsules

51. Thorazine Spansule capsules

52. Rynatan pediatric suspension

53. Procardia XL

ANSWERS AND EXPLANATIONS

1. The answer is C *[see IV.A.1.a; IV.A.3.d].*
Glucose, urea, and sucrose are nonelectrolytes. Sodium chloride is a strong electrolyte. Electrolytes are substances that form ions when dissolved in water. Thus they can conduct an electric current through the solution. Ions are particles that bear electrical charges: Cations are positively charged, and anions are negatively charged. Strong electrolytes are completely ionized in water at all concentrations. Weak electrolytes (e.g., ephedrine) are only partially ionized at most concentrations. Because nonelectrolytes do not form ions when in solution, they are nonconductors.

2. The answer is D *[see IV.A.3.b].*
The pH is a measure of the acidity, or hydrogen ion concentration, of an aqueous solution. The pH is the logarithm of the reciprocal of the hydrogen ion (H^+) concentration expressed in moles per liter. Because the logarithm of a reciprocal equals the negative logarithm of the number, the pH is the negative logarithm of the H^+ concentration. A pH of 7.0 indicates neutrality. As the pH decreases, the acidity increases. The pH of arterial blood is 7.35–7.45; of urine, 4.8–7.5; of gastric juice, approximately 1.4; and of cerebrospinal fluid, 7.35–7.40. The concept of pH was introduced by Sörensen in the early 1900s. Alkalinity is the negative logarithm of $[OH^-]$ and is inversely related to acidity.

3. The answer is B *[see IV.A.2.d].*
Osmotic pressure is an example of a colligative property. The osmotic pressure is the magnitude of pressure needed to stop osmosis across a semipermeable membrane between a solution and a pure solvent. The colligative properties of a solution depend on the total number of dissociated and undissociated solute particles. These properties are independent of the size of the solute. Other colligative properties of solutes are reduction in the vapor pressure of the solution, elevation of its boiling point, and depression of its freezing point.

4. The answer is C *[see IV.A.1.b].*
The colligative properties of a solution are related to the total number of solute particles that it contains. Examples of colligative properties are the osmotic pressure, lowering of the vapor pressure, elevation of the boiling point, and depression of the freezing, or melting, point.

5. The answer is B *[see IV.A.3.e].*
The Henderson-Hasselbalch equation for a weak acid and its salt is as follows:

$$pH = pK_a + \log \frac{[salt]}{[acid]}$$

where pK_a is the negative log of the dissociation constant of a weak acid and [salt]/[acid] is the ratio of the molar concentration of salt and acid used to prepare a buffer.

6. The answer is C *[see V.D.1].*
Although all of the mechanisms listed can be responsible, the chemical degradation of medicinal compounds, particularly esters in liquid formulations, is usually caused by hydrolysis. For this reason, drugs that have ester functional groups are formulated in dry form whenever possible. Oxidation is another common mode of degradation and is minimized by including antioxidants (e.g., ascorbic acid) in drug formulations. Photolysis is reduced by packaging susceptible products in amber or opaque containers. Decarboxylation, which is the removal of COOH groups, affects compounds that include carboxylic acid. Racemization neutralizes the effects of an optically active compound by converting half of its molecules into their mirror-image configuration. As a result, the dextrorotatory and levorotatory forms cancel each other out. This type of degradation affects only drugs that are characterized by optical isomerism.

7. The answer is C *[see V.E.3.d].*
Testing of a drug formulation to determine its shelf life can be accelerated by applying the Arrhenius equation to data obtained at higher temperatures. The method involves determining the rate constant (k) values for the degradation of a drug at various elevated temperatures. The log of k is plotted against the reciprocal of the absolute temperature, and the k value for degradation at room temperature is obtained by extrapolation.

8. The answer is E *[see IV.A.3.g].*
The solubility of a weak acid varies as a function of pH. Because pH and pK_a (the dissociation constant) are related, solubility is also related to the degree of ionization. Aspirin is a weak acid that is completely ionized at a pH that is 2 units greater than its pK_a. Therefore, it is most soluble at pH 6.0.

9. The answer is B *[see VI.B.7].*
Aluminum acetate and aluminum subacetate solutions are astringents that are used as antiperspirants and as wet dressings for contact dermatitis. Strong iodine solution and benzalkonium chloride are topical antibacterial solutions. Acetic acid is added to products as an acidifier. Aromatic ammonia spirit is a respiratory stimulant.

10. The answer is A *[see IV.B.1.a].*
A suspension is a two-phase system that consists of a finely powdered solid dispersed in a liquid vehicle. The particle size of the suspended solid should be as small as possible to minimize sedimentation, but it is usually > 0.5 μm.

11. The answer is C *[see VI.E.3.a].*
Levigation is the process of blending and grinding a substance to separate the particles, reduce their size, and form a paste. Levigation is performed by adding a small amount of suitable levigating agent (e.g., glycerin) to the solid and blending the mixture with a mortar and pestle.

12. The answer is A *[see VI.D.3].*
Acacia, or gum arabic, is the exudate obtained from the stems and branches of various species of *Acacia,* a woody plant native to Africa. Acacia is a natural emulsifying agent that provides a stable emulsion of low viscosity. Emulsions are droplets of one or more immiscible liquids dispersed in another liquid. Emulsions are inherently unstable: the droplets tend to coalesce into larger and larger drops. The purpose of an emulsifying agent is to keep the droplets dispersed and prevent them from coalescing. Polysorbate 20, polysorbate 80, and sorbitan monopalmitate are also emulsifiers, but are synthetic, not natural, substances.

13. The answer is D *[see VI.E.2].*
Ointments are typically used as emollients to soften the skin, as protective barriers, or as vehicles for medication. A variety of ointment bases are available. Vanishing cream, an emulsion type of ointment base, is an oil-in-water emulsion that contains a high percentage of water. Stearic acid is used to create a thin film on the skin when the water evaporates.

14. The answer is B *[see VI.F.2.a].*
By convention, a rectal suppository for an adult weighs approximately 2 g. Suppositories for infants and children are smaller. Vaginal suppositories typically weigh approximately 5 g. Rectal suppositories are usually shaped like an elongated bullet (cylindrical and tapered at one end). Vaginal suppositories are usually ovoid.

15. The answer is A *[see VI.F.4.c].*
In the fusion method of making suppositories, molds made of aluminum, brass, or nickel–copper alloys are used. Finely powdered drug mixed with melted cocoa butter is poured into a mold that is lubricated very lightly with mineral oil.

16. The answer is B *[see VI.G; Table 3-8].*
The *USP* defines a very fine chemical powder as one that completely passes through a standard #120 sieve, which has 125-μm openings. The *USP* classification for powdered vegetable and animal drugs differs from that for powdered chemicals. To be classified as very fine, powdered vegetable and animal drugs must pass completely through a #80 sieve, which has 180-μm openings.

17. The answer is C *[see VI.G.1.c.(3.(b)].*
Pulverization by intervention is the milling technique that is used for drug substances that are gummy and tend to reagglomerate or resist grinding (e.g., camphor, iodine). In this sense, intervention is the addition of a small amount of material that aids milling and can be removed easily after pulverization is complete. For example, camphor can be reduced readily if a small amount of volatile solvent (e.g., alcohol) is added. The solvent is then allowed to evaporate.

18. The answer is D *[see VI.G.2.c].*
The pharmacist uses geometric dilution to mix potent substances with a large amount of diluent. The potent drug and an equal amount of diluent are first mixed in a mortar by trituration. A volume of diluent equal to the mixture in the mortar is added, and the mix is again triturated. The procedure is repeated, and each time, diluent equal in volume to the mixture then in the mortar is added, until all of the diluent is incorporated.

19. The answer is A *[see VI.G.3.b.(4)].*
Hygroscopic and volatile drugs are best protected by waxed paper, which is waterproof. The packet may be double-wrapped with a bond paper to improve the appearance of the completed powder.

20. The answer is A *[see VI.H.2.c.(1)].*
Hard capsules are numbered from 000 (largest) to 5 (smallest). Their approximate capacity ranges from 600 to 30 mg; however, the capacity of the capsule depends on the density of the contents.

21. The answer is A *[see VI.H.3.a–b].*
The shells of soft gelatin capsules are plasticized by the addition of a polyhydric alcohol (polyol), such as glycerin or sorbitol. An antifungal preservative can also be added. Both hard and soft gelatin capsules can be filled with a powder or another dry substance. Soft gelatin capsules are also useful dosage forms for fluids or semisolids.

22. The answer is C *[see VI.H.4.a].*
A content uniformity test is a test of potency. To ensure that each tablet or capsule contains the intended amount of drug substance, the *USP* provides two tests: weight variation and content uniformity. The content uniformity test can be used for any dosage unit, but is required for coated tablets, for tablets in which the active ingredient makes up < 50% of the tablet, for suspensions in single-unit containers or in soft capsules, and for many solids that contain added substances. The weight variation test can be used for liquid-filled soft capsules, for any dosage form unit that contains at least 50 mg of a single drug if the drug makes up at least 50% of the bulk, for solids that do not contain added substances, and for freeze-dried solutions.

23. The answer is A *[see V.A and V.B].*
The reaction velocity, or degradation rate, of a pharmaceutical product is affected by several factors, including temperature, solvents, and light. The degradation rate increases two to three times with each 10° increase in temperature. The effect of temperature on reaction rate is given by the Arrhenius equation:

$$k = Ae^{-Ea/RT}$$

where k is the reaction rate constant, A is the frequency factor, Ea is the energy of activation, R is the gas constant, and T is the absolute temperature.

24. The answer is D *[see V.B.2.a].*
In zero-order degradation, the concentration of a drug decreases over time. However, the change of concentration with respect to time is unchanged. In the equation:

$$-\frac{dC}{dt} = k$$

the fact that dC/dt is negative signifies that the concentration is decreasing. However, the velocity of the concentration change is constant.

25. The answer is B *[see V.B.2.b.(2)].*
The half-life ($t_{1/2}$) is the time required for the concentration of a drug to decrease by one half. For a first-order degradation:

$$t_{1/2} = \frac{0.693}{k}$$

Because both k and 0.693 are constants, $t_{1/2}$ is a constant.

26. The answer is D *[see VI.F.3].*
A satisfactory suppository base should remain firm at room temperature. Preferably, it should not melt < 30°C to avoid premature softening during storage and insertion. It should also be inert, nonsensitizing, nonirritating, and compatible with a variety of drugs. Moreover, it should melt just below body temperature and should dissolve or disintegrate rapidly in the fluid of the body cavity into which it is inserted.

27. The answer is E *[see VI.F.3.c.(1)].*
Cocoa butter is a fat that is obtained from the seed of *Theobroma cacao*. Chemically, it is a mixture of stearin, palmitin, and other glycerides that are insoluble in water and freely soluble in ether and chloroform. Depending on the fusion temperature, cocoa butter can crystallize into any one of four crystal forms. Cocoa butter is a good base for rectal suppositories, although it is less than ideal for vaginal or urethral suppositories.

28. The answer is C *[see VI.I.5].*
To satisfy the *USP* standards, tablets are required to pass one of two tests. A weight variation test is used if the active ingredient makes up the bulk of the tablet. A content uniformity test is used if the tablet is coated or if the active ingredient makes up < 50% of the bulk of the tablet. Many tablets for oral administration are required to meet a disintegration test. Disintegration times are specified in the individual monographs. A dissolution test may be required instead if the active component of the tablet has limited water solubility. Hardness and friability would affect the disintegration and dissolution rates, but hardness and friability tests are in-house quality control tests, not official *USP* tests.

29. The answer is D (II, III) *[see VI.A.1].*
Water for injection *USP* is water that has been purified by distillation or by reverse osmosis. This water is used to prepare parenteral solutions that are subject to final sterilization. For parenteral solutions that are prepared aseptically and not subsequently sterilized, sterile water for injection *USP* is used. Sterile water for injection *USP* is water for injection *USP* that has been sterilized and suitably packaged. This water meets the *USP* requirements for sterility. Bacteriostatic water for injection *USP* is sterile water for injection *USP* that contains one or more antimicrobial agents. It can be used in parenteral solutions if the antimicrobial additives are compatible with the other ingredients in the solution, but it cannot be used in newborns. Purified water *USP* is not used in parenteral preparations.

30. The answer is E (I, II, III) *[see IV.B.2].*
An ideal suspension would have particles of uniform size, minimal sedimentation, and no interaction between particles. Although these ideal criteria are rarely met, they can be approximated by keeping the particle size as small as possible, the densities of the solid and the dispersion medium as similar as possible, and the dispersion medium as viscous as possible.

31. The answer is D (II, III) *[see IV.B.2].*
As Stokes's law indicates, the sedimentation rate of a suspension is slowed by reducing its density, reducing the size of the suspended particles, or increasing its viscosity by incorporating a thickening agent. Sodium benzoate is an antifungal agent and would not reduce the sedimentation rate of a suspension.

32. The answer is C (I, II) *[see VI.C.3].*
Acacia and methylcellulose are common suspending agents. Acacia is a natural product, and methylcellulose is a synthetic polymer. By increasing the viscosity of the liquid, these agents enable particles to remain suspended for a longer period.

33. The answer is E (I, II, III) *[see VI.D.3].*
Emulsifying agents provide a mechanical barrier to coalescence. They also reduce the natural tendency of the droplets in the internal phase (oil or water) of the emulsion to coalesce. Three mechanisms appear to be involved. Some emulsifiers promote stability by forming strong, pliable interfacial films around the droplets. Emulsifying agents also reduce interfacial tension. Finally, ions (from the emulsifier) in the interfacial film can lead to charge repulsion that causes droplets to repel one another, thereby preventing coalescence.

34. The answer is B (III) *[see VI.D.3].*
All of the substances listed are emulsifying agents, but only sorbitan esters are nonionic synthetic agents. Tragacanth, like acacia, is a natural emulsifying agent. Sodium lauryl sulfate is an anionic surfactant. Sorbitan esters (known colloquially as Spans because of their trade names) are hydrophobic and form water-in-oil emulsions. The polysorbates (known colloquially as Tweens) are also nonionic, synthetic sorbitan derivatives. However, they are hydrophilic and therefore form oil-in-water emulsions. Sodium lauryl sulfate, as an alkali soap, is also hydrophilic and thus forms oil-in-water emulsions.

35. The answer is C (I, II) *[see VI.F.1–2].*
Rectal suppositories are useful for delivering systemic medication under certain circumstances. Absorption of a drug from a rectal suppository involves release of the drug from the suppository vehicle, diffusion through the rectal mucosa, and transport to the circulation through the rectal veins. The rectal veins bypass the liver, so this route avoids rapid hepatic degradation of certain drugs (first-pass effect). The rectal route is also useful when a drug cannot be given orally (e.g., because of vomiting). However, the extent of drug release and absorption is variable. It depends on the properties of the drug, the suppository base, and the environment in the rectum.

36. The answer is E (I, II, III) *[see VI.G.1.c].*
Milling is the process of mechanically reducing the particle size of solids before they are formulated into a final product. To work effectively, a lubricant must coat the surface of the granulation or powder. Hence fine particle size is essential. Decreasing the particle size increases the surface area and can enhance the dissolution rate. Thermolabile drugs may undergo degradation because of the buildup of heat during milling.

37. The answer is D (II, III) *[see VI.G.2.a.(2)].*
Some solid substances (e.g., aspirin, phenylsalicylate, phenacetin, thymol, camphor) liquefy or form eutectic mixtures when in close, prolonged contact with one another. These substances are best insulated by the addition of light magnesium oxide or magnesium carbonate. Other inert diluents that can be used are kaolin, starch, and bentonite.

38. The answer is B (III) *[see VI.G.2.b].*
When powders are mixed, if comminution is especially important, a porcelain or ceramic mortar that has a rough inner surface is preferred over the smooth working surface of a glass mortar. Because a glass mortar cleans more easily after use, it is preferred for chemicals that may stain a porcelain or ceramic mortar as well as for simple mixing of substances that do not require comminution.

39. The answer is A (I) *[see VI.G.3.a–b].*
Powders for oral use can be dispensed by the pharmacist in bulk form or divided into premeasured doses (divided powders). Divided powders are traditionally dispensed in folded paper packets (chartulae) made of parchment, bond paper, glassine, or waxed paper. However, individual doses can be packaged in metal foil or small plastic bags if the powder needs greater protection from humidity or evaporation.

40. The answer is C (I, II) *[see VI.I.2.b].*
Tablets for oral ingestion usually contain excipients that are added to the formulation for their special functions. Binders and adhesives are added to promote granulation or compaction. Diluents are fillers that are added to make up the required tablet bulk. They can also aid in the manufacturing process. Disintegrants aid in tablet disintegration in gastrointestinal fluids. Lubricants, antiadherents, and glidants aid in reducing friction or adhesion between particles or between tablet and die. For example, lubricants are used in the manufacture of tablets to reduce friction when the tablet is ejected from the die cavity. Lubricants are usually hydrophobic substances that can affect the dissolution rate of the active ingredient.

41. The answer is E (I, II, III) *[see VI.2.b.(3)].*
Disintegrants are added to tablet formulations to facilitate disintegration in gastrointestinal fluids. Disintegration of the tablet in the body is critical to its dissolution and subsequent absorption and bioavailability. The binder and the compression force used during tablet manufacturing affect the hardness of the tablet as well as tablet disintegration and drug dissolution.

42. The answer is B (III) *[see VI.I.3.a.(4)].*
An enteric-coated tablet has a coating that remains intact in the stomach, but dissolves in the intestines to yield the tablet ingredients there. Enteric coatings include various fats, fatty acids, waxes, and shellacs. Cellulose acetate phthalate remains intact in the stomach because it dissolves only when the pH > 6. Other enteric-coating materials include povidone (polyvinylpyrrolidone), polyvinyl acetate phthalate, and hydroxypropyl methylcellulose phthalate.

43. The answer is A *[see VI.I.4].*

44. The answer is D *[see VI.I.4].*

45. The answer is B *[see VI.I.4].*

46. The answer is A *[see VI.I.4].*
Sticking is adhesion of tablet material to a die wall. It may be caused by excessive moisture or by the use of ingredients that have low melting temperatures. Mottling is uneven color distribution. It is most often caused by poor mixing of the tablet granulation but may also occur when a degraded drug produces a colored metabolite. Capping is separation of the top or bottom crown of a tablet from the main body. Capping implies that compressed powder is not cohesive. Reasons for capping include excessive force of compression, use of insufficient binder, worn tablet tooling equipment, and entrapment of air during processing. Picking is adherence of tablet surface material to a punch. It can be caused by a granulation that is too damp, by a scratched punch, by static charges on the powder, and particularly by the use of a punch tip that is engraved or embossed.

47. The answer is A *[see VI.G.1.c; VI.G.2].*

48. The answer is D *[see VI.G.1.c; VI.G.2].*

49. The answer is C *[see VI.G.1.c; VI.G.2].*
Comminution is the process of reducing the particle size of a powder to increase its fineness. Several comminution techniques are suitable for small-scale use in a pharmacy. Trituration is used both to comminute and to mix dry powders. If comminution is desired, the substance is rubbed in a mortar that has a rough inner surface. Pulverization by intervention is often used for substances that tend to agglomerate or resist grinding. A small amount of easily removed (e.g., volatile) solvent is added. After the substance is pulverized, the solvent is allowed to evaporate or is otherwise removed. Levigation is often used to prepare pastes or ointments. The powder is reduced by adding a suitable nonsolvent (levigating agent) to form a paste and then either rubbing the paste in a mortar with a pestle or rubbing it on an ointment slab with a spatula. Spatulation and tumbling are techniques that are used to mix or blend powders, not to reduce them. Spatulation is blending small amounts of powders by stirring them with a spatula on a sheet of paper or a pill tile. Tumbling is blending large amounts of powder in a large rotating container.

50. The answer is B *[see VI.K.3.e].*

51. The answer is E *[see VI.K.3.a].*

52. The answer is C *[see VI.K.3.f].*

53. The answer is D *[see VI.K.3.d].*
Controlled-release dosage forms are designed to release a drug slowly for prolonged action in the body. A variety of pharmaceutical mechanisms are used to provide the controlled release. Ion-exchange resins may be complexed to drugs by passing a cationic drug solution through a column that contains the resin. The drug is complexed to the resin by replacement of hydrogen atoms. Release of drug from the complex depends on the ionic environment within the gastrointestinal tract and on the properties of the resin. Coated beads (e.g., Thorazine Spansule capsules) or granules produce blood levels similar to those obtained with multiple dosing. The various coating thicknesses produce a sustained-release effect.

Matrix devices may use insoluble plastics, hydrophilic polymers, or fatty compounds. These components are mixed with the drug and compressed into a tablet. The primary dose, or the portion of the drug to be released immediately, is placed on the tablet as a layer or coat. The remainder of the dose is released slowly from the matrix. Relatively insoluble tannate-amine complexes provide for a prolonged gastrointestinal absorption phase and sustained systemic concentrations of the weak bases. Osmotic systems employ osmotic pressure to control the release of the active ingredient from the formulation. Osmotic tablet formulations provide a semipermeable membrane as a coating that surrounds the osmotically active core. The coating allows water to diffuse into the core but does not allow drug to diffuse out. As water flows into the tablet, the drug dissolves. The laser-drilled hole in the coating allows the drug solution within the tablet to flow to the outside at a rate that is equivalent to the rate of water flow into the tablet. The osmotic pressure gradient and a zero-order drug-release rate will be maintained as long as excess osmotically active solute (e.g., electrolyte) remains in the tablet core.

4
Biopharmaceutics and Drug Delivery Systems
Lawrence H. Block

I. INTRODUCTION

A. Biopharmaceutics is the study of the relation of the physical and chemical properties of a drug to its bioavailability, pharmacokinetics, and pharmacodynamic and toxicologic effects.

    1. A **drug product** is the finished dosage form (e.g., tablet, capsule, solution) that contains the active drug ingredient in association with nondrug (usually inactive) ingredients (**excipients**) that make up the **vehicle,** or **formulation matrix.**

    2. The phrase *drug delivery system* is often used interchangeably with the terms *drug product* or *dosage form.* However, a **drug delivery system** is a more comprehensive concept, which includes the drug formulation and the dynamic interactions among the drug, its formulation matrix, its container, and the patient.

    3. Bioavailability is a measurement of the rate and extent (amount) of systemic absorption of the therapeutically active drug.

B. Pharmacokinetics is the study of the time course of drug movement in the body during absorption, distribution, and elimination (excretion and biotransformation).

C. Pharmacodynamics is the study of the relation of the drug concentration or amount at the site of action (receptor) and its pharmacologic response as a function of time.

II. DRUG TRANSPORT AND ABSORPTION

A. Transport of drug molecules *across* cell membranes. Drug absorption requires the drug to be transported across various cell membranes. Drug molecules may enter the bloodstream and be transported to the tissues and organs of the body. Drug molecules may cross additional membranes to enter cells. Drug molecules may also cross an intracellular membrane, such as the nuclear membrane or endoplasmic reticulum, to reach the site of action. Figure 4-1 demonstrates some of the key transport processes involved in drug absorption.

Figure 4-1. The key drug transport processes in intestinal epithelial cells. *1,* Transcellular passive (diffusion and partitioning); *2,* paracellular transport (diffusion and convection); *3,* carrier-mediated transport; *4,* P-glycoprotein-mediated efflux. [Modified from Brayden DJ, Pharm News 4(1);1997:11–15.]

1. **General principles**
   a. A **cell membrane** is a semipermeable structure composed primarily of lipids and proteins.
   b. Drugs may be transported by **passive diffusion, partitioning, carrier-mediated transport, paracellular transport,** or **vesicular transport.**
   c. Usually, **proteins, drugs bound to proteins,** and **macromolecules** do not easily cross cell membranes.
   d. **Nonpolar lipid-soluble drugs** traverse cell membranes more easily than do **ionic** or **polar water-soluble drugs.**
   e. **Low molecular weight drugs** diffuse across a cell membrane more easily than do **high molecular weight drugs.**

2. **Passive diffusion and partitioning**
   a. *Within* the cytoplasm or in interstitial fluid, most drugs undergo transport by simple diffusion.
   b. **Fick's law of diffusion. Simple passive diffusion** involves the transfer of drugs from an area of high concentration (C_1) to an area of lower concentration (C_2) according to Fick's law of diffusion:

$$\frac{dQ}{dt} = \frac{DA}{h}(C_1 - C_2)$$

   where dQ/dt is the rate of drug diffusion, D is the diffusion coefficient for the drug, A is the surface area of the plane across which transfer occurs, h is the thickness of the region through which diffusion occurs, and $(C_1 - C_2)$ is the difference between the drug concentration in area 1 and area 2, respectively.

   c. Passive drug transport *across* cell membranes involves the successive **partitioning** of a solute between aqueous and lipid phases as well as **diffusion** within the respective phases. Modifying Fick's law of diffusion to accommodate the partitioning of drug gives the following:

$$\frac{dQ}{dt} = \frac{DAK}{h}(C_1 - C_2)$$

   The rate of drug diffusion, dQ/dt, now reflects its direct dependence on K, the oil to water partition coefficient of the drug, as well as on A and $(C_1 - C_2)$.

   d. **Ionization of a weak electrolyte** is affected by the pH of the medium in which the drug is dissolved as well as by the pK_a of the drug. The nonionized species is more lipid soluble than the ionized species, and it partitions more readily across cell membranes.

3. **Carrier-mediated transport**
   a. **Active transport** of the drug across a membrane is a carrier-mediated process that has the following characteristics.
      (1) The drug moves against a concentration gradient.
      (2) The process requires energy.
      (3) The carrier may be selective for certain types of drugs that resemble natural substrates or metabolites that are normally actively transported.
      (4) The carrier system may be saturated at a high drug concentration.
      (5) The process may be competitive (i.e., drugs with similar structures may compete for the same carrier).
   b. **Facilitated diffusion** is also a carrier-mediated transport system. However, facilitated diffusion occurs with (i.e., in the direction of) a concentration gradient and does not require energy.

4. **Paracellular transport.** Drug transport across tight (narrow) junctions between cells or trans-endothelial channels of cells is known as **paracellular transport.** It involves both diffusion and the **convective** (bulk) flow of water and accompanying water-soluble drug molecules through the paracellular channels.

5. **Vesicular transport** is the process of engulfing particles or dissolved materials by a cell. Vesicular transport is the only transport mechanism that does not require a drug to be in an aqueous solution to be absorbed. **Pinocytosis** and **phagocytosis** are forms of vesicular transport.
   a. **Pinocytosis** is the engulfment of small solute or fluid volumes.

    b. Phagocytosis is the engulfment of larger particles, or macromolecules, generally by macrophages.

    c. Endocytosis and **exocytosis** are the movement of macromolecules into and out of the cell, respectively.

6. Other transport mechanisms: transporter proteins. Various **transporter proteins** (e.g., **P-glycoprotein**) are embedded in the lipid bilayer of cell membranes in tandem in α-helical transmembrane regions or domains. These proteins are adenosine triphosphate- (ATP; energy) dependent "pumps," which can facilitate the efflux of drug molecules from the cell. Because these transmembrane efflux pumps are often found in conjunction with metabolizing enzymes such as **cytochrome P450 3A4,** their net effect is to substantially reduce intracellular drug concentrations. Thus they determine, to a large extent, the pharmacokinetic disposition and circulating plasma concentrations of drugs (e.g., cyclosporin, nifedipine, digoxin) that are substrates for these proteins.

B. Routes of drug administration

1. Parenteral administration

    a. Intravenous bolus injection. The drug is injected directly into the bloodstream, distributes throughout the body, and acts rapidly. Any side effects, including an intense pharmacologic response, anaphylaxis, or overt toxicity, also occur rapidly.

    b. Intra-arterial injection. The drug is injected into a specific artery to achieve a high drug concentration in a specific tissue before drug distribution occurs throughout the body. Intra-arterial injection is used for diagnostic agents and occasionally for chemotherapy.

    c. Intravenous infusion. The drug is given intravenously at a constant input rate. Constant-rate intravenous infusion maintains a relatively constant plasma drug concentration once the infusion rate is approximately equal to the drug's elimination rate from the body (i.e., once steady state is reached).

    d. Intramuscular injection. The drug is injected deep into a skeletal muscle. The rate of absorption depends on the vascularity of the muscle site, the lipid solubility of the drug, and the formulation matrix.

    e. Subcutaneous injection. The drug is injected beneath the skin. Because the subcutaneous region is less vascular than muscle tissues, drug absorption is less rapid. The factors that affect absorption from intramuscular depots also affect subcutaneous absorption.

    f. Miscellaneous parenteral routes

        (1) Intra-articular injection. The drug is injected into a joint.

        (2) Intradermal (intracutaneous) injection. The drug is injected into the dermis (i.e., the vascular region of the skin below the epidermis).

        (3) Intrathecal injection. The drug is injected into the spinal fluid.

2. Enteral administration

    a. Buccal and sublingual administration. A tablet or lozenge is placed under the tongue (**sublingual**) or in contact with the mucosal (**buccal**) surface of the cheek. This type of administration allows a nonpolar, lipid-soluble drug to be absorbed across the epithelial lining of the mouth. After buccal or sublingual administration, the drug is absorbed directly into the systemic circulation, bypassing the liver and any first-pass effects.

    b. Peroral (oral) drug administration. The drug is administered orally, is swallowed, and undergoes absorption from the gastrointestinal tract through the mesenteric circulation to the hepatic portal vein into the liver and then to the systemic circulation. The peroral route is the most common route of administration.

        (1) The peroral route is the most convenient and the safest route.

        (2) Disadvantages of this route include the following.

            (a) The drug may not be absorbed from the gastrointestinal tract consistently or completely.

            (b) The drug may be digested by gastrointestinal enzymes or decomposed by the acid pH of the stomach.

            (c) The drug may irritate mucosal epithelial cells or complex with the contents of the gastrointestinal tract.

            (d) Some drugs may be incompletely absorbed because of first-pass effects or presystemic elimination (e.g., the drug is metabolized by the liver before systemic absorption occurs).

            (e) The absorption rate may be erratic because of delayed gastric emptying or changes in intestinal motility.

    (3) Most drugs are **xenobiotics** or **exogenous** molecules and, consequently, are absorbed from the gastrointestinal tract by **passive diffusion** and **partitioning. Carrier-mediated transport, paracellular transport,** and **vesicular transport** play smaller, but critical, roles, particularly for endogenous molecules.

    (4) Drug molecules are absorbed throughout the gastrointestinal tract; but the **duodenal region,** which has a large surface area because of the villi and microvilli, is the primary absorption site. The large blood supply provided by the mesenteric vessels allows the drug to be absorbed more efficiently (see II.A.2).

    (5) **Altered gastric emptying** affects arrival of the drug in the duodenum for systemic absorption. **Gastric emptying time** is affected by food content, emotional state, and drugs that alter gastrointestinal tract motility (e.g., anticholinergics, narcotic analgesics, prokinetic agents).

    (6) Normal intestinal motility from **peristalsis** brings the drug in contact with the intestinal epithelial cells. A sufficient period of contact (residence time) is needed to permit drug absorption across the cell membranes from the mucosal to the serosal surface.

    (7) Some drugs, such as **cimetidine** and **acetaminophen,** when given in an immediate-release peroral dosage form to fasted subjects produce a systemic drug concentration time with two peaks. This **double-peak phenomenon** is attributed to variability in stomach emptying, variable intestinal motility, and enterohepatic cycling.

  c. Rectal administration. The drug in solution (enema) or suppository form is placed in the rectum. Drug diffusion from the solution or release from the suppository leads to absorption across the mucosal surface of the rectum. Drug absorbed in the lower two thirds of the rectum enters the systemic circulation directly, bypassing the liver and any first-pass effects.

3. Respiratory tract administration

  a. Intranasal administration. The drug contained in a solution or suspension is administered to the nasal mucosa, either as a spray or as drops. The medication may be used for local (e.g., nasal decongestants, intranasal steroids) or systemic effects.

  b. Pulmonary inhalation. The drug, as liquid or solid particles, is inhaled perorally (with a nebulizer or a metered-dose aerosol) into the pulmonary tree. In general, **particles > 60 μm** are primarily deposited in the **trachea. Particles > 20 μm** do not reach the bronchioles, and **particles < 0.6 μm** are not deposited and are **exhaled.** Particles between **2 and 6 μm** can reach the **alveolar ducts,** although only particles of **1–2 μm are retained in the alveoli.**

4. Transdermal and topical administration

  a. Transdermal (percutaneous) drug absorption is the placement of the drug (in a lotion, ointment, cream, paste, or patch) on the skin surface for systemic absorption. An occlusive dressing or film improves systemic drug absorption from the skin. Small lipid-soluble molecules, such as nitroglycerin, nicotine, scopolamine, clonidine, fentanyl, and steroids (e.g., 17-β-estradiol, testosterone), are readily absorbed from the skin.

  b. Drugs (e.g., antibacterials, local anesthetic agents) are applied **topically** to the skin for a local effect.

5. Miscellaneous routes of drug administration include **ophthalmic, otic, urethral,** and **vaginal** administration. These routes of administration are generally used for local therapeutic activity. However, some systemic drug absorption may occur.

C. Local drug activity versus **systemic drug absorption.** The route of administration, absorption site, and bioavailability of the drug from the dosage form are major factors in the design of a drug product.

1. Drugs intended for **local activity,** such as topical antibiotics, anti-infectives, antifungal agents, and local anesthetics are formulated in dosage forms that minimize systemic absorption. The concentration of these drugs at the application site affects their activity.

2. When **systemic absorption** is desired, the bioavailability of the drug from the dosage form at the absorption site must be considered (e.g., a drug given intravenously is 100% bioavailable because all of the drug is placed directly into the systemic circulation). The amount, or dose, of drug in the dosage form is based on the extent of drug absorption and the desired systemic drug concentration. The type of dosage form (e.g., immediate release, controlled release) affects the rate of drug absorption.

III. BIOPHARMACEUTIC PRINCIPLES

A. Physicochemical properties

1. **Drug dissolution.** For most drugs with limited water solubility, the rate at which the solid drug enters into solution (i.e., the rate of dissolution) is often the rate-limiting step in bioavailability. The **Noyes-Whitney** equation describes the diffusion-controlled rate of drug dissolution (dm/dt; i.e., the change in the amount of drug in solution with respect to time):

$$\frac{dm}{dt} = \frac{DA}{\delta}(C_s - C_b)$$

where D is the diffusion coefficient of the solute, A is the surface area of the solid undergoing dissolution, δ is the thickness of the diffusion layer, C_s is the concentration of the solvate at saturation, and C_b is the concentration of the drug in the bulk solution phase at time t.

2. **Drug solubility** in a saturated solution (see Chapter 3, IV) is a static (equilibrium) property. The dissolution rate of a drug is a dynamic property related to the rate of absorption.

3. **Particle size** and **surface area** are inversely related. As solid drug particle size decreases, particle surface area increases.
   a. As described by the Noyes-Whitney equation, the dissolution rate is directly proportional to the surface area. An increase in surface area allows for more contact between the solid drug particles and the solvent, resulting in a faster dissolution rate (see III.A.1).
   b. With certain **hydrophobic drugs,** excessive particle size reduction does not always increase the dissolution rate. Small particles tend to reaggregate into larger particles to reduce the high surface free energy produced by particle size reduction.
   c. To prevent the formation of aggregates, small drug particles are molecularly dispersed in polyethylene glycol (PEG), polyvinylpyrrolidone (PVP; povidone), dextrose, or other agents. For example, a molecular dispersion of griseofulvin in a water-soluble carrier such as PEG 4000 (e.g., Gris–PEG) enhances its dissolution and bioavailability.

4. **Partition coefficient and extent of ionization**
   a. The **partition coefficient** of a drug is the ratio of the solubility of the drug, at equilibrium, in a nonaqueous solvent (e.g., *n*-octanol) to that in an aqueous solvent (e.g., water; pH 7.4 buffer solution). Hydrophilic drugs with higher water solubility have a faster dissolution rate than do hydrophobic or lipophilic drugs, which have poor water solubility.
   b. **Extent of ionization.** Drugs that are weak electrolytes (acids or bases) exist in both an ionized form and a nonionized form in solution. The extent of ionization depends on the pK_a of the weak electrolyte and the pH of the solution. The ionized form is more polar, and therefore more water soluble, than the nonionized form. The **Henderson-Hasselbalch equation** describes the relation between the ionized and the nonionized forms of a drug as a function of pH and pK_a. When the pH of the medium equals the pK_a of the drug, 50% of the drug in solution is nonionized and 50% is ionized, as can be shown from the following equations:
      (1) For weak acids:

$$pH = pK_a + \log\left(\frac{salt}{nonionized\ acid}\right)$$

   (2) For weak bases:

$$pH = pK_a + \log\left(\frac{nonionized\ base}{salt}\right)$$

5. **Salt formation**
   a. The choice of salt form for a drug depends on the desired physical, chemical, or pharmacologic properties. Certain salts are designed to provide slower dissolution, slower bioavailability, and longer duration of action. Other salts are selected for greater stability, less local irritation at the absorption site, or less systemic toxicity.
      (1) Some soluble salt forms are less stable than the nonionized form. For example, sodium aspirin is less stable than aspirin in the acid form.
      (2) A solid dosage form containing buffering agents may be formulated with the free acid form of the drug (e.g., buffered aspirin).

       (a) The buffering agent forms an alkaline medium in the gastrointestinal tract, and the drug dissolves in situ.

       (b) The dissolved salt form of the drug diffuses into the bulk fluid of the gastrointestinal tract, forms a fine precipitate that redissolves rapidly, and becomes available for absorption.

   b. **Effervescent granules** or **tablets** containing the acid drug in addition to sodium bicarbonate, tartaric acid, citric acid, or other ingredients are added to water just before oral administration. The excess sodium bicarbonate forms an alkaline solution in which the drug dissolves. Carbon dioxide is also formed by the decomposition of carbonic acid.

   c. For weakly acidic drugs, potassium and sodium salts are more soluble than divalent cation salts (e.g., calcium, magnesium) or trivalent cation salts (e.g., aluminum).

   d. For weak bases, common water-soluble salts include the hydrochloride, sulfate, citrate, and gluconate salts. The estolate, napsylate, and stearate salts are less water soluble.

6. **Polymorphism** is the ability of a drug to exist in more than one crystalline form.

   a. Different polymorphs have different physical properties, including melting point and dissolution rate.

   b. **Amorphous,** or **noncrystalline, forms** of a drug have faster dissolution rates than do crystalline forms.

7. **Chirality** is the ability of a drug to exist as **optically active stereoisomers** or **enantiomers.** Individual enantiomers may not have the same pharmacokinetic and pharmacodynamic activity. Because most chiral drugs are used as racemic mixtures, the results of studies with such mixtures may be misleading because the drug is assumed to behave as a single entity. For example, ibuprofen exists as the *R*- and *S*-enantiomers; only the *S*-enantiomer is pharmacologically active. When the racemic mixture of ibuprofen is taken orally, the *R*-enantiomer undergoes presystemic inversion in the gut to the *S*-enantiomer. Because the rate and extent of inversion are site specific and formulation dependent, ibuprofen activity may vary considerably.

8. **Hydrates.** Drugs may exist in a **hydrated, or solvated, form** or as an **anhydrous molecule.** Dissolution rates differ for hydrated and anhydrous forms. For example, the anhydrous form of ampicillin dissolves faster and is more rapidly absorbed than the hydrated form.

9. **Complex formation.** A **complex** is a species formed by the reversible or irreversible association of two or more interacting molecules or ions. **Chelates** are complexes that typically involve a ring-like structure formed by the interaction between a partial ring of atoms and a metal. Many biologically important molecules (e.g., hemoglobin, insulin, cyanocobalamin) are chelates. Drugs such as tetracycline form chelates with divalent (e.g., Ca^{++}, Mg^{++}) and trivalent (e.g., Al^{+++}, Bi^{+++}) metal ions. Many drugs adsorb strongly on charcoal or clay (e.g., kaolin, bentonite) particles by forming complexes. Drug complexes with proteins, such as albumin or α_1-acid glycoprotein, often occur.

   a. Complex formation usually alters the physical and chemical characteristics of the drug. For example:

      (1) The chelate of tetracycline with calcium is less water soluble and is poorly absorbed.

      (2) Theophylline complexed with ethylenediamine to form aminophylline is more water soluble and is used for parenteral and rectal administration.

      (3) Cyclodextrins are used to form complexes with many drugs to increase their water solubility.

   b. Large drug complexes, such as drug–protein complexes, do not cross cell membranes easily. These complexes must dissociate to free the drug for absorption at the absorption site or to permit transport across cell membranes or glomerular filtration before the drug is excreted into the urine.

B. Drug product and delivery system formulation

   1. General considerations

      a. Design of the appropriate dosage form or **delivery system** depends on the

         (1) Physical and chemical properties of the drug

         (2) Dose of the drug

         (3) Route of administration

         (4) Type of drug delivery system desired

         (5) Desired therapeutic effect

         (6) Physiologic release of the drug from the delivery system

         (7) Bioavailability of the drug at the absorption site

         (8) Pharmacokinetics and pharmacodynamics of the drug

   b. Bioavailability. The more complicated the formulation of the finished drug product (e.g., controlled-release tablet, enteric-coated tablet, transdermal patch), the greater the potential for a bioavailability problem. For example, the **release** of a drug from a peroral dosage form and its subsequent bioavailability depend on a succession of rate processes (Figure 4-2). These processes may include the following:

     (1) Attrition, disintegration, or **disaggregation** of the drug product

     (2) Dissolution of the drug in an aqueous environment

     (3) Convection and **diffusion** of the drug molecules to the absorbing surface

     (4) Absorption of the drug across cell membranes into the systemic circulation

   c. The **rate-limiting step** in the bioavailability of a drug from a drug product is the slowest step in a series of kinetic processes.

     (1) For most conventional solid drug products (e.g., capsules, tablets), the dissolution rate is the slowest, or rate-limiting, step for bioavailability.

     (2) For a controlled- or sustained-release drug product, the release of the drug from the delivery system is the rate-limiting step.

2. Solutions are homogeneous mixtures of one or more solutes dispersed molecularly in a dissolving medium (solvent).

   a. Compared with other oral and peroral drug formulations, a drug dissolved in an aqueous solution is in the most bioavailable and consistent form. Because the drug is already in

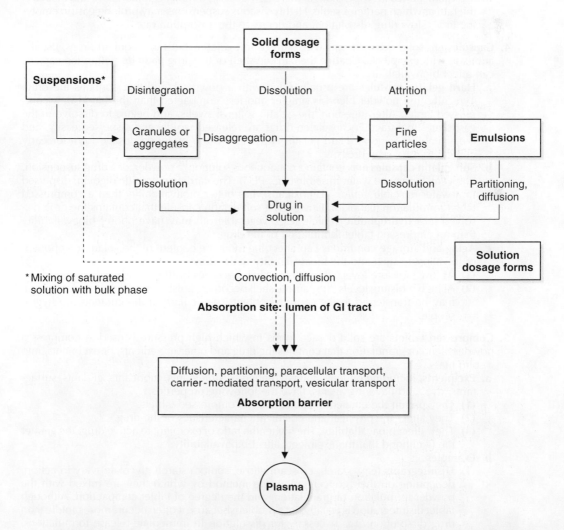

Figure 4-2. The processes involved in drug release from peroral dosage forms. *GI,* gastrointestinal.

solution, no dissolution step is necessary before systemic absorption occurs. Peroral drug solutions are often used as the reference preparation for solid peroral formulations.

b. A drug dissolved in a hydroalcoholic solution (e.g., elixir) also has good bioavailability. Alcohol aids drug solubility. However, when the drug is diluted by gastrointestinal tract fluid and other gut contents (e.g., food), it may form a finely divided precipitate in the lumen of the gastrointestinal tract. Because of the extensive dispersion and large surface area of such finely divided precipitates, redissolution and subsequent absorption occur rapidly.

c. A viscous drug solution (e.g., syrup) may interfere with dilution and mixing with gastrointestinal tract contents. The solution decreases the gastric emptying rate and the rate of transfer of drug solution to the duodenal region, where absorption is most efficient.

3. Suspensions are dispersions of finely divided solid particles of a drug in a liquid medium in which the drug is not readily soluble. The liquid medium of a suspension comprises a saturated solution of the drug in equilibrium with the solid drug.

a. The bioavailability of the drug from suspensions may be similar to that of a solution because the finely divided particles are dispersed and provide a large surface area for rapid dissolution. On the other hand, a slow dissolution rate decreases the absorption rate.

b. Suspending agents are often hydrophilic colloids (e.g., cellulose derivatives, acacia, xanthan gum) added to suspensions to increase viscosity, inhibit agglomeration, and decrease the rate at which particles settle. Highly viscous suspensions may prolong gastric emptying time, slow drug dissolution, and decrease the absorption rate.

4. Capsules are solid dosage forms with hard or soft gelatin shells that contain drugs, usually admixed with excipients. **Coating** the capsule shell or the drug particles within the capsule can affect bioavailability.

a. Hard gelatin capsules are usually filled with a powder blend that contains the drug. Typically, the powder blend is simpler and less compacted than the blend in a compressed tablet. After ingestion, the gelatin softens, swells, and begins to dissolve in the gastrointestinal tract. Encapsulated drugs are released rapidly and dispersed easily, and bioavailability is good. Hard gelatin capsules are the preferred dosage form for early clinical trials of new drugs.

b. Soft gelatin capsules may contain a nonaqueous solution, a powder, or a drug suspension. The vehicle may be water miscible (e.g., PEG). The cardiac glycoside digoxin, dispersed in a water-miscible vehicle (Lanoxicaps), has better bioavailability than a compressed tablet formulation (Lanoxin). However, a soft gelatin capsule that contains the drug dissolved in a **hydrophobic** vehicle (e.g., vegetable oil) may have poorer bioavailability than a compressed tablet formulation of the drug.

c. Aging and **storage conditions** can affect the moisture content of the gelatin component of the capsule shell and the bioavailability of the drug.

(1) At low moisture levels, the capsule shell becomes brittle and is easily ruptured.

(2) At high moisture levels, the capsule shell becomes moist, soft, and distorted. Moisture may be transferred to the capsule contents, particularly if the contents are hygroscopic.

5. Compressed tablets are solid dosage forms in which high pressure is used to compress a powder blend or granulation that contains the drug and other ingredients, or excipients, into a solid mass.

a. Excipients, including diluents (fillers), binders, disintegrants, lubricants, glidants, surfactants, dye, and flavoring agents, have the following properties.

(1) They permit the efficient manufacture of compressed tablets.

(2) They affect the physical and chemical characteristics of the drug.

(3) They affect bioavailability. The higher the ratio of excipient to active drug, the greater the likelihood that the excipients affect bioavailability.

b. Examples

(1) Disintegrants (e.g., starch, croscarmellose, sodium starch glycolate) vary in action, depending on their concentration, the method by which they are mixed with the powder formulation or granulation, and the degree of tablet compaction. Although tablet disintegration is usually not a problem because it often occurs more rapidly than drug dissolution, it is necessary for dissolution in immediate-release formulations. Inability to disintegrate may interfere with bioavailability.

(2) Lubricants are usually hydrophobic, water-insoluble substances such as stearic acid, magnesium stearate, hydrogenated vegetable oil, and talc. They may reduce wetting of the surface of the solid drug particles, slowing the dissolution and bioavailability rates of the drug. Water-soluble lubricants, such as L-leucine, do not interfere with dissolution or bioavailability.

(3) Glidants (e.g., colloidal silicon dioxide) improve the flow properties of a dry powder blend before it is compressed. Rather than posing a potential problem with bioavailability, glidants may reduce tablet-to-tablet variability and improve product efficacy.

(4) Surfactants enhance drug dissolution rates and bioavailability by reducing interfacial tension at the boundary between solid drug and liquid and by improving the wettability (contact) of solid drug particles by the solvent.

c. Coated compressed tablets have a sugar coat, a film coat, or an enteric coat with the following properties:

(1) It protects the drug from moisture, light, and air.

(2) It masks the taste or odor of the drug.

(3) It improves the appearance of the tablet.

(4) It may affect the release rate of the drug.

d. In addition, **enteric coatings** minimize contact between the drug and the gastric region by resisting dissolution or attrition and preventing contact between the underlying drug and the gastric contents or gastric mucosa. Some enteric coatings minimize gastric contact because they are insoluble at acidic pHs. Other coatings resist attrition and remain whole long enough for the tablet to leave the gastric area. By resisting dissolution or attrition, enteric coatings may decrease bioavailability. Enteric coatings are used to

(1) Minimize irritation of the gastric mucosa by the drug

(2) Prevent inactivation or degradation of the drug in the stomach

(3) Delay release of the drug until the tablet reaches the small intestine, where conditions for absorption may be optimal

6. Modified-release dosage forms are drug products that alter the rate or timing of drug release. Because modified-release dosage forms are more complex than conventional immediate-release dosage forms, more stringent quality control and bioavailability tests are required. **Dose dumping,** or the uncontrolled release of a large amount of drug, is a problem.

a. Extended-release dosage forms include **controlled-release, sustained-action,** and **long-acting drug delivery systems.** These delivery systems allow at least a twofold reduction in dosing frequency compared with conventional immediate-release formulations.

(1) The extended, slow release of controlled-release drug products produces a relatively flat, sustained plasma drug concentration that avoids toxicity (from high drug concentrations) or lack of efficacy (from low drug concentrations).

(2) Extended-release dosage forms provide an immediate (initial) release of the drug, followed by a slower sustained release.

b. Delayed-release dosage forms release active drug at a time other than immediately after administration at a desired site in the gastrointestinal tract. For example, an enteric-coated drug product does not allow for dissolution in the acid environment of the stomach but, rather, in the less acidic environment of the small intestine.

7. Transdermal drug delivery systems, or **patches,** are controlled-release devices that contain the drug for systemic absorption after topical application to the skin surface. Transdermal drug delivery systems are available for a number of drugs (nitroglycerin, nicotine, scopolamine, clonidine, fentanyl, 17-β-estradiol, and testosterone). Although the formulation matrices of these delivery systems differ somewhat, they all differ from conventional topical formulations in the following ways:

a. They have an impermeable **occlusive backing film** that prevents insensible water loss from the skin beneath the patch. This film causes increased hydration and skin temperature under the patch and enhanced permeation of the skin by the drug.

b. The formulation matrix of the patch maintains the drug concentration gradient within the device after application so that drug delivery to the interface between the patch and the skin is sustained. As a result, drug partitioning and diffusion into the skin persist, and systemic absorption is maintained throughout the dosing interval.

c. Transdermal drug delivery systems are kept in place on the skin surface by an **adhesive layer,** ensuring drug contact with the skin and continued drug delivery.

8. Targeted (site-specific) drug delivery systems are drug carrier systems that place the drug at or near the receptor site. Examples include macromolecular drug carriers (protein drug carriers), particulate drug delivery systems (e.g., liposomes, nanoparticles), and monoclonal antibodies. With targeted drug delivery, the drug may be delivered to

a. The capillary bed of the active site

b. A special type of cell (e.g., tumor cells) but not to normal cells

c. A specific organ or tissue by complexing with a carrier that recognizes the target

9. **Inserts, implants,** and **devices** are used to control drug delivery for localized or systemic drug effects. The drug is impregnated into a biodegradable or nonbiodegradable material and is released slowly. The inserts, implants, and devices are inserted into a variety of cavities (e.g., vagina, buccal cavity) or tissues (e.g., skin). For example, the leuprolide acetate implant, Viadur, is inserted beneath the skin of the upper arm. It provides palliative treatment of advanced prostate cancer for 1 year.

STUDY QUESTIONS

Directions: Each question, statement, or incomplete statement in this section can be correctly answered or completed by **one** of the suggested answers or phrases. Choose the **best** answer.

1. Which statement best describes bioavailability?

(A) relation between the physical and the chemical properties of a drug and its systemic absorption

(B) measurement of the rate and amount of therapeutically active drug that reaches the systemic circulation

(C) movement of the drug into body tissues over time

(D) dissolution of the drug in the gastrointestinal tract

(E) amount of drug destroyed by the liver before systemic absorption from the gastrointestinal tract occurs

2. The route of drug administration that gives the most rapid onset of the pharmacologic effect is

(A) intramuscular injection.

(B) intravenous injection.

(C) intradermal injection.

(D) peroral administration.

(E) subcutaneous injection.

3. The route of drug administration that provides complete (100%) bioavailability is

(A) intramuscular injection.

(B) intravenous injection.

(C) intradermal injection.

(D) peroral administration.

(E) subcutaneous injection.

4. After peroral administration, drugs generally are absorbed best from the

(A) buccal cavity.

(B) stomach.

(C) duodenum.

(D) ileum.

(E) rectum.

5. The characteristics of an active transport process include all of the following *except* for which one?

(A) Active transport moves drug molecules against a concentration gradient.

(B) Active transport follows Fick's law of diffusion.

(C) Active transport is a carrier-mediated transport system.

(D) Active transport requires energy.

(E) Active transport of drug molecules may be saturated at high drug concentrations.

6. The passage of drug molecules from a region of high drug concentration to a region of low drug concentration is known as

(A) active transport.

(B) bioavailability.

(C) biopharmaceutics.

(D) simple diffusion.

(E) pinocytosis.

7. Which equation describes the rate of drug dissolution from a tablet?

(A) Fick's law

(B) Henderson-Hasselbalch equation

(C) Law of mass action

(D) Michaelis-Menten equation

(E) Noyes-Whitney equation

8. Which condition usually increases the rate of drug dissolution from a tablet?

(A) increase in the particle size of the drug

(B) decrease in the surface area of the drug

(C) use of the free acid or free base form of the drug

(D) use of the ionized, or salt, form of the drug

(E) use of sugar coating around the tablet

9. Dose dumping is a problem in the formulation of

(A) compressed tablets.

(B) modified-release drug products.

(C) hard gelatin capsules.

(D) soft gelatin capsules.

(E) suppositories.

10. The rate-limiting step in the bioavailability of a lipid-soluble drug formulated as an immediate-release compressed tablet is the rate of

(A) disintegration of the tablet and release of the drug.

(B) dissolution of the drug.

(C) transport of the drug molecules across the intestinal mucosal cells.

(D) blood flow to the gastrointestinal tract.

(E) biotransformation, or metabolism, of the drug by the liver before systemic absorption occurs.

11. The extent of ionization of a weak electrolyte drug depends on the

(A) pH of the media and pK_a of the drug.
(B) oil to water partition coefficient of the drug.
(C) particle size and surface area of the drug.
(D) Noyes-Whitney equation for the drug.
(E) polymorphic form of the drug.

12. The rate of drug bioavailability is most rapid when the drug is formulated as a

(A) controlled-release product.
(B) hard gelatin capsule.
(C) compressed tablet.
(D) solution.
(E) suspension.

13. The amount of drug that a transdermal patch (i.e., transdermal drug delivery system) delivers within a 24-hr period depends on the

(A) patch composition, which includes an occlusive backing and an adhesive film in contact with the skin.
(B) affinity of the drug for the formulation matrix relative to its affinity for the stratum corneum.
(C) rate of drug partitioning and/or diffusion through the patch to the skin surface.
(D) surface area of the patch.
(E) All of the above

ANSWERS AND EXPLANATIONS

1. The answer is B *[see I.A.3]*.
Bioavailability is the measurement of the rate and extent (amount) of therapeutically active drug that reaches the systemic circulation. The relation of the physical and the chemical properties of a drug to its systemic absorption (i.e., bioavailability) is known as its biopharmaceutics. The movement of a drug into body tissues is an aspect of pharmacokinetics, which is the study of drug movement in the body over time. The dissolution of a drug in the gastrointestinal tract is a physicochemical process that affects bioavailability. Significant destruction of a drug by the liver before it is systemically absorbed (known as the first-pass effect because it occurs during the first passage of the drug through the liver) decreases bioavailability.

2. The answer is B *[see II.B.1.a]*.
When the active form of the drug is given intravenously, it enters the systemic circulation directly. The drug is delivered rapidly to all tissues, including the drug receptor sites. For all other routes of drug administration, except intra-arterial injection, the drug must be systemically absorbed before it is distributed to the drug receptor sites. For this reason, the onset of pharmacologic effects is slower. If the drug is a prodrug that must be converted to an active drug, oral administration, not intravenous injection, may not provide the most rapid onset of activity if conversion to the active form takes place in the gastrointestinal tract or liver.

3. The answer is B *[see II.C.2]*.
When a drug is given by intravenous injection, the entire dose enters the systemic circulation. With other routes of administration, the drug may be lost before it reaches the systemic circulation. For example, with first-pass effects, a portion of an orally administered drug is eliminated, usually through degradation by liver enzymes, before the drug reaches its receptor sites.

4. The answer is C *[see II.B.2.b.(4)]*.
Drugs given orally are well absorbed from the duodenum. The duodenum has a large surface area because of the presence of villi and microvilli. In addition, because the duodenum is well perfused by the mesenteric blood vessels, a concentration gradient is maintained between the lumen of the duodenum and the blood.

5. The answer is B *[see II.A.2–3]*.
Fick's law of diffusion describes passive diffusion of drug molecules moving from a high concentration to a low concentration. This process is not saturable and does not require energy.

6. The answer is D *[see II.A.2]*.
The transport of a drug across a cell membrane by passive diffusion follows Fick's law of diffusion: The drug moves with a concentration gradient (i.e., from an area of high concentration to an area of low concentration). In contrast, drugs that are actively transported move against a concentration gradient.

7. The answer is E *[see III.A.1]*.
The Noyes-Whitney equation describes the rate at which a solid drug dissolves. Fick's law is similar to the Noyes-Whitney equation in that both equations describe drug movement caused by a concentration gradient. Fick's law generally refers to passive diffusion, or passive transport, of drugs. The law of mass action describes the rate of a chemical reaction, the Michaelis-Menten equation involves enzyme kinetics, and the Henderson-Hasselbalch equation gives the pH of a buffer solution.

8. The answer is D *[see III.A.1–3]*.
The ionized, or salt, form of a drug has a charge and is generally more water soluble and, therefore, dissolves more rapidly than the nonionized (free acid or free base) form of the drug. The dissolution rate is directly proportional to the surface area and inversely proportional to the particle size. An increase in the particle size or a decrease in the surface area slows the dissolution rate.

9. The answer is B *[see III.B.6]*.
A modified-release, or controlled-release, drug product contains two or more conventional doses of the drug. An abrupt release of the drug, known as dose dumping, may cause intoxication.

10. The answer is B *[see III.B.1.c].*
For lipid-soluble drugs, the rate of dissolution is the slowest (i.e., rate-limiting) step in drug absorption and thus in bioavailability. The disintegration rate of an immediate-release or conventional compressed tablet is usually more rapid than the rate of drug dissolution. Because the cell membrane is a lipoprotein structure, transport of a lipid-soluble drug across the cell membrane is usually rapid.

11. The answer is A *[see III.A.4.b].*
The extent of ionization of a weak electrolyte is described by the Henderson-Hasselbalch equation, which relates the pH of the solution to the pK_a of the drug.

12. The answer is D *[see III.B.2.a].*
Because a drug in solution is already dissolved, no dissolution is needed before absorption. Consequently, compared with other drug formulations, a drug in solution has a high rate of bioavailability. A drug in aqueous solution has the highest bioavailability rate and is often used as the reference preparation for other formulations. Drugs in hydroalcoholic solution (e.g., elixirs) also have good bioavailability. The rate of drug bioavailability from a hard gelatin capsule, compressed tablet, or suspension may be equal to that of a solution if an optimal formulation is manufactured and the drug is inherently rapidly absorbed.

13. The answer is E *[see III.B.7].*
Drug delivery from a transdermal drug delivery system depends on all of the factors cited—that is, on the presence of an occlusive backing (to maintain skin hydration and elevate skin temperature slightly) and an adhesive film to maintain contact of the formulation matrix with the skin to enable drug transfer from the patch into the skin. If the drug's affinity for the formulation matrix is greater than its affinity for the stratum corneum, the drug's escaping tendency from the patch will be reduced, minimizing the gradient for drug transfer into the skin. The microviscosity of the formulation matrix, the presence of a membrane between the drug reservoir in the patch and the skin surface, and interaction of the drug with the formulation matrix affect the rate and extent of diffusion and/or partitioning of the drug through the patch to the skin surface. Finally, the extent of drug delivery from the patch is directly proportional to the surface area of the patch in contact with the skin surface.

5

Extemporaneous Prescription Compounding

Loyd V. Allen Jr.

I. INTRODUCTION

A. Definitions

1. **Compounding vs manufacturing**

2. It is important, but oftentimes difficult, to distinguish between compounding and manufacturing.

3. **Compounding** has been defined by the National Association of Boards of Pharmacy as

   the preparation, mixing, assembling, packaging, or labeling of a drug or device (i) as the result of a practitioner's prescription drug order or initiative based on the pharmacist/patient/prescriber relationship in the course of professional practice or (ii) for the purpose of, as an incident to research, teaching, or chemical analysis and not for sale or dispensing. Compounding also includes the preparation of drugs and devices in anticipation of prescription drug orders based on routine, regularly observed patterns.

4. **Manufacturing** has been defined as

   the production, preparation, propagation, conversion or processing of a drug or device, either directly or indirectly, by extraction from substances of natural origin or independently by means of chemical or biological synthesis, and includes any packaging or repackaging of the substance(s) or labeling or relabeling of its container, and the promotion and marketing of such drugs or devices. Manufacturing also includes the preparation and promotion of commercially available products from bulk compounds for resale by pharmacies, practitioners, or other persons.

5. The purpose of pharmaceutical compounding is to prepare an individualized drug treatment for a patient based on an order from a duly licensed prescriber. The fundamental difference between compounding and manufacturing is the existence of a pharmacist/prescriber/patient relationship that controls the compounding of the drug preparation. Compounded drugs are not for resale but, rather, are personal and responsive to the patient's immediate needs. They are prepared and administered by the patient's healthcare professionals, which allows for the monitoring of patient outcomes. On the other hand, drug manufacturers produce batches consisting of tens or hundreds of thousands of dosage units, such as tablets or capsules, for resale, using many personnel and large-scale manufacturing equipment. These products are distributed through the normal channels of interstate commerce to individuals unknown to the company. Manufacturers are not required to, and do not, provide oversight of individual patients. It is also acceptable and routine practice for pharmacists to compound for "office use" those preparations that are not commercially available. These preparations are "For Office Use Only" and are not for resale or to be given to the patients to take home; they are to be administered at the office.

6. The *United States Pharmacopeia* (*USP*) uses the term *preparation* to refer to compounded prescriptions and the term *products* to refer to manufactured pharmaceuticals. Also, for stability purposes, compounded preparations are assigned a "beyond-use" date and manufactured products are assigned an "expiration date."

B. Regulation

1. **Current good manufacturing practices (cGMPs)** are the standards of practice used in the pharmaceutical industry and are regulated by the Food and Drug Administration (FDA).

2. Good compounding practices (GCPs) are the standards of practice detailed in the *USP*, chapter <1075>. Community pharmacists must comply with state board of pharmacy regulations and guidelines to ensure a quality preparation, which includes using proper materials, weighing equipment, documented techniques, and dispensing and storage instructions.

3. Legal considerations
   a. Extemporaneous compounding by the pharmacist or a prescription order from a licensed practitioner, as with the dispensing of any other prescription, is controlled by the state boards of pharmacy.
   b. The legal risk (liability) of compounding is no greater than the risk of filling a prescription for a manufactured product because the pharmacist must ensure that the correct drug, dose, and directions are provided. The pharmacist is also responsible for preparing a quality pharmaceutical preparation, providing proper instructions regarding its storage, and advising the patient of any adverse effects.

4. Food and Drug Administration. The FDA has developed a list of preparations that should not be extemporaneously compounded. This list was developed primarily from commercial products that have been removed from the market owing to safety and/or efficacy concerns. This is a lengthy list and must be read carefully because, in some cases, only certain dosage forms of a specific drug are included on the list and others are not. The list is too extensive to include here but can be accessed at www.fda.gov/cder/pharmcomp/pcwd.txt.

C. Stability and quality control of compounded preparations

1. Beyond-use dates. The assignment of a beyond-use date is one of the most difficult tasks required of a compounding pharmacist. Chapters <795> and <797> of the *USP* provide guidelines for this task. Chapter <795> involves nonsterile preparations, and chapter <797> involves sterile preparations. Current *USP* criteria for nonaqueous liquids and solid formulations (for which a manufactured drug product is the source of active ingredients) include a beyond-use date not later than 25% of the time remaining until the product's expiration date or 6 months, whichever is earlier. When a *USP* or *National Formulary* (*NF*) substance is the source of active ingredient, the beyond-use date is not later than 6 months. For water-containing formulations (prepared from ingredients in solid form), the beyond-use date is not later than 14 days when stored at cold temperatures. For all other formulations, the beyond-use date is not later than the intended duration of therapy or 30 days, whichever is earlier. These beyond-use dates may be exceeded when there is supporting valid scientific stability information that is directly applicable to the specific preparation.

2. Quality control. Quality control is becoming one of the fastest growing aspects of pharmacy compounding. Pharmacists are becoming more involved in the final testing of compounded preparations or are sending them to contract laboratories for testing. For example, the following quality control tests can be considered for the respective compounded dosage forms:
   a. Ointments, creams, and gels. Theoretical weight compared to actual weight, pH, specific gravity, active drug assay, physical observations (color, clarity, texture–surface, texture–spatula spread, appearance, feel), and rheological properties.
   b. Hard gelatin capsules. Weight overall, average weight, individual weight variation, dissolution of capsule shell, disintegration of capsule contents, active drug assay, physical appearance (color, uniformity, extent of fill, locked), and physical stability (discoloration, changes in appearance).
   c. Special hard gelatin capsules. Weight overall, average weight, individual weight variation, dissolution of capsule shell, disintegration of capsule contents, active drug assay, physical appearance (color, uniformity of appearance, uniformity of extent of fill, closures), and physical stability (discoloration or other changes).
   d. Suppositories, troches, lollipops, and sticks. Weight, specific gravity, active drug assay, physical observations (color, clarity, texture of surface, appearance, feel), melting test, dissolution test, physical stability.
   e. Oral and topical liquids. Weight to volume, pH, specific gravity, active drug assay, globule size range, rheological properties/pourability, physical observations (color, clarity), and physical stability (discoloration, foreign materials, gas formation, mold growth).
   f. Parenteral preparations. Weight or volume, pH, specific gravity, osmolality, assay, physical observations, (color, clarity), particulate matter, sterility, and pyrogenicity.

3. **Quality control testing.** Pharmacists have the option of doing testing in-house or outsourcing it to laboratories.
   a. **In-house testing** can include measurements such as weight, volume, pH, specific gravity, osmolality, physical observations, sterility and endotoxins.
   b. **Out-sourced testing** can include sterility, endotoxins, potency, and dissolution.
   c. **Test results** should be kept on file with the compounding records for the individual compounded preparations.

II. REQUIREMENTS FOR COMPOUNDING

A. **Sources for chemicals and drugs.** Pharmacists can obtain small quantities of the appropriate chemicals or drugs from wholesalers or chemical supply houses. These suppliers then may act as consultants to the pharmacists by ensuring their product's purity and quality.

B. **Equipment.** The correct equipment is important when compounding. Many state boards of pharmacy have a required minimum list of equipment for compounding prescriptions. Suggested equipment, which varies according to the amount of material needed and the type of compounded prescription (e.g., parenteral), includes the following:

1. Electronic balance and/or class A prescription balance
2. Hot plate
3. Magnetic stirrer
4. Electric mixer
5. Special containers for packaging (e.g., applicator tip bottles, insufflators)
6. Graduated cylinders from 10 mL to 1000 mL
7. Glass, Wedgwood, and porcelain mortars and pestles of various sizes
8. Funnels of various sizes
9. Spatulas of various sizes, including several plastic spatulas
10. Weighing and filter papers
11. Stirring rods (glass)
12. Ointment/pill tile
13. Capsule-filling machine
14. Ointment-filling machine
15. Autoclave
16. Laminar flow clean bench
17. Special suppository, troche and medication-stick molds
18. Record-keeping system (compounding log book)
19. Glass beakers from 50 mL to 1000 mL

C. **Location of compounding area.** Many pharmacies actively involved in compounding have dedicated a separate area in the pharmacy to this process. The ideal location is away from heavy foot traffic and is near a sink where there is sufficient space to work and store all chemicals and equipment. For compounding of sterile preparations, a laminar air-flow hood (minimal) and a clean room are current practice, or isolation barrier technology equipment.

D. **Sources of information**
1. Library at a college of pharmacy
2. **References**
   a. Allen Jr LV. *The Art, Science and Technology of Pharmaceutical Compounding.* 2nd ed. Washington, DC: American Pharmaceutical Association, 2002.

    b. Anon. *Remington: The Science and Practice of Pharmacy.* 21st ed. Philadelphia: Lippincott Williams & Wilkins; 2006.

    c. Smith A, Heckelman PE, O'Neil M, Budavari S, eds. *Merck Index.* 13th ed. Whitehouse Station, NJ: Merck & Co, 2001.

    d. *The USP Pharmacists' Pharmacopeia.* Rockville, MD: U.S. Pharmacopeial Convention, Inc., 2005.

    e. Allen LV Jr, Popovich NG, Ansel HC. *Ansel's Pharmaceutical Dosage Forms and Drug Delivery Systems.* Media, PA: Lippincott Williams & Wilkins, 2005.

3. Journals
    a. *International Journal of Pharmaceutical Compounding*
    b. *U.S. Pharmacist*
    c. *Pharmacy Times*
    d. *Lippincott's Hospital Pharmacy*
    e. *American Journal of Health-System Pharmacists*

4. Manufacturers' drug product information inserts; compounding specialty suppliers

5. Web sites
    a. Compounding Today: www.CompoundingToday.com
    b. *International Journal of Pharmaceutical Compounding:* www.ijpc.com
    c. Paddock Laboratories, Inc.: www.paddocklabs.com

III. COMPOUNDING OF SOLUTIONS

A. Definition. *USP* 29 defines **solutions** as liquid preparations that contain one or more chemical substances dissolved (i.e., molecularly dispersed) in a suitable solvent or mixture of mutually miscible solvents. Although the uniformity of the dosage in a solution can be assumed, the stability, pH, solubility of the drug or chemicals, taste (for oral solutions), and packaging need to be considered.

B. Types of solutions

1. Sterile parenteral and ophthalmic solutions require special consideration for their preparation (see XI).

2. Nonsterile solutions include oral, topical, and otic solutions.

C. Preparation of solutions. Solutions are the easiest of the dosage forms to compound extemporaneously, as long as a few general rules are followed.

1. Each drug or chemical is dissolved in the solvent in which it is most soluble. Thus the solubility characteristics of each drug or chemical must be known.

2. If an alcoholic solution of a poorly water-soluble drug is used, the aqueous solution is added to the alcoholic solution to maintain as high an alcohol concentration as possible.

3. The salt form of the drug—not the free-acid or base form, which both have poor solubility—is used.

4. Flavoring or sweetening agents are prepared ahead of time.

5. When adding a salt to a syrup, dissolve the salt in a few milliliters of water first; then add the syrup to volume.

6. The proper vehicle (e.g., syrup, elixir, aromatic water, purified water) must be selected.

D. Examples

1. Example 1
    a. Medication order

Triamcinolone acetonide	100 mg
Menthol	50 mg
Ethanol	10 mL
Propylene glycol	30 mL

Glycerin	20 mL
Sorbitol 70% solution, qs	100 mL
Sodium saccharin	100 mg
Sodium metabisulfite	20 mg
Disodium EDTA	100 mg
Purified water	5 mL

b. **Compounding procedure.** Triamcinolone acetonide 0.1% mouthwash solution is prepared by dissolving the triamcinolone acetonide and menthol in the ethanol. Add the propylene glycol, glycerin, and about 10 mL of the 70% sorbitol and mix well. Dissolve the sodium saccharin, sodium metabisulfite, and disodium EDTA in the purified water. Add the aqueous solution to the drug mixture and mix well. Add sufficient 70% sorbitol solution to volume and mix well.

How much of the triamcinolone base is present in this prescription? The molecular weight of triamcinolone is 394.4 and that of triamcinolone acetonide is 434.5.

$$\frac{394.4}{434.5} \times 100 \text{ mg} = 91 \text{ mg of triamcinolone base}$$

2. **Example 2**
   a. **Medication order**

Potassium chloride	1 mEq/mL
Preserved flavored, oral vehicle, qs	100 mL

   b. **Calculations.** The molecular weight of potassium chloride is 74.5 (K = 39; Cl = 35.5). One milliequivalent (mEq) weighs 74.5 mg.

   $$100 \text{ mL} \times 74.5 \text{ mg/mL} = 7450 \text{ mg or } 7.45 \text{ g of KCl required}$$

   What is the molar concentration of this prescription?

   7.45 g per 100 mL or 74.5 g per 1000 mL
   1 mole of KCl weights 74.5 g
   It is a 1 molar solution

   c. **Compounding procedure.** The solubility of potassium chloride is 1 g in 2.8 mL water. Therefore, dissolve the 7.45 g KCl in 21 mL of purified water. Add sufficient preserved flavored oral vehicle to volume and mix well.

3. **Example 3**
   a. **Medication order**

Salicylic acid	2%
Lactic acid	6 mL
Flexible collodion, ad	30 mL

   b. **Compounding procedure.** Pharmacists must use caution when preparing this prescription because flexible collodion is extremely flammable. A 1-oz. applicator-tip bottle is calibrated, using ethanol, which is poured out and allowed to evaporate, resulting in a dry bottle. Salicylic acid (0.6 g) is added directly into the bottle, to which is added the 6 mL of lactic acid. The bottle is agitated or a glass stirring rod is used to dissolve the salicylic acid. Flexible collodion is added up to the calibrated 30-mL mark on the applicator-tip bottle.

4. **Example 4**
   a. **Medication order**

Iodine	2%
Sodium iodide	2.4%
Alcohol, qs	30 mL

   b. **Compounding procedure.** Iodine (0.6 g) and sodium iodide (0.72 g) are dissolved in the alcohol, and the final solution is placed in an amber bottle. A **rubber or plastic spatula** is used because **iodine is corrosive.**

IV. COMPOUNDING OF SUSPENSIONS

A. **Definition. Suspensions** are defined by *USP* 29 as liquid preparations that consist of solid particles dispersed throughout a liquid phase in which the particles are not soluble.

B. General characteristics

1. Some suspensions should contain an antimicrobial agent as a preservative.

2. Particles settle in suspensions even when a suspending agent is added; thus suspensions must be well shaken before use to ensure the distribution of particles for a uniform dose.

3. Tight containers are necessary to ensure the stability of the final preparation.

4. Principles to keep in mind when compounding include the following:
   a. Insoluble powders should be small and uniform in size to decrease settling.
   b. The suspension should be viscous.
   c. Topical suspensions should have a smooth, impalpable texture.
   d. Oral suspensions should have a pleasant odor and taste.

C. Formation of suspensions.
Suspensions are easy to compound; however, physical stability after compounding the final preparation is problematic. The following steps may minimize stability problems.

1. The particle size of all powders used in the formulation should be reduced.

2. A thickening (suspending) agent may be used to increase viscosity. Common thickening agents include alginic acid, bentonite, VEEGUM, methylcellulose, and tragacanth.

3. A levigating agent may aid in the initial dispersion of insoluble particles. Common levigating agents include glycerin, propylene glycol, alcohol, syrups, and water.

4. Flavoring agents and preservatives should be selected and added if the preparation is intended for oral use. Common preservatives include methylparaben, propylparaben, benzoic acid, and sodium benzoate. Flavoring agents may be any flavored syrup or flavor concentrate (Table 5-1).

5. The source of the active ingredients (e.g., bulk powders versus tablets or capsules) must be considered; if commercial dosage forms are used, the inactive ingredients must be considered and only immediate-release tablets or capsules should be used and not modified release.

D. Preparation of suspensions

1. The insoluble powders are triturated to a fine powder.

2. A small portion of liquid is used as a levigating agent, and the powders are triturated until a smooth paste is formed.

Table 5-1. Selected Flavor Applications

Drug Category	Preferred Flavors
Antibiotics	Cherry, maple, pineapple, orange, raspberry, banana-pineapple, banana-vanilla, butterscotch-maple, coconut custard, strawberry, vanilla, lemon custard, cherry custard, fruit-cinnamon
Antihistamines	Apricot, black currant, cherry, cinnamon, custard, grape, honey, lime, loganberry, peach-orange, peach-rum, raspberry, root beer, wild cherry
Barbiturates	Banana-pineapple, banana-vanilla, black currant, cinnamon-peppermint, grenadine-strawberry, lime, orange, peach-orange, root beer
Decongestants and expectorants	Anise, apricot, black currant, butterscotch, cherry, coconut custard, custard mint-strawberry, grenadine-peach, strawberry, lemon, coriander, orange-peach, pineapple, raspberry, strawberry, tangerine
Electrolyte solutions	Cherry, grape, lemon-lime, raspberry, wild cherry, black currant, grenadine-strawberry, lime, Port wine, Sherry wine, root beer, wild strawberry

3. The vehicle containing the suspending agent is added in divided portions. A high-speed mixer greatly increases the dispersion.

4. The preparation is brought to the required volume using the vehicle.

5. The final mixture is transferred to a "tight" bottle for dispensing to the patient.

6. All suspensions are dispensed with a "shake well" label.

7. Suspensions are not filtered.

8. The water-soluble ingredients, including flavoring agents, are mixed in the vehicle before mixing with the insoluble ingredients.

E. Examples

1. Example 1
a. Medication order

Propranolol HCl	4 mg/mL
Disp	30 mL
Sig:	1 mL p.o. t.i.d.

b. **Calculations.** Propranolol HCl: 4 mg/mL × 30 mL = 120 mg. Propranolol HCl is available as a powder or in immediate-release and extended-release (long-acting) dosage forms. Only the powder or the immediate-release tablets are used for compounding prescriptions; therefore, some combination of propranolol HCl tablets that yields 120 mg active drug (e.g., 3 × 40 mg tablets) may be used.

c. **Compounding procedure.** The propranolol tablets are reduced to a fine powder in a mortar. The powder or the comminuted tablets are levigated to a smooth paste, using a 2% methylcellulose solution. To this mixture, about 10 mL of a suitable flavoring agent is added. The mixture is transferred to a calibrated container and brought to the final volume with purified water or suitable suspending vehicle. A "shake well" label is attached to the prescription container.

2. Example 2
a. Medication order

Zinc oxide	10
Ppt sulfur	10
Bentonite	3.6
Purified water, ad	90 mL
Sig:	Apply t.i.d.

b. **Compounding procedure.** The powders are reduced to a fine uniform mixture in a mortar. The powders are mixed to form a smooth paste using water and transferred to a calibrated bottle. The final volume is attained with purified water. A "shake well" label is attached to the prescription container.

3. Example 3
a. Medication order

Rifampin suspension	20 mg/mL
Disp	120 mL
Sig:	u.d.

b. **Calculations.** Rifampin: 20 mg/mL × 120 mL = 2400 mg. Rifampin is available in 150-mg and 300-mg capsules. Hence, 8 capsules containing 300 mg of rifampin in each capsule or 16 capsules containing 150 mg of rifampin per capsule are needed.

c. **Compounding procedure.** The contents of the appropriate number of rifampin capsules are emptied into a mortar and comminuted with a pestle. This powder is levigated with a small amount of 1% methylcellulose solution. Then 20 mL of simple syrup are added and mixed. The mixture is brought to the final volume with simple syrup. "Shake well" and "refrigerate" labels are attached to the prescription container.

V. EMULSIONS

A. **Definition.** Emulsions are **two-phase systems** in which one liquid is dispersed throughout another liquid in the form of small droplets (see Chapter 3.VI.D).

B. **General characteristics.** Emulsions can be used **externally** as lotions and creams or **internally** to mask the taste of medications.

1. The two liquids in an emulsion are immiscible and require the use of an **emulsifying agent.**

2. Emulsions are classified as either **oil-in-water (o/w)** or **water-in-oil (w/o);** there can also be multiple emulsions, such as **oil-in-water-in-oil (o/w/o)** and **water-in-oil-in-water (w/o/w),** as well as emulsion-gels, in which the external phase of an oil in water emulsion is thickened with a gelling agent.

3. Emulsions are **unstable,** and the following steps should be taken to prevent the two phases of an emulsion from separating into two layers after preparation.
   a. The correct **proportions** of oil and water should be used during preparation. The internal phase should represent 40–60% of the total volume.
   b. An emulsifying **agent** is needed for emulsion formation.
   c. A **hand homogenizer,** which reduces the size of globules of the internal phase, may be used; if small quantities are compounded, two 60-mL syringes attached with a Leur-Lock adapter can be used and the materials pushed back and forth between the two syringes.
   d. **Preservatives** should be added if the preparation is intended to last longer than a few days. Generally, a combination of methylparaben (0.2%) and propylparaben (0.02%) may be used.
   e. A **"shake well" label** should be placed on the final preparation.
   f. The preparation should be **protected** from light and extreme temperature. Both freezing and heat may have an effect on stability.

C. **Emulsifying agents**

1. **Gums,** such as acacia or tragacanth, are used to form o/w emulsions. These emulsifying agents are for general use, especially for emulsions intended for internal administration (Table 5-2).
   a. Use 1 g of acacia powder for every 4 mL of fixed oil or 1 g to 2 mL for a volatile oil.
   b. If using tragacanth in place of acacia, 0.1 g of tragacanth is used for every 1 g of acacia.

2. **Methylcellulose and carboxymethylcellulose** are used for o/w emulsions. The concentrations of these agents vary, depending on the grade that is used. Methylcellulose is available in several viscosity grades, ranging from 15 to 4000 and designated by a centipoise number, which is a unit of viscosity.

3. **Soaps** can be used to prepare o/w or w/o emulsions for external preparations.

4. **Nonionic emulsifying agents** can be used for o/w and w/o emulsions.

D. **Formation and preparation of emulsions.** The procedure for preparing an emulsion depends on the desired emulsifying agent in the formulation.

1. A **mortar** and **pestle** are frequently all the equipment that is needed.
   a. A mortar with a **rough surface** (e.g., Wedgwood) should be used. This rough surface allows maximal dispersion of globules to produce a fine particle size.
   b. A **rapid motion** is essential when triturating an emulsion using a mortar and pestle.
   c. The mortar should be able to hold at least three times the **quantity** being made. Trituration seldom requires more than 5 min to create the emulsion.

2. **Electric mixers** and hand homogenizers are useful for producing emulsions after the coarse emulsion is formed in the mortar.

3. The **order** of mixing of ingredients in an emulsion depends on the type of emulsion being prepared (i.e., o/w or w/o) as well as the emulsifying agent chosen. Methods used for compounding include the following:
   a. **Dry gum** (continental) method is used for forming emulsions using natural emulsifying agents and requires a specific order of mixing.
   b. **Wet gum** (English) method is used for forming emulsions using natural emulsifying agents and requires a specific order of mixing.
   c. **Bottle method** is used for forming emulsions using natural emulsifying agents and requires a specific order of mixing.

Table 5-2. Agents Used in Prescription Compounding

Ointments	

Oleaginous or hydrocarbon bases
  Anhydrous
  Nonhydrophilic
  Insoluble in water
  Not water removable (occlusive)
  Good vehicles for antibiotics
Example
  Petrolatum
	Hydrous emulsion bases (w/o)
	  Hydrous
	  Hydrophilic
	  Insoluble in water
	  Not water removable (occlusive)
	Examples
	  Cold cream
	  Hydrous lanolin

Absorption, or hydrophilic, bases
  Anhydrous
  Hydrophilic
  Insoluble in water
  Not water removable (occlusive)
Examples
  Hydrophilic petrolatum
  Lanolin USP (anhydrous)
	Emulsion bases (o/w)
	  Hydrous
	  Hydrophilic
	  Insoluble in water
	  Water removable
	  Can absorb 30–50% of weight
	Examples
	  Hydrophilic ointment USP
	  Acid mantle cream

	Water soluble
	  Anhydrous or hydrous
	  Soluble in water
	  Water removable
	  Hydrophilic
	Example
	  Polyethylene glycol ointment

Suspending Agents	
Acacia 10% Alginic acid Bentonite 6% Carboxymethylcellulose 1–%	Methylcellulose 1–7% Sodium alginate 1–2% Tragacanth 1–3% VEEGUM 6%

Preservatives	
Methylparaben 0.02–0.2%	Propylparaben 0.01–0.04%

Emulsifying Agents	

Hydrophilic colloids
  Acacia
  Tragacanth
  Pectin; favor o/w
  Carboxymethylcellulose
  Methylcellulose
Proteins
  Gelatin
  Egg whites; favor o/w
Inorganic gels and magmas
  Milk of magnesia
  Bentonite; favor o/w
	Surfactants, nonionic
	  Concentrations used (1–30%)
	  Tweens (e.g., polysorbate 80)
	  Spans
	
	Soaps
	  Triethanolamine
	  Stearic acid
	Others
	  Sodium lauryl sulfate
	  Dioctyl sodium sulfosuccinate
	  Cetyl pyridinium chloride

o/w, oil-in-water; *w/o,* water-in-oil

d. Beaker method is used to prepare emulsions using synthetic emulsifying agents and produces a satisfactory preparation regardless of the order of mixing.

4. **Preservatives.** If the emulsion is kept for an extended period of time, refrigeration is usually sufficient. The preparation should not be frozen. If a preservative is used, it must be soluble in the water phase to be effective.

5. **Flavoring agents.** If the addition of a flavor is needed to mask the taste of the oil phase, the flavor should be added to the external phase before emulsification (Table 5-3).

E. Examples

1. **Example 1**
   a. **Medication order**

Mineral oil	18 mL
Acacia, qs	
Distilled water, qs ad	90.0 mL
Sig:	1 tablespoon q.d.

   b. **Compounding procedure.** With the dry gum method, an initial emulsion (primary emulsion) is formed, using 4 parts (18 mL) of oil, 2 parts (9 mL) of water, and 1 part (4.5 g) of powdered acacia. The mineral oil is triturated with the acacia in a Wedgwood mortar. The 9 mL of water is added all at once and, with rapid trituration, form the primary emulsion, which is triturated for about 5 min. The remaining water is incorporated in small amounts with trituration. The emulsion is transferred to a 90-mL prescription bottle, and a "shake well" label is attached to the container.

2. **Example 2**
   a. **Medication order**

Olive oil	30 mL
Zinc oxide	8 g
Calamine	8 g
Lime water	30 mL

   b. **Compounding procedure.** The olive oil is placed in a suitably sized beaker. Using an electric mixer, the zinc oxide, the calamine, and the lime water are added in that order. This yields a w/o emulsion. This procedure is known as the nascent soap method. The olive oil reacts with the calcium hydroxide solution (lime water) and forms a soap. For this reaction to occur, fresh lime water (calcium hydroxide solution) is required. A small quantity of oleic acid can also be added to further stabilize the emulsion.

3. **Example 3**
   a. **Medication order**

Mineral oil	50 mL
Water, qs	100 mL
Sig:	2.5 mL p.o. h.s.

   b. **Compounding procedure.** Using a combination of nonionic emulsifying agents, such as Span 40 and Tween 40, the correct hydrophilic–lipophilic balance (HLB) is obtained. Next, the mineral oil is warmed in a water bath to about 60°C, and the Span 40 is

Table 5-3. Flavor Selection Guide

Taste	Masking Flavor
Salt	Butterscotch, maple
Bitter	Wild cherry, walnut, chocolate mint, licorice
Sweet	Fruit, berry, vanilla
Acid	Citrus

dissolved in the heated mineral oil. The water is warmed to about 65°C, and the Tween 40 is dissolved in the heated water. This mixture is added to the mineral oil and dissolved Span 40 and stirred until cooled. An "external use only" label is added to the container.

VI. POWDERED DOSAGE FORMS

A. **Definition. Powders** are intimate mixtures of dry, finely divided drugs and/or chemicals that may be intended for internal (oral powders) or external (topical powders) use. The major types are powder papers, bulk powders, and insufflations.

B. **General characteristics**

1. Powder dosage forms are used when **drug stability** or **solubility** is a concern. These dosage forms may also be used when the powders are too bulky to make into capsules and when the patient has difficulty swallowing a capsule.

2. Some **disadvantages** to powders include unpleasant-tasting medications and, occasionally, the rapid deterioration of powders.

3. **Blending** of powders may be accomplished by using trituration in a mortar, stirring with a spatula, and sifting. Geometric dilution should be used if needed. When heavy powders are mixed with lighter ones, the heavier powder should be placed on top of the lighter one and then blended. When mixing two or more powders, each powder should be pulverized separately to about the same particle size before blending together.
   a. The mortar and pestle method is preferred when **pulverization** and a thorough mixing of ingredients are desired (geometric dilution). A Wedgwood mortar is preferable, but glass or porcelain may also be used.
   b. Light powders are mixed best by using the **sifting method.** The sifting is repeated three to four times to ensure thorough mixing of the powders.

C. **Preparation of powder dosage forms**

1. **Bulk powders,** which may be used internally or topically, include dusting powders, douche powders, laxatives, antacids, and insufflation powders.

2. After a bulk powder has been pulverized and blended, it should be dispensed in an appropriate container.
   a. **Hygroscopic** or **effervescent** salts should always be placed in a tight, wide-mouth jar.
   b. **Dusting** powders should be placed in a container with a sifter top.

3. **Eutectic mixtures** of powders can cause problems because they may liquefy. One remedy is to add an inert powder, such as magnesium oxide, to separate the eutectic materials.

4. **Powder papers** are also called divided powders.
   a. The entire powder is initially blended. Each dose is then individually weighed.
   b. The dosage should be weighed, then transferred onto a powder paper and folded. This technique requires practice. Hygroscopic, deliquescent, and effervescent powders require the use of glassine paper as an inside lining. Plastic bags or envelopes with snap-and-seal closures offer a convenient alternative to powder papers.
   c. The folded papers are dispensed in a powder box or other suitable container; however, these containers are not child resistant.

D. **Examples**

1. **Example 1**
   a. **Medication order**

Camphor	100 mg
Menthol	200 mg
Zinc oxide	800 mg
Talc	1.9 g
M foot powder	
Sig:	Apply to feet b.i.d.

b. **Compounding procedure.** The camphor and menthol are triturated together in a glass mortar, where a liquid eutectic is formed. The zinc oxide and talc are blended and mixed with the eutectic, using geometric dilution. This mixing results in a dry powder, which is passed through a wire mesh sieve. The final preparation is dispensed in a container with a sifter top.

2. **Example 2**
   a. **Medication order**

Citric acid	0.3 g
Sodium bicarbonate	0.25 g
Psyllium mucilloid	2 g
Powdered flavor, qs	

   M. Ft d.t.d. charts v
   Sig: Empty the contents of one chart
       into a glass of water and take h.s.

   b. **Calculations.** Calculate for one extra powder paper:

$$\text{Citric acid } 0.3 \text{ g} \times 6 \text{ doses} = 1.8 \text{ g}$$
$$\text{Sodium bicarbonate } 0.25 \text{ g} \times 6 \text{ doses} = 1.5 \text{ g}$$
$$\text{Psyllium mucilloid } 2 \text{ g} \times 6 \text{ doses} = 12 \text{ g}$$
$$\text{Total wight} = 15.3 \text{ g}$$
$$15.3 \text{ g}/6 \text{ doses} = 2.55 \text{ g/dose}$$

   Note: Also consider the weight of the powdered flavor.

   c. **Compounding procedure.** The ingredients are first pulverized and weighed. The citric acid and sodium bicarbonate are mixed together first; the psyllium mucilloid is then added along with the powdered flavor, using geometric dilution. Each dose (2.55 g) of the resultant mixture is weighed and placed into a powder paper. This preparation is an effervescent powder. When dissolved in water, the citric acid and sodium bicarbonate react to form carbonic acid, which yields carbon dioxide, making the solution more palatable.

VII. CAPSULES

A. **Definition. Capsules** are solid dosage forms in which the drug is enclosed within either a hard or soft soluble container or shell. The shells are usually made from a suitable gelatin. Hard gelatin capsules may be manually filled for extemporaneous compounding.

B. **Capsule sizes**

   1. A list of capsule sizes and the approximate amount of powder that may be contained in the capsule appear on the side of the capsule box (Table 5-4).

   2. Capsule sizes for oral administration in humans range from no. 5, the smallest, to no. 000, the largest.

Table 5-4. Approximate Amount of Powder Contained in Capsules

Capsule Size	Range of Powder Capacity (mg)
No. 5	60–130
No. 4	95–260
No. 3	130–390
No. 2	195–520
No. 1	225–650
No. 0	325–910
No. 00	390–1300
No. 000	650–2000

3. No. 0 is usually the largest oral size suitable for human patients.

4. Capsules for veterinarians are available in no. 10, no. 11, and no. 12, containing approximately 30, 15, and 7.5 g, respectively.

C. Preparation of hard and soft capsules

1. As with the bulk powders, all ingredients are triturated and blended, using geometric dilution.

2. The correct size capsule must be determined by trying different capsule sizes, weighing them, and then choosing the appropriate size.

3. Before filling capsules with the medication, the body and cap of the capsule are separated. Filling is accomplished by using the "punch" method (Alternatively, small capsule machines are commonly used to prepare up to 300 capsules at a time, extemporaneously).
  a. The powder formulation is compressed with a spatula on a pill tile or paper sheet with a uniform depth of approximately half the length of the capsule body.
  b. The empty capsule body is repeatedly pressed into the powder until full.
  c. The capsule is then weighed to ensure an accurate dose. An empty tare capsule of the same size is placed on the pan containing the weights.

4. For a large number of capsules, capsule-filling machines can be used for small-scale use to save time. Most commonly, capsules machines are used capable of preparing 100 to 300 capsules at a time.

5. The capsule is wiped clean of any powder or oil and dispensed in a suitable prescription vial.

D. Examples

1. Example 1
  a. Medication order

Rifampin	100 mg
dtd #50	
Sig:	1 cap p.o. q.d.

  b. Calculations. Compound this prescription using the commercially available 300-mg capsules as the drug source. Calculate for at least one extra capsule.

  $$51 \text{ caps} \times 100 \text{ mg/cap} = 5100 \text{ mg rifampin}$$
  $$5100 \text{ mg rifampin} \div 300 \text{ mg/cap} = 17 \text{ caps}$$

  c. Compounding procedure. Use 17 rifampin capsules, each containing 300 mg rifampin. The content of each capsule is emptied, and the powder is weighed. The powder equivalent to 100 mg rifampin is placed in a capsule (e.g., if the total contents of one capsule weigh 360 mg; then $100/300 = x/360$; $x = 120$ mg of active drug powder required from the capsule contents to provide 100 mg active drug) and sufficient lactose added to fill the capsule. The total filled capsule contents weigh 200 mg. The weight of the active drug powder is subtracted from 200 mg to obtain the amount of lactose required per capsule, which is 200 mg − 120 mg = 80 mg. This is multiplied by 51 capsules. Enough lactose (51 capsules × 80 mg/cap = 4.08 g) is added to make a total of 10.2 g of powder. The powders are combined, using geometric dilution, and 50 capsules can be punched out. Each capsule should weigh 200 mg (10.2 g/51 caps).

2. Example 2
  a. Medication order. This order is for veterinary use only.

Castor oil	8 mL
Disp	12 caps
Sig:	2 caps p.o. h.s.

  b. Calculations. No calculations are necessary.

AQ3

    c. Compounding procedure. A no. 11 veterinary capsule is used. Using a calibrated dropper or a pipette, 8 mL of the oil is carefully added to the inside of each capsule body. Next, the lower inside portion of the cap is moistened, using a glass rod or brush. The cap and body are joined together, using a twisting motion, to form a tight seal. The capsules are placed on a piece of filter paper and checked for signs of leakage. The capsules are dispensed in the appropriate size and type of prescription vial. They can be stored in a refrigerator if desired.

VIII. MOLDED TABLETS (TABLET TRITURATES)

A. Definition. Tablet triturates are small, usually cylindrical molded or compressed tablets. They are made of powders created by moistening the powder mixture with alcohol and water or by the process of sintering. They can be used for compounding potent drugs in small doses and for preparation of a rapidly disintegrating/dissolving dosage form.

B. Formulation and preparation of tablet triturates using moistened powders

1. Tablet triturates are made in special molds consisting of a pegboard and a corresponding perforated plate.

2. In addition to the mold, a diluent, usually a mixture of lactose and sucrose (80:20), and a moistening agent, usually a mixture of ethyl alcohol and water (60:40), are required.

3. The diluent is triturated with the active ingredients.

4. A paste is then made, using the alcohol and water mixture.

5. This paste is spread into the mold; the tablets are punched out and remain on the pegs until dry.

C. Example

   1. Medication order

Atropine sulfate	0.4 mg
Disp	#500 TT
Sig:	u.d.

   2. Calculations. For 500 TT: 500 × 0.4 mg = 200 mg atropine sulfate

   3. Compounding procedure. The mold prepares 70-mg tablets. The 200 mg of atropine sulfate, 6.8 g of sucrose, and 28 g of lactose are weighed and mixed by geometric dilution. The powder is wet with a mixture of 40% purified water and 60% ethyl alcohol (95%). The paste that is formed is spread onto the tablet triturate mold; the tablets are then punched out of the mold and allowed to dry on the pegs. This procedure is repeated until the required number of tablet triturates has been prepared.

D. Formulation and preparation of tablet triturates using sintering

1. These tablet triturates are made in special molds consisting of materials that can tolerate heat to about 100°C.

2. In addition to the mold, a diluent, usually a mixture of active drug and diluent, which make up approximately 65% of the tablet weight, are blended together. Mannitol is good to use in combination with lactose for particle sizes of 60–80 mesh fraction.

3. The mixture is triturated with polyethylene glycol 3350 with a particle size of 80–100 mesh fraction.

4. The powder mixture is placed into appropriate molds and lightly tamped.

5. The molds containing the powder are placed in an oven at about 90°C for 10–20 min, removed and allowed to cool. Depending on the molds used, the tablets can be dispensed in the molds or removed from the molds and packaged and labeled.

E. Example

6. Medication order

Homatropine hydrobromide	300 mg
Mannitol	3.5 g
Lactose	3.47 g
Flavor (dry powder type), qs	
Polyethylene glycol 3350	3.5 g

7. **Calculations.** As presented, this formula is for 100 rapid-dissolving tablet triturates.

8. **Compounding procedure.** Blend the homatropine hydrobromide, mannitol, lactose, and dry flavor together until fine and uniformly mixed. Separately, reduce the particle size of the polyethylene glycol 3350 to 100–200 mesh fraction. Lightly blend in the polyethylene glycol 3350 into the previously blended powders. Place 100 mg of the powder into the cavities of a mold (some blister packs work well; otherwise, obtain a tablet triturate mold or a special mold for preparing these tablets). Place the mold containing the powder in an oven at 80–90°C for 15–20 min. The time depends on the mold, formulation, oven, etc. Remove from the oven and place in a refrigerator for approximately 5 min. Remove from the refrigerator and let set at room temperature. Package and label.

IX. OINTMENTS, CREAMS, PASTES, AND GELS

A. Definitions

1. **Ointments, creams, and pastes** are semisolid dosage forms intended for topical application to the skin or mucous membranes. **Ointments** are characterized as being oleaginous in nature; **creams** are generally o/w or w/o emulsions, and **pastes** are characterized by their high content of solids (about 25%).

2. **Gels** (sometimes called jellies) are semisolid systems consisting of suspensions made up of either small inorganic particles or large organic molecules interpenetrated by a liquid.

B. General characteristics. These dosage forms are semisolid preparations generally applied externally. Semisolid dosage forms may contain active drugs intended to:

1. Act solely on the surface of the skin to produce a local effect (e.g., antifungal agent; topicals)

2. Release the medication, which, in turn, penetrates into the skin (e.g., hydrocortisone cream)

3. Release medication for systemic absorption through the skin (e.g., nitroglycerin; transdermals)

C. Types of ointment bases

1. Hydrophobic bases feel greasy and contain mixtures of fats, oils, and waxes. Hydrophobic bases cannot be washed off using water.

2. Hydrophilic bases are usually emulsion bases. The o/w-type emulsion bases can be easily washed off with water, but the w/o type is slightly more difficult to remove.

D. Preparation of ointments, creams, pastes, and gels

1. Mixing can be done in a mortar or on an ointment slab or tile.

2. Liquids are incorporated by gradually adding them to an absorption-type base and mixing.

3. Insoluble powders are reduced to a fine powder and then added to the base, using geometric dilution.

4. Water-soluble substances are dissolved with water and then incorporated into the base.

5. The final preparation should be smooth (impalpable) and free of any abrasive particles.

E. Examples

1. Example 1
a. Medication order

Sulfur
Salicylic acid, aa   600 mg
White petrolatum, ad   30 g
Sig: Apply t.i.d.

b. Compounding procedure. The particle sizes of the sulfur and salicylic acid are reduced separately in a Wedgwood mortar and then blended together. Using a pill tile, the powder mixture is levigated with the base. Using geometric dilution, the base and powders are blended to the final weight. An ointment jar or plastic tube is used for dispensing, and an "external use only" label is placed on the container.
c. Alternate method. Suppose you have sulfur 5% in white petrolatum ointment and a salicylic acid 5% ointment. **How can you prepare the prescription using these and diluting with white petrolatum?**

Using alligation

5   2 parts of the 5% ointment

2

0   3 parts of the white petrolatum or diluent (may also include other ointment)

However, since we are using two different 5% ointments, 2 parts of each, this leaves 1 part for the white petrolatum. A total of 5 parts is to be used to make 30 g (6 g per part): 2 parts (12 g) of the sulfur 5%, 2 parts (12 g) of the salicylic acid 5%, and 1 part (6 g) of the white petrolatum could be used. To check:

$$12 \text{ g} \times 0.05 = 600 \text{ mg of sulfur}$$
$$12 \text{ g} \times 0.05 = 600 \text{ mg of salicylic acid}$$
$$12 \text{ g} + 12 \text{ g} + 6 \text{ g} = 30 \text{ g}$$

2. Example 2
a. Medication order

Methylparaben   0.25 g
Propylparaben   0.15 g
Sodium lauryl sulfate   10 g
Propylene glycol   120 g
Stearyl alcohol   250 g
White petrolatum   250 g
Purified water   370 g
Disp   60 g
Sig: Apply u.d.

b. Calculations. The quantity of each ingredient required to prepare 60 g is obtained as follows. The medication order is for 1000 g; therefore, the multiplication factor is 60/1000 = 0.06.

$$0.25 \text{ g} \times 0.06 = 0.15 \text{ g methylparaben}$$
$$0.15 \text{ g} \times 0.06 = 0.009 \text{ g propylparaben}$$
$$10 \text{ g} \times 0.06 = 0.6 \text{ g sodium lauryl sulfate}$$
$$120 \text{ g} \times 0.06 = 7.2 \text{ g propylene glycol}$$
$$250 \text{ g} \times 0.06 = 15 \text{ g stearyl alcohol}$$
$$250 \text{ g} \times 0.06 = 15 \text{ g white petrolatum}$$
$$370 \text{ g} \times 0.06 = 22.2 \text{ g purified water}$$

Since the 0.009 g of propylparaben is too small to accurately weigh, a dilution can be prepared as follows, assuming a minimum weighable quantity of 120 mg. Weigh 120 mg of propylparaben and add to 40 mL of propylene glycol, resulting in a propylparaben concentration of 3 mg/mL. Take 3 mL of this solution to obtain the propylparaben and subtract the 3 mL from the quantity of propylene glycol required in the formula.

    c. Compounding procedure. The stearyl alcohol and the white petrolatum are melted on a steam bath and heated to about 75°C. The other ingredients, previously dissolved in purified water at about 78°C, are added. The mixture is stirred until it congeals. An ointment jar is used for dispensing, and an "external use only" label is placed on the jar.

3. Example 3
a. Medication order

Scopolamine hydrobromide	0.25%
Soy lecithin	12 g
Isopropyl palmitate	12 g
Pluronic F-127 20% gel, qs	100 mL
Sig:	Apply 0.1 mL t.i.d.

    b. Calculations. The quantity of scopolamine hydrobromide required for the prescription will be

$$0.0025 \times 100 \text{ mL} = 0.25 \text{ g or } 250 \text{ mg}$$

    c. Compounding procedure. Mix the soy lecithin with the isopropyl palmitate. Dissolve the scopolamine hydrobromide in about 3 mL of purified water and add to about 70 mL of the Pluronic F-127 gel. Add the soy lecithin–isopropyl palmitate mixture, and mix well. Add sufficient Pluronic F-127 gel to volume, and mix well using a shearing technique. Package and label.

X. SUPPOSITORIES

A. General characteristics

    1. Suppositories are **solid bodies** of various weights and shapes, adapted for introduction into the rectal, vaginal, or urethral orifices of the human body. They are used to deliver drugs for their local or systemic effects.

    2. Suppositories differ in **size** and **shape** and include
      a. Rectal
      b. Vaginal
      c. Urethral

B. Common suppository bases

    1. Cocoa butter (theobroma oil), which melts at body temperature, is a fat-soluble mixture of triglycerides that is most often used for rectal suppositories. Witepsol is a synthetic triglyceride. Fatty acid bases include Fattibase.

    2. Polyethylene glycol (PEG, carbowax) derivatives are water-soluble bases suitable for vaginal and rectal suppositories. Polybase is an example.

    3. Glycerinated gelatin is a water-miscible base often used in vaginal and rectal suppositories.

C. Suppository molds

    1. Suppository molds can be made of rubber, plastic, brass, stainless steel, or other suitable material.

    2. The formulation and volume of the base depend on the size of the mold used, less the displacement caused by the active ingredient.

D. Methods of preparing and dispensing suppositories

    1. Molded suppositories are prepared by first melting the base and then incorporating the medications uniformly into the base. This mixture is then poured into the suppository mold (fusion method).

2. **Hand-rolled suppositories** require a special technique. With proper technique, it is possible to make a preparation equal in quality to the molded suppositories.

3. **Containers for the suppositories** are determined by the method and base used in preparation. Hand-rolled and molded suppositories should be dispensed in special boxes that prevent the suppositories from coming in contact with each other. Suppositories made using plastic strip molds are easily dispensed in various types of packages.

4. **Storage conditions.** If appropriate, a "refrigerate" label should appear on the container. Regardless of the base or medication used in the formulation, the patient should be instructed to store the suppositories in a cool, dry place.

E. **Examples**

1. **Example 1**
    a. **Medication order**

Naproxen suppository	500 mg
Disp	#12
Sig:	Insert u.d. into rectum

    b. **Calculations.** Each standard adult suppository should weigh 2 g, but it depends on the mold used and should be calibrated before compounding. Also, the displacement must be determined for the added powder.

    2 g (total weight) − 0.540 g (weight of base displaced by the 500-mg tablet) per suppository

    = 1.46 g cocoa butter per suppository × 13 suppositories
    = 18.98 g cocoa butter

    c. **Compounding procedure.** The 13 naproxen 500-mg tablets are triturated to a fine powder, using a Wedgwood or porcelain mortar. The 18.98 g cocoa butter base is melted in a beaker, using a water bath. The temperature of the water bath should not exceed 36°C. The powder is then added and stirred until mixed. The mixture is poured into an appropriate rectal suppository mold (about 2 g per suppository) and placed into a refrigerator until the suppositories congeal. Any excess is scraped from the top of the mold, and a suppository box is used for dispensing. A "refrigerate" label is placed on the box.

2. **Example 2**
    a. **Medication order**

Progesterone	50 mg
Disp	#14
Sig:	1 per vagina once daily on days 14–28 of cycle

    b. **Calculations.** Total weight of each vaginal suppository is 1.9 g. Assuming 50 mg progesterone displaces 50 mg PEG base:

    50 mg progesterone/suppository × 15 = 750 mg progesterone
    1.9 g (total weight) − 0.050 g progesterone
    = 1.85 g PEG × 15 suppositories
    = 27.75 g PEG total

    c. **Compounding procedure.** The PEG is melted to 55–57°C, and 750 mg progesterone is added. This mixture is poured into a vaginal suppository mold, allowed to cool, cleaned, and dispensed.

XI. PARENTERAL PREPARATIONS

A. **General requirements.** The extemporaneous compounding of sterile preparations occurs in many pharmacy environments, including community, home healthcare, hospital, and nuclear. Minimum requirements include

1. Proper equipment and supplies

2. Proper facilities, including a laminar-flow clean bench and a clean room or isolation barrier technology equipment

3. Proper documentation of all preparations made

4. Quality control, including batch sterility testing

5. Proper storage both at the facility and in transport to the patient's home

6. Proper labeling of the prescription preparation

7. Knowledge of product's/preparation's stability and incompatibilities

8. Knowledge of all ancillary equipment involved in compounding or delivery of the medications

B. **Compounding of parenteral preparations**

1. Compounding of sterile preparations, including intravenous admixtures, requires special skills and training. Compounding parenteral preparations or providing this service without proper training should not be attempted.

2. These preparations must be compounded in a clean environment, using aseptic technique (i.e., working under controlled conditions to minimize contamination).

3. Dry powders of parenteral drugs for reconstitution are used for drug products or preparations that are unstable as solutions. It is important to know the correct diluents that can be used to yield a solution.

4. Solutions of drugs for parenteral administration may also be further diluted before administration. If further dilution is required, then the pharmacist must know the stability and compatibility of the drug in the diluent.

C. **Reconstitution of a dry powder from a vial**

1. Work takes place in a clean-air environment, observing aseptic technique.

2. The manufacturer's instructions should be checked to determine the required volume of diluent.

3. The appropriate needle size and syringe are chosen, keeping in mind that the capacity of the syringe should be slightly larger than the volume required for reconstitution.

4. Using the correct diluent, the surface of the container is cleaned, using an alcohol prep pad, after which the alcohol is permitted to evaporate.

5. The syringe is filled with the diluent to the proper volume.

6. The surface of the vial containing the sterile powder is cleaned, using an alcohol prep pad, after which it is permitted to dry. The diluent is injected into the vial containing the dry powder.

7. The vial is gently shaken or rolled, and the powder is allowed to dissolve.

8. After the powder has dissolved, the vial is inverted and the desired volume is withdrawn.

9. The vehicle is prepared by swabbing the medication port of the bag or bottle with an alcohol prep pad.

10. The solution in the syringe is injected into the vehicle. If a plastic container is used, care must be taken not to puncture the side walls of the container with the tip of the needle.

11. The container should be shaken or kneaded or rotated to ensure thorough mixing of the contents.

12. The contents of the container should be checked for particulate matter.

13. A sterile seal or cap is applied over the port of the container.

14. All needles and syringes should be properly discarded.

15. The bag is labeled.

D. Removing the fluid contents from an ampule

1. The ampule is held upright to open it, and the top is tapped to remove any solution trapped in this area.

2. The neck of the ampule is swabbed with an alcohol swab.

3. The ampule is grasped on each side of the neck with the thumb and index finger of each hand and quickly snapped open.

4. A 5-μm filter needle is attached to a syringe of the appropriate size.

5. The ampule is tilted, and the needle is inserted.

6. The needle is positioned near the neck of the ampule, and the solution is withdrawn from the ampule.

7. If the solution is for an intravenous push (bolus injection), the filter needle is removed from the syringe and replaced with a cap.

8. If the solution is for an intravenous infusion, then the filter needle is removed and replaced with a new needle of the appropriate size. The drug is injected into the appropriate vehicle.

9. All materials should be discarded properly, and the final product or preparation should be labeled.

E. Removing drug solution from a vial

1. The tab around the rubber closure on the vial is removed, and this surface is swabbed with an alcohol prep pad.

2. An equivalent amount of sterile air is injected into the vial to prevent a negative vacuum from being created and to allow the drug to be removed.

3. Using the appropriate needle size and syringe, the needle is inserted into the rubber closure.

4. The plunger is pushed down, and air is released into the vial; when the plunger is pulled back, the solution is withdrawn.

5. The solution is then injected into the appropriate vehicle.

F. Examples

1. Example 1
a. Medication order

Progesterone	5 g
Benzyl alcohol	10 mL
Sesame oil, qs	100 mL

b. Compounding procedure. Dissolve the progesterone in the benzyl alcohol. Add sufficient sesame oil to make 100 mL. Sterilize by filtration through a sterile 0.2-μm filter or by dry heat (170°C for 1.5 hr). Package in sterile vials and label.

2. Example 2
a. Medication order

Fentanyl (as the citrate)	2 mg
Bupivacaine hydrochloride	125 mg
0.9% sodium chloride injection, qs	100 mL

b. Calculations. Since 157 μg fentanyl citrate is equivalent to 100 μg fentanyl, the quantity of fentanyl citrate required is (157/100) × 2 mg = 3.14 mg fentanyl citrate. This is the quantity of fentanyl citrate that would be required if compounding as a high-risk preparation from bulk powders. It would also require 125 mg bupivacaine, and the remainder is the 0.9% sodium chloride injection. However, commercial products are available so we can calculate how much of each might be required using fentanyl 50 μg/mL injection and bupivacaine hydrochloride 0.5% injection.

$$2 \text{ mg fentanyl} = 2{,}000 \text{ μg}$$

$$\frac{2000 \text{ μg}}{50 \text{ μg/mL}} = 40 \text{ mL of fentanyl injection}$$

Bupivacaine hydrochloride 0.5% injection contains 500 mg/100 mL; therefore,

$$\frac{500}{100} = \frac{125}{x}; \; x = 25 \text{ mL}$$

If 40 mL of fentanyl injection is used, and 25 mL of bupivacaine hydrochloride injection is used, then 40 + 25 = 65 mL; the quantity of 0.9% sodium chloride injection required is 100 mL − 65 mL = 35 mL. Note: **If the order is to be filled in a 20-mL pump with delivery for 30 days, what is the delivery rate in μL/hr?**

$$\frac{20 \text{ mL}}{30 \text{ days}} = 0.667 \text{ mL/day}$$

$$\frac{0.667 \text{ mL/day}}{24 \text{ hr}} = 0.0277 \text{ mL/hr}$$

$$0.0277 \text{ mL} \times 1000 \text{ μL/mL} = 27.7 \text{ μL/hr}$$

   c. **Compounding procedure.** Using commercially available injections, accurately measure the volume of each and fill into a sterile ambulatory pump reservoir. An air bubble can be injected and used to thoroughly mix the solution. Remove the air from the reservoir, and tightly seal/close the outlet. Label.

3. Example 3
   a. **Medication order**

Morphine sulfate	5 g
Citric acid	100 mg
Sodium chloride, qs to isotonic	
Methylparaben	150 mg
Sterile water for injection, qs	100 mL

   b. **Calculations.** Using a sodium chloride equivalent of 0.09 for a 5% morphine sulfate solution, 0.18 for citric acid, 1 for sodium chloride, and ignoring the methylparaben, the calculations can be made as follows:

5 g morphine sulfate is equivalent to 450 mg sodium chloride (5 g × 0.09 = 450 mg). 100 mg citric acid is equivalent to 18 mg sodium chloride (100 mg × 0.18 = 18)

$$450 \text{ mg} + 18 \text{ mg} = 468 \text{ mg}$$

To be isotonic, the solution needs the equivalent of 900 mg of sodium chloride in the 100 mL: 900 mg − 468 mg = 432 mg sodium chloride needs to be added.

   c. **Compounding procedure.** Dissolve the methylparaben in about 90 mL of sterile water for injection. A small amount of heat may be required. Cool the solution to room temperature; then add the morphine sulfate, citric acid, and sodium chloride. Add sufficient sterile water for injection to volume and mix well. Sterilize by filtration through a sterile 0.2-μm filter into a sterile vial or reservoir. Package and label.

4. Example 4
   a. **Medication order**

Mefoxitin	1 g
Diluent to final concentration of 125 mg/mL	

   b. **Calculations.** A 1-g vial of Mefoxin (cefoxitin for injection) is reconstituted with 10 mL of diluent to provide for approximate withdrawal of 10.5 mL and an approximate average concentration of 95 mg/mL. **What quantity of diluent should be added to provide an approximate average concentration of 125 mg/mL?**

$$10.5 \text{ mL} - 10 \text{ mL} = 0.5 \text{ mL occupied by the powder}$$

$$\frac{1000 \text{ mg}}{125 \text{ mg/mL}} = 8 \text{ mL total volume}$$

$$8 \text{ mL} - 0.5 \text{ mL} = 7.5 \text{ mL diluent to be added}$$

   c. **Compounding procedure.** Aseptically, withdraw 7.5 mL of diluent and inject into the vial to be reconstituted, using an appropriate vented needle. Gently swirl until dissolved.

STUDY QUESTIONS

Directions for questions 1–3: Each question or incomplete statement in this section can be correctly answered or completed by **one** of the suggested answers or phrases. Choose the **best** answer.
The following medication order is given to the pharmacist by the physician.

Olive oil	60.0 mL
Vitamin A	60,000 units
Water	120.0 mL
Sig:	15 mL t.i.d.

1. The final dosage form of this prescription will be

(A) a solution.
(B) an elixir.
(C) an emulsion.
(D) a suspension.
(E) a lotion.

2. When preparing this prescription, the pharmacist needs to add

(A) Tween 80.
(B) acacia.
(C) glycerin.
(D) alcohol.
(E) propylene glycol.

3. Which of the following caution labels should the pharmacist affix to the container when dispensing this preparation?

(A) Do not refrigerate.
(B) Shake well.
(C) For external use only.
(D) No preservatives added.

Directions for questions 4–9: Each question or statement in this section can be correctly answered or completed by **one or more** of the suggested answers or phrases. Choose the correct answer, A–E:

A	if **I only** is correct
B	if **III only** is correct
C	if **I and II** are correct
D	if **II and III** are correct
E	if **I, II, and III** are correct

4. Which statements about the following prescription are correct?

Morphine	1 mg/mL
Flavored vehicle, qs ad	120 mL
Sig:	5–20 mg p.o. q 3–4 hours prn pain

I. The amount of morphine needed is 240 mg.
II. Powdered morphine alkaloid should be used when compounding this prescription.
III. The final dosage form of this prescription is a solution.

5. When preparing the following prescription, the pharmacist should

Podophyllum	5%
Salicylic acid	10%
Acetone	20%
Flexible collodion, ad	30 mL
Sig:	Apply q h.s.

I. triturate 1.5 g of podophyllum with the 8 mL of acetone.
II. add 3 g of salicylic acid to the collodion with trituration.
III. affix an "external use only" label to the container.

6. Which statements about the following prescription are correct?

Sulfur	6 g
Purified water	
Camphor water, aa qs ad	60

   I. Precipitated sulfur can be used to prepare this prescription.
   II. The sulfur can be triturated with glycerin before mixing with other ingredients.
   III. A "shake well" label should be affixed to the bottle.

7. Which statements about the following prescription are correct?

Starch	10%
Menthol	1%
Camphor	2%
Calamine, qs ad	120

   I. The powders should be blended together in a mortar, using geometric dilution.
   II. The prescription should be prepared by dissolving the camphor in a sufficient amount of 90% alcohol.
   III. A eutectic mixture should be avoided.

8. When preparing the following prescription, the pharmacist should

Salicylic acid	3 g
Sulfur ppt	7 g
Lanolin	10 g
White petrolatum	10 g

   I. reduce the particle size of the powders, using a mortar and pestle or using the pill tile with a spatula.
   II. place on an ointment tile and levigate the ingredients, using geometric dilution.
   III. package the ointment in an ointment jar or tube.

9. An equal volume of air is injected when removing drug solutions from

   I. vials.
   II. ampules.
   III. syringes.

ANSWERS AND EXPLANATIONS

1. The answer is C *[see V.B.1.].*

2. The answer is B *[see V.B.2; V.C.1].*

3. The answer is B *[see V.B.3].*
For 1–3: Because olive oil and water are two immiscible liquids, their incorporation requires a two-phase system in which one liquid is dispersed throughout another liquid in the form of small droplets. To accomplish this, an emulsifying agent is necessary. Acacia is the most suitable emulsifying agent when forming an oil-in-water emulsion that is intended for internal use.

Emulsions are physically unstable, and they must be protected against the effects of microbial contamination and physical separation. Shaking before use redistributes the two layers of emulsion. Because light, air, and microorganisms also affect the stability of an emulsion, preservatives can be added.

4. The answer is B (III) *[see III.A.C.3].*
The concentration of morphine needed for the prescription described in the question is 1 mg/mL, and because 120 mL is the final volume, 120 mg of morphine is needed to compound this prescription. Morphine alkaloid has poor solubility; therefore, one of the salt forms should be used. Because morphine is dissolved in the vehicle, resulting in a liquid preparation, the final dosage form is a solution.

5. The answer is B (III) *[see III.C.1.; III.C.5; III.D.3].*
Calculating for the amount of each ingredient of the prescription in the question requires 1.5 g of podophyllum, 3 g of salicylic acid, and 6 mL of acetone. The correct procedure would be to triturate the podophyllum with the acetone, then add the triturated salicylic acid to a calibrated bottle containing the podophyllum and acetone. Flexible collodion is then added up to the 30-mL calibration. An "external use only" label should be affixed to the container.

6. The answer is E (I, II, and III) *[see IV.B.2; IV.C.5; IV.D.1–2].*
While precipitated sulfur can be used to prepare the prescription described in the question, it is difficult to triturate; therefore, it must first be levigated with a suitable levigating agent (e.g., glycerin). All suspensions, owing to their instability, require shaking before use to redistribute the insoluble ingredients.

7. The answer is A (I) *[see VI.C.3; VI.D.1].*
The proper procedure for compounding the prescription described in the question is to first form a liquid eutectic. This is done by triturating the menthol and camphor together in a mortar. This eutectic is then blended with the powdered starch and calamine, using geometric dilution.

8. The answer is E (I, II, and III) *[see IX.D.1–3; IX.E.1].*
The proper procedure for preparing the prescription given in the question is to reduce the particle size of each powder and mix them together, using geometric dilution. This ensures the proper blending of the powders. Next, this powdered mixture is incorporated, geometrically, with the petrolatum. Then, the lanolin is added geometrically.

9. The answer is A (I) *[see XI.E.2].*
An equal volume of air must be injected when removing a drug solution from a vial. This is done to prevent the formation of a vacuum within the vial. This problem does not occur with ampules and syringes containing drug solutions; therefore, it is unnecessary to inject any air when removing them.

6
Basic Pharmacokinetics

Riccardo L. Boni

Leon Shargel

I. PHARMACOKINETICS

A. INTRODUCTION

1. **Rates and orders of reactions.** The **rate** of a chemical reaction or pharmacokinetic process is the velocity with which it occurs. **The order** of a reaction is the way in which the concentration of a drug or reactant in a chemical reaction affects the rate.

   a. **Zero-order reaction.** The drug concentration changes with respect to time at a constant rate, according to the following equation:

   $$\frac{dC}{dt} = -k_0$$

   where C is the drug concentration and k_0 is the **zero-order rate constant** expressed in units of concentration per time (e.g., milligrams per milliliter per hour). Integration of this equation yields the linear (straight-line) equation:

   $$C = -k_0 t + C_0$$

   where k_0 is the slope of the line (see Figure 3-5) and C_0 is the y intercept, or drug concentration, when time (t) equals zero. The negative sign indicates that the slope is decreasing.

   b. **First-order reaction.** The change in drug concentration with respect to time equals the product of the rate constant and the concentration of drug remaining, according to the following equation:

   $$\frac{dC}{dt} = -kC$$

   where k is the first-order rate constant, expressed in units of reciprocal time, or time^{-1} (e.g., 1/hr or hr^{-1}).

   (1) Integration of this equation yields the following mathematically equivalent equations:

   $$C = C_0 e^{-kt}$$
   $$\ln C = -kt + \ln C_0$$

   $$\log C = \frac{-kt}{2.3} + \log C_0$$

   (2) A graph of the equation in Figure 6-1 shows the linear relation of the log of the concentration versus time. In Figure 6-1, the slope of the line is equal to $-k/2.3$, and the y intercept is C_0. The values for C are plotted on logarithmic coordinates, and the values for t are shown on linear coordinates.

   (3) The **half-life ($t_{1/2}$)** of a reaction or process is the time required for the concentration of a drug to decrease by one half. For a first-order reaction or process, the half-life is a constant and is related to the first-order rate constant, according to the following equation:

   $$t_{1/2} = \frac{0.693}{k}$$

2. **Models and compartments**

   a. A **model** is a mathematic description of a biologic system and is used to express quantitative relationships.

b. A **compartment** is a group of tissues with similar blood flow and drug affinity. A compartment is not a real physiologic or anatomic region.

3. Drug distribution
  a. Drugs distribute rapidly to tissues with high blood flow and more slowly to tissues with low blood flow.
  b. Drugs rapidly cross capillary membranes into tissues because of **passive diffusion** and **hydrostatic pressure. Drug permeability** across capillary membranes varies.
    (1) Drugs easily cross the capillaries of the glomerulus of the kidney and the sinusoids of the liver.
    (2) The capillaries of the brain are surrounded by glial cells that create a **blood–brain barrier,** which acts as a thick lipid membrane. Polar and ionic hydrophilic drugs cross this barrier slowly.
  c. Drugs may accumulate in tissues as a result of their physicochemical characteristics or special affinity of the tissue for the drug.
    (1) Lipid-soluble drugs may accumulate in adipose (fat) tissue because of partitioning of the drug.
    (2) Tetracycline may accumulate in bone because complexes are formed with calcium.
  d. Plasma protein binding of drugs affects drug distribution.
    (1) A drug bound to a protein forms a complex that is too large to cross cell membranes.
    (2) Albumin is the major plasma protein involved in drug protein binding. α_1-**Glycoprotein,** also found in plasma, is important for the binding of such basic drugs as propranolol.
    (3) Potent drugs, such as phenytoin, that are highly bound ($> 90\%$) to plasma proteins may be displaced by other highly bound drugs. The displacement of the bound drug results in more free (nonbound) drug, which rapidly reaches the drug receptors and causes a more intense pharmacologic response.

B. One-compartment model

  1. Intravenous bolus injection. The entire drug dose enters the body rapidly, and the rate of absorption is neglected in calculations (Figure 6-1). The entire body acts as a single compartment, and the drug rapidly equilibrates with all of the tissues in the body.
    a. Drug elimination is a first-order kinetic process, according to the equations in I.A.1.b.
      (1) The first-order elimination rate constant (k or k_{el}) is the sum of the rate constants for removal of drug from the body, including the rate constants for renal excretion and metabolism (**biotransformation**) as described by the following equation:

$$k = k_e + k_m$$

where k_e is the rate constant for renal excretion and k_m is the rate constant for metabolism. This equation assumes that all rates are first-order processes.

      (2) The **elimination half-life ($t_{1/2}$)** is given by the following equation:

$$t_{1/2} = \frac{0.693}{k}$$

    b. Apparent volume of distribution (V_D) is the hypothetical volume of body fluid in which the drug is dissolved. This value is not a true anatomic or physical volume.
      (1) V_D is needed to estimate the amount of drug in the body relative to the concentration of drug in the plasma, as shown in the following:

$$V_D \times C_p = D_B$$

where V_D is the apparent volume of distribution, C_p is the plasma drug concentration, and D_B is the amount of drug in the body.

      (2) To calculate the V_D after an intravenous bolus injection, the equation is rearranged to give:

$$V_D = \frac{D_B^0}{C_P^0}$$

where D_B^0 is the dose (D_B) of drug given by intravenous bolus and C_P^0 is the extrapolated drug concentration at zero time on the y axis, after the drug equilibrates (Figure 6-1).

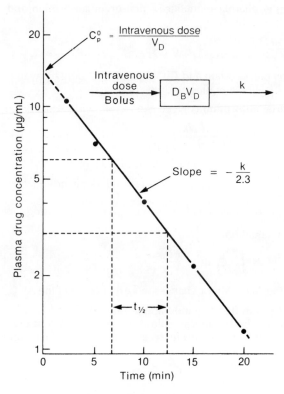

Figure 6-1. Generalized pharmacokinetic model for a drug administered by rapid intravenous bolus injection. C_P^0, extrapolated drug concentration; V_D, apparent volume of distribution; D_B, amount of drug in the body; k, elimination rate constant; $t_{1/2}$, elimination half-life. [Adapted with permission from Gibaldi M, Perrier D. Pharmacokinetics, 2nd ed. New York, Marcel Dekker, Inc., 1982. Copyright © 1982 Routledge/Taylor & Francis Group, LLC.]

(3) According to the equation, V_D is increased and C_P^0 is decreased when the drug is distributed more extravascularly into the tissues. When more drug is contained in the vascular space or plasma, C_P^0 is increased and V_D is decreased.

2. Single oral dose. If the drug is given in an oral dosage form (e.g., tablet, capsule), the drug is rapidly absorbed by first-order kinetics. Elimination of the drug also follows the principles of first-order kinetics (Figure 6-2).

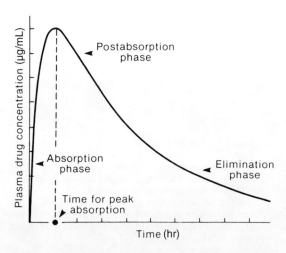

Figure 6-2. Generalized plot for a one-compartment model showing first-order drug absorption and first-order drug elimination. [Adapted with permission from Shargel L, Wu-Pong S, Yu ABC. Applied Biopharmaceutics and Pharmacokinetics, 5th ed. New York, McGraw-Hill, 2005.]

a. The following equation describes the pharmacokinetics of **first-order absorption and elimination:**

$$C_P = \frac{FD_0 k_A}{V_D(k_A - k)} (e^{-kt} - e^{-K_A t})$$

where k_A is the first-order absorption rate constant and F is the fraction of drug bioavailable. Changes in F, D_0, V_D, k_A, and k affect the plasma drug concentration.

b. The time for maximum, or **peak, drug absorption** is given by the following equations:

$$t_{max} = \frac{2.3 \log (k_A/k)}{k_A - k}$$

where t_{max} depends only on the rate constants k_A and k, not on F, D_0, or V_D.

c. After t_{max} is obtained, the peak drug concentration (C_{max}) is calculated, using the equation in I.B.2.a and substituting t_{max} for t.

d. The area under the curve (AUC) may be determined by integration of $\int_0^t C_P dt$ using the trapezoidal rule or by the following equation:

$$[AUC]_0^\infty = \int_0^\infty C_P \, dt = \frac{FD_0}{V_D k}$$

changes in F, D_0, k, and V_D affect the AUC. Minor changes in k_A do not affect the AUC.

e. To obtain $[AUC]_0^\infty$, obtain the [AUC] from 0 to t by the trapezoidal rule and add on the extrapolated section of AUC, which is the last measurable drug concentration at time t divided by the slope of the terminal elimination curve, as shown in the following equation:

$$[AUC]_0^\infty = [AUC]_0^t + \frac{C_{P,t}}{k}$$

f. **Lag time** occurs at the beginning of systemic drug absorption. For some individuals, systemic drug absorption is delayed after oral drug administration because of delayed stomach emptying or other factors.

3. Intravenous infusion

a. Intravenous infusion is an example of zero-order absorption and first-order elimination (Figure 6-3).

b. A few oral controlled-release drug products release the drug by zero-order kinetics and have **zero-order systemic absorption.**

Figure 6-3. Generalized semilogarithmic plot for a drug showing zero-order absorption and first-order elimination. C_{ss}, steady-state concentration; k, elimination rate constant. [Adapted with permission from Gibaldi M, Perrier D. Pharmacokinetics, 2nd ed. New York, Marcel Dekker, Inc., 1982. Copyright © 1982 Routledge/Taylor & Francis Group, LLC.]

c. The plasma drug concentration at any time after the start of an intravenous infusion is given by the following equation:

$$C_p = \frac{R}{V_D k}(1 - e^{-kt})$$

where R is the zero-order rate of infusion given in units as milligrams per hour or milligrams per minute.

d. If the intravenous infusion is discontinued, the plasma drug concentration declines by a first-order process. The elimination half-life, or elimination rate constant, k, may be obtained from the declining plasma drug concentration versus time curve.

e. As the drug is infused, the plasma drug concentration increases to a plateau, or **steady-state concentration (C_{ss}).**

   (1) Under steady-state conditions, the fraction of drug absorbed equals the fraction of drug eliminated from the body.

   (2) The plasma concentration at steady state (C_{ss}) is given by the following equation:

$$C_{ss} = \frac{R}{V_D k}$$

   (3) The rate of drug infusion (R) may be calculated from a rearrangement of the equation if the desired C_{ss}, the V_D, and the k are known. These values can often be obtained from the drug literature. To calculate the rate of infusion, the following equation is used:

$$R = C_{ss} V_D k$$

   where C_{ss} is the desired (target) plasma drug concentration. The product, $V_D k$, is also equal to total body clearance, Cl_T.

f. A **loading dose (D_L)** is given as an initial intravenous bolus dose to produce the C_{ss} as rapidly as possible. The intravenous infusion is started at the same time as the D_L.

   (1) The time to reach C_{ss} depends on the elimination half-life of the drug. Reaching 90%, 95%, or 99% of the C_{ss} without a D_L takes 3.32, 4.32, or 6.65 half-lives, respectively. Thus, for a drug with an elimination $t_{1/2}$ of 8 hr, it will take 3.32×8 hr, or 26.56 hr, to reach 90% of C_{ss} if no loading dose is given.

   (2) The D_L is the amount of drug that, when dissolved in the apparent V_D, produces the desired C_{ss}. Thus D_L is calculated by the following equation:

$$D_L = C_{ss} V_D \text{ and } D_L = \frac{R}{k}$$

g. An intravenous infusion provides a relatively constant plasma drug concentration and is particularly useful for drugs that have a narrow therapeutic range. The IV infusion keeps the plasma drug concentration between the minimum toxic concentration (MTC) and the minimum effective concentration (MEC).

4. Intermittent intravenous infusions

  a. Intermittent intravenous infusions are infusions in which the drug is infused for short periods to prevent accumulation and toxicity.

  b. Intermittent intravenous infusions are used for a few drugs, such as the aminoglycosides. For example, gentamicin may be given as a 1-hr infusion every 12 hr. In this case, steady-state drug concentrations are not achieved.

  c. The peak drug concentration in the plasma for a drug given by intermittent intravenous infusion may be calculated by the following equation:

$$C_{p,\,n} = \frac{R(1 - e^{-kt})(1 - e^{-nk\tau})}{Cl(1 - e^{-k\tau})}$$

where $C_{p,n}$ is the peak drug concentration, R is the rate of drug infusion, Cl is total body clearance, k is the dosage interval, n is the number of infusions, t is the time for the infusion, and τ is the dosage interval.

5. Multiple doses. Many drugs are given intermittently in a multiple-dose regimen for continuous or prolonged therapeutic activity. This regimen is often used to treat chronic disease.

  a. If drug doses are given frequently before the previous dose is completely eliminated, then plasma drug concentrations accumulate and increase to a steady-state level.

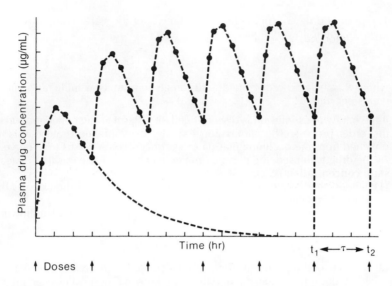

Figure 6-4. Generalized plot showing plasma drug concentration levels after administration of multiple doses and levels of accumulation when equal doses are given at equal time intervals. τ, time interval between doses (t), or the frequency of dosing. [Adapted with permission from Shargel L, Wu-Pong S, Yu ABC. Applied Biopharmaceutics and Pharmacokinetics, 5th ed. New York, McGraw-Hill, 2005]

 b. At **steady state,** plasma drug concentration fluctuates between a maximum (C_{max}^{∞}) and a minimum (C_{min}^{∞}) value (Figure 6-4).

 c. When a multiple-dose regimen is calculated, the **superposition principle** assumes that previous drug doses have no effect on subsequent doses. Thus the predicted plasma drug concentration is the total plasma drug concentration obtained by adding the residual drug concentrations found after each previous dose.

 d. When a multiple-dose regimen is designed, only the **dosing rate** (D_0/τ) can be adjusted easily.

  (1) The dosing rate is based on the **size of the dose** (D_0) and the **interval (τ) between doses,** or the **frequency of dosing.**

  (2) The dosing rate is given by the following equation:

$$\text{Dosing rate} = \frac{D_0}{\tau}$$

  (3) As long as the dosing rate is the same, the expected **average drug concentration at steady state (C_{Av}^{∞})** is the same (Figure 6-4).

   (a) For example, if a 600-mg dose is given every 12 hr, the dosing rate is 600 mg/ 12 hr, or 50 mg/hr.

   (b) A dose of 300 mg every 6 hr or 200 mg every 4 hr also gives the same dosing rate (50 mg/hr), with the same expected C_{Av}^{∞}. However, the C_{max}^{∞} and C_{min}^{∞} values will be different.

   (c) For a larger dose given over a longer interval (e.g., 600 mg every 12 hr), the C_{max}^{∞} is higher and the C_{min}^{∞} lower compared with a smaller dose given more frequently (e.g., 200 mg every 4 hr).

 e. Certain antibiotics are given by **multiple rapid intravenous bolus injections.**

  (1) The peak, or **maximum, serum drug concentration** at steady state may be estimated by the following equation:

$$C_{max}^{\infty} = \frac{\dfrac{D_0}{V_D}}{1 - e^{-k\tau}}$$

  (2) The **minimum serum drug concentration** (C_{min}^{∞}) at steady state is the drug concentration after the drug declines one dosage interval. Thus C_{min}^{∞} is determined by the following equation:

$$C_{min}^{\infty} = C_{max}^{\infty} \, e^{-kt}$$

(3) The **average drug concentration** (C_{Av}^{∞}) at steady state is estimated with the equation used for multiple oral doses:

$$C_{Av}^{\infty} = \frac{FD_O}{kV_D\tau}$$

For intravenous bolus injections, $F = 1$.

f. Orally administered drugs given in **immediate-release dosage forms** (e.g., solutions, conventional tablets, capsules) by multiple oral doses are usually rapidly absorbed and slowly eliminated $k_A \geq k$). C_{max}^{∞} and C_{min}^{∞} for these drugs are approximated by the equations shown in I.B.5.e.(1)–(2).

(1) For more exact calculations of C_{min}^{∞} and C_{max}^{∞} after multiple oral doses, the following equations are used:

$$C_{max}^{\infty} = \frac{FD_Ok_A}{V_D(k_A - k)}\left(\frac{1}{1 - e^{-k\tau}}\right) \text{ and }$$

$$C_{min}^{\infty} = \frac{FD_Ok_A}{V_D(k_A - k)}\left(\frac{1}{1 - e^{-k\tau}}\right)e^{-kt}$$

(2) The calculation of C_{Av}^{∞} is the same as for multiple intravenous bolus injections, using the equation shown in I.B.5.e.(3).

(3) The term $1/(1 - e^{-k\tau})$ is known as the **accumulation rate.**

(4) The fraction of drug remaining in the body (f) after a dosage interval is given by the following equation:

$$f = e^{-k\tau}$$

g. **Loading dose**. An initial loading dose (D_L) is given to obtain a therapeutic steady-state drug level quickly.

(1) For multiple oral doses, D_L is calculated by:

$$D_L = D_M\frac{1}{1 - e^{-k\tau}}$$

where D_M is the maintenance dose.

(2) If D_M is given at a dosage interval equal to the elimination half-life of the drug, then D_L equals twice the maintenance dose.

C. Multicompartment models

1. Drugs that exhibit multicompartment pharmacokinetics distribute into different tissue groups at different rates. Tissues with high blood flow equilibrate with a drug more rapidly than tissues with low blood flow. Drug concentration in various tissues depends on the physical and chemical characteristics of the drug and the nature of the tissue. For example, highly lipid-soluble drugs accumulate slowly in fat (lipid) tissue.

2. **Two-compartment model (intravenous bolus injection)**
   a. After an intravenous bolus injection, the drug distributes and equilibrates rapidly into highly perfused tissues (**central compartment**) and more slowly into peripheral tissues (**tissue compartment**).

b. The initial rapid decline in plasma drug concentration is known as the **distribution phase.** The slower rate of decline in drug concentration after complete equilibration is achieved is known as the **elimination phase** (Figure 6-5).

c. The **plasma drug concentration** at any time is the sum of two first-order processes, as given in the following equation:

$$C_p = Ae^{-at} + Be^{-bt}$$

where *a* and *b* are hybrid first-order rate constants and *A* and *B* are *y* intercepts.

(1) The **hybrid first-order rate constant *b*** is obtained from the slope of the elimination phase of the curve (Figure 6-5) and represents the first-order elimination of drug from the body after the drug equilibrates with all tissues.

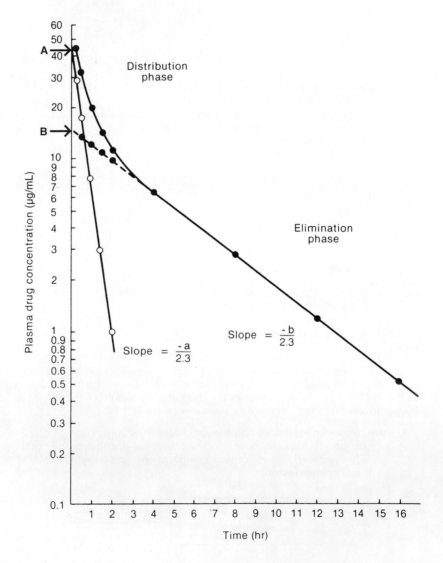

Figure 6-5. Generalized plot showing drug distribution and equilibration for a two-compartment model (intravenous bolus injection). The distribution phase is the initial rapid decline in plasma drug concentration. The elimination phase is the slower rate of decline after complete equilibration of the drug is achieved. [Adapted with permission from Shargel L, Wu-Pong S, Yu ABC. Applied Biopharmaceutics and Pharmacokinetics, 5th ed. New York, McGraw-Hill, 2005]

(2) The **hybrid first-order rate constant *a*** is obtained from the slope of the residual line of the distribution phase after the elimination phase is subtracted.

d. The **apparent volume of distribution** depends on the type of pharmacokinetic calculation. Volumes of distribution include the volume of the central compartment (V_p), the volume of distribution at steady state (V_{ss}), and the volume of the tissue compartment (V_t).

3. Two-compartment model (oral drug administration)

   a. A drug with a rapid distribution phase may not show two-compartment characteristics after oral administration. As the drug is absorbed, it equilibrates with the tissues so that the elimination half-life of the elimination portion of the curve equals $0.693/b$.

   b. Two-compartment characteristics are seen if the drug is absorbed rapidly and the distribution phase is slower.

4. Models with additional compartments

   a. The addition of each new compartment to the model requires an additional first-order plot.

   b. The addition of a third compartment suggests that the drug slowly equilibrates into a deep tissue space. If the drug is given at frequent intervals, the drug begins to accumulate into the third compartment.

   c. The terminal linear phase generally represents the elimination of the drug from the body after equilibration occurs. The rate constant from the elimination phase is used to calculate dosage regimens.

   d. Adequate pharmacokinetic description of multicompartment models is often difficult and depends on proper plasma sampling and determination of drug concentrations.

5. Elimination rate constants

   a. The elimination rate constant, k, represents drug elimination from the central compartment.

   b. The terminal elimination rate constant (b or λ in the two-compartment model) represents drug elimination after drug distribution is mostly completed.

D. Nonlinear pharmacokinetics are also known as capacity-limited, dose-dependent, or saturation pharmacokinetics. Nonlinear pharmacokinetics do not follow first-order kinetics as the dose increases (Figure 6-6). Nonlinear pharmacokinetics may result from the saturation of an enzyme- or carrier-mediated system.

   1. Characteristics of nonlinear pharmacokinetics include

   a. The AUC is not proportional to the dose.

Figure 6-6. Generalized plot showing plasma drug concentration versus time for a drug with Michaelis-Menten (nonlinear) elimination kinetics. For this one-compartment model (intravenous injection), the doses are 1 mg, 10 mg, and 100 mg; and the apparent in vivo rate constant (k_M) is 10 mg. The maximum velocity of the reaction (V_{max}) is 0.2 mg/min. [Adapted with permission from Gibaldi M, Perrier D. Pharmacokinetics, 2nd ed. New York, Marcel Dekker, Inc., 1982. Copyright © 1982 Routledge/Taylor & Francis Group, LLC.]

   b. The amount of drug excreted in the urine is not proportional to the dose.
   c. The elimination half-life may increase at high doses.
   d. The ratio of metabolites formed changes with increased dose.

2. Michaelis-Menten kinetics describe the velocity of enzyme reactions. Michaelis-Menten kinetics are used to describe nonlinear pharmacokinetics.
   a. The **Michaelis-Menten equation** describes the rate of change (velocity) of plasma drug concentration after an intravenous bolus injection, as follows:

$$\frac{dC_p}{dt} = \frac{-V_{max}C_p}{k_M + Cp}$$

   where V_{max} is the maximum velocity of the reaction, C_p is the substrate or plasma drug concentration, and k_M is the rate constant equal to the C_p at 0.5 V_{max}.

   b. At low C_p values, where $C_p << k_M$, this equation reduces to a first-order rate equation because both k_M and V_{max} are constants.

$$\frac{dC_p}{dt} = \frac{-V_{max}C_p}{k_M} = -k'C_p$$

   c. At high C_p values, where $C_p >> k_M$, the Michaelis-Menten equation is a zero-order rate equation, as follows:

$$\frac{dC_p}{dt} = -V_{max}$$

3. Drugs that follow nonlinear pharmacokinetics may show zero-order elimination rates at high drug concentrations, fractional-order elimination rates at intermediate drug concentrations, and first-order elimination rates at low drug concentrations (Figure 6-6).

E. Clearance is a measurement of drug elimination from the body. Units for clearance are volume per time (e.g., liters per hour).

1. Total body clearance (Cl_T) is the drug elimination rate divided by the plasma drug concentration. According to the concept of clearance, the body contains an apparent volume of distribution in which the drug is dissolved. A constant portion of this volume is cleared, or removed, from the body per unit time.
   a. The following equations express the measurement of total body clearance:

$$Cl_T = \frac{\text{drug elimination}}{\text{plasma drug concentration}} = \frac{(dDe/dt)}{Cp}$$

$$Cl_T = V_D k$$

$$Cl_T = \frac{FD_0}{AUC}$$

   b. For drugs that follow first-order (linear) pharmacokinetics, total body clearance is the sum of all the clearances in the body, as shown in the following equation:

$$CL_T = CL_R + Cl_{NR}$$

   where CL_R is renal clearance and Cl_{NR} is nonrenal clearance. Nonrenal clearance, Cl_{NR}, is often equated with hepatic clearance, Cl_H.

   c. The relation between Cl_T and $t_{1/2}$ is obtained by substituting $0.693/t_{1/2}$ for k in the equation in I.E.1 a to obtain the following expression:

$$t_{1/2} = \frac{0.693\,V_D}{Cl_T}$$

   where V_D and Cl_T are considered independent variables, and $t_{1/2}$ is considered a dependent variable.

   d. As clearance decreases (e.g., in renal disease), $t_{1/2}$ increases. Changes in V_D also cause proportional changes in $t_{1/2}$.

Figure 6-7. Generalized plot showing the excretion rate versus plasma drug concentration for a drug with active tubular secretion and for a drug secreted by glomerular filtration only. [Adapted with permission from Shargel L, Wu-Pong S, Yu ABC. Applied Biopharmaceutics and Pharmacokinetics, 5th ed. New York, McGraw-Hill, 2005]

2. **Renal drug excretion** is the major route of drug elimination for polar drugs, water-soluble drugs, drugs with low molecular weight (< 500), and drugs that are biotransformed slowly. The relation between the drug excretion rate and the plasma drug concentration is shown in Figure 6-7. Drugs are excreted through the kidney into the urine by glomerular filtration, tubular reabsorption, and active tubular secretion.

   a. **Glomerular filtration** is a passive process by which small molecules and drugs are filtered through the glomerulus of the nephron.
      (1) Drugs bound to plasma proteins are too large to be filtered at the glomerulus.
      (2) Drugs such as **creatinine and inulin** are not actively secreted or reabsorbed. They are used to measure the **glomerular filtration rate (GFR).**

   b. **Tubular reabsorption** is a passive process that follows Fick's law of diffusion.
      (1) Lipid-soluble drugs are reabsorbed from the lumen of the nephron back into the systemic circulation.
      (2) For weak electrolyte drugs, urine pH affects the ratio of nonionized and ionized drug.
         (a) If the drug exists primarily in the nonionized or lipid-soluble form, then it is reabsorbed more easily from the lumen of the nephron.
         (b) If the drug exists primarily in the ionized or water-soluble form, then it is excreted more easily in the urine.
         (c) Depending on the pK_a of the drug, alteration of urine pH alters the ratio of ionized to nonionized drug and affects the rate of drug excretion. For example, alkalinization of the urine by the administration of sodium bicarbonate increases the excretion of salicylates (weak acids) into the urine.
      (3) An increase in urine flow caused by simultaneous administration of a diuretic decreases the time for drug reabsorption. Consequently, more drug is excreted if given with a diuretic.

   c. **Active tubular secretion** is a carrier-mediated active transport system that requires energy.
      (1) Two active tubular secretion pathways exist in the kidney: one system for weak acids and one system for weak bases.
      (2) The active tubular secretion system shows competition effects. For example, **probenecid** (a weak acid) competes for the same system as penicillin, decreasing the rate of penicillin excretion, resulting in a longer penicillin $t_{1/2}$.
      (3) The renal clearance of drugs that are actively secreted, such as **p-aminohippurate (PAH),** is used to measure **effective renal blood flow (ERBF).**

3. **Renal clearance** is the volume of drug contained in the plasma that is removed by the kidney per unit time. **Units for renal clearance** are expressed in volume per time (e.g., milliliters per minute or liters per hour).

a. Renal clearance may be measured by dividing the rate of drug excretion by the plasma drug concentration, as shown in the following equation:

$$Cl_R = \frac{\text{rate of drug excretion}}{C_p} = \frac{\frac{dD_u}{dt}}{C_p}$$

b. Measurement of renal clearance may also be expressed by the following equation:

$$Cl_R = k_e V_D$$

where k_e is the first-order renal excretion rate constant and

$$Cl_R = \frac{D_u^{\infty}}{AUC}$$

where D_u^{∞} is the total amount of parent (unchanged) drug excreted in the urine.

c. Renal clearance is measured without regard to the physiologic mechanism of renal drug excretion. The probable mechanism for renal clearance is obtained with a **clearance ratio,** which relates drug clearance to inulin clearance (a measure of GFR).
   (1) If the clearance ratio is < 1.0, the mechanism for drug clearance may result from filtration plus reabsorption.
   (2) If the ratio is 1.0, the mechanism may be filtration only.
   (3) If the ratio is > 1.0, the mechanism may be filtration plus active tubular secretion.

4. Hepatic clearance is the volume of plasma containing drug that is cleared by the liver per unit time.
   a. Measurement of hepatic clearance. Hepatic clearance is usually measured indirectly, as the difference between total body clearance and renal clearance, as shown in the following equation:

$$Cl_H = Cl_T - Cl_R$$

where Cl_H is the hepatic clearance. Hepatic clearance is generally considered to be equivalent to Cl_{NR}, or nonrenal drug clearance. Hepatic clearance can also be calculated as the **product of the liver blood flow (Q)** and the **extraction ratio (ER),** as shown in the following equation:

$$Cl_H = Q(ER)$$

   (1) The **extraction ratio** is the fraction of drug that is irreversibly removed by an organ or tissue as the plasma-containing drug perfuses that tissue.
   (2) The extraction ratio is obtained by measuring the plasma drug concentration entering the liver and the plasma drug concentration exiting the liver:

$$ER = \frac{C_a - C_v}{C_a}$$

where C_a is the arterial plasma drug concentration entering the liver and C_v is the venous plasma drug concentration exiting the liver.

   (3) Values for the ER range from 0 to 1. For example, if the ER is 0.9, then 90% of the incoming drug is removed as the plasma perfuses the liver. If the ER is 0, then no drug is removed by the liver.

   b. Blood flow, intrinsic clearance, and **protein binding** affect hepatic clearance.
   (1) Blood flow to the liver is approximately 1.5 L/min and may be altered by exercise, food, disease, or drugs.
      (a) Blood enters the liver through the hepatic portal vein and hepatic artery and leaves through the hepatic vein.
      (b) After oral drug administration, the drug is absorbed from the gastrointestinal tract into the mesenteric vessels and proceeds to the hepatic portal vein, liver, and systemic circulation.
   (2) Intrinsic clearance, Cl_{int} describes the ability of the liver to remove the drug independently of blood flow.
      (a) Intrinsic drug clearance primarily occurs because of the inherent ability of the **biotransformation enzymes** (mixed-function oxidases) to metabolize the drug as it enters the liver.

(b) Normally, basal level mixed-function oxidase enzymes biotransform drugs. Levels of these enzymes may be increased by various drugs (e.g., phenobarbital) and environmental agents (e.g., tobacco smoke). These enzymes may be inhibited by other drugs and environmental agents (e.g., cimetidine, acute lead poisoning).

(3) **Protein binding.** Drugs that are bound to protein are not easily cleared by the liver or kidney because only the free, or nonplasma protein-bound, drug crosses the cell membrane into the tissue.

    (a) **The free drug** is available to drug-metabolizing enzymes for biotransformation.

    (b) A sudden increase in free-drug plasma concentration results in more available drug at pharmacologic receptors, producing a more intense effect in the organs (e.g., kidney, liver) involved in drug removal.

    (c) **Blood flow (Q), intrinsic clearance (Cl_{int}),** and fraction of free drug in plasma (f) are related to hepatic clearance as shown in the following equation:

$$Cl_H = Q\left(\frac{fCl_{int}}{Q + fCl_{int}}\right)$$

    (1) The hepatic clearance of drugs that have high extraction ratios and high Cl_{int} values (e.g., propranolol) is most affected by changes in blood flow and inhibitors of the drug metabolism enzymes.

    (2) The hepatic clearance of drugs that have low extraction ratios and low Cl_{int} values (e.g., theophylline) is most affected by changes in Cl_{int} and is affected only slightly by changes in hepatic blood flow.

    (3) Only drugs that are highly plasma protein bound (i.e., > 95%) and have a low intrinsic clearance (e.g., phenytoin) are affected by a sudden shift in protein binding. This shift causes an increase in free-drug plasma concentration.

c. **Biliary drug excretion,** an active transport process, is also included in hepatic clearance. Separate active secretion systems exist for weak acids and weak bases.

    (1) Drugs that are excreted in bile are usually high molecular weight compounds (i.e., > 500) or polar drugs, such as reserpine, digoxin, and various glucuronide conjugates.

    (2) Drugs may be recycled by the **enterohepatic circulation.**

        (a) Some drugs are absorbed from the gastrointestinal tract through the mesenteric and hepatic portal veins, proceeding to the liver. The liver may secrete some of the drug (unchanged or as a glucuronide metabolite) into the bile.

        (b) The bile and drug are stored in the gallbladder and will empty into the gastrointestinal tract through the bile duct and then may be reabsorbed.

        (c) If the drug is a **glucuronide metabolite,** bacteria in the gastrointestinal tract may hydrolyze the glucuronide moiety, allowing the released drug to be reabsorbed.

d. **First-pass effects (presystemic elimination)** occur with drugs given orally. A portion of the drug is eliminated before systemic absorption occurs.

    (1) First-pass effects generally result from rapid drug biotransformation by liver enzymes. Other mechanisms include metabolism of the drug by gastrointestinal mucosal cells, intestinal flora, and biliary secretion.

    (2) First-pass effects are usually observed by measuring the **absolute bioavailability** (F) of the drug (see Chapter 7). If $F < 1$, then some of the drug was eliminated before systemic drug absorption occurred.

    (3) Drugs that have a **high hepatic extraction ratio,** such as propranolol and morphine, show first-pass effects.

    (4) To obtain better systemic absorption of a drug that demonstrates high first-pass effects, then either

        (a) The drug dose could be increased (e.g., propranolol, penicillin)

        (b) The drug could be given by an alternate route of administration (e.g., nitroglycerin sublingual, insulin subcutaneous, estradiol transdermal)

        (c) The dosage form could be modified as a delayed-release drug product (e.g., enteric-coated aspirin, mesalamine) so that the drug may be absorbed more distally in the GI tract

F. Noncompartment methods. Some pharmacokinetic parameters for absorption, distribution, and elimination may be estimated with noncompartment methods. These methods usually require comparison of the areas under the curve.

1. **Mean residence time**
   a. **Mean residence time (MRT)** is the average time for the drug molecules to reside in the body. MRT is also known as the *mean transit time* and *mean sojourn time.*
   b. The MRT depends on the route of administration and assumes that the drug is eliminated from the central compartment.
   c. The MRT is the total residence time for all molecules in the body divided by the total number of molecules in the body, as shown in the following equation:

   $$MRT = \frac{\text{total residence time for all drug molecules in the body}}{\text{total number of drug molecules}}$$

   d. **MRT after IV bolus injection**
      (1) The MRT after a bolus intravenous injection is calculated by the following equation:

      $$MRT_{IV} = \frac{AUMC}{AUC_{0-\infty}}$$

      where AUMC is the area under the first moment versus time curve from $t = 0$ to $t = \text{infinity}$ and $AUC_{0-\infty}$ is the area under the plasma drug concentration versus time curve from $t = 0$ to $t = \text{infinity}$. $AUC_{0-\infty}$ is also known as the zero moment curve.

      (2) The MRT_{IV} is related to the elimination rate constant by the following expression:

      $$MRT_{IV} = 1/k$$

      (3) During MRT_{IV}, 62.3% of the intravenous bolus dose is eliminated.
      (4) The MRT for a drug given by a noninstantaneous input is longer than the MRT_{IV}.

2. **Mean absorption time (MAT)** is the difference between MRT and MRT_{IV} after an extravascular route is used.

   $$MAT = MRT_{ev} - MRT_{IV}$$

   When first-order absorption occurs, $MAT = 1/ka$.

3. **Clearance** is the volume of plasma cleared of drug per unit time and may be calculated without consideration of the compartment model.

   $$Cl = \frac{FD_0}{AUC_{0-\infty}}$$

   After an IV dose, $F = 1$.

4. **Steady-state volume of distribution (V_{ss})**
   a. The steady-state volume of distribution is the ratio of the amount of drug in the body at steady state and the average steady-state drug concentration.
   b. After an intravenous bolus injection, V_{ss} is calculated by the following equation:

   $$Vss = \frac{dose_{IV}(AUMC)}{AUC^2}$$

II. **Clinical Pharmacokinetics** is the application of pharmacokinetic principles for the rational design of an individualized dosage regimen. The two main objectives are **maintenance of an optimum drug concentration at the receptor site** to produce the desired therapeutic response for a specific period and **minimization of any adverse or toxic effects** of the drug.

III. **Toxicokinetics** is the application of pharmacokinetic principles to the design, conduct, and interpretation of drug safety evaluation studies.

   A. **Toxicokinetics** is also used to validate dose-related exposure in animals. Toxicokinetic studies are performed in animals during preclinical drug development to aid in prediction of human drug toxicity. Toxicokinetic (nonclinical) studies may continue after the drug has been tested in humans.

  B. **Clinical toxicology** is the study of adverse effects of drugs and toxic substances (poisons) in the human body. The pharmacokinetics of a drug in an overmedicated (intoxicated) patient may be very different from the pharmacokinetics of the same drug given in therapeutic doses. For example, a very high toxic dose may show nonlinear pharmacokinetics due to saturation kinetics compared to the drug given at lower therapeutic doses in which the drug levels follow linear pharmacokinetics.

IV. Population Pharmacokinetics is the study of sources and correlates of variability in drug concentrations among individuals who are the target patient population. Population pharmacokinetics is most often applied to the clinical patient who is receiving relevant doses of a drug of interest. Both pharmacokinetic and nonpharmacokinetic data may be considered, including gender, age, weight, creatinine clearance, and concomitant disease.

STUDY QUESTIONS

Directions: Each question, statement or incomplete statement in this section can be correctly answered or completed by **one** of the suggested answers or phrases. Choose the **best** answer.

1. Creatinine clearance is used as a measurement of

(A) renal excretion rate.
(B) glomerular filtration rate (GFR).
(C) active renal secretion.
(D) passive renal absorption.
(E) drug metabolism rate.

For questions 2–5: A new cephalosporin antibiotic was given at a dose of 5 mg/kg by a single intravenous bolus injection to a 58-year-old man who weighed 75 kg. The antibiotic follows the pharmacokinetics of a one-compartment model and has an elimination half-life of 2 hr. The apparent volume of distribution is 0.28 L/kg, and the drug is 35% bound to plasma proteins.

2. What is the initial plasma drug concentration (C_p^0) in this patient?

(A) 0.24 mg/L
(B) 1.80 mg/L
(C) 17.9 mg/L
(D) 56.0 mg/L
(E) 1339 mg/L

3. What is the predicted plasma drug concentration (C_p) at 8 hr after the dose?

(A) 0.73 mg/L
(B) 1.11 mg/L
(C) 2.64 mg/L
(D) 4.02 mg/L
(E) 15.10 mg/L

4. How much drug remains in the patient's body (D_B) 8 hr after the dose?

(A) 15.3 mg
(B) 23.3 mg
(C) 84.4 mg
(D) 100.0 mg
(E) 112.0 mg

5. How long after the dose is exactly 75% of the drug eliminated from the patient's body?

(A) 2 hr
(B) 4 hr
(C) 6 hr
(D) 8 hr
(E) 10 hr

For questions 6–11: A 35-year-old man who weighs 70 kg and has normal renal function needs an intravenous infusion of the antibiotic carbenicillin. The desired steady-state plasma drug concentration is 15 mg/dL. The physician wants the antibiotic to be infused into the patient for 10 hr. Carbenicillin has an elimination half-life $(t_{1/2})$ of 1 hr and an apparent volume distribution (V_D) of 9 L in this patient.

6. Assuming that no loading dose was given, what rate of intravenous infusion is recommended for this patient?

(A) 93.6 mg/hr
(B) 135.0 mg/hr
(C) 468.0 mg/hr
(D) 936.0 mg/hr
(E) 1350.0 mg/hr

7. Assuming that no loading intravenous dose was given, how long after the initiation of the intravenous infusion would the plasma drug concentration reach 95% of the theoretic steady-state drug concentration?

(A) 1.0 hr
(B) 3.3 hr
(C) 4.3 hr
(D) 6.6 hr
(E) 10.0 hr

8. What is the recommended loading dose?

(A) 93.6 mg
(B) 135.0 mg
(C) 468.0 mg
(D) 936.0 mg
(E) 1350.0 mg

9. To infuse the antibiotic as a solution containing 10 g drug in 500 mL 5% dextrose, how many milliliters per hour of the solution would be infused into the patient?

(A) 10.0 mL/hr
(B) 46.8 mL/hr
(C) 100.0 mL/hr
(D) 936.0 mL/hr
(E) 1141.0 mL/hr

10. What is the total body clearance rate for carbenicillin in this patient?

(A) 100 mL/hr
(B) 936 mL/hr
(C) 4862 mL/hr
(D) 6237 mL/hr
(E) 9000 mL/hr

11. If the patient's renal clearance for carbenicillin is 86 mL/min, what is the hepatic clearance for carbenicillin?

(A) 108 mL/hr
(B) 1077 mL/hr
(C) 3840 mL/hr
(D) 5160 mL/hr
(E) 6844 mL/hr

12. The earliest evidence that a drug is stored in tissue is

(A) an increase in plasma protein binding.
(B) a large apparent volume of distribution (V_D).
(C) a decrease in the rate of formation of metabolites by the liver.
(D) an increase in the number of side effects produced by the drug.
(E) a decrease in the amount of free drug excreted in the urine.

13. The intensity of the pharmacologic action of a drug is most dependent on the

(A) concentration of the drug at the receptor site.
(B) elimination half-life ($t_{1/2}$) of the drug.
(C) onset time of the drug after oral administration.
(D) minimum toxic concentration (MTC) of the drug in plasma.
(E) minimum effective concentration (MEC) of the drug in the body.

14. Drugs that show nonlinear pharmacokinetics have which property?

(A) A constant ratio of drug metabolites is formed as the administered dose increases.
(B) The elimination half-life ($t_{1/2}$) increases as the administered dose increases.
(C) The area under the plasma drug concentration versus time curve (AUC) increases in direct proportion to an increase in the administered dose.
(D) Both low and high doses follow first-order elimination kinetics.
(E) The steady-state drug concentration increases in direct proportion to the dosing rate.

15. The loading dose (D_L) of a drug is usually based on the

(A) total body clearance (Cl_T) of the drug.
(B) percentage of drug bound to plasma proteins.
(C) fraction of drug excreted unchanged in the urine.
(D) apparent volume of distribution (V_D) and desired drug concentration in plasma.
(E) area under the plasma drug concentration versus time curve (AUC).

16. The renal clearance of inulin is used as a measurement of

(A) effective renal blood flow.
(B) rate of renal drug excretion.
(C) intrinsic enzyme activity.
(D) active renal secretion.
(E) glomerular filtration rate (GFR).

17. All of the following statements about plasma protein binding of a drug are true *except* which one?

(A) Displacement of a drug from plasma protein binding sites results in a transient increased volume of distribution (V_D).

(B) Displacement of a drug from plasma protein binding sites makes more free drug available for glomerular filtration.

(C) Displacement of a potent drug that is normally > 95% bound may cause toxicity.

(D) Albumin is the major protein involved in protein binding of drugs.

(E) Drugs that are highly bound to plasma proteins generally have a greater V_D compared with drugs that are highly bound to tissue proteins.

18. The onset time for a drug given orally is the time for the drug to

(A) reach the peak plasma drug concentration.

(B) reach the minimum effective concentration (MEC).

(C) reach the minimum toxic concentration (MTC).

(D) begin to be eliminated from the body.

(E) begin to be absorbed from the small intestine.

19. The initial distribution of a drug into tissue is determined chiefly by the

(A) rate of blood flow to tissue.

(B) glomerular filtration rate (GFR).

(C) stomach emptying time.

(D) affinity of the drug for tissue.

(E) plasma protein binding of the drug.

20. Which tissue has the greatest capacity to biotransform drugs?

(A) brain

(B) kidney

(C) liver

(D) lung

(E) skin

21. The principle of superposition in designing multiple-dose regimens assumes that

(A) each dose affects the next subsequent dose, causing nonlinear elimination.

(B) each dose of drug is eliminated by zero-order elimination.

(C) steady-state plasma drug concentrations are reached at approximately 10 half-lives.

(D) early doses of drug do not affect subsequent doses.

(E) the fraction of drug absorbed is equal to the fraction of drug eliminated.

For questions 22–24: A new cardiac glycoside is developed for oral and intravenous administration. The drug has an elimination half-life ($t_{1/2}$) of 24 hr and an apparent volume of distribution (V_D) of 3 L/kg. The effective drug concentration is 1.5 ng/mL. Toxic effects of the drug are observed at drug concentrations > 4 ng/mL. The drug is bound to plasma proteins at approximately 25%. The drug is 75% bioavailable after an oral dose.

22. What is the oral maintenance dose, if given once a day, for a 68-year-old man who weighs 65 kg and has congestive heart failure (CHF) and normal renal function?

(A) 0.125 mg

(B) 0.180 mg

(C) 0.203 mg

(D) 0.270 mg

(E) 0.333 mg

23. What is the loading dose (D_L) for this patient?

(A) 0.270 mg

(B) 0.293 mg

(C) 0.450 mg

(D) 0.498 mg

(E) 0.540 mg

24. If the drug is available in tablets of 0.125 mg and 0.250 mg, what is the patient's plasma drug concentration if he has a dosage regimen of 0.125 mg every 12 hr?

(A) 1.39 ng/mL

(B) 1.85 ng/mL

(C) 2.78 ng/mL

(D) 3.18 ng/mL

(E) 6.94 ng/mL

Directions for question 25: The question in this section can be correctly answered by **one or more** of the suggested answers. Choose the correct answer, A–E.

A	if **I only** is correct
B	if **III only** is correct
C	if **I and II** are correct
D	if **II and III** are correct
E	if **I, II, and III** are correct

25. Which equation is true for a zero-order reaction rate of a drug?

I. $\dfrac{\mathrm{d}A}{\mathrm{d}t} = -k$

II. $t_{1/2} = \dfrac{0.693}{k}$

III. $A = A_{o}e^{-kt}$

ANSWERS AND EXPLANATIONS

1. The answer is B *[see I.E.2.a].*
A substance that is used to measure the GFR must be filtered but not reabsorbed or actively secreted. Although inulin clearance gives an accurate measurement of GFR, creatinine clearance is generally used because no exogenous drug must be given. However, creatinine formation depends on muscle mass and muscle metabolism, which may change with age and various disease conditions.

2. The answer is C *[see I.B.1.b.(2)].*

3. The answer is B *[see I.A.1.b.(1); I.B.1].*

4. The answer is B *[see I.B.1.a.(2)].*

5. The answer is B *[see I.B.1.a.(2)].*
Substituting the data for this patient in the equation for the initial plasma drug concentration (C_P^0) gives

$$C_P^0 = \frac{D_o}{V_D} = \frac{5 \text{ mg}}{0.28 \text{ L/kg}} = 17.9 \text{ mg/L}$$

To obtain the patient's plasma drug concentration (C_p) 8 hr after the dose, the following calculation is performed:

$$C_p = C_P^0 e^{-kt}$$

$$k = \frac{0.693}{t_{1/2}} = \frac{0.963}{2} = 0.347 \text{ hr}^{-1}$$

$$C_p = 17.9e^{-(0.347)(8)}$$
$$C_p = (17.9)(0.0623) = 1.11 \text{ mg/L}$$

The amount of drug in the patient's body at 8 hr is calculated as follows:

$$D_B = C_p V_D = (1.11)(0.28)(75) = 23.3 \text{ mg}$$

For any first-order elimination process, 50% of the initial amount of drug is eliminated at the end of the first half-life, and 50% of the remaining drug (i.e., 75% of the original amount) is eliminated at the end of the second half-life. Because the drug in the current case has an elimination half-life ($t_{1/2}$) of 2 hr, 75% of the dose is eliminated in two half-lives, or 4 hr.

6. The answer is D *[see I.B.3.e.(3)].*

7. The answer is C *[see I.B.3.c].*

8. The answer is E *[see I.B.3.f.(2)].*

9. The answer is B *[see I.B.3.e.(3)].*

10. The answer is D *[see I.B.3.e.(3); I.E.1.a].*

11. The answer is B *[see I.E.4.a].*
The equation for the plasma concentration at steady state (C_{ss}) provides the formula for calculating the rate of an intravenous infusion (R). The equation is

$$C_{ss} = \frac{R}{kV_D}$$

where k is the first-order elimination rate constant and V_D is the apparent volume of distribution. Rearranging the equation and substituting the data for this patient give the following calculations:

$$R = C_{ss}kV_D = \frac{15 \text{ mg}}{100 \text{ mL}} \times \frac{0.693}{1 \text{ hr}} \times 9000 \text{ mL}$$

$$R = 936 \text{ mg/hr}$$

The time it takes for an infused drug to reach the C_{ss} depends on the elimination half-life of the drug. The time required to reach 95% of the C_{ss} is equal to 4.3 times the half-life, whereas the time required to reach 99% of the C_{ss} is equal to 6.6 times the half-life. Because the half-life in the current case is 1 hr, the time to reach 95% of the C_{ss} is 4.3 × 1 hr, or 4.3 hr.

The loading dose (D_L) is calculated as follows:

$$D_L = C_{ss}V_D = \frac{15 \text{ mg}}{100 \text{ mL}} \times 9000 \text{ mL} = 1350 \text{ mg}$$

The answer to question 6 shows that the infusion rate should be 936 mg/hr. Therefore, if a drug solution containing 10 g in 500 mL is used, the required infusion rate is

$$\frac{936 \text{ mg}}{1 \text{ hr}} \times \frac{500 \text{ mL}}{10{,}000 \text{ mg}} = 46.8 \text{ mL/hr}$$

The patient's total body clearance (Cl_T) is calculated as follows:

$$Cl_T = kV_D$$

$$Cl_T = \frac{0.693}{1} \times 9000 \text{ mL} = 6237 \text{ mL/hr}$$

The hepatic clearance (Cl_H) is the difference between total clearance (Cl_T) and renal clearance (Cl_R):

$$Cl_H = Cl_T - Cl_R$$
$$Cl_H = 6237 - (86 \text{ mL/min} \times 60 \text{ min/hr}) = 1077 \text{ mL/hr}$$

12. The answer is B *[see I.B.1.b.(1)].*
A large apparent volume of distribution (V_D) is an early sign that a drug is not concentrated in the plasma, but is distributed widely in tissue. An increase in plasma protein binding suggests that the drug is located in the plasma rather than in tissue. A decrease in hepatic metabolism, an increase in side effects, or a decrease in urinary excretion of free drug is caused by a decrease in drug elimination.

13. The answer is A *[see I.A.3.d.(3)].*
As more drug is concentrated at the receptor site, more receptors interact with the drug to produce a pharmacologic effect. The intensity of the response increases until it reaches a maximum. When all of the available receptors are occupied by drug molecules, additional drug does not produce a more intense response.

14. The answer is B *[see I.D].*
Nonlinear pharmacokinetics is a term used to indicate that first-order elimination of a drug does not occur at all drug concentrations. With some drugs, such as phenytoin, as the plasma drug concentration increases, the elimination pathway for metabolism of the drug becomes saturated and the half-life increases. The area under the plasma drug concentration versus time curve (AUC) of the drug is not proportional to the dose; neither is the rate of metabolite formation. The metabolic rate is related to the effects of the drug.

15. The answer is D *[see I.B.1.b.(2); I.B.5.g.(1)].*
A loading dose (D_L) of a drug is given to obtain a therapeutic plasma drug level as rapidly as possible. The D_L is calculated on the basis of the apparent volume of distribution (V_D) and the desired plasma level of the drug.

16. The answer is E *[see I.E.3.c].*
Inulin is neither reabsorbed nor actively secreted. Therefore, it is excreted by glomerular filtration only. The inulin clearance rate is used as a standard measure of the GFR, a test that is useful both in a clinical situation and in the development of new drugs.

17. The answer is E *[see I.A.3.d].*
Drugs that are highly bound to plasma proteins diffuse poorly into tissue and have a low apparent volume of distribution (V_D).

18. The answer is B *[see I.B.3.g].*
The onset time is the time from the administration of the drug to the time when absorbed drug reaches

the MEC. The MEC is the drug concentration in the plasma that is proportional, but not necessarily equal, to the minimum drug concentration at the receptor site that elicits a pharmacologic response.

19. The answer is A *[see I.A.3.a].*
The initial distribution of a drug is chiefly determined by blood flow, whereas the affinity of the drug for tissue determines whether the drug concentrates at that site. The GFR affects the renal clearance of a drug, not its initial distribution. The gastric emptying time and degree of plasma protein binding affect drug distribution but are less important than the rate of blood flow to tissue.

20. The answer is C *[see I.E.4.b.(2)].*
The kidney, lung, skin, and intestine all have some capacity to biotransform, or metabolize, drugs; but the brain has little capacity for drug metabolism. The liver has the highest capacity for drug metabolism.

21. The answer is D *[see I.B.5.c].*
The superposition principle, which underlies the design of multiple-dose regimens, assumes that earlier drug doses do not affect subsequent doses. If the elimination rate constant or total body clearance of the drug changes during multiple dosing, then the superposition principle is no longer valid. Changes in the total body clearance (Cl_T) may be caused by enzyme induction, enzyme inhibition, or saturation of an elimination pathway. Any of these changes would cause nonlinear pharmacokinetics.

22. The answer is D *[see I.B.5.e.(3)].*

23. The answer is E *[see I.B.5.g.(1)]*

24. The answer is A *[see I.B.5.d.(2); I.B.5.e.(3)].*
The oral maintenance dose (D_o) should maintain the patient's average drug concentration at the effective drug concentration. The bioavailability of the drug (F), the apparent volume of distribution (V_D), the dosage interval (τ), and the excretion rate constant (k) must be considered in calculating the dose. The equation used is

$$C_{Av}^{\infty} = FD_o / kV_D\tau$$

For this drug, $F = 0.75$, $k = 0.693/24$ hr, $V_D = 3$ L/kg $\times$ 65 kg, $\tau = 24$ hr, and $C_{Av}^{\infty} = 1.5$ ng/mL, or 1.5 μg/L. Therefore, by substitution, $D_o = 270$ μg, or 0.270 mg. When the maintenance dose is given at a dosage frequency equal to the half-life, then the loading dose is equal to twice the maintenance dose, in this case 540 μg, or 0.540 mg. To determine the plasma drug concentration for a dosage regimen of 0.125 mg every 12 hr, the C_{Av}^{∞} formula is used. This time, $F = 0.75$, $D_o = 0.125$ mg, $k = 0.693/24$ hr, $V_D = 3$ L/kg $\times$ 65 kg, and $\tau = 12$ hr. Therefore, $C_{Av}^{\infty} = 1.39$ ng/mL. For cardiac glycosides, the peak (C_{max}) and trough (C_{min}) concentrations are calculated, and plasma drug concentrations are monitored after dosing. The loading dose (D_L) may be given in small increments over a specified period, according to the dosage regimen suggested by the manufacturer.

25. The answer is A (I) *[see I.A.1.a].*
The first equation in the question describes a zero-order reaction (dA/dt) in which the reaction rate increases or decreases at a constant rate (k). A zero-order reaction produces a graph of a straight line with the equation of $A = -kt + A_o$ when A is plotted against time (t). The other equations in the question represent first-order reactions.

7

Bioavailability and Bioequivalence

Leon Shargel

I. DEFINITIONS[1]

A. Bioavailability is a measurement of the rate and extent (amount) to which the active ingredient or active moiety becomes available at the site of action. Bioavailability is also considered a measure of the rate and extent of therapeutically active drug that is systemically absorbed. For drug products that are not intended to be absorbed into the bloodstream, bioavailability may be assessed by measurements intended to reflect the rate and extent to which the active ingredient or active moiety becomes available at the site of action.

B. Bioequivalent drug products. A generic drug product is considered bioequivalent to the **reference listed drug (RDL) product** if both products are pharmaceutical equivalents and the generic drug product's rate and extent of systemic drug absorption (bioavailability) do not show a statistically significant difference when administered in the same molar dose of the active ingredient, in the same chemical form, in a similar dosage form, by the same route of administration, and under the same experimental conditions. The RDL is generally the brand product.

C. Generic drug product

1. The generic drug product requires an **abbreviated new drug application** (ANDA) for approval by the U.S. Food and Drug Administration (FDA) and may be marketed after patent expiration of the reference drug product (see Chapter 1).

2. The generic drug product must be a **therapeutic equivalent** to the reference drug product but may differ in certain characteristics, including shape, scoring configuration, packaging, and excipients (such as colors, flavors, preservatives, expiration date, and minor aspects of labeling).

D. Pharmaceutical equivalents are drug products that contain the same therapeutically active drug ingredient(s); contain the same salt, ester, or chemical form; are of the same dosage form; and are identical in strength, concentration, and route of administration. Pharmaceutical equivalents may differ in characteristics such as shape, scoring configuration, release mechanisms, packaging, and excipients (including colors, flavoring, and preservatives).

E. The reference listed drug product is usually the currently marketed, brand-name product with a full **new drug application (NDA)** approved by the FDA. The RLD is the reference drug product identified by FDA (see "Electronic Orange Book" at www.fda.gov/cder/ob/default.htm).

F. Therapeutic equivalent drug products are pharmaceutical equivalents that can be expected to have the same clinical effect and safety profile when administered to patients under the same conditions specified in the labeling. Therapeutic equivalent drug products have the following criteria:

1. The products are safe and effective.

2. The products are pharmaceutical equivalents that contain the same active drug ingredient in the same dosage form, given by the same route of administration; meet compendial or other applicable standards of strength, quality, purity, and identity; and meet an acceptable in vitro standard.

---

[1]The U.S. Food and Drug Administration (FDA) annually publishes the book *"Approved Drug Products with Therapeutic Equivalence Evaluation* also know as the "Electronic Orange Book" (available online at www.fda.gov/cder/ob/default.htm). This source should be consulted for the latest definitions of therapeutic equivalence–related terms

3. The drug products are bioequivalent in that they do not present a known potential problem and are shown to meet an appropriate bioequivalence standard.

4. The drug products are adequately labeled.

5. The drug products are manufactured in compliance with current good manufacturing practice regulations.

G. **Pharmaceutical alternatives** are drug products that contain the same therapeutic moiety but are different salts, esters, or complexes (e.g., tetracycline hydrochloride versus tetracycline phosphate) or are different dosage forms (e.g., tablet versus capsule; immediate-release dosage form versus controlled-release dosage form) or strengths.

II. BIOAVAILABILITY AND BIOEQUIVALENCE.
These may be determined directly using pharmacokinetic studies (e.g., plasma drug concentration versus time profiles, urinary drug excretion studies), measurements of an acute pharmacodynamic effect, comparative clinical studies, or in vitro studies. The choice of study used is based on the site of action of the drug and the ability of the study design to compare drug delivered to that site by the two products.

A. **Acute pharmacodynamic effects,** such as changes in heart rate, blood pressure, electrocardiogram (ECG), clotting time, or forced expiratory volume in 1 sec (FEV_1) can be used to measure bioavailability when no assay for plasma drug concentration is available or when the plasma drug concentration does not relate to the pharmacological response (e.g., a bronchodilator such as albuterol given by inhalation). Quantitation of the pharmacological effect versus time profile can be used as a measure of bioavailability and/or bioequivalence (Figure 7-1).

1. **Onset time.** As the drug is systemically absorbed, the drug concentration at the receptor rises to a **minimum effective concentration** (MEC) and a pharmacological response is initiated. The time from drug administration to the MEC is known as the onset time.

2. **Intensity.** The intensity of the pharmacological effect is proportional to the number of receptors occupied by the drug up to a *maximum* pharmacological effect. The maximum pharmacological effect may occur before, after, or at peak drug absorption.

3. **Duration of action.** As long as the drug concentration remains above the MEC, pharmacological activity is observed. The duration of action is the time for which the drug concentration remains above the MEC.

Figure 7-1. Generalized plasma drug concentration versus time curve after oral drug administration. *MEC,* minimum effective concentration; *MTC,* minimum toxic concentration. [Adapted with permission from Shargel L, Wu-Pong S, Yu ABC: Applied Biopharmaceutics and Pharmacokinetics, 5th ed. New York, McGraw-Hill, 2005, p. 6.]

Figure 7-2. Generalized plasma drug concentration versus time curve, showing peak time and peak concentration. *AUC,* area under the curve; *MEC,* minimum effective concentration; *MTC,* minimum toxic concentration. [Adapted with permission from Shargel L, Wu-Pong S, Yu ABC: Applied Biopharmaceutics and Pharmacokinetics, 5th ed. New York, McGraw-Hill, 2005, p. 7.].

4. **Therapeutic window.** As the drug concentration increases, other receptors may combine with the drug to exert a toxic or adverse response. This drug concentration is the **minimum toxic concentration** (MTC). The drug concentration range between the MEC and the MTC is the therapeutic window.

B. **Plasma drug concentration**. The plasma drug concentration versus time curve is most often used to measure the systemic bioavailability of a drug from a drug product (Figure 7-2).

1. **Time for peak plasma drug concentration** (T_{max}) relates to the rate constants for systemic drug absorption and elimination. If two oral drug products contain the same amount of active drug but different excipients, the dosage form that yields the faster rate of drug absorption has the shorter T_{max}.

2. **Peak plasma drug concentration** (C_{max}). The plasma drug concentration at T_{max} relates to the intensity of the pharmacological response. Ideally, C_{max} should be within the therapeutic window.

3. **Area under the plasma drug concentration versus time curve** (AUC) relates to the amount or extent of drug absorption. The amount of systemic drug absorption is directly related to the AUC. The AUC is usually calculated by the **trapezoidal rule** and is expressed in units of concentration multiplied by time (e.g., $\frac{\mu g}{mL} \times$ hr).

C. **Urinary drug excretion.** Measurement of urinary drug excretion can determine bioavailability from a drug product. This method is most accurate if the active therapeutic moiety is excreted unchanged in significant quantity in the urine (Figure 7-3).

1. **The cumulative amount of active drug excreted in the urine** (D_U^∞) is directly related to the extent of systemic drug absorption.

2. **The rate of drug excretion in the urine** (dD_U/dt) is directly related to the rate of systemic drug absorption.

3. **The time for the drug to be completely excreted** (t^∞) corresponds to the total time for the drug to be systemically absorbed and completely excreted after administration.

D. **Comparative clinical trials** to a drug can be used to measure bioavailability quantitatively. Clinical studies are highly variable and less precise than other methods because of individual differences in drug pharmacodynamics and subjective measurements.

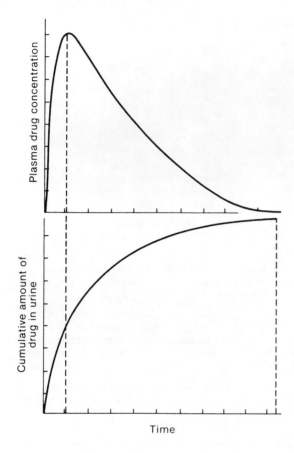

Figure 7-3. These corresponding plots show the relationship of the plasma drug concentration versus time curve to the cumulative amount of drug in the urine versus time curve. [Adapted with permission from Shargel L, Wu-Pong S, Yu ABC: Applied Biopharmaceutics and Pharmacokinetics, 5th ed. New York, McGraw-Hill, 2005, p. 463.]

E. **In vitro measurements of bioequivalence.** Bioequivalence may sometimes be demonstrated using an in vitro bioequivalence standard, especially when such an in vitro test has been correlated with human in vivo bioavailability data. For example, the rate of drug dissolution in vitro for certain drug products correlates with drug bioavailability in vivo. If the dissolution test in vitro is considered statistically adequate to predict drug bioavailability, then, in some cases, dissolution may be used in place of an in vivo bioavailability study.

III. RELATIVE AND ABSOLUTE BIOAVAILABILITY

A. **Relative bioavailability** is the systemic availability of the drug from a dosage form as compared to a reference standard given by the same route of administration. Relative bioavailability is calculated as the ratio of the AUC for the dosage form to the AUC for the reference dosage form given in the same dose. A relative bioavailability of 1 (or 100%) implies that drug bioavailability from both dosage forms is the same but does not indicate the completeness of systemic drug absorption. The determination of relative bioavailability is important in generic drug studies (e.g., bioequivalence studies).

B. **Absolute bioavailability** (*F*) is the fraction of drug systemically absorbed from the dosage form. *F* is calculated as the ratio of the AUC for the dosage form given orally to the AUC obtained after intravenous (IV) drug administration (adjusted for dose). A parenteral drug solution given by IV administration is considered to have 100% systemic absorption (i.e., *F* = 1). An *F* value of 0.80 (or 80%) indicates that only 80% of the drug was systemically available from the oral dosage form.

IV. BIOEQUIVALENCE STUDIES FOR SOLID ORAL DRUG PRODUCTS

A. Design of bioequivalence studies

1. The FDA's Division of Bioequivalence, Office of Generic Drugs provides guidance for the performance of in vitro dissolution and in vivo bioequivalence studies. These guidances are available at www.fda.gov/cder/guidances.

2. **Fasting study.** Bioequivalence studies are usually evaluated by a single-dose, two-period, two-treatment, two-sequence, open-label, randomized crossover design, comparing equal doses of the test (generic) and reference (brand) products in fasted, adult, healthy subjects.
   a. Both men and women may be used in the study.
   b. Blood sampling is performed just before the dose (zero time) and at appropriate intervals after the dose to obtain an adequate description of the plasma drug concentration versus time profile.

3. **Food intervention study.** If the bioavailability of the active drug ingredient is known to be affected by food, the generic drug manufacturer must include a single-dose, randomized, crossover, food effects study comparing equal doses of the test product and reference products given immediately after a standard high-fat–content breakfast.

4. **Other study designs.** Crossover studies may not be practical in drugs with a long half-life in the body, and a parallel study design may be used instead. Alternate study methods, such as in vitro studies or equivalence studies with clinical or pharmacodynamic end points, are used for drug products where plasma concentrations are not useful to determine delivery of the drug substance to the site of activity (such as inhalers, nasal sprays, and topical products applied to the skin).

5. **Waiver of an in vivo bioequivalence study**
   a. A comparative in vitro dissolution (drug-release) study between the test and the reference products may be used in lieu of an in vivo bioequivalence study for some immediate-release (conventional) oral drug products.
   b. No bioequivalence study is required for certain drug products given as a solution such as oral, parenteral, ophthalmic, or other solutions because bioequivalence is self-evident. In this case, the drug is in a pure aqueous solution and there is no drug dissolution rate consideration.

B. Pharmacokinetic evaluation of the data. Pharmacokinetic analysis includes calculation for each subject of the AUC to the last quantifiable concentration (AUC_{0-t}) and to infinity ($AUC_{0-\infty}$), T_{max}, and C_{max}. In addition, the elimination rate constant (k), the elimination half-life ($t_{1\backslash2}$), and other parameters may be estimated.

C. Statistical evaluation of the data

1. The statistical methodology for analyzing bioequivalence studies is called the two one-sided test procedure. Two situations are tested with this statistical methodology.
   a. The first of the two one-sided tests determines whether a generic product (test), when substituted for a brand-name product (reference) is significantly less bioavailable.
   b. The second of the two one-sided tests determines whether a brand-name product (reference) when substituted for a generic product (test) is significantly less bioavailable.
   c. Based on the opinions of FDA medical experts, a difference of $> 20\%$ for each of the above tests was determined to be significant and, therefore, undesirable for all drug products.

2. An analysis of variance (ANOVA) should be performed on the log transformed AUC and C_{max} values obtained from each subject. The 90% confidence intervals for both pharmacokinetic parameters, AUC and C_{max}, must be entirely within the 80% to 125% boundaries based on log transformation of the data. The ratio of the means of the study data (test to reference) should lie in the center of the 90% confidence interval, or close to 100% (equivalent to a test to reference ratio of 1) (Table 7-1).

3. Different statistical criteria are sometimes used when bioequivalence is demonstrated through comparative clinical trials, pharmacodynamic studies, or comparative in vitro methodology.

Table 7-1. Bioavailability Comparison of a Generic (Test) and Brand (Reference) Drug Product[a]

Parameter	Units	Test (T)	Ratio Reference (R)	(%) T/R	90% Confidence Limits
AUC_{0-t}	μg hr/mL	1466	1494	98.1	93.0–102.5
$AUC_{0-\infty}$	μg hr/mL	1592	1606	99.1	94.5–104.1
C_{max}	μg mL	11.6	12.5	92.8	88.5–98.6
T_{max}	hr	1.87	2.10	89.1	

AUC, area under the curve; C_{max}, peak plasma drug concentration; T_{max}, time for peak plasma drug concentration.
[a]The results were obtained from a two-way crossover, single-dose, fasting study in 24 healthy adult volunteers. Mean values are reported. No statistical differences were observed between AUC and C_{max} values for the test and reference products.

4. The bioequivalence methodology and criteria described above simultaneously control for both differences in the average response between test and reference products as well as the precision with which the average response in the population is estimated. This precision depends on the within-subject (normal volunteer or patient) variability in the pharmacokinetic parameters (AUC and C_{max}) of the two products and on the number of subjects in the study. The width of the 90% confidence interval is a reflection in part of the within-subject variability of the test and reference products in the bioequivalence study.

V. BIOEQUIVALENCE ISSUES

A. **Problems in determining bioequivalence** include lack of an adequate study design; inability to accurately measure the drug analytes, including metabolites and enantiomers (chiral drugs); and lack of systemic drug absorption (Table 7-2.)

B. **Bioequivalence studies** for which objective blood drug concentrations cannot be obtained require either a pharmacodynamic study, a clinical trial, or an in vitro study that has been correlated with human in vivo bioavailability data.

1. Pharmacodynamic measurements are more difficult to obtain, and the data tend to be variable, requiring a larger number of subjects compared to the bioequivalence studies for systemically absorbed drugs.
   a. A bioequivalence study using pharmacodynamic measurements tries to obtain a pharmacodynamic effect versus time profile for the drug in each subject.

Table 7-2. Problem Issues in the Determination of Bioequivalence

Problem Issues	Example
Drugs with highly variable bioavailability[a]	Propranolol, verapamil
Drugs with active metabolites	Selegiline
Chiral drugs	Ibuprofen, albuterol
Drugs with nonlinear pharmacokinetics	Phenytoin
Orally administered drugs that are not systemically absorbed	Cholestyramine resin, sucralfate
Drugs with long elimination half-lives	Probucol
Variable-dosage forms	Dyazide, conjugated estrogens
Nonoral drug delivery	
Topical drugs	Steroids, antifungals
Transdermal delivery systems	Estrogen patch
Drugs given by inhalation aerosols	Bronchodilators, steroids
Intranasal drugs	Intranasal steroids
Biotechnology derived drugs	Erythropoietin, interferon
Bioavailable drugs that should not reach peak drug levels	Potassium supplements, hormone replacement therapy
Target population used in the bioequivalence studies	Pediatric patients; renal disease

[a]These drugs have high intrasubject variability.

b. The area under the effect versus time profile, peak effect, and time for peak effect are obtained for the test and reference products and are then statistically analyzed.

2. Comparative clinical trials are more difficult to run, do not have easily quantifiable observations, and are quite costly.

3. In vitro studies may require the development of a reliable surrogate marker that may be correlated with human in vivo bioavailability data. For example, the penetration of drug into layers of skin with respect to time (*dermatopharmacokinetics*) has been suggested as a method for measuring the bioequivalence of topical drug products intended for local activity.

VI. DRUG PRODUCTION SELECTION

A. Generic drug substitution

1. **Generic drug substitution** is the process of dispensing a generic drug product in place of the prescribed drug product (e.g., generic product for brand-name product, generic product for another generic product, brand-name product for generic product). The substituted product must be a therapeutic equivalent to the prescribed product.

2. Generic drug products that are classified as therapeutic equivalents by the FDA are expected to produce the same clinical effect and safety profile as the prescribed drug.

3. **Prescribability** refers to the measurement of average bioequivalence in which the comparison of population means of the test and reference products falls within acceptable statistical criteria. Prescribability is the current basis for FDA approval of therapeutic equivalent generic drug products.

4. **Switchability** refers to the measurement of individual bioequivalence, which requires knowledge of individual variability (intrasubject variability) and subject-by-formulation effects. Switchability ensures that the substituted generic drug product produces the same response in the individual patient.

B. Therapeutic substitution

1. Therapeutic substitution is the process of dispensing a therapeutic alternative in place of the prescribed drug product. For example, amoxicillin is dispensed for ampicillin.

2. The substituted drug product is usually in the same therapeutic class (e.g., calcium channel blocker) and is expected to have a similar clinical profile.

C. Formulary issues

1. A **formulary** is a list of drugs. A **positive** formulary lists all the drugs that may be substituted, whereas a **negative** formulary lists drugs for which the pharmacist may not substitute. A **restrictive** formulary lists only those drugs that may be reimbursed without justification by the prescriber; for drugs not listed in the restrictive formulary, the prescriber must justify the need for the nonlisted drug.

2. Many states have legal requirements that address the issue of drug product selection. States may provide information and guidance in drug product selection through positive, negative, or restrictive formularies.

3. The FDA annually publishes *Approved Drug Products with Therapeutic Equivalence Evaluations* (the "Orange Book"). This publication is also reproduced in the *United States Pharmacopeia* (*USP*), DI Vol. III, *Approved Drug Products and Legal Requirements,* published annually by the USP Convention. The "Electronic Orange Book" may be found at www.fda.gov/cder/ob/default.htm.

   a. The "Orange Book" provides therapeutic evaluation codes for drug products (Table 7-3).

      (1) "A-"rated" drug products are drug products that contain active ingredients and dosage forms that are *not* regarded as presenting either actual or potential bioequivalence problems or drug quality standards issues. However, all oral dosage forms must meet an appropriate in vitro bioequivalence standard that is acceptable to the FDA to be approved as therapeutically equivalent and may be interchanged.

Table 7-3. Therapeutic Equivalence Evaluation Codes

A Codes	Drug products that are considered to be therapeutically equivalent to other pharmaceutically equivalent products
AA	Products in conventional dosage forms not presenting bioequivalence problems
AB	Products meeting bioequivalence requirements
AN	Solutions and powders for aerosolization
AO	Injectable oil solutions
AP	Injectable aqueous solutions
AT	Topical products

B Codes	Drug products that the FDA does not at this time consider to be therapeutically equivalent to other pharmaceutically equivalent products
BC	Extended-release tablets, extended-release capsules, and extended-release injectables
BD	Active ingredients and dosage forms with documented bioequivalence problems
BE	Delayed-release oral dosage forms
BN	Products in aerosol-nebulizer drug delivery systems
BP	Active ingredients and dosage forms with potential bioequivalence problems
BR	Suppositories or enemas for systemic use
BS	Products with drug standard deficiencies
BT	Topical products with bioequivalence issues
BX	Insufficient data

FDA, U.S. Food and Drug Administration.

      (2) "B"-rated" drug products are drug products for which actual or potential bioequivalence problems have not been resolved by adequate evidence of bioequivalence. These products often have specific dosage form problems rather than a problem with the active ingredients (e.g., two different nicotine patches). "B-"rated drug products are *not* considered therapeutically equivalent to other pharmaceutically equivalent products and are *not* interchangeable.

      (3) Certain products present special situations that deserve a more complete explanation than can be provided by the two-codes used in the "Orange Book." These drugs have particular problems with standards of identity, analytical methodology, or bioequivalence that are considered individually. For these drugs, consult the "Orange Book."

   b. For some drug products, bioequivalence has not been established or no generic product is currently available.

 4. Various hospitals, institutions, insurance plans, health maintenance organizations (HMOs), and other third-party plans may have a formulary that provides guidance for drug product substitution.

STUDY QUESTIONS

Directions for questions 1–3: Each of the questions, statements, or incomplete statements in this section can be correctly answered or completed by **one** of the suggested answers or phrases. Choose the **best** answer.

1. The parameters used to describe bioavailability are

   (A) C_{max}, AUC_{0-t}, and $AUC_{0-\infty}$.
   (B) C_{max}, AUC_{0-t}, $AUC_{0-\infty}$, and T_{max}.
   (C) C_{max}, AUC_{0-t}, $AUC_{0-\infty}$, and $t_{1\backslash 2}$.
   (D) C_{max} and AUC_{0-t}.
   (E) C_{max}, AUC_{0-t}, $AUC_{0-\infty}$, and T_{max}, and $t_{1\backslash 2}$.

2. To determine the absolute bioavailability of a drug given as an oral extended-release tablet, the bioavailability of the drug must be compared to the bioavailability of the drug from

   (A) an immediate-release oral tablet containing the same amount of active ingredient.
   (B) an oral solution of the drug in the same dose.
   (C) a parenteral solution of the drug given by intravenous (IV) bolus or IV infusion.
   (D) a reference (brand) extended-release tablet that is a pharmaceutical equivalent.
   (E) an immediate-release hard gelatin capsule containing the same amount of active drug and lactose.

3. A single-dose, two-way crossover, fasting, comparative bioavailability study was performed in 24 healthy, adult male subjects. Plasma drug concentrations were obtained for each subject, and the results shown in Table 7-Q3 were obtained. The relative bioavailability of the drug from the generic tablet compared to the reference tablet is

   (A) 82.3%.
   (B) 69.8%.
   (C) 91.7%.
   (D) 96.2%.
   (E) 103.9%

Table 7-Q3

Drug Product	Dose (mg)	C_{max} (µg/mL)	T_{max} (hr)	$AUC_{0-\infty}$ (µg hr/mL)
IV bolus injection	100			1714
Oral solution	200	21.3	1.2	3143
Generic tablet	200	17.0	2.1	2822
Reference tablet	200	16.5	1.9	2715

IV, intravenous.

Directions for questions 4–5: The questions and incomplete statements in this section can be correctly answered or completed by **one or more** of the suggested answers. Choose the answer, **A–E.**

A	if **I only** is correct
B	if **III only** is correct
C	if **I and II** are correct
D	if **II and III** are correct
E	if **I, II, and III** are correct

4. For two drug products, generic (test) and brand (reference), to be considered bioequivalent

I. there should be no statistical difference between the extent of bioavailability of the drug from the test product compared to the reference product.

II. the 90% confidence intervals about the ratio of the means of the C_{max} and AUC values for the test product to reference product must be within 80%–125% of the reference product.

III. there should be no statistical differences between the mean C_{max} and AUC values for the test product compared to the reference product.

5. For which of the following products is measuring plasma drug concentrations not appropriate for estimating bioequivalence?

I. metered-dose inhaler containing a bronchodilator

II. antifungal agent for the treatment of a vaginal infection

III. enteric-coated tablet containing a nonsteroidal anti-inflammatory agent

ANSWERS AND EXPLANATIONS3

1. The answer is B *[see II.B].*
AUC relates to the extent of drug absorption. C_{max} and T_{max} relate to the rate of drug absorption. The elimination $t_{1/2}$ of the drug is usually independent of the route of drug administration and is not used as a measure of bioavailability. For the FDA, only the C_{max} and AUC parameters must meet 90% confidence intervals of 80–125% of the reference (brand) product (Table 7.1).

2. The answer is C *[see III.B].*
After an IV bolus injection or IV infusion, all the dose is absorbed into the body. The ratio of the AUC of the drug given orally to the AUC of the drug given by IV injection is used to obtain the absolute bioavailability (F) of the drug.

3. The answer is E *[see III.A].*
The relative bioavailability is determined from the ratio of the AUC of the generic (test) product to the AUC of the reference standard. Thus the relative bioavailability can exceed 100%, whereas the absolute bioavailability cannot exceed 100%. $\dfrac{AUC_{generic}}{AUC_{reference}} = \dfrac{2822}{2715} = 1.039$ or 103.9%.

4. The answer is E *[see IV.C].*
Although T_{max} is an indication of rate of drug absorption, it is a discrete measurement and usually too variable to use for statistical comparisons in bioequivalence studies. Statistical comparisons use AUC and C_{max} values from test and reference drug products as the basis of bioequivalence.

5. The answer is C *[see IV.A].*
Although some systemic absorption may be demonstrated after administering a metered dose inhaler containing a bronchodilator or a vaginal antifungal agent, bioequivalence can be determined only by using a clinical response measurement.

8
Functional Group Chemistry and Biochemistry

Marc W. Harrold

I. FUNCTIONAL GROUP CHEMISTRY

A. Introduction. Drug molecules can be viewed as a collection of functional groups (i.e., groups of atoms present within the drug that confer specific chemical and physical properties [Figure 8-1]). Functional groups determine such characteristics as ionization, solubility in aqueous and lipid environments (aka polarity), reactivity, chemical stability, and in vivo metabolic stability. Additionally, these functional groups are **capable of forming specific bonds** (primarily noncovalent) with their receptors and are thus extremely important in drug activity and potency.

1. Functional groups that impart **hydrophilicity** are likely to increase the drug's water solubility, while functional groups that impart **lipophilicity** (hydrophobicity) are likely to increase the drug's tendency to cross cellular membranes through passive diffusion. See Chapter 12 VIII B 1 for a further discussion of water and lipid solubility.
   a. Acidic and basic functional groups allow for **drug ionization** and, in most cases, impart enhanced water solubility to the molecule. One notable exception to this is seen in **amphoteric drugs** (i.e., those compounds possessing both acidic and basic functional groups). As exemplified by ampicillin in Figure 8-2, amphoteric compounds can form **zwitterions,** or **internal salts.** Since the zwitterion form of ampicillin has a net overall charge of zero, it has difficulty dissolving in aqueous environments such as the gastrointestinal (GI) tract.
   b. Neutral functional groups (i.e., those that are incapable of ionization) can enhance either water or lipid solubility depending on their ability to form **hydrogen bonds with water.** Hydrogen bonding is the primary mechanism for increasing the water solubility of non-electrolytes (i.e., compounds that do not possess acidic, basic, or quaternary ammonium functional groups).

2. Functional group **reactivity** affects **drug shelf life, stability,** and **storage.** There are a number of functional groups that will degrade, primarily through air oxidation and hydrolysis, under **normal environmental conditions.** Two examples of this latter concern are seen with aspirin and nitroglycerin. Both compounds are subject to rapid hydrolysis if exposed to moist environments.

3. Functional groups also affect **in vivo stability** and the duration of drug action. The susceptibility of a given drug to metabolic biotransformation depends in part upon the functional groups that are present (see Chapter 17 II, III).
   a. Drugs that contain a large number or percentage of hydrophilic functional groups are often eliminated from the body unchanged or with minimal metabolism.
   b. Drugs that contain a large number or percentage of lipophilic functional groups often require extensive metabolism.

Figure 8-1. Ibuprofen, a nonsteroidal anti-inflammatory agent, is comprised of an ionizable, hydrophilic carboxylic acid and three hydrophobic functional groups: an isobutyl alkyl chain, an ethyl alkyl group, and an aromatic ring.

Figure 8-2. Ampicillin is an amphoteric compound. It contains an acidic carboxylic acid and a basic amine and exists in vivo as a zwitterion. The proton from the carboxylic acid binds to the basic amine, producing a molecule with an overall net charge equal to zero.

B. Acidic functional groups

1. **Types.** Shown in Figure 8-3 are examples of the six most common acidic functional groups. In general, carboxylic acids tend to be more acidic than any of the other five functional groups. The tetrazole ring provides the best charge delocalization since resonance allows the charge to be equally shared among all five atoms in the ring.

2. **Common attributes**
   a. Acidic functional groups impart **hydrophilicity** to a drug molecule due to their potential for ionization.
   b. Acidic functional groups can form **ionic, ion–dipole, and hydrogen bonds** with receptors, enzymes, transport proteins, and other macromolecules.
   c. Acidic functional groups can form **salts when combined with bases.**
   d. **Carboxylic acids** are often **esterified** for the purposes of prodrug formation (see Chapter 17, section VI for additional information). They can also undergo acid- or enzyme-catalyzed **decarboxylation** reactions.
   e. **Metabolism.** Acidic functional groups can undergo **conjugation** with glucuronic acid, glycine, and glutamine.

Figure 8-3. Examples of drugs that contain an acidic functional group as part of their chemical structure.

C. Basic functional groups

1. Types

   a. Aliphatic and alicyclic amines are the most common basic functional groups. As shown in Figure 8-4, these amines can be **primary, secondary, or tertiary,** depending on the number of substituents attached to the nitrogen.

   b. Aromatic amines, such as that seen in procainamide (Figure 8-4), are much less basic and for all intents and purposes can be considered neutral.

   c. Aromatic, heterocyclic nitrogens vary in their basicity, but in general are much less basic than aliphatic and alicyclic amines (Figure 8-5).

   d. Additional basic functional groups include **imines, hydrazines, amidines,** and **guanidines** (Figure 8-6). Imines tend to be less basic than aliphatic and alicyclic amines, whereas guanidines tend to be much more basic. The basicity of the other two functional groups lies somewhere in between.

2. Common attributes

   a. Basic functional groups impart **hydrophilicity** to a drug molecule due to their potential for ionization and their ability to form hydrogen bonds.

   b. Basic functional groups can form **ionic, ion–dipole, and hydrogen bonds** with receptors, enzymes, transport proteins, and other macromolecules.

   c. Basic functional groups can form **salts when combined with acids.**

   d. Metabolism. Common metabolic pathways for primary amines are **oxidative deamination, acetylation, and N-oxidation.** Common pathways for secondary and tertiary amines are **acetylation** (secondary amines only), **oxidative N-dealkylation,** and **N-oxidation.** Aromatic amines can be **acetylated,** while aromatic heterocyclic nitrogens can undergo **N-oxidation or N-dealkylation.** Imine, hydrazine, amidine, and guanidine groups can undergo similar reactions as those listed for primary, secondary, and tertiary amines. Additionally, amines can be **glucuronidated, sulfated,** and **methylated** by **phase II conjugation** reactions.

D. Additional hydrophilic functional groups

1. Similar to amines, **hydroxyl groups (or alcohols)** may be classified as **primary, secondary, or tertiary,** depending on the number of substituents attached to their respective carbons. A good example of this is seen with the glucocorticoid fludrocortisone (Figure 8-7).

   a. Hydroxyl groups can form **ion–dipole and hydrogen bonds** with receptors, enzymes, transport proteins, and other macromolecules.

Gabapentin
(primary amine)

Albuterol
(secondary amine)

Lidocaine
(tertiary amine)

Ticlopidine
(alicyclic tertiary amine)

Procainamide
(aromatic amine)

Figure 8-4. Examples of drugs that contain a primary, secondary, tertiary, or aromatic amine as part of their chemical structure. Whenever an amine is part of a nonaromatic ring (e.g., ticlopidine), it is referred to as an alicyclic amine. Whenever an amine amino is part of a side chain or is attached to a nonaromatic ring, it is referred to as an aliphatic or alkyl amine. Whenever an amine is directly attached to an aromatic ring (e.g., procainamide), it is referred to as an aromatic amine.

Quinidine
(quinoline nitrogen)

Serotonin
(indole nitrogen)

Prazosin
(heterocyclic guanidine group)

Figure 8-5. Examples of drugs that contain aromatic, heterocyclic nitrogens as part of their chemical structure.

b. Hydroxyl groups **enhance water solubility** due to their ability to form hydrogen bonds with water.

c. Hydroxyl groups are often **esterified** in order to produce prodrugs. See Chapter 17 VI for additional information on prodrugs.

d. Metabolism. Primary hydroxyl groups are initially **oxidized to aldehydes** and then to **carboxylic acids.** Secondary hydroxyl groups are **oxidized to ketones,** while tertiary hydroxyl groups are not usually oxidized. Hydroxyl groups may also undergo **phase II glucuronide or sulfate conjugation.**

Lorazepam
(imine nitrogen)

Tetrahydrozoline
(amidine group)

Hydralazine
(hydrazine nitrogen)

Guanethidine
(guanidine group)

Figure 8-6. Examples of drugs that contain a basic imine, hydrazine, amidine, or guanidine functional group as part of their chemical structure.

Figure 8-7. Examples of drugs that contain a hydroxyl group, phenol, catechol, or quaternary ammonium functional group as part of their chemical structure. Fludrocortisone contains a primary, secondary, and tertiary hydroxyl group. This designation is similar to that used for amines and depends on the number of substituents attached to the respective carbons. As illustrated with levodopa, a catechol is simply two phenol groups that are *ortho* to one another.

2. **Phenols,** as exemplified by estradiol (Figure 8-7), are hydroxyl groups that are directly attached to an aromatic ring.
    a. Due to resonance stabilization of the aromatic ring, phenols can be ionized in basic environments; however, most phenols are **primarily unionized** at physiological pH and as such should be treated as **neutral,** nonionizable functional groups.
    b. Similar to alcohols, phenols primarily form **ion–dipole and hydrogen bonds.** They can also **enhance water solubility** and be esterified to form prodrugs (see Chapter 17 VI).
    c. Drug molecules containing phenols or **catechols** (see **levodopa** in Figure 8-7) are susceptible to **air oxidation** and to **oxidation on contact with ferric ions.**
    d. **Metabolism.** Phenols undergo **sulfation, glucuronidation, aromatic hydroxylation,** and **O-methylation.**
3. **Quaternary ammonium salts,** as exemplified by ipratropium bromide (Figure 8-7), are neither acidic nor basic but contain a **permanent positive charge.**
    a. These salts **enhance water solubility;** however, due to the permanence of the positive charge, compounds containing this functional group often have **difficulty passing through lipid membranes.**
    b. Similar to amines, quaternary ammonium salts can participate in **ionic** and **ion–dipole bonds.**
    c. Quaternary ammonium salts are generally not metabolized; however, **N-dealkylation** could occur in some cases.

E. **Functional groups with intermediate polarity**
    1. **Ketones** are less prevalent than alcohols and phenols in the structures of drug molecules. One example is seen in the oral hypoglycemic agent, acetohexamide, shown in Figure 8-8.
        a. Ketones are primarily lipid soluble; however, they are able to form **hydrogen bonds** with alcohols and certain amines. They can also form **ion–dipole** bonds.

Figure 8-8. Examples of drugs that contain a ketone, ester, amide, lactone, or lactam as part of their chemical structure.

   b. Metabolism. Ketones are very stable. Their primary route of metabolism is **reduction to an alcohol.**

2. Compounds containing **esters, amides** and their respective cyclic forms, **lactones, and lactams** can be seen in Figure 8-8.
   a. These functional groups are capable of forming **hydrogen bonds** with receptors, enzymes, transport proteins, other macromolecules, and water. Similar to ketones, esters and lactones can function as **hydrogen-bond acceptors,** while amides and lactams can function as either **hydrogen-bond donors or acceptors.**
   b. Metabolism. Enzymatic **hydrolysis** is the primary route of metabolism for these functional groups. Esters and lactones are hydrolyzed to alcohols and carboxylic acids, while amides and lactams are hydrolyzed to amines and carboxylic acids. Esters and lactones are more susceptible to hydrolysis than are amides and lactams. Additionally, some lactams may undergo **N-dealkylation** prior to or in place of hydrolytic cleavage.

F. Lipophilic functional groups

1. **Alkyl groups** are **saturated hydrocarbon chains, links, and rings** that can vary in size from single-carbon **methyl** and **methylene** groups to large chains. Similar to the designations previously given for amines, the designation **alicyclic** refers to alkyl groups that are part of a nonaromatic ring, while the designation **aliphatic** refers to those that are part of a side chain or that function to connect, or bridge, other functional groups. Examples of alkyl groups are illustrated in Figure 8-9.
   a. Alkyl groups can participate in **van der Waals interactions** (i.e., induced dipole–induced dipole bonds) and **hydrophobic bonding.**
   b. Metabolism. Oxidation is the major route of metabolism. Alkyl side chains are usually oxidized at either the **terminal (ω)** or **penultimate (ω-1)** carbon atoms.

2. **Alkenes,** also known as **olefins,** are **unsaturated** analogs of alkyl groups (see Figure 8-9).
   a. The binding ability of alkenes is similar to that of saturated alkyl groups.

Figure 8-9. Examples of drugs that contain alkyl groups and alkenes as part of their chemical structure. For the sake of clarity, only certain functional groups have been highlighted.

   b. Metabolism. Alkenes are somewhat more reactive than alkyl groups and are subject to metabolic **hydration, epoxidation, peroxidation,** and **reduction.**

3. Most **aromatic hydrocarbons** are analogs of either **benzene** or **naphthalene** (see Figure 8-10 for examples). When attached to a drug molecule, benzene is referred to as a **phenyl group.**
   a. Similar to alkyl groups and alkenes, aromatic hydrocarbons can participate in **van der Waals interactions** and **hydrophobic bonding.** Additionally, aromatic rings can participate in **charge-transfer interactions.** Electron-rich aromatic rings (i.e., those with electron-donating groups) can form dipole-like interactions with electron-poor aromatic rings (i.e., those with electron-withdrawing groups).
   b. Metabolism. Oxidation is the primary route of metabolism for aromatic hydrocarbons, with **hydroxylation, epoxidation,** and **diol formation** comprising the three most common pathways.

4. **Ether** functional groups contain an oxygen atom bound on both sides by either alkyl or aromatic carbons. They can be present as either a terminal functional group, such as the **methoxy group** of naproxen, or as part of a central chain/backbone, such as that seen in gemfibrozil (Figure 8-10).
   a. The contribution of ethers to drug binding is minimal; however, these functional groups can participate in **dipole–induced dipole interactions** and can serve as **hydrogen-bond acceptors.**
   b. Metabolism. Methyl and ethyl ethers can undergo ***O*-dealkylation,** while those larger do not generally undergo metabolism. While ethers used as organic solvents (e.g., diethylether) can form **peroxides and may explode,** this property is generally not present in drug molecules.

5. **Alkyl and aromatic halides** are **electron-withdrawing** functional groups. They are often used to "lock" a drug molecule in a desired conformation and/or to decrease aromatic oxidation of the drug. Fluorine is the smallest halogen, with its size very similar to that of hydrogen. Chlorine is the second smallest, followed by bromine and iodine, respectively. See Figure 8-10 for specific examples.

Figure 8-10. Examples of drugs that contain an aromatic hydrocarbon, ether, and/or alkyl or aromatic halide as part of their chemical structure. For the sake of clarity, only certain functional groups have been highlighted.

    a. With the exception of fluorine, which can serve as a hydrogen-bond acceptor, halides do not directly participate in the binding of drugs to their receptors or other macromolecules.

    b. Metabolism. Aromatic halides are not normally metabolized. Alkyl halides can undergo **oxidative dehalogenation** to form aldehydes.

II. BIOCHEMISTRY

    A. Introduction. Biochemistry is the study of chemical principles that support life processes. It influences drug metabolism, therapeutic effectiveness, and biotransformation. Biochemically significant molecules include amino acids, carbohydrates, lipids, pyrimidines, purines, and biopolymers—proteins and enzymes, which are built from amino acids; polysaccharides, which are built from carbohydrates; and nucleic acids, which are built from pyrimidines and purines.

    B. Amino acids are the monomeric units of proteins and enzymes and have the following general formula:

$$R-CH-COOH$$
$$|$$
$$NH_2$$

    1. With the exception of glycine, naturally occurring amino acids are L, α-amino acids. Proteins are made up of the 20 different amino acids, which differ in the side chain (R) attached to

the α-carbon. The 20 different side chains vary in size, shape, charge, hydrogen-bonding capacity, and chemical reactivity. A protein can be hydrolyzed into its component α-amino acids by acids, bases, or enzymes.
   a. Amino acids with **acidic side chains** include aspartic acid and glutamic acid.
   b. Amino acids with **basic side chains** include arginine, lysine, and histamine.
   c. Amino acids with **polar, nonionic side chains** include glycine, serine, cysteine, threonine, tyrosine, asparagine, and glutamine.
   d. Amino acids with **nonpolar, hydrophobic side chains** include alanine, valine, leucine, isoleucine, phenylalanine, methionine, proline, and tryptophan.

2. Amino acids have a **zwitterion structure,** which accounts for their high melting point and low water solubility. Amino acids in solution have the following general formula:

$$R—CH—COO^-$$
$$\overset{|}{NH_3^+}$$

3. **Ionization** of amino acids to the zwitterion form or other forms depends on pH (Figure 8-11).

C. Carbohydrates. These are polyhydroxy aldehydes or ketones. Three major classes of carbohydrates exist.

1. **Monosaccharides** (simple sugars), such as glucose or fructose, consist of a single polyhydroxy aldehyde or ketone unit.
   a. Aldehydic monosaccharides are reducing sugars.
   b. Monosaccharides can be linked together by **glycosidic bonds,** which are hydrolyzed by acids but not by bases.

2. **Oligosaccharides,** such as sucrose, maltose, and lactose, consist of short chains of monosaccharides joined covalently.
   a. Sucrose cannot be absorbed by the intestine until it is converted by sucrase into its components, glucose and fructose.
   b. Maltose is hydrolyzed by maltase into two molecules of glucose.
   c. Lactose (or milk sugar) cannot be absorbed by the intestine until it is converted by lactase into its components, galactose and glucose.

3. **Polysaccharides,** such as **cellulose** and **glycogen,** consist of long chains of monosaccharides.

D. Pyrimidines and purines. These are bases that, when bonded with ribose, form nucleosides, which when subsequently bonded to phosphoric acid form nucleotides—the structural building blocks of nucleic acids.

1. **Pyrimidine bases** include:
   a. Cytosine (C), found in deoxyribonucleic acid (DNA) and ribonucleic acid (RNA)
   b. Uracil (U), found in RNA only
   c. Thymine (T), found in DNA only

Figure 8-11. Amino acid ionization in solution. The carboxyl and amino groups are either in ionized or unionized form depending on the pH of the solution.

   2. Purine bases include:
   a. **Adenine** (A), found in DNA and RNA
   b. **Guanine** (G), found in DNA and RNA

   3. Pyrimidines and purines exhibit **tautomerism** (a form of stereoisomerism) and can exist in either **keto** (lactam) or **enol** (lactim) forms.

E. Biopolymers

1. Proteins are polymers of amino acids that are linked together by **peptide bonds** (i.e., links between carbonyl carbons and amino nitrogens [Figure 8-12]). Proteins have four structural levels.
   a. **Primary** structure refers to the sequence of amino acids and location of disulfide bonds in the protein.
   b. **Secondary** structure refers to the spatial arrangement of sequenced amino acids (for example, α–conformation [helical coil] or β-conformation [pleated sheet]).
   c. **Tertiary** structure refers to the three-dimensional structure of a single protein.
   d. **Quaternary** structure refers to the arrangement of individual subunit chains into complex molecules.

2. Enzymes are proteins capable of acting as catalysts for biologic reactions. They may be simple or complex and may require cofactors or coenzymes for biologic activity.
   a. An enzyme enhances the rate of a specific chemical reaction by lowering the **activation energy** of the reaction. It does not change the reaction's equilibrium point, and it is not used up or permanently changed by the reaction.
   b. A cofactor may be an **inorganic component** (usually a metal ion) or a **nonprotein organic molecule.** A cofactor may be biologically inactive without an apoenzyme (the protein portion of a complex enzyme). A cofactor firmly bound to the apoenzyme is called a **prosthetic group.** An organic cofactor that is not firmly bound but is actively involved during catalysis is called a **coenzyme.**
   c. A complete, catalytically active enzyme system is referred to as a **holoenzyme.**
   d. Enzymes fall into six major classes.
      (1) Oxidoreductases (e.g., dehydrogenases, oxidases, peroxidases) are important in the oxidative metabolism of drugs.
      (2) Transferases catalyze the transfer of groups, such as phosphate and amino groups.
      (3) Hydrolases (e.g., proteolytic enzymes, amylases, esterases) hydrolyze their substrates.
      (4) Lyases (e.g., decarboxylases, deaminases) catalyze the removal of functional groups by means other than hydrolysis.
      (5) Ligases (e.g., DNA ligase, which binds nucleotides together during DNA synthesis) catalyze the coupling of two molecules.
      (6) Isomerases catalyze various isomerizations, such as the change from D to L forms or the change from cisisomers to transisomers.

3. Polysaccharides (also called glycans) are long-chain polymers of carbohydrates and may be linear or branched. They are classified as homopolysaccharides or heteropolysaccharides.
   a. **Homopolysaccharides** (e.g., starch, glycogen, cellulose) contain only one type of monomeric unit.
      (1) Starch (a reserve food material of plants) is composed of two glucose polymers—amylose (linear and water soluble) and amylopectin (highly branched and water insoluble). It yields mainly maltose (a glucose disaccharide) after enzymatic hydrolysis with salivary or pancreatic amylase; only glucose after complete hydrolysis by strong acids.

Figure 8-12. Peptide bond formation occurs as a result of the condensation of the carboxyl group of one amino acid with the amino group of another. Water is eliminated during this process.

(2) Glycogen, like amylopectin, is a highly branched, compact chain of D-glucose. The main storage polysaccharide of animal cells, it is found mostly in liver and muscle and can be hydrolyzed by salivary or pancreatic amylase into maltose and D-glucose.

(3) Cellulose (a water-insoluble structural polysaccharide found in plant cell walls) is a linear, unbranched chain of D-glucose. It cannot be digested by humans because the human intestinal tract secretes no enzyme capable of hydrolyzing it.

  b. Heteropolysaccharides (e.g., heparin, hyaluronic acid) contain two or more types of monomeric units.

(1) Heparin (an acid mucopolysaccharide) consists of sulfate derivatives of N-acetyl-D-glucosamine and D-iduronate. It can be isolated from lung tissue and is used medically to prevent blood clot formation.

(2) Hyaluronic acid, a component of bacterial cell walls as well as of the vitreous humor and synovial fluid, consists of alternating units of N-acetyl-D-glucosamine and N-acetyl-muramic acid.

4. Nucleic acids are linear polymers of nucleotides—pyrimidine and purine bases linked to ribose or deoxyribose sugars (nucleosides) and bound to phosphate groups. The backbone of the nucleic acid consists of alternating phosphate and pentose units with a purine or pyrimidine base attached to each.

  a. Nucleic acids are closely associated with **cellular cations** and such basic proteins as **histones** and **protamines.**

  b. The two main types of nucleic acids are **DNA** and **RNA.** RNA exists in three forms.

(1) Ribosomal RNA (rRNA) functions as a framework to bind both messenger and transfer RNA. It is comprised of numerous subunits with the 40S and 60S being the most well known. Ribosomal RNA is also thought to have other functions; however, these have not been fully elucidated.

(2) Messenger RNA (mRNA) serves as the template for protein synthesis and specifies a polypeptide's amino acid sequence.

(3) Transfer RNA (tRNA) carries activated amino acids to the ribosomes, where the amino acids are incorporated into the growing polypeptide chain.

  c. In both DNA and RNA, the successive nucleotides are joined by **phosphodiester bonds** between the 5'-hydroxy group of one nucleotide's pentose and the 3'-hydroxy group of the next nucleotide's pentose.

  d. DNA differs from RNA in that it **lacks a hydroxyl group** at the pentose's C_2' position, and it contains T rather than U.

  e. DNA structure consists of two α-helical DNA strands coiled around the same axis to form a double helix. The strands are antiparallel—the 5', 3'-internucleotide phosphodiester links run in opposite directions.

(1) Hydrogen bonding between specific base pairs A–T and C–G holds the two DNA strands together. The strands are complementary (the base sequence of one strand determines the base sequence of the other).

(2) The **hydrophobic bases** are on the inside of the helix; the hydrophilic deoxyribose–phosphate backbone is on the outside.

III. BIOCHEMICAL METABOLISM

A. Overview. Biochemical metabolism is the review of pathways that lead to the synthesis or breakdown of compounds important to the life of an organism.

1. Control of metabolism. Metabolism is controlled by substrate concentration, enzymes (constitutive or induced), allosteric (regulatory) enzymes, hormones, and compartmentation.

2. Catabolism is the sum of degradation reactions that usually release energy for useful work (e.g., mechanical, osmotic, biosynthetic).

3. Anabolism is the sum of biosynthetic (build-up) reactions that consume energy to form new biochemical compounds (metabolites).

4. Amphibolic pathways are those that may be used for both catabolic as well as anabolic purposes. **Krebs cycle** breaks down metabolites primarily to release 90% of the total energy of an organism. It also draws off metabolites to form compounds such as amino acids (e.g., aspartic, glutamic, alanine). Hemoglobin has its heme moiety formed from succinyl coenzyme A (succinyl CoA) and glycine followed by a complex set of reactions.

B. Bioenergetics

1. **Substrate level phosphorylation** entails the formation of one unit of adenosine triphosphate (ATP) per unit of metabolite transformed (e.g., succinyl CoA to succinate, phosphoenolpyruvate to pyruvate). These reactions do not need oxygen.

2. **Oxidative phosphorylation** entails the formation of one-and-a-half or two-and-a-half units of ATP per unit of metabolite transformed by oxidoreductase enzymes (e.g., dehydrogenases); these enzymes use flavin A dinucleotide (FAD) formed from the vitamin riboflavin, or nicotinamide A dinucleotide (NAD^+) from the vitamin nicotinamide as cofactors. The reactions are coupled to the electron transport system, and the energy released is used to form ATP in the mitochondria.

C. Carbohydrate metabolism

1. **Catabolism.** This process releases stored energy from carbohydrates.
   a. **Glycogenolysis** is the breakdown of glycogen into glucose phosphate in the liver and skeletal muscle. It is controlled by the hormones glucagon and epinephrine.
   b. **Glycolysis** is the breakdown of sugar phosphates (e.g., glucose, fructose, glycerol) into pyruvate (aerobically) or lactate (anaerobically).

2. **Anabolism.** This process consumes energy to build up complex molecules from simpler molecules.
   a. **Glycogenesis** is the formation of glycogen in the liver and muscles from glucose consumed in the diet; its synthesis is controlled by the pancreatic hormone insulin.
   b. **Gluconeogenesis** is the formation of glucose from noncarbohydrate sources, such as lactate, alanine, pyruvate, and Krebs cycle metabolites; fatty acids cannot form glucose.

D. Krebs cycle. This pathway is also known as the citric acid cycle, serves both breakdown and synthetic purposes, and occurs in the mitochondrial compartment.

1. **Catabolism.** This pathway converts pyruvate (glycolysis), acetyl CoA (fatty acid degradation), and amino acids to carbon dioxide and water with a release of energy. The cycle is strictly oxygen-dependent (aerobic). Mature red blood cells lack mitochondria; hence, there is no Krebs cycle activity.

2. **Anabolism.** This pathway forms amino acids such as aspartate and glutamate from cycle intermediates; also, the porphyrin ring of heme (e.g., hemoglobin, myoglobin, cytochromes) is formed from a cycle intermediate.

3. **Anaplerotic reactions.** Because metabolites are used to make amino acids or heme (e.g., succinyl CoA), the metabolite must be replaced by intermediates from other sources (e.g., glutamate from the breakdown of protein forms α-ketoglutarate).

4. **Electron transport.** The electron transport system accepts electrons and hydrogen from the oxidation of Krebs cycle metabolites and couples the energy released to synthesize ATP in the mitochondria.

E. Lipid metabolism

1. **Catabolism. Triglycerides** (triacylglycerols) stored in fat cells (adipocytes) are hydrolyzed by hormone-sensitive lipases into three fatty acids and glycerol.
   a. **Fatty acids** are broken down by beta oxidation to acetyl CoA (two carbon units), which enter the Krebs cycle to complete the oxidation to carbon dioxide and water with release of considerable energy. Too rapid breakdown of fatty acids leads to ketone bodies (ketogenesis) as in diabetes mellitus.
   b. **Glycerol** enters glycolysis and is oxidized to pyruvate and, via the Krebs cycle, to carbon dioxide and water.
   c. **Steroids** may be converted to other compounds such as bile acids, vitamin D, or steroidal hormones (e.g., cortisone, estrogens, androgens); they are not broken down completely.

2. **Anabolism. Biosynthesis** forms fatty acids, steroids, and other terpene-related metabolites.
   a. **Fatty acids** are formed in the cytoplasm, and unsaturation occurs in the mitochondria

or endoplasmic reticulum. Humans cannot make linoleic acid; thus, it is important that it be included in the diet (essential fatty acid).
   b. Terpene compounds are derived from acetyl CoA via mevalonate and include:
      (1) Cholesterol and other steroids
      (2) Fat-soluble vitamins (i.e., A, D, E, K)
      (3) Bile acids
   c. Sphingolipids contain sphingenine formed from palmitoyl CoA and serine. Sphingenine forms a ceramide backbone when joined to fatty acids. The addition of sugars, sialic acid, or choline phosphate forms compounds such as cerebrosides, gangliosides, or sphingomyelin found in nerve tissues and membranes.
   d. Phosphatidyl compounds, such as phosphatidyl choline (lecithin), phosphatidyl serine, or ethanolamine, are also important parts of membranes.

F. Nitrogen metabolism. Nitrogen metabolism involves amino acid metabolism and nucleic acid metabolism (see Chapter 9 for a discussion of the nucleic acid role in cell activity).

   1. Catabolism
      a. Amino acids. The amino group is removed by a transaminase enzyme. The carbon skeleton is broken down to acetyl CoA (ketogenic amino acids) or to citric acid cycle intermediates (glycogenic amino acids) and oxidized to carbon dioxide and water for energy. Glycogenic amino acids form glucose as needed via gluconeogenesis; some amino acids are both ketogenic and glycogenic (e.g., tyrosine).
      b. Purines are salvaged (90%), and the remaining 10% are degraded in a sequence that includes xanthine oxidase forming uric acid in humans.
      c. Pyrimidines are catabolized to β-alanine, ammonia, and carbon dioxide.

   2. Anabolism
      a. Amino acids are formed from the citric acid cycle intermediates (see III D 2); others must be eaten daily in dietary proteins. The latter are called essential amino acids (phenylalanine, valine, tryptophan [PVT]; threonine, isoleucine, methionine [TIM]; histidine, arginine in infants, lysine, leucine [HALL]).
      b. Purines are formed by complex reactions using carbamoyl phosphate, aspartate, glutamine, glycine, carbon dioxide, and formyl tetrahydrofolate.
      c. Pyrimidines are formed from aspartate and carbamoyl phosphate in a multistep process.

G. Nitrogen excretion. Excess nitrogen must be eliminated because it is toxic. Humans primarily excrete urea but also excrete uric acid.

   1. Urea synthesis. The **Krebs-Henseleit pathway** is used to form urea principally in the liver. The ammonia is removed from amino acids by amino acid transferases (transaminases) that use pyridoxal phosphate (vitamin B_6) as a coenzyme. **Glutamine** is formed from glutamate (an intermediate) and ammonia; glutamine and carbon dioxide form carbamoyl phosphate, which enters the urea cycle and after several steps forms urea.

   2. Uric acid synthesis. Although most purines are salvaged, humans excrete the remaining purines as uric acid.

STUDY QUESTIONS

Directions: Each of the numbered items or incomplete statements in this section is followed by answers or by completions of the statement. Select the **one** lettered answer or completion that is **best** in each case.

1. Which of the following functional groups can react with hydrochloric acid to form a salt?

(A) Tertiary amines
(B) Carboxylic acids
(C) Amides
(D) Ethers
(E) Secondary alcohols

2. The compound shown contains all of the following functional groups EXCEPT:

(A) a phenol
(B) a substituted phenyl ring
(C) an ester
(D) an alicyclic nitrogen
(E) a ketone

3. Which of the following functional groups is most susceptible to hydrolysis?

(A) $R-CO-R$
(B) $R-COOR$
(C) $R-O-R$
(D) $R-NH-CH_3$
(E) $R-COOH$

4. Monomer units of proteins are known as

(A) monosaccharides
(B) prosthetic groups
(C) amino acids
(D) purines
(E) nucleosides

5. Which of the following formulas represents the zwitterion form of an amino acid?

(A) $H_2N-CH-COO^-$
   $\quad\quad\quad |$
   $\quad\quad\quad R$

(B) $\overset{+}{H_3N}-CH-COOH$
   $\quad\quad\quad\quad |$
   $\quad\quad\quad\quad R$

(C) $H_2N-CH-COOH$
   $\quad\quad\quad |$
   $\quad\quad\quad R$

(D) $\overset{+}{H_3N}-CH-COO^-$
   $\quad\quad\quad\quad |$
   $\quad\quad\quad\quad R$

(E) $H_2N-CH-CONH-CH-COOH$
   $\quad\quad\quad |\quad\quad\quad\quad\quad |$
   $\quad\quad\quad R\quad\quad\quad\quad\quad R$

6. Glucose is a carbohydrate that cannot be hydrolyzed into a simpler substance. It is best described as

(A) a sugar
(B) a monosaccharide
(C) a disaccharide
(D) a polysaccharide
(E) an oligosaccharide

7. All of the following carbohydrates are considered to be polysaccharides EXCEPT

(A) heparin
(B) starch
(C) glycogen
(D) maltose
(E) cellulose

8. Which of the following compounds are considered the building blocks of nucleic acids?

(A) Nucleotides
(B) Nucleosides
(C) Monosaccharides
(D) Purines
(E) Amino acids

9. Which of the following terms best describes a cofactor that is firmly bound to an apoenzyme?

(A) Holoenzyme
(B) Prosthetic group
(C) Coenzyme
(D) Transferase
(E) Heteropolysaccharide

10. Enzymes that uncouple peptide linkages are best classified as

(A) hydrolases
(B) ligases
(C) oxidoreductases
(D) transferases
(E) isomerases

11. The sugar that is inherent in the nucleic acids RNA and DNA is

(A) glucose
(B) sucrose
(C) ribose
(D) digitoxose
(E) maltose

Directions: Each item below contains three suggested answers of which **one or more** is correct. Choose the answer

A	if **I only** is correct
B	if **III only** is correct
C	if **I and II** are correct
D	if **II and III** are correct
E	if **I, II, and III** are correct

12. Which of the following functional groups can form a hydrogen bond?

I. An aromatic amine
II. A tertiary hydroxyl
III. An aromatic hydrocarbon

13. Which of the following functional groups commonly undergoes conjugation with glucuronic acid?

I. A carboxylic acid
II. A primary amine
III. A phenol

Questions 14–16

The following questions refer to the drug molecule shown below.

14. The functional groups that enhance this compound's ability to cross cell membranes include:

I. the phenyl rings
II. the central alkyl chain
III. the secondary and tertiary hydroxyls

15. Based upon the functional groups present, this drug would be expected to be able to form:

I. van der Waals interactions
II. ionic bonds
III. hydrogen bonds

16. Possible metabolic pathways for this drug include:

I. reduction of the carboxylic acid
II. hydrolytic cleavage
III. aromatic oxidation

ANSWERS AND EXPLANATIONS

1. The answer is A *[I C 2 c].*
Substances that react with acids to form salts must be bases. Only organic compounds that contain the nitrogen-containing amine group are bases. While amides contain nitrogen, the adjacent carbonyl group decreases the basicity; therefore, they are essentially neutral.

2. The answer is C *[Figures 8-4, 8-7, 8-8, 8-10].*
As shown in Figure 8-8, esters have a carbonyl atom directly bonded to an oxygen atom. This structural feature is not present in this compound. However, the compound does have three substituted phenyl rings, two phenols, a tertiary alicyclic nitrogen, a ketone, and an ether.

3. The answer is B *[I E 2 b].*
Hydrolysis is a double decomposition reaction in which water is one of the reactants. Esters, particularly simple esters, commonly undergo hydrolysis. Certain types of ethers such as glycosides also undergo hydrolysis, but they usually require strongly alkaline conditions or a catalyst such as an enzyme. Ketones, amines, or carboxylic acids do not undergo hydrolysis.

4. The answer is C *[II B 1, II E 1].*
Proteins are large molecules with molecular weights ranging from 5000 to more than 1 million daltons. All proteins are composed of chains of amino acids and can be hydrolyzed to yield a mixture of their respective amino acids. There are 20 α-amino acids, which are commonly found in proteins. All the naturally occurring amino acids in proteins are L-enantiomers, with the exception of glycine. All have at least one amino group and one carboxyl group. The amino acids are linked together through the amino group of one amino acid and the carboxyl group of another amino acid with the splitting out of a water molecule to form an amide linkage, which in a protein is referred to as a peptide.
Monosaccharides are simple, nonhydrolyzable sugars. Purines and pyrimidines are organic bases, while a prosthetic group is a cofactor that is firmly bound to an apoenzyme.

5. The answer is D *[I A 1 a, II B 2, 3, II E 1, Figures 8-2, 8-11, 8-12].*
A zwitterion is a single species containing both negative and positive charges. It sometimes is referred to as an internal salt. Amino acids have an amino group and a carboxyl group in the same molecule. The amino group, which is basic, attracts the proton from the carboxyl group and becomes positively charged, while the carboxyl group becomes negatively charged when it donates its proton to the amino group. Amino acids exist as zwitterions at near neutral pH such as occurs within a cell or in the bloodstream.

6. The answer is B *[II C 1].*
While glucose is a sugar, it is more specifically a simple sugar that cannot be hydrolyzed into more simple sugars—thus, it is classified as a monosaccharide. Sugars may be simple, such as glucose, or complex, such as sucrose, and are classified as disaccharides or oligosaccharides, respectively. Polysaccharides consist of long chains of monosaccharides such as cellulose and glycogen.

7. The answer is D *[II C 2 b, 3, E 3 a, b].*
Polysaccharides are long-chain polymers of sugars. As the prefix "poly" indicates, there are many sugar units in the molecule. Maltose is composed of two molecules of glucose and is classified as a disaccharide or an oligosaccharide.

8. The answer is A *[II D, E 4].*
Nucleic acids are linear polymers of nucleotides that consist of three different molecules that are covalently linked to form one unit: (1) an organic base of either a purine or a pyrimidine; (2) a 5-carbon sugar (e.g., pentose); and (3) a phosphoric acid group. A nucleoside consists of the organic base and the pentose. A monosaccharide is a simple nonhydrolyzable carbohydrate, which may be considered a building block of polysaccharides. Purines are heterocyclic bases. Adenine and guanine are the two purines found in deoxyribonucleic acid (DNA) and ribonucleic acid (RNA). Amino acids are the building blocks of protein.

9. The answer is B *[II E 2 b–d].*
Complex, or conjugated, enzymes contain a nonprotein group called a cofactor, which is required for biologic activity. In many cases, the cofactor is quite firmly bound to the protein. In others, the binding occurs only during the reaction that the enzyme catalyzes. Cofactors that are firmly bound to the protein are known as prosthetic groups, whereas those that are actively bound to the protein only during catalysis are referred to as coenzymes.

A holoenzyme is a complete, catalytically active enzyme system. A transferase is an enzyme that catalyzes the transfer of groups from one substance to another, such as catechol-*O*-methyl transferase (COMT). A heteropolysaccharide is a polysaccharide that contains two or more different monomeric units, such as heparin.

10. The answer is A *[II E 2 d].*
A peptide linkage is an amide functional group formed from the loss of a molecule of water from two amino acids. Uncoupling this linkage is the reverse of this reaction, a hydrolysis reaction. A hydrolase is an enzyme that catalyzes hydrolysis reactions. More specific terms for an enzyme that catalyzes the hydrolysis of proteins are amidase or peptidase. A ligase catalyzes the coupling of two molecules. An oxidoreductase catalyzes oxidation reactions. A transferase catalyzes the transfer of groups from one substance to another. An isomerase catalyzes the interconversion of one isomer to another.

11. The answer is C *[II E 4].*
Nucleic acids are biopolymers consisting of long chains of nucleotides. Nucleotides contain a pentose monosaccharide as one of their three constituents. RNA contains, as the name suggests, the monosaccharide ribose, whereas DNA contains deoxyribose. The only difference between these two sugars is the absence of oxygen in the 2 position of the ribose ring. Glucose, also known as dextrose, is a hexose. Digitoxose is a deoxyhexose present in the digitalis glycosides. Sucrose and maltose are disaccharides.

12. The answer is C (I, II) *[I C 2 b, D 1 a, F 3 a].*
Hydrogen bonds are a specialized type of dipole bond in which a hydrogen atom serves as a bridge between two electronegative atoms. Hydrogen-bond donors include hydroxyl groups, phenols, amines, and amides. Hydrogen-bond acceptors include hydroxyl groups, phenols, unionized nitrogen atoms, ketones, and ethers. Hydrocarbons, regardless if they are aliphatic, alicyclic, or aromatic, are not capable of forming hydrogen bonds.

13. The answer is E (I, II, and III) *[I B 2 e, C 2 d, D 2 d].*
Glucuronide conjugation is the most common phase II metabolic pathway for two reasons: (1) The body has a readily available supply of glucuronic acid, and (2) there are a large number of functional groups that can react with this compound. Included among these functional groups are carboxylic acids, primary, secondary and tertiary amines, and phenols.

14–16. The answers are: 14-C (I, II) *[I A 1, D 1 b, F 1, 3],* **15-E (I, II, and III)** *[I B 2 b, C 2 b, D 1 a, F 1 a, 3 a],* **16-B (III)** *[I B 2 e, E 2 b, F 3 b].*
Lipophilic functional groups increase a drug's ability to cross cell membranes. The three aromatic phenyl rings, as well as the aliphatic butyl chain connecting the central phenyl ring to the nitrogen of the piperadine ring, are all lipophilic (i.e., hydrophobic) and contribute to the drug's passage through cell membranes. The hydroxyl groups, as well as the acidic carboxylic acid and the basic alicyclic amine, are all hydrophilic and enhance the overall water solubility of the compound.

The phenyl rings, as well as the central alkyl chain and the methyl groups, are capable of forming van der Waals interactions with aromatic and aliphatic hydrocarbon regions on receptor molecules. The carboxylic acid and the basic nitrogen are capable of forming both ionic and hydrogen bonds, while the hydroxyl groups are also capable of forming hydrogen bonds.

Of the metabolic pathways listed, aromatic oxidation is the only plausible choice. The two unsubstituted phenyl rings are very susceptible to hydroxylation, epoxidation, and/or diol formation. Carboxylic acids are not normally reduced, but rather conjugated with either glucuronic acid, glycine or glutamine. Esters, amides and their cyclic derivatives, lactones and lactams, are the primary functional groups that undergo hydrolysis. None of these functional groups are present in the compound shown.

9
Microbiology
Gail Goodman-Snitkoff

I. SCOPE OF MICROBIOLOGY. Microbiology is the study of organisms from three domains as well as acellular entities that are not considered to be living in the biological sense.

A. Domains of living organisms

1. **Archaea** include prokaryotes with cell walls that are biochemically different from bacteria and that inhabit extreme environments of heat, cold, pH, or salts. Archaea are not a medically important domain of microorganisms.

2. **Eukarya** contains some microorganisms—for example, fungi (yeasts and molds), protozoa, and algae—along with macroscopic organisms such as mushrooms, plants, and animals. **Dimorphic fungi** are those that can exist in either the unicellular (yeast) or the filamentous (mold) phase, depending on the incubation temperature (e.g., *Histoplasma* and *Blastomyces*).

   a. **Fungi** are classified into phyla based on the type of reproductive structures observed or the lack of observable sexual reproductive structures.
   - (1) **Ascomycota** (ascus) (e.g., *Candida* and *Histoplasma*)
   - (2) **Basidiomycota** (basidium) (e.g., *Cryptococcus*)
   - (3) **Zygomycota** (zygote) (e.g., *Rhizopus*)
   - (4) **Deuteromycota** (asexual, also called fungi imperfecti) (e.g., *Coccidioides*). Recently, some sexual reproductive states have been identified in fungi classified as belonging to Deuteromycota.

   b. **Protozoa,** unicellular, nonphotosynthetic eukaryotes characterized by mode of motility, include the following:
   - (1) **Mastigophora** (flagellates) (e.g., *Giardia*)
   - (2) **Sarcodina** (amoebae) (e.g., *Entamoeba*)
   - (3) **Ciliophora** (ciliates) (e.g., *Balantidium*)
   - (4) **Sporozoa** (nonmotile) (e.g., *Plasmodium*)

3. **Bacteria** contain a wide variety of prokaryotes, including gram-positive and gram-negative bacteria. Sections II–VII characterize bacteria in more detail.

B. Nonliving, but medically significant entities are the following

1. **Viruses** (see VIII), which are classified by:
   a. **Capsid structure,** which is the protein coating around the nucleic acid
   b. **Type and strandedness of nucleic acid,** which could be DNA or RNA, either single or double stranded
   c. Presence or absence of a **lipid envelope** surrounding the protein capsid
   d. Presence of **enzymes,** which may be either incorporated into the lipid envelope or found in the capsid near the nucleic acid

2. **Prions, infectious proteins,** are implicated in some spongiform encephalopathies (e.g., mad cow disease, Creutzfeldt-Jakob disease, and kuru).

II. TAXONOMY AND NOMENCLATURE OF BACTERIA

A. Taxonomy is classification or ordering into groups based on degree of relatedness. Bacteria are **prokaryotes** that belong to the Bacteria domain and the Eubacteria kingdom and are grouped and named primarily by morphology, biochemical and metabolic differences, and immunologic and genetic relationships. DNA technology has lead to the reclassification of some organisms based on DNA sequences and homology. Bacteria are named using the **Linnaean** or **binomial** system as a genus and species (e.g., *Homo sapiens* is the genus and species for humans).

B. Morphology is the classification of bacteria by shape and structure.

1. **Cultural morphology** is based on the size, shape, and texture of colonies that are grown in pure culture on an agar plate. Each colony originates from a **colony-forming unit (CFU),** consisting of a single cell or group of adherent cells.

2. **Microscopic morphology** describes bacteria on the basis of the size, shape, and arrangement of the cells (see II.C–D).

C. Stains. Because of their small size and relative transparency, bacteria must be stained to be visible under the light microscope. Staining is also used as a classification system. The major types of staining reactions are the following:

1. **Simple stain.** A single dye (e.g., Gentian violet, safranin) that colors the cells.

2. **Gram stain.** A differential staining procedure that divides bacterial cells into either gram-positive (purple) or gram-negative (pink).

3. **Acid-fast stain.** A procedure that stains cells that have an outer layer of a waxy lipid (acid-fast) but not cells that lack that layer (non-acid-fast).

4. **Spore stain.** A procedure that uses heat to help dye enter the spore.

5. **Capsule stain.** Two dyes are used to stain the cell and the background, allowing visualization of the unstained capsular material.

D. Bacterial cell shape and arrangement

1. **Cocci** are spherical and exist in chains (*Streptococcus pyogenes*), pairs or diplococci (*Streptococcus pneumoniae, Neisseria gonorrhoeae*), clusters (staphylococci), and packets of four or eight (sarcinae).

2. **Bacilli** are cylindrical and rod-shaped organisms (pseudomonads, *Escherichia*).

3. **Coccobacilli** are short rounded rods (*Brucella*).

4. **Spirochetes and spirilla** are helical, like a corkscrew (*Treponema pallidum*); spirilla are rigid helices, whereas spirochetes are flexible helices.

5. **Fusobacteria** have tapered ends and are slightly curved (i.e., fusiform; *Fusobacterium mortiferum*).

6. **Filamentous** organisms are branching organisms and are associated with mold-like bacteria (*Actinomyces bovis*).

7. **Vibrios** are comma shaped rods (*Vibrio cholerae*).

8. **Pleomorphic** organisms exist in varied forms (*Haemophilus, Legionella, Corynebacteria*).

E. Other classification parameters

1. **Presence or absence** of
   a. **Spores** used for survival (*Bacillus anthracis*).
   b. **Capsules** or **slime layers** used for adherence. Capsules are also antiphagocytic (*Streptococcus pneumoniae, Neisseria meningitidis*).

2. **Motility** and the type of **flagella**
   a. **Monotrichous.** A single flagellum
   b. **Lophotrichous.** A tuft of flagella at either or both poles
   c. **Amphitrichous.** A flagellum at both poles
   d. **Peritrichous.** Flagella distributed evenly over the entire cell
   e. **Axial filaments.** Periplasmic flagella wrapped around spirochetes
   f. **Gliding motility.** As demonstrated by slime molds

III. STRUCTURE OF THE PROKARYOTIC CELL

A. Overview. Prokaryotic cells (bacteria) are **small** and relatively **simple** (Figure 9-1). They have the following characteristics:

1. **Contain no internal membrane bound organelles** but have complex cell wall structures

2. Lack a true nucleus, a nuclear membrane, and intracytoplasmic membranous organelles (e.g., plastids, endoplasmic reticulum, vacuoles)

3. Multiply asexually by **binary fission** rather than by mitosis or meiosis

4. **Protein synthesis** is mediated by 70s rather than by 80s ribosomes.

5. Bacterial genetic information is arranged on a single supercoiled circular strand of double-stranded DNA; the **nucleoid** is the area of the cell containing the tightly coiled chromosome.

6. Some bacteria contain storage granules, or inclusion bodies, the staining of these granules may also be useful in identifying the bacteria.

B. External structures

1. **Capsule and slime layer**
   a. The **capsule** is an adherent, surface coat made up of long chain repeats of carbohydrates or peptides. The capsule differs in composition among bacteria of different genus and species. Antigenic differences among capsules can be used to identify strains within a single species of bacteria (*Streptococcus pneumoniae*). Capsules are usually polysaccharide in nature; however, the capsule of *Bacillus* is polypeptide. The capsule has several functions:
      (1) Increases the **virulence** (degree of organism pathogenicity) of a microorganism
      (2) Prevents **phagocytosis** of the organism by macrophages and neutrophils
      (3) Aids in **adherence** of the organism to host cells
   b. If the polysaccharide is nonadherent, it is called a **slime layer.**

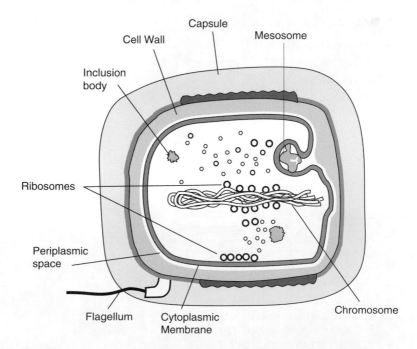

Figure 9-1. Structure of a procaryote cell. [Adapted with permission from Winn WC Jr, Allen SD, Janda WM, et al. Koneman's Color Atlas and Textbook of Diagnostic Microbiology, 6th ed. Philadelphia: Lippincott Williams & Wilkins, 2006.]

    c. Transformation from smooth to rough colonies on media indicates **capsule loss.** Concurrently, there is a loss of virulence. This capsular material is immunogenic, thereby inducing the production of **antibodies,** which act as opsonins to enhance phagocytosis (**opsonization**).

2. Flagella are proteinaceous, helically coiled organs used for movement that extend outward from the cytoplasm through the cell wall into the environment (Figure 9-2). Flagella rotate either clockwise or counterclockwise, allowing a series of runs and tumbles in response to chemicals in the environment. The direction of movement is controlled by a complex mechanism involving chemoreceptors and an intracellular cascade of methylation and phosphorylation reactions, causing bacteria to move toward nutrient chemoattractants and away from repellants.

  a. Structure

    (1) Flagella are composed of **flagellin,** a protein called **H antigen,** which is antigenically distinct from other flagella in eucaryotes.

    (2) Flagella have **three parts**:

      (a) Basal body

        (i) Attaches the flagella to the cytoplasmic membrane and cell wall

Figure 9-2. Structure of a procaryote flagella from a Gram-negative organism. [Adapted with permission from Winn WC Jr, Allen SD, Janda WM, et al. Koneman's Color Atlas and Textbook of Diagnostic Microbiology, 6th ed. Philadelphia : Lippincott Williams & Wilkins, 2006.]

        (ii) The number of rings that make up the basal body differ in gram-positive (two) and gram-negative (four) organisms. The L and D rings are absent in Gram-positive organisms.

    (b) Hook

    (c) Filament

  b. Periplasmic flagella, also called **axial filaments,** occur in spirochetes and are embedded into the cell wall's outer membrane. Because they cause a corkscrew type of motion on contraction, these organisms are not hindered by the viscosity of media.

3. Pili (fimbriae) are proteinaceous, hair-like extensions that are shorter than flagella and composed of regularly arranged protein subunits called **pilin** or **fimbrilin.** They are more common in gram-negative organisms but can be found in gram-positive organisms. There are two morphological and functional varieties:

  a. Common (attachment) pili

    (1) Appear in greater numbers than sex pili

    (2) Have adhesive properties, which are important in the formation of biofilms

    (3) Are lectins, which are responsible for trophism, the ability of the organism to bind to specific receptors on host cells

  b. Sex (conjugative or F) pili

    (1) Are longer than common pili

    (2) Form in groups of < 10

    (3) Are involved in the transport of DNA between donor and recipient cells

C. The cell wall, periplasmic space, and cytoplasmic membrane

1. The **cell wall** is rigid. Although it provides the general shape of the cell, its function is to protect the cell from osmotic shock. If the cell wall is destroyed, the bacterial cells are susceptible to alterations in the tonicity of the environment. The wall is composed of a basic **peptidoglycan layer,** which in turn is composed of repeating disaccharide units (a polymer of *N*–acetylglucosamine and *N*–acetylmuramic acid), with a four-amino-acid side chain that is covalently linked to amino acids from neighboring disaccharide units, forming a stable cross-linked structure. Most bacteria are designated as either gram-positive or gram-negative, based on fundamental differences in the components of the cell wall. Owing to the uniqueness and the importance of the cell wall to bacterial viability, it is the target of many antibiotic agents.

  a. Gram-positive organisms have a thick cell wall, which is 90% peptidoglycan, with extensive cross-linking that is approximately 40 layers thick and forms a layered network around the cytoplasmic membrane. Within the cell wall, a variety of elements serve to stabilize the cell wall, maintain its association with the cytoplasmic membrane, and act as receptors and antigenic determinants. These elements include proteins, polysaccharides and teichoic acid (glycerol or ribitol phosphodiesters).

    (1) Teichoic acids (glycerol or ribitol phosphodiesters)

      (a) Membrane-associated teichoic acids (lipoteichoic acid) are covalently linked to glycolipids of the cytoplasmic membrane.

      (b) Wall-associated teichoic acids are covalently linked to the glycan chain of peptidoglycan.

  b. Gram-negative organisms' cell walls are multilayered with a thin peptidoglycan layer that has no teichoic acids. External to this is the **outer membrane,** a complex cell wall layer, which is linked to the peptidoglycan layer by the **lipoprotein** layer. The outer membrane acts as a hydrophobic diffusion barrier and consists of

    (1) Phospholipid, a bilayer similar to the cytoplasmic membrane with protein channels, called **porins,** for nutrient transport. The phospholipid layer of the outer membrane faces the cytoplasmic membrane.

    (2) The **lipopolysaccharide (LPS)** component projects from the cell surface and is both toxic and antigenic (**O antigen**). In a gram-negative organism, the LPS **blocks diffusion** of low molecular weight substances into the cell, so antibiotics and chemicals that attack the cell wall (e.g., lysozyme, penicillin) cannot easily pass through. LPS, also known as **endotoxin,** is toxic to humans and is composed of three parts:

      (a) Lipid A: toxic portion that can either slough off intact cells or be released into circulation upon lysis of the cell, causing nonspecific inflammation, including diarrhea, fever, and septic shock

   (b) Core polysaccharide: similar within genera
   (c) O-specific side chain: species specific
  (3) Protein

 2. The **periplasmic space,** an area between the cell wall and the cytoplasmic membrane, contains a gel of several types of molecules (e.g., hydrolytic enzymes, periplasmic-binding proteins) that process molecules before they enter the cytoplasm. It also contains proteins that act as chemoreceptors for chemotaxis, others that act as carriers of nutrients (similar to carriers in the cytoplasmic membrane), and antibiotic-inactivating enzymes.

 3. The **cytoplasmic membrane** is a phospholipid bilayer matrix of a fatty acid core (hydrophobic) and glycerol phosphate (hydrophilic). In the presence of proteins embedded in the matrix, these membranes are actively and passively engaged in several **cellular functions.**
  a. Transportation of nutrients through
   (1) Passive diffusion
   (2) Facilitated diffusion
   (3) Active transport (this method is the only one that actively uses energy because molecules are moving into the cell against a concentration gradient)
  b. The site of **respiration proteins** used for **electron transport** and energy formation
  c. Enzymes involved in the assembly of the cell wall components
  d. Secretion of exotoxins and other substances for the breakdown of macromolecules

D. Internal structures

 1. Storage granules are inclusion bodies used for food or energy storage (e.g., polyphosphate complexes, carbohydrate).

 2. Ribosomes are cellular units that synthesize protein by the translation of messenger RNA (mRNA) base sequences into amino acid protein sequences. These ribosomes, unlike those in eukaryotic cells, are 70s units and are not associated with membranes such as mitochondria or rough endoplasmic reticulum.

 3. The **nuclear region** of bacteria is a condensed area (a nucleoid) containing the bacterial chromosome, which lacks a nuclear membrane and consists of a long, double-stranded, supercoiled, circular DNA molecule.

 4. Some organisms contain **plasmids,** circular double-stranded pieces of DNA that are found outside of the bacterial chromosome. These structures are autonomous (not controlled by the bacterial chromosome), contain information for heavy metal and antibiotic resistance, are conjunctive, and carry genetic elements called **transposons.**

IV. MICROBIAL PHYSIOLOGY

A. Nutritional types

 1. Autotrophs use carbon dioxide as their sole or main carbon source.
  a. Photoautotrophs use light as an energy source.
  b. Chemoautotrophs oxidize organic or inorganic compounds to produce energy.

 2. Heterotrophs use organic compounds as their main carbon source.
  a. Photoheterotrophs use light as an energy source.
  b. Chemoheterotrophs oxidize organic and inorganic compounds to produce energy.

 3. Prototrophs are parent cells that have no special nutritional requirements. They require the same nutrients as the major number of the natural members of the species.

 4. Auxotrophs are mutated so that they cannot synthesize the same essential nutrients (usually amino acids) as their parent cell.

 5. Subsets
  a. Holophytic. Organisms whose nutrients must be in a soluble, diffusible form
  b. Holozoic. Organisms that need complex nutrients, often solid materials that are ingested and then broken down
  c. Saprophytic. Organisms whose nutrients are obtained from dead or decaying organic matter

    d. Parasitic. Organisms whose nutrients are obtained from and at the expense of a living organism (human pathogens)

B. Nutritional requirements. Bacteria use a wide variety of nutrients to obtain energy and to construct new cellular components. The six elements used as the main components of carbohydrates, lipids, proteins, and nucleic acids are carbon, oxygen, hydrogen, nitrogen, phosphorus, and sulfur. Several minor and trace elements as well as cations play various roles in the microorganisms.

C. Temperature relations

    1. **Psychrophile,** an organism that grows well at 0°C, has optimal growth at 15°C or less, and a maximum growth temperature of 20°C

    2. **Mesophile:** an organism with optimal growth at 20°–45°C, minimum growth temperatures between 15° and 20°C, and a maximum growth temperature of approximately 45°C (human pathogens)

    3. **Thermophile:** an organism that can grow at 55°C or greater, with a minimum growth temperature of approximately 45°C.

D. Oxygen requirements. How organisms use oxygen can be a major factor in their classification.

    1. **Aerobes** have the ability to grow in the presence of atmospheric oxygen.
      a. Obligate aerobes depend completely on oxygen for growth. Oxygen serves as terminal electron acceptor in aerobic respiration.
      b. Facultative aerobes have the ability to grow with or without molecular oxygen.

    2. **Anaerobes** have the ability to grow without oxygen.
      a. Obligate anaerobes do not tolerate oxygen at all and die in its presence. Many strains lack catalase and superoxide dismutase, which protect cells from the destructive oxidizing capabilities of hydrogen peroxide and superoxide ions, which are normally produced under aerobic conditions.
      b. Facultative anaerobes do not require oxygen but grow better in its presence.

    3. **Microaerophiles** require oxygen levels below normal atmospheric pressures for growth (e.g., *Helicobacter pylori*)

    4. **Capnophiles** require higher levels of carbon dioxide than are found at normal atmospheric pressures for growth (e.g., *Neisseria* sp. and *Streptococcus pneumoniae*).

E. Bacterial growth curve. Bacterial growth is defined as an increase in the number of cells present. Because bacteria reproduce by **binary fission,** growth can be plotted as the log of the cell number versus time to produce a curve with four distinct phases (Figure 9-3).

    1. **Lag phase.** A transition period during which the bacteria are replicating DNA and the enzymes needed for the new environment are being induced. The cells are increasing in size but not in number. During this phase of growth, the cells are most permeable.

    2. **Logarithmic (log) phase.** Division occurs at constant and maximal rate, and the number of cells increases in a geometric progression. The generation time, which varies among species, is usually 15–20 minutes (*Escherichia*), but may be hours (*Mycobacterium*). Because the cell wall is being synthesized so rapidly, bacterial cells are most susceptible to cell wall inhibitors during this phase.

    3. **Stationary phase.** The growth rate tapers off and growth and death rates are nearly equal. A fairly constant population of viable cells results. During this phase, cellular metabolites are polluting the environment.

    4. **Death phase.** When the concentration of viable cells decreases because of the accumulation of toxic wastes and autolytic enzymes.

V. METABOLISM AND ENERGY PRODUCTION. Microorganisms derive energy from nutrients by a series of chemical reactions by which the energy stored in chemical bonds is transferred to newly formed chemical bonds to provide energy storage in a useful form, such as adenosine triphosphate (ATP).

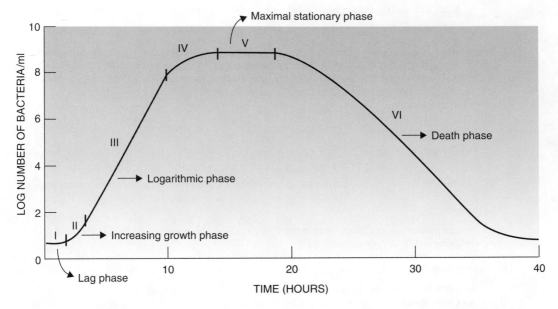

Figure 9-3. Growth curve of bacterial culture. [Reprinted with permission from Winn WC Jr, Allen SD, Janda WM, et al. Koneman's Color Atlas and Textbook of Diagnostic Microbiology, 6th ed. Philadelphia: Lippincott Williams & Wilkins, 2006.]

A. ATP generation

1. **Substrate-level phosphorylation** releases energy through direct transfer of high-energy phosphate groups from an intermediate metabolic compound to adenosine diphosphate (ADP). No molecular oxygen or other inorganic final electron acceptor is required.

2. **Oxidative phosphorylation** removes electrons from organic compounds and passes these electrons through a series of electron acceptors along an electron transport chain, with molecular oxygen or some other inorganic compound as the final acceptor.

B. Fermentation refers to energy-producing oxidative sequences, in which organic compounds serve as both electron donors and acceptors. This process occurs in the absence of external electron acceptors.

1. **Glycolysis** is the first step in fermentation and respiration and causes the oxidation of glucose to pyruvic acid with a yield of two moles of ATP. There are different pathways for pyruvic acid production in microorganisms:
   a. The **Embden–Meyerhof (glycolytic) pathway** is the major pathway.
   b. The **Entner–Doudoroff pathway** is an alternate.
   c. The **hexose monophosphate shunt** used with the glycolytic pathway is an alternative.

2. **Secondary fermentation process.** Many bacteria use pyruvate to oxidize **reduced nicotinamide adenine dinucleotide (NADH),** produced in glycolysis, to manufacture a variety of final products.
   a. **Lactic acid fermentation.** The simplest process, which converts pyruvate to lactate (*Lactobacillus, Streptococcus*).
   b. **Alcohol fermentation.** Pyruvate is converted to ethanol and carbon dioxide (*Saccharomyces*).
   c. **Mixed acid fermentation.** A combination of lactic, formic, and acetic acids is produced with ethanol, hydrogen, and carbon dioxide (*Escherichia coli*).
   d. **Butanediol fermentation.** Pyruvate is converted to acetoin, which is reduced to 2,3-butanediol (*Enterobacter*).
   e. **Butyric acid fermentation.** Butanol, isopropanol, and acetone are produced (*Clostridium*).

f. Propionic acid fermentation. Pyruvate is converted to oxaloacetate with the addition of carbon dioxide and then to propionic acid (*Propionibacterium*).

C. Respiration refers to energy-producing oxidative sequences, in which inorganic compounds act as the last electron acceptor in a series of reactions. This process includes **glycolysis,** the **tricarboxylic acid (TCA) cycle,** and the **electron transport system,** which yields ATP when coupled with oxidative phosphorylation.

1. **Aerobic respiration.** Oxygen serves as the final electron acceptor.
   a. Pyruvate is converted to **acetyl coenzyme A** and carbon dioxide and water through the **TCA cycle.**
   b. The **electron transport system** plays a role in the transport of electrons along a series of carriers found in the cytoplasmic membrane, each with successively higher oxidation potentials. Major components of the electron transport system include
      (1) Cytochromes
      (2) Flavoproteins
      (3) Ubiquinones

2. **Anaerobic respiration.** An inorganic electron acceptor other than oxygen (e.g., nitrate, sulfate, carbonate) serves as the final electron acceptor.

VI. GENETICS

A. Definition and terms. Genetics is the study of what genes are, how they carry information, and how they are replicated and passed on.

1. **Chromosomes** are bodies composed of DNA that contain genetic information. Bacteria have only one chromosome—a single, continuous (closed), double-stranded, circular piece of DNA.
   a. **Duplication** occurs by semiconservative replication, in which the two strands of the helix separate (**origin**) and at this point (**two replication forks**) new strands are synthesized, bidirectionally, with the originals serving as templates.
   b. **Structure.** The cell membrane is attached to the chromosome; as the cell grows, it separates the daughter chromosomes. Therefore, each daughter cell has one original and one new strand.

2. **Genes** are DNA segments that are processed in two steps to produce various proteins. A normal bacterial cell is **haploid.**

B. Regulation and expression of genetic information

1. **DNA** has many **functions.**
   a. It is **duplicated** for transfer to progeny during cell division.
   b. It is **transcribed** into RNA, which can be translated into a protein.
   c. It contains **control signals,** which ultimately control the synthesis of protein.
   d. It can be **mutated** to alter specific characteristics encoded by genes.
   e. It can be duplicated and transferred to **other bacterial cells** in processes other than cell division (e.g., conjugation).

2. **DNA replication, transcription,** and **translation** affect cellular growth and development.
   a. Bacterial **replication** involves accurate duplication of chromosomal DNA, which enables the formation of two identical daughter cells.
   b. **Transcription** of information from DNA to RNA is the first of two steps needed to produce necessary proteins. One gene can be transcribed into many copies of RNA. Simplistically, RNA polymerase locates the beginning of the gene (promotor), and this area undergoes localized unwinding to allow RNA polymerase to **transcribe** RNA (called **mRNA**) from the DNA template. The RNA is not processed, as in eukaryotes. There are no introns and exons, no capping of the 5′ end, and no polyadenine tails added to the 3′ end.
   c. **Translation** is the processing of genetic information to synthesize proteins. Before transcription is completed, a ribosome will attach to the 5′ end of the message. The 70s

bacterial **ribosome** is composed of two subunits, 30s and 50s. The ribosome **translates** the message into protein by reading the **triplet codon** (three nucleotides) as a specific amino acid. This amino acid is carried to the site by **transfer RNA (tRNA)** and pairs with the codon by an **anticodon.** Amino acids are joined, and the ribosome moves to the next codon. This continues until the complete protein is synthesized.

3. **Regulation.** The products of cellular growth must be produced in correct proportions for the cell to live and function. The two most common mechanisms of metabolic and genetic regulation are as follows:
   a. **Feedback inhibition** of enzyme activity (metabolic regulation) inhibits the synthesis of the cell growth product. The product binds with an allosteric site on the enzyme, thereby inactivating the active site.
   b. **Repression** of enzyme activity (genetic regulation) inhibits the synthesis of the enzyme at the transcriptional level.
   c. **Induction** of enzyme activity activates the synthesis of the enzyme at the transcription level.

C. **Other methods of DNA transfer.** Microorganisms can change their genetic constitution by the transfer of genetic material from a donor chromosome to a recipient chromosome (recombination). Recombination occurs between homologous segments (those that have similar nucleotide sequences). There are three general mechanisms:

1. **Transformation** involves the recipient cell taking up cell-free, fragmented (i.e., naked) DNA and recombining genetic elements.
   a. This process is **primitive** and occurs naturally within only a few genera.
   b. Requirements include competent recipient cells (exhibiting DNA receptors) or a **"leaky" bacterial cell wall,** so that DNA can be introduced into the cell.
   c. It is generally associated with **recombinant DNA technology** or **cloning,** a technique to amplify a specific gene in preparation for analysis. In this process, the bacterial cell walls are made leaky by chemical treatment.
      (1) Cloning involves splicing a gene into a plasmid DNA (**vector**). All vectors share several common characteristics:
         (a) Typically small, well-characterized molecules of DNA
         (b) Contain at least one replicon and can be replicated within the host even when the vectors contain foreign DNA
         (c) Code for a phenotypic trait that can be used to detect the presence of foreign DNA, which can often be used to distinguish parental from recombinant vectors
      (2) **Selectable markers** are used to find cells that contain these vectors.
      (3) **Plasmids** cannot maintain stability unless they are beneficial to the host, so the plasmid should contain a gene essential for cellular survival—either an enzyme required in a metabolic pathway or a gene that resists certain antibiotics (see III.D.4).

2. **Conjugation** is an important means of gene transfer, particularly among gram-negative organisms. This process involves two mating types—the donor (**F⁺**) and recipient (**F⁻**) cells—and the extrachromosomal piece known as the sex or fertility factor (**F factor**). The F factor (e.g., F plasmid or episome) is not under the control of the chromosome and can replicate autonomously. Plasmid-mediated exchange of genetic information can occur only through the expression of transfer genes. The genes encoded on the plasmid result in the transfer of a single strand of DNA through the sex pilus into the recipient cell. The F factor has several genes that code for formation and aid in donor attachment of sex pili. During this process, a copy is made, a single strand is transferred, and the recipient becomes F^+. R plasmids also exist, which encode for resistance to certain antibiotics or heavy metals. When an F plasmid integrates into the cellular chromosome, the bacterial strain is said to be a **high-frequency recombination (Hfr)** strain. During the conjugal transfer involving an Hfr strain, depending on the amount of time, the whole bacterial chromosome may be transferred. Antibiotic-resistance genes are often parts of **transposons** (see III.D.4), which are responsible for additions, deletions, and inversions of large (4–80 kilobases) sequences. When different transposons ''jump'' into transferable plasmids, contagious resistance to multiple antibiotics can occur.

3. **Transduction** is the transfer of genetic material by **bacteriophages** (viruses that infect bacteria). Such viruses can be classified into two groups:

a. **Lytic phages** enter the cell, replicate, and package their DNA; they then lyse the cell to release mature infective virions.

b. **Lysogenic (temperate) phages** can alternate between two pathways:
(1) The lytic pathway
(2) Integrating into the host DNA and remaining dormant
(a) The viral DNA does not replicate but is integrated into the host genome and is known as **prophage.**
(b) The prophage suppresses the lytic state by synthesizing a protein known as a repressor, which protects the cell from further infection by a virus.
(c) Some prophages can change the cell's phenotype (**phage** or **lysogenic conversion**), which allows the organism to elaborate materials (exotoxins or virulence factors) that are detrimental to the human host. Lysogenic conversion thereby increases the virulence or the symptoms of a specific pathogen—for example, *Corynebacterium diphtheriae* (diphtheria toxin), *Streptococcus pyogenes* (erythrogenic toxin in scarlet fever), and *Clostridium tetani* (tetanus toxin).

VII. EXAMPLES OF UNIQUE BACTERIA

A. *Chlamydia* are obligate intracellular parasites that

1. **Lack the ability to generate ATP;** hence they must obtain it from the host cell

2. Have a **two-phase life cycle**
a. The infectious form, or **elementary body,** is a dense, nonreplicating cell that is resistant to drying in the environment.
b. The **reticulate body** forms from engulfed elementary body and undergoes binary fission. After multiple divisions, the reticulate bodies become the dense, elementary bodies, which are released from the host cell (e.g., *Chlamydia trachomatis,* which causes blindness and sexually transmitted diseases).

B. *Rickettsia,* obligate intracellular parasites transmitted by arthropods, appear to have the ability to generate ATP, but instead **use the host cell products, including ATP, amino acids, nicotinamide adenine dinucleotide (NAD), and coenzyme A** (e.g., *Rickettsia rickettsii,* which causes Rocky Mountain spotted fever).

C. *Mycoplasma,* the smallest bacteria, are unique in that

1. They **lack a cell wall.**

2. The plasma membrane contains **sterols** for added strength (e.g., *Mycoplasma pneumonia,* which causes an atypical or walking pneumonia).

VIII. VIRUSES

A. **Viral structure**

1. The basic structure of a virus is the **virion** or **nucleocapsid.** This structure is composed of a protein coat, which surrounds the viral genome. The shape of the nucleocapsid is one component that determines the classification of the virus. As noted in I.B.1.b, the viral genome is composed of either RNA or DNA and may be single or double stranded. The nucleocapsid of viruses that infect humans has two basic shapes.
a. **Icosahedral.** A regular **geometric** structure with 12 or more faces; resembles a soccer ball
b. **Helical.** The proteins that make up the structure wrap in a helical fashion. Helical capsids often have cone or bullet shapes.

Table 9-1. The Multiplication of Animal Viruses

Number	Step	Action(s)
1	Attachment (adsorption)	Virus attaches to a protein or polysaccharide molecule (receptor) on the surface of a cell
2	Penetration	Entire virus enters the cell, in some cases because it was phagocytized by the cell
3	Uncoating	Viral nucleic acid escapes from the capsid
4	Biosynthesis	Viral genes are expressed, resulting in the production of pieces or parts of viruses (i.e., viral DNA and viral proteins)
5	Assembly	Viral pieces are assembled to create complete virions
6	Release	Complete virions escape from the bacterial cell by lysis or budding

Reprinted by permission from Burton GRW, Engelkirk PG. Microbiology for the Health Sciences, 7th ed. Philadelphia: Lippincott Williams & Wilkins, 2004.

2. The virion may have a **lipid envelope,** which is produced when the virus buds from the host cell. The envelope is composed of the host cell plasma membrane and virally coded glycoproteins.

B. **Viral replication.** Viruses are nonliving entities that must enter a host cell to **replicate.** Once in the host cell, the virus is able to replicate its genome and produce more viruses, which will infect other cells. The steps in the multiplication of animal viruses are outlined in Table 9-1 and involve

1. The virus attaches (**attachment**) to the host cell using viral proteins or glycoproteins, which bind to receptors on the host cell surface.

2. The virion then **enters (penetration)** the host cell. Entry may be accomplished by fusion of a viral envelope with the cell membrane or by uptake of the virion into an endocytic vesicle. If the virus enters the cell through an endocytic vesicle, there are several ways for it to leave the endocytic vesicle and enter the cytoplasm of the host cell.

3. Once in the host cell, the virus **uncoats**, and the nucleic acid is released from the capsid. The free nucleic acid then is able to begin the process of reproduction.

4. **Protein synthesis** occurs in two stages. **Early proteins** are necessary for the synthesis of a new viral genome and are synthesized immediately after infection. **Late proteins** are synthesized after the viral genome has been copied; these are the proteins necessary for the assembly of the capsid, glycoproteins for the envelope, and any enzymes included in the nucleocapsid.
   a. For viruses with a **single-stranded RNA genome,** the RNA may be a plus (+) strand or a minus (−) strand. Plus-strand RNA genomes are mRNAs and are translated directly to proteins. Minus-strand RNA genomes have an RNA-dependent RNA polymerase that copies the genome into a strand of mRNA for transcription.
   b. **Double-stranded RNA genomes** use an RNA-dependent RNA polymerase to transcribe the minus strand of RNA into a message for translation.
   c. Some plus-strand RNA viruses are members of the **retrovirus** family (e.g., human immunodeficiency virus). These viruses have an enzyme called reverse polymerase, which transcribes the RNA to double-stranded DNA. The double-stranded DNA is integrated into the host cell chromosome (a **provirus**) and then transcribed to mRNA using host cell enzymes. The viral mRNA is then translated into viral proteins.
   d. In viruses with a **DNA genome,** the DNA may be double stranded or single stranded. In either case, the DNA is transcribed to mRNA and then translated into proteins.

5. After genome and protein synthesis, the virus is **assembled** into new virions.

6. After assembly, the virions are **released** from the host cell. For nonenveloped viruses, the virions are released when the host cell lyses. Enveloped viruses are released from the host cells by budding out of the host cell membrane.

IX. TRANSMISSION OF INFECTIOUS AGENTS

A. Infections agents are found in a number of different environments, called **reservoirs.**

1. **Humans** are **reservoirs** for diseases that are obligate human pathogens, which include almost all viral infections and many bacterial diseases. When humans are the reservoir for the disease, they are said to be **carriers.**
   a. **Asymptomatic carriers** harbor an infection but have no symptoms. Some asymptomatic carriers carry the infectious agent as part of their normal flora (*Streptococcus pyogenes*).
   b. **Symptomatic carriers** have obvious signs and symptoms of disease.

2. An **animal reservoir** exists when the primary host is an animal. Such animals may be wild (e.g., foxes, raccoons) or domesticated (livestock and pets).

3. **Environmental reservoirs** include soil, lakes, and plants.

B. The **transmission of infectious agents** depends on the source of infection. For diseases with human reservoirs, the mechanisms of transmission include

1. **Contact**
   a. **Direct contact** requires physical contact between an infected individual and a susceptible individual (sexually transmitted diseases).
   b. **Indirect contact** involves a susceptible individual coming in contact with a contaminated surface (many viruses and bacteria). **Fomites** are surfaces that can be and frequently are contaminated with microorganisms (door knobs, counters and other surfaces, computer keyboards, toys).

2. **Droplet transmission.** Infected droplets are formed when an infected individual coughs or sneezes. The infected droplets transmit the disease to a susceptible individual when they come in contact with the mucous membranes of the individual's nose, mouth, or eyes (measles).

3. **Airborne transmission.** When small contaminated dust particles or the residue from dried droplets (droplet nuclei) remain suspended in the air for long periods of time, they can transmit disease (influenza, pneumonia, tuberculosis). These small nuclei can infect both the upper and the lower respiratory tract.

4. **Food and water contamination.** Food or water contaminated with bacteria from human or animal feces leads to transmission of disease through the fecal–oral route.

C. **Vectors** are animals capable of transmitting diseases. The most common vector for disease is the mosquito (malaria), but other insects (fleas, ticks and flies) are also vectors (Rocky Mountain spotted fever). In addition, mammals (dogs, mice and rats) can be vectors for disease.

D. **Entry into a host.** Bacteria can enter a host through ingestion of food or water, inhalation of droplets or dust particles, injection by an insect vector, or by contamination of a wound.

X. MECHANISMS OF PATHOGENICITY

A. Microorganisms cause disease in different ways. Although signs and symptoms of the disease are often the result of the host response, microorganisms can damage tissue through the production of exotoxins and endotoxins, and by direct effects. In addition, microbial virulence factors contribute to the ability of a microorganism to infect a host and cause disease.

1. **Virulence factors** are the characteristics of an organism that allow it to either damage the host or evade host defenses.
   a. **Exotoxins** are toxins that are secreted by the microorganism either into the environment or after colonization of a host.
      (1) Exotoxins secreted into food or water that are then ingested by a host cause intoxication (botulism and staphylococcal food poisoning).
      (2) Exotoxins produced after infection and colonization interfere with cell function or physically damage the cell (*Bordetella pertussis, Corynebacterium diphtheriae, Vibrio cholera*).

Table 9-2. Important Human Pathogens and Their Diseases

Infectious Agent	Typical Infection
Bacteria	
Gram-positive cocci	
Staphylococcus aureus	Abscess, skin infections, toxic shock
Streptococcus pyogenes	Strep throat, erysipelas, rheumatic fever
Streptococcus pneumoniae	Pneumonia
Gram-positive rods	
Bacillus	Anthrax
Clostridium	Gas gangrene, tetanus
Corynebacterium	Diphtheria
Acid-fast rods	
Mycobacterium tuberculosis	Tuberculosis
Mycobacterium leprae	Leprosy
Nocardia	Nocardiosis
Gram-negative cocci	
Neisseria gonorrhoeae	Gonorrhea
Neisseria meningitidis	Meningitis
Gram-negative rods	
Bordetella	Pertussis
Brucella	Brucellosis
Escherichia coli	Sepsis, diarrhea, urinary tract infection
Haemophilus influenzae	Meningitis
Legionella	Legionnaires disease
Pseudomonas	Opportunistic lung and burn infections
Salmonella	Typhoid fever, salmonellosis
Shigella	Dysentery
Vibrio cholerae	Cholera
Yersinia pestis	Plague
Spirochetes	
Borrelia	Lyme disease
Treponema pallidum	Syphilis
Mycoplasma	Pneumonia, urinary infections
Rickettsia	Rocky Mountain spotted fever
Chlamydia	Urethritis, vaginitis
Fungi	
Systemic mycoses	
Aspergillus	Aspergillosis
Blastomyces	Blastomycosis
Candida albicans	Candidiasis
Coccidioides immitis	Valley fever
Cryptococcus neoformans	Cryptococcosis
Pneumocystis (carinii) jiroveci	Pneumonia (PCP)
Sporothrix schenckii	Sporotrichosis
Protozoa	
Entamoeba histolytica	Amoebiasis
Giardia lamblia	Giardiasis
Plasmodium	Malaria
Toxoplasma gondii	Toxoplasmosis
Trichomonas vaginalis	Trichomoniasis
Trypanosoma brucei	Sleeping sickness
Helminths	
Ascaris	Acariosis
Cestodes	Tapeworm
Schistosoma	Shchistosomiasis
Various fluke infections	
Various roundworm infections	

Adapted with permission from Cowan MK, Talaro KP. Microbiology: A Systems Approach. 1st ed.: McGraw-Hill, 2005. With permission of The McGraw-Hill Companies, Inc.

Table 9-3. Important Human Virus Families and Their Diseases

Family	Virus	Disease
DNA viruses		
Poxviridae	Variola and vaccinia	Smallpox, cowpox
Herpesviridae	Herpes simplex 1 virus (HSV-1)	Fever blister, cold sores
	Herpes simplex 2 virus (HSV-2)	Genital herpes
	Varicella zoster virus (VZV)	Chickenpox, shingles
	Human cytomegalovirus (CMV)	CMV infections
Adenoviridae	Human adenoviruses	Adenovirus infection
Papovaviridae	Human papillomavirus (HPV)	Several types of warts
	JC virus (JCV)	Progressive multifocal leukoencephalopathy (PML)
Hepadnaviridae	Hepatitis B virus (HBV; of Dane particle)	Serum hepatitis
Parvoviridae	Parvovirus B19	Erythema infectiosum
RNA viruses		
Picornaviridae	Poliovirus	Poliomyelitis
	Coxsackievirus	Hand-foot-mouth disease
	Hepatitis A virus (HAV)	Short-term hepatitis
	Human rhinovirus	Common cold, bronchitis
Calciviridae	Norwalk virus	Viral diarrhea, Norwalk virus syndrome
Togaviridae	Eastern equine encephalitis virus	Eastern equine encephalitis (EEE)
	Western equine encephalitis virus	Western equine encephalitis (WEE)
	Yellow fever virus	Yellow fever
	St. Louis encephalitis virus	St. Louis encephalitis
	Rubella virus	Rubella (German measles)
Flaviviridae	Dengue fever virus	Dengue fever
	West Nile fever virus	West Nile fever
Bunyaviridae	Bunyamwera viruses	California encephalitis
	Sin Nombre virus	Respiratory distress syndrom
	Rift Valley fever virus	Rift Valley fever
	Crimean-Congo hemorrhagic fever virus (CCHF)	Crimean-Congo hemorrhagic fever
Filoviridae	Ebola, Marburg virus	Ebola fever
Reoviridae	Colorado tick fever virus	Colorado tick fever
	Human rotavirus	Rotavirus gastroenteritis
Orthomyxoviridae	Influenza virus, type A (Asian, Hong Kong, swine)	Influenza, flu
Paramyxoviridae	Parainfluenza virus, types 1–5	Parainfluenza
	Mumps virus	Mumps
	Measles virus	Measles (red)
	Respiratory syncytial virus (RSV)	Common cold syndrome
Rhabdoviridae	Rabies virus	Rabies (hydrophobia)
Retroviridae	Human T-cell leukemia virus (HTLV)	T-cell leukemia
	HIV (1 and 2)	AIDS
Arenaviridae	Lassa virus	Lassa fever
Coronaviridae	Infectious bronchitis virus (IBV)	Bronchitis
	Enteric corona virus	Coronavirus enteritis
	SARS virus	Severe acute respiratory syndrome

Adapted with permission from Cowan MK, Talaro KP. Microbiology: A Systems Approach. 1st ed.: McGraw-Hill, 2005. With permission of The McGraw-Hill Companies, Inc.

    b. Endotoxins (see III.C.1.b) are integral parts of the outer membrane of gram-negative bacteria. During an infection, endotoxins are able to induce fever and shock in the host.

    c. Capsules (see III. B.1) are used for adherence to host surfaces and help the bacteria evade phagocytosis by the host cells.

  2. Mechanisms of disease. There are three main patterns by which microorganisms cause disease:

    a. Intoxication [see X.A.1.a.(1)]

    b. Infection is sufficient to cause disease for some microorganisms, especially for diseases such as pneumonia, in which the capsule surrounding the bacteria stimulates a strong inflammatory response. This response is responsible for many of the symptoms of the disease. In some cases, infection may be followed by toxin production (see X.A.1.a.(2)), as in diphtheria.

    c. Invasion of host tissues and then growth in the tissue is the mechanism of disease infection by viruses and bacteria such as *Mycobacteria*. Some bacteria (e.g., *Shigella* sp.) are able to produce toxins after the invasion of host tissue.

XI. DISEASES CAUSED BY INFECTIOUS AGENTS

A. Diseases caused by bacteria, fungi, protozoa, and helminths (Table 9-2)

B. Diseases caused by viruses (Table 9-3)

STUDY QUESTIONS

Directions for questions 1–12: Each question, statement, or incomplete statement in this section can be correctly answered or completed by **one** of the suggested answers or phrases. Choose the **best** answer.

1. Cell walls of both gram-positive and gram-negative bacteria are composed of complex macromolecules. Which of the following statements describes both types of cell walls?

(A) They contain significant amounts of teichoic acid.
(B) They contain pores made from proteins.
(C) Their antigenic specificity is determined by the polysaccharide O antigen.
(D) They contain peptidoglycan.

2. Which of the following descriptions best characterizes sex pili?

(A) They enable DNA transport between bacteria during conjugation.
(B) They play a role in the adhesion of bacteria to their target cells.
(C) They are numerous on the bacterial cell surface.
(D) They are found only on gram-positive organisms.

3. The mode of gene transfer in which naked DNA is taken up is called

(A) transformation.
(B) transduction.
(C) conjugation.
(D) cell fusion.

4. Bacteria that make either a fermentative or respiratory set of enzymes are known as

(A) obligate anaerobes.
(B) obligate aerobes.
(C) microaerophiles.
(D) facultative organisms.

5. Which of the following statements describes plasmids?

(A) They are single-stranded DNA molecules.
(B) They carry optional genes.
(C) They carry genes essential for growth.
(D) They are always found in linear form.

6. All of the following statements describe the nuclear body *except* which one?

(A) It is referred to as nucleoid.
(B) It is free of ribosomes.
(C) It is composed of ribosomes.
(D) It lacks a nuclear membrane.

7. Bacteria that grow at temperatures as high as 55°C are known as

(A) psychrophiles.
(B) thermophiles.
(C) mesophiles.
(D) auxotrophs.

8. Which of the following organisms can use only molecular oxygen as the final acceptor?

(A) obligate anaerobes
(B) facultative anaerobes
(C) obligate aerobes
(D) strict anaerobes

9. Viruses are classified by all of the following *except* by

(A) structure of capsid.
(B) type of nucleic acid.
(C) oxygen requirements.
(D) presence of lipid envelope.

10. Protozoa are classified by

(A) shape.
(B) cell wall type.
(C) sexual reproductive structures.
(D) mode of motility.

11. Which of the following is *not* part of the viruses infectious cycle?

(A) attachment
(B) unwrapping
(C) replication of the genome
(D) protein synthesis
(E) release

12. Infectious agents are transmitted to people from reservoirs. These reservoirs include

(A) asymptomatic carriers.
(B) animals.
(C) lakes.
(D) soil.
(E) all of the above.

Directions for questions 13–20: The questions and incomplete statements in this section can be correctly answered or completed by **one or more** of the suggested answers. Choose the correct answer, A–D.

A   if **I, II, and III** are correct
B   if **I and III** are correct
C   if **II and IV** are correct
D   if **IV only** is correct

13. Gram-negative and gram-positive cell walls share which of the following characteristics?

I. peptide cross-links between polysaccharides
II. hydrolysis by lysozyme
III. rigid polysaccharide framework
IV. a wide variety of complex lipids

14. A declining growth rate occurs during which of the following phases of bacterial cell growth?

I. lag phase
II. exponential phase
III. stationary phase
IV. death phase

15. The peptidoglycan backbone of a bacterial cell contains

I. dipeptide chains.
II. *N*-acetylmuramic acid.
III. teichoic acid.
IV. *N*-acetylglucosamine.

16. Entities that are acellular do not fit the classical definition of living things. They are

I. bacteria.
II. viruses.
III. fungi.
IV. prions.

17. Dimorphic fungi have

I. a yeast phase.
II. a sexual phase.
III. a mold phase.
IV. basidium.

18. Transmission of an infectious disease by the fecal–oral route occurs when

I. infectious agents are deposited on surfaces such as door knobs.
II. an individual coughs or sneezes and droplets with infectious agents are expelled.
III. an insect such as a mosquito injects an infectious agent into an individual.
IV. food or water is contaminated with human or animal feces.

19. Virulence factors that enhance microbial pathogenicity include

I. capsules.
II. endotoxins.
III. exotoxins.
IV. peptidoglycans.

20. On Friday, January 13, a number of patrons of Mom's Diner became ill 2–6 hr after eating at the restaurant. The health department was called in to investigate. During the investigation, it was found that all the individuals who became ill had eaten banana cream pie, Mom's speciality, but had not eaten anything else in common. The investigators found no viable pathogens in the pie, but tests indicated the presence of staphylococcal contamination of the cream pie. Illness resulting from this contamination would be considered an

I. infection.
II. incrimination.
III. invasion.
IV. intoxication.

ANSWERS AND EXPLANATIONS

1. The answer is D *[see III.C.1]*.
The cell wall of gram-positive bacteria is a thick layer of peptidoglycan with a large amount of teichoic acids (surface antigens). Gram-negative bacteria have only a small amount of peptidoglycan, no teichoic acid, and an outer membrane composed of lipoprotein and lipopolysaccharide, of which the polysaccharide makes up the O antigen.

2. The answer is A *[see III.B.3.b]*.
Sex pili are found only on gram-negative organisms and in very small numbers (< 10). They act as fragile transport tubes for DNA exchange. Common pili are adhesions.

3. The answer is A *[see VI.C.1]*.
Of the three methods of DNA transfer, only transformation takes up DNA without an intermediary.

4. The answer is D *[see IV.D.1.b]*.
Facultative organisms can grow without air and make either a fermentative or a respiratory set of enzymes, depending on the conditions.

5. The answer is B *[see III.D.4; VI.C.2]*.
The chromosome carries all of the genes essential for growth, whereas plasmids are extrachromosomal, double-stranded, circular pieces of DNA that carry optional genes that add extra properties.

6. The answer is C *[see III.D.2–3]*.
Ribosomes are found in the cytoplasm, not in the nucleoid (a long, circular, double-stranded DNA without a nuclear membrane).

7. The answer is B *[see IV.C.1–3]*.
Thermophiles grow at 55°C and are found in hot springs and compost piles. Mesophiles grow at approximately 37°C, psychrophiles grow at 15°C and lower, and auxotrophs are mutant organisms.

8. The answer is C *[see IV.D.1–2]*.
Obligate aerobes require oxygen and lack an alternative fermentative pathway. Obligate anaerobes are strict anaerobes that cannot live in the presence of oxygen. Facultative anaerobes can use oxygen as the final acceptor or to provide an alternate fermentative pathway.

9. The answer is C *[see I.B.1; VIII.A]*.
Viruses are classified by the structure of the capsid, the type and strandedness of the nucleic acid, the presence of a lipid envelope, and the presence of enzymes. Viruses do not generate their own energy, hence there is no need for oxygen. Viruses use the energy in the host cell.

10. The answer is D *[see I.A.2.b]*.
Protozoa are unicellular, nonphotosynthetic eukaryotes that are classified by their mode of motility or lack of motility. The types of motility are flagella, cilia, and amoeboid movement.

11. The answer is B *[see VIII.B.1–6]*.
The viral infectious cycle consists of attachment, entry, uncoating (not unwinding), protein synthesis, genome replication, assembly, and release.

12. The answer is E *[see IX.A.1–3]*.
Infectious agents can be found in many different environments, including people, animals, and the natural environment.

13. The answer is A (I, II, III) *[see III.C.1–2]*.
Peptidoglycan is the basic layer of the cell wall in both gram-positive and gram-negative organisms. It provides a rigid framework that is susceptible to the action of lysozyme. Gram-positive cells are deficient in lipids; however, gram-negative cells are rich in complex lipids (e.g., lipopolysaccharide). Both types of cell walls have cross-links between polysaccharides.

14. The answer is D (IV) *[see IV.E.1–4]*.
During the lag phase, the cells prepare for growth, so there is no actual growth. Growth is maximal during the exponential phase and levels out during the stationary phase with no net increase in cell number. There is a decline in organism number during the death phase because there are more organisms dying than are being produced.

15. The answer is C (II, IV) *[see III.C.1]*.
The cell wall of both gram-positive and gram-negative organisms is composed of repeating disaccharide units. These units contain *N*-acetylglucosamine and *N*-acetylmuramic acid, to which tetrapeptide chains are cross-linked. Only gram-positive organisms have teichoic acid.

16. The answer is C (II, IV) *[see I.B.1–2]*.
Viruses are basically proteins and nucleic acids, whereas prions are proteins, neither of which are cells. Bacteria are prokaryotic cells, and fungi are eukaryotic cells.

17. The answer is B (I, III) *[see I.A.2.a.(1)–(4)]*.
Dimorphic fungi like *Blastomyces, Coccidioides,* and *Histoplasma* can be grown in either a yeast (unicellular) or mold (filamentous) phase, depending on the temperature of incubation. Fungi are placed in phyla based on the type of sexual reproduction observed: either ascus, basidium, or zygote. Fungi imperfecti consist of species without observable sexual reproductive structures.

18. The answer is D (IV) *[see IX.B.1–4]*.
The fecal–oral route of transmission involves contamination of food or water with animal feces.

19. The answer is A (I, II, III) *[see X.A.1]*.
Capsules act as virulence factors by inhibiting phagocytosis and acting to attach microorganisms to host surfaces. Exotoxins are secreted by microorganisms and either alter cell functions or cause cell death. Endotoxins induce shock in mammalian hosts through the lipid A component of the molecule. Peptidoglycan is the backbone of the bacterial cell wall.

20. The answer is D (IV) *[see X.A.1.a.(1); X.A.2]*.
Staphylococcus aureus can produce an exotoxin, which results in gastrointestinal disease. When there is disease in the absence of infection or invasion of the tissues by a live organism, the disease is called an intoxication.

10
Immunology
Gail Goodman-Snitkoff

I. THE PHYSIOLOGY OF THE IMMUNE SYSTEM

A. Immunogens, antigens, and haptens

1. **Immunogens** are chemical compounds that cause a specific immune response.

2. **Antigens** are chemical compounds that bind to products of an immune response. When the antigens are recognized by antibody or activated cells, they can be eliminated by a specific immune response.

3. **Immunogen–antigens.** Compounds associated with or secreted by parasitic bacteria, protozoa, fungi, and viruses and of molecular weight (mol wt) > 5000 daltons may act as both immunogens and antigens.
   a. Molecular complexity is as important as molecular weight in determining the status of a compound as an immunogen. For a molecule to be immunogenic, it must contain protein or peptide. Therefore, proteins, glycoproteins, lipoproteins, and nucleoproteins are the most potent immunogen–antigens.
   b. Drugs of sufficient molecular weight (e.g., insulin) can act as immunogen–antigens. The cells of another individual and the cells of one's own body (see III) can act as immunogen–antigens. Immunogen–antigens can be contacted environmentally (e.g., pollens).

4. **Haptens** are low molecular weight compounds that act as immunogens after covalently binding to a larger molecule or cell surface. After they stimulate the immune system in this complex, these compounds can act as antigens in the unbound or bound state.
   a. Haptens may be present in the environment (e.g., pentadecyl catechol of poison ivy).
   b. Several types of drugs act as haptens (e.g., penicillin).

5. **Tolerogens** are chemical compounds that elicit specific nonresponsiveness. This specific nonresponsiveness may be caused by the ability of the compound to be broken down by the body or by the route of administration of the compound (e.g., oral administration often causes specific nonresponsiveness).

6. In this chapter, the term *antigen* is used for compounds and cells that are both immunogens and antigens.

B. Cells of the immune system

1. **B lymphocytes and T lymphocytes** are the primary cells of specific immune responses. All B and T lymphocytes are antigen specific because they have specific antigen receptors as part of their plasma membranes. In this chapter, the terms *B cell* and *T cell* are used instead of B lymphocyte and T lymphocyte.

2. **Antigen receptors of B cells** are antibody molecules.
   a. B cells have thousands of identical antibodies in their membranes that allow them to bind to a small group of chemically related antigens. This group defines the antigen specificity of each B cell. Different B cells have different antigen specificities, but each B cell has only one specificity. B cells that recognize specific antigens divide to form new B cells (**memory B cells**) and **plasma cells (antibody-forming cells),** which secrete free, soluble (humoral) antibody molecules into extracellular fluids (Figure 10-1).
   b. Virgin B cells have not responded to an antigen since their release into the circulation from bone marrow. Their membrane antibodies are of the immunoglobulin M (IgM) and D (IgD) classes (see I.D).
   c. Memory B cells are derived by cell division from another B cell that has responded to an antigen. Their membrane antibodies are of immunoglobulin classes A (IgA), E (IgE), or G (IgG; see I.D).

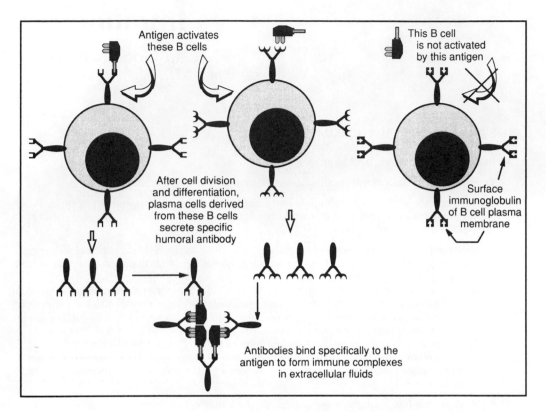

Antigen activates
these B cells

This B cell
is not activated
by this antigen

After cell division
and differentiation,
plasma cells derived
from these B cells
secrete specific
humoral antibody

Surface
immunoglobulin
of B cell plasma
membrane

Antibodies bind specifically to the
antigen to form immune complexes
in extracellular fluids

Figure 10-1. B cells: antigen specificity and activation.

3. **Antigen receptors of T cells** have two membrane proteins (α and β or γ and δ), which define the antigen specificity of each T cell, and several other integral membrane proteins known as **CD3 complex.** Therefore, T cells are **CD3$^+$.** Each T cell has thousands of identical antigen receptors in its membrane. Different T cells of different antigen specificities differ in the conformation of their antigen receptors.

    a. **Major histocompatibility complex (MHC) proteins.** The antigen receptors of T cells do not recognize antigens alone. Rather, they normally recognize **peptide epitopes** (fragments of antigen) that are chemically combined with MHC proteins on the surface of other body cells (Figure 10-2). MHC proteins are divided into **two major classes:**

        (1) **Class I proteins,** which are present on the surfaces of almost all body cells

        (2) **Class II proteins,** which are present only on the surfaces of special **antigen-presenting cells (APCs)**

    b. **Thymus gland.** T cells do not enter the circulation directly from bone marrow but first enter the thymus gland to mature. Most developing T cells die in the thymus. The cells that die either do not recognize normal self-antigens or produce a response against normal self-antigens.

        (1) T cells that are released from the thymus into the circulation are **virgin T cells.**

        (2) T cells that originate through cell division from the responses of other T cells are **memory T cells or effector T cells.**

    c. **Glycoproteins.** Most T cells can be classified by the presence of a membrane glycoprotein known as **CD4**—the **helper,** or **T$_H$ cell**—or the presence of **CD8**—the **cytotoxic T lymphocyte (CTL),** or **T$_C$ cell.**

        (1) **T$_H$ cells** can be divided into two functional groups: **T$_H$1** and **T$_H$2.** These cells have different functions in the immune response and regulate immune responses through the production of interleukins (IL; also called lymphokines), which are proteins that act on cells in an autocrine, paracrine, or endocrine manner.

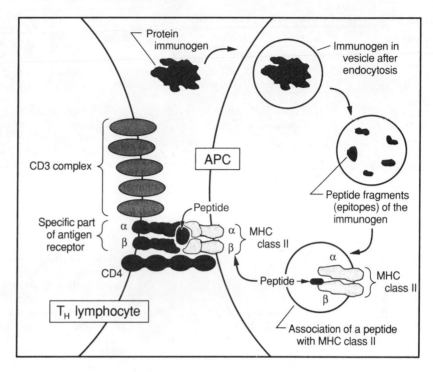

Figure 10-2. Helper T cell (T_H cell) antigen recognition. *MHC,* major histocompatibility complex; *APC,* antigen-presenting cell.

(a) **T_H1 cells** activate other cells, including some T_H cells, T_C cells, and macrophages. In addition, they can decrease antibody (Ab) production by inhibiting the formation of T_H2 cells.

(b) **T_H2 cells** activate B cells to divide and produce Ab. They can also inhibit the formation of T_H1 cells.

(2) **T_C cells** are able to kill cells that are infected by viruses. They do this through direct binding with the infected cell or through the release of cytotoxins.

(3) **T_r cells,** or T regulatory cells, have recently been described. Most of these cells are $CD4^+$, although there is a $CD8^+$ subset as well. All of these cells suppress immune responses through the secretion of IL-10 and transforming growth factor β (TGF-β); in addition, cells designated $CD4^+CD25^+$ are also able to inhibit other T cells through direct contact.

(4) Interleukins are part of a larger network of regulatory **cytokines.** This network includes secretions of other cell types in addition to those of lymphocytes. Table 10-1 lists the sources and actions of important cytokines that regulate the immune system and inflammation.

4. **Natural killer (NK) cells** are large, granular lymphocytes without a specific T or B cell antigen receptor. Their cytotoxicity is similar to that of CTL (T_C) cells. NK cells recognize and destroy tumors.

5. **APCs** are essential for most immune responses and are found in the sites at which these responses originate.

   a. The best understood APCs are the **macrophages** and **dendritic cells** of the **lymph nodes, spleen,** and **other lymphoid tissue.** Most immune responses within these organs begin when these cells present epitopes bound to their surface MHC class II molecules to T_H cells and secrete cytokines as accessory signals (Figure 10-2). APCs, especially macrophages, are able to control the type of immune response generated. They do this by secreting different cytokines in response to different types of pathogens (e.g., extracellular bacteria, intracellular bacteria, viruses).

Table 10-1. Major Cytokines and Their Actions

Cytokine	Sources of Secretion[a]	Major Actions
IL-1	Macrophages, APCs, others	T and B cell activation, pyrogenic, proinflammatory
TNF-α, TNF-β	Macrophages, T_H1 cells, T_C cells	Similar to IL-1, but including cytotoxicity
IL-2	T_H0 cells, T_H1 cells	T cell, B cell, and NK cell activation
IFN-γ	T_H1 cells	Induction of MHC, activation of macrophages and NK cells, formation of memory B cells, antiviral
IFN-α, IFN-β	Leukocytes, fibroblasts	Induction of MHC, antiviral, and growth inhibition
IL-3	Macrophages, T_H cells	Proliferation of multilineage marrow stem cells
IL-4	T_H2 cells	B cell activation and memory B cell formation, increased mast cell precursors, activation of mast cells
IL-5	T_H2 cells	Memory B cell formation, eosinophil production
IL-6	T_H2 cell, other types	Plasma cell maturation, others similar to IL-1
IL-7	Bone marrow stroma	Lymphocyte maturation
IL-8 (CXCL8)	Monocytes, macrophages, endothelial, fibroblasts cells	Chemokine, attraction and activation of neutrophils, attraction of T cells
IL-9	T_H1 cells	Proliferation and differentiation of bone marrow cells and thymocytes
IL-10	Macrophages, T_H2 cells CD8$^+$ T cells, B cells	Increased humoral (antibody), decreased cell-mediated immunity, mast cell growth
IL-11	Bone marrow stroma	Proliferation and differentiation of bone marrow cells and thrombocytes
IL-12	Macrophages, B cells	Promotion of cell-mediated immunity, activation of T_C and NK cells, suppression of humoral immunity
IL-13	T_H cells	IL-4-like effects on B cells, inhibition of production of inflammatory cytokines by monocytes
IL-14	T_H cells	Important for the generation of B memory cells
IL-15	Endothelial cells, epithelial monocytes, muscle cells	IL-2-like effects
GM-CSF	T_H1 cells, macrophages	Marrow proliferation of myeloid precursors
G-CSF	Fibroblasts, endothelial cells	Proliferation and survival of neutrophil precursors
M-CSF	Fibroblasts, endothelial cells	Survival of monocyte macrophages

APC, antigen-presenting cell; *G-CSF*, granulocyte colony-stimulating factor; *GM-CSF*, granulocyte-macrophage colony-stimulating factor; *IFN*, interferon; *IL*, interleukin; *M-CSF*, macrophage colony-stimulating factor; *MHC*, major histocompatibility complex; *NK cell*, natural killer cell; *$T_C$cell*, T cytotoxic cell; *$T_H$cell*, T helper cell; *TNF*, tumor necrosis factor.
[a]Not all sources are listed.

    b. Any cell in the body can act as an APC for immune responses involving CTL cells. Nucleated cells can present fragments of antigens bound to their surface MHC class I molecules to T_c (CD8$^+$) lymphocytes.

    c. Both T and B cells continually circulate from the blood through the lymph nodes, spleen, and other secondary lymphoid tissue and then back into the blood. If there is antigen present in the secondary lymphoid tissue that binds specifically to the receptor on the T or B cell, then an immune response can begin.

6. **Neutrophils, macrophages, eosinophils, basophils, platelets,** and **mast cells** assist in elimi-nating antigens from the body. Their functions may be phagocytic, proinflammatory, cyto-toxic, regulatory, or a combination of these.

C. Humoral immunity: primary and memory responses that produce antibodies

1. **Overview.** In most humoral immune responses, antigens are recognized by antigen-specific B cells and T_H cells (non-antigen-specific B and T_H cells do not respond). Initially, B and T_H2 cells divide to increase their cell numbers. Responding B cells produce both memory B cells and plasma cells, aided by cytokines secreted by T_H2 cells. **T-independent responses** to certain bacterial polysaccharide antigens do not require T_H cells. During T-independent responses, a subclass of B cells (B1 B cells) responds alone and produces plasma cells that secrete IgM antibodies, but no memory B cells are produced.

2. **Primary immune response.** The first time a specific antigen is encountered, only **virgin B cells** and **virgin T_H cells** are present to respond to the antigen. Initially, the T_H cells become T_H effector cells, and the B cells produce plasma cells that secrete IgM antibody. Later in the immune response, plasma cells producing other classes of antibody develop. The primary immune response is detected in the serum after 4 days and peaks in 7–11 days. In a primary immune response, IgM is produced first and is followed by IgG. Memory B and T_H2 cells are also produced. Memory B cells can also be activated to produce the other classes of antibody in subsequent immune responses.

3. **Memory immune responses.** The second or subsequent encounter with the same antigen or a closely related antigen produces responses by memory B cells and memory T_H2 cells. These responses are more rapid because memory cells require less antigen for stimulation and are of greater magnitude because there are more antigen-specific B and T cells to respond. Most serum antibody produced is IgG, with smaller amounts of IgA and IgE. Significant amounts of antibodies are produced as rapidly as 2–3 days after the reencounter with antigen, and the absolute amount of antibody (measured in milligrams per deciliter of serum) is greater than in primary immune responses. The duration of memory varies among antigens and probably among individuals. Some, but not all, memory is lifelong.

4. **Major roles of antibodies**
   a. The first function of an antibody is to act as an **antigen receptor** for B cells so that the B cells can recognize and respond to antigens.
   b. The second function of an antibody is to aid in the **elimination of antigen.** Elimination occurs through nonspecific functions, such as phagocytosis or complement activation. The mechanism of elimination depends on the class of antibody involved.
   c. The third function of an antibody is **neutralization of toxins.** Neutralization occurs when an antibody binds to the toxin and prevents it from reaching the target cell or receptor.

D. Immunoglobulins: antigen binding and class-specific functions. The terms *antibody* and *immu-noglobulin* are used interchangeably.

1. **Structure.** The standard immunoglobulin unit has four polypeptide chains: two identical light (L) polypeptide chains and two identical heavy (H) polypeptide chains. The structure is represented as H_2L_2. Each chain can be divided into a **C-terminal constant region** and an **N-terminal variable region** of amino acids (Figure 10-3). The N-terminal variable region formed from the H and L variable domains is responsible for antigen binding by the immuno-globulin. The C-terminal constant regions of the H chain determine the class of the immuno-globulin.

2. **Class.** There are five general heavy-chain, constant-region amino acid sequences. These determine the **five general classes of immunoglobulins: IgM, IgG, IgE, IgA,** and **IgD.** Within some classes, variants of the heavy-chain sequence yield subclasses: IgM1–2, IgG1–4, and IgA1–2. The class of an immunoglobulin defines its nonspecific antigen elimination or inflammatory function. These functions are activated only after antigen–antibody complexes are formed, not by unbound antibodies.
   a. **IgM** is the first immunoglobulin secreted during primary immune responses. It plays a minor role in memory responses. It does not leave the blood in significant amounts because of its pentameric structure and large size (mol wt 900,000 daltons). It accounts for approximately 20% of the adult serum immunoglobulin. IgM is the most potent **activator of the complement system** (see I.E.2). Its serum half-life is 9–11 days.

Figure 10-3. Immunoglobulin molecule. *Fc,* fragment, crystallizable.

b. IgG is the predominant serum immunoglobulin secreted at the end of the primary immune responses and during memory responses. It can diffuse from blood into other extracellular fluids, particularly in inflamed microvasculature, and it crosses the placenta to enter the fetal circulation. It accounts for approximately 70% of adult serum immunoglobulin. It **opsonizes antigens** for **phagocytosis and activates the complement system.** Its serum half-life is 25–35 days.

c. IgE is secreted during memory responses and may also be secreted late during a primary response. It normally accounts for < 1% of serum immunoglobulin. It **binds to IgE receptors located on the cell surfaces of blood basophils and on connective tissue mast cells** to trigger the secretion of inflammatory mediators from these cells in the presence of specific antigens. IgE mediates allergic reactions. Its serum half-life is 2–3 days, but its mast cell–bound half-life is several months to years.

d. IgA is secreted during memory responses and may also be secreted late during a primary response. It accounts for 10% of serum immunoglobulin. However, it is **secreted in large quantities across mucosal surfaces into gastrointestinal, respiratory, lachrymal, mammary, and genitourinary secretions, where it protects mucosa from colonization** by bacteria and other microorganisms. Its serum half-life is approximately 5 days.

e. IgD accounts for < 1% of serum immunoglobulin and has no known function as a secreted immunoglobulin.

3. Specificity. The specificity of each immunoglobulin for antigen binding resides in the two identical antigen-binding sites, each formed by the combination of the variable regions of heavy and light chains. IgG, IgE, and IgD as well as serum IgA have two antigen-binding sites. IgM antibodies have 10 identical antigen-binding sites through the combination of five H_2L_2 units with a joining polypeptide chain to form a pentamer. Likewise, secreted IgA typically exists as a dimer with four binding sites.

4. **Quantitation of immunoglobulin: antigen binding and cross-reactivity.** Between 10^8 and 10^{11} unique immunoglobulins with different antigen-binding specificities are formed by the immune system.
   a. Each immunoglobulin specificity can bind to several different, but closely structurally related, antigens. This ability illustrates the phenomenon of cross-reactivity of a single antibody for multiple antigens. Each immunoglobulin–antigen interaction is quantitated by its **association constant (K_a).**
   b. Cross-reactivity may also occur through the sharing of some, but not all, antigens by two strains of bacteria, viruses, or other microorganisms.
   c. Because each microorganism has several antigens, each elicits the production of multiple antibodies with unique specificities by the immune system. This response is known as a **polyclonal response** and results in a combination of antibodies known as a **polyclonal antiserum** and defines the serotype of the immunizing organism.

5. **Fragments of immunoglobulin for clinical use.** Immunoglobulins can be enzymatically cleaved into fragments—for example, **Fab** and **F(ab′)$_2$** (antigen-binding fragments), **Fc** (crystallizable fragment), and **Fv** (variable region fragment). Fab and F(ab′)$_2$ fragments are clinically useful because they retain antigen specificity, but not class-specific (e.g., inflammatory) functions, and are readily excreted renally. Conversely, this characteristic limits their effectiveness in certain situations.

E. **Antigen elimination and acute inflammatory mechanisms of humoral immunity**

1. **Opsonization** is the preparation of any extracellular antigen for phagocytosis through binding of antibody. Neutrophils and macrophages have a variety of receptors for the constant region of IgG antibodies ($F_C\gamma R$), which bind antigen–antibody complexes. When the antigen is soluble, the immune complexes must be sufficiently large to induce this reaction. This binding triggers phagocytosis of the antigen–antibody complex and activates the metabolism of the phagocyte, shifting it toward the production of bactericidal oxygen radicals (e.g., superoxide anion, hydrogen peroxide).

2. **Complement** is a group of approximately 20 serum proteins that, when activated, form a proteolytic cascade similar to the clotting and fibrinolytic sequence. Within this complex of proteins, there are some that inhibit complement activation. Complement is responsible for increasing the inflammatory response, phagocytosis of antigen, lysis of cells (usually pathogens), and clearance of immune complexes.
   a. In the **classic activation pathway,** immune complexes of IgM or IgG antibodies bound to antigen bind subunits of complement component 1 (C1) and trigger an initial series of proteolytic cleavages.
   b. In the **alternative activation pathway,** the cell walls of certain microorganisms (e.g., gram-negative bacteria) are able to bind C3b and other complement proteins that initiate a different sequence of proteolytic cleavages, leading to the same end point as the classic activation pathway.
   c. In the **mannose-binding pathway,** mannose-binding protein (MBP) is produced by the liver during the acute-phase response. MBP binds to mannose on the surface of bacteria and, in conjunction with associated serum proteases, triggers proteolytic cleavages identical to those seen in the classic pathway of complement.
   d. C3b, C4b, and associated degradation products provide opsonization, via complement receptors on cells such as macrophages and neutrophils, in addition to that provided by IgG in immune complexes.
   e. **Proinflammatory fragments** of certain complement proteins act both by **direct activity on the microvasculature,** promoting arteriole dilation and increased vascular permeability, and by triggering the release of histamine and other proinflammatory mediators from mast cells and basophils.
   f. A complex of complement proteins known as the **membrane attack complex (MAC)** can insert into any lipid bilayer membrane, forming a large channel through which ions and water diffuse. Many bacteria, enveloped viruses, and some human or mammalian cells are subject to this osmotic lysis.

3. **Circulating basophils and connective tissue mast cells** are mainly proinflammatory cells that rapidly initiate acute inflammation. Triggers of secretion include mechanical and thermal trauma and immunologic triggers, complement, and IgE.
   a. **IgE antibodies,** regardless of antigen specificity, equilibrate between serum and binding noncovalently to high-affinity IgE receptors on mast cell and basophil surfaces. This activity arms the mast cells and basophils, but the triggering of secretion by these cells requires that antigen bind to and cross-link antigen-specific IgE molecules already affixed to their receptors.
   b. Mast cells and basophils, when triggered, immediately secrete the contents of their storage granules, including histamine, tumor necrosis factor α (TNF-α), proteases, and chemotactic proteins for neutrophils and eosinophils. In addition, activation of phospholipase A_2 releases arachidonic acid from membrane phospholipids and results in the synthesis of various leukotrienes, prostaglandins, and thromboxanes. The primary effects of these mediators are
      (1) Vascular dilation
      (2) Increased vascular permeability
      (3) Contraction of respiratory and gastrointestinal smooth muscle
      (4) Neutrophil and eosinophil chemotaxis

4. **Antibody-dependent cell-mediated cytotoxicity** is mediated by cells with cytotoxic potential as well as receptors for IgG. These cells, NK cells, macrophages, and some T_C cells, bind to and lyse target cells coated with IgG.

5. **Acute inflammation** allows increased ease of movement of crucial components of the blood into the tissues, including phagocytes (especially neutrophils), IgG antibodies, complement, clotting proteins, and kinins. The adaptive result is the isolation and removal of invading microorganisms and necrotic tissues, followed by tissue repair and regeneration.

F. **Cell-mediated immune** responses (**cell-mediated immunity**) are those in which **antibody is not involved in the elimination of antigen.**

1. **Nonviral intracellular parasites** of macrophages, such as *Mycobacteria, Listeria,* and certain protozoa, are primarily eliminated by T cell–macrophage immunity. CD4$^+$ T_H1 cells recognize infected macrophages and secrete lymphokines, particularly interferon γ (IFN-γ). These lymphokines activate macrophages to produce more bactericidal oxygen radicals (e.g., superoxide anion, hydrogen peroxide) and also to increase the secretory function of the macrophages and inhibit phagocytosis, enabling the macrophages to kill the parasites in the **extracellular** environment.

2. **Viruses** must be eliminated from both extracellular sites and infected cells.
   a. **Antibodies** opsonize virus particles in blood and tissue fluids for phagocytosis, but antibodies are generally ineffective against infected cells.
   b. **CTL cells** recognize infected cells and directly kill them in an antigen-specific manner, secreting lymphokines, such as TNF-β as well as granzymes and granulysins. In addition, CTL can induce apoptosis via FAS ligand binding to FAS on the target cells. Often, the cells are killed before infectious virus particles are assembled. When killed cells release infectious viral particles, they may be opsonized by an antibody. Cell-mediated immunity and humoral immunity must function in concert to provide optimal antiviral defenses.
   c. **NK cells** kill infected (and tumor) cells in a non-antigen-specific manner, binding to MHC-like molecules using a variety of receptors. NK cells kill their target cells using mechanisms similar to those used by CTLs.
   d. **IFN-γ** (secreted by CTL, NK, and T_H1 cells) and **IFN-α** and **IFN-β** (secreted by macrophages and other cells) provide additional antiviral immunity by binding to receptors on other cells and inducing synthesis of kinases and endonucleases (i.e., antiviral proteins), which inhibit viral and cellular growth. Interferons also upregulate class I MHC proteins, which make infected cells more visible to CTL cells.

3. **Tumors** are modified host cells and must be eliminated by the immune system, usually by cell-mediated immunity.
   a. **NK cells** are primarily responsible for killing tumor cells. They act by recognizing changes in cell-surface proteins or by **antibody-dependent cell-mediated cytotoxicity.**

    b. CTL cells recognize tumor cells in an antigen-specific manner and kill them by secreting lymphokines, such as TNF-β, and by inducing apoptosis through the binding of FAS and FAS-ligand.

    c. Macrophages also kill tumor cells in a nonspecific manner, through the release of TNF-α.

  4. Graft rejection (see V)

II. Hypersensitivity Reactions are exaggerated, inappropriate, or prolonged immune responses that cause damage to otherwise normal tissue.

Four types of hypersensitivity reactions are recognized, primarily on the basis of the mechanisms of pathogenesis (Figure 10-4). Many different diseases are included within each type. **Allergens** are broadly defined as antigens or haptens that induce hypersensitivity reactions, and they are usually nonpathogenic, nontoxic agents.

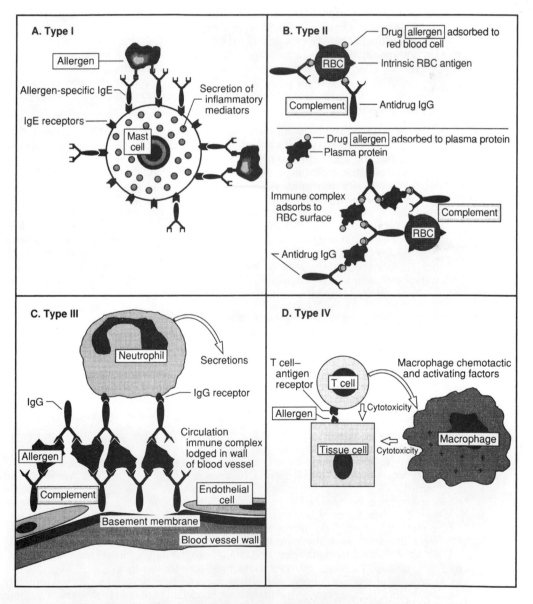

Figure 10-4. The four main types of hypersensitivity reactions. *RBC,* red blood cell.

A. IgE-mediated type I hypersensitivity reaction (immediate hypersensitivity)

1. A type I hypersensitivity reaction is caused by **inappropriate production and hypersecretion of IgE** to specific allergens plus auxiliary factors, such as increased mucosal permeability to irritants (e.g., SO_2, NO_2, diesel fumes). The **tendency to hypersecrete IgE is inheritable;** a child's probability of being a hypersecretor is 50% if one parent is a hypersecretor and 75% if both parents are hypersecretors. These individuals are considered to be atopic.

   a. IgE is produced locally after nonsystemic exposure to an antigen.
      (1) In normosecretors (1–10 μg/dL of IgE), arming of local mast cells occurs (see I.B.6).
      (2) In hypersecretors (typically 100 μg–1 mg/dL of IgE), IgE spillover occurs, arming basophils and nonlocal mast cells and causing increased occupancy of mast cell and basophil IgE receptors by IgE.
   b. Because there is a lag period for IgE synthesis and cell arming, a type I reaction usually does not occur on the first (or first seasonal) exposure to a specific allergen.

2. **Common allergens**
   a. **Respiratory allergens** include pollens of various plants (e.g., ragweed, grasses, trees), fungi, animal fur, carpet mites, and other shed allergens.
   b. **Gastrointestinal allergens** include dairy products, shellfish, tree nuts, and peanuts.
   c. **Skin and mouth allergens** include topically applied drugs (e.g., procaine).
   d. **Intravenous allergens** include insect venoms and drugs that act as cell or plasma protein-bound haptens (e.g., penicillin, cephalosporins, vaccines). These drugs may cause type II or III hypersensitivity reactions in people who do not hypersecrete IgE in response to these drugs.

3. **Activation of mast cell and basophil secretion** by an allergen requires two or more receptor-bound IgE molecules to be cross-linked by a specific allergen. Hapten-size drugs that provoke this reaction both sensitize the immune system and trigger mast cells when the drug is bound to a larger molecule (e.g., a protein). Activation leads to a transient increase in the cyclic adenosine monophosphate (cAMP) level, followed by an increase in the level of cyclic guanosine monophosphate (cGMP) relative to cAMP. This is followed by phospholipase C producing second messengers, which lead to a rapid increase in cytoplasmic calcium ions (Ca^{++}). With the increase in cytoplasmic Ca^{++}, there is immediate fusion of vesicles containing inflammatory mediators with the cell membrane and release of these mediators into the extracellular milieu. In addition, after degranulation, mast cells produce additional cytokines, leukotrienes, and prostaglandins. These activate the late-phase response, which further activates the local inflammatory response. Prolonged increases in cAMP levels inhibit mast cell activation.

4. **Effects of mediators secreted from mast cells and basophils**
   a. Vasodilation and increased capillary permeability are caused by histamine; the leukotrienes C4, D4, and E4; and prostaglandin D_2 (PGD_2) secreted by mast cells.
   b. Gastrointestinal and respiratory smooth muscle constriction is caused primarily by the leukotrienes C4, D4, and E4; PGD_2; and platelet-activating factor secreted by mast cells and other leukocytes.
   c. Eosinophil and neutrophil infiltration is caused by chemotactic factors secreted by mast cells.

5. **Local symptoms of pathogenesis** include inflammation of the upper (rhinitis) and lower respiratory tract (asthma), gastrointestinal tract, and skin.
   a. Common clinical symptoms include urticaria, pruritus (itching), nasal congestion, bronchoconstriction, mucus and lachrymal hypersecretion, laryngeal edema, vomiting, and diarrhea.
   b. Symptoms may be confined to the portal of allergen entry (e.g., respiratory allergen: respiratory symptoms) or may be more widespread as a result of allergen spillover into the circulation (e.g., food allergen: gastrointestinal, skin, respiratory symptoms).
   c. **Atopic dermatitis** typically includes severe pruritic dermatitis, and may also include rhinitis or asthma, food allergies, and changes in the cell-mediated immune system.
   d. The local introduction of allergen sometimes leads to anaphylaxis.
   e. Approximately 50% of patients with asthma hypersecrete IgE. This tendency is probably contributory, but ancillary, to the underlying bronchial hyperreactivity present in these patients (see Chapter 48).

6. **Systemic anaphylactic manifestations of pathogenesis.** In sensitized individuals, intravenous injection of an allergen (e.g., bee venom) or absorption across the mucous membranes (e.g., peanuts) can cause systemic edema and hypovolemic shock, with cardiac arrhythmia, asphyxiation as a result of bronchoconstriction and mucous hypersecretion, and urticaria. Death usually occurs because of asphyxiation. While other sensitized individuals may have only mild local symptoms upon encountering the allergen, these results demonstrate differing host responses to identical proteins.

7. **Time course.** Immediate hypersensitivity reactions have two phases. The **early reaction,** resulting from mediator secretion by mast cells, begins within 1–2 min after allergen contact and peaks within 1–2 hr. The **late-phase reaction** begins 6–12 hr after contact with the allergen and lasts for several hours. The late-phase reactions are initiated by newly synthesized leukotrienes and prostaglandins along with cytokines, chemokines, and other inflammatory mediators. The late-phase reaction is characterized by increased numbers of eosinophils and is maintained by the products of these cells.

8. **Diagnosis.** In scratch tests, a variety of allergens are injected intradermally to screen for the presence of a wheal and flare (i.e., edema and erythema) response in the skin. **Radioallergosorbent (RAST)** and **radioimmunosorbent (RIST) assays** use radiolabeled reagents to detect serum IgE concentrations. The results of these assays do not always agree with each other or with clinical manifestations of type I hypersensitivity.

9. **Prophylaxis**
   a. Identifying and avoiding allergens is the most important form of prophylaxis.
   b. **Hyposensitization (desensitization)** is performed by injecting weekly, increasing doses of allergen intramuscularly to elicit an allergen-specific IgG response and decrease the allergen-specific IgE. Once desensitization has been achieved, monthly injections are used to maintain the IgG levels. IgG is able to bind to the allergen and inhibit its binding to the mast-cell bound IgE.

10. **Therapy**
   a. **Competitive H$_1$-antagonists** of histamine are useful in local forms but do not completely reverse the inflammation because histamine is not the only inflammatory mediator in the reaction. Competitive H$_1$-antagonists have little effect on anaphylaxis.
   b. **Epinephrine** reverses anaphylaxis through its α-agonist and β-agonist effects. Patients with systemic allergies are given epinephrine self-administration kits. β$_2$-agonists (e.g., albuterol) are able to promote bronchodilation, and α$_1$-agonists (e.g., phenylpropanolamine) decrease nasal congestion.
   c. **Cromolyn sodium** (cromoglycate) is a locally administered inhibitor of mast cell degranulation. **Glucocorticoids** are able to block the late phase of the reaction but are less effective during the early phase. **Antileukotriene therapies** are also able to block the late phase of the reaction.
   d. **Topical steroids** inhibit inflammation and immune responses. Topical application via spray or inhaler limits the side effects seen when glucocorticoids are administered systemically. In addition to using topical steroids alone, they are also combined with long-acting β$_2$-agonists as therapy for asthma.
   e. **Anti-IgE therapy** is composed of a high-affinity monoclonal antibody to the Fc region of IgE. It is able to bind IgE and prevent sensitization of mast cells and basophils. This therapy is useful in highly atopic individuals and is used for individuals with severe asthma for whom other therapies have proven ineffective.

B. **Non-IgE-mediated type I hypersensitivity reactions** are probably the result of several poorly understood causes and are sometimes called **anaphylactoid reactions.** The following factors may contribute to and exacerbate non-IgE-mediated type I reactions.

5. Respiratory β$_2$-receptor unresponsiveness, which leads to a diminished bronchodilatory effect of the sympathetic nervous system.

6. Hyperreactivity of mast cells through H$_2$-receptor unresponsiveness. This decreases the negative feedback of histamine on the activation of mast cells.

C. **Type II hypersensitivity reactions**

1. **Pathogenesis.** Antibody-mediated cytotoxicity occurs through the production of IgM or IgG. These antibodies are able to bind to specific allergens located on cell surfaces.
   a. These allergens may be intrinsic to the cell (i.e., natural cell-surface components) or extrinsic compounds (i.e., drugs) adsorbed to the cell surface.
   b. Cytotoxicity may result from activation of complement, phagocytosis of the IgG opsonized cell, or both.
   c. A third cytotoxic mechanism, known as antibody-dependent, cell-mediated cytotoxicity, involves the direct killing of antibody-coated cells by NK cells, macrophages, or eosinophils.
   d. Type II reactions may exhibit anaphylactic signs and symptoms if enough complement is activated; however, they usually do not progress to this stage.

2. **Common allergens.** Type II allergens are diverse. It is the pathogenic mechanism that is common to all the reactions.
   a. Foreign blood surface antigens may act as allergens to produce **transfusion mismatches** or **Rh disease.**
   b. Drug allergens (or drug metabolite allergens) acting as haptens are the **leading cause of hemolytic anemia.**
      (1) These allergens may directly adsorb to cell surfaces and be specifically bound by antibodies (e.g., penicillins, cephalosporins, quinidine).
      (2) Alternately, they may form serum-phase immune complexes, which adsorb nonspecifically to blood cell surfaces. This makes the cell susceptible to lysis owing to the "innocent bystander" effect (e.g., rifampin, sulfonamides, chlorpromazine).
   c. **Self-antigens** are the allergen in certain autoimmune diseases (e.g. myasthenia gravis, autoimmune hemolytic anemia; see III) Autoimmune hemolytic anemia is sometimes associated with administration of α-methyldopa, which induces autoantibodies against the red blood cell surface.
   d. **Hyperacute rejection** of transplanted tissue (see V)

3. **Chemical mediators.** Complement proteins produce cytotoxicity and inflammation, which stimulate **macrophages and granulocytes** to secrete cytokines and enzymes, which in turn enhance inflammation.

4. **Clinical symptoms** depend on the type of antigen or allergen involved (see II.D.2). Hemolytic anemia and thrombocytopenia are the major clinical signs of type II hypersensitivity reactions. In hyperacute graft rejection, the transplanted tissue does not successfully perfuse because of antibody-mediated cytotoxicity to the transplanted vasculature.

5. **Time course**
   a. In the first sensitization to a drug allergen, the blood cell lysis and inflammation begin 7–10 days after initiation of drug therapy. The second exposure to the drug causes symptoms within 3 days.
   b. **Transfusion mismatch.** Hemolysis begins 1–2 hr after transfusion. Peak effects occur after approximately 12 hr.
   c. **Rh disease** does not occur in the first RhD^+ pregnancy of an RhD^- mother. Maternal IgG is produced in the second and subsequent pregnancies after transplacental maternal sensitization to the RhD^+ fetal red blood cells. This sensitization usually takes place in the third trimester. Maternal anti-RhD IgG crosses the placenta, binds to the fetal red blood cells, and activates the fetal complement system prenatally, which leads to perinatal hemolytic anemia.

6. **Prophylaxis and therapy.** In drug-induced hypersensitivity reactions, withdrawing the drug usually reverses the lysis. Preventing recontact is the best prophylaxis. In Rh disease, anti-RhD is administered during pregnancy and within 72 hr postpartum for each Rh^+ pregnancy. The simplest explanation for the efficacy of anti-RhD is that this passive immunization (see VI.B.2.d) binds to fetal red blood cells in the maternal circulation and prevents sensitization of the maternal immune system.

D. **Type III hypersensitivity reactions** involve the persistence of immune complexes in the circulation or at local tissue sites when they are not removed after production of specific antibodies and antigen–antibody complexes. The subtypes of type III hypersensitivity reactions have diverse causes, and only the pathogenic mechanism is common to them all.

1. **Pathogenesis.** Immune complexes activate complement, cause inflammation, and induce positive chemotaxis in neutrophils. Persistence of immune complexes may be caused by the following:

   a. A **high concentration of antigen or antibody,** which leads to a disparity in the molar ratio of antigen to antibody and the production of small immune complexes.

   b. **Chronic formation of immune complexes** in the circulation as a result of **persistence of antigen** as with some chronic infections.

   c. Other factors that cause insoluble immune complexes to form and precipitate intravascularly or on basement membranes.

2. **Common allergens**

   a. **Self-antigens in most non-organ-specific** (rheumatologic) **autoimmune disorders** (e.g., systemic lupus erythematosus, rheumatoid arthritis)

   b. **Bacterial or protozoan antigens in persistent or chronic infections** and in the initial stages of viremia for certain viral infections (e.g., prodrome of hepatitis B virus infection).

   c. **Drugs** (e.g., penicillin, sulfonamides, thiouracil).

   d. **Antisera** from another species (e.g., horse), can cause serum sickness when used for passive immunization.

   e. **Fungal and bacterial spores** in the local respiratory form of the reaction

3. **Chemical mediators. Complement proteins** cause inflammation and **stimulate mast cell and basophil secretions,** which enhance inflammation. The increased vascular permeability allows immune complexes to leave the circulation and attach to basement membranes, which underlay the endothelial lining of blood vessels. The kidney glomerulus and small arteries are particularly susceptible. Complement and mast cell proteins attract neutrophils; these cells can phagocytize immune complexes and release enzymes that damage local tissue, thus intensifying inflammation. In addition, platelet aggregation and microthrombus formation may occur.

4. **Clinical symptoms** depend on the severity and systemic or local nature of immune complex deposition and persistence.

   a. The first symptoms of systemic reactions are lymphadenopathy, splenomegaly, fever, and rash. These are common in drug-induced and viremia-induced type III hypersensitivity reactions.

   b. More serious symptoms include vasculitis and glomerulonephritis, both of which may become necrotizing. These symptoms often occur with systemic lupus erythematosus (SLE). Arthralgia and arthritis occur in both systemic and local reactions.

   c. The most common types of local type III hypersensitivity reactions are pneumonitis from inhaled fungi and bacteria to which the patient is occupationally exposed (e.g., moldy hay in **farmer's lung**) and reactions to spores borne in aerosol microdroplets from dirty ultrasonic humidifiers (e.g., **humidifier lung**). The cause of these diseases is not completely understood, but both IgE and IgG are involved. IgE causes the initial inflammation and trapping of antigen, and IgG is responsible for the long-term effects. Symptoms include

      (1) Nasal congestion and bronchoconstriction

      (2) Joint pain and inflammation of rheumatoid arthritis caused by joint-localized immune complexes involving rheumatoid factor and neutrophil phagocytosis (see Chapter 49)

5. **Time course**

   a. **Systemic.** In patients with no prior exposure to the allergen, the symptoms appear in 1–2 weeks (possibly longer) after exposure. In patients with preexisting antibodies, symptoms appear within several hours to 1 day after exposure. Severe symptoms, such as glomerulonephritis, usually require 2 weeks or more to appear.

   b. **Local.** In patients with preexisting antibodies, hypersensitivity pneumonitis symptoms appear 6–8 hr after exposure to the antigen.

6. **Prophylaxis and therapy.** In drug-induced reactions, **withdrawing the drug** usually reverses the reaction. Treatment includes antihistamines or corticosteroids. Transient infectious forms resolve spontaneously as immune complexes are removed by phagocytes.

E. **Type IV hypersensitivity reactions**

   1. **Pathogenesis.** Type IV reactions include prolonged inappropriate and appropriate immune responses mediated by antigen-specific T_H1 cells in concert with activated macrophages.

The T$_H$1 cells infiltrate tissues in which the antigen is presented and recruit and activate macrophages. The release of enzymes and cytokines by these cells results in inflammation and disruption of tissue structure in the absence of antibody.

    a. Reactions to infections involve a T$_H$1 response against specific intracellular bacterial (e.g., *Mycobacteria*) and protozoan parasites. When the response is prolonged and ineffective, granuloma formation will occur.

    b. Contact dermatitis is an inappropriate skin reaction to haptens (e.g., pentadecyl catechols of poison ivy), which bind to epidermal cell surfaces and elicit a CTL and T$_H$1 cell response.

    c. Tuberculin reaction is observed in the dermis and is an appropriate reaction to mycobacterial antigens. This reaction indicates a state of active T$_H$1 immunity (owing to an active infection) or T cell memory to the organism. (In patients who had a positive tuberculin reaction, a subsequent negative reaction would indicate immunologic anergy or unresponsiveness).

2. Common antigens

    a. Infectious agents include *Mycobacterium tuberculosis, M. leprae, Listeria monocytogenes, trypanosomes,* and viruses.

    b. Hapten allergens, such as pentadecyl catechols from poison ivy, poison oak, chromates, nickel ions (leached from watch backs and other jewelry), acrylates, hair dyes that contain *p*-phenylene diamine, para-aminobenzoic acid, and certain antibiotic ointments (e.g., topical neomycin), may induce **contact dermatitis.**

    c. Antigens that induce a tuberculin reaction include purified protein derivative (PPD), tuberculin (Mantoux reaction), *Candida,* mumps, and other antigens from microorganisms.

3. Chemical mediators are important in type IV reactions. These mediators are cytokines produced by activated T$_H$1 cells. The cytokines attract and activate macrophages to the site(s) where the pathogen/allergen is located. In turn, the activated macrophages secrete cytokines, which are responsible for inflammation and cytotoxicity (e.g., TNF-α).

4. Clinical symptoms depend on the subtype of reaction.

    a. Granulomas are local aggregations of T$_H$1 cells, macrophages, and giant epithelioid cells (derived from fusion of activated macrophages). They occur at sites of chronic infection and serve to restrict the spread of the infection.

    b. In contact sensitivity, cellular infiltration of the epidermis by CTL, T$_H$1 cells, and macrophages produces microvesicle formation with spongiosis.

    c. Tuberculin tests cause erythema and induration as a result of cellular infiltration of the dermis, but no epidermal spongiosis is observed.

5. Time course

    a. Granulomas form at various times after the onset of a chronic immune response but generally require a minimum of 2 weeks.

    b. Contact sensitivity may not occur with the first transient exposure. However, in a sensitized individual, skin inflammation will appear 12–24 hr after contact with the antigen and peaks between 48 and 72 hr after exposure.

    c. Tuberculin reactions follow the same time course as contact sensitivity. This reaction is often called **delayed cutaneous hypersensitivity,** or delayed-type hypersensitivity.

6. Prophylaxis and therapy. Treatment of granulomas depends on the organism involved. Proper treatment to resolve the infection will also aid in resolving the chronic immune response. For contact sensitivity, it is necessary to identify the antigen/allergen involved. Removal and avoidance of the allergen is important for prophylaxis. For treatment, topical corticosteroids suppress T cell and macrophage function. In severe cases, oral corticosteroid therapy may be required.

III. Autoimmunity is a tissue-damaging immune response directed specifically and inappropriately against one or more self-antigens.

    A. The **origin** of autoreactive immune responses is not generally known, but it requires loss of self-tolerance and deregulation of the control networks that normally prevent development of autoimmune disease. Such deregulation may include lack of regulation of T$_H$ and T$_C$ cells, cross-reactivity with antigens from microorganisms, loss of self-tolerance or failure to develop tolerance, and aberrant presentation of self-antigen on specific HLA molecules.

B. Epidemiology

1. **Familial clustering** is evident for many, if not most, autoimmune reactions representing a complex inherited predisposition toward autoimmunity. In most cases, this predisposition is associated with specific MHC types, usually class II molecules (e.g., rheumatoid arthritis with the MHC class II molecule HLA-DR4).

2. These reactions are more common in women. The female-to-male ratio in myasthenia gravis is approximately 2:1 and in SLE is approximately 10:1. In contrast, Sjögren disease and Goodpasture syndrome are more common in men than in women.

C. Pathogenesis

1. **Overview.** In a specific autoimmune disorder, the primary pathogenic mechanism may be humoral (mediated by antibodies with or without a contribution by complement), T cell mediated, or involve both humoral and cell-mediated components. These diseases are commonly associated with exacerbation and remission of the disease.

2. **Environmental factors** are thought to contribute to pathogenesis. However, specific associations have been found in only a few cases; these include *Streptococcus* group A pharyngitis, rheumatic fever, exposure to organic solvents, Goodpasture syndrome, ultraviolet irradiation, and SLE. It is likely that environmental factors act in concert with genetic predisposition to induce disease.

3. **Organ-specific and systemic (non-organ-specific) disorders**
   a. **Organ-specific disorders** (e.g., antithyroid autoimmunity) are limited to and directed specifically against self-antigen in a single organ. Lesions and clinical symptoms are limited primarily to that organ. Cellular damage may be mediated through antibody-mediated and complement-mediated cytotoxicity (type II hypersensitivity) and/or through cell-mediated cytotoxicity (type IV hypersensitivity).
   b. **Systemic disorders** (e.g., SLE)
      (1) These disorders are also known as connective tissue, collagen vascular, or rheumatologic disorders. Autoantibodies are formed against antigens found in most or all tissues, especially those located in the nuclei of cells and containing DNA, RNA, or nuclear-associated proteins (**antinuclear antibodies**). Pathologic changes occur systematically, primarily in the connective tissue and are at least partially caused by type III hypersensitivity reactions. Symptoms may be seen in the blood vessels, kidney glomeruli, skin, joints, and serous membranes.
      (2) Non-organ-specific disorders are sometimes difficult to distinguish from one another because of the similarities in autoantigens and pathogenesis. For example, most patients with SLE have circulating antinuclear antibodies; however, these also occur in 50–65% of patients with Sjögren syndrome and rheumatoid arthritis as well as in a small percentage of clinically normal individuals. By contrast, rheumatoid factor (anti-IgG) is seen in 75–90% of patients with rheumatoid arthritis or Sjögren syndrome as well as in 35% of patients with SLE. The synovitis of rheumatoid arthritis is often a clinical finding in SLE, and the vasculitis of SLE is found in rheumatoid arthritis (see Chapter 49).

D. Organ-specific autoimmunities

1. **Rheumatic fever** is not technically an autoimmune response because antibodies are produced against group A streptococci and cross-react with cardiac muscle fibers that are damaged by complement. Increased risk is related to a strong immune response to streptococcal M antigen.

2. **Antithyroid autoimmunities** (see Chapter 52). Aspects of several subtypes may occur in the same patient. Increased risk is associated with MHC class II types DR3 and DR5.
   a. **Primary autoimmune myxedema.** Antibodies against the thyroid-stimulating hormone (TSH) receptor on thyroid follicle cells act as antagonists to the stimulation of growth of the follicle cells normally provoked by TSH. The result is thyroid atrophy with hypothyroidism.

    b. Hashimoto thyroiditis. Antibodies against thyroid peroxidase on follicle cells cause cytotoxicity and inflammation through the activation of complement. Antibodies against thyroglobulin (colloid) also may be present. Cell-mediated immunity may cause some cytotoxic damage. The resulting hypothyroidism is treated with synthetic thyroid hormone.

    c. Graves disease. Antibodies act as agonists of TSH, binding to the TSH receptor and stimulating hypersecretion of thyroid hormone (thyroid-stimulating immunoglobulins). The result is hyperthyroidism, which is treated by antithyroid drugs (e.g., propylthiouracil) or thyroid ablation with surgery or radiation.

3. Myasthenia gravis

    a. Pathogenesis. Antibodies against the nicotinic acetylcholine receptor on skeletal muscle plasma membrane at neuromuscular junctions act as competitive antagonists of **acetylcholine** binding. This activity causes weakness and fatigue in skeletal muscles. In addition to this direct blockage of neuromuscular transmission, down regulation of receptors and complement damage to muscle fibers occur. Many patients have swallowing and respiratory muscle dysfunction that may be caused by penicillamine therapy. Increased risk is associated with MHC class I type B8.

    b. Therapy. Anticholinesterase therapy (e.g., neostigmine) increases acetylcholine synaptic concentrations (preservation of endogenous acetylcholine). Immunosuppression with corticosteroids is used in severe cases; plasmapheresis to remove autoreactive antibodies from the blood is also helpful. Thymectomy helps many patients.

4. Autoimmune pernicious anemia

    a. Pathogenesis. Antibodies against intrinsic factor are secreted into the stomach lumen, where they inhibit the association of intrinsic factor with vitamin B_{12}. Thus the absorption of vitamin B_{12} is decreased. This condition also can result from antibodies against gastrin receptors on parietal cells of the stomach mucosa that block stimulation of the cells by gastrin and decrease their secretion of intrinsic factor.

    b. Therapy is intramuscular injection of cyanocobalamin or oral administration of concentrated intrinsic factor preparations.

5. Goodpasture syndrome

    a. Pathogenesis. Antibodies against **glomerular capillary basement membrane (GBM)** activate complement and neutrophil-mediated damage. This activation leads to glomerulonephritis, with rapid deterioration of renal function. These antibodies cross-react with pulmonary capillary basement membrane, producing pulmonary hemorrhage in smokers. Increased risk is associated with MHC class II type DR2.

    b. Therapy. Immunosuppressive therapy includes corticosteroids, with plasmapheresis to remove autoreactive antibodies.

6. Autoimmune hemolytic anemia (red blood cell), thrombocytopenia (platelet), neutropenia (neutrophil), and lymphopenia (lymphocyte)

    a. Pathogenesis. Antibodies against membrane antigens of one or more of the indicated cell types may activate complement and opsonize the cells for rapid splenic phagocytosis. It may also occur as part of the spectrum of autoimmunity in non-organ-specific disorders, particularly SLE. These autoimmune varieties must be distinguished from those precipitated by responses to external antigens (e.g., drugs) but the clinical effects are similar.

    b. Therapy. These disorders are often acute and self-limiting, but therapy is required when they are chronic. In adults, treatment begins with corticosteroids. Additional options are cyclophosphamide, chlorambucil, and intravenous immune globulin (IVIG).

7. Insulin-dependent diabetes mellitus (IDDM; see Chapter 51). Progressive and ultimately complete destruction of pancreatic B-islet cells occurs in diabetes. Although they are predictively useful, antibodies against insulin and surface cytoplasmic antigens of the B-islet cell are present before clinical onset. The main cytotoxic mechanisms appear to be mediated by T cells and macrophages. This view is supported by the beneficial effects of cyclosporine therapy in patients with early-stage IDDM at levels that have little effect on antibody production. Increased risk is associated with MHC class II types DR3 and DR4.

8. Multiple sclerosis (MS)

    a. Pathogenesis. T cells and macrophages, which are thought to be cytocidal for oligodendrocytes, infiltrate the central nervous system (CNS) and **attack the basic protein of myelin** as an autoantigen. The immunologic component may be secondary to other, unknown initiating agents. **CNS demyelination with sclerotic plaques** leads to spasticity. Increased risk is associated with MHC class II type DR2. Guillain-Barré syndrome is a related condition that involves peripheral nervous system (PNS) demyelination that, unlike MS, can be acute.

   b. **Therapy.** Spasticity is treated with **baclofen** with variable effectiveness. The peripheral skeletal muscle relaxant **dantrolene** is effective in some patients. **Adrenocorticotropic hormone (ACTH),** rather than corticosteroids, is the favored immunosuppressive therapy. Recombinant IFN-β-1b (Betaseron), IFN-β-1a, and glatiramer acetate are approved by the U.S. Food and Drug Administration (FDA) as a treatment for MS.

E. Non-organ-specific autoimmunities. The similarities and differences in this class of disorders are shown by a comparison of Sjögren syndrome and SLE. Rheumatoid arthritis is discussed in Chapter 48.

 1. Sjögren syndrome

   a. **Diagnosis** is usually based on lymphocytic infiltration and the presence of autoantibodies against salivary gland antigens and exocrine glands of the eyes, gastrointestinal and respiratory systems, and vagina. Hypergammaglobulinemia (50%) as a result of hyperactive B cells, antinuclear antibodies (50–65%), and rheumatoid factors (anti-IgG; 75–90%) are present in the indicated percentages of patients.

   b. **Pathogenesis.** Primary symptoms include **inhibition of exocrine gland secretion,** with dryness of the eyes, mouth, and gastrointestinal, respiratory, and vaginal mucous membranes; and pain and edema in the salivary glands. Patients with hypergammaglobulinemia often have type III hypersensitivity reactions (e.g., vasculitis with CNS involvement and kidney disease; see II.D).

   c. **Therapy.** Mild cases are treated with **artificial tears** and frequent drinking of water. For more serious cases (e.g., vasculitis), treatment is similar to that for SLE (**systemic corticosteroids**).

 2. SLE

   a. **Diagnosis** is complicated and depends on the presence of 4 or more of 11 criteria. The most useful criterion is a high concentration of antinuclear antibodies directed against double-stranded DNA and the Smith (Sm) nuclear antigen, both of which are considered specific for SLE. Other diagnostic criteria include the presence of the lupus erythematosus cell (a neutrophil that has phagocytosed nuclei); a discoid erythematous facial rash; photosensitivity; oral ulcers; arthritis; persistent proteinuria; and anticardiolipin, antierythrocyte, or antileukocyte antibodies.

   b. **Pathogenesis** is that of **type III hypersensitivity.** Patients have **hyperactivity of B cells** of unknown origin. This hyperreactivity causes hypergammaglobulinemia, with circulating immune complexes of DNA and other nuclear antigens that precipitate onto vascular basement membranes and activate complement.

      (1) Mild arthritis, fever, rash, and fatigue occur.

      (2) Progressive necrotizing vasculitis with CNS involvement and glomerulonephritis are the most serious consequences, occurring in approximately 50% of patients.

      (3) Hypertension may develop secondary to kidney disease.

      (4) Hemolytic anemia and thrombocytopenia are common.

      (5) Behavioral changes occur in approximately 25% of patients.

      (6) Several drugs (e.g., **procainamide, hydralazine, quinidine, methyldopa, isoniazid, phenytoin, chlorpromazine**) provoke a lupus-like syndrome that usually resolves when the drug is withdrawn. The basis for this syndrome is not understood. No renal disorder occurs in drug-induced SLE.

   c. **Therapy.** Mild disease (e.g., low-grade fever, arthritis) is managed with nonsteroidal anti-inflammatory drugs (NSAIDs). Therapy for patients with severe symptoms is usually oral methylprednisolone. Cyclophosphamide may also be used, and plasmapheresis to remove circulating immune complexes may be helpful.

F. Prospects for more specific immunologic therapies. Current therapies involve approaches that suppress all immune responses; however, current clinical trials seek to suppress only lymphocytes that are activated—for example:

 1. Feeding autoantigens to patients to induce immunologic suppression

 2. Vaccination with autoreactive T cells to induce immunologic suppression

3. Administration of **anti-T$_H$** monoclonal antibodies (particularly anti-CD4) to eliminate autoreactive T cells

4. Administration of **conjugates of IL-2 and toxins** from plants or bacteria to eliminate autoreactive T cells without generalized T cell suppression

IV. **Immunodeficiency** is either primary or secondary. **Primary immunodeficiencies** are either **hereditary** or **congenital,** and at least one element basic to the immune system does not function properly or is absent. **Secondary immunodeficiencies** are the **result of another systemic** disorder or are **iatrogenic in patients given immunosuppressive therapy.** They usually develop in patients who previously showed normal immune function. The expected clinical outcome of an immunodeficiency is governed by the specific portion of the immune system that is affected (e.g., B and T cells, phagocytic cells, and complement).

A. **Primary immunodeficiencies** are, with one exception, rare. Examples are the following:

1. **X-linked agammaglobulinemia** (hypogammaglobulinemia) is an inherited deficiency in antibody production (humoral immunity) in which T cell function is relatively normal, but B cells do not fully mature because of a failure of B cell signaling. Serum immunoglobulin levels are low. Because this disorder is linked to the X chromosome, it occurs primarily in men.
   a. **Pathogenesis** occurs 6–9 months after birth and represents situations in which antibody function is deficient but T-cell function is intact, such as recurrent infections with extracellular pyogenic bacteria (e.g., streptococci, pneumococci, *Haemophilus*). Immunity to fungi and most viruses is generally functional.
   b. **Clinical symptoms** include pneumonia, sinusitis, otitis, meningitis, and septicemia.
   c. **Therapy** is **passive immunization with human intravenous immunoglobulin** (IVIG; see VI.B.1.c).

2. **Common variable immunodeficiency** is an acquired deficiency of B cell maturation to plasma cells. It can occur at any age and in either sex. Symptoms and treatment are similar to those for X-linked agammaglobulinemia; the pathogenesis and origin vary significantly.

3. **Selective IgA deficiency** is the most common primary immunodeficiency, affecting approximately 0.5% of the U.S. population. It appears to be inherited. The low secretory IgA (sIgA) concentration predisposes patients to extracellular bacterial infections of the mucosal surfaces, leading to respiratory, urogenital, and gastrointestinal infections. Some affected individuals are asymptomatic for unknown reasons. Certain autoimmunities may be more prevalent. There is no specific immunologic therapy.

4. **DiGeorge syndrome** results from developmental failure of the thymus and parathyroid glands, accompanied by cardiovascular and other developmental anomalies. Patients have a decrease in total T cell numbers but relatively normal immunoglobulin levels.
   a. **Pathogenesis** in severe cases (i.e., little functional thymic tissue) represents conditions involving T cell deficiency, such as recurrent infections of the skin, lungs, genitourinary tract, and blood with opportunistic pathogens, particularly viruses (e.g., herpes viruses), fungi (e.g., *Candida*), and protozoa (e.g., *Pneumocystis carinii*); increased incidence of certain cancers; graft-versus-host (GVH) disease (see V.C) after transfusion of whole blood; and death in infancy or early childhood.
   b. **Therapy** for severe T cell deficiencies is bone marrow transplantation, although thymus grafts may be attempted in DiGeorge syndrome (see V.C).

5. **Nezelof syndrome** is probably inherited and causes lymphopenia and thymic abnormalities but normal or elevated serum immunoglobulin levels. Gram-negative sepsis may occur in addition to the opportunistic infections associated with T cell deficiency.

6. **Severe combined immunodeficiency disorders (SCIDs)** are a heterogeneous group of inherited disorders with deficiencies in T cells, B cells (variable), and serum immunoglobulin. Infections with opportunistic organisms occur in the first few months postnatally, and survival for longer than 1 year is rare without successful bone marrow transplantation. Three forms involve failure of DNA biosynthesis or repair, and a fourth defect is the result of deficiency of the γ chain of the IL-2 receptor.

7. **Chronic granulomatous disease (CGD)** is a defect in the ability of phagocytes to kill bacteria. The disease is caused by a genetic defect in the production of oxygen radicals that are important for intracellular and extracellular killing of bacteria. The defect can occur in any of the four proteins essential for producing oxygen radicals, but the most common defect is X-linked. CGD is characterized by chronic infection with organisms such as *Staphylococcus aureus* and is usually fatal.

8. **Leukocyte adhesion deficiency (LAD)** is associated with a defect in the phagocytic cells. These cells lack intercellular adhesion molecules, the proteins necessary for binding to the endothelial cells of the blood vessels and other cell membranes. This defect leads to an inability of phagocytic cells to exit the blood and enter the tissues. In addition, the phagocytes have a decreased ability to bind to activated components of complement on a bacterial surface, leading to a decrease in phagocytosis. Patients have severe bacterial infections, especially in the mouth and gastrointestinal tract.

9. **Chédiak–Higashi syndrome** is a deficiency in the fusion of lysosomes with phagocytic vesicles. The cause is unknown, but this syndrome leads to bacterial survival in the phagocyte, with an increase in bacterial infections.

10. **Defects in complement** may be the result of defects in the activation pathways, membrane attack complex, or regulatory proteins. Defects in the activation pathways and in the membrane attack complex are associated with increased infections owing to pyogenic bacteria and with increased rates of immune complex diseases, such as SLE. Defects in regulation can be observed as angioneurotic edema and nocturnal hemoglobinuria.

B. **Secondary immunodeficiencies** involve decreased immunologic responsiveness.

1. **Cytotoxic drugs** prevent the division of responding lymphocytes, suppress the production of blood cells in bone marrow, and may directly kill cells. Patients who receive chemotherapy and exhibit a significant loss of neutrophils may be treated with filgrastim or recombinant granulocyte colony-stimulating factor (G-CSF; Neupogen), to restore the white blood cell count to normal levels. Treatment to increase neutrophil levels in these patients results in decreased morbidity rates from bacterial infection. Corticosteroids broadly suppress immune system cells, including decreased division, cytokine secretion, and chemotaxis (emigration from the blood into tissues).

2. **Leukemias, lymphomas, and myelomas** are associated with decreased immune responsiveness, at least some of which results from destruction of the architecture of lymphoid organs (e.g., spleen, lymph nodes). Malignancy-related immunodeficiency also occurs in other cancers.

3. **Protein–calorie malnutrition** significantly decreases immune competence, particularly in children.

4. **Aging** is associated with decreased immunologic competence.

5. **Acute infections** produce a transient immunodeficiency.

6. **AIDS** is a secondary immunodeficiency that is usually persistent and is an indirect consequence of infection by **HIV-1** or **HIV-2.** HIV-1 is the more common subtype in the United States and western Europe.
   a. **Pathogenesis.** The viral envelope glycoprotein 120 (gp120) has a strong affinity for CD4 (see I.B.3.c), allowing the virus to directly infect T_H cells. In addition, these proteins use one of two chemokine receptors: CCR5 to gain entry to macrophages and dendritic cells and CXCR4 to gain entry into $CD4^+$ T cells. Because it is a retrovirus, viral entry and uncoating release the viral RNA genome and the associated reverse transcriptase enzyme, which synthesizes a double-stranded DNA copy of the genome (provirus). The proviral copy is integrated into the genome of the infected cell, and the virus enters a period of latency, during which it is essentially hidden from the immune system.
      (1) During **initial infection,** there may be an acute illness that lasts an average of 3 weeks and resembles mononucleosis; some individuals have no symptoms.
      (2) **Seroconversion** (i.e., the appearance of antiviral antibodies) occurs 3 weeks to 6 months after the initial exposure to HIV-1. A period of **asymptomatic infection** typically follows seroconversion.

(3) Infected T_H cells are killed when **viral genes are reactivated from latency** and viruses bud from the cell. In addition, infected T_H cells may fuse to form syncytia. This fusion may hasten the spread of virus to uninfected T_H cells and contribute to cell killing. A **progressive depletion of T_H** cells occurs (normal count: 800–1000/mm³). However, even before an obvious loss of $CD4^+$ T cells occurs, there is evidence of a defect in $CD4^+$ T cell function. The functional defect is a failure of these cells to respond to antigens to which they were previously sensitized (e.g., tetanus toxoid). The defect in responsiveness may be a function of the $CD4^+$ T cells, the APCs, or both.

(4) Macrophages may produce new virus without being killed and may spread the virus to uninfected T_H cells and other cell types. $CD4^+$ cell lines that are susceptible to HIV infection include neurons, liver, and fibroblasts. In direct cell-to-cell transfer of the virus, minimal exposure to the extracellular immune system (e.g., antibody) may occur.

(5) **APCs** are also affected by the infection. There is a loss of follicular dendritic cells and interdigitating cells in the lymphoid tissue. This loss leads to decreased antigen presentation to the $CD4^+$ T cells. In addition, the cytokines produced by the APCs may produce $CD4^+$ T cells that increase B cell activation but do not produce the appropriate cytokines for T cell proliferation. This activity changes the T_H cell ratios.

b. Clinical symptoms

(1) **Persistent generalized lymphadenopathy** (extrainguinal) is an indicator of impending progression to full disease. Unexplained fever, night sweats, diarrhea, and other symptoms known as **AIDS-related complex (ARC)** may occur.

(2) Progression to full-blown AIDS may occur 8 years or longer after the initial infection. Depletion of the T_H cell level to < 200/mm³ and oral candidiasis suggest imminent disease. Because $CD8^+$ T cells are not significantly affected, the ratio of circulating $CD4^+$ to $CD8^+$ cells is inverted. In addition, the number of virgin T_H cells relative to memory T_H cells increases. T_H cells are lost, and memory T_H cells are lost in relatively larger numbers. There is also a shift in the type of T_H cell help being generated.

(3) A diagnosis of AIDS involves the occurrence of **opportunistic infections** or **neoplasms as a result of the progressive immunodeficiency** caused by severe depletion of T_H cell (CD4) function. Also included in this diagnosis are the HIV wasting syndrome and encephalopathy.

(a) Opportunistic infections are the major consequence of AIDS, particularly by *P. carinii* (as many as 80% of patients), *Candida albicans, Mycobacterium avium-intracellulare,* herpes simplex virus (HSV), cytomegalovirus (CMV), and others. Tuberculosis occurs as a reactivation of a latent infection in carriers. Cumulatively, **these opportunistic infections are the primary cause of death.**

(b) **Kaposi sarcoma,** an otherwise rare cancer, occurs in fewer than one half of patients with AIDS. Non-Hodgkin lymphoma is also more common in these individuals than in the general population.

(4) **HIV-associated dementia complex (HADC)** affects more than one half of patients with AIDS. In HADC, macrophages infiltrate the brain and are the most productively infected cell in comparison to neurons or glia. Some patients show demyelination.

(5) Other immune system abnormalities include polyclonal B cell activation and hypergammaglobulinemia with a concomitant decreased ability to mount humoral immune responses to specific antigens. Chemotaxis, cytokine secretion, and cytotoxic ability of monocyte–macrophages are all diminished. These problems are consequences of impaired T cell regulation.

c. Therapy

(1) Current therapy includes prophylactic use of antibiotics and antifungal agents. Optimal anti-HIV therapy is combination therapy with three antiretroviral drugs. At present, there are three classes of antiretroviral drugs approved by the FDA. These are nucleoside reverse-transcriptase inhibitors (NRTIs; e.g., zidovudine-AZT, lamivudine, stavudine, zalcitabine-ddC, didanosine-ddI, and abacavir), nonnucleoside reverse-transcriptase inhibitors (NNRTIs; e.g., nevirapine, delavirdine, efavirenz), and protease inhibitors (e.g., saquinavir, indinavir, ritonavir, nelfinavir). IFN-α is recommended for the treatment of Kaposi sarcoma. Other drugs and immunomodulators are currently under development and testing.

(2) An effective active vaccine is necessary to limit the spread of HIV infection. Because of viral antigenic variation, cell-to-cell transmission, and the uncertain role of antibodies in protection, the process of vaccine development is difficult. A live, attenuated vaccine (see VI.C.2) is considered too great a risk. Trials of subunit vaccines are under way.

V. GRAFT REJECTION

A. Overview. Individual differences in the molecular structures of cells and tissues occur, except in identical twins, because of the genetic variation inherent in humans. Because of these molecular differences, transplanted tissues or organs (i.e., grafts) are likely to be antigenically different from the recipient and therefore may stimulate an immune response.

1. Although MHC class I and II glycoproteins play an essential role in all T cell immune responses (see I.B.3.a), these molecules are particularly antigenic and variant in structure among different humans (polymorphic).

2. Each person's set of MHC glycoproteins is called his or her **human leukocyte antigen (HLA),** or **histocompatibility, type.** Class I glycoproteins are known as HLA-A, -B, and -C antigens. Class II glycoproteins are known as HLA-DR, -DP, and -DQ antigens. Each person receives one set of genes (a haplotype) encoding these protein antigens from each parent.

3. Identical twins have the same histocompatibility type. For other siblings, the probability is approximately 25% (0.25) that two siblings with the same parents are HLA identical, or matched, and approximately 50% that they are one half HLA matched, or haploidentical. Parents and children are almost always haploidentical. Some transplanted tissues are rejected because of HLA incompatibility. In other cases, the reason for rejection is the result of minor histocompatibility antigens or is unknown. HLA matching is not always a factor in rejection.

B. Common solid-organ transplants are kidney, heart, liver, heart–lung, and pancreas. Organs are obtained from cadavers or living donors. The probability of an exact HLA match in a cadaver graft is approximately 1 in 10 million.

1. **HLA matching**
   a. The primary problem with organ donation is rejection of the transplanted organ by the host's immune response. Donation of an organ by an HLA-matched sibling is the best way to avoid this problem.
   b. Although HLA-DR and HLA-B matching decreases the rejection reaction in renal and cardiac grafts, rejection does occur in HLA-matched situations. HLA matching is not important in liver transplantation.

2. **Types of rejection of organ grafts**
   a. **Hyperacute rejection** is mediated by preexisting antibody in the recipient, usually against ABO mismatches. Complement is activated, clotting occurs, and the vasculature of the transplanted organ is occluded. Rejection occurs within 2 days after transplantation. An ABO-mismatched graft is rarely attempted. Rejection is essentially untreatable.
   b. **Acute rejection** is a T cell–macrophage-mediated attack on the graft based on HLA and other tissue antigen mismatches. T cells and macrophages infiltrate the graft and, in 10–14 days, cause cellular necrosis and inflammation perivascularly. The entire graft begins to necrose if untreated.
   c. **Chronic rejection** occurs several months to several years after transplantation. It causes fibrosis and occlusion of small arteries and arterioles in the kidneys and atherosclerosis in the heart. It is controlled by immunologic injury and mediated primarily antibody and includes the release of inflammatory cytokines by macrophages. Despite the high success rate of MHC-matched, pharmacologically treated grafts in the first year after transplantation (85–90% kidney grafts), the rejection rate after 5 years is nearly 50%. This form of rejection is relatively resistant to therapy, although treatment with corticosteroids can be helpful.

C. Bone marrow transplantation is sometimes attempted in patients with immunodeficiency diseases, aplastic anemias, some leukemias, and certain genetic diseases. The graft contains a high proportion of donor lymphocytes that respond to the host HLA and other antigens. This response causes graft-versus-host (GVH) disease.

1. Graft T cell recognition of the host is important in GVH disease, as shown by the decreased incidence of GVH disease after procedures that purge mature T cells from the donor marrow.

2. **Clinical symptoms** of GVH disease are seen in the skin (e.g., rash, desquamation), gastrointestinal tract (e.g., pain, vomiting, intestinal bleeding), and liver (e.g., necrosis indicated by increased serum bilirubin levels). Death commonly occurs.

3. HLA matching is important in bone marrow transplantation, but the failure rate even of matched grafts as a result of GVH disease is high.

4. Because the recipient of the marrow (host) is immunosuppressed, owing to primary immunodeficiency or by drugs or radiation, host rejection of transplanted bone marrow is less important.

D. **Prophylaxis and treatment of graft rejection**

1. **Immunosuppression of the graft recipient**
   a. **Corticosteroids** (e.g., methylprednisolone, prednisone) are administered just before transplantation and rapidly tapered because of their side effects. Corticosteroids are used in combination with azathioprine, cyclosporine, or **antilymphocyte globulins/ antithymocyte globulins (ALGs/ATGs).**
   b. **Azathioprine** is given before transplantation. Maintenance doses are given afterward.
   c. **Methotrexate** is used primarily for bone marrow transplantation in combination with ALG/ATG. It is administered either a few days before or at the time of transplantation.

2. **Specific suppression of T cells**
   a. **Cyclosporine A** (cyclosporin) binds to an intracellular protein known as cyclophilin and blocks the transcription of cytokine genes in a T cell that has recognized antigens. In this way, it inhibits T_H cell secretion of IL-2 and production of the high-affinity IL-2 receptor and prevents complete T cell activation. It is administered prophylactically because it is more effective if it is present before rejection begins. Cyclosporine A is commonly combined with other agents. The major side effect is nephrotoxicity.
   b. **Tacrolimus (FK-506)** is an immunosuppressive agent that inhibits T_H cell function in the same way as cyclosporine A. Both drugs function through the same pathway and are not used together.
   c. **Rapamycin** (sirolimus) inhibits T_H cell response to IL-2 and prevents T_H cell activation. It works through a different pathway than either cyclosporine or tacrolimus and is especially effective in combination with the other drugs.
   d. **ALG** and **ATG** are antisera derived from animals. They contain a variety of antibody specificities against T cell antigens. They are used both prophylactically and therapeutically in bone marrow and organ transplantation.
   e. **Muromonab-CD3** (OKT3) is a mouse monoclonal antibody specific for the CD3 antigen, which is present on all peripheral T cells. OKT3 is used therapeutically to halt and reverse acute rejection as soon as it is diagnosed.
      (1) Its main action is the opsonization of T cells for enhanced phagocytosis. It is administered daily for 10–14 days. Only one course is typically used because it causes an immune response against the foreign mouse antibody.
      (2) Acute side effects are common, probably because of nonspecific T cell activation that causes the release of cytokines. Side effects include high fever, chills, blood pressure changes, vomiting, diarrhea, and respiratory distress. OKT3 is contraindicated in patients who have fluid overload because it may cause fatal pulmonary edema.
      (3) OKT3 may also be used in vitro to purge donor bone marrow of T cells to reduce the risk of GVH disease.

3. **Investigational agents** being tested to prevent or reverse graft rejection include anti–T cell immunotoxins (see VII.C.1), conjugates of IL-2 and a toxin, and other monoclonals that prevent T cells from adhering to foreign graft cells. These agents are administered to the graft recipient. In addition, monoclonal antibodies are used to mask HLA antigens on the graft tissue before it is transplanted into the recipient.

VI. VACCINATION

A. Overview

1. **Passive vaccination** is the intramuscular or intravenous injection of antibody preparations to enhance a patient's immune competence. Protection depends on the serum half-life of the injected antibody and is limited to several weeks to several months for each administration of human sera.

2. **Active vaccination** is the intramuscular, subcutaneous, or oral introduction of one or more antigens designed to stimulate the immune system to produce a specific immune response. This response generates antibody, activated T cells, and specific memory. Protection through memory varies with the vaccine, but immunity is long lasting.

B. Passive vaccination (Table 10-2)

1. **Preparations.** Doses of intramuscular preparations are sometimes given in units per kilogram and sometimes in milliliters per kilogram. The dose varies with the vaccine and patient population. Intravenous preparations are commonly used in high doses.

   a. **Standard human serum immunoglobulin for intramuscular vaccination** is a polyclonal antiserum prepared from pooled plasma of donors. It contains 165 mg/mL human immu-

Table 10-2. Passive Vaccines

Illness	Vaccine	Rationale
Intramuscular		
Hepatitis B (HBV)	Hepatitis B immunoglobulin (HBIG)	Prophylaxis
Hepatitis A (HAV)	Immunoglobulin, intramuscular (IGIM)	Prophylaxis
Non-A, non-B hepatitis	IGIM	Prophylaxis, therapy
Measles	IGIM	Prophylaxis, therapy
Rabies	Rabies immunoglobulin (RIG)	Prophylaxis
Rubella	IGIM	Fetal prophylaxis in exposed mother
Varicella	Varicella zoster immunoglobulin (VZIG)	Prophylaxis and therapy in immunocompromised individual
Tetanus	Tetanus immunoglobulin (TIG)	Prophylaxis
Hypogammaglobulinemia	IGIM	Therapy for antibody deficiency
Rh disease	Rho (D) immunoglobulin (RhoGAM)	Prophylaxis during pregnancy and after delivery of Rh$^+$ fetus by Rh$^-$ mother
Botulism	Botulism antiserum (equine)	Prophylaxis, therapy
Snakebite	Polyvalent antivenin (equine)	Prophylaxis, therapy
Black widow bite	Black widow antivenin (equine)	Prophylaxis, therapy
Intravenous[a]		
Hypogammaglobulinemia	Intravenous immunoglobulin (IVIG)	Therapy for antibody deficiency
Idiopathic thrombocytopenic purpura (ITP)	IVIg	Therapy
Chronic lymphocytic leukemia	IVIg	Therapy for antibody deficiency
Cytomegalovirus (CMV) infection	CMV IVIG	Therapy in renal transplant patients
Acute renal rejection	Muromonab-CD3 (murine)	Reversal of acute rejection

[a]U.S. Food and Drug Administration–approved uses; many others currently in trials result from vaccine preparation in cells of nonhuman origin. The valence of a vaccine indicates the number of strains of organism included (e.g., trivalent polio vaccine includes three strains of poliovirus).

noglobulin, predominantly the four subclasses of IgG. Side effects are rare, minimal, and usually confined to minor inflammation and pain at the site of injection. This preparation is unsuitable for intravenous injection because antibody aggregates form and may activate complement and platelets.

b. Special intramuscular immunoglobulins (IGIMs) are individual sera prepared from plasma lots of subjects actively immunized against or recovering from specific diseases. Each serum is enriched for antibodies of the desired specificity (e.g., tetanus immunoglobulin contains more antibodies against tetanus toxin than would be found in IGIM).

c. IVIGs are prepared from pooled human serum and modified to minimize antibody aggregation. Chills, nausea, and abdominal pain occur in approximately 10% of patients. Side effects are diminished by reducing the rate of intravenous infusion. Premedication with corticosteroids is recommended, and intravenous epinephrine is used if anaphylaxis occurs.

d. Animal antisera. Equine (horse) antisera are used in certain situations (Table 10-2). Mouse monoclonal antibody (muromonab-CD3) is used in acute renal rejection (see V.D.2.e). The half-lives of animal antibodies are shorter in humans.

2. Rationales for passive vaccination

a. Prophylaxis of infectious disease. Antibodies are given prophylactically to prevent clinical symptoms of a viral or bacterial infectious process, particularly in a patient without previous exposure and therefore without immunologic memory. The vaccine protects the recipient during the incubation period for infection. For example:

(1) *Clostridium tetani* infection has an incubation period of approximately 5 days before significant quantities of tetanus toxin are produced. A primary immune response of 7–10 days is too slow. Passive vaccination with tetanus immunoglobulin (TIG) binds the toxin and prevents disease.

(2) Hepatitis B immunoglobulin (HBIG) is administered to individuals as soon as possible after exposure to prevent viral infection.

b. Prophylaxis or therapy prevents or attenuates the effects of infection in special populations. Examples are the use of **varicella zoster immunoglobulin (VZIG)** in immunocompromised patients and the use of IGIM in pregnant women who are exposed to rubella and have not been actively vaccinated.

c. Treatment of antibody deficiency. Individuals who are deficient in antibody production, either because of primary immunodeficiency (see IV) or as a result of chronic lymphocytic leukemia, receive intravenous immunoglobulin (IVIG) or IGIM every 2–4 weeks to maintain humoral immunity. IVIG is preferred.

d. Other situations. IVIG is used for idiopathic (autoimmune) thrombocytopenia purpura. Intramuscular $Rh_o(D)$ immunoglobulin (RhoGAM) is used prophylactically for Rh disease (see II.C.5.c). Muromonab-CD3 (see V.D.2.e) is used for acute renal graft rejection.

C. Active vaccination (Table 10-3) is used for prophylaxis.

1. Overview

a. Contents. Active vaccines contain one or more subunits of a pathogen or whole pathogenic organisms but may also contain preservatives, low doses of antibiotics, and other compounds that do not affect the immune response.

b. Administration. Active vaccines are administered subcutaneously, intramuscularly, intradermally, orally, or intranasally. Some are introduced adsorbed to aluminum hydroxide or aluminum phosphate adjuvants. An adjuvant increases the antigenicity of the vaccine.

c. Seroconversion. For most active vaccines, the success of the series of vaccinations is indicated by seroconversion of the patient. Seroconversion indicates that a person who previously did not have specific serum antibodies (i.e., seronegative) now has these antibodies (i.e., seropositive). Seroconversion does not indicate established immunity for certain vaccines (e.g., bacillus Calmette-Guérin vaccine for tuberculosis).

d. A schedule of active vaccination is recommended for infants and children (Table 10-3). The first vaccination is given after the infant is 6 weeks old because responses are normally inadequate in newborns and because maternal antibodies remain in the newborn circulation; some vaccines (e.g., hepatitis B virus; HBV), however, may be given immediately after birth. Some vaccines are intended for use primarily in noninfant populations.

Table 10-3. Commonly Administered U.S. Food and Drug Administration–Approved Active Vaccines

Vaccine	Target Popluation[a]	Number of Vaccinations	Schedule	Notes
Live, attenuated viral				
Oral polio (OPV; trivalent)	Infants, children, healthcare and day-care workers	4	2, 4, 15–18 months; 1 at school entry	Approximately 1 in 2.6 million risk of vaccine-induced paralysis; no longer recommended because of risks; substitute killed vaccine
Measles, mumps, rubella (MMR)	Infants, children	2	15 months (< 12 months if high risk); 1 at school entry	Generally affords lifelong immunity
Rubella	Adolescent girls not previously vaccinated	1	Postpuberty	Protects future fetus from congenital rubella injury
Varicella	Children, other at-risk individuals	1 (if ≥13 years old, 2)	1 between 12 and 18 months or 2–3 years; after 13 years old, 2–4 weeks apart	Duration of immunity or effect on development of shingles unknown
Influenza (trivalent)	Individuals between 5 and 59 years old at risk for infection	1 per year	Annually for maximum protection	Administered intranasally
Bacterial				
BCG tuberculosis	Individuals exposed to sputum-positive tuberculosis patients	Varies	Depends on success or initial vaccination	Unpredictable effectiveness; induces cell-mediated immunity
Killed, inactivated viral or viral subunit				
Influenza (trivalent or polyvalent)	Geriatric patients, healthcare workers, individuals at risk for complications	1 per year	Annually for maximum protection	Variant strains may appear each year; vaccine must be updated annually
Hepatitis B (HBV)	All	3	Between 1 and 2 months, 2 and 3 months, after 6 months	Recombinant, subunit
Inactivated polio (IPV; trivalent)	All children; as booster in healthcare and day-care workers	4	2, 4, 15–18 months; 1 at school entry	No sIgA; thus reduced protection; no paralysis risk

(Continued on next page)

Table 10-3. Continued.

Vaccine	Target Population[a]	Number of Vaccinations	Schedule	Notes
Killed, inactivated viral or viral subunit				
Rabies (HDCV)	Animal-care workers	4 or 5[b], with boosters	7 days apart; boosters as required to maintain immunoglobulin	Two doses to exposed, already immune individual
Bacterial, subunit				
Diphtheria, tetanus, pertussis (DTP)	Infants, children	4, with boosters	2,4, 15–18 months; 1 at school entry	Tetanus toxoid (Td) booster every 10 years or on exposure through a wound
Tetanus and diphtheria toxoids (Td)	Children ≥ 7 years old; adults with no vaccination	3, with boosters	Second dose in 4–8 weeks; third dose 6 months later	Td booster every 10 years or on exposure through a wound if more than 10 years or vaccine history unavailable
Haemophilus b (Hib)	Infants, children, HIV-infected adults	Depends on formulation	Depends on formulation	Polysaccharide capsule is poor antigen; conjugate vaccines enhance potency
Pneumococcus (polyvalent)	At-risk adults or children ≥ 2 years old (e.g., immunocompromised patients, geriatric patients)	1 or 1 per year	As necessary in at-risk patients; not given during active infection; 1 per year in geriatric patients	Poor response to polysaccharide antigen in children < 5 years old
Meningococcus (quadrivalent A, C Y, W-135)	College freshmen living in dormitories; high-risk adults or children ≥ 2 years old, including individuals with complement component deficiencies or anatomic or functional asplenia	1, subcutaneously	As necessary in at-risk individuals at 3- to 5-year intervals	Polysaccharide vaccine give poor response in children < 2 years old; does not protect against serotype B, which accounts for 46% of cases

BCG, bacille Calmette-Guérin; *HDCV*, human diploid cell vaccine; *sIgA*, secretory immunoglobulin A.
[a]Entire target population is not listed in all cases.
[b]Five doses to already exposed individuals.

e. Most vaccines require **a series of vaccinations;** others are effective with a single vaccination. For those that require a series, intervals between vaccinations greater than those recommended do not generally diminish protection. The duration of memory varies with each vaccine, and **booster vaccinations** are often necessary.

f. **Side effects** include inflammation at the site of vaccination, malaise, mild fever, chills, headache, myalgia, and arthralgia. More severe side effects include febrile illness, somnolence, seizures, or anaphylactic hypersensitivity to vaccine antigens or accessory components (e.g., antibiotic, chicken protein). Severe reactions contraindicate continuation of a series. A person with severe febrile illness should not be actively vaccinated until the illness resolves.

2. **Types of active vaccines**

   a. **Live, attenuated vaccines** consist of whole organisms (usually viruses). These organisms multiply after vaccination, but are attenuated to reduce their pathogenicity.

      (1) A small dose produces a strong immune response because the antigen concentration increases when the organism multiplies. Some vaccines elicit lifelong immunity in two doses—for example, the measles, mumps, rubella (MMR) vaccine. Because of their relative genetic instability, viruses can revert to virulence and cause the disease against which the patient is vaccinated. This is a particular problem with one of the serotypes of the oral polio vaccine (OPV).

      (2) Live, attenuated viral vaccines are not recommended for pregnant women or those intending to become pregnant within 3 months of vaccination. Live, attenuated viral or bacterial vaccines are not given to immunocompromised individuals.

   b. **Killed, inactivated vaccines** may contain whole killed cells (e.g., phenol-killed *Bordetella pertussis*) or any antigenic fraction isolated from the organism. They are usually given adsorbed to adjuvant.

   c. Some isolated antigens (**subunit vaccines**) may require inactivation before they are used in a vaccine —for example, formaldehyde-modified toxin of *Clostridium tetani,* known as **tetanus toxoid (Td)** after modification. Inactivation eliminates pathogenicity, but preserves some antigenicity. Other subunit vaccines include proteins and glycoproteins of an organism that are produced by recombinant DNA technology in bacteria, yeast, or mammalian cells and are then used as the antigens for vaccination. The HBV vaccine contains proteins produced by recombinant genetic technologies and is approved by the FDA for use in humans.

      (1) Because no live organisms are present, reversion to pathogenicity is not a problem. However, doses of cells or antigens must be higher than in live, attenuated vaccines, and hypersensitivity reactions to vaccine components are more common. Minimum effective doses are usually measured in numbers of cells or micrograms of antigen.

      (2) Vaccines in which the antigenic fragment is a polysaccharide (e.g., *Haemophilus* b) are usually poor at eliciting immune responses and memory, probably because they do not evoke T cell activation. These vaccines have been improved by conjugating the polysaccharide to another antigenic compound (e.g., Td). These are known as **conjugate vaccines.**

4. **Experimental vaccines** include other subunit vaccines; peptides produced by chemical, cell-free synthesis; recombinant DNA viruses containing genes for the antigens of multiple organisms; and anti-idiotype antibodies used for active vaccination.

5. **Specific vaccines** in common use and recommended administration schedules are listed in Table 10-3.

D. **Simultaneous administration of active and passive vaccines.** Sometimes active and passive vaccines against a pathogenic organism are administered simultaneously to maximize postexposure prophylaxis. The immunoglobulin offers immediate protection, and the active vaccine stimulates an immune response. These vaccines are given at separate sites to prevent antibody (passive) and antigen (active) from reacting and inactivating one another.

1. Infants with **HBV** who are born to mothers who have the hepatitis B surface antigen (HBsAg) are significantly protected from becoming chronic carriers by this combined prophylaxis.

2. **Rabies.** Postexposure prophylaxis typically includes the combined use of active and passive vaccines because of the lethal nature of the unchecked infection. The exception is patients with a previous active vaccination who have sufficient existing serum antibody concentration.

3. Tetanus. Combined prophylaxis is sometimes used, depending on the type of wound and the patient's history of active vaccination. Recommended guidelines are as follows:

   a. A tetanus-prone wound is one that produces anaerobic conditions (e.g., deep puncture) or one in which exposure to *Clostridium* or its spores is probable (e.g., contaminated with animal feces). If the patient's history of active vaccination is uncertain or includes fewer than three doses, both TIG and Td are administered. The patient returns to complete the toxoid series.

     (1) If the wound is tetanus-prone but the patient received a full series of active vaccination, no treatment is necessary if the last Td dose was received within the last 5 years.

     (2) If the last dose was received more than 10 years ago, Td, but not TIG, is given to boost memory immunity and antibody production.

   b. For a **clean, minor wound,** if the patient's history of active vaccination is uncertain or includes fewer than three doses, Td is administered.

     (1) If the patient received a full series of active vaccinations, no treatment is necessary if the last Td dose was received within 10 years.

     (2) If the last dose was received more than 10 years ago, Td, but not TIG, is given to boost memory immunity and antibody production.

VII. PROSPECTS FOR IMMUNOMODULATION

A. Fab antidigoxin antibody preparations obtained from sheep are approved for the reversal of toxicity associated with toxic digoxin serum levels. The antibody binds digoxin and prevents it from binding to its normal receptor site. The Fab–digoxin complex is excreted renally.

B. Monoclonal antibodies are generally produced through the in vitro fusion of a cancerous plasma cell (myeloma) with an activated mouse B cell. The resulting **hybridoma** secretes murine (mouse) antibodies of a single defined specificity and has the immortality characteristic of the myeloma. Techniques for the production of human monoclonal antibodies and a variety of hybrid mouse–human monoclonal antibodies are also available.

   1. Monoclonal antibodies—for example, whole antibodies or Fab or $F(ab')_2$ fragments—are routinely used for in vitro diagnostic tests (e.g., blood group and tissue typing for HLA), screening for cancer-related antigens (e.g., carcinoembryonic antigen; CEA), urine testing for drugs and metabolites, and testing for HIV infection. In these and many other diagnostic applications, monoclonal antibodies are often conjugated to enzymes, radioisotopes, or fluorescent dyes.

   2. Muromonab-CD3 is used to treat acute graft rejection. Other monoclonal antibodies are used for treatment of breast cancer and leukemia.

   3. In clinical trials, the use of **monoclonal antibodies against T cells** causes improvement in certain autoimmune disorders.

   4. Monoclonal antibodies against neoplastic cells show some success, and are useful in treating certain leukemias and lymphomas, as well as breast and colon cancers.

C. Monoclonal antibodies are conjugated to enzymes, drugs, prodrugs, radioisotopes, or plant and bacterial toxins to provide specific delivery of the conjugated agent to one or more focused in vivo sites of action. Several problems are associated with the use of these agents.

   1. Immunotoxins are usually produced by the conjugation of a monoclonal antibody to a biologic polypeptide toxin (e.g., diphtheria toxin) that is modified to reduce nonspecific toxicity.

   2. Although they are being tested for graft rejection and autoimmunity, immunotoxins are primarily used as antineoplastic agents. Clinical trials show moderate success in treating leukemia and lymphoma, with lower success rates against tumors such as breast carcinoma.

   3. Monoclonal antibodies conjugated to radioisotopes (e.g., ^{90}Y) cause remissions in patients with Hodgkin disease and acute T cell leukemia.

   4. Monoclonal antibodies conjugated to enzymes that activate a prodrug to the active drug at a specific tissue site (e.g., neoplastic cell surface) are in human trials.

D. **Immunostimulation** has been attempted with a variety of compounds, ranging from cytokines to bacterial products (Table 10-1).

1. IFN-α has many subtypes. Two are currently FDA approved. Because it inhibits cell growth, it is used to treat hairy cell leukemia, Kaposi sarcoma in patients with AIDS, and genital warts. At low doses, interferons stimulate immune cellular function (e.g., T cells, NK cells, macrophages), but at high doses, they are immunosuppressive. The use of IFN-α against other cancers produces variable results.

2. IFN-γ provides greater immunostimulation in the intact immune system, but its effects depend on dose and timing. The combined use of IFN-α and IFN-γ yields better results. The most common side effects of interferon therapy are influenza-like symptoms. IFN-γ is approved for use as a macrophage-activating factor in chronic granulomatous disease.

3. Several protocols using **IL-2** show promising results, with apparently complete remissions in some patients with melanoma. With this technique, known as adoptive immunotherapy, a patient's peripheral blood lymphocytes, or tumor-infiltrating lymphocytes, are removed. They are cultured with IL-2 and reinfused with additional IL-2. These IL-2–responsive cells are likely T cells and NK cells. Severe capillary leakage syndrome, occasionally leading to death, is a problematic side effect.

4. **Hormones of the thymus** that induce T cell maturation and other functions are used to increase certain cell-mediated immune functions, with variable results.

5. Sulfur-containing compounds, such as **levamisole** (a phenylimidothiazole anthelmintic) and diethyldithiocarbamate (**Imuthiol**), have immunostimulatory activity. Their effect is greater on cell-mediated immunity than on humoral immunity. Levamisole is approved as an oral agent for use in colon cancer in combination with fluorouracil.

6. **Inosine pranobex** is licensed for use in many countries as an immunostimulant. It induces T cell differentiation and augments cell-mediated immune functions, with minimal toxicity.

7. As a component of mycobacterial cell walls, **muramyl dipeptide (MDP)** stimulates macrophage activation and may be used as an adjuvant, given with antigen (see I), or given alone as an immunostimulant.

STUDY QUESTIONS

Directions: Each of the question, statement, or items or incomplete statement in this section can be correctly answered or completed by **one** of the suggested answers or phrases. Choose the **best** answer.

1. A man has symptoms of a viral infection of about 4 days' duration. To confirm the diagnosis, the physician draws a blood sample and requests the antibody titer (level) for the suspected agent. The first blood sample shows a low titer of antibody. A week later, another blood sample is drawn, and the titer against the virus is much higher. This situation is an example of

(A) an inflammatory response to the viral infection.
(B) a primary immune response to the viral infection.
(C) a secondary immune response to the viral infection.
(D) a cellular response to the viral infection.

2. Which class of antibody has the longest serum half-life and opsonizes antigens for phagocytosis through two different pathways?

(A) Immunoglobulin G (IgG)
(B) Immunoglobulin M (IgM)
(C) Immunoglobulin A (IgA)
(D) Immunoglobulin E (IgE)

3. Urticaria that appears rapidly after the ingestion of food usually indicates which type of hypersensitivity reaction?

(A) Type I
(B) Type II
(C) Type III
(D) Type IV

4. In which autoimmune disorder is the mechanism of pathogenesis classified as type II hypersensitivity?

(A) Systemic lupus erythematosus (SLE)
(B) Insulin-dependent diabetes mellitus (IDDM)
(C) Graves disease
(D) Hashimoto thyroiditis

5. A patient receives long-term, high-dose therapy with a sulfonamide. After approximately 3 weeks of therapy, the patient has a low-grade fever, rash, and muscle and joint pain. Which type of hypersensitivity accounts for these symptoms?

(A) Type I
(B) Type II
(C) Type III
(D) Type IV

6. In which type IV hypersensitivity reaction is the tissue-damaging disorder considered an inappropriate response by the immune system?

(A) Poison ivy dermatitis
(B) Chronic tuberculosis
(C) Acute graft rejection
(D) Tuberculin test

7. Which agent is commonly used to treat multiple sclerosis (MS)?

(A) Neostigmine
(B) Cyanocobalamin
(C) IFN-β-1b
(D) Propylthiouracil

8. The therapeutic role of muromonab-CD3 in acute renal graft rejection is probably based on

(A) activation of T cell function and secretion of cytokines.
(B) destruction of T cells by complement.
(C) opsonization of T cells for phagocytosis.
(D) selective inhibition of T_H cell function.

9. Which is a current clinical application of intravenous human immunoglobulin (IVIG)?

(A) Prophylaxis after hepatitis B virus (HBV) exposure
(B) Treatment of humoral immunodeficiency
(C) Prophylactic infant immunization for polio
(D) Prophylaxis for Rh disease by infant immunization

10. Which cytokine is approved for the treatment of certain forms of cancer?

(A) Interleukin 2 (IL-2)
(B) Interferon α (IFN-α)
(C) Interferon δ (IFN-δ)
(D) Imuthiol

For questions 11 and 12: A 6-year-old child has a deep puncture wound. The parent is unsure of the child's history of vaccination.

11. If no other information is available, what should the physician recommend?

(A) No vaccination
(B) Tetanus immunoglobulin (TIG)
(C) Tetanus toxoid (Td)
(D) Both TIG and Td at separate sites

12. If the child received a full series of diphtheria, pertussis, tetanus (DPT) vaccinations, the last at entry into school, what should the physician recommend?

(A) No vaccination
(B) Tetanus immunoglobulin (TIG)
(C) Tetanus toxoid (Td)
(D) Both TIG and Td at separate sites

13. Persistent infections by opportunistic pathogens, such as *Candida albicans* and *Pneumocystis carinii,* could indicate all of the following *except*

(A) inherited T cell immunodeficiency.
(B) humoral immunodeficiency.
(C) AIDS.
(D) combined immunodeficiency.

14. Which statement about HIV infection is *not* correct?

(A) Individuals who become infected with HIV-1 always show overt symptoms shortly after infection.
(B) Seroconversion to positive status for anti-HIV-1 antibodies is the primary criterion for diagnosis of a viral carrier.
(C) The incubation period for the pathogenesis of AIDS is believed to be 8 years or longer after the initial infection with HIV.
(D) CD4$^+$ T cells and macrophages may be able to spread HIV to uninfected CD4$^+$ cells without releasing any extracellular virus particles.

Directions: The questions and incomplete statements in this section can be correctly answered or completed by **one or more** of the suggested answers. Choose the answer, A–E.

> **A** if **I only** is correct
> **B** if **III only** is correct
> **C** if **I and II** are correct
> **D** if **II and III** are correct
> **E** if **I, II, and III** are correct

15. Which statements about the currently approved sheep Fab fragment used to counteract digoxin overdose are true?

I. It is obtained by the immunization of sheep with a digoxin–protein conjugate and subsequent proteolytic cleavage of the collected antibody.
II. It specifically binds digoxin, preventing its activity.
III. It has a serum half-life of approximately 3 weeks.

16. CD4$^+$ T cells specifically recognize antigens in which form?

I. Bound to major histocompatibility (MHC) class I molecules on the surface of any body cell
II. In free, soluble form in extracellular fluids
III. Bound to MHC class II molecules on the surface of special antigen-presenting cells (APCs)

17. What is a normal outcome of the activation of the complement system by either the classic or alternative pathway?

I. Acute inflammation
II. Opsonization of immune complexes
III. Cytolytic action

18. In antiviral immunity, what directly recognizes and kills viral-infected cells?

I. Cytotoxic T cells (CTLs)
II. Antiviral antibodies
III. Interferons

19. A patient is treated with penicillin and produces antibodies against the drug. They are still mostly present. An emergency situation requires administration of an intravenous dose of penicillin. If the patient has a type I penicillin hypersensitivity reaction, which pathologic consequence would be expected, and within what time course of clinical onset?

   I. Hemolytic anemia, with an onset of 1–2 hr after the intravenous dose
   II. Anaphylaxis, with an onset of a few minutes after the intravenous dose
   III. Cutaneous urticaria and pruritus, with an onset of a few minutes after the intravenous dose

20. Which situation occurs in all type IV hypersensitivity reactions?

   I. Infiltration of the affected tissue by mononuclear cells
   II. A delay of 12 hr or longer in the onset of clinical symptoms after allergen contact
   III. Significant beneficial effect of the administration of H_1-antagonists

21. Which immunologic finding is *not* unique to systemic lupus erythematosus (SLE)?

   I. Hypergammaglobulinemia
   II. The presence of circulating antinuclear antibodies
   III. The presence of circulating rheumatoid factors

22. An organ donor who is human leukocyte antigen (HLA) matched with the recipient of a graft is sought. Which individual is at least somewhat likely to provide a total HLA match?

   I. A sibling of the graft recipient
   II. A parent of the graft recipient
   III. A cadaver

23. Graft-versus-host (GVH) disease is associated primarily with which type of transplantation?

   I. Kidney
   II. Heart
   III. Bone marrow

24. The prophylactic use of cyclosporine in graft rejection is probably based on its ability to

   I. inhibit synthesis of antibodies, thereby preventing hyperacute rejection.
   II. inhibit activation of T cells, thereby preventing acute rejection.
   III. block transcription of the interleukin 2 (IL-2) gene and synthesis or secretion of IL-2.

25. Which is a valid comparison of live, attenuated and killed, inactivated active vaccines?

   I. Replication of the organisms in a live, attenuated vaccine increases the stimulation of the immune system and a lower dose is often required.
   II. Attenuated vaccines often require multiple doses.
   III. A killed, inactivated vaccine probably produces lifelong immunity in one or two doses.

26. Which active vaccine is recommended for healthcare workers but is not routinely given to infants?

   I. Measles, mumps, rubella (MMR) vaccine
   II. Influenza polyvalent
   III. Tetanus toxoid (Td)

27. Which statement about pneumococcus and meningococcus vaccines is true?

   I. They are composed of purified polysaccharides.
   II. They are recommended for children < 2 years of age.
   III. The vaccines protect against all serotypes of disease causing pneumococcus or meningococcus.

ANSWERS AND EXPLANATIONS

1. The answer is B *[see 1.C.2–3].*
A primary immune response to an infection is characterized by the initial production of IgM, beginning about 4 days after antigen is encountered. A switch to a different immunoglobulin isotype (i.e., IgG, IgE, or IgA) occurs before the peak of antibody production is reached. The peak primary immune response occurs 10–14 days after the antigen is encountered, and the serum contains both IgM and IgG.

2. The answer is A *[see I.D.2.b; I.E].*
IgG has a serum half-life of 25–35 days, longer than that of any other class, although mast cell–bound IgE has the longest half-life. In general, immune complexes containing IgG are opsonized for phagocytosis through binding to the IgG receptors on neutrophils and macrophages and additionally through the activation of complement. IgM also opsonizes, but only through the activation of complement.

3. The answer is A *[see II.A.5.a–b].*
Food allergies are usually type I reactions. In a patient with preexisting hypersecreted IgE specific to a food allergen and bound to mast cells, the allergic response usually occurs shortly after ingestion. Mast cell secretions lead to vomiting. Systemic spillover of allergen into the circulation may lead to milder effects in other tissues (e.g., urticaria).

4. The answer is D *[see II.C.1–2.c; III.D.2.b].*
Antithyroid peroxidase antibodies produce complement-mediated cytotoxicity to thyroid follicle cells (a type II pathogenic mechanism). In SLE, persistent circulating immune complexes are responsible for much of the pathogenesis (type III). In Graves disease, an antibody acting as a TSH agonist hyperstimulates the thyroid. In IDDM, T cell cytotoxicity to beta islet cells is probably responsible for the major pathogenesis (type IV).

5. The answer is C *[see II.D.2.c; II.D.4.a–b; II.D.5.a].*
One of the most common causes of type III hypersensitivity is the response to drugs. This type of reaction is often seen after long-term, high-dose therapy. The treatment of choice is to discontinue treatment and substitute an unrelated drug.

6. The answer is A *[see II.E.1].*
Poison ivy contains a hapten, pentadecyl catechol, which is not known to be toxic. Therefore, its capacity to elicit an immune response is inappropriate because it serves no useful function. In chronic tuberculosis, the immune response is attempting, although unsuccessfully, to eliminate the mycobacterial pathogen. Acute graft rejection is also appropriate, but unfortunate, because it is a response against foreign tissue. A tuberculin test is an appropriate manifestation of the existence of active immunity or memory to *Mycobacterium.*

7. The answer is C *[see III.D.8.b].*
Treatment with IFN-β-1b lowers the frequency of attacks by 33–50% at 2 years in MS patients. Neostigmine is used as an anticholinergic agent in myasthenia gravis. Cyanocobalamin is administered in autoimmune pernicious anemia to replace nonabsorbed vitamin B_{12}. Propylthiouracil is used as an antithyroid in Graves disease.

8. The answer is C *[see V.D.2.e].*
Muromonab-CD3 is a mouse anti-CD3 monoclonal antibody that binds to all T cells because CD3 is a constant part of the antigen receptor of each T cell. The binding of muromonab-CD3 opsonizes the T cells for phagocytosis. Therefore, the total number of T cells is reduced. Mouse antibodies are inefficient at activating human complement. Some T cell activation with cytokine secretion occurs, but it is an undesirable side effect of muromonab-CD3 administration.

9. The answer is B *[see VI.B.1.c; Table 10-2].*
IVIGs are used to replace antibody in immunodeficient individuals. Hepatitis B immunoglobulin (HBIG) is administered intramuscularly. Anti-Rh antibody is also administered intramuscularly to the mother immediately postpartum (sometimes during pregnancy), but not to the infant. Prophylactic infant immunization for polio is provided through active, not passive, vaccination.

10. The answer is B *[see VII.D].*
IFN-α is approved for use in patients with hairy cell leukemia and in patients with AIDS and Kaposi sarcoma. Some of its beneficial effects probably derive from its ability to inhibit growth. The other cytokines are in various stages of clinical trials as antineoplastic therapies, although IFN-γ is approved for use in patients with chronic granulomatous disease. Imuthiol is not a cytokine but a synthetic drug.

11. The answer is D *[see VI.D.3.a; Table 10-3].*

12. The answer is A *[see VI.D.3.a; Table 10-3].*
A patient with an uncertain history of vaccination and a tetanus-prone wound requires both active and passive vaccination. TIG provides immediate protection if the individual does not have memory. Td begins the series that leads to the establishment of memory. A tetanus-prone wound in an individual with a full series of active vaccinations requires no treatment if the last vaccination in the series was administered less than 5 years earlier. These recommendations are general guidelines.

13. The answer is B *[see IV.A; IV.B.6].*
Opportunistic infections by fungi, viruses, and parasites other than extracellular pyogenic bacteria suggest a deficiency of T cell function. Inherited T cell immunodeficiency and AIDS are inherited and acquired T cell deficiencies, respectively. Combined immunodeficiency includes both humoral and T cell deficiency. Only humoral immunodeficiency is a primarily humoral deficiency in which the expected signs are recurrent infections by extracellular pyogenic bacteria.

14. The answer is A *[see IV.B.6.a.(1)].*
It is not known what percentage of individuals shows overt symptoms after initial infection. Those who do, however, generally show mononucleosis-like symptoms for approximately 3 weeks. Some individuals display no overt symptoms.

15. The answer is C (I, II) *[see I.A.4; I.D.2; I.D.5; VII.A].*
Digoxin is a hapten, a molecule that is too small to stimulate responses (be an immunogen) in its free form, but can be recognized by antibodies. To obtain sheep antidigoxin antibodies, the sheep is immunized with digoxin that has been coupled to a larger molecule, in this case, a protein. The antibodies obtained from the sheep are cleaved with proteolytic enzymes to yield the Fab fragment. This fragment is specific to and can bind digoxin, blocking its biologic activity. Animal antibodies have a shorter serum half-life when injected into humans, and all Fab fragments, even human, have a short half-life compared to complete antibody molecules. Only complete human IgG has a half-life of approximately 1 month.

16. The answer is B (III) *[see I.B.3; I.B.5].*
CD4$^+$, or helper, T cells have receptors that recognize fragments (epitopes) of immunizing antigens (immunogens) only when the fragments are bound to an MHC class II molecule on the surface of APCs. As a result, T cells cannot be activated inappropriately by soluble antigens. CD8$^+$ T cells recognize fragments bound to MHC class I molecules.

17. The answer is E (I, II, III) *[see I.E.2].*
When complement is activated, different proteins of the complement sequence have functions that lead to all three actions. Acute inflammation allows greater movement of plasma proteins and phagocytes from blood to tissue. Opsonization of immune complexes enhances their phagocytosis. Cytolysis of microorganisms often results in their killing.

18. The answer is A (I) *[see I.F.2].*
Antiviral antibodies are probably most important in extracellular immunity to viruses, binding virus particles for opsonization and preventing additional infection of cells. Interferons are secreted from viral-infected and other cells (e.g., macrophages, T cells) and, after binding to receptors, induce the appearance of antiviral proteins in other cells. CTLs recognize viral-infected cells and cause direct cytotoxicity.

19. The answer is D (II, III) *[see II.A.2.d; II.A.6–7; II.C.1.b; II.C.5].*
If the patient produced antibodies that are still present and the hypersensitivity reaction is type I, these antibodies are IgE, mostly bound to mast cell and basophil IgE receptors. Their half-life is several months to years. Intravenous introduction of penicillin causes rapid activation of and secretion by blood basophils. Symptoms of type I hypersensitivity occur within minutes. These symptoms may be severe (anaphylaxis) or less severe (cutaneous, gastrointestinal, or respiratory), depending on the individual. Hemolytic anemia is an expected result of a type II hypersensitivity reaction to penicillin, based on the presence of IgM or IgG antibodies in the serum. The onset is delayed by a few hours in a patient with preexisting antibodies.

20. The answer is C (I, II) *[see II.E.3–6].*
Type IV hypersensitivity reactions are delayed after the introduction of allergen because allergen-specific T cells become activated and attract other cells, such as macrophages, to the site of allergen introduction (e.g., the epidermis of the skin in contact sensitivity, the lungs in tuberculosis). These sites are infiltrated by mononuclear cells. Inflammation is primarily caused by tissue disruption and necrosis as well as by secretion of cytokines by the infiltrating cells. Although histamine secretion can also occur from local mast cells, H_1-antagonists of histamine usually do not have significant effects because T cell and macrophage activation, migration, and secretion are not greatly affected by these drugs.

21. The answer is E (I, II, III) *[see III.C.3.b].*
All three findings are common to more than one non-organ-specific autoimmune disorder, but they occur in different percentages of patients with specific disorders. For example, antinuclear antibodies are probably present in all patients with SLE but are found in only a fraction of patients with rheumatoid arthritis and Sjögren syndrome. Rheumatoid factors are more common in rheumatoid arthritis than in SLE or Sjögren syndrome, and hypergammaglobulinemia is more prevalent in SLE than in Sjögren syndrome.

22. The answer is A (I) *[see V.A.3; V.B].*
Parents and children are rarely HLA matched but are usually half matched. An HLA match from a cadaver-derived organ is unlikely. The probability that two siblings are HLA matched is 25%; the probability that they are half matched is 50%.

23. The answer is B (III) *[see V.C.1].*
In bone marrow transplantation, marrow containing competent lymphocytes is transplanted to a generally immunosuppressed host. The greatest problem is an immune response by the graft against HLAs and other tissue antigens of the host. In renal and cardiac transplantation, the greatest problem is rejection of the foreign organ by the immune system of the host (HVG disease).

24. The answer is D (II, III) *[see V.B.2; V.D.2.a].*
Cell-mediated immune mechanisms are thought to be more important in acute graft rejection, and the inhibition of T cell activation appears to be the key element in immunosuppression. Responding T cells require signaling from IL-2 to reach full activation and progress to cell division. IL-2 is produced by activated T cells and can act in an autocrine manner. Cyclosporine blocks transcription of the IL-2 gene during T cell activation, inhibits the synthesis of IL-2, and prevents full T cell activation and division. Its effects are limited to activated T cells. Because it has no direct effect on antibody synthesis, it is not useful in the hyperacute rejection phenomena that are based on antibody-mediated mechanisms. Hyperacute rejection is essentially untreatable because it depends on the presence of antibodies in the graft recipient.

25. The answer is A (I) *[see VI.C.2.a–b].*
Live, attenuated vaccines introduce organisms that are competent to replicate. This replication stimulates the immune response. For this and probably other reasons, a live, attenuated vaccine (but not a killed, inactivated vaccine) probably provides lifelong immunity in one or two doses.

26. The answer is D (II, III) *[see VI.C.1.d; Table 10-3].*
The MMR vaccine is administered to infants within or shortly after the 1st year of life. A second dose is recommended at school entry. Influenza active vaccine is targeted toward specific adult populations. Healthcare workers are included in this target population, as are infants and children at risk; however, the vaccine is not routinely administered to infants. Td is not routinely administered to infants, who instead receive DTP. Td is used primarily for initial vaccinations in adults who were not previously vaccinated and for 10-year booster vaccinations in all individuals, including healthcare workers.

27. The answer is A (I) *[see VI.C.2; Table 10-3]*.
The pneumococcal and meningococcal vaccines are multivalent and contain purified polysaccharide from a number of different serotypes. However, these vaccines do not contain polysaccharide from all the relevant infectious agents. Purified polysaccharides do not stimulate immune responses in children younger than 2 years of age. For polysaccharide vaccines to be effective in young children, the polysaccharide must be conjugated to a protein as in the Hib vaccine.

11
Biotechnology Drug Products

Godwin W. Fong

Charles Lee

I. INTRODUCTION. Advances in biotechnology have made many formerly unstable or difficult-to-produce biologic products available for therapeutic use. Some life-threatening diseases are now treated with biotechnology products.

   A. Interferon (INF) is an example of a drug that was genetically engineered to inhibit certain types of cancer cells and some viruses.

   B. Cellular hormones known as **interleukins,** lymphotoxins, and tumor necrosis factor are now used to treat cancer and immunodeficiency diseases.

   C. Monoclonal antibodies (MAbs) can deliver toxins specifically to cancer cells and destroy them. MAbs are also used with radioisotopes to diagnose and visualize cancer cells. Monoclonal antibodies have been developed to target signaling pathways associated with immune response and are being used to treat various immunological disorders, such as rheumatoid arthritis, inflammatory bowel disease, psoriasis, and moderate to severe asthma.

   D. Many biopharmaceutical products derived from the body tissues (through cell lines) are now produced on a large scale. Modified natural products also may be further improved.

   E. A synthetic analogue of thyrotropin-releasing hormone prevents paralysis after spinal cord injuries in animal studies.

   F. Superoxide dismutase may be useful in preventing damage to tissues that are deprived of oxygen.

   G. New biotechnologic treatments have been developed for emphysema, congestive heart failure, ulcers, atherosclerosis, and an increasing number of medical conditions. Table 11-1 lists the biotechnology products that are approved for human use.

II. BASIC TERMINOLOGY

   A. An **antigen** is a substance that stimulates the production of antibodies.

   B. An **antibody** is an immunoglobulin produced by the body in response to stimulation from an antigen.

   C. Antisense DNA is a complementary strand of DNA that is specifically synthesized to attach to the sense DNA and prevent genetic transcription. The sense DNA that carries the information that affects the disease process is usually elucidated before an antisense drug is designed.

   D. Colony-stimulating factors (CSFs) are a class of glycoprotein hormones. CSFs regulate the differentiation and formation of blood cells from precursor cells.

   E. Cytokines are a group of special proteins (nonantibodies) released by cells to trigger action in other cells.

   F. DNA is the molecule that contains the genetic instructions of a cell. DNA consists of deoxyribose, phosphate, and repeating bases as building blocks. The four bases are adenine, guanine, thymine, and cytosine.

227

Table 11-1. Approved Recombinant Therapeutics and Vaccines

Drug (Trade Name)	Indication(s)	Company; Year Introduced
Human insulin (Humulin)	Diabetes	Eli Lilly, Genentech; 1982
Somatrem for injection (Protropin)	Human growth hormone deficiency in children	Genentech; 1985
Interferon α-2a (Roferon-A)	Hairy cell leukemia	Hoffmann-La Roche; 1986
Interferon α-2b (Intron A)	Hairy cell leukemia	Schering-Plough, Biogen; 1986
	Extension of therapy for chronic hepatitis C from 6 months to 18–24 months	1997
	Follicular lymphoma in conjunction with chemotherapy	1997
Hepatitis B vaccine recombinant (Recombivax HB)	Prevention of hepatitis B	Merck, Chiron; 1986
Muromonab-CD3 (Orthoclone OKT3)	Reversal of acute kidney transplant rejection	Ortho Biotech; 1986
Somatropin for injection (Humatrope)	Human growth hormone deficiency in children	Eli Lilly; 1987
Alteplase (Activase)	Acute myocardial infarction	Genentech; 1987
	Acute pulmonary embolism	1990
	Restoration of function to central venous access devices (as assessed by the ability to withdraw blood)	2001
Interferon α-2a (Roferon-A)	AIDS-related Kaposi sarcoma	Hoffmann-La Roche; 1988
Interferon α-2b (Intron A)	AIDS-related Kaposi sarcoma	Schering-Plough, Biogen; 1988
	Genital warts	1991
	Hepatitis C	
Interferon n3 (Alferon N injection)	Genital warts	Interferon Sciences; 1989
Hepatitis B vaccine (Engerix-B)	Hepatitis B prevention	SmithKline Beecham, Biogen; 1989
	Chronic hepatitis C infection	1998
Erythropoietin (Epogen)	Anemia associated with chronic renal failure	Amgen, Johnson & Johnson, Kirin; 1989
Erythropoietin (Procrit)	Anemia associated with AIDS or zidovudine administration	Amgen, Ortho Biotech; 1990
	Anemia associated with chronic renal failure	1990
	Chemotherapy-associated anemia in patients with nonmyloid malignancy	1993
	Anemia associated with cancer and chemotherapy	
PEG-adenosine (ADAGEN)	ADA-deficient severe combined immunodeficiency	Enzon, Eastman Kodak; 1990
Interferon γ-1b (Actimmune)	Management of chronic granulomatous disease	Genentech; 1990
	Delaying time to disease progression in patients with severe, malignant osteopetrosis	InterMune Pharmaceuticals (2000)
CMV immunoglobulin (CytoGam)	Prevention of CMV in kidney transplant recipients	Medimmune; 1990
Filgrastim; G-CSF	Chemotherapy-induced neutropenia	Amgen; 1991
	Acute myeloid leukemia	1998

Product	Indication	Manufacturer; Year
Glucocerebrosidase (Ceredase)	Type I Gaucher disease[a]	Genzyme; 1991
Glucocerebrosidase (Cerezyme)	Type I Gaucher disease[a]	Genzyme; 1994
Sargramostim (GM-CSF) (Prokine)	Autologous bone marrow transplantation	Hoechst-Roussel, Immunex; 1991
Sargramostim (GM-CSF) (Leukine)	Neutrophil recovery after bone marrow transplantation	Immunex, Hoechst-Roussel; 1991
Antihemophilic factor (Mononine)	Hemophilia B	Armour; 1992
Antihemophilic factor (Recombinate)	Hemophilia A	Genetics Institute, Baxter Healthcare; 1992
Interleukin 2 (Proleukin)	Renal cell carcinoma	Chiron; 1992
	Metastatic melanoma	1998
111Indium-labeled antibody (OncoScint CR103)	Detection, staging, and follow-up of colorectal cancer	Cytogen, Knoll; 1992
111Indium-labeled antibody (OncoScint OV103)	Detection, staging, and follow-up of ovarian cancer	1992
Interferon β-1b (Betaseron)	Relapsing/remitting multiple sclerosis	Chiron, Berlex; 1993
DNase alfa (Pulmozyme)	Cystic fibrosis	Genentech; 1993
Factor VIII (Kogenate)	Hemophilia A	Genentech, Miles; 1993
Filgrastim (G-CSF) (Neupogen)	Bone marrow transplant	Amgen; 1994
PEG-i-asparaginase (Oncaspar)	Refractory childhood acute lymphoblastic leukemia	Enzon; 1994
Human growth hormone (Nutropin)	Short stature caused by human growth hormone deficiency	Genentech; 1994
Abciximab (ReoPro)	Antiplatelet prevention of blood clots	Centocor; 1994
	Treatment of a broader range of patients undergoing percutaneous coronary intervention; revised dosage and patient management to reduce bleeding	
	Unstable angina that does not respond to conventional medical therapy when percutaneous coronary intervention is planned within 24 hr	
Live varicella virus vaccine (Varivax)	Active immunization of persons 12 months of age and older	Merck; 1995
RSV immunoglobulin (RespiGam)	Prevention of serious lower respiratory tract infection in children younger than 24 months old	Massachusetts Public Health Biologic Labs; 1996
Inactivated hepatitis A vaccine (Vaqta)	Immunization against hepatitis A in children older than 6 years of age	Merck; 1996
Interferon β-1a (Avonex)	Multiple sclerosis	Biogen; 1996
Human antihemophilic factor	Hemophilia A	Centeon; 1996
Haemophilus b conjugate (meningococcal protein conjugate) and hepatitis B (recombinant vaccine) (Comvax)	Immunization of individuals 6 weeks to 15 months of age born of HBsAg-negative mothers	Merck; 1996
Cryoprecipitated antihemophilic factor A	Control of bleeding associated with Factor VIII deficiency	Blood Bank of the Redwoods; 1996
Reteplase (Retavase)	Acute myocardial infarction in adults	Boehringer Mannheim; 1996

(Continued on next page)

Table 11-1. Continued.

Drug (Trade Name)	Indication(s)	Company; Year Introduced
DTaP vaccine (Infanrix)	Primary and booster immunization of infants and children except as a fifth dose in children who previously received four doses of DTaP	SmithKline Beecham; 1997
Recombinant coagulation Factor IX (BeneFix)	Control and prevention of hemorrhagic episodes in patients with hemophilia B, including perioperative management of patients with hemophilia B who are undergoing surgery	Genetics Institute; 1997
Autologous cultured chondrocytes (Carticel SM Service)	Repair of clinically significant, symptomatic, cartilaginous defects of the femoral condyle (medial, lateral, or trochlear) caused by acute or repetitive trauma	Genzyme Tissue Repair; 1997
Interferon alfacon-1 (Infergen)	Treatment of chronic HCV infection in patients 18 years of age or older who have compensated liver disease and anti-HCV serum antibodies or HCV RNA	Amgen; 1997
	Subsequent treatment of HCV-infected patients who tolerated an initial course of interferon therapy	1997
Rabies vaccine (RabAvert)	Preexposure and postexposure immunization of children and adults	Chiron; 1997
Oprelvekin (Neumega)	Prevention of severe thrombocytopenia and reduction of the need for platelet transfusions after myelosuppressive chemotherapy in patients with nonmyeloid malignancies who are at high risk for severe thrombocytopenia	Genetics Institute; 1997
Rituximab (Rituxan)	Treatment of patients with relapsed or refractory low-grade or follicular B cell non–Hodgkin lymphoma	Genentech; 1997
Daclizumab (Zenapax)	Prophylaxis of acute organ rejection in patients receiving renal transplants; part of an immunosuppressive regimen that includes cyclosporine and corticosteroids	Hoffman-La Roche; 1997
Becaplermin (Regranex)	Lower-extremity diabetic neuropathic ulcers that extend into the subcutaneous tissue or beyond and have an adequate blood supply	OMJ Pharmaceuticals; 1997
HTLV-I and -II (Vironostika HTLV-I and -II MicroELISA System)	Detection of antibodies to HTLV-I and -II in human serum or plasma	Organon Teknika; 1998
Fibrin sealant (Tisseel VH kit)	Adjunct to hemostasis in surgeries that involve cardiopulmonary bypass	Osterreichisches Institut fur Haemoderivate; 1998
	Treatment of splenic injuries caused by blunt or penetrating trauma to the abdomen when control of bleeding by conventional surgical techniques, including suture, ligature, and cautery, is ineffective or impractical	

Product	Indication	Company; Year
Pooled plasma, solvent detergent treated (VIPLAS/SD)	Closure of colostomies Documented deficiencies of coagulation factors for which there are no concentrate preparations available, including congenital single-factor deficiencies of Factors I, V, VII, XI, and XIII and acquired multiple coagulation factor deficiencies Reversals of warfarin effect Thrombotic thrombocytopenic purpura	V.I. Technologies; 1998
Basiliximab (Simulect)	Prophylaxis of acute organ rejection in patients undergoing renal transplantation Part of an immunosuppressive regimen that includes cyclosporine and corticosteroids	Novartis; 1998
	Use in renal transplantation in combination with triple immunosuppressive therapy Use in pediatric renal transplantation Use of an IV bolus injection	2001
Palivizumab (Synagis)	Prophylaxis of serious lower respiratory tract disease caused by RSV in pediatric patients at high risk of RSV disease	Medimmune; 1998
Sacrosidase (Sucraid)	Congenital sucrose isomaltase deficiency	Orphan Medical; 1998
Eptifibatide (Integrilin)	Acute coronary syndrome Treatment of patients undergoing percutaneous coronary intervention	COR Therapeutics; 1998
Diphtheria and tetanus toxoids and acellular pertussis vaccine adsorbed (Certiva)	Active immunization of individuals 6 weeks to 7 years of age (before the 7th birthday)	North American Vaccine; 1998
Infliximab (Remicade)	Treatment of moderately to severely active Crohn disease to reduce the signs and symptoms in patients who have an inadequate response to conventional therapies Treatment of patients with fistulizing Crohn disease to reduce the number of draining enterocutaneous fistula(s)	Centocor; 1998
	For reduction in signs and symptoms of rheumatoid arthritis in patients who have had an inadequate response to methotrexate	1999
	Inhibition of progression of structural damage in patients with rheumatoid arthritis who have had an inadequate response to methotrexate	2000
	Improving physical function in patients with moderately to severely active rheumatoid arthritis who have had an inadequate response to methotrexate	2002

(*Continued on next page*)

Table 11-1. Continued.

Drug (Trade Name)	Indication(s)	Company; Year Introduced
	Reducing signs and symptoms, and inducing and maintaining clinical remission in patients with moderately to severely active Crohn disease who have had an inadequate response to conventional therapy	2002
	Reducing the number of draining enterocutaneous and rectovaginal fistulas and maintaining fistula closure in patients with fistulizing Crohn disease	2003
	Improving physical function in patients with moderately to severely active rheumatoid arthritis who have had an inadequate response to methotrexate	2003
Rotavirus vaccine, live, oral, tetravalent (RotaShield)	Primary immunization of infants at 2, 4, and 6 months of age	Wyeth-Ayerst Laboratories; 1998
Trastuzumab (Herceptin)	Metastatic breast cancer in patients whose tumors overexpress the HER-2 protein and who have received one or more chemotherapy regimens for metastatic disease	Genentech; 1998
	Median survival	2001
(Etanercept) Enbrel	Reduction in signs and symptoms of moderately to severely active rheumatoid arthritis in patients who have had an inadequate response to one or more DMARDs	Immunex; 1998
	Reducing the signs and symptoms and delaying structural damage in patients with moderately to severely active rheumatoid arthritis, including those who have not previously failed treatment with a DMARD	2000
	Reducing signs and symptoms of active arthritis in patients with psoriatic arthritis	2002
Recombinant OspA (LYMErix)	Active immunization against Lyme disease in people 15–70 years old	SmithKline Beecham; 1998
Vitravene (Fomivirsen)	Local treatment of CMV retinitis in patients with AIDS who are intolerant of or have a contraindication to other treatments for CMV retinitis or who were insufficiently responsive to previous treatments	Isis Pharmaceuticals, Ciba Vision; 1998
Antithymocyte globulin (Thymoglobulin)	Acute rejection in renal transplant patients	Pasteur-Mérieux Serums et Vaccines—France; 1998
Denileukin diftitox (Ontak)	Treatment of patients with persistent or recurrent cutaneous T cell lymphoma whose malignant cells express the CD25 component of the interleukin 2 receptor	Seragen; 1999

Product	Indication	Company; Year
Hepatitis B immunoglobulin (Nabi-HB)	Treatment of acute exposure to HBsAg, perinatal exposure of infants born to HBsAg-positive mothers; Sexual exposure to HBsAg-positive individuals; Household exposure of infants to people with acute hepatitis B virus infection	Nabi; 1999
Recombinant coagulation factor VIIa (NovoSeven)	Treatment of bleeding episodes in hemophilia A or B with inhibitors to Factor VIII or Factor IX	Novo Nordisk A/S—Denmark; 1999
Interferon α-n1, lymphoblastoid (Wellferon)	Chronic HCV infection in patients 18 years of age or older who do not have decompensated liver disease	GlaxoWellcome; 1999
Antihemophilic factor/von Willebrand factor complex (Humate-P)	Used in adult patients for treatment and prevention of bleeding hemophilia A (classic hemophilia); Used in adult and pediatric patients for treatment of spontaneous and trauma-induced bleeding episodes in severe von Willebrand disease; Used in mild and moderate von Willebrand disease when use of desmopressin is known or suspected to be inadequate	Centeon Pharma—Germany; 1999
Hetastarch (Hextend)	Plasma volume expander for treatment of hypovolemia during surgery	BioTime; 1999
Pneumococcal 7-valent conjugate vaccine (diphtheria CRM197 protein) (Prevnar)	Immunization of infants 2, 4, 6, and 12–15 months of age to prevent invasive pneumococcal disease; Immunization of infants and toddlers against otitis media caused by vaccine serotypes	Lederle Laboratories Division American Cyanamid; 2000 2002
Antihemophilic factor (recombinant) (ReFacto)	Control and prevention of hemorrhagic episodes and for short-term routine and surgical prophylaxis in patients with hemophilia A	Genetics Institute; 2000
BCG, live (PACIS)	Treatment of CIS in the absence of associated invasive cancer of the bladder	BioChem Pharma—Canada; 2000
Tenecteplase (TNKase)	Reduction of mortality associated with AMI	Genentech; 2000
Crotalidae polyvalent immune Fab (ovine) (CroFab)	Treatment of minimal and moderate North American Crotalidae envenomation	Protherics; 2000
Botulinum toxin type B (MYOBLOC)	Treatment of cervical dystonia to reduce the severity of abnormal head position and neck pain	Elan Pharmaceuticals; 2000
Botulinum toxin type A (BOTOX or BOTOX COSMETIC)	Treatment of cervical dystonia; Temporary improvement in the appearance of moderate to severe glabellar lines associated with corrugator and/or procerus muscle activity in adult patients ≥ 65 years of age	Allergan; 2002

(Continued on next page)

Table 11-1. Continued.

Drug (Trade Name)	Indication(s)	Company; Year Introduced
Peginterferon α-2b (PEG-Intron)	Treatment of chronic hepatitis C in patients not previously treated with interferon-α who have compensated liver disease and are at least 18 years of age	Schering; 2001
Alemtuzumab (Campath)	Treatment of patients with B cell chronic lymphocytic leukemia who have been treated with alkylating agents and who have failed fludarabine therapy	Millennium and ILEX Partners; 2001
Hepatitis A inactivated and hepatitis B (recombinant) vaccine (TWINRIX)	Active immunization of people 18 years of age or older against disease caused by hepatitis A virus and infection by all known subtypes of hepatitis B virus	SmithKline Beecham Biologicals; 2001
Digoxin immune Fab (ovine) (DigiFab)	Treatment of patients with life-threatening or potentially life-threatening digoxin toxicity or overdose	Protherics; 2001
Darbepoetin α (Aranesp)	Treatment of anemia associated with chronic renal failure, including patients on dialysis and patients not on dialysis	Amgen; 2001
	Treatment of anemia in patients with nonmyeloid malignancies when anemia is the result of the effect of concomitantly administered chemotherapy	2002
Hepatitis B immunoglobulin (human) (Nabi-HB)	Treatment of acute exposure to HBsAg after acute exposure to blood containing HBsAg, perinatal exposure of infants born to HBsAg-positive mothers, sexual exposure to HBsAg-positive persons, and household exposure of infants to people with acute hepatitis B virus infection	Nabi; 2001
Anakinra (Kineret)	Reduction in signs and symptoms of moderately to severely active rheumatoid arthritis, in patients 18 years of age or older who have failed one or more DMARD	Amgen; 2001
Drotrecogin α (activated) (Xigris)	Reduction of mortality in adult patients with severe sepsis (sepsis associated with acute organ dysfunction) who have a high risk of dying from sepsis, as measured by a scoring system based on their general health and the severity of their illness (e.g., by APACHE II)	Eli Lilly; 2001
Pegfilgrastim (Neulasta)	To decrease the incidence of infection, as manifested by febrile neutropenia, in patients with nonmyeloid malignancies receiving myelosuppressive anticancer drugs associated with a clinically significant incidence of febrile neutropenia	Amgen; 2002
Ibritumomab tiuxetan (Zevalin)	Treatment of patients with relapsed or refractory low-grade, follicular, or transformed B-cell non–Hodgkin lymphoma, including patients with rituximab (Rituxan) refractory follicular non–Hodgkin lymphoma	IDEC Pharmaceuticals; 2002

Biotechnology Drug Products 235

Drug	Indication	Company; Year
Interferon β-1a (Rebif)	The therapeutic regimen includes rituximab, [111]indium ibritumomab tiuxetan, and [90]yttrium ibritumomab tiuxetan. Treatment of patients with relapsing forms of multiple sclerosis to decrease the frequency of clinical exacerbations and delay the accumulation of physical disability	Serono; 2002
DTaP vaccine adsorbed (DAPTACEL)	Active immunization of infants and toddlers at 2, 4, 6, and 17–20 months of age against diphtheria, tetanus, and pertussis	Aventis Pasteur—Canada; 2002
Rasburicase (Elitek)	Initial management of plasma uric acid levels in pediatric patients with leukemia, lymphoma, and solid tumor malignancies who are receiving anticancer therapy expected to result in tumor lysis and subsequent elevation of plasma uric acid	Sanofi-Synthelabo; 2002
Peginterferon α-2a (PEGASYS)	Treatment of adults with chronic hepatitis C who have compensated liver disease and who have not been previously treated with interferon α	Hoffman-La Roche; 2002
	Combination therapy with ribavirin, USP (Copegus), for the treatment of chronic HCV infection	2002
Peginterferon α-2a co-packaged with ribavirin (Pegasys Copegus Combination Pack)	Prefilled syringes of Pegasys (peginterferon α-2a) for the treatment of chronic hepatitis C, as a subcutaneous injection taken once a week	2004
Urokinase (Abbokinase)	For adults for the lysis of acute massive pulmonary emboli, defined as obstruction of blood flow to a lobe or multiple segments. For the lysis of pulmonary emboli accompanied by unstable hemodynamics (i.e., failure to maintain blood pressure without supportive measures)	Abbott Laboratories; 2001
Adalimumab (Humira)	For reducing signs and symptoms and inhibiting the progression of structural damage in adult patients with moderately to severely active rheumatoid arthritis who have had an inadequate response to one or more DMARDs. Can be used alone or in combination with methotrexate (MTX) or other DMARDs	Abbott Laboratories; 2002
Laronidase (Aldurazyme)	For patients with Hurler and Hurler-Scheie forms of MPS-I and for patients with the Scheie form who have moderate to severe symptoms	Biomarin Pharmaceutical; 2003
Alefacept (Amevive)	Treatment of adult patients with moderate to severe chronic plaque psoriasis who are candidates for systemic therapy or phototherapy	Biogen; 2003

(Continued on next page)

Table 11-1. Continued.

Drug (Trade Name)	Indication(s)	Company; Year Introduced
Agalsidase beta (Fabrazyme)	For use in patients with Fabry disease to reduce GL-3 deposition in capillary endothelium of the kidney and certain other cell types	Genzyme; 2003
Tositumomab and ^{131}iodine tositumomab (Bexxar)	Treatment of patients with CD20 positive, follicular, non–Hodgkin lymphoma, with and without transformation, whose disease is refractory to rituximab and has relapsed after chemotherapy	Corixa; 2004
Omalizumab (Xolair)	For adults and adolescents (≥ 12 years of age) with moderate to severe persistent asthma who have a positive skin test or in vitro reactivity to a perennial aeroallergen and whose symptoms are inadequately controlled with inhaled corticosteroids	Genentech; 2004
Bevacizumab (Avastin)	First-line treatment for patients with metastatic colorectal cancer	Genentech; 2004
Cetuximab (Erbitux)	A monoclonal antibody that targets the protein EGFR	Imclone Systems; 2004
^{99m}Technetium fanolesomab (NeutroSpec)	For scintigraphic imaging of patients with equivocal signs and symptoms of appendicitis aged 5 years or older	Palatin Technologies; 2004
Natalizumab (Tysabri)	Treatment of patients with relapsing forms of multiple sclerosis to reduce the frequency of clinical exacerbations	Biogen Idec; 2004
Palifermin (Kepivance)	Decreases the incidence and duration of severe oral mucositis in patients with hematologic malignancies receiving myelotoxic therapy requiring hematopoietic stem cell support	Amgen; 2004
Galsulfase (Naglazyme)	Treatment of patients with MPS-VI	Biomarin Pharmaceuticals; 2005

ADA, adenosine deaminase; *AMI*, acute myocardial infarction; *CIS*, carcinoma-in-situ; *CMV*, cytomegalovirus; *DMARD*, disease-modifying antirheumatic drug; *DTaP*, diphtheria and tetanus toxoids and acellular pertussis; *EGFR*, epidermal growth factor receptor; *G-CSF*, granulocyte colony-stimulating factor; *GL*, globotriaosylceramide; *GM-CSF*, granulocyte-macrophage colony-stimulating factor; *HBsAg*, hepatitis B surface antigen; *HCV*, hepatitis C virus; *HER-2*, human epidural growth factor receptor 2; *HTLV*, human T lymphotropic virus; *MPS*, mucopolysaccharidosis; *PEG*, polyethylene glycol; *RSV*, respiratory syncytial virus.
[a]Gaucher disease is an autosomal dominant or recessive disorder caused by an excess of glucocerebroside in the reticuloendothelial cells because of the lack of the metabolic enzyme cerebrosidase. Proliferation of abnormal cells leads to splenomegaly, hepatomegaly, skeletal lesions, and other symptoms.
Data from Biotechnology in the U.S. Pharmaceutical Industry. Research Triangle Park, NC, Institute for Biotechnology Information, 1995; and www.fda.gov.

G. **DNA ligase** is an enzyme that seals single-stranded nicks between nucleotides in double-stranded DNA. DNA ligase enables DNA fragments from different sources to be joined.

H. **DNA polymerase** is an enzyme that catalyzes the synthesis of DNA. It uses a single strand of DNA as the template and nucleotides as the substrates.

I. An **enzyme** is a protein that catalyzes a substrate during its conversion to a product.

J. A **gene** is a segment of DNA that codes for a specific polypeptide.

K. A **genome** is the genetic information content of a cell.

L. A **hormone** is an endogenous substance that is secreted by one type of cell and acts on another type of cell.

M. A **hybridoma** is a hybrid cell produced by the fusion of a myeloma cell and a specific antibody-producing B lymphocyte. A single hybridoma produces a single type of antibody.

N. **Interferon (INF)** is any of a class of glycoproteins produced by animal cells in response to viral infection.

O. **Interleukin** is a group of proteins synthesized by macrophages and T lymphocytes in response to antigen and other stimulation.

P. A **lymphokine** is any of a class of soluble proteins produced by some white blood cells. These proteins stimulate other white blood cells as part of the immune response.

Q. A **plasmid** is a circular piece of duplex DNA that is not part of a chromosome and can replicate independently. Plasmids are used as vectors for the transfer of DNA in recombinant DNA technology.

R. **RNA** is a macromolecule that contains information for protein synthesis. The three types of RNA are ribosomal (rRNA), transfer (tRNA), and messenger (mRNA). RNA is also the genetic material of some viruses.

S. **Recombinant DNA (rDNA)** is a hybrid DNA that is formed when pieces of DNA from different sources are joined. The process is also known as gene splicing.

T. A **restriction endonuclease** is an enzyme that cleaves DNA at sequence-specific sites.

U. **Tumor necrosis factor (TNF)** is a lymphokine produced by macrophages. It can be activated to kill tumor cells.

V. **Reverse transcriptase** is an enzyme present in RNA viruses that catalyzes the formation of DNA from the viral RNA.

III. **PROTEINS AND PEPTIDES.** Proteins and peptides play essential roles in all aspects of cellular function. Many **endogenous** substances synthesized in the body are essential proteins. Many enzymes that catalyze vital reactions in the body are proteins.

A. **Hemoglobin (Hb)** is a large protein involved in oxygen transport.

B. **Globulins** are special proteins in the plasma that are involved in immunogenic response and antibody formation.

C. **Albumin** is a plasma protein that binds to many drugs and is used as a carrier for new drugs.

D. Other well-known proteins include insulin and the enzymes involved in digestion.

Table 11-2. Immunoglobulin Applications

Gammaglobulinemia
Hepatitis A prophylaxis
Measles and rubella prophylaxis
Multiple myeloma with specific antibody
   deficiency
Prophylaxis in infants and children with HIV
   exposure
Chronic inflammatory demyelinating neuropathy
Acquired hemophilia
Orphan drug for the treatment of juvenile
   rheumatoid arthritis
Respiratory tract infections
Immune thrombocytopenic purpura
Orphan drug for the treatment of polymyositis
   and acute myocarditis
Acute exposure to hepatitis B surface antigen
Kawasaki disease in conjunction with high-dose
   aspirin

    E. Protein is an important component of **keratin** in hair and **myosin** in muscles.

    F. **Albumin (human) 5% USP** is used to reverse hypovolemia in shock patients, burn patients, and those with chronic hypoalbuminemia.

IV. **Immunoglobulin (Ig)** is an important class of globulin proteins involved in immunity and the allergic response. **IgG** is used therapeutically to modulate or replace antibody in various **immunodeficiency** and disease states. Intramuscular and intravenous preparations are available from a variety of manufacturers (Tables 11-2 and 11-3). Most of these products must be stored under refrigeration (2–8°C) and have a limited shelf life.

V. RECOMBINANT HUMAN GRANULOCYTE COLONY-STIMULATING FACTOR (G-CSF)

    A. CSFs are **glycoproteins** that regulate the production of many types of blood cells and components in the body. These include **macrophages, eosinophils, neutrophils, basophils,** and **platelets.** Natural and modified CSFs are used to treat a number of congenital disorders and several forms of cancer.

    B. **Lenograstim** is a **recombinant human granulocyte CSF** (rhG-CSF) derived from Chinese hamster ovary cells. It is glycosylated at the same site as natural hG-CSF (threonine-133) and consists of 174 amino acids.

    C. **Filgrastim** is an *Escherichia coli*–derived glycoprotein. It is not glycosylated, and it differs in structure from natural hG-CSF. Like natural hG-CSF and **filgrastim,** lenograstim selectively promotes the proliferation, differentiation, and maturation of blood cell precursors. Dose-

Table 11-3. Immunoglobulin Products

Gamimune-N	Nabi-HB
Gammagard	RespiGam
Polygram	Sandoglobulin
Gammar	Polygam
Iveegam	Venoglobulin

related increases in blood neutrophil counts are observed after lenograstim administration. Lenograstim reduces the duration of **neutropenia** and the severity of infection in patients who are receiving **cytotoxic chemotherapy** for **nonmyeloid malignancy.** Colony-forming assays show that lenograstim is approximately three times as potent as filgrastim. These agents were similarly potent in cell-proliferation assays. Both natural and recombinant G-CSF products stimulate the release of mature neutrophils from hematopoietic tissue, prolong their survival, and enhance their phagocytic and cytotoxic activity.

D. Other actions of rhG-CSF include synergism with **interleukin 3** (IL-3) to induce megakaryocyte formation and with granulocyte-macrophage CSF (GM-CSF) to stimulate granulocyte- macrophage colonies.

VI. GLYCOPROTEINS

A. Many special proteins acquire biologic activity as a result of their covalent linking with a polymer of sugar or **carbohydrate.** The covalently linked protein–carbohydrate molecule is a **glycoprotein.** Glycoproteins form natural structural membranes in the cells of unicellular (e.g., bacteria) and multicellular (e.g., humans, animals) organisms.

B. **N-acetylglucosamine (NAG)** forms the cell membrane in bacteria. It is an example of a carbohydrate chain linked to a protein through a chain of amino acids. Bacterial resistance to penicillin is linked to the integrity of **NAG** in the cell membrane.

C. The extent and site of **glycosylation** of a protein molecule may affect the physicochemical properties, stability, and specificity of a surface receptor in a cell. Glycoproteins on the surface of red blood cells are involved in recognizing the specific blood type.

D. The charge at the site of a glycoprotein molecule may play a role in the orientation and interaction of the receptor. The charge may be modified by **sialic acid, sulfate,** and **phosphate groups.** The protein molecule presents potential sites for **N-glycosylation** and **O-glycosylation.** Change in glycosylation is a powerful tool for use in engineering the preferred configuration and stability when designing recombinant glycoprotein for therapeutic use.

E. **Carbohydrates** contribute to activities in a number of ways, including recognition of the terminal sialic acids of glycoproteins by various viruses and bacteria, recognition of polylactosamines on **erythrocytes** by autoimmune antibodies, and recognition of sialylated, fucosylated lactosaminoglycans on leukocytes by E-selectin of endothelial cells.

VII. DNA

A. DNA is the genetic material of all organisms except some viruses, whose genetic material is in the form of RNA. Most organisms have double-stranded DNA. Some viruses contain single-stranded DNA. This type of virus replicates itself by entering a host cell, where it makes a complementary copy of itself and temporarily forms a double strand.

B. All DNA molecules consist of many covalently linked subunits called nucleotides. The nucleotides consist of deoxyribose, phosphate, and one of the nitrogen-containing bases (adenine, guanine, thymine, or cytosine). DNA encodes information to produce all of the proteins needed by the organism. The DNA sequence may be modified or recombined with new strands. This recombinant technology may be used to correct genetic defects in living organisms.

VIII. ANTISENSE DRUGS

A. Many diseases occur because of genetic defects or errors in the gene involved in producing essential enzymes or proteins. Genetic information resides in **chromosomes** that house helical strands of DNA within the nucleus. The **Human Genome Initiative** was created several years ago to study all human genes. This national effort is now yielding information on many serious diseases that involve congenital defects, cancer, infection, AIDS, and other disorders of the immune system.

B. Strategies are now available to moderate many disease processes by altering or blocking the **transcription** of DNA. If the DNA sequence is altered so that the **complementary strand** is transcribed instead of the normal "sense" gene, then the DNA cannot make a copy of the normal RNA that participates in protein synthesis. The aberrant copies of RNA may pair up (**hybridize**) with other RNA strands that complement it and thereby block protein synthesis. This technique involves targeting DNA or RNA with **antisense** drugs.

C. Many oligonucleotides are designed to target viral disease and cancer cells. To further stabilize the drug, phosphodiesters are chemically converted to phosphothioates.

D. Antisense drugs against cytomegalovirus (CMV), HIV, and other viruses are in various phases of clinical trials. The first antisense drug, Vitravene, was approved by the U.S. Food and Drug Administration (FDA) in 1998. Vitravene is a potent biotechnology drug that is indicated for the local treatment of CMV retinitis in patients with AIDS who are intolerant of other treatments, who have a contraindication to other treatments, or who were insufficiently responsive to previous treatments. The recommended labeled dosage is an induction dose on days 1 and 15, followed by a monthly intravitreal injection of 330 μg.

E. When the **nucleotide** base sequence of a gene that controls a specific body function is known, the antisense DNA strand can be synthesized. If necessary, the DNA strand can be modified to provide increased stability and potency. These strands can then be introduced into cells, where they attach themselves to the **complementary** sense DNA strands and depress transcription of these genes. This technique was performed successfully in cell culture for the gene that produces human **squamous cell carcinoma** of the **larynx.**

F. If a duplicate copy of a gene is inserted into a chromosome in **reverse orientation** to the normal gene, then the antisense DNA strand of this gene is transcribed. This process yields an antisense mRNA strand that is complementary to the mRNA strand transcribed for the normal gene. The two complementary RNA strands bind to each other, thereby preventing the **translation** of the normal RNA strand that may control protein synthesis.

IX. GENE THERAPY. The first example of human gene therapy is from 1990, when the FDA approved PEG-ADA (Enzon) for **adenosine deaminase** deficiency. This rare, but serious, genetic disorder weakens the immune system and causes increased susceptibility to infection. Two girls were reinfused with their own genetically altered white blood cells. The altered cells live and function normally, and the two girls were living a relatively normal life after 5 years.

X. MISCELLANEOUS BIOTECHNOLOGIC PRODUCTS

A. Alteplase (Activase, Genentech) is a **thrombolytic** agent formerly known as **tissue-plasminogen activator.** Intravenous alteplase effectively produces recanalization of occluded coronary arteries after acute **myocardial infarction.** Intravenous alteplase is also effective in the treatment of acute massive **pulmonary embolism.** Adverse effects, including bleeding complications, **reperfusion arrhythmias,** and reinfarction, are the primary concerns with this therapy. Systemic fibrinolysis is less than that seen with streptokinase. The recommended dose to produce **recanalization** after myocardial infarction is 100 mg in divided doses. The recommended dose to treat pulmonary embolism is 100 mg infused intravenously over 2 hr.

B. Antithrombin III (heparin cofactor, human antithrombin III, ATnativ, Pharmacia) is designated an orphan product. It is used as replacement therapy to prevent or treat thromboembolic episodes in congenital deficiency states. The amount of intravenous antithrombin III concentrate to be administered is based on antithrombin III levels. In patients who have congenital or acquired **antithrombin III deficiency,** the goal is to maintain levels between 80% and

120% of normal. Once-daily doses of antithrombin III should maintain serum levels above 80% of normal. Levels should be monitored twice daily until they stabilize, then daily thereafter immediately before the next dose is administered.

C. **IL-3** is a **hematopoietic growth factor** used to treat patients with bone marrow failure. Recombinant human IL-3 (rhIL-3) alone improves neutrophil and platelet counts in patients who have **chemotherapy-related bone marrow failure** and myelodysplastic syndromes. However, only minimal improvements in hematopoiesis are seen in patients who have aplastic anemia. Enhanced responses are seen with the sequential combined use of rhIL-3 and other hematopoietic growth factors (e.g., GM-CSF). Recombinant human IL-3 is given subcutaneously or intravenously. Intravenous doses range from 30 to 1000 $\mu g/m^2$/day infused over 4 hr.

D. **Aldesleukin,** a lymphokine, is a hrIL-2 product that is used to treat **metastatic renal cell carcinoma.** The starting dose is 0.037 mg/kg every 8 hr by a 15-min intravenous infusion. Aldesleukin is absorbed erratically after intramuscular or subcutaneous injection. It follows two-compartment pharmacokinetics, with an α-half-life of 13 min and a β-half-life of 85 min. It is eliminated renally. The principal side effects are hypotension and flulike symptoms. Most adverse effects are dose related.

E. **Abciximab** (c7E3 Fab, ReoPro) is a chimeric monoclonal antibody Fab fragment that is specific for platelet glycoprotein IIb–IIIa receptors. Abciximab is extremely effective in reducing fatalities ($> 50\%$) in subjects who have **unstable angina** after they undergo **angioplasty.** The recommended dosage is an intravenous bolus of 0.25 mg/kg administered 10–60 min before the start of angioplasty, followed by a continuous infusion of 10 μg/min for 12 hr. Platelet aggregation is almost completely inhibited 2 hr after the initiation of abciximab therapy. The major complication of abciximab infusion is dose-related bleeding.

F. **Campath-1** is a MAb that targets human lymphocytes and monocytes. It is used for **immunosuppression** in patients who undergo organ transplant. The intravenous dose is 25 mg once or twice daily. Campath-1 is also used to treat refractory **autoimmune disorders,** including rheumatoid arthritis. It is used experimentally to treat vasculitis. Campath-1 antibodies are used to prevent graft-versus-host disease and to treat **lymphoid malignancy** caused by immunosuppression in patients who undergo organ transplant.

G. **Edobacomab** is an immunoglobulin directed against **gram-negative bacterial endotoxins.** For **septic shock,** single doses of 2–15 mg/kg intravenously every 24 hr are used. The volume of distribution ranges from 4 to 8 L. The elimination half-life is 10–18 hr. The main side effects are hypersensitivity reactions and antibody production. The drug is also being investigated for the treatment of gram-negative sepsis and septic shock.

H. **Muromonab-CD3** is an immunosuppressive agent with specific targeting. It is effective in reversing **acute renal allograft rejection.** The usual dose is 5 mg/day intravenously for 10–14 days after the initial signs and symptoms of rejection. The volume of distribution is approximately 6.5 L, and the half-life is 18 hr. Side effects include flulike symptoms, which appear to be associated with the release of cytokines. Symptoms may be self-limiting or severe and life threatening.

I. **Nebacumab** is an immunoglobulin directed against gram-negative bacterial endotoxins. The drug is being investigated for the treatment of **gram-negative sepsis** and **septic shock.** Signs and symptoms of septic shock usually resolve during the first 7 days after treatment. Its half-life is 15.9 hr, and the volume of distribution is 48.5 mL/kg.

J. **Satumomab pendetide** is an MAb conjugate produced from the murine MAb B72.3. It requires radiolabeling to form [111]indium chloride satumomab pendetide. It is used as a **diagnostic imaging agent** in the staging of patients with known **colorectal** and **ovarian carcinoma.** The metabolic fate of this agent is unclear. The antibody conjugate is cleared slowly. It has a terminal half-life of approximately 56 hr. Approximately 10% of an administered dose appears in the urine.

K. **Zolimomab aritox** (Orthozyme-CD5, Xoma/Ortho Biotech) is an immunoconjugate of monoclonal anti-CD5 murine IgG and the ricin A-chain toxin. Its primary use is in the treatment of steroid-resistant graft-versus-host disease after **allogeneic bone marrow transplant** for hematopoietic neoplasms (e.g., acute myelogenous leukemia). Other potential uses include the treatment of **rheumatoid arthritis** and insulin-dependent diabetes mellitus. After therapeutic doses, peak serum levels range from 1 to 5 μg/mL. The serum half-life is 1.5–4 hr. The dose varies, depending on the indications.

L. Betaseron (INF-β, Berlex Laboratories) is a glycoprotein with antiviral, antiproliferative, and immunomodulatory activity. Many of its effects are similar to those of INF-α. Its uses include the treatment of multiple sclerosis, AIDS, malignant melanoma, herpesvirus, and papillomavirus infections. It is also recommended at a dose of 8 million units subcutaneously every other day to reduce exacerbations in patients who have relapsing-remitting multiple sclerosis. It is administered intravenously, intramuscularly, subcutaneously, intrathecally, topically, or intralesionally for a variety of indications. Its biologic activity is evident in the absence of detectable serum levels. Serum concentrations are not consistently detectable after subcutaneous or intramuscular administration. Interferon β may cross the disrupted blood–brain barrier. The compound does not appear in urine after systemic administration. Adverse effects include flulike symptoms, bone marrow suppression, neurotoxic effects with high doses, anorexia and other gastrointestinal symptoms, and elevations of liver enzymes and serum creatinine.

STUDY QUESTIONS

Directions: Each of the question, statement, or items or incomplete statement in this section can be correctly answered or completed by **one** of the suggested answers or phrases. Choose the **best** answer.

1. Which type of cell contains double-stranded DNA?

(A) Human cells
(B) Bacteria cells
(C) HIV cells
(D) Viruses

2. Which enzyme is used by the human immuno-deficiency virus (HIV) to form DNA in the host cell?

(A) Restrictive endonuclease
(B) DNA-directed polymerase
(C) Reverse transcriptase
(D) Both A and B
(E) None of the above

3. Gammaglobulin is considered to be

(A) DNA.
(B) RNA.
(C) a protein.
(D) None of the above

4. Glycoprotein is considered to be a protein linked to

(A) a carbohydrate.
(B) a hormone.
(C) a lipid.
(D) DNA.
(E) None of the above

5. An enzyme that cleaves DNA at a specific site is called a

(A) restriction endonuclease.
(B) restrictive ribonuclease.
(C) trypsin.
(D) None of the above

6. An example of a cytokine is

(A) interleukin.
(B) insulin.
(C) gonadotropin.
(D) thyroxine.
(E) None of the above

7. A common storage condition for most biotech-nology products after reconstitution is

(A) at room temperature.
(B) in a cool place.
(C) in a warm place.
(D) no excessive heat.
(E) in a freezer.

8. What drug is used to prevent embolism in the lung and during myocardial infarction?

(A) Alteplase
(B) Human growth hormone
(C) Granulocyte-macrophage colony-stimulating factor (GM-CSF)
(D) Epogen (EPO)
(E) None of the above

9. What base is found in DNA?

(A) Cytosine
(B) Adenine
(C) Guanine
(D) Thymine
(E) All of the above

ANSWERS AND EXPLANATIONS

1. The answer is A *[see VII.A].*
Human cells contain double-stranded DNA, whereas lower organisms (e.g., bacteria, viruses) do not.

2. The answer is C *[see II.V].*
Reverse transcriptase is the enzyme that a virus uses to assemble its DNA from RNA. Unlike higher organisms, viral particles have genetic material in the RNA and need a host cell for reproduction.

3. The answer is C *[see III.C; Table 11-2].*
Gammaglobulin is a subclass of immunoglobulin protein involved in immunity and allergic response.

4. The answer is A *[see III.B; VI].*
Glycoprotein consists of a carbohydrate linked to a protein.

5. The answer is A *[see II.T].*
A restriction endonuclease is an enzyme that specifically cleaves DNA molecules. Ribonuclease will cleave RNA only, and trypsin is a digestive enzyme found in the gastrointestinal tract.

6. The answer is A *[see II.O;, X.C].*
Interleukin is a "messenger" substance synthesized by the cell (cytokine) to communicate and trigger cellular response.

7. The answer is B *[see I].*
Most biologic compounds are heat labile and must be stored at low temperature.

8. The answer is A *[see X.A; Table 11-1].*
Alteplase is a thrombolytic agent formerly known as tissue-plasminogen activator.

9. The answer is E *[see VII.B].*
All DNA molecules consist of nucleotides, which consist of deoxyribose, phosphate, and one of the following nitrogen-containing bases: adenine, guanine, thymine, and cytosine.

12
Principles of Pharmacodynamics and Medicinal Chemistry

Marc W. Harrold

Nelson S. Yee

I. INTRODUCTION. Pharmacodynamics is a branch of pharmacology that focuses on the study of the biochemical and physiological effects of drugs and the mechanisms by which they produce such effects. Analysis of drug action provides the basis for rational design of therapeutic agents and provides insight into the regulation of cellular functions.

II. EFFECTS OF DRUGS

A. Perturbation of normal physiological processes. The actions of drugs are the consequences of the dynamic interactions between drug molecules and cellular components. Such interactions lead to alteration in the functions of these components, called **receptors.** The resulting biochemical and physiologic changes form the basis of the cellular response to the drug. Drugs act by modulating the ongoing processes inside the cells.

B. Agonists and antagonists

1. Potentially, any macromolecular component may act as a **drug receptor.** For example, c-Kit tyrosine kinase can be inhibited by imatinib mesylate (Gleevec), cyclooxygenase-2 is blocked by celecoxib (Celebrex), and chromosomal DNA is cross-linked by cisplatin (Platinol).

2. Certain drug receptors normally serve as receptors for endogenous ligands and thus are **physiological receptors.** For example, adrenergic receptors are physiological receptors for catecholamines.

3. Drugs whose responses resemble the effects of the endogenous molecules are receptor **agonists.** For example, bethanechol directly stimulates cholinergic receptors and is thus an agonist.

4. **Pharmacological antagonists** are drugs that lack **intrinsic activity** and produce effects by **competitively** or **noncompetitively** inhibiting the action of the endogenous molecules at the receptor.
   a. A **competitive antagonist** acts by interfering with binding of the endogenous ligand to the receptor in a reversible manner. For example, propanolol competes with catecholamines for binding with adrenergic β-receptors.
   b. A **noncompetitive antagonist** acts by interacting with the nonligand binding site of the receptor (e.g., through covalent modification), such that normal binding of the endogenous ligand to the receptor is irreversibly inhibited. For instance, monoamine oxidase (MAO) inhibitors such as tranylcypromine (Parnate) initially interact with MAO in a reversible manner but then form covalent adducts that irreversibly inhibit MAO.

5. **Partial antagonists** inhibit the endogenous ligand from binding the receptor but possess some intrinsic activity. Nalorphine is a partial antagonist for the opiate receptor.

6. **Physiological antagonism** occurs when the drugs act independently at different receptor sites, often yielding opposing actions. For example, epinephrine and acetylcholine act on the sympathetic and parasympathetic autonomic nervous system, respectively, and their effects are antagonistic to each other.

7. **Neutralizing antagonism** occurs when two drugs bind with each other to form an inactive compound. For example, digoxin-binding antibody used in digoxin overdose acts by sequestering the drug, resulting in the formation of an inactive complex.

III. MECHANISMS OF DRUG ACTION

A. Cell surface receptors

1. Receptors can be **proteins or glycoproteins.** For example, cellular determinants such as CD20 antigen on B lymphocytes can bind with rituximab (Rituxan), a chimeric monoclonal antibody targeted against the CD20 antigen.

2. The binding of drugs to receptors is highly specific and can involve a variety of interactions, including hydrophobic interactions and van der Waals forces with ionic, hydrogen, and covalent bonds. The type of interaction and the binding affinity can influence the duration and reversibility of the drug action.

3. The interaction and binding affinity are related to the chemical structure of both the drug and the ligand. Chemical modification of the structure of the drug molecule can change the pharmacological and pharmacokinetic properties of drugs.

4. Through structure–activity relationship studies, synthetic drug analogs can be developed to achieve a high selectivity of drug action—a desirable ratio of therapeutic to toxic effect with a better-tolerated side effect profile.

B. Signal transduction by cell-surface receptors

1. Cell-surface receptors are composed of extracellular domains that bind the ligands (drugs or physiological molecules). For example, epidermal growth factor (EGF) receptor normally binds EGF and transforming growth factor α, and it is the target of the monoclonal antibody cetuximab (Erbitux), which competitively binds to the EGF receptor.

2. The ligand binding serves as a triggering signal that can be propagated in the target cell through intracellular regulatory molecules, known as **second messengers** or **effectors.** For example, isoproterenol binds with the β-adrenergic receptor, which is functionally coupled to adenylate cyclase via the stimulatory G protein (G_s). As a result, adenylate cyclase is activated, and the cyclic adenosine monophosphate (cAMP) level increases.

3. Ligand binding of receptors often leads to interaction of the receptors with the cytoplasmic effectors, which in turn become activated. Integration of the multiple signal transducing events along the receptor–effector system might change the cellular phenotype or gene expression, leading to new protein synthesis. For example, binding of the ligands to the EGF receptor leads to activation of the tyrosine kinase of the intracellular domain of the receptor, which then activates downstream signaling pathways that results in cellular proliferation. The monoclonal antibody erlotinib (Tarceva) binds to the adenosine triphosphate (ATP) pocket of the tyrosine kinase of the EGF receptor and inhibits normal ATP binding, thus inhibiting the activity of the tyrosine kinase.

C. Signaling mediated by intracellular receptors.
Thyroid hormone, steroid hormones, vitamin D, and the retinoids act through binding cytoplasmic receptors, which translocate into the nucleus. These receptors are soluble, DNA-binding proteins that regulate the transcription of specific genes. For example, all-trans-retinoic acid (ATRA; Vesanoid) binds to retinoic acid receptor in the cytosol, resulting in up-regulation of target gene expression and differentiation of leukemic promyelocytes.

D. Target cell desensitization and hypersensitization

1. Cells have the ability to **respond** to endogenous regulatory molecules or exogenously added drugs over a wide range of concentrations. However, protective mechanisms are available for maintaining homeostatic control to prevent overstimulation or understimulation of the target cells.

2. Cell **regulation** can occur at different levels along the signal transduction pathway. Regulation can involve changes in the level of the receptors or alterations in the downstream effector molecules.

3. The expression of receptors is normally under homeostatic control through receptor internalization, recycling, and de novo synthesis.

4. **Down-regulation and desensitization**
   a. **Down-regulation** of receptors is caused by continuous prolonged exposure of receptors to drugs that disrupt the homeostatic equilibrium and result in altered levels of the receptors. This disruption involves endocytosis of ligand-bound receptors, resulting in sequestration of receptors from the cell surface and possibly accelerated degradation of the receptors or inactivation of the receptors.
   b. **Desensitization** is the result of down-regulation. The target cells become desensitized, and the effect of subsequent exposure to the same concentration of the drug is reduced. Therefore, an increased concentration of the drug is required to produce an effect of the same magnitude as the initial exposure with a smaller drug concentration.
   c. Repeated doses of bronchodilator such as albuterol inhaler for the treatment of asthma can lead to down-regulation of β-adrenergic receptors in the bronchial cells. The patient develops tolerance and requires increased dosage of the drug to achieve relief of the initial extent. In this case, the target cells become desensitized only to ligands that bind to those receptors; this is called **homologous desensitization.**

5. **Heterologous desensitization.** Some forms of desensitization involve alteration of components in the signaling pathway, such as a G protein. When cultured fibroblasts are exposed to prostaglandin E_1 (PGE_1), which normally activates adenylate cyclase through a G_s, the cells lose responsiveness not only to PGE_1 but also to other ligands binding to other receptors that act through the G_s–adenylate cyclase pathway.

6. **Hyperreactivity** or **supersensitivity** to receptor agonists is expected when target cells are subject to long-term exposure to receptor antagonists followed by abrupt cessation of administration of the drug. This can involve receptor **up-regulation** through synthesis of new receptors.

E. **Pharmacological effects not mediated by receptors.** The effects of some drugs do not involve binding with specific receptors because of interaction with molecules or ions, which are not typically defined as receptors.

1. **Colligative** drug effects are characterized by a lack of requirement for highly specific chemical structure.
   a. Volatile general **anesthetic** agents with diverse structures are lipophilic and interact with the lipid bilayer of cell membranes, resulting in depressed excitability.
   b. **Cathartics,** such as magnesium sulfate and sorbitol, act by increasing the osmolarity of intestinal fluids and thus changing the distribution of water.

2. Methotrexate, cytarabine, and 5-fluorouracil are examples of **antimetabolites.** Antimetabolites are structural analogs of endogenous molecules and are incorporated into cellular components that interfere with the normal cellular functions.

3. Certain drugs interact with specific ions normally found in body fluids. For example, **antacids** such as aluminum hydroxide, calcium carbonate, and magnesium hydroxide act by neutralizing gastric acid.

IV. RELATIONSHIP BETWEEN DRUG CONCENTRATION AND EFFECT

A. **Dose–response relationship.** In general, the larger the drug dose, the higher the drug concentration at its site of action and the greater the effect of the drug, up to a maximum effect. Higher drug concentrations (or doses) will not produce an effect greater than the maximum effect.

B. **A quantal dose–response curve** describes the relationship between the number of patients exhibiting a defined response (e.g., a 50% increase in peak flow) and the specified dose of the drug (e.g., minimum dose of albuterol for 50% increase in peak flow). This relationship often follows a gaussian (bell-shaped) distribution (Figures 12-1 and 12-2).

C. **A graded dose–response curve** describes the relationship between the magnitude of the effect of a drug (e.g., reduction of blood pressure by nifedipine) in an individual and the dose of the drug (Figure 12-3).

Figure 12-1. Frequency distribution curve, plotting the number of patients showing a quantal response to a drug against the minimum dose needed to produce the response.

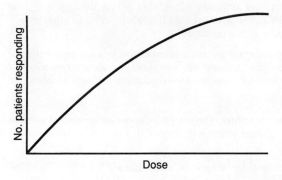

Figure 12-2. Quantal dose–response curve, cumulating the data used to plot Figure 12-1.

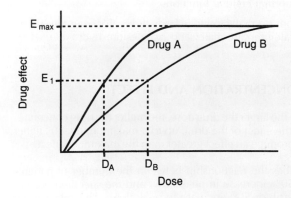

Figure 12-3. Graded dose–response curves for two drugs, A and B. D_A and D_B, amount (dose) of drug A and drug B, respectively, needed to produce the drug effect, E_1; E_{max}, maximum effect.

Figure 12-4. Log dose–response curves for two drugs, A and B. ED_{50}, smallest dose showing an effect that is 50% of the maximum effect (E_{max}).

1. Generally, as the dose of a drug increases, the effect produced will reach a maximum level.

2. Graded dose–response curves for different drugs allow comparison of their efficacies and potencies.
   a. **Efficacy** of a drug is measured by its maximum effect (E_{max}).
   b. **Potency** of a drug is a relative measure that compares the different doses (molar doses) of different drugs needed to produce the same effect. From a clinical viewpoint, potency is considered in drug selection (e.g., triazolam is preferred for the treatment of insomnia instead of diazepam).
   c. In clinical situations, a drug with greater efficacy might be needed to achieve the therapeutic outcome (e.g., hydromorphone is preferred to acetaminophen for controlling bone pain in a patient with metastatic breast cancer).

D. A **log dose–response curve** describes the relationship between the drug effect and the log of the dose. This curve facilitates comparison of potency and efficacy among different drugs with the same mechanism of action (which thus have the same slopes) (Figure 12-4).

1. The **efficacy** of a drug is determined by the **height** of its log dose–response curve (**E_{max}**); the higher the curve, the greater the E_{max} and efficacy.

2. The **potency** of two drugs can be compared by determining their **ED_{50}**. The ED_{50} is the **dose** of each drug producing 50% of the corresponding maximum effect (50% of E_{max}). The smaller the ED_{50}, the greater the potency.

3. A **competitive antagonist** shifts the log dose–response curve to the **right,** and the shift is **parallel.** A greater concentration of the agonist is required to produce the same response than when the competitive antagonist is absent. Even in the presence of the antagonist, the **same E_{max}** can be achieved if enough agonist is added (Figure 12-5).

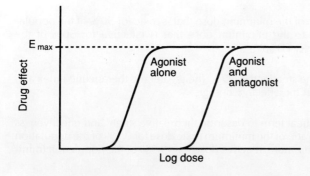

Figure 12-5. Shift in the log dose-response curve that occurs when an agonist is administered in the presence of a competitive antagonist. E_{max}, maximum effect.

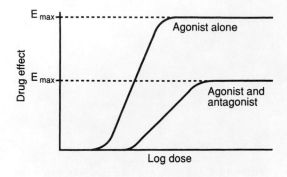

Figure 12-6. Shift in the log dose–response curve and lowering of the maximum effect (E_{max}) that occur when an agonist is given in the presence of a noncompetitive antagonist.

4. A **noncompetitive antagonist** binds to the same receptor or binds to another site that prevents the agonist from producing a response. The shift of the log dose–response curve is to the **right** and **nonparallel,** resulting in a **lower E_{max}**. The action of the antagonist cannot be overcome even if more agonist is present (Figure 12-6).

V. ENHANCEMENT OF DRUG EFFECTS

A. **Addition** occurs when two different drugs with the same effect are given together, resulting in a drug effect that is equal in magnitude to the sum of the individual effects of the two drugs. For example, trimethoprim and sulfamethoxazole inhibit different steps in the synthesis of folic acid, resulting in the suppression of bacterial growth.

B. **Synergism** occurs when two drugs with the same effect are given together, producing a drug effect that is greater in magnitude than the sum of the individual effects of the two drugs. For example, penicillin and gentamicin are synergistic in their antipseudomonal activities.

C. **Potentiation** occurs when one drug, lacking an effect of its own, increases the effect of another drug that is active. For example, carbidopa is an inactive analog of dopa. When carbidopa blocks the degradation of dopa and is given with dopa, it prolongs the half-life of dopa and the duration of the anti-Parkinsonian effect.

VI. SELECTIVITY OF DRUG ACTION

A. The **therapeutic index** and the **margin of safety** are the relationship (ratio) between the dose of a drug required to produce undesired effects (toxic or lethal) and the dose required to produce the desired effects (therapeutic).

1. The **therapeutic index** of a drug is a relative measure of the safety and effectiveness in laboratory studies.

2. The **therapeutic index** is the ratio of the minimum dose that is toxic for 50% of the population (**median toxic dose; TD_{50}**) to the minimum dose that is effective for 50% of the population (**median effective dose; ED_{50}**).

B. In general, the greater the TD_{50} or the smaller the ED_{50}, the greater the therapeutic index and thus the safer the drug when used at the effective dosage.

C. The **margin of safety** is a more practical term to describe the relative safety and effectiveness of a drug. The margin of safety is the ratio of the minimum toxic dose for 0.1% of the population (**minimal toxic dose; $TD_{0.1}$**) to the minimum effective dose for 99.9% of the population (**minimal effective dose; $ED_{99.9}$**).

VII. DRUG SOURCES AND MAJOR CLASSES

A. **Natural products** are drugs obtained from plant and animal sources.

   1. **Alkaloids** are nitrogen-containing compounds obtained primarily from plants through extraction and purification, which possess pharmacological activity. The majority of alkaloids are basic compounds (e.g., **morphine,** from the opium poppy; **atropine,** from the belladonna plant); although some are neutral amides (e.g., **colchicine,** from the autumn crocus). All alkaloids end in the suffix *-ine;* however, it is important to note that not all drugs that end in *-ine* are alkaloids (e.g., meperidine).

   2. **Peptides and polypeptides** are polymers of amino acids, are obtained from either human or animal sources and are smaller than **proteins.** The amino acid length distinctions between these three classifications are vague and often vary from one source to another. Naturally occurring peptides have little to no oral activity and short half-lives (e.g., **somatostatin,** a 14–amino acid peptide; **glucagon,** a 29–amino acid polypeptide).

   3. **Steroids** are chemical derivatives of cyclopentanoperhydrophenanthrene and can be obtained from either human or animal sources (e.g., **estradiol, testosterone, hydrocortisone**).

   4. **Hormones** are chemical substances that are formed in one organ or part of the body and carried in the blood to another organ or part. They are principally proteins or steroids and can be obtained either synthetically, through recombinant DNA technology (e.g., **insulin**), or from animal sources (e.g., **thyroid hormones** and **conjugated estrogens**).

   5. **Glycosides** are organic substances consisting of a sugar moiety bound to a nonsugar (aglycone) moiety by means of a glycosidic bond (i.e., a bond between the anomeric carbon of the sugar and a hydroxy group on the aglycone). They can be of either plant (e.g., **digitoxin**) or microbial (e.g., **streptomycin, doxorubicin**) origin.

   6. **Vitamins** are organic substances that are present in foods and are essential to normal metabolism.
      a. **Water-soluble vitamins** are thiamine (B_1), riboflavin (B_2), niacin (B_3), pyridoxine (B_6), cyanocobalamin (B_{12}), ascorbic acid (C), folic acid, pantothenic acid, and biotin (H).
      b. **Lipid-soluble vitamins** are retinol (A), ergocalciferol (D), α-tocopherol (E), and phytonadione (K).

   7. **Polysaccharides** are polymers of sugars that can be obtained from either human or animal sources. These compounds can be used either directly (e.g., **heparin**), after partial depolymerization (e.g., **tinzaparin, enoxaparin**), or after structural modification (e.g., **sucralfate**).

   8. **Antibiotics** are chemical substances produced by microorganisms that either suppress or kill other microorganisms (e.g., **penicillin, tetracycline, doxorubicin**).

B. **Synthetic products** are drugs synthesized from organic compounds.

   1. Synthetic products can have **chemical structures closely resembling those of active natural products** (e.g., **hydroxymorphone,** which resembles morphine; **ampicillin,** which resembles penicillin).

   2. Synthetic products can contain similar spacing of functional groups but lack the general structure of a naturally occurring compound. **Peptidomimetics** are molecules with no peptide bonds, a molecular weight < 700, and activity similar to the original peptide (e.g., **losartan** is a peptidomimetic and an angiotensin II receptor antagonist).

   3. Synthetic products also can be **completely new products,** obtained by screening synthesized materials for drug activity (e.g., **barbiturates, antibacterial sulfonamides, thiazide diuretics, phenothiazine antipsychotics, benzodiazepine anxiolytics**).

C. **Major chemical and pharmacologic classes of drugs** (Table 12-1; Figures 12-7, 12-8, 12-9, 12-10, and 12-11)

Table 12-1. Major Chemical and Pharmacological Classes of Drugs

Classification[a]	Acid/Base Character[b]	Example[c] (Structure)
1. Polyhalogenated ethers and hydrocarbons General anesthetics	Nonelectrolyte	Isoflurane (**1**)
2. Barbiturates Sedative/hypotonics; anticonvulsants	Acidic	Phenobarbital (**2**)
3. Benzodiazepines Anxiolytic agents; sedative/hypnotics	Basic	Diazepam (**3**)
4. Hydantoins Anticonvulsants	Acidic	Phenytoin (**4**)
5. Succinimides Anticonvulsants	Acidic or nonelectrolyte	Methsuximide (**5**)
6. Phenothiazines Antipsychotics; antihistamines; antiemetics	Basic	Chlorpromazine (**6**)
7. Thioxanthenes Antipsychotics	Basic	Thiothixene (**7**)
8. Butyrophenones Antipsychotics	Basic	Haloperidol (**8**)
9. Tricyclic antidepressants Antidepressant agents	Basic	Imipramine (**9**)
10. Selective serotonin reuptake inhibitors Anxiolytic agents	Basic	Fluoxetine (**10**)
11. Benzazepines Atypical antipsychotics	Basic	Olanzapine (**11**)
12. Methylxanthines CNS stimulants; bronchodilators	Basic (weak)	Theophylline (**12**)
13. Opioids Narcotic analgesics; antitussives	Basic	Codeine (**13**)
14. 4-Phenylpiperidines Narcotic analgesics	Basic	Meperidine (**14**)
15. Phenylpropylamines Narcotic analgesics	Basic	Methadone (**15**)
16. Direct-acting cholinergics GI smooth-muscle stimulant; cataract therapy	Quaternary ammonium salt	Bethanechol (**16**)
17. Aminoalkyl esters Anticholinergic agents	Basic or quaternary ammonium salt	Dicyclomine (**17**)
18. Aminoalkyl ethers Anticholinergic agents; antihistamines (H_1-antagonists)	Basic	Benztropine (**18**)
19. Aminoalcohols Anticholinergic agents	Basic or quaternary ammonium salt	Biperiden (**19**)
20. Ethylenediamines Antihistamines (H_1-antagonists)	Basic	Tripelennamine (**20**)
21. Alkylamines (propylamines) Antihistamines (H_1-antagonists)	Basic	Chlorpheniramine (**21**)
22. Piperazines Antihistamines (H_1-antagonists); antivertigo; antiemetics	Basic	Cyclizine (**22**)
23. Mast cell degranulation inhibitors Antiallergenics	Acidic	Cromolyn sodium (**23**)
24. Phenylethylamines Sympathomimetics (α- and β-adrenergic agonists)	Basic	Albuterol (**24**)
25. Adrenergic α_2-agonists Antihypertensive agents	Basic	Guanabenz (**25**)

(*Continued on next page*)

Table 12-1. Continued.

Classification[a]	Acid/Base Character[b]	Example[c] (Structure)
26. Adrenergic α_1-agonists Antihypertensive agents	Basic	Terazosin (**26**)
27. Aryloxypropanolamines β-adrenergic blockers	Basic	Propranolol (**27**)
28. Prostaglandins Eicosanoids	Acidic	Misoprostol (**28**)
29. Salicylates NSAIDs	Acidic	Aspirin (**29**)
30. Fenamates NSAIDs	Acidic	Mefenamic acid (**3**)
31. Pyrazolidinediones NSAIDs	Acidic	Phenylbutazone (**31**)
32. Arylacetic acids (includes indoleacetic acids, pyrrolacetic acids, and propionic acids) NSAIDs	Acidic	Tolmetin (**32**)
33. Selective COX-2 inhibitors NSAIDs	Acidic (weak) or nonelectrolyte	Rofecoxib (**33**)
34. Triptans 5-HT$_{1B/1D}$ agonists	Basic	Sumatriptan (**34**)
35. Serotonin 5-HT$_3$ antagonists Antiemetic agents	Basic	Ondansetron (**35**)
36. Coumarins Oral anticoagulants	Acidic	Warfarin (**36**)
37. Sulfated polysaccharides Anticoagulants	Acidic	Heparin (**37**)
38. Benzothiadiazides (thiazides) Diuretics; saluretics	Acidic	Chlorothiazide (**38**)
39. High-ceiling (loop) diuretics Diuretics; saluretics	Acidic	Furosemide (**39**)
40. Organic nitrates Antianginal agents	Nonelectrolyte	Isosorbide dinitrate (**40**)
41. Dihydropyridines Antihypertensives; antianginal agents; antiarrhythmics	Basic (weak)	Nifedipine (**41**)
42. Angiotensin II receptor antagonists Antihypertensive agents	Acidic	Losartan (**42**)
43. ACE inhibitors Antihypertensive agents	Amphoteric	Enalapril (**43**)
44. HMG-CoA reductase inhibitors Cholesterol-lowering agents	Acidic	Pravastatin (**44**)
45. Bile acid sequestrants Cholesterol-lowering agents	Basic or quaternary ammonium salt	Cholestyramine (**45**)
46. Fibrates Cholesterol- and triglyceride-lowering agents	Acidic	Gemfibrozil (**46**)
47. Steroids Estrogens; progestins; androgens; adrenocorticoids	Nonelectrolyte	Dexamethasone (**47**)
48. Selective estrogen receptor modulators Estrogen receptor agonists and antagonists	Basic	Raloxifene (**48**)
49. 5α-reductase inhibitors Antiandrogen	Nonelectrolyte	Finasteride (**49**)
50. Androgen receptor antagonists Antiandrogen	Nonelectrolyte	Nilutamide (**50**)

(*Continued on next page*)

Table 12-1. Continued.

Classification[a]	Acid/Base Character[b]	Example[c] (Structure)
51. Sulfonylureas Oral hypoglycemics	Acidic	Tolbutamide (**51**)
52. Meglitinides Oral hypoglycemics	Acidic	Repaglinide (**52**)
53. Thiazolidinediones (glitazones) Insulin sensitizers; antidiabetic agents	Amphoteric (acid stronger than base)	Pioglitazone (**53**)
54. α-Glucosidase inhibitors Antidiabetic agents	Basic	Miglitol (**54**)
55. H_2-receptor antagonists Antiulcer agents	Basic	Cimetidine (**55**)
56. Proton pump inhibitors Antiulcer agents	Basic	Omeprazole (**56**)
57. Nitrosoureas Antineoplastic agents	Nonelectrolyte	Carmustine (**57**)
58. β-Chloroethylamines (nitrogen mustards) Antineoplastic agents	Basic	Mechlorethamine (**58**)
59. Folate antimetabolites Antineoplastic agents; antibacterial agents; antifungals	Amphoteric	Methotrexate (**59**)
60. Purine antimetabolites Antineoplastic agents; Antiviral agents	Basic	6-Mercaptopurine (**60**)
61. Pyrimidine antimetabolites Antineoplastic agents; antiviral agents	Basic	Cytarabine (**61**)
62. Anthracyclines Antineoplastic agents	Basic	Doxorubicin (**62**)
63. Topoisomerase inhibitors Antineoplastic agents	Basic	Topotecan (**63**)
64. HIV protease inhibitors Antiretroviral agents	Basic	Saquinavir (**64**)
65. Sulfanilamides Antibacterial agents	Acidic	Sulfamethoxazole (**65**)
66. Penicillins Antibacterial agents	Acidic	Ampicillin (**66**)
67. Cephalosporins Antibacterial agents	Acidic	Cefoxitin (**67**)
68. Tetracyclines Antibacterial agents	Amphoteric	Tetracycline (**68**)
69. Aminoglycosides Antibacterial agents	Basic	Gentamicin (**69**)
70. Macrolides Antibacterial agents	Basic	Erythromycin (**70**)
71. 4-Quinolones Antibacterial agents	Amphoteric	Enoxacin (**71**)
72. Allylamines Antifungal agents	Basic	Terbinafine (**72**)
73. Polyenes Antifungal agents	Amphoteric	Amphotericin B (**73**)
74. Imidazoles Antifungal agents	Basic	Oxiconazole (**74**)

ACE, angiotensin-converting enzyme; *COX,* cyclooxygenase; *5-HT,* 5-hydroxytryptamine (serotonin), *GI,* gastrointestinal; *HMG-CoA,* β-hydroxy-β-methylglutaryl coenzyme A; *NSAID,* nonsteroidal anti-inflammatory drug.
[a]Organized according to chemical structure. Not an inclusive list; includes only classifications that contain multiple compounds with a similar structure. In some instances (e.g., direct-acting cholinergic agonists and H_2-receptor antagonists), drugs are chemically similar but are usually denoted only by pharmacological classifications.
[b]A general notation; some specific singular agents fall outside these general notations (e.g., ampicillin is amphoteric, whereas the penicillins are generally acidic).
[c]Structures are given in Figures 12-7–12-11.

Figure 12-7. Chemical structures (**1–19**) representing the major chemical classes of drugs listed in Table 12-1.

Figure 12-8. Chemical structures (**20–37**) representing the major chemical classes of drugs listed in Table 12-1.

VIII. DRUG ACTION AND PHYSICOCHEMICAL PROPERTIES

A. Drug action results from the interaction of drug molecules with either normal or abnormal physiological processes. Drugs normally interact with receptors, which can be either proteins, enzymes, cell lipids, or pieces of DNA or RNA.

Figure 12-9. Chemical structures (**38–53**) representing the major chemical classes of drugs listed in Table 12-1.

1. Systemically active drugs must **enter** and **be transported by body fluids.**
   a. The drug must **pass various membrane barriers, escape excessive distribution** into sites of loss, and **penetrate to the active site.**
   b. At the active site, the drug molecules must orient themselves and interact with the receptors to **alter function.**

Figure 12-10. Chemical structures (**54–68**) representing the major chemical classes of drugs listed in Table 12-1.

    c. The drug must be removed from the active site and **metabolized** to a form that is easily **excreted** by the body.

2. Drug absorption, metabolism, utilization, and excretion all depend on the **drug's physico-chemical properties** and the **host's physiological** and **biochemical properties.** A drug's physicochemical properties can be altered via the synthesis of chemical analogs, whereas the host's properties usually cannot be altered.

Figure 12-11. Chemical structures (**69–74**) representingthe major chemical classes of drugs listed in Table 12-1.

B. Two of the most important **physicochemical properties** of a drug molecule are its polarity and its acid–base nature.

   1. **Drug polarity** is a relative measure of a drug's lipid and water solubility and is usually expressed in terms of a **partition coefficient.**
      a. The partition coefficient (*P*) of a drug is defined as the ratio of the solubility of the compound in an organic solvent to the solubility of the same compound in an aqueous environment:

$$P = \frac{[\text{Drug}]_{\text{lipid}}}{[\text{Drug}]_{\text{aqueous}}}$$

The partition coefficient is often expressed as a log value.

      b. **Water solubility** (or **hydrophilicity**) depends primarily on two factors: ionic character and hydrogen-bonding capabilities. The presence of oxygen- and nitrogen-containing functional groups usually enhances water solubility. Water solubility is required for:
         (1) Dissolution in the gastrointestinal (GI) tract
         (2) Preparation of parenteral solutions (as opposed to suspensions)
         (3) Preparation of ophthalmic solutions
         (4) Adequate urine concentrations (pertains primarily to antibiotics)
      c. **Lipid solubility** (or **lipophilicity**) is enhanced by nonionizable hydrocarbon chains and ring systems. Lipid solubility is required for:
         (1) Penetration through the lipid bilayer in the GI tract
         (2) Penetration through the blood–brain barrier
         (3) Preparation of intramuscular (IM) depot injectable formulations
         (4) Enhanced pulmonary absorption within the respiratory tract
         (5) Enhanced topical potency (seen with many topical glucocorticoids)
         (6) Enhanced plasma protein binding

   2. Ionization of **acids** and **bases** plays a role with substances that dissociate into ions.
      a. The **ionization constant (K_a)** indicates the relative strength of the acid or base. An acid

with a K_a of 1×10^{-3} is stronger (more ionized) than one with a K_a of 1×10^{-5}, whereas a base with a K_a of 1×10^{-7} is weaker (less ionized) than one with a K_a of 1×10^{-9}.

b. The **negative log** of the **ionization constant (pK$_a$)** also indicates the relative strength of the acid or base. An acid with a pK$_a$ of 5 ($K_a = 1 \times 10^{-5}$) is weaker (less ionized) than one with a pK$_a$ of 3 ($K_a = 1 \times 10^{-3}$), whereas a base with a pK$_a$ of 9 ($K_a = 1 \times 10^{-9}$) is stronger (more ionized) than one with a pK$_a$ of 7 ($K_a = 1 \times 10^{-7}$).

c. Strong acids—for example, **hydrochloric acid** (HCl), sulfuric acid (H_2SO_4), nitric acid (HNO_3), hydrobromic acid (HBr), iodic acid (HIO_3), and perchloric acid ($HClO_4$)—are completely ionized. Almost all other acids, including organic acids, are weak. **Organic acids** contain one or more of these functional groups:
   (1) Carboxylic acid group (—COOH)
   (2) Phenolic group (Ar—OH)
   (3) Sulfonic acid group (—SO_3H)
   (4) Sulfonamide group (—SO_2NH—R)
   (5) Imide group (—CO—NH—CO—)
   (6) β-Carbonyl group (—CO—CHR—CO—)
   (7) Tetrazole ring (five-member CHN_4 ring; see Figure 12-9, **42,** for example)

d. **Strong bases**—for example, sodium hydroxide (NaOH), potassium hydroxide (KOH), magnesium hydroxide ($Mg(OH)_2$), calcium hydroxide ($Ca(OH)_2$), barium hydroxide ($Ba(OH)_2$), and quaternary ammonium hydroxides—are also completely ionized. Almost all other bases, including organic bases, are weak.
   (1) **Organic bases** contain a primary, secondary, or tertiary aliphatic or alicyclic amino group (—NH_2, —NHR, or —NR_2).
   (2) Most aromatic or unsaturated heterocyclic nitrogens are so weakly basic that they do not readily form salts with acids. Saturated heterocyclic nitrogens, in contrast, are similar to aliphatic amines.
   (3) Additional basic functional groups include imine nitrogens (—N≡C—), hydrazine nitrogens (—NH—NH_2), amidine nitrogens (—NH—C≡N—), and guanidine nitrogens (four atom functional group, CH_4N_3; see Figure 12-8, **25,** for example).

e. **Weak acids.** Ionization of a weak acid (e.g., acetic acid, which has a pK$_a$ of 4.76) takes place as follows:

$$CH_3COOH \rightleftharpoons CH_3COO^- + H^+$$

   (1) When a weak acid (such as acetic acid) is placed in an **acid medium,** the equilibrium shifts to the left, suppressing ionization. This decrease in ionization conforms to **Le Chatelier's principle,** which states that when a stress is placed on an equilibrium reaction, the reaction will move in the direction that tends to relieve the stress.
   (2) When a weak acid is placed in an **alkaline medium,** ionization increases. The H^+ ions from the acid and the OH^- ions from the alkaline medium combine to form water, shifting the equilibrium to the right.
   (3) **Weakly acidic drugs** are less ionized in acid media than in alkaline media. When the pK$_a$ of an acidic drug is greater than the pH of the medium in which it exists, it will be > 50% in its nonionized (molecular) form and thus more likely to cross lipid cellular membranes.

f. **Weak bases.** Ionization of a weak base is the opposite of that for a weak acid.
   (1) Weak bases are less ionized in a **basic (alkaline) medium** and more ionized in an **acid medium.**
   (2) **Weakly basic** drugs are less ionized in alkaline media than in acid media. When the pK$_a$ of a basic drug is less than the pH of the medium in which it exists, it will be > 50% in its nonionized (molecular) form and thus more likely to cross lipid cellular membranes.

g. **Percent ionization** can be approximated by using the **rule of nines.** If the |pH − pK$_a$| = 1, then a 90:10 ratio (note that there is one nine in the ratio) exists. If the |pH − pK$_a$| = 2, the ratio becomes 99:1 (two nines in the ratio), and if the |pH − pK$_a$| = 3, the ratio is 99.9:0.1 (three nines in the ratio). The predominant form, ionized or unionized, in these ratios can easily be determined (see VIII.B.2.e.(3); VIII.B.2.f.(2)).

3. A **salt** is the combination of an acid and a base.
   a. With a few minor exceptions (mercuric and cadmium halides and lead acetate), **all salts are strong electrolytes.**

   b. Because the vast majority of drugs are organic molecules, drug salts can be divided into two classes based on the chemical nature of the substance forming the salt.

     (1) **Inorganic salts** are made by combining drug molecules with inorganic acids and bases, such as hydrochloric acid, sulfuric acid, potassium hydroxide, and sodium hydroxide. The salt form of the drug has increased water solubility in comparison with the parent molecule. Inorganic salts are generally used to increase the aqueous dissolution of a compound.

     (2) **Organic salts** are made by combining drug molecules with either **small, hydrophilic** organic compounds (e.g., succinic acid, citric acid) or **lipophilic** organic compounds (e.g., procaine). Water-soluble organic salts are used to increase dissolution and bioavailability as well as to aid in the preparation of parenteral and ophthalmic formulations (e.g., timolol maleate). Lipid-soluble organic salts are primarily used to make depot injections (e.g., procaine penicillin).

   c. **Amphoteric compounds** contain both acidic and basic functional groups and are capable of forming **internal salts,** or zwitterions, which often have dissolution problems.

   d. **Dissolution of salts** can alter the pH of an aqueous medium.

     (1) Salts of **strong acids** (e.g., HCl, H_2SO_4) and **basic drugs** (e.g., cimetidine) dissociate in an aqueous medium to yield an **acidic solution.**

     (2) Salts of **strong bases** (e.g., NaOH, KOH) and **acidic drugs** (e.g., phenobarbital) dissociate in an aqueous medium to yield a **basic solution.**

     (3) Salts of **weak acids** and **weak bases** dissociate in an aqueous medium to yield an **acidic, basic,** or **neutral solution,** depending on the respective ionization constants involved.

     (4) Salts of **strong acids** and **strong bases** (e.g., NaCl) do not significantly alter the pH of an aqueous medium.

  4. A **neutralization reaction** might occur when an acidic solution of an organic salt (a solution of a salt of a strong acid and a weak base) is mixed with a basic solution (a solution of a salt of a weak acid and a strong base). The nonionized organic acid or the nonionized organic base is likely to **precipitate** in this case. This reaction is the basis for many **drug incompatibilities,** particularly when intravenous solutions are mixed. Neutralization reactions can be avoided by knowing how to predict the approximate pH of the aqueous solutions of common drug salts.

   a. Generally, a drug's **salt form** can be recognized when the generic or trade name consists of two separate words, indicating a **cation** and an **anion.**

   b. Drugs with **nitrate, sulfate,** or **hydrochloride** notations (e.g., pilocarpine nitrate, morphine sulfate, meperidine hydrochloride) are salts of **strong acids.** Thus these drugs (e.g., pilocarpine, morphine, meperidine) must be **bases.**

   c. Drugs with **sodium** or **potassium cations** (e.g., warfarin sodium, potassium penicillin G) are salts of **strong bases.** Thus these drugs (e.g., warfarin, penicillin G) must be **acids.**

   d. Drugs whose cation name ends with the suffix **"-onium"** or **"-inium"** and whose anion is a chloride, bromide, iodide, nitrate, or sulfate (e.g., benzalkonium chloride, cetylpyridinium chloride), are known as quaternary ammonium salts and form **neutral aqueous solutions.**

IX. STRUCTURAL FEATURES AND PHARMACOLOGIC ACTIVITY. Drugs can be classified as structurally nonspecific or structurally specific.

  A. **Structurally nonspecific drugs** are those for which the drug's interaction with the cell membrane depends more on the drug molecule's physical characteristics than on its chemical structure. Usually, the interaction is based on the **cell membrane's lipid nature** and the **drug's lipid attraction.** Most **general anesthetics,** as well as some **hypnotics** and some **bactericidal agents,** act through this mechanism.

  B. **Structurally specific drugs** are those for which pharmacological activity is determined by the drug's ability to bind to a **specific endogenous receptor.**

   1. **Receptor-site theory** describes the pharmacological activity of such drugs.

    a. The **lock-and-key theory** postulates a completely complementary relationship between the drug molecule and a specific area on the surface of the receptor molecule (i.e., the

active, or **catalytic, site**). This theory does not account for conformational changes in either drug or receptor molecules and is an oversimplification of a complex process.

  b. The **induced-fit theory** also postulates a complementary relationship between the drug molecule and its active site; however, it provides for **mutual conformational changes** between the drug and its receptor. Conformational changes in the receptor molecule are then translated into biological responses. This theory explains many more phenomena (e.g., **allosteric inhibitors**) than the lock-and-key model.

  c. The **occupational theory of response** further postulates that, for a structurally specific drug, the intensity of the pharmacological effect is directly proportional to the number of receptors occupied by the drug.

2. **Receptor-site binding.** The **ability to bind to a specific receptor,** although not independent of the drug's physical characteristics, is primarily determined by the drug's **chemical structure.**

  a. In such an interaction, the drug's **chemical reactivity** plays an important role, reflected in its **bonding ability** and in the **exactness of its fit** to the receptor.

  b. **Drug interaction** with a specific receptor is analogous to the fitting together of jigsaw-puzzle pieces. Only drugs of similar shape (i.e., similar chemical structure) can bind to a specific receptor and initiate a biological response.

  c. Often, only a **critical portion of the drug molecule** (rather than the whole molecule) is involved in receptor-site binding.

    (1) The functional group making up this critical portion is known as a **pharmacophore.**

    (2) Drugs with **similar critical regions** but differences in other parts may have similar qualitative (although not necessarily quantitative) pharmacological activity.

  d. In general, the **better a drug fits** the receptor site, the **higher the affinity** between the drug and the receptor and the **greater** the observed biological response. A drug that binds to a receptor and elicits a biological response is called an **agonist.**

  e. Some drugs, lacking the specific pharmacophore for a particular receptor, can nonetheless bind to that receptor. Such a drug will have little or no pharmacological effect and might also prevent a molecule having the specific pharmacophore from binding, blocking the expected biological response. A drug that blocks a natural agonist and prevents it from binding to its receptor is called an **antagonist.**

3. The **stereochemistry** of both the receptor-site surface and the drug molecule helps determine the nature and efficiency of the drug–receptor interaction. Stereoisomers can be divided into three main groups: **optical isomers, geometric isomers,** and **conformational isomers.**

  a. **Optical isomers** contain at least one asymmetric, or chiral, carbon atom (i.e., a carbon atom that is covalently bonded to four different substituents). Each asymmetric carbon atom can exist in one of two nonsuperimposable isomeric forms (Figure 12-12).

    (1) **Enantiomers** are optical isomers that are mirror images of one another. Enantiomers have identical physical and chemical properties except that one rotates the plane of polarized light in a clockwise direction (**dextrorotatory;** designated D or +) and the other in a counterclockwise direction (**levorotatory;** designated L or –).

    (2) An equal mixture of D and L enantiomers is called a **racemic mixture** and is optically inactive.

    (3) Enantiomers can have large differences in potency, receptor fit, biological activity, transport, and metabolism. These differences result when the drug molecule has an asymmetric interaction with a receptor, a transport protein, or a metabolizing enzyme. For example, **levorphanol** has narcotic, analgesic, and antitussive properties, whereas its mirror image, **dextrorphanol,** has only antitussive activity.

    (4) **Diastereomers** are stereoisomers, which are neither mirror images nor superimposable. A drug must have at least two chiral centers to exist in diastereomers. Unlike enantiomers, in which all stereochemical centers are opposite, diastereomers have

Figure 12-12. The two enantiomers of 2-hydroxybutane. The chiral, or asymmetric, carbon is bonded to four different groups: a methyl group, an ethyl group, a hydroxy group, and a hydrogen. The structures shown are mirror images, which cannot be superimposed.

Figure 12-13. Epimerization of tetracycline to 4-epi-tetracycline. The stereochemistry of the 4-dimethylamino group is inverted; however, the stereochemistry of all other chiral centers remains unchanged.

some stereochemical centers that are identical and some that are opposite. Diastereomers possess different physicochemical properties and thus differ in properties such as solubility, volatility, and melting point.

(5) **Epimers** are a special type of diastereomers because all epimers are also diastereomers; however, the opposite is not true. Epimers are compounds that are structurally identical in all respects except for the stereochemistry of one chiral center. The process of **epimerization** (in which the stereochemistry of one chiral center is inverted) is important in drug degradation and inactivation (Figure 12-13).

b. **Geometric isomers (*cis–trans* isomers)** occur as a result of restricted rotation around a chemical bond, owing to double bonds or rigid ring systems in the molecule.

(1) ***Cis–trans* isomers** are not mirror images and have different physicochemical properties and pharmacologic activity.

(2) Because the functional groups of these isomers are separated by different distances, they generally do not fit the same receptor equally well. If these functional groups are pharmacophores, the isomers will **differ in biological activity.** For example, *cis*-diethylstil-bestrol has only 7% of the estrogenic activity of *trans*-diethylstilbestrol (Figure 12-14).

c. **Conformational isomers,** also known as **rotamers** or **conformers,** are nonsuperimposable orientations of a molecule that result from the rotation of atoms around single bonds. Almost every drug can exist in more than one conformation, and this ability allows many drugs to bind to multiple receptors and receptor subtypes. For example, the *trans* conformation of acetylcholine binds to the muscarinic receptor, whereas the *gauche* conformation binds to the nicotinic receptor (Figure 12-15).

d. **Bioisosteres** are molecules containing groups that are spatially and electronically equivalent and thus are interchangeable without significantly altering the molecules' physicochemical properties. **Isosteric replacement** of functional groups can increase potency,

Figure 12-14. The presence of the double bond in diethylstilbestrol allows for the formation of *cis* and *trans* geometric isomers. Only the *trans* isomer has estrogenic activity.

Figure 12-15. The *trans* (**A**) and *gauche* (**B**) conformations of acetylcholine occur as the result of rotation around the carbon–carbon single bond.

decrease side effects, separate biological activities, and increase the duration of action by altering metabolism. In addition, **isosteric analogs** may act antagonistically to the parent molecule.

(1) **Procainamide,** an amide, has a longer duration of action than **procaine,** an ester, because of the isosteric replacement of the ester oxygen with a nitrogen atom (Figure 12-16).

(2) **Alloxanthine** is an inhibitor of xanthine oxidase. It is also an isostere of **xanthine,** the normal substrate for the enzyme (Figure 12-16).

X. MECHANISMS OF DRUG ACTION

A. Interaction with receptors (see IX.B.1–2)

1. **Agonists** interact with specific cellular constituents, known as receptors, and elicit an observable biological response. Agonists have both **affinity** for the receptor and **intrinsic activity.**

Procainamide

Procaine

Alloxanthine

Xanthine

Figure 12-16. Bioisosteric pairs procainamide/procaine and alloxanthine/xanthine. The isosteric replacements are boxed.

2. **Partial agonists** interact with the same receptors as full agonists but are unable to elicit the same maximum response. Partial agonists have lower intrinsic activity than full agonists; however, their affinity for the receptor can be greater than, less than, or equal to that of full agonists.

3. **Antagonists** inhibit the actions of agonists.
   a. **Pharmacological antagonists** bind to the same receptor as the agonist, either at the same site or at an allosteric site. They have affinity for the receptor but lack intrinsic activity. Pharmacological antagonists can be subdivided into reversible, irreversible, competitive, and noncompetitive categories similar to enzyme inhibitors (see X.B.2).
   b. **Chemical antagonists** react with one another, resulting in the inactivation of both compounds.
      (1) The anticoagulant **heparin,** an acidic polysaccharide, is chemically antagonized by **protamine,** a basic protein, via an acid–base interaction.
      (2) **Chelating agents** can be used as **antidotes for metal poisoning. Ethylenediaminetetraacetic acid** (EDTA) chelates calcium and lead; **penicillamine** chelates copper; and **dimercaprol** chelates mercury, gold, antimony, and arsenic.
   c. **Functional (or physical) antagonists** produce antagonistic physiological actions through binding at separate receptors. The adrenergic and cholinergic nervous systems frequently produce this type of antagonism. **Acetylcholine** constricts the pupil by acting on receptors that control the circular muscles of the eye, whereas **norepinephrine** dilates the pupil by acting on receptors that control ocular dilator muscles.

B. **Interaction with enzymes**

1. **Activation,** or **increased enzyme activity,** can result from induction of enzyme protein synthesis by such drugs as barbiturates, phenytoin and other antiepileptics, rifampin, antihistamines, griseofulvin, and oral contraceptives.
   a. **Allosteric binding.** A drug can enhance enzyme activity by allosteric binding, which triggers a conformational change in the enzyme system and thus alters its affinity for substrate binding.
   b. **Coenzymes** play a role in optimizing enzyme activity. Coenzymes include **vitamins** (particularly the **vitamin B complex**) and **cofactors**—mainly metallic ions such as sodium (Na^+), potassium (K^+), magnesium (Mg^{++}), calcium (Ca^{++}), zinc (Zn^{++}), and iron (Fe^{++}). Coenzymes activate enzymes by complexation and stereochemical interaction.

2. **Inhibition,** or **decreased enzyme activity,** can result from drugs that interact with the apoenzyme, the coenzyme, or even the whole enzyme complex. The drug might modify or destroy the apoenzyme's protein conformation, react with the coenzyme (thus reducing the enzyme system's capacity to function), or bind with the enzyme complex (rendering it unable to bind with its substrate).
   a. **Reversible inhibition** results from a **noncovalent interaction** between the enzyme and the drug. The drug is free to associate and dissociate with the enzyme, and an equilibrium exists between bound and free drug.
   b. **Irreversible inhibition** results from a stable, **covalent interaction** between the enzyme and the drug. Once bound to the enzyme, the drug is not able to dissociate.
   c. **Competitive inhibition** occurs when there is **mutually exclusive binding** of the substrate and the inhibitor. While it is possible for competitive inhibitors to bind to allosteric sites, these inhibitors are usually structurally similar to the natural substrates and compete with the substrates for common binding sites. Competitive inhibition can be overcome by increasing the concentration of the substrate.
   d. **Noncompetitive inhibition** occurs when a drug binds to an **allosteric site** on the enzyme. This binding induces a conformational change in the enzyme that inhibits enzyme action, even if a substrate is bound to the enzyme. Increasing substrate concentration does not overcome this type of inhibition.

C. **Interaction with DNA/RNA formation and function**

1. **Inhibition of nucleotide biosynthesis** occurs when folate, purine, and pyrimidine **antimetabolites** interfere with the biosynthesis of purine and pyrimidine building blocks.
   a. **Folic acid analogs** (e.g., methotrexate, trimetrexate) inhibit purine and thymidylate synthesis by inhibiting dihydrofolate reductase.

    b. Purine analogs (e.g., 6-mercaptopurine, thioguanine) act as antagonists in the synthesis of purine bases. These analogs do not act as active inhibitors until they are converted to their respective nucleotides.

    c. Pyrimidine analogs (e.g., 5-fluorouracil) inhibit the synthesis of thymidylic acid by inhibiting thymidine synthetase. As with purine analogs, pyrimidine analogs are not active until they are converted to their respective nucleotides.

2. Inhibition of DNA or RNA biosynthesis occurs when drugs interfere with nucleic acid synthesis. These drugs are used primarily as antineoplastic agents for cancer chemotherapy.

    a. Drugs that interfere with DNA replication and function include intercalating agents (e.g., the **anthracyclines, dactinomycin**), alkylating agents (e.g., **nitrogen mustards, nitrosoureas**), and antimetabolites.

    b. Drugs that can damage and destroy DNA include compounds that produce free radicals (e.g., **bleomycin,** the **anthracyclines**) and compounds that inhibit topoisomerases (e.g., **epipodophyllotoxins, mitoxantrone, irinotecan, topotecan**).

    c. Drugs that interfere with microtubule assembly in the metaphase of **cell mitosis** include the **vinca alkaloids** and **paclitaxel.**

D. Inhibition of protein synthesis

1. Tetracyclines interfere with protein synthesis by inhibiting transfer RNA (tRNA) binding to the ribosome and blocking the release of completed peptides from the ribosome.

2. Chloramphenicol and **erythromycin** (which compete for the same binding site) bind to the ribosome and inhibit peptidyl transferase, blocking formation of the peptide bond and interrupting formation of the peptide chain.

3. Aminoglycosides decrease the fidelity of transcription by binding to the ribosome, which permits formation of an abnormal initiation complex and prohibits addition of amino acids to the peptide chain. In addition, aminoglycosides cause misreading of the messenger RNA (mRNA) template, so that incorrect amino acids are incorporated into the growing polypeptide chain.

4. Quinupristin and dalfopristin, in combination, constrict the exit channel on ribosomal RNA (rRNA). This action prevents newly synthesized polypeptides from being released and in turn inhibits further protein synthesis.

E. Interaction with cell membranes

1. Digitalis glycosides inhibit the cell membrane's sodium–potassium pump, inhibiting the influx of K^+ and the outflow of Na^+.

2. Quinidine affects the membrane potential of myocardial membranes by prolonging both the polarized and depolarized states.

3. Local anesthetics block impulse conduction in nerve cell membranes by interfering with membrane permeability to Na^+ and K^+.

4. Polyene antifungal drugs (e.g., amphotericin B, nystatin) affect cell membrane permeability, causing leakage of cellular constituents.

5. Certain antibiotics (e.g., polymyxin B, colistin) affect cell membrane permeability through an unknown mechanism.

6. Acetylcholine increases membrane permeability to cations.

7. Omeprazole and **lansoprazole** inhibit the H^+/K^+ pump (located in parietal cell membranes), thus decreasing the efflux of protons into the stomach.

8. Several **antineoplastic** agents exert their actions by initially binding to **cellular determinants (CDs)** expressed by tumor cells.

    a. Gemtuzumab ozogamicin binds with CD33 expressed by leukemic cells and immature myelomonocytic cells.

    b. Alemtuzumab, a monoclonal antibody, binds to the CD52 antigen expressed on B lymphocytes, T lymphocytes, and various other cells.

F. Nonspecific action

1. Structurally nonspecific drugs form a monomolecular layer over entire areas of certain cells. Because they involve such large surfaces, these drugs are usually given in relatively large doses.

2. Drugs that act by nonspecific action include the **volatile general anesthetic gases** (e.g., ether, nitrous oxide), some **depressants** (e.g., ethanol, chloral hydrate), and many antiseptic compounds (e.g., phenol, rubbing alcohol).

STUDY QUESTIONS

Directions: Each of the questions, statements, or incomplete statements in this section can be correctly answered or completed by **one** of the suggested answers or phrases. Choose the **best** answer.

1. A 40-year-old man complains of dysuria and urinary urgency and is diagnosed to have uncomplicated gonococcal urethritis. He is given procaine penicillin G intramuscularly. In addition, probenecid is given to prolong the duration of action of penicillin. This type of combined drug effect is known as

(A) synergism.
(B) competitive antagonism.
(C) addition.
(D) potentiation.
(E) noncompetitive antagonism.

2. A 40-year-old teacher was prescribed lovastatin for the treatment of hypercholesterolemia. She wanted to know the mechanism of the drug before taking it. Her pharmacist explained to her that lovastatin acts by blocking the substrate-binding site of the enzyme β-hydroxy-β-methylglutaryl-coenzyme A (HMG-CoA) reductase, which catalyzes the rate-limiting step in cholesterol biosynthesis. Such drug effect is known as

(A) addition.
(B) synergism.
(C) noncompetitive antagonism.
(D) potentiation.
(E) competitive antagonism.

3. A 70-year-old man had prolonged bleeding during an elective knee surgery. Subsequently, the patient admitted to the surgeon that he had been self-administering 81 mg aspirin daily. The consultant pharmacist explained to the patient that, although aspirin has a short plasma half-life, it can irreversibly inhibit platelet function by acetylating the nonsubstrate-binding site of the platelet cyclooxygenase, resulting in prolonged effect on platelet aggregation. This drug effect is known as

(A) potentiation.
(B) competitive antagonism.
(C) synergism.
(D) addition.
(E) noncompetitive antagonism.

4. A 65-year-old woman with intractable pain secondary to bony metastasis of breast cancer had been receiving escalating doses of morphine sulfate intravenously. At 10 A.M., she was found to be unresponsive, her respiratory rate was 4 breaths per minute, and her pupils were pin-pointed. Naloxone, a competitive antagonist of the opiate receptor, was given intravenously and repeated once. She gradually became conscious and began to complain of pain unrelieved by morphine given at the previous dose. This is most likely because

(A) naloxone directly aggravates the pain caused by the bony metastasis.
(B) naloxone reduces the E_{max} for morphine.
(C) naloxone reduces the ED_{50} for morphine.
(D) naloxone increases the E_{max} for morphine.
(E) naloxone increases the ED_{50} for morphine.

5. Which of the following statements regarding signal transduction is *incorrect*?

(A) Thyroxine-bound receptors act on DNA and regulate specific transcription of genes.
(B) Cyclic adenosine monophosphate can act as a second messenger.
(C) The level of drug receptors at the cell surface increases with chronic stimulation by receptor agonists.
(D) Binding of ligand to cell-surface receptors can lead to synthesis of proteins.
(E) Antacids act by interacting with small ions normally found in the gastrointestinal tract.

6. A pharmacist is consulted about selecting a drug that is relatively safe and effective for treating the patient. He searches the literature and obtains the following data that may help guide his decision. The $TD_{0.1}$ and $ED_{99.9}$ for drug A are 20 mg and 0.4 mg, respectively; whereas the $TD_{0.1}$ and $ED_{99.9}$ for drug B are 15 mg and 0.2 mg, respectively. Which of the following statements is true?

(A) Drug A has a higher $TD_{0.1}$ and thus should be the drug of choice.
(B) Both drugs have the same margin of safety, so more information is needed.
(C) Drug B has a higher margin of safety and thus is preferred to drug A.
(D) Drug A is preferred because it has a greater margin of safety than drug B.
(E) The information obtained is irrelevant.

7. Which of the following statements concerning a drug receptor is true?

(A) It mediates the nonspecific action of volatile anesthetics.
(B) Its expression is induced only by exogenously added drugs.
(C) It can bind endogenous ligand to produce physiological activity.
(D) It mediates the cathartic activity of magnesium citrate.
(E) Down-regulation of receptor level can lead to sensitization of the target cell to the receptor agonist.

8. Which of the following statements concerning morphine and hydromorphone is true?

(A) Hydromorphone is a more effective analgesic because it has a smaller ED_{50} than morphine.
(B) Morphine and hydromorphone are equally potent because they have the same E_{max}.
(C) Morphine has a greater ED_{50} and is thus a less effective analgesic than hydromorphone.
(D) Hydromorphone is a more potent analgesic because it has a greater E_{max} than morphine.
(E) Hydromorphone has a smaller ED_{50} and thus is a more potent analgesic than morphine.

9. A 72-year-old man with hypertension has been taking high-dose propranolol for 20 years. He left home for a week and forgot to bring his medication with him. One day, he was found collapsed on the floor and was brought to the emergency room. His blood pressure was 300/180, heart rate was 180 beats per minute, and retinal hemorrhage was observed. Which of the following best explains this situation?

(A) The β-adrenergic receptors in the cardiac muscles underwent spontaneous mutation and became hyperactive.
(B) Reduction in the chronic antagonism of the β-adrenergic receptor led to down-regulation of the β-adrenergic receptor.
(C) The propranolol that he had previously ingested remained in his body and acted as a receptor agonist.
(D) Long-term administration of propranolol results in desensitization of cardiac muscles to endogenous β-adrenergic stimulation.
(E) Reduction in the chronic level of receptor blockade results in supersensitivity to stimulation with endogenous catecholamines.

10. A 42-year-old man with chronic lymphocytic leukemia undergoing therapy mentioned to his pharmacist that his doctor had prescribed rituximab for treating his cancer. The patient asked what rituximab is and how it works. His pharmacist explained to him that rituximab is a monoclonal antibody that

(A) inhibits DNA synthesis.
(B) blocks cell cycle progression.
(C) binds to cell surface molecules.
(D) boosts the immune response.

11. A 65-year-old woman experienced anginal pain with ST segment elevation on EKG. She was treated with IV heparin, nitroglycerin, and atenolol for acute myocardial infarction. Then 2 hr later, when her nurse replaced her Foley bag, she noticed frank blood draining out of the Foley catheter. The physician checked the patient's partial thrombin time which was > 150 s. The patient was then administered protamine, which acts by

(A) promoting thrombosis.
(B) reacting with heparin and thus neutralizing the effect of heparin.
(C) directly inhibiting bleeding.
(D) enhancing secretion of procoagulants.

12. A 45-year-old man with acute promyelocytic leukemia is being treated with all-*trans*-retinoic acid (ATRA). He asks the pharmacist if ATRA works like vitamin A as a health supplement. The pharmacist explained that ATRA is a form of vitamin A that acts by

(A) improving immune functions.
(B) inhibiting leukemic cell secretion.
(C) limiting leukemic cell growth.
(D) inducing differentiation of leukemic cells.

13. A 55-year-old man with a history of heavy smoking had been diagnosed with non-small-cell lung cancer, which was treated with chemotherapy; his disease progressed. He is now receiving erlotinib, and he asks his pharmacist how erlotinib works. The pharmacist explains that erlotinib acts by

(A) inhibiting protein tyrosine kinase activity of tumor cells.
(B) decreasing level of protein tyrosine kinase of tumor cells.
(C) increasing ligand binding of protein tyrosine kinase of tumor cells.
(D) inducing tumor cell differentiation.

14. Which of the following acids has the highest degree of ionization in an aqueous solution?

(A) Aspirin; $pK_a = 3.5$
(B) Indomethacin; $pK_a = 4.5$
(C) Warfarin; $pK_a = 5.1$
(D) Ibuprofen; $pK_a = 5.2$
(E) Phenobarbital; $pK_a = 7.4$

15. Which of the following salts will most likely yield an aqueous solution with a pH < 7?

(A) Sodium salicylate
(B) Potassium chloride
(C) Magnesium sulfate
(D) Potassium penicillin
(E) Atropine sulfate

16. Which of the following chemical/pharmacological classes of agents is *incorrectly* matched with its acid–base nature?

(A) Adrenergic β_2-agonists: basic
(B) Prostaglandins: acidic
(C) Organic nitrates: nonelectrolytes
(D) Meglitinides: acidic
(E) 4-Quinolones: basic

17. All of the following medicinal agents are classified as natural products *except*

(A) atropine.
(B) diazepam.
(C) digitoxin.
(D) penicillin.
(E) morphine.

18. All of the following statements about a structurally specific agonist are true *except* which one?

(A) Activity is determined more by its chemical structure than by its physical properties.
(B) The entire molecule is involved in binding to a specific endogenous receptor.
(C) The drug cannot act unless it is first bound to a receptor.
(D) A minor structural change in a pharmacophore can produce a loss in activity.
(E) The higher the affinity between the drug and its receptor, the greater the biological response.

19. The dextro (D) form of β-methacholine (structure shown) is approximately 500 times more active than the levo (L) enantiomer. The observed difference in pharmacological activity between the two isomers is most likely the result of differences in

(A) receptor selectivity.
(B) dissolution.
(C) distribution.
(D) interatomic distance between pharmacophore groups.
(E) solubility.

20. The compound shown below can be classified as a

(A) penicillin.
(B) thiazide.
(C) coumarin.
(D) phenothiazine.
(E) hydantoin.

21. Which of the following statements concerning the structure shown below is *not* correct?

(A) The compound is an acid.
(B) The compound can be used to treat arthritis.
(C) The compound is a fenamate.
(D) The compound increases prostaglandin production.
(E) The compound is a nonsteroidal anti-inflammatory drug (NSAID).

22. All of the following classes of drugs are used to treat hypertension *except*

(A) aryloxypropanolamines.
(B) thiazides.
(C) fibrates.
(D) dihydropyridines.
(E) angiotensin-converting enzyme (ACE) inhibitors.

23. Flurazepam has pK_a of 8.2. What percentage of flurazepam will be ionized at a urine pH of 5.2?

(A) 0.1%
(B) 1%
(C) 50%
(D) 99%
(E) 99.9%

Directions for questions 24–28: The questions and incomplete statements in this section can be correctly answered or completed by **one or more** of the suggested answers. Choose the answer, A–E.

A	if **I only** is correct
B	if **III only** is correct
C	if **I and II** are correct
D	if **II and III** are correct
E	if **I, II, and III** are correct

24. Drugs that act systemically must

I. undergo biotransformation into an active form after reaching their active site.
II. be in a form capable of passage through various membrane barriers.
III. be in or be converted to a form that is readily excreted from the body.

25. Examples of strong electrolytes (i.e., completely dissociated in an aqueous solution) include

I. acetic acid.
II. pentobarbital sodium.
III. diphenhydramine hydrochloride.

26. Precipitation may occur when mixing aqueous solutions of meperidine hydrochloride with which of the following solutions?

I. Sodium bicarbonate injection
II. Atropine sulfate injection
III. Sodium chloride injection

27. Drugs classified as antimetabolites include which of the following?

I. 5-fluorouracil
II. sulfisoxazole
III. digoxin

28. The excretion of a weakly acidic drug is generally more rapid in alkaline urine than in acidic urine. This process occurs because

I. a weak acid in alkaline media will exist primarily in its ionized form, which cannot be reabsorbed easily.
II. a weak acid in alkaline media will exist in its lipophilic form, which cannot be reabsorbed easily.
III. all drugs are excreted more rapidly in an alkaline urine.

Questions 29–32, refer to the drug meperidine (structure shown).

29. Functional groups present in the molecule shown include

 I. an ester.
 II. a tertiary amine.
 III. a carboxylic acid.

30. Meperidine is classified as a

 I. weak acid.
 II. salt.
 III. weak base.

31. Assuming that meperidine is absorbed after oral administration and that a large percentage of the dose is excreted unchanged, the effect of alkalinization of the urine will increase its

 I. duration of action.
 II. rate of excretion.
 III. ionization in the glomerular filtrate.

32. The appropriate chemical classification for meperidine is

 I. phenylpropylamine.
 II. piperazine.
 III. 4-phenylpiperidine.

Directions for questions 33–37: The relationship of each pair of structures shown in this section is most closely associated with **one** of the following terms. The terms may be used more than once or not at all. Choose the **best** answer, **A–E.**

A	Geometric isomers
B	Enantiomers
C	Diastereomers
D	Bioisosteres
E	Conformational isomers

33.

34.

35.

36.

37.

ANSWERS AND EXPLANATIONS

1. The answer is D *[see V.C].*
Probenecid alone is inactive against gonococci. However, it can compete with penicillin for urinary excretion. Thus probenecid can reduce the elimination rate of penicillin, whose duration of action becomes prolonged. Therefore, probenecid potentiates the activity of penicillin when the two are given together.

2. The answer is E *[see II.B.4.a; IV.D.3].*
Lovastatin reversibly binds to the substrate-binding site of the enzyme HMG-CoA reductase, which catalyzes the rate-limiting step in the synthesis of cholesterol, thus lowering the cholesterol level. Therefore, lovastatin inhibits the enzyme by competitive antagonism.

3. The answer is E *[see II.B.4.b; IV.D.4].*
Aspirin can covalently modify the platelet cyclooxygenase through acetylation of the enzyme other than the substrate-binding site, causing irreversible inhibition of platelet aggregation. Therefore, aspirin inhibits platelet function by noncompetitive antagonism of cyclooxygenase.

4. The answer is E *[see IV.D.3].*
Naloxone is a competitive antagonist of opiate receptor. If one compares the log dose–response curve of both morphine and naloxone to that of morphine alone, the morphine–naloxone curve is shifted to the right. As a result, the ED_{50} for morphine is increased. This means that a larger than previous dose of morphine is required for achieving the same analgesic effect.

5. The answer is C *[see III.D.4].*
The level of drug receptors at the cell surface usually decreases when the target cells are chronically stimulated by receptor agonists. Down-regulation of receptors is a protective mechanism that can prevent the target cells from being overstimulated.

6. The answer is C *[see VI.C].*
The margin of safety of the two drugs can be helpful in guiding selection of a drug. Margin of safety is the ratio of $TD_{0.1}$ to $ED_{99.9}$. Thus the margin of safety for drug A is 20 mg $\div$ 0.4 mg, or 50, whereas the margin of safety for drug B is 15 mg $\div$ 0.2 mg, or 75. Because drug B has a greater margin of safety than drug A, drug B is relatively safe at the dosage given to produce the desired effect.

7. The answer is C *[see II.B.2; III.D.4; III.E.1.a–b].*
A drug receptor, such as muscarinic cholinergic receptor, which can bind atropine, normally binds endogenous acetylcholine to produce the physiological responses controlled by the parasympathetic autonomic nervous system. Volatile anesthetics act colligatively as solutes in the lipid bilayer of the cell membrane. Drug receptors are endogenously expressed, but their level can be modulated by exogenously added drugs. The cathartic activity of magnesium citrate is a consequence of increase in the osmolarity of the gastrointestinal fluids. Down-regulation of receptor level can lead to desensitization, not sensitization, of the target cell to the receptor agonist.

8. The answer is E *[see IV.D.1–2].*
The efficacy of a drug is determined by its E_{max}, whereas its potency is measured by the ED_{50}. Hydromorphone has a smaller ED_{50} and thus is a more potent analgesic than morphine. Hydromorphone and morphine are both agonists for opiate receptors, and they have the same analgesic efficacy (i.e., they have the same E_{max}) if sufficient amounts of both drugs are used.

9. The answer is E *[see III.D.6].*
A chronic level of blocking the β-adrenergic receptors by propranolol results in up-regulation of the receptor level. When the patient ceased taking the drug, the cardiac muscles became supersensitive to stimulation with endogenous catecholamines. This resulted in the hypertensive crisis that caused cerebral hemorrhage and loss of consciousness.

10. The answer is C *[see III.A.1].*
Rituximab is a monoclonal antibody that specifically binds to CD20 antigen on malignant and normal B lymphocytes, leading to their destruction.

11. The answer is B *[see X.A.3.b.(1)].*
Protamine is a chemical antagonist of heparin that acts via an acid–base interaction.

12. The answer is D *[see III.C].*
ATRA binds to retinoic acid receptor on the cell membrane, leading to expression of target genes and resulting in differentiation of leukemic promyelocytes.

13. The answer is A *[see III.B.3].*
Erlotinib binds to the ATP pocket of the tyrosine kinase of the EGF receptor and thus inhibits tyrosine kinase activity.

14. The answer is A *[see VIII.B.2.b].*
The pK_a (the negative log of the acid ionization constant) indicates the relative strength of an acidic drug. The lower the pK_a of an acidic drug, the stronger it is as an acid. A strong acid is defined as one that is completely ionized or dissociated in an aqueous solution; therefore, the stronger the acid, the greater the ionization.

15. The answer is E *[see VIII.B.3.d].*
The solution must contain an acidic substance to have a pH < 7. Atropine sulfate is a salt of a weak base and a strong acid; therefore, its aqueous solution is acidic. Sodium salicylate and potassium penicillin are both salts of strong bases and weak acids; therefore, their aqueous solutions are alkaline. Magnesium sulfate and potassium chloride are salts of strong bases and strong acids; therefore, their aqueous solutions are neutral.

16. The answer is E *[see Table 12-1; Figures 12-8, 12-9, and 12-11].*
4-Quinolones are amphoteric compounds. All compounds in this chemical class contain a carboxylic acid as well as a basic nitrogen. Most 4-quinolones contain a basic piperazine ring and basic heterocyclic rings; however, some of the older compounds in this class only have the basic heterocyclic rings. All other compounds are correctly matched with their acid–base nature.

17. The answer is B *[see VII.A–B].*
Diazepam is a benzodiazepine anxiolytic, which—although it is a heterocyclic nitrogen-containing molecule—is not an alkaloid and is prepared synthetically. Natural products refer to substances biosynthesized in plants or animals. Natural products include alkaloids, such as atropine and morphine; peptides, such as glucagon; steroids, such as estradiol; hormones, such as insulin; glycosides, such as digitoxin; vitamins, such as riboflavin; polysaccharides, such as heparin; and antibiotics, such as penicillin.

18. The answer is B *[see IX.B].*
The binding of a drug to its receptor usually involves only specific functional groups. These groups make up what is known as the pharmacophore of the drug molecule. Although the entire drug molecule is present at the receptor site, only a portion of it, the pharmacophore, is required for a biological response.

19. The answer is A *[see IX.B.3.a; Figure 12-12].*
The term *enantiomer* and the D and L indicate that the β-methacholine has a chiral center and exhibits optical isomerism. Because the optical isomers have different orientations in space, one orientation will give a better fit than the other and will most likely have greater biological activity than the other. Dissolution, distribution, interatomic distances, and solubility are all related to the physical and chemical properties of the two compounds, which are identical because the compounds are enantiomers.

20. The answer is B *[see Table 12-1; Figures 12-7 to 12-10].*
Key structural features of a thiazide—a benzothiadiazine ring with an electron-withdrawing chloride atom and a sulfonyl group on the benzene ring—identify this compound as a thiazide.

21. The answer is D *[see Table 12-1; Figure 12-8].*
The carboxylic acid identifies this compound as an acid. Other structural features identify it as a fenamate. Fenamates are NSAIDs that can be used for inflammatory disorders (e.g., arthritis, bursitis). The mechanism of action of NSAIDs is inhibition of cyclooxygenase, which results in a decrease in the production of prostaglandins.

22. The answer is C *[see Table 12-1].*
Fibrates decrease cholesterol and triglyceride levels. All of the other chemical classes can be used to treat hypertension. Aryloxypropanolamines are β-blockers, thiazides are diuretics, dihydropyridines are calcium channel blockers, and ACE inhibitors decrease the synthesis of angiotensin II, a potent vasoconstrictor.

23. The answer is E *[see VIII.B.2.f–g; Table 12-1].*
Flurazepam (take note of the suffix, which helps classify the compound) is a benzodiazepine and thus a basic compound. Because the pH is less than the pK_a, flurazepam is in an acidic environment and, therefore, exists primarily in the ionized form. The percent ionized can be easily calculated by using the rule of nines. The $|pH - pK_a|$ is 3, so the ratio is 99.9%:0.01% in favor of the ionized form.

24. The answer is D (II, III) *[see VIII.A.1–2].*
Generally, drugs must be lipophilic to pass through lipoprotein membranes and hydrophilic to be excreted by the kidney. Drugs do not have to be converted into an active form at their active site, although most drugs must be in their active form when they reach their active site. Many drugs are active in the form in which they are administered. Some drugs, usually referred to as prodrugs, are biotransformed into their active form after administration. Theoretically, drugs that reach their active site and then are metabolically activated should be more specific in their action and have fewer side effects. Currently, research efforts are under way to develop site-specific delivery systems and processes.

25. The answer is D (II, III) *[see VIII.B.2.c; VIII.B.3.a; VIII.B.4.a].*
Almost all salts (with very few exceptions) are strong electrolytes, and the terminology *pentobarbital sodium* and *diphenhydramine hydrochloride* indicate that each compound is salt. Acetic acid is a weak acid; therefore, it is a weak electrolyte.

26. The answer is A (I) *[see VIII.B.3–4].*
When meperidine hydrochloride solution is mixed with the alkaline solution of sodium bicarbonate, a neutralization reaction occurs with the possible precipitation of the water-insoluble free base meperidine. A neutralization reaction occurs when acidic solutions are mixed with basic solutions, or conversely. No reaction, in terms of acid–base, occurs when solutions are mixed with other acidic or neutral solutions or when basic solutions are mixed with other basic or neutral solutions. There should be no reaction, then, when the meperidine hydrochloride solution, which is acidic, is mixed with the acidic solution of atropine sulfate or the neutral solution of sodium chloride.

27. The answer is C (I, II) *[see IX.B.3.d; X.C.1; X.E.1].*
Both sulfisoxazole and 5-fluorouracil compete with and antagonize isosteric normal biological molecules and thus are antimetabolites. Digoxin is a drug that is thought to inhibit Na^+/K^+–ATPase or to affect intracellular influx or use of calcium ion (Ca^{++}). Because digoxin is steroidal, it is not isosteric with either an enzyme, which is a protein, or an ion; therefore, it is not classified as an antimetabolite.

28. The answer is A (I) *[see VIII.B.1; VIII.B.2.e].*
A weakly acidic drug will be more ionized in an alkaline urine; therefore, it will be more polar and thus more soluble in the aqueous urine. It would also be less liposoluble, less likely to undergo tubular reabsorption, and thus be more likely to be excreted.

29. The answer is C (I, II) *[see VIII.B.2–3; Figure 12-7].*

30. The answer is B (III) *[see VIII.B.2–3; Figure 12-7].*

31. The answer is A (I) *[see VIII.B.2–3; Figure 12-7].*

32. The answer is B (III) *[see VIII.B.2–3; Figure 12-7].*

The molecule contains a basic nitrogen, which is bonded to three carbon atoms (i.e., a tertiary amine), and an ethyl carboxylate, which is an ester group. An ester is the product of the reaction of an alcohol with a carboxylic acid that forms an alkyl carboxylate. There is no free carboxylic acid present. However, if this molecule is subjected to hydrolysis, it forms a carboxylic acid and ethyl alcohol.

Because meperidine contains a tertiary amine, it is classified as a base; because it is an organic base, it is considered weak. The nitrogen is not protonated. It is not ionic and, therefore, is not a salt.

Alkalinization of the urine decreases the ionization of meperidine, making it more liposoluble and thus more likely to undergo reabsorption in the kidney tubule. This results in a decreased rate of excretion and an increased duration of action. The six-member, nonaromatic ring is a piperidine ring that is substituted at the 4-position (nitrogen is position 1) with a phenyl ring. The compound does not contain a piperazine ring or a propyl group.

33. The answer is C (I, II) *[see IX.B.3.a.4; Figure 12-13].*

These molecules are isomers that have two asymmetric carbon atoms. They are not superimposable and are not mirror images; therefore, they are known as diastereomers.

34. The answer is B (I, II) *[see IX.B.3.a.1; Figure 12-12].*

These molecules are isomers that have one asymmetric carbon atom. They are nonsuperimposable mirror images; therefore, they are enantiomers.

35. The answer is A (I, II) *[see IX.B.3.b; Figure 12-14].*

These molecules have different spatial arrangements; however, these molecules do not have an asymmetric center. The presence of the double bond, which restricts the rotation of the groups on each carbon atom involved in the double bond, characterizes this type of isomerism as geometric.

36. The answer is D (I, II) *[see IX.B.3.d; Figure 12-16].*

These molecules are neither isomers nor the same compound because one contains three oxygens, whereas the other contains two oxygens and a sulfur. Because oxygen and sulfur are in the same periodic family, they are isosteric and are known as bioisosteres.

37. The answer is E (I, II) *[see IX.B.3.c; Figure 12-15].*

These structures are actually two views of the same compound. Rotation around the side chain single bonds connecting the ring nitrogen to the tertiary nitrogen produces these two different conformations. Thus these are conformational isomers.

13

Medicinal Chemistry and Pharmacology: Drugs Affecting the Nervous System

Habiba O. U. Vongtau

Ashiwel S. Undie

I. INTRODUCTION. Drugs affecting the nervous system modulate neurotransmission in the **central nervous system (CNS),** which consists of the brain and the spinal cord, or in the **peripheral nervous system (PNS),** which is made up of the **autonomic nervous system (ANS)** and the somatic system that innervates the skeletal muscles. The ANS in turn consists of sympathetic (or adrenergic) and parasympathetic (or cholinergic) branches. Agents acting in the ANS include adrenergic agonists and antagonists, cholinergic agonists and antagonists, and indirectly acting agents that could affect one or both ANS systems. Drugs affecting the PNS are useful for treating a variety of ailments, including blood pressure disturbances, bronchial asthma, cardiac dysfunctions, anaphylactic reactions, nasal congestion, and skeletal muscle spasticity. Drugs affecting the CNS provide anesthesia and sedation, relieve pain and anxiety, suppress movement disorders and epileptic seizures, and treat psychotic and affective disorders. These drugs include general and local anesthetics, anxiolytics and sedative hypnotics, opioid analgesics, antiparkinsonian agents, antiepileptics, antipsychotics, and antidepressants.

II. GENERAL MECHANISMS OF DRUG ACTION IN THE NERVOUS SYSTEM. Drugs acting in the nervous system achieve their pharmacological effects by modifying the synaptic concentrations or receptor actions of neurotransmitters. Other drugs modulate the intracellular response pathways by which the receptor actions of the transmitters are conveyed to yield the ultimate physiological response. The major neurotransmitters in the nervous system, their primary receptor subtypes, and the predominant effects of receptor stimulation on neurotransmission are shown in Table 13-1. Some general mechanisms by which diverse drugs modulate the activity of the nervous system are summarized in Table 13-2, with examples drawn from the adrenergic and cholinergic components of the PNS. In addition, there are various classes of drugs that modulate neural function by interacting with the pores of ion channels or by binding to allosteric sites on the protein subunits that constitute the channel.

III. ADRENERGIC AGONISTS

A. **Chemistry**

1. **Direct-acting adrenergic agonists** interact directly with adrenergic receptors to elicit a response. These agonists include norepinephrine and epinephrine, which are endogenous, or naturally occurring catecholamines. The catecholamines are biosynthesized from tyrosine, an amino acid (Figure 13-1). Examples of other direct-acting adrenergic agonists are naphazoline, terbutaline, and dobutamine (Figure 13-2). The classification of adrenergic agonists and antagonists shown in Table 13-3 provides a broad perspective on the variety of agents that act on this system to produce their pharmacological and therapeutic effects.
   a. The ethylamine chain common to these agonists is essential to their activity.
   b. N-substituents alter drug activity. Small substituents (e.g., hydrogen, α-methyl group) produce α-receptor activity, as with norepinephrine; larger substituents (e.g., an isopropyl group) produce β-receptor activity, as with isoproterenol.
   c. Removal of the *para* (4) hydroxyl group leaves only α-receptor activity, as with phenylephrine.

Table 13-1. Major Neurotransmitters in the Nervous System, Their Major Postsynaptic Receptors, and Receptor Effects on Ionic Conductance and Second Messenger (Signaling) Pathways

Neurotransmitter	Primary Receptor Subtypes	Effects of Receptor Stimulation
Acetylcholine	Muscarinic M_1 (and M_3, M_5)	Excitatory ($\uparrow$ IP3/DAG)
	Muscarinic M_2 (and M_4)	Inhibitory ($\downarrow$ cAMP)
	Nicotinic (N_1 and N_2)	Excitatory ($\uparrow$ cation conductance)
Dopamine	D_1 (and D_5)	Excitatory ($\uparrow$ cAMP; $\uparrow$ IP3/DAG)
	D_2 (and D_3, D_4)	Inhibitory ($\downarrow$ cAMP; $\uparrow K^+$ conductance)
GABA	$GABA_A$	Inhibitory ($\uparrow$ Cl$^-$ ion conductance)
	$GABA_B$	Mixed (cAMP modulation; $\downarrow$ Ca^{++}; $\uparrow$ K$^+$ fluxes)
Glutamate	Ionotropic–NMDA	Excitatory ($\uparrow$ Ca^{++} ion conductance)
	Ionotropic–AMPA/kainate	Excitatory ($\uparrow$ cation conductance)
	Metabotropic	Excitatory ($\uparrow$ IP3/DAG; cAMP modulation)
Histamine	H_1	Excitatory ($\uparrow$ IP3/DAG)
	H_2	Excitatory ($\uparrow$ cAMP)
Norepinephrine	α_1	Excitatory ($\uparrow$ IP3/DAG)
	α_2	Inhibitory ($\downarrow$ cAMP)
	β_1	Excitatory ($\uparrow$ cAMP)
	β_2	Inhibitory in ANS ($\uparrow$ cAMP)
	β_3	Excitatory ($\uparrow$ cAMP)
Serotonin	5-HT$_1$	Inhibitory ($\downarrow$ cAMP)
	5-HT$_2$	Excitatory ($\uparrow$ IP3/DAG)
	5-HT$_{(3/4/5/6/7)}$	Mixed (type 4,6,7 $\uparrow$ cAMP)
Opioid peptides	μ	Mixed ($\downarrow$ cAMP; Ca^{++} and K$^+$ channel effects)
	δ	Mixed ($\downarrow$ cAMP; Ca^{++} and K$^+$ channel effects)
	κ	Mixed ($\downarrow$ cAMP; Ca^{++} and K$^+$ channel effects)

AMPA, α-amino-3-hydroxy-5-metnylisoxazole-4-propionic acid; *ANS,* autonomic nervous system; *cAMP,* cyclic adenosine monophosphate; *DAG,* d–– a–– g––; *5-HT,* 5-hydroxytryptamine (serotonin); *GABA,* γ-aminobutyric acid; *IP$_3$,* inositol triphosphate; *NMDA,* N-methyl-d-aspartate.

Table 13-2. Some General Mechanisms of Drug Action in the Nervous System Exemplified by the Adrenergic and Cholinergic Neurotransmitter Systems

Mechanism	Adrenergic System	Cholinergic System
Ganglionic stimulation	Nicotine	
Ganglionic blockade	Hexamethonium, trimethaphan	
Inhibition of neurotransmitter synthesis	Metyrosine, carbidopa	Hemicholinium
Inhibition of neurotransmitter release	Bretylium, guanethidine	Botulinum toxin
Facilitation of neurotransmitter release	Amphetamine, tyramine	α-Latrotoxin
Depletion of vesicular transmitter storage	Reserpine	Vesamicol
Blockade of neurotransmitter reuptake	Cocaine, desipramine	See note[a]
Inhibition of neurotransmitter metabolism	Clorgyline (inhibits MAO-A) Selegiline (inhibits MAO-B) Tolcapone (inhibits COMT)	Neostigmine and other AChE inhibitors
Direct interaction with postsynaptic receptors	Adrenoceptor agonists	Cholinergic agonists
	Adrenoceptor antagonists	Cholinergic antagonists

AChE, acetylcholinesterase; *COMT,* catechol-*O*- methyltransferase; *MAO,* monoamine oxidase.
[a]Reuptake is not a major mechanism for termination of acetylcholine's action; most of the released transmitter is metabolized by AChE.

Figure 13-1. Synthesis of catecholamines from the amino acid tyrosine. In the presence of tyrosine hydroxylase, (**A**) tyrosine is converted to (**B**) dihydroxyphenylalanine (dopa). Further substitutions permit the synthesis of (**C**) dopamine, (**D**) norepinephrine, and (**E**) epinephrine.

Figure 13-2. Structural formulas of representative direct-acting sympathomimetic amines. **A.** Naphazoline. **B.** Terbutaline. **C.** Dobutamine.

Table 13-3. Classification of Adrenoceptor Agonists and Antagonists[a]

Class	Adrenoceptor Agonist	Adrenoceptor Antagonist
A. Nonselective		
A.1. Indirect acting	Tyramine	
	Ephedrine	
	Amphetamine	
	Cocaine	
A.2. Direct acting	Norepinephrine	Labetalol
	Epinephrine	Carvedilol
B. α-Receptor selective		
B.1. Nonselective α	Oxymetazoline	Phenoxybenzamine
	Xylometazoline	Phentolamine
	Tetrahydrozoline	
B.2. Selective α_1	Phenylephrine	Prazosin
	Methoxamine	Terazosin
	Metaraminol	Doxazosin
		Indoramin
B.3. Selective α_2	Clonidine	Rauwolscine
	Guanabenz	Yohimbine
	Guanfacine	Tolazoline
	Rilmenidine	
	Moxonidine	
	α-Methyldopa	
C. β-Receptor selective		
C.1. Nonselective β	Isoproterenol	Propranolol
		Nadolol
		Pindolol
		Carteolol
		Timolol
		Sotalol
		Penbutolol
C.2. Selective β_1	Xamoterol	Acebutolol
		Atenolol
		Betaxolol
		Celiprolol
		Esmolol
		Metoprolol
C.3. Selective β_2	Metaproterenol	Butoxamine
	Fenoterol	
	Terbutaline	
	Albuterol (Salbutamol)	
	Ritodrine	
	Salmeterol	
	Formoterol	
	Pirbuterol	
	Bitolterol	
C.4. Selective β_3	BRL37344; CL316243	

[a]To describe the classification of a particular drug, the receptor selectivity class in the left column is combined with the receptor activity descriptor on the top of the column—for example, tyramine is an indirect-acting adrenoceptor agonist, and tolazoline is a selective α_2-adrenoceptor antagonist.

d. The *meta* (3) hydroxyl group is essential for direct α- and β-activity. However, drugs in which the *meta* hydroxyl is replaced by a sulfonamide or a hydroxymethyl group retain activity.

e. Catecholamines are inactivated by methylation of the *meta* hydroxyl group (catalyzed by catechol-*O*-methyltransferase; COMT) and by oxidative deamination (catalyzed by monoamine oxidase; MAO).

2. Indirect-acting adrenergic agonists are chemically related to the catecholamines, but they do not interact directly with adrenergic receptors. These mostly synthetic compounds induce their pharmacological effects by enhancing the release of the endogenous neurotransmitters. Physiologically, therefore, they have effects similar to the catecholamine neurotransmitters; hence their nickname *sympathomimetic amines.* Examples include amphetamine, ephedrine, and tyramine (Figure 13-3).

a. Indirect-acting sympathomimetic amines may have two, one, or no hydroxyl groups. The fewer the hydroxyl groups, the higher the lipophilicity, and the greater the absorption and the duration of activity after oral administration. Faster and greater absorption also implies less intestinal destruction of the drug.

b. Alkyl substitution at the α-carbon (adjacent to the amino group) retards destruction of phenol and phenyl compounds and increases lipophilic character, contributing to prolonged activity.

c. N-substitution with bulky groups increases direct β-receptor activity, as with the direct-acting agents.

B. Pharmacology

1. Adrenergic peripheral responses are mediated by both α- and β-adrenoceptors (Table 13-4). Adrenergic (and other ANS) receptors may be located at the cell membranes of nerve terminals (prejunctional receptors) or at the membranes of postjunctional cells, which receive the neural input from the nerve terminals. Prejunctional and postjunctional receptors are also called presynaptic and postsynaptic receptors, respectively; both the prejunctional cell and the postjunctional cell are nerve cells separated by a synaptic space.

a. α-Receptors fall into two principal groups.

(1) Postjunctional α₁-adrenergic receptors are found in the radial smooth muscle of the iris; in the arteries, arterioles, and veins; in the pilomotor smooth muscle of hair follicles; in the heart; and in the sphincters of the gastrointestinal (GI) tract. Drugs that are **α₁-selective agonists** cause excitatory responses such as vasoconstriction and smooth muscle contraction and include phenylephrine and methoxamine.

(2) Prejunctional α₂-adrenergic receptors mediate the inhibition of adrenergic neurotransmitter release. Drugs that are **α₂-selective agonists** also inhibit lipolysis in fat cells and promote platelet aggregation. Examples of such drugs include clonidine and guanabenz.

Figure 13-3. Chemical structures of some indirect-acting sympathomimetic amines. **A.** Hydroxyamphetamine (Paredrine). **B.** Ephedrine or pseudoephedrine (Sudafed). **C.** Methamphetamine (methedrine). **D.** Tyramine.

Table 13-4. Adrenoceptor-Mediated Responses to Adrenergic Agonists

Organ/Tissue	Receptor Type	Response
Heart	β_1	Increases conduction velocity (dromotropic)
		Increases contraction force (inotropic)
		Increases contraction rate (chronotropic)
Arterioles	α_1	Constricts cerebral arterioles
		Constricts cutaneous arterioles
		Constricts visceral arterioles
	β_2	Dilates skeletal muscle arterioles
Eye	α_1	Contracts iris sphincter muscle, producing mydriasis
Lung	β_2	Relaxes tracheal and bronchial muscles
Intestine	α, β	Decreases peristalsis
	α_1	Contracts sphincters
Urinary bladder	α_1	Contracts trigone and sphincter muscles, inhibiting micturition
Uterus	β_1	Relaxes detrusor muscle
	α_1	Excites uterine contractions
	β_2	Inhibits uterine contractions
Adipose tissue	β_3	Causes adipolysis; mobilizes fatty acids

  b. β-Receptors fall into three principal groups.

    (1) Postjunctional β_1-adrenergic receptors are found mainly in the myocardium, where their stimulation increases myocardial conduction speed (dromotropic effect) and the force (inotropic effect) and rate (chronotropic effect) of myocardial contraction. Drugs that are **β_1-selective agonists** include xamoterol and to some extent dobutamine.

    (2) Postjunctional β_2-adrenergic receptors are found in bronchiolar and vascular smooth muscle, where their stimulation causes smooth muscle dilatation or relaxation. Drugs that are **β_2-selective agonists** include albuterol and terbutaline.

    (3) Postjunctional β_3-adrenergic receptors are expressed on fat cells, and their stimulation causes lipolysis. A number of β_3-agonists, such as BRL37344 and CL316243, are under development as potential treatments for obesity, non-insulin-dependent diabetes mellitus, and frequent urination.

  2. Direct-acting adrenergic agonists (e.g., norepinephrine, phenylephrine, clonidine, terbutaline) produce their effects primarily by direct stimulation of adrenergic receptors. They may be receptor selective, as with the drugs listed earlier, or they may be nonselective. For example, the adrenergic neurotransmitter norepinephrine affects all adrenergic receptors, especially α_1-, α_2-, and β_1-receptors, whereas the adrenal medullary hormone epinephrine affects α_1-, α_2-, β_1-, and β_2-receptors. Isoproterenol affects both β_1- and β_2-receptors but not α-receptors.

  3. Indirect-acting adrenergic agonists work through other primary mechanisms, which ultimately lead to receptor effects. For example, tyramine acts by releasing norepinephrine from storage sites in adrenergic neurons, and cocaine blocks the reuptake of norepinephrine, thereby increasing the duration and activity of the transmitter at the synapse.

  4. Certain agonists (e.g., ephedrine, metaraminol, mephentermine) produce their effects through both direct and indirect mechanisms.

C. Therapeutic indications

  1. Epinephrine, an α- and β-adrenergic agonist, is indicated to treat bronchospasm and hypersensitivity reactions and is the agent of choice for anaphylactic reactions. It is used to prolong the activity of local anesthetic solutions and to restore cardiac activity in cardiac arrest. Epinephrine is also used topically in the treatment of glaucoma, presumably decreasing intraocular pressure by enhancing the outflow of aqueous humor and through vasoconstriction-induced decrease in production of aqueous humor. Local application of epinephrine is used to arrest blood flow in epistaxis and gingival surgery.

2. **Phenylephrine,** an α_1-selective agonist, is used to provide pressor activity in hypotensive emergencies, to prolong the activity of local anesthetic solutions, and to relieve paroxysmal atrial tachycardia. Phenylephrine or phenylpropanolamine is given systemically for nasal decongestion. Oxymetazoline and xylometazoline, also α-receptor agonists, are applied locally to relieve nasal congestion.

3. **Clonidine** and related α_2-selective agonists (e.g., methyldopa, guanfacine, guanabenz) are used as antihypertensives based on their inhibition of central sympathetic outflow. Apraclonidine is used topically in the eye to decrease intraocular pressure during surgery.

4. **Isoproterenol,** a β-adrenergic agonist, is used as a bronchodilator and as a cardiac stimulant in shock and cardiac arrest.

5. **Dobutamine,** a relatively β_1-selective agonist, is used to improve myocardial function in congestive heart failure, especially in emergency situations.

6. **Terbutaline** and other β_2-selective agonists (e.g., metaproterenol, albuterol, bitolterol, salmeterol) are used as systemic or local bronchodilators in the treatment of bronchospastic conditions such as asthma.

7. The β_2-selective agonist **ritodrine** is used preferentially to relax uterine smooth muscle in the treatment of premature labor.

D. **Adverse effects.** Adrenergic agonists may cause cardiac dysrhythmias, cerebral hemorrhage, pulmonary hypertension and edema, anxiety, headache, and rebound nasal congestion.

IV. ADRENERGIC ANTAGONISTS

A. **Chemistry**

1. **α-Adrenergic antagonists** (α-blockers) have varied structures and bear little resemblance to the adrenergic agonists. Antagonists include the ergot alkaloids (e.g., ergotamine), the dibenzamines (e.g., phenoxybenzamine), the benzolines (e.g., tolazoline), and the quinazolines (e.g., prazosin) (Figure 13-4).

2. **β-Adrenergic antagonists** (β-blockers) are structurally similar to β-agonists (Figure 13-5). The **catechol ring** can be replaced by a variety of other ring systems without loss of antagonistic activity. The length of the side chain is important, and the side chain hydroxyl as well as a propyl or other bulky substitution on the chain nitrogen are essential for interaction with β-receptors.

Figure 13-4. The structural formulas of representative α-blockers. **A.** Phenoxybenzamine (Dibenzyline). **B.** Prazosin (Minipress).

Figure 13-5. The structural formulas of representative β-blockers. **A.** Propranolol (Inderal). **B.** Pindolol (Visken). **C.** Atenolol (Tenormin). **D.** Timolol (Blocadren).

B. Pharmacology

1. Adrenergic antagonists inhibit or block adrenergic receptor-mediated responses.

2. β-Adrenergic antagonists may be α_1-selective (e.g., prazosin) or nonselective (e.g., phenoxybenzamine). Phenoxybenzamine is an irreversible antagonist because it forms covalent bonds with α-receptors, thereby inactivating the receptors.

3. β-Adrenergic antagonists may be β_1-selective (e.g., metoprolol) or nonselective (e.g., propranolol). However, β_1-selective agents may lose their selectivity at higher doses and thus block β_2-receptors as well.

C. Therapeutic indications

1. Prazosin and related α_1-selective antagonists (e.g., doxazosin, terazosin, trimazosin, alfuzosin) produce vasodilation (by blocking basal vascular tone maintained by circulating catecholamine activation of vascular α_1-receptors). They are thus important antihyperten-

$$\underset{\text{CH}_3\overset{\text{C}}{\overset{\|}{\text{O}}}\text{COCH}_2\text{CH}_2\overset{+}{\text{N}}(\text{CH}_3)_3}{} \ \ \text{Cl}^-$$

Figure 13-6. The structural formula of acetylcholine.

sive agents. They are also useful in the symptomatic treatment of benign prostatic hyperplasia.

2. **Phenoxybenzamine** and **phentolamine** (nonselective α-blockers) can be used to relieve vasospasm in Raynaud syndrome and for acute hypertensive emergencies resulting from pheochromocytoma or from intake of MAO inhibitors or sympathomimetics. Tolazoline, a similar agent, is used to treat persistent neonatal pulmonary hypertension.

3. **Labetalol,** an agent that possesses both selective α_1-blocking activity and nonselective β-blocking activity, is used in the treatment of hypertension.

4. Propranolol, a nonselective β-antagonist, is used for the prophylaxis of angina pectoris, supraventricular and ventricular dysrhythmias, and migraine headache. It is also used as an antihypertensive, a negative inotropic agent in hypertrophic obstructive cardiomyopathy, and a negative chronotropic agent in anxiety and hyperthyroidism.

5. β_1-Selective antagonists (e.g., metoprolol, betaxolol, atenolol, acebutolol) are used in the treatment of hypertension, tachyarrhythmias, and angina.

6. Both β_1-selective (betaxolol) and β_1-nonselective (timolol) blockers decrease ciliary body production of aqueous humor and may be used in the topical treatment of glaucoma.

D. **Adverse effects**

1. **Prazosin** can cause sudden syncope with the first dose, orthostatic hypotension, dizziness, headache, drowsiness, palpitations, fluid retention, and priapism.

2. **Phenoxybenzamine** can cause orthostatic hypotension, tachycardia, inhibition of ejaculation, miosis, and nasal congestion.

3. **Propranolol** can cause bradycardia and congestive heart failure, increased airway resistance, increased serum triglycerides, decreased high-density lipoprotein cholesterol, blood dyscrasias, psoriasis, depression, hallucinations, and transient hearing loss. Sudden withdrawal can be cardiotoxic owing to rebound sympathomimetic activity.

4. **Metoprolol** has adverse effects similar to those of propranolol, except that it is less likely to increase airway resistance given its β_1-selectivity.

V. CHOLINERGIC AGONISTS

A. **Chemistry**

1. **Acetylcholine,** the natural endogenous mediator and the most potent cholinergic agonist, is an ester of acetic acid and choline, a quaternary amino alcohol (Figure 13-6). Acetylcholine is unstable and quickly inactivated through hydrolysis by acetylcholinesterase. Thus it is extremely short acting and usually is not a satisfactory therapeutic agent.

2. **Therapeutically useful cholinergic agonists** may be direct acting or indirect acting.
   a. **Direct-acting agonists** may be produced by replacing the acetyl group of acetylcholine with a carbamoyl group or by substituting a methyl group of the β-carbon. These substitutions produce compounds that are more resistant to acetylcholinesterase and thus have longer durations of action. Such stable agonists include methacholine (Provocholine) and bethanechol (Urecholine) (Figure 13-7).

$$\underset{\text{CH}_3\overset{\text{O}}{\overset{\|}{}}\text{COCH}_2\underset{\underset{\text{CH}_3}{|}}{\text{CH}}\overset{+}{\text{N}}(\text{CH}_3)_3}{} \ \ \text{Cl}^- \qquad\qquad \underset{\text{NH}_2\overset{\text{O}}{\overset{\|}{}}\text{COCH}_2\underset{\underset{\text{CH}_3}{|}}{\text{CH}}\overset{+}{\text{N}}(\text{CH}_3)_3}{} \ \ \text{Cl}^-$$

A   **B**

Figure 13-7. Clinically useful direct-acting cholinergic agonists. **A.** Methacholine chloride (Provocholine). **B.** Bethanechol chloride (Urecholine).

Figure 13-8. The structural formula of neostigmine bromide (Prostigmin), a reversible acetylcholinesterase inhibitor.

    b. Indirect-acting agonists are generally acetylcholinesterase inhibitors and are divided into two major classes.

        (1) Reversible (short-acting) agents are principally carbamates (carbamic acid esters), such as physostigmine (eserine) and neostigmine (Prostigmin) (Figure 13-8).

        (2) Irreversible (long-acting) agents are principally organophosphate esters, such as isoflurophate (Floropryl) and echothiophate (phospholine) (Figure 13-9).

B. Pharmacology

1. Cholinergic responses are mediated by both muscarinic and nicotinic receptors (Table 13-5).

    a. PNS muscarinic receptors are present at parasympathetic postjunctional neuroeffector sites.

    b. PNS nicotinic receptors are present at the ganglia of both the parasympathetic and the sympathetic branches of the ANS and at the neuromuscular junctions of the somatic nervous system.

2. Cholinergic agonists act by mimicking the activity of endogenous acetylcholine at muscarinic and nicotinic receptor sites.

    a. Direct-acting agonists interact directly with these receptors.

    b. Indirect-acting agonists inhibit or block the activity of cholinesterase enzymes (e.g., acetylcholinesterase, butyrylcholinesterase), which metabolize endogenous acetylcholine to inactive metabolites. Thus, after the physiological release of endogenous acetylcholine from nerve terminals, these agents allow the neurotransmitter to accumulate at cholinergic synapses, thereby enhancing cholinergic receptor stimulation. Organophosphate cholinesterase inhibitors, such as certain agricultural insecticides and the so-called nerve gases, can be extremely toxic because they bind to the enzyme to form an irreversible or long-lasting enzyme inhibitor complex.

C. Therapeutic indications

1. Direct-acting agonists are indicated to:

    a. Initiate micturition in acute nonobstructive urinary retention (e.g., bethanechol)

    b. Produce miosis in the treatment of glaucoma (e.g., pilocarpine)

2. Indirect-acting agonists are indicated to:

    a. Produce miosis in the treatment of glaucoma (e.g., physostigmine, isoflurophate, echothiophate)

    b. Aid in the differential diagnosis of myasthenia gravis (a disease caused by nicotinic receptor hypofunction at the neuromuscular junction) and hypercholinergic crisis (which produces depolarization blockade of the neuromuscular junction; e.g., edrophonium)

    c. Treat myasthenia gravis (e.g., ambenonium, neostigmine, pyridostigmine)

    d. Counteract intoxication or adverse effects from compounds with anticholinergic activity (e.g., physostigmine)

D. Adverse effects

Figure 13-9. The structural formula of isoflurophate (Floropryl), an irreversible acetylcholinesterase inhibitor.

Table 13-5. Cholinoceptor-Mediated Responses to Cholinergic Agonists

Organ	Response
Heart	
Atrioventricular node	Decreased conduction velocity (negative dromotropy)
Atria, ventricles	Decreased contraction force (negative inotropy)
Sinoatrial node	Decreased contraction rate (negative chronotropy)
Eye	
Sphincter muscle	Contraction, producing miosis
Ciliary muscle	Contraction, accommodates for near vision
Lung	
Bronchial muscle	Contraction (bronchoconstriction)
Bronchial glands	Increased secretion
Gastrointestinal tract	
Intestine	Increased motility (peristalsis)
Sphincters	Relaxation of sphincters
Glands	Increased secretions
Urinary bladder	
Detrusor muscle	Contraction
Trigone and sphincter	Relaxation
Glands (sweat, salivary, nasopharyngeal, lacrimal)	
	Increased glandular secretion

1. **Topical adverse effects** include congested conjunctivae, myopic accommodation, and transient lenticular opacity.

2. **Systemic adverse effects** include headache, syncope, nausea, vomiting, bradycardia, hypotension, bronchospasm, abdominal cramps, diarrhea, epigastric distress, salivation, sweating, lacrimation, flushing, and tremors.

VI. Cholinergic Antagonists block the actions of acetylcholine at muscarinic or nicotinic cholinoceptors.

A. Chemistry

1. **Atropine,** an alkaloid obtained from the belladonna plant, is the prototypical cholinergic antagonist (anticholinergic agent). A portion of the atropine molecule is structurally similar to acetylcholine (Figure 13-10), permitting the molecule to bind to postjunctional receptors. However, the molecule has no intrinsic activity, and its bulky shape prevents acetylcholine from binding to the receptor.

2. **Synthetic anticholinergic agents**—for example, dicyclomine (Bentyl), glycopyrrolate (Robinul), propantheline (Pro-Banthine)—are also available. These agents, like atropine, are bulky analogs of acetylcholine (Figure 13-11).

3. An important factor that determines the pharmacological spectrum of anticholinergic agents is the presence of a **quaternary nitrogen** (as in propantheline, glycopyrrolate, and ipratropium), which reduces passage across the blood–brain barrier, or a **tertiary nitrogen** (as in dicyclomine, pirenzepine, tropicamide, and benztropine), which permits a broader volume of distribution.

Figure 13-10. Structural formula of atropine, a cholinergic antagonist.

B. Pharmacology

1. Cholinergic antagonists **competitively inhibit** the activity of endogenous acetylcholine.

2. Antagonists that inhibit muscarinic receptor-mediated responses are called **antimuscarinic agents;** those that inhibit nicotinic receptor-mediated responses at the ganglia are called **ganglionic-blocking agents,** whereas those that inhibit nicotinic receptor-mediated responses at the neuromuscular junction are called **neuromuscular blockers.**

C. Therapeutic indications

1. **Antimuscarinic agents** are indicated to:
   a. Reduce glandular and bronchiolar secretions before anesthesia (e.g., atropine, glycopyrrolate)
   b. Induce sedation (e.g., scopolamine)
   c. Alleviate motion sickness (e.g., scopolamine)
   d. Reduce vagal stimulation of the myocardium (e.g., atropine)
   e. Produce ophthalmic mydriasis and cycloplegia (e.g., homatropine)
   f. Reduce GI smooth muscle spasms (e.g., propantheline)
   g. Treat bronchospasm associated with chronic obstructive pulmonary disease (e.g., ipratropium)
   h. Control Parkinson disease symptoms and some neuroleptic-induced extrapyramidal reactions (e.g., benztropine, trihexyphenidyl)
   i. Treat intoxication by cholinergic agonists or by acute mushroom poisoning (e.g., atropine)

2. **Ganglionic-blocking agents** are indicated to treat hypertensive crisis (e.g., trimethaphan, mecamylamine, hexamethonium). By blocking ganglionic transmission, these agents reduce sympathetic activity, resulting in a hypotensive effect.

D. Adverse effects

1. **Topical adverse effects** include hyperopic accommodation and increased intraocular pressure.

2. **Systemic adverse effects** include headache, nervousness, drowsiness, dizziness, palpitations, tachycardia, dry mouth, mydriasis, blurred vision, nausea, vomiting, constipation, urinary retention, and fever.

Figure 13-11. Structural formula of propantheline bromide (Pro-Banthine), a synthetic cholinergic antagonist.

Figure 13-12. Structural formula of tubocurarine chloride (Tubarine), a competitive nondepolarizing agent.

VII. NEUROMUSCULAR BLOCKING AGENTS

A. Chemistry

1. **Neuromuscular blocking agents** can be competitive (as with the prototypical curare alkaloids) or depolarizing (as with succinylcholine). They act by blocking the effects of acetylcholine at the nerve–muscle junction of skeletal muscles.

2. The **competitive nondepolarizing agents** include the naturally occurring alkaloids of **curare,** which are bulky and rigid molecules, as well as several synthetic analogs.
   a. The **principal active alkaloid** in curare is tubocurarine (Figure 13-12). A closely related trimethylate derivative is metocurine (Metubine). Their most important structural feature is the presence of a tertiary–quaternary amine in which the distance between the two cations is rigidly fixed at abou t 14Å, twice the length of the critical receptor-binding moiety of acetylcholine.
   b. A number of **potent synthetic analogs** have been developed. These include the structurally similar **isoquinolines** atracurium (Tracrium), doxacurium (Nuromax), and mivacurium (Mivacron) as well as the **steroid derivatives** pancuronium (Pavulon), vecuronium (Norcuron), and pipecuronium (Arduan).

3. The **noncompetitive depolarizing agents** include succinylcholine (Anectine) and gallamine (Flaxedil; Figure 13-13).
   a. Unlike the large, bulky competitive agents, noncompetitive agents are slender aliphatic molecules.
   b. **Succinylcholine** has a short duration of action compared with the other neuromuscular blocking agents. This results from its simple ester functional group, which is rapidly hydrolyzed by plasma and liver pseudocholinesterase (butyrylcholinesterase). Its action may be prolonged, however, in patients with an abnormal genetic variant of pseudocholinesterase, which has only about 20% the activity of normal pseudocholinesterase.

B. Pharmacology

1. The **competitive nondepolarizing agents** compete with acetylcholine for nicotinic receptors at the neuromuscular junction. These agents decrease the end-plate potential so that the depolarization threshold is not reached. Competitive nondepolarizing agents produce a surmountable blockade of neuromuscular transmission in that administration of cholinesterase

Figure 13-13. Structural formula of succinylcholine chloride, a noncompetitive depolarizing agent.

inhibitors or prejunctional release of a large quantity of acetylcholine can relieve the blockade.

2. The **noncompetitive depolarizing agents** desensitize the nicotinic receptors at the neuromuscular junction. These agents react with the nicotinic receptors, decreasing receptor sensitivity in a manner similar to that of excess released acetylcholine. They depolarize the excitable membrane for a prolonged period (2–3 min); the membrane then becomes unresponsive (desensitized).

C. **Therapeutic indications.** Neuromuscular blocking agents, which cause only skeletal muscle paralysis (the patient remains conscious and capable of sensation), are used to:

1. Promote skeletal muscle relaxation and facilitate endotracheal intubation, as an adjunct to surgical anesthesia

2. Limit trauma associated with skeletal muscle contraction during electroconvulsive shock therapy

3. Relax the skeletal muscles and facilitate bone placement and manipulations during orthopedic procedures

D. **Adverse effects**

1. **Competitive nondepolarizing agents** can cause respiratory paralysis, histamine release, bronchospasm, and hypotension (e.g., tubocurarine) or respiratory paralysis, tachycardia, and hypertension (e.g., pancuronium).

2. **Noncompetitive depolarizing agents** (e.g., succinylcholine, gallamine) can cause respiratory paralysis, muscle fasciculation with pain, extraocular muscle contraction with increased intraocular pressure, and increased intragastric pressure. In addition, succinylcholine may cause muscarinic responses such as bradycardia, increased glandular secretions, and cardiac arrest. In combination with the anesthetic halothane, succinylcholine may cause malignant hyperthermia in genetically predisposed individuals.

VIII. **General Anesthetics** induce a combined state of analgesia, amnesia, loss of consciousness, inhibition of sensory and autonomic reflexes, and skeletal muscle relaxation. Ideal general anesthetics induce anesthesia rapidly and smoothly and permit rapid recovery of the patient once administration of the agent ceases.

A. **Chemistry**

1. **Volatile or inhalation anesthetics** are drugs inhaled as gases or vapors. These diverse drugs are relatively simple lipophilic molecules. They include the inorganic agent nitrous oxide (N_2O) and the **nonflammable** halogenated hydrocarbons (e.g., halothane) and ethers (e.g., methoxyflurane, isoflurane, desflurane, sevoflurane).

2. **Nonvolatile or intravenous anesthetics** are administered intravenously or occasionally intramuscularly and come as aqueous solutions, aqueous propylene glycol solutions, or emulsions.
   a. The **water-soluble** and relatively short-acting agents include ultra-short-acting barbiturates (e.g., thiopental, methohexital, thiamylal), cyclohexylamines (e.g., ketamine), benzodiazepines (e.g., diazepam, midazolam), butyrophenones (e.g., droperidol), and opioid analgesics (e.g., morphine, fentanyl).
   b. The imidazole etomidate is prepared as an **aqueous propylene glycol solution,** which is compatible with many preanesthetics.
   c. The dialkylphenol propofol is administered as an **emulsion,** which should not be mixed with other therapeutic agents before administration (Figure 13-14).

B. **Pharmacology**

1. **General anesthetics** depress the CNS, producing a reversible loss of consciousness and loss of all forms of sensation.

Figure 13-14. Structural formulas of nonvolatile general anesthetics: **A.** Thiopental sodium (pentothal). **B.** Ketamine hydrochloride (Ketaject). **C.** Fentanyl citrate (Sublimaze). **D.** Midazolam (Versed). **E.** Etomidate (Amidate). **F.** Propofol (Diprivan).

2. **Inhalational anesthetics** are absorbed and primarily excreted through the lungs. Frequently, these drugs are supplemented with analgesics, a skeletal muscle relaxant, and an antimuscarinic agent.
   a. **Analgesics** permit a reduction in the required concentration of inhalational anesthetic.
   b. **Skeletal muscle relaxants** cause adequate muscle relaxation during surgery.
   c. **Antimuscarinic agents** decrease buccal and bronchiolar secretions.

3. **Nonvolatile anesthetics** are usually administered intravenously (e.g., thiobarbiturates, benzodiazepines), but some agents may also be given intramuscularly (e.g., ketamine).

C. **Therapeutic indications**

1. **Inhalational anesthetics** are indicated to provide general surgical anesthesia.

2. **Nonvolatile anesthetics** (e.g., thiopental, diazepam, midazolam) are indicated to induce drowsiness and provide relaxation before the induction of inhalational general anesthesia.

3. Use of some previously popular volatile anesthetics has been discontinued because of serious toxicity (e.g., chloroform) or because of the flammable and explosive properties of the compounds (e.g., cyclopropane, diethylether).

D. Adverse effects. General anesthetics depress respiration, circulation, and the CNS. They can also decrease hepatic and kidney function (e.g., methoxyflurane) and cause cardiac dysrhythmias as a result of increased myocardial sensitivity to catecholamines (e.g., halothane).

IX. LOCAL ANESTHETICS

A. Chemistry. Most local anesthetics are structurally similar to the alkaloid cocaine (Figure 13-15). These drugs consist of a hydrophilic amino group linked through an ester or amide connecting group to a lipophilic aromatic moiety. A few phenols and aromatic alcohols also have local anesthetic activity.

1. Ester-type agents are generally short acting owing to rapid hydrolysis by plasma esterases. These agents include cocaine, procaine, chloroprocaine, benzocaine, butamben, and tetracaine.

2. Amide-type agents are generally longer acting and are metabolized in the liver. Examples of the amide-type local anesthetics include lidocaine, dibucaine, prilocaine, mepivacaine, bupivacaine, and etidocaine.

3. The drug's pK_a influences its chemical state, which in turn determines the anesthetic effectiveness of the compounds. The site of anesthetic action is at the inner surface of the cell membrane. At tissue pH, the drug is in the form of a lipophilic, uncharged, secondary or tertiary amine and thus diffuses across connective tissue and cell membranes and enters nerve cells, where it is ionized to a charged ammonium cation. The cationic form of the drug is the active form of the drug that blocks the generation of action potentials at the membrane receptor complex. Also, because of its charged ammonium cation, the ionized molecule poorly penetrates the cell membranes and remains trapped within the cell, thereby enhancing its duration of action.

B. Pharmacology

1. Local anesthetics **reversibly block nerve impulse conduction** and **produce reversible loss of sensation** at their administration site. They do not produce a loss of consciousness.
   a. Small, nonmyelinated nerve fibers that conduct pain and temperature sensations are affected first.
   b. Local anesthetics appear to become entrapped within the nerve membrane or to bind to specific membrane sodium ion (Na^+) channels, restricting Na^+ permeability in response to partial depolarization.

2. Local anesthetic solutions frequently contain the vasoconstrictor **epinephrine,** which reduces vascular blood flow at the administration site. This prolongs the duration of action and reduces systemic absorption and hence systemic toxicity.

A   **B**

Figure 13-15. Structural formulas of local anesthetics structurally similar to cocaine. **A.** Procaine (Novocaine) and **B.** lidocaine (Xylocaine).

C. Therapeutic indications. Local anesthetics are indicated to:

1. Produce regional nerve block for the relief of pain when injected close to the innervating nerve

2. Provide anesthesia for minor operations when infiltrated around the tissue site

3. Provide anesthesia for surgery of the lower limbs and pelvis and for obstetric surgery when injected into the epidural space or the subarachnoid space of the spinal cord

4. Provide anesthesia of the skin and mucous membranes when applied locally, including two miscellaneous local anesthetics: **dyclonine,** used primarily in throat lozenges and sprays, and **pramoxine,** used primarily in antihemorrhoidal preparations

D. Adverse effects

1. Ester-type local anesthetics can cause hypersensitivity reactions in susceptible individuals.

2. Systemic absorption of toxic concentrations of local anesthetics can cause seizures; CNS, respiratory, and myocardial depression; and circulatory collapse.

X. ANTIPSYCHOTICS. The classic antipsychotic agents are the phenothiazines, thioxanthenes, and butyrophenones. Chemical classes of newer compounds with antipsychotic activity include the dihydroindolones (e.g., molindone), dibenzoxazepines (e.g., loxapine), dibenzodiazepines (e.g., clozapine), diphenylbutylpiperidines (e.g., pimozide), and benzisoxazoles (e.g., risperidone).

A. Chemistry

1. **Phenothiazines** (e.g., chlorpromazine, triflupromazine, thioridazine, prochlorperazine, trifluoperazine, fluphenazine) must have a **nitrogen-containing side chain substituent** on the ring nitrogen for antipsychotic activity (Table 13-6). The ring and side chain nitrogens must be separated by a three-carbon chain; phenothiazines in which the ring and side chain nitrogens are separated by a two-carbon chain have only antihistaminic or sedative activity.
   a. The side chains are either aliphatic, piperazine, or piperidine derivatives. Piperazine side chains confer the greatest potency and the highest pharmacological selectivity.
   b. Fluphenazine and long-chain alcohols form stable, **highly lipophilic esters** (e.g., enanthate, decanoate), which possess markedly prolonged activity.

2. **Thioxanthenes** (e.g., chlorprothixene, thiothixene) lack the ring nitrogen of phenothiazines and have a side chain attached by a double bond (Figure 13-16).

3. **Butyrophenones** (e.g., haloperidol) are chemically unrelated to phenothiazines but have similar activity (Figure 13-17).

4. Newer agents derive from diverse chemical classes and include clozapine, olanzapine, loxapine, pimozide, molindone, quetiapine, risperidone, sertindole, and remoxipride.

B. Pharmacology

1. Antipsychotics have generally **similar** pharmacodynamic effects in the treatment of psychotic illness. Their antipsychotic action (i.e., improvement of cognitive and behavioral abnormalities) results primarily from their blockade of dopamine receptors in cortical and limbic areas of the brain, whereas their adverse extrapyramidal effects such as parkinsonian reactions result from antagonism of dopamine receptors in the basal ganglia.

2. Other effects vary among the classes of antipsychotics and include antiemetic activity and blockade of muscarinic, serotonergic, α_1-adrenergic, and H_1-histaminergic receptors.

3. The atypical antipsychotics (e.g., clozapine) are newer agents that show strong antagonistic properties at serotonin receptors in addition to their blockade of dopamine receptors. Compared to the phenothiazines, butyrophenones, and other classic antipsychotic drugs, the atypical agents are effective in ameliorating a wider range of symptoms, including negative symptoms, and they also are less likely to induce extrapyramidal side effects.

Table 13-6. Antipsychotic Phenothiazines

General Phenothiazine Structure[a]		

Drug	X-Substituent	R-Substituent[a]
Chlorpromazine (Thorazine)	—Cl	—$(CH_2)_3$—$N(CH_3)_2$
Triflupromazine (Vesprin)	—CF_3	—$(CH_2)_3$—$N(CH_3)_2$
Thioridazine (Mellaril)	—SCH_3	—$(CH_2)_2$— (piperidine with N—CH_3)
Prochlorperazine (Compazine)	—Cl	—$(CH_2)_3$—N(piperazine)N—CH_3
Trifluoperazine (Stelazine)	—CF_3	—$(CH_2)_3$—N(piperazine)N—CH_3
Fluphenazine (Prolixin)	—CF_3	—$(CH_2)_3$—N(piperazine)N—$(CH_2)_2$—OH

[a]Antipsychotic phenothiazines have the general structure shown. Substituents at positions marked X and R result in different drugs.

Figure 13-16. A. Thioxanthenes, similar to phenothiazines, have substituents at the X and R positions that alter drug activity. Chlorprothixene (Taractan) has a —Cl substituent at X and CH—$(CH_2)_2$—$N(CH_3)_2$ at R. **B.** Thiothixene (Navane) has a —SO_2 $N(CH_3)_2$ substituent at X and the structure shown at R.

Figure 13-17. Structural formula of haloperidol (Haldol), a butyrophenone antipsychotic.

Figure 13-18. A. Phenelzine (Nardil), a hydralazine derivative MAO inhibitor. **B.** Tranylcypromine (Parnate), a cyclopropylamine derivative MAO inhibitor.

C. Therapeutic indications. Antipsychotics are indicated primarily for the treatment of psychosis associated with schizophrenia (e.g., haloperidol, clozapine), paranoia, and Tourette syndrome (e.g., pimozide).

D. Adverse effects

1. **Centrally mediated adverse effects** include drowsiness; extrapyramidal symptoms such as akathisia, acute dystonia, akinesia, and tardive dyskinesia; alteration of temperature-regulating mechanisms including poikilothermy; increased appetite and weight gain; and alterations in hypothalamic and endocrine function, such as increased release of corticotropin, gonadotropins, prolactin, growth hormone, and melanocyte-stimulating hormone.

2. **Peripheral adverse effects** include postural hypotension and reflex tachycardia, hepatotoxicity and jaundice, failure of ejaculation, bone marrow depression, photosensitivity, xerostomia, and blurred vision.

XI. Antidepressive and Antimanic Agents may be broadly classified into five structurally and mechanistically unrelated groups: the MAO inhibitors, classical or tricyclic antidepressants, selective serotonin reuptake inhibitors (SSRIs), third-generation or atypical antidepressants, and antimanic antidepressants or mood stabilizers.

A. Chemistry

1. **MAO inhibitors** may be weakly potent **hydralazines** (e.g., phenelzine) or extremely potent **phenylcyclopropylamines,** which are ring-closed amphetamine derivatives (e.g., tranylcypromine; Figure 13-18).

2. **Tricyclic** antidepressants, which are used commonly, are secondary or tertiary amine derivatives of molecules that have a fused three-ring system.
   a. The principal tricyclic antidepressants are derivatives of dibenzazepine (e.g., imipramine, desipramine, clomipramine, trimipramine) and dibenzocycloheptadiene (e.g., amitriptyline, nortriptyline, protriptyline; Figures 13-19 and 13-20).
   b. Other closely related tricyclic antidepressants include doxepin, a dibenzoxepin, and amoxapine, a dibenzoxazepine.

Figure 13-19. Structural formulas of tricyclic antidepressants derived from dibenzazepine **A.** Imipramine (Tofranil). **B.** Desipramine (Norpramin).

Figure 13-20. Structural formulas of tricyclic antidepressants derived from dibenzocycloheptadiene. **A.** Amitriptyline (Elavil). **B.** Nortriptyline (Aventyl).

3. **Atypical** antidepressants have varied structures, ranging from the simple phenethylamine venlafaxine and the phenylpiperazine nefazodone to the aminoketone bupropion and the complex heterocyclics maprotiline and mirtazapine.

4. **SSRIs** have varied chemical structures and are related only by their pharmacologically common ability to inhibit the reuptake of serotonin from the synaptic cleft. These compounds include fluoxetine, paroxetine, sertraline, and fluvoxamine (Figure 13-21).

5. **Lithium** is an element that is used in the form of the carbonate salt in the treatment of manic depression or bipolar disease. Other agents in this therapeutic category include the organic compounds **valproic acid** and **carbamazepine.**

B. Pharmacology

1. **MAO inhibitors** appear to produce their antidepressant effects by blocking the intraneuronal oxidative deamination of brain biogenic amines (e.g., dopamine, norepinephrine, serotonin). This action increases the availability of biogenic amines at central aminergic synapses and hence the probability of interaction with postsynaptic receptors to elicit the desired therapeutic effects. Other biochemical events (e.g., the down-regulation of central β-adrenergic and serotonergic receptors) that result from chronic inhibition of MAO and reuptake blockade can also explain the therapeutic action of antidepressants. This explanation is suggested by the latency period of MAO inhibitors, which take 2–4 weeks to become effective.

2. **Tricyclic** antidepressants appear to act principally by reducing CNS neuronal reuptake of the biogenic amines norepinephrine and serotonin. This prolongs the synaptic availability of biogenic amines and hence their action at central aminergic receptors.

3. **SSRIs and atypical** antidepressants have various effects on reuptake of biogenic amines. The SSRIs selectively inhibit serotonin reuptake into the nerve terminal, thus prolonging

A

B

Figure 13-21. Structural formulas of atypical antidepressants. **A.** Trazodone (Desyrel). **B.** Fluoxetine (Prozac).

the synaptic activity of the amine. Trazodone and other heterocyclics also inhibit amine transmitter reuptake. Although bupropion appears to selectively inhibit dopamine reuptake, its mechanism may involve additional currently unknown actions because some other inhibitors of dopamine reuptake may not exhibit antidepressive effects.

4. **Lithium** appears to interfere with transmembrane Na^+ exchange, alters the release of aminergic neurotransmitters, and blocks inositol metabolism, ultimately leading to depletion of cellular inositol and inhibition of phospholipase C-mediated signal transduction. The relevance of these actions to the mood-stabilizing effects of lithium, however, has not been established. Carbamazepine and valproic acid are known to interfere with ionic conductances in nerve cells and to modulate other intracellular signaling cascades, but the contributions of these actions to their clinical effectiveness in bipolar disorder remain unclear.

C. Therapeutic indications

1. **MAO inhibitors** are indicated to treat depression, phobic anxiety, and narcolepsy that has not responded to other treatments. However, their use is limited by their adverse effects (see XI.D.1).

2. **Tricyclic and atypical** antidepressants and the SSRIs are the agents of choice for endogenous depression. In addition, imipramine is used to treat enuresis; clomipramine, fluoxetine, and fluvoxamine are used in obsessive–compulsive disorder; and doxepin is used for anxiety.

3. **Lithium and valproic acid** are indicated for the treatment of manic–depression (or bipolar disease). The antiepileptic drug, carbamazepine, has also been used as a mood stabilizer in bipolar illness.

D. Adverse effects

1. **MAO inhibitors** interact with sympathomimetic drugs and with foods that have a high tyramine concentration, such as cheese, wine, and sausage. Hypertensive crises can result. In addition, MAO inhibitors can cause a wide range of adverse effects, including
   a. CNS effects, such as CNS stimulation, tremors, agitation, overactivity, hyperreflexia, mania, and insomnia followed by weakness, fatigue, and drowsiness
   b. Cardiovascular effects, such as postural hypotension
   c. GI effects, such as nausea, abdominal pain, and constipation
   d. Antimuscarinic effects, such as dry mouth, urinary retention, and constipation

2. **Tricyclic** antidepressants can cause adverse effects, including
   a. CNS effects, such as drowsiness, dizziness, weakness, fatigue, and confusion
   b. Cardiovascular effects, such as orthostatic hypotension, tachycardia, and interference with atrioventricular conduction
   c. Antimuscarinic effects, such as dry mouth, urinary retention, and constipation
   d. GI effects, such as nausea, vomiting, diarrhea, and anorexia
   e. Bone marrow depression
   f. Mania (in patients with manic–depressive illness)

3. **Atypical** antidepressants can cause adverse effects, including
   a. CNS effects, such as dizziness, nightmares, confusion, drowsiness, fatigue, headache, insomnia, impaired memory, akathisia, numbness, and tonic–clonic seizures
   b. Cardiovascular effects, such as hypertension, hypotension, tachycardia, chest pain, and syncope
   c. GI effects, such as nausea, vomiting, diarrhea, and constipation
   d. Blurred vision and tinnitus
   e. Antimuscarinic effects, such as urinary retention, dry mouth, and constipation
   f. Bone marrow depression
   g. Sexual dysfunction and menstrual irregularities

4. **Lithium** therapy may be associated with development of fine hand tremors and increased urination; these side effects, however, usually diminish with continued therapy.

XII. ANXIOLYTICS AND SEDATIVE HYPNOTICS.
Antianxiety and sedative–hypnotic agents in current use comprise the highly effective benzodiazepines (e.g., alprazolam, diazepam,

flurazepam) and the atypical azaspirodecanediones (e.g., buspirone) and imidazopyridines (e.g., zolpidem). Diverse classes of agents previously used as anxiolytics and sedative hypnotics (e.g., barbiturates, meprobamate, and hydroxyzine) are no longer favored because of their liability to produce tolerance, physical dependence, severe withdrawal reactions, and serious toxicity with overdosage.

A. Chemistry

1. **Benzodiazepines** (e.g., alprazolam, chlordiazepoxide, clonazepam, clorazepate, diazepam, lorazepam, and oxazepam) have various durations of action, which can be correlated with their structures in some cases (Table 13-7).
   a. Agents with a 3-hydroxyl group are easily metabolized by phase II glucuronidation and are short acting (see R_3-substituent in Table 13-7).
   b. Agents lacking a 3-hydroxyl group must undergo considerable phase I metabolism, including 3-hydroxylation. These agents are long acting. Most long-acting agents form the intermediate metabolite desmethyldiazepam, which has a long half-life. Thus these agents can have a cumulative action.
   c. Triazolobenzodiazepines (e.g., alprazolam) undergo a different pattern of metabolism and are intermediate in activity.
   d. Agents lacking an amino side chain are not basic enough to form water-soluble salts with acids. For example, intravenous solutions of diazepam contain propylene glycol as a solvent. Precipitation can occur if these solutions are mixed with aqueous solutions.

2. **Azaspirodecanediones or azapirones** (e.g., buspirone, gepirone, ipsapirone, tiospirone) are chemically unrelated to the benzodiazepines. Represented by buspirone, these agents have anxiolytic activity resembling that of the benzodiazepines. Unlike the benzodiazepines, buspirone lacks CNS depressant activity and is considered an atypical anxiolytic (Figure 13-22).

3. The **imidazopyridine** zolpidem is a nonbenzodiazepine sedative hypnotic with actions generally resembling those of the benzodiazepines.

4. **Barbiturates** are 5,5-disubstituted derivatives of barbituric acid, a saturated triketopyrimidine (Table 13-8).
   a. Two side chains in position 5 are essential for sedative–hypnotic activity.
   b. Long-acting agents have a phenyl and an ethyl group in position 5.
   c. Branched side chains, unsaturated side chains, or side chains longer than an ethyl group increase lipophilicity and metabolism rate. Increased lipophilicity leads to a shorter onset of action, a shorter duration of action, and increased potency.
   d. Replacement of the position 2 oxygen with sulfur produces an extremely lipophilic molecule that distributes rapidly into lipid tissues outside the brain.
      (1) These ultra-short-acting barbiturates are not useful as sedative hypnotics but are effective in facilitating the induction of anesthesia (see XII.C.4). The action of these drugs is terminated quickly.
      (2) The prototype ultra-short-acting barbiturate is thiopental (pentothal), the 2-thio isostere of pentobarbital.
   e. The barbiturates and many of their metabolites are weak acids, and changes in urinary pH greatly influence their excretion. This is particularly true with overdoses, when a relatively large amount of unchanged drug appears in the glomerular filtrate.
   f. Phenobarbital is one of the most powerful and versatile agents that can induce certain enzyme systems (e.g., the cytochrome P450 metabolic system). This increases the potential for drug interactions and includes interaction with any drug metabolized by this system. Other barbiturates have less enzyme-inducing effect, except when they are used continuously in higher-than-normal doses.

5. **Piperidinediones** (e.g., glutethimide, methyprylon) and **aldehydes** (e.g., paraldehyde, chloral hydrate) differ structurally (Figure 13-23) and are used less commonly than the benzodiazepines as sedative hypnotics.

B. Pharmacology

1. **Benzodiazepines** appear to produce their calming and hypnotic effects by depressing the limbic system and reticular formation through potentiation of the inhibitory neurotransmitter γ-aminobutyric acid (GABA).
   a. Anxiolytic activity correlates with the drug's binding affinity to a macromolecular complex consisting of $GABA_A$ receptors and chloride channels.

Table 13-7. Benzodiazepine Anxiolytics and Sedative Hypnotics

General Benzodiazepine Structure[a]

R_1, R_2, R_3, R_7, X (general benzodiazepine ring structure)

Drug	R_1-Substituent	R_2-Substituent	R_3-Substituent	X (R_2'-Substituent)	Comments
Diazepam (Valium)	—CH3	=O~~	—H	—H	
Chlordiazepoxide (Librium)	= (ring double bond)	—NH—CH_3	—H	—H	—O (N-oxide) at position 4
Halazepam (Paxipam)	—CH_2CF_3	=O	—H	—H	
Clorazepate (Tranxene)	—H	=OH (—OK)	—COOH (—COOK)	—H	
Oxazepam (Serax)	—H	=O	—OH	—H	
Lorazepam (Ativan)	—H	=O	—OH	—Cl	
Alprazolam (Xanax)	R_1—C(CH_3)=N—N=R_2 (fused R_1-R_2 triazolo ring)		—H	—H	
Flurazepam (Dalmane)	$CH_2CH_2N(C_2H_5)_2$	=O	—H	—F	
Quazepam (Doral)	—CH_2CF_3	=S	—H	—F	
Triazolam (Halcion)	R_1—C(CH_3)=N—N=R_2 (fused R_1-R_2 triazolo ring)		—H	—H	
Temazepam (Restoril)	—CH_3	=O	—OH	—H	

[a]Benzodiazepine anxiolytics and sedative hypnotics have the general structure shown. Substituents at the positions marked R_1, R_2, R_3, R_7, and X (R_2') and the ring nitrogen at the position 2 result in different drugs and clinical properties. All compounds shown have Cl substitution at position R_7. Clonazepam, not shown, has an NO_2 substituent at R_7 and is used primarily as an anticonvulsant.

Figure 13-22. Structural formula of buspirone (BuSpar), the prototypical azaspirodecanedione anxiolytic.

    b. The interaction of benzodiazepines with GABA causes an increase in the frequency of chloride channel opening events, leading to a facilitation of chloride ion conductance, membrane hyperpolarization, and ultimately synaptic inhibition.

    c. In addition to their anxiolytic properties, most benzodiazepines have other significant CNS actions, including hypnotic, anesthetic, anticonvulsant, and muscle relaxant effects at appropriate doses.

    d. Benzodiazepines increase the depressant effects of alcohol and other CNS depressant drugs.

  2. Azaspirodecanediones have multiple biochemical actions, but their principal mechanism of anxiolytic effect is still unknown.

    a. Buspirone binds to central dopamine and serotonin receptors rather than to GABA-chloride ionophore receptor complexes. Interactions of azapirones with serotonin

Table 13-8. Barbiturate Sedative Hypnotics

General Barbiturate Structure[a]

Drug	R_1-Substituent	R_2-Substituent	Duration of Action
Phenobarbital (luminal)	$-CH_2CH_3$	(phenyl)	Long
Amobarbital (Amytal)	$-CH_2CH_3$	$-CH_2CH_2CH(CH_3)_2$	Intermediate

Butabarbital (Butisol)	$-CH_2CH_3$	$-CHCH_2CH_3$
		    $\vert$
		    CH_3
			Intermediate

Pentobarbital (Nembutal)	$-CH_2CH_3$	$-CHCH_2CH_2CH_3$
		    $\vert$
		    CH_3
			Short

Secobarbital (Seconal)	$-CH_2CH=CH_2$	$-CHCH_2CH_2CH_3$
		    $\vert$
		    CH_3
			Short

[a]Barbiturate sedative hypnotics have the general structure shown. Substituents at the R_1 and R_2 positions result in different drugs with different durations of action.

$Cl_3C—CH(OH)_2$

B

Figure 13-23. A. Structural formula of glutethimide (Doriden), a piperidinedione sedative hypnotic. **B.** Structural formula of chloral hydrate (Noctec), an aldehyde sedative hypnotic.

(5-HT) receptors may be agonistic when acting at somatodendritic 5-HT_{1A} autoreceptors or antagonistic when acting at postsynaptic 5-HT_{1A} receptors.
  b. Buspirone possesses no hypnotic or anticonvulsant properties and does not appear to enhance the depressant effects of alcohol or other CNS depressant drugs.
  c. Buspirone has minimal abuse liability and does not produce rebound anxiety after abrupt discontinuation.

3. **The imidazopyridines** have strong sedative effects with minimal clinical anxiolytic actions.
  a. Zolpidem is as effective as the benzodiazepines in shortening sleep latency and in prolonging total sleep time in patients with insomnia.
  b. Zolpidem is rarely associated with physical dependence, rebound insomnia, or respiratory depression even in overdosage.

4. **Barbiturates** are less selective than benzodiazepines and produce generalized CNS depression.
  a. Barbiturates bind to a site that is distinct from the benzodiazepine binding site on a macromolecular GABA-chloride ionophore receptor complex. Barbiturate binding induces an increase in the duration of channel opening events and thus mimics or enhances the inhibitory actions of GABA.
  b. Barbiturates have a wide range of dose-dependent pharmacological actions related to CNS depression, including sedation, hypnosis, and anesthesia. They also act as potent respiratory depressants and inducers of hepatic microsomal drug-metabolizing enzyme activity.

5. **Piperidinediones, aldehydes,** and other nonbarbiturate sedative hypnotics have similar pharmacological actions related to CNS depression.
  a. Chloral hydrate is commonly used to induce sleep in pediatric or geriatric patients. Its low cost is the major factor accounting for its preferred use in institutional settings.
  b. Chloral hydrate is biotransformed to trichloroethanol, which is responsible for the pharmacological activity of the drug. Chloral hydrate induces hepatic microsomal drug-metabolizing enzyme activity.

C. **Therapeutic indications**

1. **Benzodiazepines and the azaspirodecanedione buspirone** are indicated to treat anxiety. Buspirone is more effective in patients with generalized anxiety of mild to moderate severity. The antianxiety effects of buspirone may require up to a week to be established.

2. **Benzodiazepines and the imidazopyridine** are indicated to produce drowsiness and promote sleep.

3. **Benzodiazepines** are indicated for use as a preanesthetic medication, as anticonvulsants, and during acute alcohol withdrawal.

4. **Barbiturates** are no longer considered appropriate as anxiolytics or sedative hypnotics in view of the availability of the safer benzodiazepines. Long-acting barbiturates continue to be widely used as antiepileptics, and the ultra-short-acting barbiturates are used for the induction of general anesthesia and as general anesthetics for short surgical procedures.

5. Chloral hydrate is indicated for use as a pediatric or geriatric hypnotic and as a preanesthetic agent for minor surgical and dental procedures.

D. Adverse effects

1. Adverse effects associated with **benzodiazepines** include
   a. CNS effects, such as CNS depression, drowsiness, sedation, ataxia, confusion, and dysarthria
   b. GI effects, such as nausea, vomiting, and diarrhea
   c. Psychiatric effects (rare), such as paradoxical excitement, insomnia, paranoia, and rage reactions
   d. Potential for abuse and dependence

2. Adverse effects of **buspirone** are limited to restlessness, dizziness, headache, nausea, diarrhea, and paresthesias.

3. **Barbiturates** can cause a variety of adverse effects, including
   a. CNS effects, such as drowsiness, confusion, nystagmus, dysarthria, depressed sympathetic ganglionic transmission, hyperalgesia, impaired judgment, impaired fine motor skills, paradoxical excitement (in geriatric patients), and potentiation of other CNS depressant drugs
   b. Respiratory and cardiovascular effects, such as respiratory depression, bradycardia, and orthostatic hypotension
   c. GI effects, such as nausea, vomiting, constipation, diarrhea, and epigastric distress
   d. Exfoliative dermatitis and Stevens-Johnson syndrome
   e. Headache, fever, hepatotoxicity, and megaloblastic anemia (with the chronic use of phenobarbital)

4. **Trichloroethanol,** the active metabolite of **chloral hydrate,** is metabolized to trichloroacetic acid, which is highly toxic and tends to accumulate with repeated administration of chloral hydrate. Use of chloral hydrate is associated with the following adverse effects.
   a. GI effects, such as GI irritation and upset, nausea, and vomiting
   b. CNS effects, such as CNS depression, disorientation, incoherence, drowsiness, ataxia, headache, and potentiation of other CNS depressants (particularly alcohol)
   c. Leukopenia

XIII. ANTIEPILEPTICS

A. Chemistry. Antiepileptics (anticonvulsants) vary widely in structure (Figure 13-24).

1. **Older agents,** which are still widely used, include derivatives of the long-acting barbiturates (e.g., phenobarbital, mephobarbital, metharbital, primidone), hydantoins (e.g., phenytoin, ethotoin), succinimides (e.g., ethosuximide, phensuximide), oxazolidinediones (e.g., trimethadione, dimethadione), and dialkylacetates (e.g., valproic acid).

2. **Newer agents,** which are more structurally diverse, include the iminostilbenes (e.g., carbamazepine), benzodiazepines (e.g., diazepam, clonazepam, clorazepate), GABA-analog GABApentin, phenyltriazine derivative lamotrigine, and dicarbamate felbamate.

B. Pharmacology

1. Antiepileptics prevent or reduce excessive discharge and reduce the spread of excitation from CNS seizure foci.

2. The mechanisms of action of antiepileptics appear to be alteration of Na^+ neuronal concentrations by promotion of Na^+ efflux (e.g., hydantoins) and restoration or enhancement of GABAergic inhibitory neuronal function (e.g., barbiturates, benzodiazepines, valproic acid).

C. Therapeutic indications. These agents are generally categorized by the type of seizure against which they are effective.

Figure 13-24. Structural formulas of the antiepileptic agents. **A.** Primidone (Mysoline). **B.** Phenytoin (Dilantin). **C.** Ethosuximide (Zarontin). **D.** Trimethadione (Tridione). **E.** Clonazepam (Klonopin). **F.** Carbamazepine (Tegretol). **G.** Valproic acid (Depakene).

1. Drugs that are indicated for the treatment of **tonic–clonic (grand mal) seizures** include phenobarbital, phenytoin, primidone, and carbamazepine.

2. Drugs that are indicated for the treatment of **absence (petit mal) seizures** include phenobarbital, ethosuximide, trimethadione, clonazepam, and valproic acid.

3. Clonazepam is indicated for the treatment of **myoclonic seizures.**

4. Agents that are effective against **partial seizures** include clorazepate, felbamate, gabapentin, and lamotrigine.

5. Phenytoin, phenobarbital, primidone, and carbamazepine are effective against **psychomotor seizures.**

6. Intravenous diazepam, phenytoin, and phenobarbital are indicated for the treatment of **status epilepticus.**

D. Adverse effects

1. **Barbiturates** (see XII.D.3) and **benzodiazepines** (see XII.D.1) used as antiepileptics have the same adverse effects as when used for anxiolytic or sedative–hypnotic purposes. Intravenous use of these agents could cause cardiovascular collapse and respiratory depression.

2. Antiepileptic agents generally have the propensity to cause the following side effects:
   a. GI irritation, nausea, and vomiting
   b. CNS sedation, diplopia, nystagmus, ataxia, dizziness, and confusion
   c. Blood dyscrasias, including aplastic anemia and bleeding disorders
   d. Allergic-type reactions, including Stevens-Johnson syndrome
   e. Various organ-system toxicities, including renal and liver failure, pancreatitis, and cardiotoxicity

3. The hydantoins (e.g., phenytoin) can also cause specific arrhythmias and gingival hyperplasia.

4. Antiepileptics as a class also have the potential to cause various **birth defects,** including cleft palate (e.g., carbamazepine, phenytoin) and neural tube defects (e.g., valproic acid). These effects present a unique problem in treating pregnant women with convulsive disorders. Discontinuation of anticonvulsant therapy can result in a seizure state that could harm the fetus. However, continued therapy can increase the risk of birth defects and place the mother at risk of bleeding disorders during delivery. Moreover, pregnancy by itself can either increase or decrease seizure incidence of the mother. Risk–benefit evaluation of therapy should be made on individual cases based on the patient's history.

XIV. ANTIPARKINSONIAN AGENTS

A. **Chemistry.** The principal antiparkinsonian agents are either **dopaminergic agonists** or **cholinergic antagonists.**

1. Some **anticholinergic antiparkinsonian** agents are structurally related to **atropine** (e.g., benztropine, trihexyphenidyl). Other antiparkinsonian anticholinergic agents are procyclidine (Kemadrin), orphenadrine (Norflex), and biperiden (Akineton).

2. The prototypical **dopaminergic** antiparkinsonian agent is the **catecholamine levodopa** (Figure 13-25), a prodrug that must be converted in vivo to dopamine by **dopa decarboxylase.** Direct receptor-acting dopaminergics include **ergolines,** such as bromocriptine (Parlodel) and pergolide (Permax); the phenanthrene **apomorphine;** and the newer nonergoline dopamine agonists **pramipexole** (Mirapex) and **ropinirole** (Requip).

3. Three agents are available that improve the therapeutic efficacy and safety of levodopa.
   a. **Carbidopa,** a levodopa analog that does not cross the blood–brain barrier, is a **decarboxylase inhibitor** that diminishes the decarboxylation and subsequent inactivation of levodopa in **peripheral tissues.** A combination of levodopa and carbidopa (Sinemet) is available for clinical use.
   b. **Selegiline (deprenyl),** is a **selective MAO-B inhibitor** that inhibits the intracerebral degradation of endogenous or levodopa-derived dopamine.
   c. **Tolcapone** or **entacapone** are selective inhibitors of COMT, thus reducing the conversion of levodopa to 3-*O*-methyldopa, an inactive metabolite that also inhibits levodopa uptake into the brain.

B. **Pharmacology.** Antiparkinsonian agents act by restoring the striatal balance of dopaminergic and cholinergic neurotransmission, which is deranged in parkinsonism as a result of degeneration of dopaminergic neurons that supply dopamine to the **striatum (caudate-putamen).**

1. **Levodopa,** which can cross the blood–brain barrier, is the immediate precursor of the striatal neurotransmitter dopamine and is converted to dopamine in the body.

2. **Amantadine,** an antiviral agent, appears to stimulate the release of dopamine from intact striatal dopaminergic terminals.

3. **Apomorphine, bromocriptine, pergolide, pramipexole, and ropinirole,** which are direct dopaminergic receptor agonists, mimic the activity of dopamine in the caudate-putamen.

Figure 13-25. Structural formulas of antiparkinsonian agents. **A.** Benztropine (Cogentin). **B.** Trihexy-phenidyl (Artane). **C.** Ethopropazine (Parsidol). **D.** Levodopa (Larodopa).

4. **Selegiline,** an inhibitor of the central MAO-B isoenzyme, blocks the central catabolism of dopamine, increasing its availability in the caudate-putamen.

5. **Anticholinergics,** such as trihexyphenidyl, benztropine, and orphenadrine, block the excitatory cholinergic system, thus reducing the functional imbalance between dopamine and acetylcholine in the striatum.

6. The enzyme inhibitors, **carbidopa and tolcapone,** increase the transport and bioavailability of levodopa in the brain and are thus given as adjunctive treatments with levodopa.

C. Therapeutic indications

1. **Levodopa,** currently the most effective treatment for parkinsonism, is indicated to treat the idiopathic, postencephalitic, or arteriosclerotic form of the disease.

2. **Amantadine** is indicated to treat idiopathic, postencephalitic, or arteriosclerotic parkinsonism as well as extrapyramidal symptoms induced by antipsychotic drugs (with the exception of tardive dyskinesia).

3. **Apomorphine** (Apokyn) has been approved for treating the rigidity and akinesia or immobility associated with Parkinson disease.

4. **Bromocriptine** is indicated to treat idiopathic or postencephalitic parkinsonism.

5. **Selegiline, anticholinergics,** and **antihistamines** are indicated for use as adjunctive therapy for all types of parkinsonism, including drug-induced extrapyramidal symptoms (with the exception of tardive dyskinesia).

D. Adverse effects

1. **Levodopa** is associated with the following adverse effects:
   a. GI effects, such as GI upset, nausea, vomiting, anorexia, and excessive salivation
   b. Cardiovascular effects, such as orthostatic hypotension, tachycardia, and dysrhythmias
   c. CNS effects, such as headache, dizziness, and insomnia

    d. Abnormal involuntary movements, such as dyskinesia and choreiform or dystonic movements

    e. Psychiatric effects, such as delusions, hallucinations, confusion, psychoses, and depression

2. Apomorphine can cause nausea and vomiting, somnolence, dizziness, and hallucinations and may exacerbate existing dyskinesia. The drug has a reasonable potential for abuse, primarily because of its perceived prolibido effects.

3. Amantadine is associated with the following adverse effects:
    a. CNS effects, such as drowsiness, insomnia, dizziness, slurred speech, and nightmares
    b. Urinary retention and ankle edema
    c. Livedo reticularis (mottling of skin on the extremities)
    d. Psychiatric effects, such as hallucinations and confusion

4. Bromocriptine and related ergolines are associated with nausea, hypotension, psychiatric effects such as confusion and hallucinations, livedo reticularis, and abnormal involuntary movements such as dyskinesia and choreiform of dystonic movements.

5. Selegiline is associated with adverse effects that are similar to those of bromocriptine, including dyskinesias and hallucinations.

6. Anticholinergic antiparkinsonian agents have the same adverse effects as other cholinergic antagonists (see VI.D).

XV. OPIOID ANALGESICS AND ANTAGONISTS. Analgesic opioids are opioid receptor agonists that consist of natural opiate alkaloids and their synthetic derivatives.

A. Chemistry. The opiate alkaloids are derived from opium, which is considered the oldest drug on record. **Opium** (the dried exudate of the poppy seed capsule) contains about 25 different alkaloids. Of these, morphine is the most important, both quantitatively and pharmacologically (Figure 13-26).

1. Morphine's phenolic hydroxyl group is extremely important for activity; however, analgesic activity appears to depend on a *p*-phenyl-*N*-alkylpiperidine moiety, in which the piperidine ring is in the chair form and is perpendicular to the aromatic ring. The alkyl group is usually methyl. The **morphine molecule** can be altered in a variety of ways; related compounds also can be synthesized from other starting materials.

2. Natural or synthetic opioids may be classified into four chemical groups (Figure 13-27):
    a. Phenanthrenes (e.g., morphine and hydromorphone; codeine and hydrocodone; nalbuphine and buprenorphine; nalorphine, naltrexone, and naloxone). Methylation of the phenolic 3-hydroxyl group with or without modification of the 6-hydroxyl group of morphine yields agents with reduced agonist potency but enhanced oral bioavailability (e.g., codeine, hydrocodone, oxycodone).
    b. Phenylheptylamines (e.g., methadone and propoxyphene) are bisphenyl derivatives of heptylamine that have strong (methadone) or moderate (propoxyphene) agonist potency and excellent oral bioavailability.
    c. Phenylpiperidines include meperidine, fentanyl, and sufentanil, which are strong agonists that are more effective when given parenterally, and the moderate agonists diphenoxylate and loperamide.
    d. The **morphinan** levorphanol is a strong agonist with high oral bioavailability.

Figure 13-26. Structural formula of morphine.

Figure 13-27. Structural formulas of selected opioid agonists. Morphine analogs: (**A**) codeine, (**B**) heroin, (**C**) hydromorphone (Dilaudid), and (**D**) oxycodone (Percodan). Piperidine analgesics: (**E**) meperidine (Demerol) and (**F**) diphenoxylate (Lomotil). Methadone analgesics: (**G**) methadone (Dolophine) and (**H**) propoxyphene (Darvon).

Figure 13-28. Structural formulas of opioid antagonists. **A.** Naloxone (Narcan). **B.** Pentazocine (Talwin). **C.** Butorphanol (Stadol).

3. **Opioid antagonists** are derived by replacing the methyl group on the nitrogen atom with more bulky substitutions. Thus nalbuphine and buprenorphine are phenanthrene **mixed agonist–antagonists;** naltrexone and naloxone are phenanthrene **pure antagonists;** and butorphanol and levallorphan are morphinan-derived antagonists (Figure 13-28).

4. Agents having both a free phenolic hydroxyl group and a tertiary amine function (e.g., morphine and nalbuphine) are chemically amphoteric. Amphotericity probably accounts for the erratic absorption of morphine when administered orally.

5. Some newer opioid analgesic agents, such as **tramadol,** are chemically unrelated to the natural, semisynthetic, and synthetic opiate derivatives.

6. Numerous analog of endogenous opioid peptides have been synthesized and are being used in research.

B. Pharmacology

1. **Opioid analgesics** mimic the actions of endogenous opioid peptides at CNS opioid receptors, raising the pain threshold and increasing pain tolerance. The analgesic actions are mediated primarily through the μ-subtype of opioid receptors.

2. Other actions attributable to stimulation of opioid receptors include induction of euphoria, sedation, cough suppression, and chemoreceptor trigger-zone stimulation leading to nausea and vomiting.

3. **Tramadol** appears to act via a metabolite, which is selective for the μ-opioid receptor and also inhibits reuptake of norepinephrine and serotonin. Its nonopiate character appears to confer no clear benefits over the opiates.

4. **Pure opioid antagonists** such as naloxone block the actions of opioid agonists. **Mixed agonist–antagonists** such as nalbuphine, buprenorphine, butorphanol, and pentazocine block the actions of agonists at some receptor subtypes while directly stimulating other receptor subtypes to produce agonistic effects.

C. Therapeutic indications

1. Opioid analgesics are indicated to relieve **moderate to severe pain,** such as the pain associated with myocardial infarction, cancer, and labor. In the latter use, meperidine is preferred to morphine because meperidine is less likely to induce **neonatal respiratory depression.**

2. Opioids are used also as **preanesthetic medications,** as **analgesic adjuncts during anesthesia,** and occasionally as a primary anesthetic agent.

3. Mild to moderate agonistic opioids are used as **antitussives** (e.g., codeine and dextromethorphan) and as **antidiarrheals** (e.g., diphenoxylate and loperamide).

4. Pure opioid antagonists are used as antidotes to reverse the adverse effects of opioid agonists or opioid agonist–antagonists (e.g., respiratory depression, cardiovascular depression, sedation). Naltrexone is an orally active compound that possesses pure antagonistic activity and is used in the treatment of opioid addiction.

D. Adverse effects

1. Opioid analgesics are associated with the following adverse effects:

a. CNS effects, including CNS depression, miosis, dizziness, sedation, confusion, disorientation, and coma

b. GI effects, including nausea, vomiting, constipation, biliary spasm, and increased biliary tract pressure

c. Cardiovascular effects, such as orthostatic hypotension, peripheral circulatory collapse, dysrhythmias, and cardiac arrest

d. Respiratory depression

e. Bronchoconstriction

f. Psychiatric effects, such as euphoria, dysphoria, and hallucinations

g. Abuse potential and dependence

h. Precipitation of withdrawal symptoms in opioid-dependent patients (when opioid agonist–antagonists, such as pentazocine or nalbuphine, are used as analgesics)

i. Classic opioid analgesics can also prompt the release of histamine, causing intense pruritus, vasodilation, and bronchoconstriction, which can be confused with a true allergic reaction.

j. Tramadol appears to have significantly fewer respiratory depressant effects than the classic opioids. It also does not appear to cause the release of histamine. It has fewer cardiovascular effects with the exception of orthostatic hypotension, which is produced. Tramadol does possess the typical μ receptor-mediated side effects of constipation, nausea, vomiting, and sedation.

2. Opioid antagonists are associated with the following adverse effects:

a. Pure opioid antagonists can precipitate a withdrawal syndrome in opioid-dependent patients. Pure antagonists, given in the absence of opioid agonists or agonist–antagonists, produce no clinically significant effects.

b. In the absence of opioids, mixed agonist–antagonists produce opioid-like effects, such as respiratory depression.

STUDY QUESTIONS

Directions for questions 1–14: Each of the questions, statements, or incomplete statements in this section can be correctly answered or completed by **one** of the suggested answers or phrases. Choose the **best** answer.

1. Which of the following drugs would most likely be used in the treatment of bronchospasm that is associated with chronic obstructive pulmonary disease?

   (A) edrophonium
   (B) ipratropium
   (C) ambenonium
   (D) propantheline
   (E) homatropine

2. All of the following adverse effects are manifestations of cholinergic agonists *except*

   (A) bradycardia.
   (B) bronchoconstriction.
   (C) xerostomia.
   (D) lacrimation.
   (E) myopic accommodation.

3. Which of the following drugs is considered to be the agent of choice for anaphylactic reactions?

   (A) clonidine
   (B) isoproterenol
   (C) epinephrine
   (D) phenylephrine
   (E) terbutaline

4. Which of the following neuromuscular blocking agents can cause muscarinic responses such as bradycardia and increased glandular secretions?

   (A) tubocurarine
   (B) succinylcholine
   (C) pancuronium
   (D) decamethonium
   (E) gallamine

5. Which of the following agents would *not* be appropriate in the treatment of glaucoma?

   (A) atropine
   (B) pilocarpine
   (C) physostigmine
   (D) timolol
   (E) epinephrine

6. Adverse reactions to atropine include all of the following *except*

   (A) photophobia.
   (B) dry mouth.
   (C) sedation.
   (D) diarrhea.
   (E) tachycardia.

7. Which of the following drugs is a volatile substance that is administered by inhalation?

   (A) thiopental
   (B) halothane
   (C) alprazolam
   (D) buspirone
   (E) phenytoin

8. The structure of prochlorperazine is shown. Which of the following medications, because of its chemical relationship to prochlorperazine, would most likely cause similar side effects?

   (A) fluphenazine
   (B) thioridazine
   (C) alprazolam
   (D) buspirone
   (E) pentobarbital

9. The brief duration of action of an ultra-short-acting barbiturate is the result of a

   (A) slow rate of metabolism in the liver.
   (B) low lipid solubility, resulting in a minimal concentration in the brain.
   (C) high degree of binding to plasma proteins.
   (D) rapid rate of redistribution from the brain owing to its high liposolubility.
   (E) slow rate of excretion by the kidneys.

10. Which of the following mechanisms of action is true and most likely contributes to the treatment of parkinsonism?

(A) The direct-acting dopaminergic agonist amantadine mimics the activity of striatal dopamine.
(B) The antimuscarinic activity of diphenhydramine contributes to the restoration of striatal dopaminergic–cholinergic neurotransmitter balance.
(C) Striatal H_1-receptors are blocked by the antihistaminic trihexyphenidyl.
(D) The ergoline bromocriptine stimulates the release of striatal dopamine from intact terminals.
(E) The ability of dopamine to cross the blood–brain barrier allows it to restore striatal dopaminergic–cholinergic neurotransmitter balance.

11. All of the following adverse effects are associated with the use of levodopa *except*

(A) sialorrhea.
(B) orthostatic hypotension.
(C) delusions, confusion, and depression.
(D) dyskinesia and dystonia.
(E) livedo reticularis.

12. The activity of which of the following drugs depends on a *p*-phenyl-*N*-alkylpiperidine moiety?

(A) phenobarbital
(B) chlorpromazine
(C) diazepam
(D) imipramine
(E) meperidine

13. Opioids are used as all of the following agents *except*

(A) antitussives.
(B) analgesics.
(C) anti-inflammatories.
(D) antidiarrheals.
(E) preanesthetic medications.

14. Which of the following agents would *not* be an alternative to phenobarbital in the treatment of partial seizures?

(A) trimethadione
(B) gabapentin
(C) felbamate
(D) lamotrigine
(E) None of the above

Directions for questions 15–19: The questions and incomplete statements in this section can be correctly answered or completed by **one or more** of the suggested answers. Choose the answer, A–E.

A   if **I only** is correct
B   if **III only** is correct
C   if **I and II** are correct
D   if **II and III** are correct
E   if **I, II, and III** are correct

15. Cholinesterase inhibitors can be used therapeutically

I. as miotic agents in the treatment of glaucoma.
II. to increase skeletal muscle tone in the treatment of myasthenia gravis.
III. to decrease gastrointestinal (GI) and urinary bladder smooth muscle tone.

16. Antimuscarinic agents are used in the treatment of Parkinson disease and in the control of some neuroleptic-induced extrapyramidal disorders. These agents include

I. ipratropium.
II. benztropine.
III. trihexyphenidyl.

17. Certain drugs are sometimes incorporated into local anesthetic solutions to prolong their activity and reduce their systemic toxicity. These drugs include

I. dobutamine.
II. phenylephrine.
III. epinephrine.

18. Improper administration of local anesthetics can cause toxic plasma concentrations that may result in

I. seizures and central nervous system (CNS) depression.
II. respiratory and myocardial depression.
III. circulatory collapse.

19. In addition to their anxiolytic properties, ben-
    zodiazepines are indicated for use

    I. as preanesthetic medications.
    II. as anticonvulsants.
    III. during acute withdrawal from alcohol.

For questions 20–22: A 58-year-old white male who has a history of essential hypertension and bronchial asthma has recently been diagnosed with prostatic hypertrophy. His medication history includes the following drugs:

(A) propranolol, for hypertension
(B) ipratropium, for asthma
(C) metaproterenol, for asthma
(D) finasteride (Proscar), for prostatic hypertrophy
(E) prazosin, for hypertension

Directions: The following questions can be answered by **one** of the listed drugs. Choose the **best** answer, **A–E.**

20. Which of these agents and uses could worsen the urinary retention he is experiencing as a result of his prostate problems?

21. Which agent and use could worsen or cause an acute asthma attack?

22. Which agent acts selectively at β_2-receptors?

For questions 23–25: A 55-year-old black female has a history of moderate hypertension, glaucoma, and mild osteoarthritis. Her medication history includes the following drugs:

(A) metoprolol, for hypertension
(B) pilocarpine gel, for glaucoma
(C) epinephrine drops, for glaucoma
(D) isoflurophate, for glaucoma
(E) timolol, for glaucoma

Directions: The following questions can be answered by **one or more** of the listed drugs. Choose the **best** answers, **A–E.**

23. Which of her glaucoma medicines acts via an indirect mechanism?

24. Which two agents could have an additive effect to produce excessive bradycardia?

25. Which two glaucoma agents could lessen the effects of the other?

Directions for questions 26–28: Each statement in this section describes **one** of the following drugs. Choose the **best** answer, **A–E.**

(A) tranylcypromine
(B) imipramine
(C) buspirone
(D) fluoxetine
(E) phenelzine

26. An anxiolytic drug that does not possess either hypnotic or anticonvulsant properties

27. A prototype tricyclic antidepressant with antimuscarinic properties that make it useful in the treatment of enuresis

28. An antidepressant that inhibits serotonin reuptake and may cause adverse effects such as impaired memory, akathisia, and menstrual irregularities

Directions for questions 29–31: Each structure in this section can be described by **one** of the following pharmacological categories. Choose the **best** answer.

(A) general anesthetic
(B) local anesthetic
(C) antidepressant
(D) anxiolytic
(E) opioid antagonist

29.

NH₂———⟨○⟩———COOCH₂CH₂N(CH₂CH₃)₂

31.

CH₂CH₂CH₂NH—CH₃

30.

For questions 32–33: A 38-year-old man has a history of affective disorders, including schizophrenia, depression, obsessive–compulsive disorder, and situational anxiety. His past medications include thiothixene, chlorpromazine, amitriptyline, and diazepam. His current medication profile includes two of the following drugs:

(A) clozapine
(B) fluoxetine
(C) buspirone
(D) risperidone

Directions: The following questions can be answered by **one** of the listed drugs. Choose the **best** answer, A–D.

32. Which agent is most likely being used to treat his schizophrenic psychosis?

33. Which agent is most likely being used to treat depression and obsessive–compulsive disorder?

Directions for questions 34–40: Each of the questions, statements, or incomplete statements in this section can be correctly answered or completed by **one** of the suggested answers or phrases. Choose the **best** answer.

34. Tyramine exemplifies the pharmacologic mechanism of

(A) ganglionic blockade.
(B) inhibition of transmitter release.
(C) facilitation of transmitter release.
(D) interference with vesicular storage.
(E) blockade of transmitter reuptake.

35. Considering the general chemical structures of sympathomimetic amines, deletion of the 3-hydroxy group on the phenyl ring of norepinephrine would likely produce

(A) increased α-receptor potency.
(B) increased β-receptor potency.
(C) indirect sympathomimetic activity.
(D) decreased transport through the blood–brain barrier.
(E) loss of any biological activity in the nervous system.

36. Sometimes combination treatment of Parkinson disease is warranted. Which of the following drug combinations could work cooperatively to enhance a clinical antiparkinsonian response?

(A) amphetamine and reserpine
(B) levodopa and carbidopa
(C) carbidopa and tolcapone
(D) amantadine and haloperidol
(E) dopamine and tyramine

37. Terazosin is able to facilitate micturition when used in the treatment of benign prostatic hypertrophy (BPH) because the drug

(A) relaxes the prostate gland.
(B) constricts the neck of the bladder.
(C) prevents penile erections associated with BPH.
(D) blocks seminal fluid production.
(E) blocks prostate cell growth.

38. BRL37344 is a β_3-agonist. It might be of interest to develop this agent into a clinically usable drug because of the expectation that β_3-agonists would

(A) constrict blood vessels and increase blood pressure in shock patients.
(B) induce lipolysis and decrease lipocyte mass in obese patients.
(C) increase glycogenolysis and prevent glycogen storage in liver cirrhosis.
(D) enhance renal vasodilation and increase urinary elimination of ethanol in alcoholics.
(E) cause bronchodilation and counteract the negative effects of asthma treatment agents.

39. The pharmacologic profile of carvedilol is most similar to that of

(A) esmolol.
(B) labetalol.
(C) metoprolol.
(D) nadolol.
(E) timolol.

40. Besides both of them being phenanthrene derivatives, apomorphine and morphine also have the common property of

(A) stimulating brain neurogenesis and hence antidepressant activity.
(B) eliciting a potent nerve blockade and hence anesthetic activity.
(C) stimulating μ-opioid receptors and hence analgesic efficacy.
(D) improving immobility and hence antiparkinsonian activity.
(E) inducing rewarding stimuli and hence addiction liability.

ANSWERS AND EXPLANATIONS

1. The answer is B *[see V.C.2.b–c; VI.C.1.e–g].*
Ipratropium is a newly approved antimuscarinic agent used to treat bronchospasm. Propantheline and homatropine are antimuscarinic agents used as a GI antispasmodic and as a mydriatic, respectively. Edrophonium and ambenonium are indirect-acting cholinergic agonists and, as such, would be expected to induce bronchospasm.

2. The answer is C *[see VI.D].*
Xerostomia, or dry mouth, results from reduced salivary secretions and, therefore, is not a manifestation of cholinergic agonist activity. All of the other effects listed in the question are extensions of therapeutic effects of cholinergic agonists to the point of being adverse effects.

3. The answer is C *[see III.C.1].*
Of the adrenergic agonists listed, only epinephrine—because of its broad, nonselective α- and β-activity—is an agent of choice for anaphylactic reactions. Epinephrine improves circulatory and respiratory function and counteracts the vascular effects of histamine-related anaphylaxis.

4. The answer is B *[see VII.D.2].*
Neuromuscular blocking agents interact with nicotinic receptors at the skeletal neuromuscular junction. Succinylcholine is also capable of eliciting autonomic muscarinic responses, such as bradycardia, increased glandular secretions, and cardiac arrest.

5. The answer is A *[see V.B–D].*
Both direct-acting (e.g., pilocarpine) and indirect-acting (e.g., physostigmine) cholinergics may be used in glaucoma to increase cholinergic activity and facilitate outflow of aqueous humor. Similarly, both β-agonists (e.g., epinephrine) and β-antagonists (e.g., timolol) may be used, respectively, to increase outflow and decrease production of aqueous humor. Atropine is contraindicated in glaucoma because its anticholinergic effects can block the outflow of aqueous humor and consequently increase intraocular pressure.

6. The answer is D *[see VI.D].*
Classic signs and symptoms of muscarinic blockade, as with atropine, include mydriasis, which may cause light sensitivity (photophobia), dry mouth, and constipation by decreasing secretory activity and motility in the GI tract and may cause tachycardia by inhibiting the normal inhibitory cholinergic control of the cardiac system. Diarrhea is one of the common signs of cholinergic agonists (such as salivation, lacrimation or tearing, urination, and diarrhea).

7. The answer is B *[see VIII.A.1].*
The general anesthetics are divided into two major classes of drugs: those that are gases or volatile liquids, which are administered by inhalation, and those that are nonvolatile salts, which are administered as intravenous solutions. Halothane is a halogenated hydrocarbon, which belongs to the former class. It has the advantage over older volatile anesthetics (e.g., ethyl ether, cyclopropane) of being nonflammable. Thiopental sodium, alprazolam, buspirone, and phenytoin are all nonvolatile substances that are administered orally or parenterally. Thiopental is a general anesthetic and is sometimes referred to as a basal anesthetic because it does not produce significant third-stage surgical anesthesia. Alprazolam and buspirone are anxiolytics, whereas phenytoin is an anticonvulsant.

8. The answer is A *[see X.A.1; Table 13-6].*
Fluphenazine, like prochlorperazine, is a piperazinyl phenothiazine antipsychotic and would be likely to cause similar side effects. Whereas thioridazine is also a phenothiazine antipsychotic, it is a piperidyl derivative rather than a piperazinyl derivative. Alprazolam, phenytoin, and pentobarbital are not phenothiazines; therefore, structurally, they are not similar to prochlorperazine.

9. The answer is D *[see XII.A.4.c–d; Figure 13-14].*
Ultra-short-acting barbiturates are characterized by having branched or unsaturated 5,5-side chains and by having a sulfur atom in place of oxygen in the 2 position of the barbituric acid molecule. These modifications of barbituric acid result in an extremely liposoluble molecule that is soluble in lipid tissues. After administration, an ultra-short-acting barbiturate readily crosses the blood–brain barrier but then is quickly redistributed into extracerebral tissue, resulting in a rapid loss of activity. Whereas these agents do remain in the body for a long time and seem to have slow rates of metabolism and excretion, their long retention time is owing more to their slow rate of leaching out of lipid tissue.

10. The answer is B *[see XIV.B].*
The H$_1$-antagonist diphenhydramine possesses antimuscarinic activity, which allows it to be of use in the restoration of striatal dopaminergic–cholinergic neurotransmitter balance. Amantadine appears to stimulate the release of striatal dopamine; it does not mimic the action of dopamine. Trihexyphenidyl is an antimuscarinic, not antihistaminic, agent; it blocks cholinergic, not H$_1$, receptors. Bromocriptine is a dopaminergic agonist and mimics the activity of striatal dopamine. The neurotransmitter dopamine is not able to cross the blood–brain barrier and is, therefore, not effective as an antiparkinsonian drug.

11. The answer is E *[see XIV.D.1].*
Livedo reticularis is a circulatory disorder characterized by large, bluish areas on the extremities. It is an adverse effect associated with the use of amantadine and bromocriptine but not with the use of levodopa.

12. The answer is E *[see XV.A.1–2; Figure 13-27E].*
The p-phenyl-N-alkylpiperidine moiety is common to the structurally specific opioid analgesics. Meperidine is an opioid analgesic and is an N-methyl-p-phenylpiperidine derivative. Its chemical name is ethyl 1-methyl-4-phenylpiperidine-4-carboxylate. Phenobarbital is a barbiturate sedative. Chlorpromazine is a phenothiazine antipsychotic. Diazepam is a benzodiazepine anxiolytic. Imipramine is a tricyclic dibenzazepine antidepressant.

13. The answer is C *[see XV.C].*
Unlike the salicylates, opioids do not possess anti-inflammatory activity. Opioids do suppress the cough reflex and are preeminent analgesics. Opioids cause constipation and are thus effective antidiarrheal agents. When used as preanesthetic medication, opioids permit a reduction in the amount of general anesthetic required for surgical anesthesia.

14. The answer is A *[see XIII.A.1; XII.C.2].*
Whereas many analeptics are useful in controlling more than one seizure type, trimethadione is effective primarily against absence (petit mal) seizures. In addition, its side effect profile is more extensive than the newer agents (e.g., lamotrigine, gabapentin, felbamate) that are effective in treating partial seizures.

15. The answer is C (I, II) *[see V.C.2].*
Cholinesterase inhibitors are indirect-acting cholinergic agonists useful in treating myasthenia gravis and glaucoma. Their effects on GI and urinary bladder smooth muscle would be to increase smooth muscle tone, not decrease it.

16. The answer is D (II, III) *[see VI.C.1.g–h].*
All three compounds are antimuscarinic agents; however, only benztropine and trihexyphenidyl are used to control parkinsonism and some neuroleptic-induced extrapyramidal disorders. Ipratropium is a newly approved agent for the treatment of bronchospasm.

17. The answer is D (II, III) *[see III.B.1.b; II.C.1–2].*
Dobutamine is a β$_1$-selective adrenergic agonist. It would be inappropriate to use dobutamine to decrease blood flow at the site of local anesthetic administration. Epinephrine is a nonselective α- and β-agonist, and phenylephrine is an α$_1$-selective agonist; both of these drugs can be used to limit the systemic absorption of local anesthetics and prolong their activity.

18. The answer is E (I, II, III) *[see IX.D.2].*
Careful administration of a local anesthetic by a knowledgeable practitioner is essential to prevent systemic absorption and consequent toxicity. This is especially important when the patient has cardiovascular disease, poorly controlled diabetes, thyrotoxicosis, or peripheral vascular disease.

19. The answer is E *[see XII.C.1–3].*
Benzodiazepines can serve as induction agents for general anesthesia; they also have anxiolytic properties. In addition, intravenous diazepam is used to treat status epilepticus, whereas clonazepam is used orally for myoclonic and absence (petit mal) seizures. Benzodiazepines also diminish alcohol withdrawal symptoms.

20. The answer is B *[see VI.D].*
This anticholinergic, if absorbed systemically, could cause classic anticholinergic effects, which include urinary retention.

21. The answer is A *[see IV.C.4].*
Because this is a nonselective β-blocker, there could be some inhibition of β_2-receptors in the bronchial tree, causing bronchoconstriction and possible complication of his asthma.

22. The answer is C *[see III.C.6].*
Propranolol is a nonselective β-blocker, and prazosin is a selective α_1-blocker. Neither ipratropium nor Proscar works through the adrenergic system. Metaproterenol is a selective β_2-agonist.

23. The answer is D *[see V.A.2; V.C.2].*
Pilocarpine acts directly at the muscarinic receptor, whereas epinephrine and timolol both act directly at β-receptors. Isoflurophate inhibits the metabolism of acetylcholine, indirectly increasing levels of the endogenous neurotransmitter.

24. The answer is A, E *[see IV.B.3; IV.D.4].*
Metoprolol, a β_1-selective agent, can cause bradycardia alone. The addition of topical timolol, while limiting systemic absorption, could have an additive β-blocking effect to decrease heart rate (negative chronotropy).

25. The answer is B, D *[see V.C.1–2].*
Pilocarpine and isoflurophate could limit the effects of each other, because ultimately both act via cholinergic receptors. Pilocarpine acts directly on the receptor, while isoflurophate indirectly increases acetylcholine levels. Pilocarpine and acetylcholine could compete for each other at the receptor site, effectively decreasing the effects of both. Epinephrine is a β-agonist and timolol is a β-antagonist. Although both agents are effective in treating glaucoma alone, the use of both concomitantly could result in a pharmacological antagonism, effectively decreasing the effects of both.

26. The answer is C *[see XII.B.2].*
Buspirone's mechanism of anxiolytic action is unknown. Unlike the benzodiazepines, buspirone lacks hypnotic and anticonvulsant properties. The tricyclic antidepressant imipramine is useful in the treatment of enuresis, because the compound blocks muscarinic receptors mediating micturition. Trazodone is categorized as an atypical antidepressant that selectively blocks serotonin reuptake.

27. The answer is B *[see XI.C.2].*
Buspirone's mechanism of anxiolytic action is unknown. Unlike the benzodiazepines, buspirone lacks hypnotic and anticonvulsant properties. The tricyclic antidepressant imipramine is useful in the treatment of enuresis, because the compound blocks muscarinic receptors mediating micturition. Trazodone is categorized as an atypical antidepressant that selectively blocks serotonin reuptake.

28. The answer is D *[see XI.B.3; XI.D.3].*
Buspirone's mechanism of anxiolytic action is unknown. Unlike the benzodiazepines, buspirone lacks hypnotic and anticonvulsant properties. The tricyclic antidepressant imipramine is useful in the treatment of enuresis, because the compound blocks muscarinic receptors mediating micturition. Trazodone is categorized as an atypical antidepressant that selectively blocks serotonin reuptake.

29. The answer is B *[see IX.A; Figure 13-15].*
The structure shown is that of procaine, which is a diethylaminoethyl *p*-aminobenzoate ester. It contains a hydrophilic amino group in the alcohol portion of the molecule and a lipophilic aromatic acid connected by the ester linkage. The procaine molecule is typical of ester-type local anesthetics.

30. The answer is D *[see XII.A; Table 13-7].*
The structure is that of diazepam, which has a benzo-1,4-diazepine as its base nucleus. The widely used benzo-1,4-diazepine derivatives have significant anxiolytic, hypnotic, and anticonvulsant activities.

31. The answer is C *[see XI.A.2; Figure 13-19].*
The structure is that of desipramine, which has a dibenzazepine as its base nucleus. Dibenzazepine derivatives that have a methylaminopropyl or dimethylaminopropyl group attached to the ring nitrogen have significant antidepressant activity. Similarly substituted dibenzocycloheptadienes also have antidepressant activity. Together, these two chemical classes make up the majority of the tricyclic antidepressants.

32. The answer is A *[see X.C].*
Clozapine, while therapeutically defined as a general antipsychotic, is used almost exclusively in the treatment of schizophrenia.

33. The answer is B *[see XI.A.3; XI.C.2].*
Fluoxetine is most likely being used in this patient in an attempt to treat his depression and obsessive–compulsive disorder with the same drug. Clinical trials have shown fluoxetine to improve both conditions. The use of a single agent for both conditions will minimize the risk of drug–drug interactions as well as reduce the chances of adverse effects.

34. The answer is C *[see III.A.2; III.B.3; Table 13-2].*
Tyramine is an indirectly acting sympathomimetic amine that enters the nerve terminal and displaces norepinephrine from the storage vesicles, thus increasing the quanta of the transmitter released.

35. The answer is C *[see III.A.1–2].*
Both aromatic hydroxyl functions are important for both α- and β-receptor binding. However, removal of one or both of the groups would increase uptake of the resulting compound into the brain and adrenergic nerve terminals, resulting in transmitter displacement from vesicular storage and increased transmitter release.

36. The answer is B *[see XIV.A.2–3].*
Although levodopa can cross the blood–brain barrier to gain access into the brain, a significant portion of an orally administered dose gets converted into dopamine and norepinephrine at peripheral sites, leading to peripheral side effects and decreased brain bioavailability. Carbidopa, a dopa-decarboxylase inhibitor that does not cross the blood–brain barrier, is coadministered with levodopa to decrease its peripheral conversion and increase the central delivery of the drug and hence the therapeutic response.

37. The answer is A *[see IV.C.1].*
Terazosin blocks α-receptors on the prostate gland to cause a relaxant effect, which reduces the pressure exerted by the prostate on the urethra, thus easing urinary voidance.

38. The answer is B *[see III.B.1.b].*
Stimulation of β_3-receptors induces the metabolic breakdown of fat stores into free fatty acids that can be further catabolized by the body. The hope is that this category of pharmacologic agents could, with repeated use, lead to a decrease in the content and number of fat cells and hence have an antiobesity effect.

39. The answer is B *[see IV.C.3; Table 13-3].*
Like labetalol, carvedilol is a nonselective α- and β-receptor antagonist used in the treatment of hypertension. Blockade of vascular α_1-receptors would cause vasodilatation and decreased peripheral vascular resistance, whereas blockade of myocardial β_1-receptors would decrease cardiac contractility. The resultant decrease in cardiac output would produce a fall in blood pressure (blood pressure equals cardiac output times peripheral resistance).

40. The answer is E *[see XIV.A.2; XIV.D.2; XV.A.2; XV.C].*
Despite the similarities in their names and chemical structures, these two agents have different pharmacological effects and therapeutic uses. The one commonality among them is that both produce rewarding effects and thus abuse liability—morphine primarily through its euphoriant CNS effects and apomorphine primarily through its prolibido (erectile) effects in males.

14
Autacoids and Their Antagonists, Nonnarcotic Analgesic–Antipyretics, and Nonsteroidal Anti-inflammatory Drugs

Scott F. Long

I. INTRODUCTION

A. Autacoids, also called autopharmacological agents or local hormones, have widely differing structures and pharmacological actions. Although the term remains poorly defined, the currently accepted criterion that defines a substance as an autacoid is local release and action limited to a specific site. Two of most extensively investigated autacoids are **histamine** and the **prostaglandins.** However, **serotonin, bradykinin,** and **kallidin** also function in a similar manner. While some autacoids (histamine and serotonin) function as neurotransmitters, their autacoid function is the focus of this chapter. Currently, there are no agents that specifically modulate the function of bradykinin or kallidin; however, drugs or analogs that mimic, block, or modulate other autacoid functions have important therapeutic roles.

B. Nonnarcotic analgesic-antipyretics have dissimilar structures but share certain therapeutic actions, including relief of pain, fever, and sometimes inflammation. Mechanistically, these agents act by inhibiting synthesis of prostaglandins.

C. Nonsteroidal anti-inflammatory drugs (NSAIDs) differ in structure and activity from the nonnarcotic analgesic-antipyretics, but possess anti-inflammatory properties. In addition, many of these agents also exhibit antipyretic and analgesic activity. NSAIDs also act by inhibition of prostaglandin synthesis.

II. AUTACOIDS AND THEIR ANTAGONISTS

A. Histamine and antihistaminics

1. Chemistry
   a. Histamine is a bioamine derived principally from dietary histidine, which is decarboxylated by L-histidine decarboxylase (Figure 14-1).
   b. Antihistaminics (histamine antagonists) can be classified as H_1- or H_2-receptor antagonists.
   (1) **H_1-receptor antagonists,** the classic antihistaminic agents, are chemically classified as **ethylenediamines** (e.g., pyrilamine), **alkylamines** (e.g., brompheniramine [Dimetapp], chlorpheniramine [Chlor-Trimeton]), **ethanolamines** (e.g., diphenhydramine [Benadryl], clemastine [Tavist]), **piperazines** (e.g., hydroxyzine [Atarax, Vistaril], cet-

Figure 14-1. Structural formula of histamine, an autacoid.

Figure 14-2. Structural formulas of representative H_1-receptor antagonists. **A.** Chlorpheniramine (alkylamine). **B.** Diphenhydramine (ethanolamine). **C.** Promethazine (phenothiazine). **D.** Loratadine (nonsedating piperidine).

irizine [Zyrtec]), **phenothiazines** (e.g., promethazine [Phenergan]), **dibenzocyclohep-tenes** (cyproheptadine [Periactin]), **phthalazinones** (azelastine [Optivar, Astelin]), and **piperidines** (e.g., azatadine [Optimine], loratadine [Claritin], desloratadine [Clarinex], and fexofenadine [Allegra]). Cetirizine, azelastine, loratadine, desloratadine, and fexofenadine make up the second-generation antihistaminics, which are less sedating than the older, first-generation drugs, owing to their limited ability to cross the blood–brain barrier (Figure 14-2).

(2) **H_2-receptor antagonists** are heterocyclic congeners of histamine. These include **cimetidine** (Tagamet), **ranitidine** (Zantac), **famotidine** (Pepcid), and **nizatidine** (Axid) (Figure 14-3).

(3) **Alternatives** to the H_2-receptor antagonists include **omeprazole** (Prilosec), **lansoprazole** (Prevacid), **rabeprazole** (AcipHex), **pantoprazole** (Protonix), and **esomeprazole**

Figure 14-3. Structural formulas of (**A**) cimetidine, an H_2-receptor antagonist, and (**B**) omeprazole, a proton pump inhibitor.

(Nexium); **specific inhibitors of H$^+$/K$^+$-ATPase** (proton pump inhibitors, or PPIs), the ultimate mediator of gastric acid secretion. Structurally, these agents are substituted **benzimidazoles** linked to a pyridine ring by a sulfinyl bridge, which is required for H$^+$/K$^+$-ATPase inhibition.

2. **Pharmacology**
    a. **Histamine** has powerful pharmacological actions, mediated by two specific receptor types (Table 14-1). A third histamine receptor has been identified. Its function has yet to be elucidated, but it is believed to act, at least in part, as an autoreceptor.
        (1) **H$_1$-receptors mediate** typical allergic and anaphylactic responses to histamine, such as bronchoconstriction, vasodilation, increased capillary permeability, and spasmodic contractions of gastrointestinal (GI) smooth muscle.
        (2) **H$_2$-receptors mediate** other responses to histamine, such as increased secretion of gastric acid, pepsin, and Castle's factor (intrinsic factor).
    b. **H$_1$-receptor antagonists** competitively block H$_1$-receptors, thus limiting the histamine's effects on bronchial smooth muscle, capillaries, and GI smooth muscle. These antagonists also prevent histamine-induced pain and itching of the skin and mucous membranes.
    c. **H$_2$-receptor antagonists** competitively block H$_2$-receptors, thus limiting the effects of histamine on gastric secretions.
    d. The **PPIs** irreversibly inhibit the proton pump H$^+$/K$^+$-ATPase by covalently binding to the protein.

3. **Therapeutic indications**
    a. **Exogenous histamine** can be used as a **diagnostic agent** for testing gastric function. However, other stimulants of gastric secretion (pentagastrin) are more suitable and safer.
    b. **H$_1$-receptor antagonists** are used to provide symptomatic relief of **allergic symptoms,** such as seasonal rhinitis, conjunctivitis, and the symptoms of rhinoviral infections (common cold). Their antihistaminic effects also make them useful for symptomatic relief of urticaria. Agents with a high degree of anticholinergic activity (e.g., diphenhydramine) are sometimes used to treat nausea and vomiting associated with motion sickness and vertigo. In addition, promethazine (which also has a high degree of anticholinergic activity) is sometimes used as an antiemetic, and hydroxyzine pamoate is occasionally employed as a mild anxiolytic. The second-generation drugs (i.e., loratadine, desloratadine,

Table 14-1. Selected Actions of Endogenous Histamine

Site	Action	Receptor Type
Cardiovascular		
Vascular	Arterial contraction	H$_1$
	Arteriolar relaxation	H$_1$ and H$_2$
	Venule contraction	H$_1$
	Venule relaxation	H$_2$
	Endothelial cells, release of EDRF	H$_1$
	Endothelial cells, contraction	H$_1$
Heart	Increased heart rate	H$_2$
	Increased force of contraction	H$_2$
	Slowed atrioventricular conduction	H$_1$
Respiratory		
	Bronchiolar smooth-muscle contraction	H$_1$
Gastrointestinal (GI)		
Gastric mucosa	Increased secretion of acid and pepsin	H$_2$
GI smooth muscle	Contraction	H$_1$
Various		
Cutaneous nerves	Pain and itch	H$_1$

EDRF, endothelium-derived relaxing factor.

fexofenadine, acrivastine, cetirizine, and azelastine) provide the added advantage of little to negligible sedation, owing to their relative inability to cross the blood–brain barrier.

   c. H$_2$-receptor antagonists are used to treat **gastric hypersecretory** conditions, such as duodenal ulcer and Zollinger-Ellison syndrome. They are effective in reducing pain associated with gastroesophageal reflux disease, but note that they do not prevent actual reflux.

   d. The **proton pump inhibitors** are used to treat **duodenal ulcers** and are the drugs of choice for the treatment of **Zollinger-Ellison syndrome.**

4. Adverse effects

   a. Histamine may cause numerous adverse effects related to its basic pharmacology (see II.A.2.a).

   b. H$_1$-receptor antagonists are associated with the following **adverse effects:**

     (1) Central nervous system (CNS) effects, such as CNS depression, sedation, fatigue, tinnitus, hallucinations, and ataxia

     (2) GI effects, such as nausea and vomiting

     (3) Antimuscarinic effects, such as dry mouth, urinary retention, and constipation

     (4) Teratogenic effects (possible with piperazine compounds)

   c. Nonsedating H$_1$-receptor antagonists, because they possess little anticholinergic activity and do not cross the blood–brain barrier, are relatively free of side effects.

   d. H$_2$-receptor antagonists are associated with the following adverse effects:

     (1) CNS effects, such as confusion and dizziness

     (2) Hepatic and renal dysfunction

     (3) Inhibition of the hepatic microsomal drug-metabolizing enzyme system (with cimetidine)

     (4) Androgenic effects (with high doses of cimetidine), such as impotence and gynecomastia in men and galactorrhea in women

   e. The **H$^+$/K$^+$-ATPase inhibitors** have been reported to cause diarrhea, GI pain, and headache as their most frequent adverse effects. In addition, they may interfere with the metabolism of diazepam, warfarin, phenytoin, and theophylline.

B. Serotonin

1. Chemistry

   a. Serotonin (5-hydroxytryptamine) is a bioamine that is synthesized from the amino acid tryptophan by a two-step enzymatic process catalyzed by tryptophan hydroxylase and L-amino acid decarboxylase (Figure 14-4).

   b. Serotonin agonists

     (1) 5-HT$_1$-receptor agonists (i.e., sumatriptan [Imitrex], rizatriptan [Maxalt], naratriptan [Amerge], zolmitriptan [Zomig], almotriptan [Axert], eletriptan [Relpax], and frovatriptan [Frova]) are indole derivatives structurally similar to serotonin (Figure 14-4).

     (2) Tegaserod (Zelnorm), an **indole** derivative, acts as 5-HT$_4$-receptor agonist (Figure 14-4).

     (3) Ergot alkaloids (ergotamine [Ergomar]) have some activity as a serotonin agonist/partial agonist.

   c. Serotonin antagonists

     (1) Ergot alkaloids and derivatives with antagonist/partial agonist activity include **ergonovine** (Ergotrate), **dihydroergotamine, methysergide,** and **bromocriptine** (Parlodel).

     (2) 5-HT$_3$-antagonists may be either **indole** derivatives (ondansetron [Zofran]) or **benzimidazoles** (granisetron [Kytril]). Other drugs of the class include **dolasetron** (Anzemet), **palonosetron** (Aloxi) and **alosetron** (Lotronex) (Figure 14-4).

2. Pharmacology

   a. Serotonin exerts a wide range of effects via a family of receptors that includes at least seven types and several subtypes. Major physiological effects of serotonin include vasoconstriction (5-HT$_2$); platelet aggregation (5-HT$_2$); increased release of acetylcholine in the enteric region (5-HT$_4$); nausea/emesis (5-HT$_3$); and numerous behavioral actions that influence anxiety, depression, aggression, impulsivity, and appetite (5-HT$_1$, 5-HT$_2$, 5-HT$_3$). In addition, the 5-HT$_1$-receptor acts as an autoreceptor to inhibit presynaptic activity at both serotonergic and adrenergic neurones in the CNS. Furthermore, it directly contributes to vascular tone through vasoconstriction. Serotonin may also produce numerous other effects, including the opposite of those just stated, depending on the specific receptor that mediates the event.

Figure 14-4. Structures of (**A**) serotonin and representative serotonin agonists (**B**) sumatriptan, (**C**) tegaserod, and (**D**) the serotonin antagonist ondansetron.

b. Serotonin agonists

(1) **5-HT$_1$-agonists** mimic the actions of serotonin at this receptor to decrease presynaptic neurotransmitter release. Direct vasoconstriction, decreased release of inflammatory and vasodilating substances (neurokinin A, substance P), and a direct antinociceptive activities are thought to contribute to the efficacy of these drugs.

(2) **Tegaserod** activates the serotonergic receptor (5-HT$_4$), causing the release of acetylcholine, other neurotransmitters, and calcitonin gene-related peptide. These, in turn, increase gastric and intestinal motility and tone. In addition, direct actions on the gastrointestinal smooth muscle is thought to contribute it its effect, thus accounting for both the direct and indirect actions of tegaserod.

(3) **Ergot alkaloids** produce a wide range of pharmacological effects, including both agonistic and antagonistic activity at adrenergic, dopaminergic, and serotonergic receptors. Specific actions dependent on drug and animal models.

c. Serotonin antagonists such as **ondansetron** and related drugs block the ion-channel coupled 5-HT$_3$-receptor, thus inhibiting the ability of serotonin to cause nausea and/or emesis. This action appears to occur both locally at the GI tract and centrally in the area postrema. In addition, activation of peripheral 5-HT$_3$-receptors will increase pain, abdominal distention, and motor responses of the intestinal tract. Blockade of these actions, thus slowing GI motility, by **alosetron** is responsible for its usefulness in certain cases of irritable bowel syndrome (IBS).

3. Therapeutic indications

a. Serotonin agonists

(1) Numerous CNS active drugs use the serotonergic system to modulate behavior, such as the anorexiants (dexfenfluramine), anxiolytics (buspirone), and selective serotonin reuptake inhibitors for depression (fluoxetine). These drugs are acting more on the neurotransmitter function of serotonin and are discussed here.

(2) Some **ergot alkaloids, sumatriptan,** and similar drugs act to modulate the autacoid function of serotonin. They are used to prevent and treat pain associated with migraine headaches by altering serotonin's actions that result in changes in vascular tone.

(3) In addition, some **ergot alkaloids** are used to prevent postpartum hemorrhaging (through both vasoconstrictive and uterine contractile actions) and to prevent postpartum breast engorgement (**bromocriptine,** through dopaminergic activity).

(4) Tegaserod is used in the treatment of IBS that is constipation predominant.

b. Serotonin antagonists. These agents (e.g., **ondansetron, granisetron, dolasetron, palonosetron**) are used to prevent and treat nausea and emesis secondary to antineoplastic therapy by blocking the actions of serotonin at the 5-HT$_3$-receptor. **Alosetron** is used for the treatment of IBS that is diarrhea predominant.

4. Adverse effects

    a. Serotonin agonists

      (1) 5-HT$_1$-agonists may produce feelings of warmth, paresthesias, dizziness, and tightness or heaviness in the chest. Rarely, patients may experience chest pain. Because these agents may cause coronary vasoconstriction, they are contraindicated in angina patients and should be used cautiously in patients with hypertension or other risk factors for ischemic heart disease.

      (2) Tegaserod may produce diarrhea, abdominal cramping and pain, dizziness, and headache as side effects.

      (3) Ergot alkaloids may cause GI upset and cold extremities. As toxicity progresses, the patient may experience emesis, diarrhea, peripheral pain secondary to local ischemia, and hallucinations or delusions.

    b. Serotonin antagonists. The 5-HT$_3$-antagonists will produce headache, constipation, and dizziness. In addition, granisetron has been reported to produce somnolence and diarrhea. The use of **alosetron** in patients with diarrhea-associated IBS has resulted in some cases of ischemic colitis and life-threatening complications from severe constipation. Subsequent to a series of adverse drug reactions in this manner, alosetron is generally prescribed only by physicians who have been enrolled in a prescribing programme.

C. Prostaglandins

1. Chemistry

    a. Prostaglandins (PGs) are **derivatives** of prostanoic acid, a 20-carbon fatty acid containing a 5-carbon ring (Figure 14-5). In the body, prostaglandins are principally synthesized from arachidonic acid, which is formed from the membrane phospholipids by action of phospholipase A$_2$. Specifically, prostaglandins are synthesized from arachidonic acid by the enzyme cyclooxygenase (COX), which exists as three isozymes: COX 1, 2, and 3. COX 1 appears to function constantly. Its role seems to be the daily synthesis of prostaglandins, which contribute to normal homeostasis, and includes protection of the gastric mucosa through the prostaglandins and hemostasis through the synthesis of thromboxane. COX 2 is expressed primarily in response to inflammation or injury, contributing to the inflammatory response. It is also important in normal (noninjury) regulation of cardiac and perhaps other functions. COX 3 is thought to be predominantly active within the CNS, contributing to normal thermoregulatory control and pain perception, through the synthesis of prostaglandins, centrally. Note that the products of cyclooxygenase are then converted into either prostaglandins by prostaglandin synthase or thromboxanes by thromboxane synthase. The thromboxanes differ from the prostaglandins mainly by the substitution of a tetrahydropyran ring structure for the pentane ring found in prostaglandins. The only clinically relevant thromboxane currently identified is thromboxane A$_2$ (TxA$_2$), which causes platelet aggregation.

    b. Classification of prostaglandins as prostaglandin A (PGA), prostaglandin B (PGB), prostaglandin E (PGE), and so forth relates to the presence or absence of keto or hydroxyl

Figure 14-5. Structural formula of prostanoic acid, from which the prostaglandins are derived.

Figure 14-6. Structural formula of misoprostol (Cytotec), a derivative of prostaglandin E_1 (PGE_1).

groups at positions 9 and 11 (Figure 14-5). Subscripts relate to the number and position of double bonds in the aliphatic chains (Figure 14-6).

2. Pharmacology
   a. Endogenous prostaglandins appear to affect numerous body functions. They are released in response to many chemical, bacterial, mechanical, and other insults; and they appear to contribute to the signs and symptoms of the inflammatory process, including pain and edema.
   b. Physiological responses to prostaglandins include vasodilation in most vascular beds, although vasoconstriction can occur in isolated areas. PGI inhibits platelet aggregation and stimulates gastric release of bicarbonate and mucus, both of which serve to protect the gastric epithelium. The PGEs inhibit platelet aggregation, relax bronchial and GI smooth muscle, contract uterine smooth muscle, and inhibit gastric acid secretion. Alternatively, the PGDs and PGFs contract bronchial and GI smooth muscle. Prostaglandins also increase renal blood flow, promote diuresis, natriuresis, and kaliuresis; but paradoxically they increase renin secretion. They also possess diverse endocrine and metabolic effects.

3. Therapeutic indications
   a. PGE_1 analogs
      (1) Alprostadil (Prostin VR Pediatric) is used for temporary maintenance of a patent ductus arteriosus when awaiting corrective surgery for congenital heart defects.
      (2) Alprostadil (Caverject) is used in treating impotence owing to erectile dysfunction.
      (3) Misoprostol (Cytotec) is used for the prevention of NSAID-induced GI ulcers (Figure 14-6).
   b. PGE_2 analogs and derivative dinoprostone (Prostin E_2, Prepidil, Cervidil) are used for their abortifacient effects and to induce cervical-ripening in pregnancy.
   c. $PGF_{2\alpha}$ analogs
      (1) Carboprost (Hemabate), was used for its abortifacient effects. A high incidence of cardiovascular collapse caused its removal from the U.S. market.
      (2) Latanoprost (Xalatan), **travoprost** (Travatan), **bimatoprost** (Lumigan), and **unoprostone** (Rescula) are used topically to lower intraocular pressure in glaucoma.
   d. PGI analog epoprostenol (prostacyclin, [Flolan]) is used primarily for the treatment of emergent pulmonary hypertension.

4. Adverse effects associated with PGE include the following:
   a. CNS effects, such as CNS irritability, fever, seizures, and headache
   b. Cardiovascular effects, such as hypotension, dysrhythmias, vasodilation, flushing, and cardiac arrest
   c. Respiratory effects, such as respiratory depression and distress
   d. Hematological effects, such as anemia, thrombocytopenia, and disseminated intravascular coagulation (DIC)
   e. Diarrhea
   f. Decreased renal function
   g. Spotty bleeding and menstrual irregularities, abortion, and penile pain

D. Leukotrienes

1. Chemistry
   a. Leukotrienes. The leukotrienes (LTs) are 20-carbon derivatives of the fatty acids that are formed via the enzymatic pathway catalyzed by lipoxygenase. Unlike the prostaglandins, they contain no ring structure and are covalently linked to two or three amino acids.

The two important leukotrienes identified to date (LTC_4 and LTD_4) differ only by the presence of glutamine. The nomenclature of the leukotrienes is similar to that used for the prostaglandins.

  b. Leukotriene antagonists

    (1) Lipoxygenase inhibitors such as **zileuton** (Zyflo) are benzothiophene derivatives.

    (2) Leukotriene antagonists such as **zafirlukast** (Accolate) and **montelukast** (Singulair) represent a diverse chemical group that is peptidomimetic-like in its structure.

  2. Pharmacology

    a. Leukotrienes play a role in numerous physiological functions. They have been identified as the slow-reacting substance of anaphylaxis. Specific actions of the leukotrienes include the following:

      (1) Heart

        (a) Negative inotropy

        (b) Smooth-muscle chemotaxis

      (2) GI tract. Neutrophil chemotaxis that has been correlated with inflammatory bowel disease

      (3) Pulmonary. The actions of the leukotrienes within the pulmonary system appear to be major. These actions are the most important pharmacologically.

        (a) Bronchoconstriction

        (b) Increased permeability

        (c) Increased mucus secretion

      (4) Blood/lymph. As noted previously, the leukotrienes act as chemotactic agents for neutrophils and eosinophils and act to modify lymphocyte proliferation and differentiation.

    b. Leukotriene antagonists

      (1) The lipoxygenase inhibitor zileuton prevents the synthesis of leukotrienes by inhibiting the enzyme responsible for their formation—namely lipoxygenase. This action prevents the formation of all leukotrienes, thus preventing their contribution to various inflammatory processes.

      (2) The leukotriene antagonists **zafirlukast** and **montelukast** nonselectively and competitively inhibit the endogenous leukotrienes at their various receptor sites. This action blocks the effects of histamine, most notably the bronchoconstriction and pulmonary edema associated with asthma and allergic reactions.

  3. Therapeutic indications for zileuton, zafirlukast, and montelukast are limited to the treatment of asthma. These agents reduce bronchospasm and associated symptoms that are mediated through the leukotrienes.

  4. Adverse Effects

    a. Zileuton presents with relatively few side effects, predominantly gastrointestinal in nature (i.e., dyspepsia and nausea). However, it does cause transient increases in hepatic enzymes. This potential for hepatotoxicity has limited its use.

    b. Zafirlukast may produce GI upset and liver dysfunction (not as great as with zileuton), and may inhibit the metabolism of theophylline, warfarin, and potentially other drugs. Sudden withdrawal of corticosteroids in patients taking zafirlukast has precipitated a Churg-Strauss syndrome of eosinophilic vasculitis. Patients should be counseled to take zafirlukast with food to enhance its absorption.

    c. Montelukast presents with a side-effect profile similar to that for zafirlukast but typically with less incidence than with zafirlukast. Churg-Strauss syndrome has not been reported; however, this may simply reflect the relatively recent appearance of the drug on the market. Montelukast may be taken without regard to food.

III. NONNARCOTIC ANALGESIC-ANTIPYRETICS AND NSAIDS

  A. Salicylates

    1. Chemistry

      a. Salicylates are **derivatives of salicylic acid,** which is found as the glycoside salicin in willow bark. The prototypical drug is **aspirin,** the acetyl ester of salicylic acid (Figure

Figure 14-7. Structural formula of aspirin, the prototypical salicylate analgesic-antipyretic.

14-7). A simple ester, aspirin hydrolyzes easily, is unstable in aqueous media, and is affected by moisture.
   b. **More stable** salicylates include **diflunisal** (Dolobid) and the topical agent **methyl salicylate** (wintergreen oil) (Figure 14-8). Other salicylates are **salsalate** (Disalcid); **sodium thiosalicylate** (Resolute; injectable); **choline salicylate** (Trilisate; oral liquid); and the salicylate **derivatives mesalamine** (Asacol), **olsalazine** (Dipentum), and **sulfasalazine** (Azulfidine).
   c. Most salicylates are **weak acids.** Their excretion is influenced by changes in urinary pH.

2. **Pharmacology**
   a. Salicylates **inhibit** the enzyme cyclooxygenase and thus inhibit local prostaglandin synthesis (see II.C.1.a). As a result, they are analgesic for low-intensity integumental pain, antipyretic, and anti-inflammatory. Note that aspirin is the only salicylate that irreversibly inhibits cyclooxygenase by covalent acetylation of the enzyme.
   b. Salicylates also **block** platelet cyclooxygenase and subsequent formation of thromboxane A_2. As a result, they inhibit platelet aggregation and eventual thrombus formation.

3. **Therapeutic indications**
   a. Salicylates are indicated for use as:
      (1) **Analgesics,** for relief of musculoskeletal pain, headache, neuralgias, myalgias, and spasmodic dysmenorrhea
      (2) **Anti-inflammatory agents,** for relief of various arthritis symptoms and acute rheumatic fever
      (3) **Antipyretic agents,** for relief of fever. (Children with varicella or influenza-type viral infections should not be given salicylates because of the observed association between salicylate use in these situations and Reye syndrome.)
   b. **Aspirin** is also indicated for **prophylaxis of myocardial infarction.**
   c. **Methyl salicylate** (wintergreen oil) is used topically as a **counterirritant.**
   d. **Sulfasalazine, olsalazine,** and **mesalamine** are used to reduce the inflammation associated with inflammatory bowel disease and Crohn disease.

4. **Adverse effects**
   a. **Salicylates** are associated with the following effects:
      (1) GI effects, such as nausea; vomiting; and GI irritation, discomfort, ulceration, and hemorrhage
      (2) Increased depth of respirations
      (3) Excessive bleeding associated with inhibition of thromboxane synthesis
      (4) Uncoupling of oxidative phosphorylation, hyperglycemia, glycosuria, and reduced lipogenesis

A

B

Figure 14-8. Structural formulas of salicylate derivatives. **A.** Diflunisal. **B.** Methyl salicylate.

Figure 14-9. Structural formula of acetaminophen, the prototypical *p*-aminophenol derivative.

(5) Delayed onset of labor

(6) **Low daily doses** of salicylates (2 g) decrease renal urate excretion and increase serum uric acid levels. **High daily doses** (5 g) have the opposite effect.

b. **Sulfasalazine** has also been shown to have male reproductive effects, causing infertility.

c. **Salicylism** (salicylate toxicity, usually marked by tinnitus, nausea, and vomiting)

d. **Ingestion** of 1 teaspoon of the topical agent **methyl salicylate** (wintergreen oil) can cause **fatal intoxication.**

B. *p*-Aminophenol derivatives

1. **Chemistry.** The prototypical *p*-aminophenol derivative is **acetaminophen** (Tylenol), an active metabolite of phenacetin and acetanilid (Figure 14-9).

2. **Pharmacology**
   a. *p*-Aminophenol derivatives inhibit central prostaglandin synthesis (see II.C.I.a), presumably through a selectivity for COX 3 with relatively little or no activity on COX 1 or COX 2. They are analgesic for low-intensity pain and are antipyretic.
   b. Because they are less effective than salicylates in blocking peripheral prostaglandin synthesis, they have no anti-inflammatory activity and do not affect platelet function.

3. **Therapeutic indications**
   a. **Acetaminophen** is primarily used for its **analgesic** and **antipyretic activity,** particularly in a patient unable to tolerate salicylates.
   b. **Acetaminophen** may be safely used as an **alternative antipyretic** in children with varicella or an influenza-type viral infection (see III.A.3.a.(3)).

4. **Adverse effects**
   a. When given in therapeutic doses, adverse effects are limited to:
      (1) Skin rash
      (2) Hemolytic anemia (with long-term phenacetin use)
      (3) Methemoglobinemia
      (4) Renal dysfunction and tubular necrosis
   b. Acute acetaminophen overdose causes severe hepatotoxicity with necrosis and liver failure.

C. Pyrazolone derivatives

1. **Chemistry.** The most important pyrazolone derivatives are **phenylbutazone,** its metabolite **oxyphenbutazone,** and the uricosuric agent **sulfinpyrazone** (Anturane). Phenylbutazone is the prototypical agent (Figure 14-10).

Figure 14-10. Structural formula of phenylbutazone, a pyrazolone derivative.

2. Pharmacology
   a. **Phenylbutazone, oxyphenbutazone,** and **azapropazone** inhibit prostaglandin synthesis (see II.C.l.a) and stabilize lysosomal membranes. As a result, they have analgesic, antipyretic, and anti-inflammatory effects. They also have good uricosuric activity.
   b. **Sulfinpyrazone** inhibits proximal tubular absorption of urate and has a uricosuric effect. However, it is devoid of analgesic, antipyretic, or anti-inflammatory effects.

3. Therapeutic indications
   a. **Phenylbutazone** and **oxyphenbutazone** are used for short-term treatment of acute rheumatoid arthritic conditions and acute gout. However, they should be given only after other therapeutic measures have failed.
   b. **Sulfinpyrazone** is used to control hyperuricemia in the treatment of intermittent and chronic gout.
   c. These agents are rarely used, having been replaced with relatively safer compounds.

4. Adverse effects
   a. The adverse effects of **phenylbutazone, oxyphenbutazone,** and **azapropazone** (to a much less extent) often limit their use and include
      (1) GI effects, such as discomfort, nausea, vomiting, dyspepsia, and peptic ulceration
      (2) Blood dyscrasias, such as agranulocytosis, aplastic anemia, hemolytic anemia, thrombocytopenia, and petechiae
      (3) Cardiovascular effects, such as congestive heart failure with edema and dyspnea
      (4) Renal effects, such as nephrotic lithiasis, renal necrosis, impaired renal function, and renal failure
      (5) CNS effects, such as drowsiness, agitation, confusion, headache, lethargy, numbness, weakness, tinnitus, and hearing loss
      (6) Hyperglycemia
      (7) Skin rash
   b. **Sulfinpyrazone** is associated with the following adverse effects:
      (1) GI effects, such as discomfort and upset
      (2) Blood dyscrasias, as with phenylbutazone and oxyphenbutazone
      (3) Renal failure

D. Agents used for the treatment of gout

1. Chemistry
   a. Acute attacks of gout result from an inflammatory response to joint depositions of sodium urate crystals. Therapeutic agents counter this response by reducing plasma uric acid concentrations or inhibiting the inflammatory response.
   b. Agents used for the treatment of gout have widely varying structures and include the pyrazolone derivative sulfinpyrazone (see III.C.2.b; III.C.3.b; III.C.4.b); the alkaloid **colchicine;** isopurines, such as **allopurinol** (Zyloprim); and benzoic acid derivatives, such as **probenecid** (Benemid) (Figure 14-11).

2. Pharmacology
   a. **Colchicine's** mechanism of action is presumed to be related to its antimitotic activity. It inhibits tubulin synthesis, which is required for the movement of inflammatory cells.

Figure 14-11. Structural formulas of agents used in the treatment of gout. **A.** Allopurinol. **B.** Probenecid.

Through its ability to prevent tubulin polymerization, colchicine appears to inhibit chemotaxis of leukocytes and other inflammatory cells in the affected joint, thus reducing the inflammatory response to deposited urate crystals by inhibiting leukocyte migration and phagocytosis. It also interferes with kinin formation and reduces leukocyte lactic acid production.

   b. Allopurinol reduces serum urate levels by blocking uric acid production. It competitively inhibits the enzyme xanthine oxidase, which converts xanthine and hypoxanthine to uric acid.

   c. Probenecid, a uricosuric agent, inhibits the proximal tubular reabsorption of uric acid, increasing uric acid excretion, thus reducing plasma uric acid concentrations.

3. Therapeutic indications
   a. Colchicine is used principally for the treatment of acute gout attacks.
   b. Allopurinol, which reduces uric acid synthesis and facilitates the dissolution of tophi (chalky urate deposits), is used to prevent the development or progression of chronic tophaceous gout.
   c. Probenecid is used to treat chronic tophaceous gout. It is also used in smaller doses to prolong the effectiveness of penicillin-type antibiotics by inhibiting their tubular secretion.

4. Adverse effects
   a. Chronic use of **colchicine** is associated with these adverse effects:
     (1) Agranulocytosis, aplastic anemia, myopathy, hair loss, and peripheral neuritis
     (2) Nausea, vomiting, abdominal pain, and diarrhea (indications of impending toxicity)
   b. Allopurinol is associated with the following adverse effects:
     (1) GI effects, such as GI distress, nausea, vomiting, and diarrhea
     (2) Skin rash, Stevens-Johnson syndrome, and hepatotoxicity
     (3) Precipitation of an acute gout attack (with initial allopurinol therapy owing to initial mobilization of stored urate)
   c. Probenecid is associated with the following adverse effects:
     (1) Headaches, nausea, vomiting, urinary frequency, sore gums, and dermatitis
     (2) Dizziness, anemia, hemolytic anemia, and renal lithiasis

E. NSAIDs

1. Chemistry
   a. The classic **NSAIDs** consist of many structurally diverse acids. These include **propionic acid** derivatives (fenoprofen [Nalfon], flurbiprofen [Ocufen], ibuprofen [Motrin], ketoprofen [Orudis], naproxen [Anaprox, Naprosyn], and oxaprozin [Daypro]), **acetic acid** derivatives (diclofenac [Voltaren], etodolac [Lodine], indomethacin [Indocin], ketorolac [Toradol], sulindac [Clinoril], and tolmetin [Tolectin] and the subclass of the fenamates or anthranilic acid derivatives meclofenamate and mefenamic acid [Ponstel]), and the **enolic acid** derivatives (piroxicam [Feldene], meloxicam [Mobic], and nabumetone [Relafen]) (Figure 14-12).
   b. Selective COX 2 inhibitors celecoxib (Celebrex) and **rofecoxib** (Vioxx), and **valdecoxib** (Bextra) are pyrazole derivatives (Figure 14-13).

2. Pharmacology
   a. Nonspecific NSAIDs have anti-inflammatory effects, resulting from their ability to inhibit the cyclooxygenase enzyme system and thus reduce local prostaglandin synthesis (see II.C.1.a).
   b. NSAIDs also have analgesic and antipyretic effects. In addition, some NSAIDs have mild uricosuric activity. Some agents also have weak inhibitory activity for lipoxygenase, mild selectivity for COX 2, and weak to moderate ability to inhibit leukocyte proliferation and migration and to stabilize lysosomal membranes. The clinical relevance of these secondary actions has not been elucidated.
   c. COX 2 inhibitors exert anti-inflammatory effects by specifically inhibiting prostaglandin synthesis associated with the inflammatory response. Their ability to decrease pain and inflammation associated with arthritic diseases is approximately equal to that produced by the nonselective NSAIDs. Moreover, by virtue of their selectivity, their actions on gastric mucosa and platelet aggregation are theorized to be less than the nonselective NSAIDs.

Figure 14-12. Structural formulas of representative nonsteroidal anti-inflammatory drugs (NSAIDs). **A.** Ibuprofen (propionic acid derivative). **B.** Indomethacin (acetic acid derivative). **C.** Mefenamic acid (anthranilic acid derivative). **D.** Piroxicam (enolic acid derivative).

3. Therapeutic indications

  a. NSAIDs, like aspirin, are agents of choice for the treatment of rheumatoid arthritis, osteo-arthritis, and ankylosing spondylitis. They may also be used as secondary treatments in gouty arthritis.

  b. COX 2 inhibitors are approved for use in both rheumatoid arthritis and osteoarthritis.

4. Adverse effects

  a. NSAIDs are associated with the following adverse effects:

  (1) GI effects, such as GI distress and irritation, erosion of gastric mucosa, nausea, vomit-ing, and dyspepsia

  (2) CNS effects, such as CNS depression, drowsiness, headache, dizziness, visual distur-bances, ototoxicity, and confusion

  (3) Hematologic effects, such as thrombocytopenia, altered platelet function, and pro-longed bleeding time

Celecoxib (Celebrex)

Figure 14-13. Structural formula of celecoxib, a COX 2 specific inhibitor.

        (4) Skin rash

        (5) Nephrotoxicity

  b. **COX 2 inhibitors** do not appear to cause as great an incidence of GI ulceration or antiplatelet effects as the nonselective NSAIDs. The most commonly reported side effects include GI upset at a lower incidence level. Despite the promise of minimal GI ulceration, many patients experienced gastrointestinal bleeding with these drugs soon after their release. This is thought to have been an instance of overuse/overdosing of the drug. This risk of gastric damage and potential ulceration appears to increase with chronic, high dose use of these drugs. The potential for nephrotoxicity does exist for these drugs, and patients should be monitored for changes in renal function. More recent adverse drug reactions associated with these drugs include an increased risk of thrombotic events, leading to myocardial infarction and stroke, which could be potentially fatal. This is likely the result of an inhibition of cardiovascular COX 2 and subsequent clot formation. This has lead to the voluntary removal of some of these drugs from the market and cautious, closely supervised use of the others.

STUDY QUESTIONS

Directions: Each of the questions, statements, or incomplete statements in this section can be correctly answered or completed by **one** of the suggested answers or phrases. Choose the **best** answer.

1. A 45-year-old long-haul trucker suffers from seasonal allergies. He asks advice on which over-the counter product is best to relieve his symptoms. Which of the following choices is the best recommendation for this patient?

(A) diphenhydramine
(B) promethazine
(C) clemastine
(D) chlorpheniramine
(E) loratadine

2. Which of the following choices would be most appropriate in treating nausea and vomiting associated with motion sickness?

(A) diphenhydramine
(B) brompheniramine
(C) ondansetron
(D) omeprazole
(E) ranitidine

3. Esomeprazole would be effective in the treatment of

(A) gastroesophageal reflux disease.
(B) peptic ulcer disease.
(C) Zollinger-Ellison syndrome.
(D) All of the above
(E) None of the above

4. Which of the following antiulcer medications is most like to cause drug interactions and endocrine side effects?

(A) ranitidine
(B) omeprazole
(C) lansoprazole
(D) cimetidine
(E) famotidine

5. A patient has just been diagnosed with recurrent migraine headaches. Which of the following preexisting conditions would preclude the use of sumatriptan for this patient?

(A) liver disease
(B) renal failure
(C) ischemic heart disease
(D) irritable bowel syndrome (IBS)
(E) gouty arthritis

6. Which of the following is an appropriate indication for the drug tegaserod?

(A) a female patient with constipation-related irritable bowel syndrome (IBS)
(B) a female patient with diarrhea-related IBS
(C) a male patient with Crohn disese
(D) a male patient with diarrhea-related IBS
(E) a patient with Zollinger-Ellison syndrome

7. Which of the following prostaglandin analogs is used specifically for the treatment of glaucoma?

(A) alprostadil
(B) latanoprost
(C) carboprost
(D) dinoprostone
(E) epoprostenol

8. The use of misoprostol to prevent nonsteroidal anti-inflammatory drug–induced ulcers could cause which of the following side effects?

(A) fever
(B) gastrointestinal cramping and diarrhea
(C) headache/pain
(D) All of the above
(E) None of the above

9. Which of the following asthma therapies has been associated with an acute vascular syndrome that is associated with sudden withdrawal of corticosteroid anti-inflammatory drugs?

(A) zafirlukast
(B) zileuton
(C) montelukast
(D) All of the above
(E) None of the above

10. Which of the following asthma therapies is effective by decreasing the amounts of released leukotrienes?

(A) zafirlukast
(B) zileuton
(C) montelukast
(D) All of the above
(E) None of the above

11. Rizatriptan is effective in treating migraine headache by

(A) directly vasoconstricting involved blood vessels.
(B) inhibiting the release of inflammatory neurotransmitters.
(C) directly blocking pain transmission.
(D) All of the above
(E) None of the above

12. Which of the following drugs, based on its mechanism of action, is effective in treating diarrhea-predominant irritable bowel syndrome (IBS)?

(A) tegaserod
(B) naratriptan
(C) alosetron
(D) All of the above
(E) None of the above

13. Which of the following salicylates has been linked to male reproductive toxicity with chronic dosing?

(A) aspirin
(B) diflunisal
(C) sodium thiosalicylate
(D) olsalazine
(E) sulfasalazine

14. Aspirin exerts its anti-platelet effect by inhibiting

(A) cyclooxygenase (COX) 1.
(B) COX 2.
(C) COX 3.
(D) prostaglandin synthesis.
(E) leukotriene synthesis.

15. Acetaminophen has advantages over aspirin or other nonsteroidal anti-inflammatory drugs by virtue of its

(A) relative lack of anti-platelet effects.
(B) relative lack of gastrointestinal ulcerative effects.
(C) being a safe alternative for children with viral infections.
(D) All of the above
(E) None of the above

16. Acetaminophen toxicity is characterized by

(A) profound vasoconstriction and pain.
(B) severe abdominal cramping and diarrhea.
(C) central nervous system stimulation and seizures.
(D) profound liver damage and failure.
(E) All of the above

17. Which of the following antigout medications is specifically used in acute attacks?

(A) colchicine
(B) allopurinol
(C) probenecid
(D) All of the above
(E) None of the above

18. Which of the following antigout medications acts by decreasing serum levels but increasing urine levels of uric acid, thus increasing the risk of kidney stone development?

(A) colchicine
(B) allopurinol
(C) probenecid
(D) All of the above
(E) None of the above

19. The nonsteroidal anti-inflammatory drugs, as a class, are anti-inflammatory primarily through their ability to inhibit

(A) cyclooxygenase (COX) 1.
(B) COX 2.
(C) COX 3.
(D) leukotriene synthesis.
(E) thromboxane synthesis.

20. The selective cyclooxygenase (COX) 2 inhibitors have been associated with which of the following adverse drug reactions?

(A) severe ischemic colitis
(B) torsade des pointes
(C) cardiovascular thrombotic events
(D) acute liver failure
(E) Churg-Strauss syndrome

ANSWERS AND EXPLANATIONS

1. The answer is E *[see II.A.1.b.(1); II.A.3.b].*
Diphenhydramine, promethazine, and clemastine all possess moderate to strong anticholinergic activity. This will increase the risk of sedation, which could prove dangerous in this patient. Chlorpheniramine, while the least sedating of the first-generation drugs, still may cross the blood–brain barrier and cause some sedation. Loratadine, as a second-generation drug that has minimal anticholinergic activity and does not cross the blood–brain barrier (thus producing no central effects), is least likely to cause sedation and thus affect his job.

2. The answer is A *[see II.A.3.b].*
While ondansetron is used for nausea associated with chemotherapy and anaesthetics, it is not typically used for nausea associated with motion or vertigo. Diphenhydramine, which possesses a high degree of anticholinergic activity, is effective in reducing nausea and vomiting associated with vestibulocochlear activity, vertigo, and motion sickness. None of the other choices directly reduces nausea or vomiting, therefore, diphenhydramine is the best choice.

3. The answer is D *[see II.A.1.b.(3); II.A.3.d].*
Because all three of these disease states represent some action of excessive acid secretion, esomeprazole, which also blocks the proton or acid pump, would be effective in reducing the acid-induced pain and damage associated with gastroesophageal reflux disease (GERD), peptic ulcer disease (PUD), and Zollinger-Ellison syndrome.

4. The answer is D *[see II.A.4.d].*
Of the drugs listed, and specifically, of the H_2-antagonists, cimetidine is the only drug that inhibits the hepatic microsomal metabolizing system (specifically the 3A4 isozyme) and the only drug that exhibits weak androgenic activity. The former is responsible for numerous drug interactions and some side effects, whereas the latter is responsible for endocrine (specifically androgen-like) side effects.

5. The answer is C *[see II.B.2.a; II.B.4.a.(1)].*
Sumatriptan (and other drugs in the class) specifically cause vasoconstriction. This effect, when present in coronory vessels, can cause chest tightness of pain as a normal side effect of the drug. However, in patients with ischemic heart disease, angina, or a risk for coronary artery disease, this action could precipitate attacks of angina or potentially cause myocardial infarction and should not be used in those patients.

6. The answer is A *[see II.B.1.b.(2); II.B.2.b.(2); II.B.3.a.(4)].*
Currently, drugs are available specifically for women with IBS characterized by either constipation or diarrhea. The intestinal stimulant action of tegaserod makes it useful for those patients with constipation-associated IBS. Although tegaserod (and alosetron) is (are) being evaluated for use in men with IBS, the current recommendation is primarily for women. Tegaserod, as a prokinetic agent, would worsen IBS that presents primarily with diarrhea. Because it has no anti-inflammatory effect, it would not be effective in treating the primarily inflammatory nature of Crohn disease. Tegaserod has no effect on gastric acid secretion and would, therefore, not be useful in Zollinger-Ellison syndrome.

7. The answer is B *[see II.C.3.c.(2)].*
Although most prostaglandin analogs are nonspecific in their sites of action and may produce similar physiological effects, latanoprost is specifically formulated and marketed for use in the treatment of glaucoma. Its relative selectivity for the $PGF_{2\alpha}$ receptor is responsible for its ability to lower intraocular pressure and, therefore, its benefit in treating glaucoma.

8. The answer is D *[see II.C.2.b; II.C.4].*
As noted in the answer to question 7, most prostaglandin analogs have activity at receptors throughout the body, causing a prostaglandin-like effect on numerous organ systems. Misoprostol, as a relatively nonselective agonist, would cause contraction of gastrointestinal smooth muscle, stimulate pain fibers, and reset the thermoregulatory center of the CNS, thus causing all the potential side effects listed.

9. The answer is A *[see II.D.4].*
Zafirlukast is the only drug that has been associated with Churg-Strauss syndrome, a condition of eosinophilic vasculitis that occurs when a patient who is on both zafirlukast and corticosteroid therapy suddenly discontinues the corticosteroid. This effect has not been observed with the pharmacologically similar drug montelukast. Note that slow withdrawal of the corticosteroid (which should be done anyway, to minimize acute adrenal insufficiency) will prevent this adverse drug reaction.

10. The correct answer is B *[see II.D.2.b].*
Zafirlukast and montelukast exert their effect by blocking leukotrienes at their receptor. Zileuton, which acts by inhibiting lipo-oxygenase, will decrease the synthesis of these inflammatory mediators. Therefore, it is the only drug listed that will decrease the synthesis and, consequently, the release of leukotrienes.

11. The answer is D *[see II.B.1.b.(1); II.B.2.b.(1)].*
Rizatriptan (and other drugs in the class) are acting as $5-HT_1$-agonists. This mechanism results in three distinct and beneficial pharmacodynamic effects. First, it causes direct vasoconstriction, which returns the blood vessel to its preheadache diameter. Second, by acting on neuronal receptors, it inhibits the release of additional vasodilating and pain-transmitting substances, such as neurokinin A and substance P. Third, this action has been shown to have a direct antinociceptive action, preventing the firing of pain neurones directly. Therefore all three answers correctly describe the benefit of rizatriptan.

12. The correct answer is C *[see II.B.1.c.(2); II.B.2.c; II.B.3.b].*
Alosetron is the agent useful in treating diarrhea-predominant IBS. By blocking the $5-HT_3$-receptor, it inhibits the serotonin-induced increase in intestinal motility, thus slowing peristalsis and gut movement. Tegaserod would worsen diarrhea-predominant IBS, because its serotonergic actions are agonistic and would stimulate GI smooth muscle contraction. Naratriptan, acting as a $5-HT_1$-agonist, has little effect on GI motility.

13. The correct answer is E *[see III.A.4.b].*
Of the salicylates, sulfasalazine has been most associated with this particular toxicity. It is a toxicity that occurs with chronic use of the drug in men with Crohn disease or other inflammatory conditions of the intestine. Withdrawal of the drug may allow reproductive function to return, although this is not always the case. In addition, it may take an extended period of time, after cessation of therapy, for function to return.

14. The correct answer is A *[see II.C.1.a; III.A.2.a].*
Recall that in prostaglandin and thromboxane synthesis, COX 1 is responsible for much of the daily production of maintenance eicosanoids. COX 2, while also contributing to daily production of prostaglandins and thromboxanes, is more important in inflammation. COX 3 is the central source of prostaglandins that contribute to CNS function of the eicosanoids. Also recall that it is thromboxane that specifically has platelet-aggregating ability. Therefore, it is through inhibition of COX 1 and the subsequent decrease in thromboxane (not prostaglandin or leukotriene) synthesis that the antiplatelet effect of aspirin is effected.

15. The correct answer is D *[see II.C.1.a; III.B.3].*
The roles of COX 1, 2, and 3 are reviewed in the answer to question 14. Because, mechanistically, acetaminophen is thought to be relatively selective for COX 3, it would not possess any antiplatelet activity, nor would it reduce the synthesis of gastric cytoprotective prostaglandins. Therefore, it would not interfere with platelet function or other antiplatelet therapies and it would not be prone to cause gastric ulceration. In addition, the relationship between aspirin and Reye syndrome in children with viral infections does not apparently exist with acetaminophen, making it a safe antipyretic to use in those patients.

16. The correct answer is D *[see III.B.4.b].*
Acetaminophen toxicity is characterized by a profound hepatoxicity, which is mediated by a reactive intermediary formed on saturation and depletion of the normal metabolic pathways. This does not affect the vasculature (as with the ergot derivatives), thus no vasoconstriction is observed. Neither is severe GI upset evident (although mild GI upset may occur early in toxicity). Nor does profound CNS stimulation occur, as it does with aspirin toxicity. Therefore answer D is correct.

17. The correct answer is A *[see III.D.1.a; III.D.2.a; III.D.3.a]*
Allopurinol and probenecid, while effective in preventing attacks of gouty arthritis by lowering circulating levels of uric acid, are not effective in treating the acute inflammatory situation that characterizes an acute attack. Colchicine, by inhibiting the migration of proinflammatory cells into the affected joint, will reduce the inflammatory process, thus alleviating the pain and edema associated with acute attacks of gouty arthritis.

18. The correct answer is C *[see III.D.2.c; III.D.3.c; III.D.4.c.(2)]*
Probenecid, as a uricosuric and promoting the excretion of uric acid, will effectively lower plasma concentration of urate. However, it also increases the urinary levels of uric acid. If this concentration exceeds the solubility constant of uric acid in the urine, then it may crystallize and precipitate out, causing stone formation or urinary lithiasis. For this reason, patients taking probenecid should always be counseled to drink copious amounts of water.

19. The correct answer is B *[see II.C.1.a; III.E.2]*
The roles of COX 1, 2, and 3 are reviewed in the answer to question 14. It is through their inhibition of inflammatory prostaglandin synthesis by inhibiting COX 2, that the NSAIDs exert their anti-inflammatory actions.

20. The correct answers is C *[see III.E.4.b]*
The primary side effects that have been associated with the COX 2 specific inhibitors are gastrointestinal bleeding and, more recently, potentially fatal thrombotic events. The latter is thought to reflect a toxicodynamic effect that results from inhibition of vascular COX 2, which contributes to the daily control of platelet and/or vascular function. Severe ischemic colitis has been reported with alosetron; torsade des points, with older, second-generation antihistaminics; and cisapride which are no longer available for use; acute liver failure, with acetaminophen overdose; and Churg-Strauss syndrome with zafirlukast and corticosteroid withdrawal. None of these adverse drug reactions has been associated with the COX 2 specific inhibitors.

15
Medicinal Chemistry and Pharmacology: Cardiovascular and Diuretic Drugs

J. Edward Moreton

I. INTRODUCTION. Many categories of drugs affect the cardiovascular (CV) and renal systems. Certain drugs can be used to treat heart failure (e.g., cardiac glycosides and diuretics), relieve angina pectoris (e.g., antianginal agents), and control dysrhythmias (e.g., antiarrhythmic agents). Others can reduce hypertension (e.g., antihypertensives, including a variety of diuretics, β-blocking agents, and arteriolar smooth muscle dilators), treat the hyperlipidemias (e.g., antihyperlipidemic agents), reduce clotting and treat such conditions as venous thrombosis and pulmonary embolism (e.g., anticoagulants, thrombolytics), and treat anemias (e.g., antianemic agents).

II. CARDIAC GLYCOSIDES AND POSITIVE INOTROPES

A. Chemistry

1. Almost all of the cardiac glycosides (also called **cardiotonics**) are naturally occurring steroidal glycosides obtained from plant sources. **Digitoxin** is obtained from *Digitalis purpurea,* **digoxin** from *Digitalis lanata,* and **ouabain** from *Strophanthus gratus.*

2. The cardiac glycosides are closely related structurally, consisting of one or more sugars (i.e., **glycone portion**) and a steroidal nucleus (i.e., **aglycon or genin portion**) bonded through an **ether (glycosidic) linkage.** These agents also have an **unsaturated lactone substituent (cyclic ester)** on the genin portion. The prototypical agent is **digitoxin** (Figure 15-1).
   a. **Digoxin** (Lanoxin) has an additional hydroxyl group at position 12 (Figure 15-1).
   b. **Ouabain** has a rhamnose glycone portion and additional hydroxyl groups at positions 1, 5, 11, and 19 (Figure 15-1).

3. Removing the glycone portion causes decreased activity and increased toxicity from changes in polarity that cause erratic absorption from the gastrointestinal (GI) tract.

4. The **duration of action** of a cardiac glycoside is **inversely proportional to the number of hydroxyl groups,** which increase polarity. Increased polarity results in decreased protein binding, decreased liver biotransformation, and decreased renal tubular reabsorption.
   a. **Digitoxin** has a long duration of action and may accumulate.
   b. **Ouabain,** in contrast, has an extremely short duration of action and is effective only when given intravenously.

Figure 15-1. Structural formula of digitoxin (Crystodigin), the prototypical cardiac glycoside.

Figure 15-2. Structural formulas of bipyridine derivatives. **A.** Amrinone (Inocor). **B.** Milrinone (Primacor).

5. **Amrinone, inamrinone, and milrinone** are bipyridine derivatives with positive inotropic action (Figure 15-2).

B. **Pharmacology.** Cardiac glycosides increase myocardial contractility and efficiency, improve systemic circulation, improve renal perfusion, and reduce edema. The electrophysiological effects of cardiac glycosides are summarized in Table 15-1. Angiotensin-converting enzyme (ACE) inhibitors and perhaps AT_1 angiotensin-receptor antagonists; vasodilators such as nitroprusside, nitroglycerin, and hydralazine; and diuretics may be important adjuncts to cardiac glycosides. ACE inhibitors may be considered as first-line treatment.

1. When given in therapeutic doses, cardiac glycosides produce positive inotropic effects by inhibiting membrane-bound Na^+/K^+-activated adenosine triphosphatase (ATPase). These effects of cardiac glycosides increase the rate of tension development, the contractility, and the rate of relaxation of cardiac muscle. The effects include
   a. Increase in intracellular sodium concentration
   b. Reduction in calcium transport from the cell by the sodium–calcium exchanger
   c. Facilitation of calcium entry via voltage-gated membrane channels
   d. Increased release of calcium from sarcoplasmic reticulum

2. Therapeutic doses of cardiac glycosides also cause
   a. A negative chronotropic effect from increased vagal tone of the sinoatrial (SA) node
   b. Diminished central nervous system (CNS) sympathetic outflow from increased carotid sinus baroreceptor sensitivity
   c. Systemic arteriolar and venous constriction, which increases venous return and thus increases cardiac output

3. Amrinone and milrinone produce positive inotropic effects and vasodilation via selective inhibition of type III phosphodiesterase (PDE) isozyme, leading to an increase in cyclic adenosine monophosphate (cAMP) in cardiac and smooth muscle. Inhibition of type III PDE produces

Table 15-1. Effects of Cardiac Glycosides on the Heart

Effects	Atria	AV Node	Ventricles
Direct	Contractility ↑ ERP ↑ Conduction velocity ↓	ERP ↑ Conduction velocity ↓	Contractility ↑ ERP ↓ Automaticity ↑
Indirect	ERP ↓ Conduction velocity ↑	ERP ↑ Conduction velocity ↓	No effect
On electrocardiogram	P changes	PR interval ↑	QT ↓ T and ST depressed
Adverse	Extrasystole	AV depression or block	Fibrillation
	Tachycardia		Extrasystole Tachycardia

AV, atrioventricular; *ERP,* effective refractory period; ↑, increased; ↓, decreased.
Reprinted with permission from Jacob LS, Pharmacology, 3rd ed. Malvern, PA, Harwal, 1992:96.

   a. Vasodilation and fall in vascular resistance

   b. Increased force of cardiac contraction

   c. Increased velocity of cardiac relaxation

C. Therapeutic indications

   1. Heart failure (stage C only)

   2. Atrial fibrillation

   3. Atrial flutter

   4. Paroxysmal atrial tachycardia

   5. Amrinone and milrinone are indicated for short-term treatment of congestive heart failure only.

D. Adverse effects

   1. Early adverse effects of cardiac glycosides represent the early stages of toxicity, including
      a. GI effects, such as anorexia, nausea, vomiting, and diarrhea
      b. CNS effects, such as headache, visual disturbances (green or yellow vision), confusion, delirium, neuralgias, and muscle weakness

   2. Later adverse effects represent intoxication and include such serious cardiac disturbances as premature ventricular contractions, paroxysmal and nonparoxysmal atrial tachycardia, atrioventricular (AV) dissociation or block, ventricular tachycardia, and ventricular fibrillation.

III. DRUGS FOR TREATMENT OF MYOCARDIAL ISCHEMIA

A. Chemistry

   1. Antianginal agents include **nitrites** (i.e., organic esters of nitrous acid) such as amyl nitrite, **nitrates** (i.e., organic esters of nitric acid) such as nitroglycerin and isosorbide, **β-blockers** such as propranolol, and **calcium antagonists** such as verapamil and nifedipine (Figure 15-3).
      a. Amyl nitrite is a volatile and flammable liquid administered by inhalation. It requires special precautions (especially restriction of smoking) during administration.
      b. Nitroglycerin is also a volatile and flammable liquid and requires great care during storage. It must be dispensed from its original glass containers and protected from body heat.
         (1) When given intravenously, nitroglycerin requires the use of special plastic administration sets to avoid absorption and loss of potency.
         (2) Nitroglycerin is metabolically unstable and undergoes extensive first-pass metabolism.

   2. Peripheral vasodilators include the dipiperidino-dipyrimidine dipyridamole (Figure 15-3).

B. Pharmacology

   1. Nitrites and nitrates are fast-acting antianginal agents that directly relax vascular smooth muscle by formation of the free radical nitric oxide (NO), which is identical to endothelium-derived relaxing factor (EDRF). NO activates guanylyl cyclase to increase synthesis of cyclic guanosine monophosphate (cGMP) within smooth muscle, resulting in dephosphorylation of light chain myosin and muscle relaxation. This causes peripheral pooling of the blood, diminished venous return (reduced preload), decreased systemic vascular resistance, and decreased arterial pressure (reduced afterload). These vascular effects:
      a. Reduce myocardial oxygen demand
      b. Cause redistribution of coronary blood flow along the collateral coronary arteries, improving perfusion of the ischemic myocardium

   2. β-Adrenergic blockers decrease sympathetic-mediated myocardial stimulation (see Chapter 13, IV.A.2, IV.C.4). The resulting negative inotropic and negative chronotropic effects reduce myocardial oxygen requirements.

Figure 15-3. Structural formulas of antianginal agents. **A.** Nitroglycerin (Nitrostat). **B.** Isosorbide dinitrate (Isordil). **C.** Nifedipine (Procardia). **D.** Dipyridamole (Persantine).

3. **Calcium antagonists** (also known as **calcium channel blockers**) block calcium entry through the membranous calcium ion (Ca^{++}) channels of coronary and peripheral vascular smooth muscle.
   a. Peripheral arterioles dilate and total peripheral resistance decreases, reducing afterload and reducing myocardial oxygen requirements.
   b. Calcium antagonists also increase oxygen delivery to the myocardium by dilating coronary arteries and arterioles.

4. **Dipyridamole** relaxes smooth muscles, decreasing coronary vascular resistance and increasing coronary blood flow.

C. **Therapeutic indications**

1. **Nitrites and nitrates** are used to relieve acute anginal attacks, as prophylaxis during anticipation of an acute anginal attack, and for long-term management of recurrent angina pectoris.

2. **β-Adrenergic blockers** are used for adjunctive prophylaxis of chronic stable angina pectoris in combination with nitrites or nitrates. They have also been shown to increase survival time in heart failure and after myocardial infarction (MI). Three β-blockers are proven to reduce mortality in heart failure and are now class I recommendations for heart failure.

3. **Calcium antagonists** are used to treat chronic stable angina pectoris and variant (Prinzmetal) angina.

4. **Dipyridamole** is now used primarily as a platelet aggregation inhibitor.

D. Adverse effects

1. **Nitrites and nitrates** are associated with:
   a. CNS effects, such as headache, apprehension, dizziness, and weakness
   b. CV effects, such as hypotension, tachycardia, palpitations, and syncope
   c. Skin effects, such as rash and dermatitis
   d. Methemoglobinemia

2. **β-Adrenergic blockers** are associated with:
   a. Worsening of congestive heart failure
   b. Bradycardia and hypotension
   c. Reduced kidney blood flow and decreased glomerular filtration

3. **Calcium antagonists** generally produce only mild adverse effects.
   a. When given in conjunction with β-adrenergic blockers, the CV effects of calcium antagonists may be enhanced, resulting in bradycardia, hypotension, peripheral edema, congestive heart failure, AV block, and asystole.
   b. **Verapamil** may also cause sleeplessness, muscle fatigue, nystagmus, and emotional depression. During the first week of therapy, verapamil increases serum digitalis concentrations and may cause digitalis toxicity.

4. **Dipyridamole** is associated with:
   a. GI effects, such as nausea, vomiting, and diarrhea
   b. CNS effects, such as headache and dizziness
   c. CV effects, such as hypotension (with excessive doses)
   d. Bleeding

IV. ANTIARRHYTHMIC AGENTS

A. **Chemistry.** Antiarrhythmic agents have widely diverse chemical structures. They include representatives of the following groups:

1. **Cinchona alkaloids**—such as quinidine (an optical isomer of quinine)

2. **Amides**—such as procainamide (Pronestyl), flecainide (Tambocor), and disopyramide (Norpace)

3. **Xylyl derivatives**—such as lidocaine (Xylocaine) and mexiletine (Mexitil)

4. **Quaternary ammonium salts**—such as bretylium (Bretylol)

5. **Diiodobenzyloxyethylamines**—such as amiodarone (Cordarone)

6. **β-Blockers**—such as, nadolol (Corgard), propranolol (Inderal), esmolol (Brevibloc), and acebutolol (Sectral)

7. **Calcium antagonists**—such as diltiazem (Cardizem) and verapamil (Calan)

8. **Hydantoins**—such as phenytoin (Dilantin)

B. **Pharmacology.** Antiarrhythmic agents are classified according to their ability to alter the action potential of cardiac cells (Tables 15-2 and 15-3). The myocardial action potential curve is shown in Figure 15-4.

1. **Class IA drugs** (e.g., quinidine, procainamide, disopyramide) produce state-dependent sodium channel blockade to slow the rate of rise of phase 0 (the phase of rapid depolarization and reversal of transmembrane voltage) and prolong repolarization and effective refractory period.

2. **Class IB drugs** (e.g., lidocaine, tocainide, mexiletine, phenytoin) have a minimal effect on the rate of rise of phase 0 and shorten repolarization.

3. **Class IC drugs** (e.g., flecainide, propafenone) have a marked effect in slowing the rate of rise of phase 0 and in slowing conduction. They have little effect on repolarization. Encainide was withdrawn from the market but is available on a limited basis.

Table 15-2. Major Effects of Antiarrhythmic Drugs on Electrocardiogram

Drug	QRS	QT	PR[a]
Quinidine	↑	↑	→↑
Procainamide			
Amiodarone			
Disopyramide	↑	↑	→
Lidocaine	→	↓	→↑↓
Phenytoin			
Tocainide			
Mexiletine			
Propranolol	→	↓	→↑

↑, increased; ↓, decreased; →, no change.
[a]All antiarrhythmic drugs have a variable response, usually with little observable effect. However, lidocaine hardly ever affects the PR interval, whereas phenytoin and propranolol usually increase the PR interval.
Reprinted with permission from Jacob LS. Pharmacology, 3rd ed. Malvern, PA, Harwal, 1992:102.

Table 15-3. Effects of Antiarrhythmic Drugs on Electrophysiologic Properties of the Heart

| Drug Class | Automaticity | | Effective Refractory Period | | Membrane Responsiveness |
	SA Node	Purkinje Fibers	AV Node	Purkinje Fibers	Purkinje Fibers
IA	→↑	↓→	↑→↓	↑↓	↓
IB	→	↓	→↓	↓	→↓
IC	→	↓	↑	↓	↓
II	↓	↓	↑	↓→↑	↓
III	↑↓	↑↓	↓→↑	↑	→
IV	↓	→↓	↑	→	→

↑, increased; ↓, decreased; →, no change.

Figure 15-4. Myocardial action potential curve. This curve represents ventricular depolarization/repolarization. *0,* phase 0 (rapid depolarization); *1,* phase 1 (early rapid repolarization); *2,* phase 2 (plateau); *3,* phase (final rapid repolarization); *4,* phase 4 (slow depolarization).

4. **Class II drugs** (e.g., propranolol, nadolol, esmolol, acebutolol) are β-adrenergic antagonists that competitively block catecholamine-induced stimulation of cardiac β-receptors and depress depolarization of phase 4.

5. **Class III drugs** (e.g., bretylium, amiodarone, sotalol, ibutilide, dofetilide) increase action potential duration by prolonging repolarization via blockade of the delayed rectifier potassium current I_{Kr}.

6. **Class IV drugs** (e.g., verapamil, diltiazem, bepridil) are calcium antagonists that block the slow inward current carried by calcium during phase 2 (i.e., long-sustained depolarization or the plateau of the action potential), increase the effective refractory period, and depress phase 4 depolarization.

7. **Digoxin and adenosine.** Digitalis glycosides (digoxin) elicit a vagotonic response that increases AV nodal refractoriness. Adenosine acts at G-protein-coupled adenosine receptors to increase AV nodal refractoriness.

8. **Moricizine** is a type I antiarrhythmic but not A, B, or C. It exhibits potent local anesthetic activity and myocardial membrane stabilizing activity. Moricizine reduces fast inward sodium current, decreasing the action potential duration and effective refractory period, and increases the PR, QRS, and QT_e interval.

C. **Therapeutic indications.** Antiarrhythmic agents are used to reduce abnormalities of impulse generation (ectopic pacemaker automaticity) and to modify the disturbances of impulse conduction within cardiac tissue. (Indications for specific agents are given in Table 15-4.)

Table 15-4. Use of Antiarrhythmic Drugs in Common Cardiac Arrhythmias

Arrhythmia	Treatment of Choice	Alternatives
I. Supraventricular		
Atrial fibrillation or flutter	Digital to control ventricular rate, DC shock for conversion	Quinidine to suppress recurrences after DC shock
Paroxysmal atrial or nodal tachycardia	Vagotonic maneuver; digitalis	Verapamil (quinidine, procainamide, disopyramide, and β-adrenergic antagonists may all be useful, especially prophylactically)
II. Ventricular		
Ventricular premature depolarization	Lidocaine	Procainamide, quinidine, or disopyramide for prolonged suppression
Ventricular tachycardia	DC shock	Lidocaine, procainamide, or mexiletine
III. Digitalis-induced		
	Lidocaine or phenytoin	Procainamide is somewhat useful; β-adrenergic antagonists are useful but have a high incidence of adverse effects

DC, direct current.
Reprinted with permission from Jacob LS. Pharmacology, 3rd ed. Malvern, PA, Harwal, 1992:102.

D. Adverse effects

1. **Class IA drugs** are associated with CV effects (e.g., myocardial depression, AV block, ventricular dysrhythmias, asystole, and hypotension) and with GI effects (e.g., GI upset, nausea, vomiting, and diarrhea). In addition:
   a. **Quinidine** can cause cinchonism, with tinnitus, confusion, photophobia, headache, and psychosis.
   b. **Procainamide** can cause systemic lupus erythematosus– (SLE-) like syndrome.
   c. **Disopyramide** can cause congestive heart failure and antimuscarinic effects.

2. **Class IB drugs** are associated with CNS effects (including CNS depression, drowsiness, disorientation, and paresthesias), CV effects (including hypotension and circulatory collapse), and hepatitis. In addition:
   a. **Lidocaine** can cause seizures and respiratory arrest.
   b. **Tocainide** can cause pneumonitis and blood dyscrasias.
   c. **Mexiletine** can cause hepatic injury and blood dyscrasias.
   d. **Phenytoin** can cause nystagmus, decreased mental function, and blood dyscrasias.

3. **Class IC drugs** are associated with:
   a. CV effects, including worsening of arrhythmias in patients with ventricular arrhythmias, particularly patients with a history of MI. They can worsen sinus node dysfunction and heart failure.
   b. Visual disturbances such as blurred or double vision

4. **Class II drugs** are associated with:
   a. CV effects, such as hypotension, AV block, and asystole
   b. Respiratory effects, such as bronchospasm

5. **Class III drugs** are associated with:
   a. CV effects, such as hypotension and initially increased dysrhythmias
   b. GI effects, such as nausea and vomiting

6. **Class IV drugs** are associated with CV adverse effects, such as hypotension, bradycardia, AV block, congestive heart failure, and asystole.

7. **Cardiac glycosides** (see II.D). **Adenosine** causes asystole lasting less than 5 sec and is the therapeutic objective.

8. Because of its proarrhythmic activity, **moricizine** is reserved for patients with life-threatening ventricular arrhythmias.

V. ANTIHYPERTENSIVE AGENTS

A. **Chemistry.** Antihypertensive agents vary so widely in chemical structure that they are usually classified by mechanism of action rather than chemical class (Table 15-5).

B. **Pharmacology.** Antihypertensive agents lower blood pressure by reducing total peripheral resistance or cardiac output through a variety of mechanisms (Table 15-5).

1. **Diuretics** such as thiazides create a negative sodium balance, reduce blood volume, and decrease vascular smooth muscle responsiveness to vasoconstrictors (see VI.C).

2. **Vasodilators** such as diazoxide and minoxidil are potassium channel activators that produce membrane hyperpolarization, whereas hydralazine may stimulate formation of EDRF (NO) to decrease arterial resistance. Human brain natriuretic peptide (BNP) via receptor stimulation and sodium nitroprusside via release of NO activate guanylyl cyclase, forming cGMP to relax both arterioles and veins.

3. **Peripheral sympatholytics** interfere with adrenergic function by blocking postganglionic adrenergic receptors (e.g., propranolol, prazosin), limiting the release of neurotransmitters from adrenergic neurons (e.g., guanethidine), or depleting intraneuronal catecholamine storage sites (e.g., reserpine).

4. **Central α_2-sympathomimetics** (e.g., clonidine, methyldopa) appear to mediate their effects by stimulating presynaptic α_2-inhibitory receptors, resulting in a negative sympathetic outflow and lowered peripheral resistance.

Table 15-5. Classification of Antihypertensive Agents by Their Mechanism of Action

Mechanism of Action	Drug
Vasodilators	
Arteriolar	Diazoxide (Hyperstat IV)
	Hydralazine (Apresoline)
	Minoxidil (Loniten)
Arteriolar and venous	Nitroprusside (Nipride)
Peripheral sympatholytics	Acebutolol (Sectral)
	Atenolol (Tenormin)
	Betaxolol (Kerlone)
	Bisoprolol (Zebeta)
	Carteolol (Cartrol)
	Carvedilol (Coreg)
	Doxazosin (Cardura)
	Guanadrel (Hylorel)
	Guanethidine (Ismelin)
	Labetalol (Trandate)
	Metoprolol (Lopressor)
	Nadolol (Corgard)
	Penbutolol (Levatol)
	Pindolol (Visken)
	Prazosin (Minipress)
	Propranolol (Inderal)
	Reserpine (Serpasil)
	Terazosin (Hytrin)
	Timolol (Blocadren)
Central α_2-sympathomimetics	Clonidine (Catapres)
	Guanabenz (Wytensin)
	Guanfacine (Tenex)
	Methyldopa (Aldomet)
Calcium channel blockers	Amlodipine (Norvasc)
	Diltiazem (Cardizem) SR
	Felodipine (Plendil)
	Isradipine (DynaCirc)
	Nicardipine (Cardene)
	Nifedipine (Procardia) SR
	Verapamil (Calan)
Angiotensin II receptor antagonists	Candesartan (Atacand)
	Irbesartan (Avapro)
	Losartan (Cozaar)
	Telmisartan (Micardis)
	Valsartan (Diovan)
Angiotensin-converting enzyme inhibitors	Benazepril (Lotensin)
	Captopril (Capoten)
	Enalapril (Vasotec)
	Fosinopril (Monopril)
	Lisinopril (Prinivil)
	Moexipril (Univasc)
	Perindopril (Aceon)
	Quinapril (Accupril)
	Ramipril (Altace)
	Trandolapril (Mavik)
Endothelin receptor antagonist	Bosentan (Tracleer)

5. **Calcium channel blockers** (e.g., amlodipine, diltiazem, felodipine, isradipine, nicardipine, nifedipine, verapamil) lower vascular resistance and blood pressure via blockade of voltage-gated calcium channels. Arterioles are more sensitive than veins.

6. **ACE inhibitors** (e.g., captopril) block the conversion of inactive angiotensin I to the potent vasoconstrictor angiotensin II. The reduced angiotensin II concentration also lowers aldosterone concentration, which limits sodium retention.

7. **Angiotensin II receptor antagonists** (e.g., losartan) are nonpeptide antagonists of the AT_1 angiotensin II receptor subtype located in vasculature, myocardium, brain, kidney, and adrenal glomerulosa. They produce vasodilation, cause loss of salt and water to decrease plasma volume, and decrease myogenic activity.

8. **Endothelin receptor antagonists** (e.g., bosentan) are potent orally active nonpeptide endothelin receptor antagonists.

C. Therapeutic indications

1. Antihypertensive agents are used separately or in combination to **treat high blood pressure.**

2. These agents may also be administered parenterally to **treat hypertensive emergencies** such as malignant hypertension, eclampsia, or the severe hypertension associated with excess catecholamines. Parenteral therapy may include some combination of the following agents:
   a. **Arteriolar and venous vasodilator** such as nitroprusside or bosentan (i.e., pulmonary arterial hypertension)
   b. **Arteriolar vasodilator** such as diazoxide or hydralazine
   c. **Dual α-adrenergic- and β-adrenergic-receptor blockers** such as labetalol
   d. **β-Blocking agent** such as propranolol
   e. **Ganglionic-blocking agent** such as trimethaphan

D. Adverse effects

1. **Diuretics (thiazides)** can cause
   a. Fluid and solute imbalances, such as hypokalemia, hypercalcemia, hyperuricemia, hypomagnesemia, hyponatremia, and hyperglycemia
   b. Increased serum low-density lipoprotein (LDL) cholesterol and triglyceride concentrations
   c. Other effects (see VI.C.4)

2. **Vasodilators** are associated with:
   a. GI upset
   b. CNS effects, such as headache and dizziness
   c. CV effects, such as tachycardia, fluid retention, and worsening of angina
   d. Other effects, such as nasal congestion, hepatitis, glomerulonephritis, and SLE-like syndrome

3. **Peripheral sympatholytics** are associated with a variety of adverse effects, depending on the specific agent.
   a. **β-Blockers** (e.g., propranolol) are associated with:
      (1) CV effects, such as bradycardia, congestive heart failure, and Raynaud phenomenon
      (2) GI upset
      (3) Blood dyscrasias
      (4) CNS effects, such as depression, hallucinations, organic brain syndrome, and transient hearing loss
      (5) Other effects, such as increased airway resistance, increased serum triglyceride concentrations, decreased high-density lipoprotein (HDL) cholesterol concentrations, and psoriasis
      (6) Cardiac arrhythmias if withdrawal is abrupt
   b. **Prazosin** is associated with:
      (1) CV effects, such as sudden syncope with the first dose, palpitations, and fluid retention
      (2) CNS effects, such as headache, drowsiness, weakness, dizziness, and vertigo
      (3) Antimuscarinic effects and priapism

    c. Guanethidine is associated with:
      (1) CV effects, such as bradycardia, orthostatic hypotension, and sodium and water retention
      (2) Diarrhea
      (3) Aggravation of bronchial asthma
    d. Reserpine is associated with:
      (1) CNS effects, such as nightmares, depression, and drowsiness
      (2) CV effects, such as bradycardia
      (3) GI effects, such as GI upset and activation of peptic ulcer
      (4) Nasal stuffiness

4. Central α_2-sympathomimetics also have adverse effects that vary with the specific agent.
    a. Clonidine is associated with:
      (1) CNS effects, such as sedation and drowsiness
      (2) Dry mouth and severe rebound hypertension
      (3) Insomnia, headache, and cardiac dysrhythmias (with sudden withdrawal)
    b. Methyldopa is associated with:
      (1) CV effects, such as orthostatic hypotension and bradycardia
      (2) CNS effects, such as sedation and fever
      (3) GI effects such as colitis
      (4) Other effects, such as hepatitis, cirrhosis, Coombs-positive hemolytic anemia, and SLE-like syndrome

5. Calcium channel blockers are associated with CV effects, resulting in hypotension, dizziness, headache, and flushing. When given with β-adrenergic blockers, their effects may be enhanced, resulting in bradycardia, hypotension, peripheral edema, congestive heart failure, AV block, and asystole. Long-term administration is associated with risk of gingival hyperplasia and Barrett esophagus.

6. ACE inhibitors are associated with:
    a. CV effects, such as hypotension and syncope
    b. Hematologic effects, such as neutropenia and agranulocytosis
    c. Other effects, such as chronic cough, anorexia, polyuria, oliguria, acute renal failure, cholestatic jaundice, and (rarely) angioedema

7. Angiotensin II receptor antagonists are associated with adverse effects similar to ACE inhibitors, except that cough and angioedema, which are independent of angiotensin antagonism, occur less frequently.

8. Endothelin receptor antagonists (Bosentan) have the potential for serious liver injury and damage to a fetus.

VI. DIURETICS

A. Osmotic diuretics

1. Chemistry. Osmotic diuretics (e.g., mannitol, urea, glycerin, isosorbide) are highly polar, water-soluble agents with a low renal threshold (Figure 15-5).

Figure 15-5. Structural formulas of osmotic diuretics. **A.** Mannitol (Osmitrol). **B.** Urea (Ureaphil).

2. Pharmacology
   a. Osmotic diuretics are relatively inert chemicals that are freely filtered at the glomerulus and poorly reabsorbed from the renal tubule. By increasing the osmolarity of the glomerular filtrate, they **limit tubular reabsorption of water** and thus **promote diuresis.**
   b. Because these agents increase water, sodium, chloride, and bicarbonate excretion, they cause an **increase in urinary pH.**

3. Therapeutic indications. Osmotic diuretics are used to:
   a. Help prevent and treat oliguria and anuria
   b. Reduce cerebral edema and decrease intracranial pressure
   c. Reduce intraocular pressure

4. Adverse effects. Osmotic diuretics are associated with:
   a. Headache and blurred vision
   b. Increased blood volume that worsens congestive heart failure

B. Carbonic anhydrase inhibitors

1. Chemistry. Carbonic anhydrase inhibitors are aromatic or heterocyclic sulfonamides with a prominent thiadiazole nucleus. **Acetazolamide** is the prototypical agent (Figure 15-6).

2. Pharmacology
   a. Carbonic anhydrase inhibitors **noncompetitively inhibit the enzyme carbonic anhydrase.** This prevents the enzyme from providing the tubular hydrogen ions needed for exchange with sodium in the proximal tubule, resulting in sodium bicarbonate diuresis.
   b. Because these agents increase water, sodium, potassium, and bicarbonate excretion, they cause an **alkaline urinary pH.**

3. Therapeutic indications. Carbonic anhydrase inhibitors are used to:
   a. Reduce edema (as adjunct diuretic therapy)
   b. Reduce intraocular pressure (retard aqueous humor formation)
   c. Alkalinize the urine, enhancing excretion of acidic drugs and their metabolites
   d. Treat motor disorders such as petit mal epilepsy, paroxysmal chorea and dystonia, periodic ataxia, and some cases of essential tremor

4. Adverse effects. Carbonic anhydrase inhibitors are associated with:
   a. CNS effects, such as CNS depression, drowsiness, sedation, fatigue, disorientation, and paresthesia
   b. GI effects, such as GI upset, nausea, vomiting, and constipation
   c. Hematologic effects, such as bone marrow depression, thrombocytopenia, hemolytic anemia, leukopenia, and agranulocytosis
   d. Hyperchloremic metabolic acidosis
   e. Sulfonamide-type hypersensitivity reactions

C. Benzothiadiazide diuretics

1. Chemistry
   a. The commonly used thiazide diuretics are primarily closely related **benzothiadiazides with variable substituents.** The prototypical agent is chlorothiazide (Figure 15-7A).
   b. Optimal diuretic activity depends on certain **structural features.**
      (1) The benzene ring must have a **sulfonamide** group (preferably unsubstituted) in position 7 and a **halogen** (usually a chloro group) or a **trifluoromethyl group** in position 6 (Figure 15-7).
      (2) **Saturation of the 3,4-double bond** increases potency, as with hydrochlorothiazide (Figure 15-7B).

Figure 15-6. Structural formula of acetazolamide (Diamox), the prototypical carbonic anhydrase inhibitor.

Figure 15-7. Structural formula of (**A**) chlorothiazide (Diuril), the prototypical benzothiadiazide diuretic, and (**B**) hydrochlorothiazide (HydroDIURIL). Structural formulas of (**C**) cyclothiazide (Anhydron) and (**D**) quinethazone (Hydromox), related compounds with substituents that prolong activity and enhance potency.

    (3) **Lipophilic substituents** at position 3 or **methyl groups** at position 2 enhance potency and prolong activity, as with cyclothiazide (Figure 15-7*C*) and bendroflumethiazide.

    (4) **Replacement of the sulfonyl group** in position 1 by a **carbonyl group** prolongs activity, as with quinethazone (Figure 15-7*D*).

  c. A few **sulfamoylbenzamides** (e.g., indapamide, chlorthalidone) have activity similar to that of the benzothiadiazides (Figure 15-8).

  d. **Benzothiadiazines without the sulfonamide group** (e.g., diazoxide) exhibit antihypertensive activity but lack diuretic activity (Figure 15-9).

2. Pharmacology

  a. Benzothiadiazides **directly inhibit sodium and chloride reabsorption** on the luminal membrane of the early segment of the distal convoluted tubule.

  b. These agents increase water, sodium, chloride, potassium, and bicarbonate excretion and decrease calcium excretion and uric acid secretion. They may cause an **alkaline urinary pH** by inhibiting carbonic anhydrase.

Figure 15-8. Structural formula of indapamide (Lozol), a sulfamoylbenzamide with pharmacological activity similar to that of the benzothiadiazide diuretics.

Figure 15-9. Structural formula of diazoxide (Hyperstat), a benzothiadiazine lacking a sulfonamide group and diuretic action.

3. **Therapeutic indications.** Benzothiadiazides are used to treat:
   a. Chronic edema
   b. Hypertension
   c. Congestive heart failure (as adjunctive edema therapy)

4. **Adverse effects.** Benzothiadiazides are associated with:
   a. CNS effects, such as headache, dizziness, paresthesias, drowsiness, and restlessness
   b. GI effects, such as GI irritation, nausea, vomiting, abdominal bloating, and constipation
   c. CV effects, such as orthostatic hypotension, palpitations, hemoconcentration, and venous thrombosis
   d. Hematologic effects, such as blood dyscrasias, leukopenia, thrombocytopenia, agranulocytosis, aplastic anemia, hemolytic anemia, and rash
   e. Fluid and electrolyte imbalances, such as hypokalemia, hyponatremia, and hypercalcemia
   f. Muscular cramps
   g. Hyperuricemia and acute gout attacks
   h. Hypercholesterolemia and hypertriglyceridemia
   i. Sulfonamide-type hypersensitivity reaction

D. **Loop diuretics**

1. **Chemistry.** Loop diuretics are anthranilic acid derivatives with a sulfonamide substituent (e.g., furosemide, bumetanide) or aryloxyacetic acids without a sulfonamide substituent (e.g., ethacrynic acid; Figure 15-10).

2. **Pharmacology**
   a. These agents act principally at the thick ascending limb of the loop of Henle, where they **inhibit the cotransport of sodium, potassium, and chloride from the luminal filtrate.**
   b. Loop diuretics increase excretion of water, sodium, potassium, calcium, and chloride; decrease uric acid secretion; and cause **no change in urinary pH.**

3. **Therapeutic indications.** Loop diuretics are used to treat
   a. Edema from congestive heart failure, hepatic cirrhosis, and renal disease
   b. Pulmonary edema and ascites

4. **Adverse effects.** Loop diuretics are associated with:
   a. Fluid and solute imbalances, such as dehydration, hypokalemia, hyperuricemia, hypercalciuria, and azotemia
   b. CNS effects, such as headache, vertigo, blurred vision, tinnitus, and (rarely) irreversible hearing loss
   c. Hematologic effects, such as thrombocytopenia and agranulocytosis

A **B**

Figure 15-10. Structural formulas of loop diuretics. **A.** Furosemide (Lasix). **B.** Ethacrynic acid (Edecrin).

   d. CV effects, such as orthostatic hypotension
   e. GI effects, such as nausea, vomiting, and diarrhea
   f. Leg cramps
   g. Hypercholesterolemia and hypertriglyceridemia
   h. Sulfonamide-type hypersensitivity reaction

E. Potassium-sparing diuretics

1. **Chemistry.** The potassium-sparing diuretics are pteridine or pyrazine derivatives (e.g., tri-amterene, amiloride) or steroid analog antagonists of aldosterone (e.g., spironolactone; Figure 15-11).

2. **Pharmacology**
   a. **Spironolactone** and **eplerenone** act as **competitive inhibitors of aldosterone** at mineral-ocorticoid receptors in the late distal tubule and collecting duct. They interfere with aldosterone-mediated sodium–potassium exchange, decreasing potassium secretion.
   b. **Triamterene and amiloride,** which are not aldosterone antagonists, act directly on the late distal tubule and collecting duct. They disrupt sodium exchange with potassium and hydrogen by blocking sodium channels and decreasing the driving force for secretion of potassium and hydrogen.
   c. The potassium-sparing diuretics increase bicarbonate excretion and cause an **alkaline urinary pH.**

3. **Therapeutic indications.** Potassium-sparing diuretics are used
   a. As adjunctive therapy to treat edema from congestive heart failure, hepatic cirrhosis, nephrotic syndrome, and hyperaldosteronism (primary and secondary)
   b. As adjunctive therapy (with thiazides and loop diuretics) to treat hypertension
   c. To treat or prevent hypokalemia

4. **Adverse effects**
   a. **Spironolactone** is associated with:
      (1) Hyperkalemia
      (2) GI effects, such as GI upset, GI bleeding, gastritis, nausea, abdominal cramps, and diarrhea
      (3) Endocrine effects, such as gynecomastia, menstrual irregularities, and hirsutism
      (4) CNS effects, such as mental confusion and lethargy
   b. **Triamterene** and **amiloride** are associated with:
      (1) Hyperkalemia
      (2) GI effects, such as GI upset, GI bleeding, nausea, and vomiting
      (3) CNS effects, such as headache and dizziness
      (4) Increased uric acid concentration in patients with gouty arthritis (with triamterene)
      (5) Methemoglobinemia in patients with alcoholic cirrhosis (with triamterene, which inhibits dihydrofolate reductase)

Figure 15-11. Structural formulas of potassium-sparing diuretics. **A.** Triamterene (Dyrenium). **B.** Spironolactone (Aldactone).

VII. ANTIHYPERLIPIDEMIC AGENTS

A. **Chemistry.** Antihyperlipidemic agents vary in chemical structure and are usually classified by their site of action—locally in the intestine (nonabsorbable agents) or systemically (absorbable agents).

1. **Nonabsorbable agents** are **bile acid sequestrants.** These agents are hydrophilic, water-insoluble resins that bind to bile acids in the intestine. Examples include colesevelam hydrochloride; **cholestyramine chloride,** a basic anion-exchange resin consisting of tri-methylbenzylammonium groups in a large copolymer of styrene and divinylbenzene; **colestipol hydrochloride,** a copolymer of diethylpentamine and epichlorohydrin (Figure 15-12), and **ezetimibe,** a 2-azetidinone blocker of the gastrointestinal cholesterol transporter.

2. **Absorbable agents** include **nicotinic acid** (but not the structurally similar nicotinamide), the aryloxyisobutyric acid derivatives **fenofibrate** (prodrug) and **gemfibrozil,** the 3-hydroxy-3-methylglutaryl-coenzyme A (HMG-CoA) reductase inhibitor **lovastatin,** and the fatty fish oils containing large amounts of **eicosapentaenoic acid (EPA)** and **docosahexaenoic acid (DHA;** Figure 15-13).

B. **Pharmacology.** Antihyperlipidemic agents **increase catabolism** or **reduce lipoprotein production** (e.g., lovastatin, gemfibrozil) or **increase the efficiency of lipoprotein removal** (e.g., cholestyramine, colestipol).

C. **Therapeutic indications.** These agents are used (in conjunction with appropriate diet and exercise) to reduce plasma lipoprotein concentrations.

D. **Adverse effects**

1. **Nonabsorbable agents** (e.g., cholestyramine, colestipol) are associated with GI distress, including abdominal bloating, nausea, dyspepsia, steatorrhea, and constipation or diarrhea.

2. **Absorbable agents** (e.g., statins, fibrates) are associated with GI distress, skin rash, and leukopenia.

Figure 15-12. Structural formulas of nonabsorbable antihyperlipidemic agents. **A.** Cholestyramine chloride (Questran). **B.** Colestipol hydrochloride (Colestid).

Figure 15-13. Structural formulas of absorbable antihyperlipidemics. **A.** Nicotinic acid (niacin). **B.** Gemfibrozil (Lopid). **C.** Lovastatin (Mevacor). **D.** Eicosapentaenoic acid (found in Promega, Proto-Chol, and others). **E.** Docosahexaenoic acid (found in Promega, Proto-Chol, and others).

> **a. Lovastatin** and other statins (e.g., simvastatin, pravastatin, fluvastatin, atorvastatin,) may increase blood transaminase and creatinine phosphokinase activity associated with myopathy, especially when combined with fibrates or cyclosporins.
> **b. Gemfibrozil** may also cause skeletal muscle pain, blurred vision, and anemia.
> **c. Nicotinic acid** produces flushing associated with pruritus, which may be alleviated by one aspirin per day. Tolerance to nicotinic acid develops in 1–2 weeks. High doses of nicotinic acid (2 g/day) may produce hepatic damage.

VIII. ANTICOAGULANT, ANTIPLATELET, AND THROMBOLYTIC AGENTS

A. **Anticoagulants.** The major anticoagulant agents are **heparin, low molecular weight heparin (LMWH)** and the **oral** anticoagulants.

    1. **Chemistry**
        a. **Heparin** is a large, highly acidic mucopolysaccharide composed of sulfated D-glucosamine and D-glucuronic acid molecules extracted from bovine lung and porcine intestine (Figure 15-14).
        b. **LMWH fragments** (1–10 kDa) **enoxaparin, dalteparin, tinzaparin,** and **ardeparin** are produced through controlled depolymerization of heparin, but they are not interchangeable with heparin in their actions and use.
           (1) Because they are highly acidic, heparin and LMWH fragments exist as anions at physiologic pH and are poorly absorbed from the GI tract. Thus they are usually administered parenterally as the sodium salt.

Figure 15-14. Structural formula of heparin, a mucopoly-saccharide anticoagulant agent.

(2) The action of heparin and LMWH fragments is quickly terminated by **protamine sulfate,** a highly basic protein that combines chemically with them in approximately equal amounts (mg:mg).

c. **Low molecular weight heparinoids (danaparoid)** are **glycosaminoglycans** extracted from porcine mucosa.

d. **Lepirudin** is a recombinant-DNA-derived 65 amino acid polypeptide nearly identical to **hirudin,** which belongs to the group of isopolypeptides of the leech *Hirudo medicinalis.*

e. **Argatroban** is an L-arginine-based structure.

f. **Bivalirudin** is a 20 amino acid peptide. Lepirudin, bivalirudin, and argatroban are synthetic thrombin inhibitors.

g. **Drotrecogin α** is a recombinant form of human-activated protein C that inactivates factors Va and VIIIa.

h. **Fondaparinux** is a pentasaccharide that resembles the antithrombin binding region of heparin.

i. **Coumarin derivatives,** which are highly effective, and the relatively unimportant **indanedione derivatives** are oral anticoagulants.

   (1) The **coumarin derivatives** (e.g., **warfarin, dicumarol**) are water insoluble, weakly acidic 4-hydroxycoumarin lactones (Figure 15-15).

   (a) These agents are **chemically related to vitamin K,** and their mechanism of action is directly related to their antagonism of the reductase responsible for reducing vitamin K epoxide to the reduced hydroquinone.

   (b) These agents are also highly protein bound and extensively metabolized in the liver. These characteristics, in addition to a relatively narrow therapeutic index, make the coumarin derivatives susceptible to significant drug interactions.

   (2) **Phenindione** represents a typical **indanedione derivative** (Figure 15-16).

2. **Pharmacology**

a. **Heparin** catalyzes the inhibition of thrombin by antithrombin III (heparin cofactor), preventing the conversion of fibrinogen to fibrin.

Figure 15-15. Structural formulas of coumarin-derivative oral anticoagulants. **A.** Warfarin (Coumadin). **B.** Dicumarol.

Figure 15-16. Structural formula of the indanedione-derivative oral anticoagulant phenindione (Hedulin).

b. **LMWH** fragments are unable to catalyze inhibition of thrombin, but they catalyze inhibition by antithrombin III of factor Xa, which is responsible for conversion of prothrombin to thrombin. Heparin prolongs blood clotting time both in vivo and in vitro, whereas LMWH fragments have minimal in vitro effect.

c. **Glycosaminoglycans (Danaparoid)** inhibit fibrin formation by inhibition of clotting factors Xa and IIa (lesser effect).

d. **Lepirudin, desirudin, argatroban,** and **bivalirudin** bind to and block the catalytic activity of thrombin.

e. **Drotrecogin** inhibits proteolytic inactivation of factors Va and VIIIa.

f. **Fondaparinux** facilitates inhibition of factor Xa by antithrombin by 300-fold but has no direct effect on thrombin.

g. **Oral anticoagulants interfere with the vitamin K–dependent hepatic synthesis of the active clotting factors** II (prothrombin), VII, IX, and X and the anticoagulant proteins C and S. These agents prolong blood clotting time in vivo only.

3. **Therapeutic indications**
   a. **Heparin** is indicated
      (1) For the prophylaxis and treatment of venous thrombosis, pulmonary embolism, peripheral arterial embolism, and atrial fibrillation with embolization
      (2) To prevent clotting during arterial surgery and cardiac surgery
      (3) To diagnose and treat disseminated intravascular coagulation (DIC)
      (4) To prevent postoperative venous thrombosis and pulmonary embolism (in low-dose form)
      (5) To prevent cerebral thrombosis during an evolving stroke
      (6) As adjunct therapy to prevent coronary occlusion with acute MI
   b. **LMWH** fragments are approved for treatment of thromboembolic complications associated with surgery, unstable angina, and MI.
   c. **Danaparoid** is approved for prevention of deep vein thrombosis.
   d. **Lepirudin** and **argatroban** are indicated for treatment of patients experiencing heparin-induced thrombocytopenia.
   e. **Desirudin** is approved of treatment of deep vein thrombosis.
   f. **Drotrecogin** α is approved for reduction of mortality in adult patients with severe sepsis associated with acute organ dysfunction.
   g. **Fondaparinux** is approved for the prophylaxis of deep vein thrombosis in patients undergoing hip fracture surgery and hip or knee replacement surgery. There is no antidote for **fondaparinux**-induced bleeding.
   h. **Warfarin sodium** is an oral anticoagulant indicated
      (1) For the prophylaxis and treatment of venous thrombosis, pulmonary embolism, and atrial fibrillation with embolization
      (2) As adjunct therapy to prevent coronary occlusion with acute MI

4. **Adverse effects**
   a. **Heparin**
      (1) Heparin is associated with:
         (a) Hematologic effects, such as hemorrhage, local irritation, thrombocytopenia, hematoma, ulceration, erythema, and pain
         (b) Other effects, such as hypersensitivity reactions, fever, chills, and urticaria
      (2) Severe adverse effects may be treated by administering protamine sulfate, the specific antidote for heparin.
   b. **LMWH** fragments are absorbed more uniformly than heparin, have a longer biological half-life, and may be associated with a lower incidence of side effects than heparin.

    c. Danaparoid is contraindicated in various bleeding disorders and patients hypersensitive to pork products. Danaparoid contains sodium sulfite, which may cause life-threatening allergic reactions.

    d. Lepirudin may be associated with cerebral bleeding and allergic, skin, and anaphylactic reactions.

    e. Desirudin when employed with epidural/spinal anesthesia or spinal puncture may lead to epidural or spinal hematoma, resulting in long-term or permanent paralysis.

    f. Drotrecogin α–induced bleeding is the most common serious adverse reaction.

    g. Fondaparinux when employed with epidural/spinal anesthesia or spinal puncture may lead to epidural or spinal hematoma, resulting in long-term or permanent paralysis. The most common adverse reactions associated with **fondaparinux** are bleeding complications.

    h. Warfarin

        (1) The oral anticoagulant warfarin sodium is associated with the following adverse effects:

            (a) Hemorrhage

            (b) Anorexia, urticaria, purpura, and alopecia

        (2) Bleeding may be treated by administering vitamin K (phytonadione), the specific antidote for warfarin sodium.

B. Antiplatelet agents

    1. Chemistry. Antiplatelet drugs include aspirin, a salicylate; ticlopidine, a thienopyridine; dipyridamole, a dipiperidino-dinitro pyrimidine; prostacyclin analogs, and the Fab fragments of human monoclonal antibody to the glycoprotein IIb/IIIa (GPIIb/IIIa) receptor.

    2. Pharmacology

        a. Aspirin in low doses inhibits platelet cyclooxygenase production of thromboxane A_2, preventing platelet aggregation. Cyclooxygenase is permanently inhibited for the life of the platelet (7–10 days).

        b. Ticlopidine and **clopidogrel** interfere with adenosine diphosphate– (ADP-) induced membrane-mediated platelet–fibrinogen binding, leading to inhibition of platelet–platelet aggregation.

        c. Fab fragments (e.g., abciximab) are monoclonal antibodies against the GPIIb/IIIa receptor that permanently inhibit platelet–platelet interaction.

        d. GPIIb/IIIa-receptor antagonists (e.g., tirofiban, eptifibatide) are reversible antagonists of fibrinogen, von Willebrand factor, and other adhesion ligands at the GPIIb/IIIa receptor, leading to inhibition of platelet aggregation.

        e. Anagrelide decreases platelet production.

        f. Cilostazol and its metabolites are type III PDE inhibitors that increase cAMP, leading to vasodilation and decreased platelet aggregation.

        g. Treprostinil is a prostacyclin analog of prostaglandin I_2 (PGI_2), which is a direct vasodilator and inhibitor of platelet aggregation.

        h. Dipyridamole may inhibit platelet aggregation via inhibition of:

            (1) Red blood cell adenosine, which acts on thromboxane A_2 receptors of platelets

            (2) Phosphodiesterase to increase intracellular concentrations of cAMP

            (3) Thromboxane A_2 formation

    3. Therapeutic indications

        a. Aspirin is indicated for reduction of mortality in post-MI, prophylactic treatment of MI to prevent reinfarction, and prophylaxis after transient ischemic attacks and minor stroke.

        b. Ticlopidine is approved to reduce the risk of thrombotic stroke in patients with demonstrated risk but who cannot tolerate aspirin. **Clopidogrel** is approved to reduce MI, stroke, and vascular deaths.

        c. Abciximab is indicated for use with aspirin and heparin in patients undergoing percutaneous transluminal coronary angioplasty (PTCA) or atherectomy.

        d. Tirofiban and eptifibatide are approved for treatment of acute coronary syndrome and patients undergoing PTCA.

        e. Anagrelide is approved to reduce platelet count in patients with essential thrombocythemia.

        f. Cilostazol is approved for treatment of intermittent claudication.

  g. Treprostinil is approved for treatment of pulmonary arterial hypertension.
  h. Dipyridamole is indicated for prophylaxis against thromboembolism after cardiac valve replacement.

4. **Adverse effects**
   a. **Aspirin** in doses used for treatment of thrombotic disease is associated with epigastric pain, heartburn, nausea, rash, nasal polyps, gout, and anaphylactic reactions in sensitive individuals.
   b. **Ticlopidine** is associated with a high incidence of adverse reactions, including diarrhea, rash, nausea, vomiting, GI pain, and neutropenia.
   c. **Abciximab** is associated with major and minor bleeding events, thrombocytopenia, human antichimeric antibody formation, cardiac arrhythmias, AV block, bradycardia, diarrhea, abnormal thinking, and dizziness.
   d. **Tirofiban and eptifibatide** are associated with bleeding events and bleeding complications, nausea, fever, and headaches; in the case of eptifibatide, with hypotension.
   e. **Anagrelide** carries a warning for use in patients with heart disease and may lead to serious adverse effects, including congestive heart failure, MI, heart block, fibrillation, and others.
   f. **Cilostazol** is contraindicated in patients with congestive heart failure. In dogs, cilostazol produced cardiovascular lesions, including endocardial hemorrhage and hemosiderin deposition, necrosis of smooth muscle, intimal thickening, and arteritis in the coronary artery.
   g. **Treprostinil** may produce hypotension and bleeding when combined with vasodilators and antiplatelet drugs. Injections may be extremely painful and associated with infusion site erythema, induration, rash, bleeding and bruising.
   h. **Dipyridamole** is associated with nausea, epigastric pain, dizziness, headache, and rash.

C. **Thrombolytic agents**

1. **Chemistry**
   a. **Alteplase, reteplase,** and **tenecteplase** are recombinant DNA-derived **tissue plasminogen activators (t-PAs)** consisting of 527, 355, and 527 amino acids, respectively, of the natural t-PA, which catalyzes conversion of plasminogen to plasmin.
   b. **Streptokinase** is a nonenzymatic 47-kDa protein derived from cultures of Group C β-hemolytic streptococci.
   c. **Anistreplase** (anisoylated plasminogen streptokinase activator complex; APSAC) is a complex of human lys-plasminogen and streptokinase with an anisoyl group blocking the catalytic site.
   d. **Urokinase** is a two-chain serine protease obtained from cultured human kidney cells.

2. **Pharmacology.** Thrombolytic agents facilitate the conversion of plasminogen to plasmin, which subsequently hydrolyzes fibrin to dissolve clots.
   a. **Alteplase** and **reteplase** are referred to as clot selective because conversion of plasminogen to plasmin by t-PA is enhanced several hundred-fold in the presence of fibrin.
   b. **Streptokinase,** which has no enzymatic activity, forms a one-to-one complex with plasminogen, resulting in a conformational change that exposes the catalytic site of plasminogen. The stable activated complex subsequently cleaves free plasminogen to form plasmin.
   c. **Anistreplase** is a prodrug activated in vivo by deacylation of the anisole moiety from the active site of the plasminogen–streptokinase complex. The activated complex converts plasminogen to plasmin in the bloodstream or thrombus.
   d. **Urokinase,** in contrast to streptokinase, is enzymatic and directly converts plasminogen to plasmin.

3. **Therapeutic indications**
   a. **Alteplase** and **reteplase** are indicated for treatment of acute MI and acute massive pulmonary embolism.
   b. **Streptokinase** is indicated for acute MI, deep vein thrombosis, arterial thrombosis, and arterial emboli, except those originating from the left side of the heart.
   c. **Anistreplase** is indicated for treatment of acute MI and lysis of coronary arterial thrombi.
   d. **Urokinase** is indicated for treatment of coronary artery thrombosis and pulmonary emboli.

4. Adverse effects
  a. t-PAs are associated with:
   (1) Internal bleeding of the GI and genitourinary tract, retroperitoneal bleeding, and intracranial bleeding
   (2) Superficial bleeding at catheter insertion sites, arterial punctures, and surgical sites
   (3) Other adverse effects, including hypersensitivity reactions, nausea, vomiting, hypotension, and fever
  b. Streptokinase may be associated with:
   (1) Internal and superficial bleeding [see VIII.C.4.a.(1)–(2)]
   (2) Allergic reactions, including bronchospasm, angioneurotic edema, urticaria, headache, and delayed hypersensitivity reactions
  c. Anistreplase may be associated with:
   (1) Internal and superficial bleeding [see VIII.C.4.a.(1)–(2)]
   (2) Cardiac arrhythmias and hypotension
   (3) Allergic type reactions such as bronchospasm, angioneurotic edema, urticaria, and delayed purpuric rash
  d. Urokinase may be associated with:
   (1) Internal and superficial bleeding [see VIII.C.4.a.(1)–(2)]
   (2) Allergic reactions leading to bronchospasm and skin rash

IX. ANTIANEMIC AGENTS

A. Chemistry. The major antianemic agents are iron preparations, cyanocobalamin (vitamin B_{12}), folic acid, and hematopoietic growth factors (**erythropoietin, colony-stimulating factors,** and **interleukin 11**).

1. Most iron preparations consist of ferrous salts, which are better absorbed from the GI tract than ferric salts or elemental iron. Parenteral iron preparations—including **sodium ferric gluconate** complex in sucrose (**Ferrlecit**), **iron sucrose (Saccharate),** and **iron dextran (INFeD, Dexferrum)**—should be employed only when clearly indicated.
  a. Typical oral preparations include **ferrous sulfate** (Feosol), **ferrous gluconate** (Fergon), and **ferrous fumarate** (Feostat).
  b. When parenteral administration is indicated, **sodium ferric gluconate** is preferred over **iron dextran** because it is associated with a lower risk of anaphylactic reaction. **Iron sucrose** may also have a better safety and adverse effect profile than iron dextran.

2. Cyanocobalamin (vitamin B_{12}) is a nucleotide-like macromolecule with a modified porphyrin unit (a corrin ring) containing a trivalent cobalt atom. A cyanide ion is also coordinated to the cobalt atom, as is a benzimidazole group. The benzimidazole group is bonded to an α-ribosyl phosphate.

3. Folic acid consists of three major components: a pteridine nucleus bonded to the nitrogen of *p*-aminobenzoic acid, which is bonded through an amide linkage to glutamic acid (Figure 15-17).

4. Epoetin α and **darbepoetin α** are glycoproteins produced via recombinant DNA technology. Epoetin α (165 amino acids; 30.4 kDa) is identical to natural erythropoietin.

5. Colony-stimulating factors **filgrastim** and **pegfilgrastim** (granulocyte colony-stimulating factor; G-CSF) and **sargramostim** (granulocyte-macrophage colony-stimulating factor; GM-CSF) are glycoproteins produced via recombinant DNA technology.

Figure 15-17. Structural formula of folic acid, an antianemic agent.

6. Oprelvekin (interleukin 11) is a recombinant DNA-produced nonglycosylated polypeptide growth factor that differs from the natural cytokine by one amino acid.

B. Pharmacology

1. Iron preparations (ferrous salts) are readily absorbed from the GI tract and stored in the bone marrow, liver, and spleen as **ferritin** and **hemosiderin.** They are subsequently incorporated as needed into hemoglobin, where the iron reversibly binds molecular oxygen. A lack of body iron causes iron-deficiency anemia with hypochromic, microcytic red blood cells, which transport oxygen poorly.

2. Cyanocobalamin is readily absorbed from the GI tract in the presence of intrinsic factor (Castle factor), a glycoprotein produced by gastric parietal cells that is necessary for GI absorption of cyanocobalamin.

    a. Cyanocobalamin is transported to tissue by transcobalamin II. It is essential for cell growth, for maintaining normal nerve cell myelin, and for the metabolic functions of folate.

    b. Lack of dietary cyanocobalamin (or lack of intrinsic factor) causes a vitamin B_{12} deficiency and megaloblastic anemia with hyperchromic, macrocytic, immature red blood cells. Demyelination of nerve cells also occurs, causing irreversible CNS damage.

3. Folic acid is readily absorbed from the GI tract, transported to tissue, and stored intracellularly. It is a precursor of several coenzymes (derivatives of tetrahydrofolic acid) that are involved in single carbon atom transfers. A lack of dietary folic acid causes folic acid deficiency and megaloblastic anemia with hyperchromic, macrocytic, immature red blood cells. Folic acid deficiency causes no neurologic impairment, but folic acid deficiency is associated with birth defects (e.g., spina bifida).

4. Endogenous erythropoietin, whose production in the kidneys is stimulated by blood loss, anemia, and hypoxia, is mimicked by **epoetin α** and **darbepoetin α** to increase proliferation and differentiation of erythroid progenitor cells.

5. Filgrastim and **pegfilgrastim** increase proliferation, differentiation, and activation of neutrophils in patients exhibiting neutropenia after undergoing myelosuppressive chemotherapy. **Sargramostim** stimulates maturation of granulocytes and macrophages and activation of mature cells via cell surface receptors.

6. Oprelvekin increases platelet production via stimulation of hematopoietic stem cells, megakaryocytes progenitor cells, and maturation of megakaryocytes.

C. Therapeutic indications

1. Iron preparations (ferrous salts) are used to treat iron-deficiency anemia.

2. Cyanocobalamin is used to treat megaloblastic anemia resulting from vitamin B_{12} deficiency.

3. Folic acid is used to treat megaloblastic anemia resulting from folic acid deficiency.

4. Epoetin α and **darbepoetin α** are approved for treatment of anemia resulting from chronic renal failure.

5. Filgrastim and **pegfilgrastim** are approved for treatment of chronic and chemotherapy-induced neutropenia. **Sargramostim** is approved for myeloid reconstitution in patients with non-Hodgkin or Hodgkin disease or who have undergone bone marrow transplantation.

6. Oprelvekin is approved for prevention of chemotherapy-related thrombocytopenia.

D. Adverse effects

1. Iron preparations given orally are associated with GI effects, such as GI distress, nausea, heartburn, diarrhea, and constipation. Parenteral iron administration may be associated with fatal **anaphylactic** and anaphylactoid reactions.

2. Cyanocobalamin only rarely produces adverse effects.

3. Folic acid is associated with only rare allergic reactions after parenteral administration.

4. **Epoetin α** and **darbepoetin α** may increase blood pressure, which should be monitored and effectively managed.

5. **Filgrastim** may produce allergic reactions involving skin, respiratory, or cardiovascular systems after initial or subsequent dosing. **Filgrastim** and **pegfilgrastim** are contraindicated in patients allergic to *Escherichia coli*–derived proteins.

6. **Oprelvekin** produces fluid retention, which may lead to peripheral edema and dyspnea.

STUDY QUESTIONS

Directions for questions 1–7: Each of the questions, statements, or incomplete statements in this section can be correctly answered or completed by **one** of the suggested answers or phrases. Choose the **best** answer.

1. Calcium channel blockers have all of the following characteristics *except*

(A) they block the slow inward current carried by calcium during phase 2 of the cardiac action potential.

(B) they dilate peripheral arterioles and reduce total peripheral resistance.

(C) they constrict coronary arteries and arterioles and decrease oxygen delivery to the myocardium.

(D) they are useful in treating stable angina pectoris and Prinzmetal angina.

(E) adverse effects include aggravation of congestive heart failure.

2. The termination of heparin activity by protamine sulfate is the result of

(A) a chelating action.

(B) the inhibition of gastrointestinal absorption of heparin.

(C) the displacement of heparin–plasma protein binding.

(D) an acid–base interaction.

(E) the prothrombin-like activity of protamine.

3. Which of the following cardiovascular agents is classified chemically as a glycoside?

(A) Nifedipine

(B) Digoxin

(C) Flecainide

(D) Cholestyramine

(E) Warfarin

4. Cardiac glycosides may be useful in treating all of the following conditions *except*

(A) atrial flutter.

(B) paroxysmal atrial tachycardia.

(C) congestive heart failure.

(D) ventricular tachycardia.

(E) atrial fibrillation.

5. Ingestion of which of the following vitamins should be avoided by a patient taking an oral anticoagulant?

(A) Vitamin A

(B) Vitamin B

(C) Vitamin D

(D) Vitamin E

(E) Vitamin K

6. The structure shown is characteristic of which of the following agents?

(A) Osmotic diuretics

(B) Carbonic anhydrase inhibitors

(C) Thiazides

(D) Loop diuretics

(E) Potassium-sparing diuretics

7. Which of the following diuretics is most similar in chemical structure to the antihypertensive agent diazoxide?

(A) Furosemide

(B) Spironolactone

(C) Mannitol

(D) Acetazolamide

(E) Chlorothiazide

Directions for questions 8–11: The questions and incomplete statements in this section can be correctly answered or completed by **one or more** of the suggested answers. Choose the answer, **A–E.**

A	if **I only** is correct
B	if **III only** is correct
C	if **I and II** are correct
D	if **II and III** are correct
E	if **I, II, and III** are correct

8. In the oral treatment of iron-deficiency anemias, iron is preferably administered as

   I. ferrous iron.
   II. ferric salts.
   III. elemental iron.

9. Parenterally administered antihypertensive agents used in treating hypertensive emergencies include the

   I. centrally acting antiadrenergic clonidine.
   II. arteriolar and venous vasodilator nitroprusside.
   III. ganglionic-blocking agent trimethaphan.

10. Certain factors contribute to the longer duration of action of digitoxin when compared with that of digoxin. These include

    I. greater protein binding.
    II. reduced polarity.
    III. greater tubular reabsorption.

11. Oral anticoagulants have which of the following properties?

    I. They interfere with vitamin K–dependent synthesis of active clotting factors II, VII, IX, and X.
    II. They have adverse effects that include hemorrhage, urticaria, purpura, and alopecia
    III. They prolong the clotting time of blood both in vivo and in vitro.

Directions for questions 12–14: Each group of adverse effects in this section is most closely related to **one** of the following drug classes. The drug classes may be used more than once or not at all. Choose the **best** answer, **A–E.**

(A) Cardiac glycosides
(B) Calcium channel blockers
(C) Angiotensin-converting enzyme (ACE) inhibitors
(D) β-Adrenergic blockers
(E) Nitrites and nitrates

12. Bradycardia, hypotension, increased airway resistance, and congestive heart failure

13. Visual disturbances (yellow or green vision), confusion, anorexia, vomiting, atrioventricular (AV) block, and ventricular tachycardia

14. Hypotension, acute renal failure, cholestatic jaundice, and agranulocytosis

Directions for questions 15–17: Each statement in this group is most closely characterized by **one** of the following drugs. The drugs may be used more than once or not at all. Choose the **best** answer, **A–E.**

(A) Furosemide
(B) Hydrochlorothiazide
(C) Spironolactone
(D) Mannitol
(E) Acetazolamide

15. It interferes with distal tubular aldosterone-mediated sodium–potassium exchange; renders the urine alkaline; and may cause hyperkalemia, gynecomastia, and menstrual irregularities.

16. Freely filtered, this drug limits tubular reabsorption of water and is useful in reducing cerebral edema and intracranial pressure.

17. The principal site of action of this drug is on the thick ascending limb of the loop of Henle; it is useful in treating pulmonary edema and ascites.

ANSWERS AND EXPLANATIONS

1. The answer is C *[see III.B.3; III.C.3; III.D.3].*
Calcium channel blockers are used in the treatment of angina because they dilate coronary arteries and arterioles, thus decreasing coronary vascular resistance and increasing coronary blood flow.

2. The answer is D *[see VIII.A.1; VIII.A.4; Figure 15-14].*
Heparin is a highly acidic mucopolysaccharide, whereas protamine is a highly basic protein. When administered after heparin, protamine chemically combines with it (presumably by an acid–base interaction) and inactivates its anticoagulant effect. Hence it is an effective antidote for heparin. Caution must be employed when using protamine because an excess of protamine can cause an anticoagulant effect itself.

3. The answer is B *[see II.A.1].*
Most glycosides are natural products obtained from plant material. Although there are very few medicinal agents that are glycosides, the group known as the cardiac glycosides is extremely important and is widely used for treating congestive heart failure. Digoxin is a cardiac glycoside obtained from *Digitalis lanata*. Other cardiac glycosides include digitoxin, which is obtained from *Digitalis purpurea*, and ouabain, which is obtained from *Strophanthus gratus*.

4. The answer is D *[see II.C; Table 15-4].*
Ventricular tachycardia is produced by toxic cardiac glycoside dosage and would not be a therapeutic indication for the agents. Cardiac glycosides increase systolic contraction velocity and increase the refractory period of the AV node. They also have a positive inotropic effect.

5. The answer is E *[see VIII.A.2.e; VIII.4.e].*
The oral anticoagulants, such as warfarin, act by inhibiting the liver biosynthesis of prothrombin, which is the precursor of the enzyme thrombin that catalyzes the conversion of soluble fibrinogen to the insoluble polymer fibrin, which results in clot formation. One of the principal factors in the biosynthesis of prothrombin is vitamin K, with which warfarin competes to inhibit this process. Because this is a reversible competition, vitamin K acts as an antagonist to the oral anticoagulants.

6. The answer is C *[see VI.A; Figure 15-7].*
The structure can be recognized as a benzothiadiazine, which is known also as a thiazide. It represents the structure of hydrochlorothiazide, a sulfonamide diuretic. Other sulfonamide diuretics include the carbonic anhydrase inhibitors, such as acetazolamide, and the loop diuretics, such as furosemide. Neither of these subclasses contains drugs with a benzothiadiazine nucleus.

7. The answer is E *[see VI.C; Figures 15-7 and 15-9].*
Diazoxide is a benzothiadiazine derivative; therefore, it would be most similar to chlorothiazide, which is also a benzothiadiazine. Although both the thiazides and the diazoxides have antihypertensive activity, only the thiazides have significant diuretic activity. One of the structural requirements of the thiazide diuretics is an electron-withdrawing group, such as a halogen, ortho to the sulfonamide group on the benzene nucleus. The diazoxide molecule lacks such a group.

8. The answer is A (I) *[see IX.A.1].*
Absorption of orally administered iron is significantly improved with ferrous iron than with either ferric salts or elemental iron, presumably because of its better solubility characteristics. Iron preparations (ferrous salts) are more readily absorbed from the gastrointestinal tract and are stored in the bone marrow, liver, and spleen as ferritin and hemosiderin.

9. The answer is D (II, III) *[see V.B.4; V.C.2.a; V.C.2.e].*
Clonidine is not recognized as a drug of choice for hypertensive emergencies, possibly because of its central mechanism of action and the latent period required for its effect, compared with other peripheral agents.

10. The answer is E (I, II, III) *[see II.A; Figure 15-1].*
Structurally, digitoxin has only one alcohol group on its steroidal nucleus, whereas digoxin has two. This slight difference in structure has a significant effect on the polarity of the molecule. Owing to its greater liposolubility, digitoxin is more likely to undergo tubular reabsorption, to undergo enterohepatic

cycling, to penetrate into the liver microsomes and undergo metabolism, and to be protein bound, all of which contribute to its longer duration of action and potential cumulative effects.

11. The answer is C (I, II) *[see VIII.A.2.e, VII.4.e.(1)]*.
Oral anticoagulants are effective only in vivo because they block hepatic synthesis of vitamin K–dependent coagulation factors (factors II, VII, IX, and X). This also explains the latency period associated with initiation of oral anticoagulant therapy.

12. The answer is D *[see III.D.2]*.

13. The answer is A *[see II.D]*.

14. The answer is C *[see V.D.6]*.
Nonselective β-adrenergic blockers (e.g., propranolol) produce adverse effects associated with their mechanism of action on the autonomic nervous system. Thus bronchospasm, lowering of blood pressure, and reduced heart rate result from blockade of autonomic β-adrenergic receptors. Visual disturbances (yellow or green vision) are peculiar to cardiac glycoside overdose. AV dissociation and ventricular tachycardia are obviously more significant adverse effects. ACE inhibitors reportedly may cause blood dyscrasias in addition to cholestatic jaundice and acute renal failure.

15. The answer is C *[see VI.E.2.a; VI.E.4.a]*.

16. The answer is D *[see VI.A.3.a; VI.A.3.b]*.

17. The answer is A *[see VI.D.2.a; VI.D.3.a]*.
Spironolactone interferes with aldosterone-mediated sodium–potassium exchange, reducing the amount of potassium excreted and is often used with other diuretics that promote the excretion of potassium, such as the benzothiadiazides. Mannitol increases the osmolarity of the glomerular filtrate because it is reabsorbed poorly. By increasing the osmolarity of the glomerular filtrate, mannitol limits tubular reabsorption of water, thus promoting diuresis. In this way, it reduces cerebral edema and decreases intracranial pressure. Furosemide is a diuretic of choice for treating acute congestive heart failure because it promotes a significant rapid excretion of water and sodium.

16
Medicinal Chemistry and Pharmacology: Endocrinology and Related Drugs

Marc W. Harrold

Jennifer L. Whetstone

Pui-Kai Li

I. INTRODUCTION. Hormones are substances secreted by specific tissues and transported to other specific tissues, where they exert their effects. They can be classified pharmacologically as drugs. Hormones can be obtained from natural substances (animal preparations), or they may be synthetic or semisynthetic compounds resembling the natural products. They are often used for replacement therapy (e.g., exogenous insulin for treatment of diabetes mellitus). However, they can also be used for a variety of other therapeutic and diagnostic purposes. Certain drugs (e.g., thyroid-hormone inhibitors, oral antidiabetic agents), although not hormones themselves, influence the synthesis or secretion of hormones. Therapeutically useful hormones and related drugs include the pituitary hormones, the gonadal hormones, the adrenocorticosteroids, the thyroid hormones and inhibitors, and the antidiabetic agents.

II. PITUITARY HORMONES

A. Chemistry. Pituitary hormones are divided into two groups by their site of secretion.

1. **Posterior pituitary hormones.** The two posterior pituitary hormones, **oxytocin** (Pitocin) and **vasopressin** (Pitressin), are closely related octapeptides. They differ from each other in only 2 of their 8 amino acids but have different biological actions.

2. **Anterior pituitary hormones**
   a. **Protein molecules** are anterior pituitary hormones that are used therapeutically.
      (1) **Corticotropin** (Acthar), known as **adrenocorticotropic hormone (ACTH),** is a single-chain polypeptide containing 39 amino acids. It has a molecular weight (mol wt) of 4600.
      (2) **Thyrotropin** (Thytropar), known as **thyroid-stimulating hormone (TSH),** is a glyco-protein with a mol wt of 28,000.
      (3) **Thyrotropin-releasing hormone** (**TRH;** Relefact), known as protirelin, is a tripeptide with a mol wt of 363.
      (4) **Growth hormone** (Asellacrin), known as somatotropin, consists of 191 amino acids and has a mol wt of 21,500.
   b. **Pituitary gonadotropins** are anterior pituitary hormones that are not available for thera-peutic use. These include **follicle-stimulating hormone (FSH), luteinizing hormone (LH),** and **prolactin** or **luteotropic hormone (LTH).** However, several related nonpituitary go-nadotropins have FSH-like or LH-like actions and are used therapeutically. These include the following:
      (1) **Menotropins** (Pergonal), known as human menopausal gonadotropin (hMG), are high in FSH-like and LH-activity and are obtained from the urine of postmenopausal women.
      (2) **Urofollitropin** (Metrodin) is high in FSH-like activity and is obtained from the urine of postmenopausal women.
      (3) **Human chorionic gonadotropin** (**hCG;** Follutein) has LH-like activity and is obtained from the urine of pregnant women.

B. Pharmacology. The therapeutically important pituitary hormones include the **anterior pituitary agents** (corticotropin), **growth hormone** (somatotropin), and **menotropins** (gonadotropin), and the **posterior pituitary agents** (vasopressin and oxytocin).

1. **Corticotropin** is secreted from the anterior pituitary, stimulating the adrenal cortex to produce and secrete adrenocorticosteroids (see IV).

2. **Growth hormone** stimulates protein, carbohydrate, and lipid metabolism to promote increased cell, organ, connective tissue, and skeletal growth, causing a rapid increase in the overall rate of linear growth.

3. **Menotropins** produce ovarian follicular growth and induce ovulation by means of FSH-like and LH-like actions.

4. **Vasopressin** has vasopressor and antidiuretic hormone (ADH) activity. It acts primarily on the distal renal tubular epithelium, where it promotes the reabsorption of water.

5. **Oxytocin** stimulates uterine contraction and plays an important role in the induction of labor.

C. Therapeutic indications

1. **Corticotropin** is used principally for the diagnosis and differentiation of primary and secondary adrenal insufficiency.

2. **Growth hormone** is used for the long-term treatment of children whose growth failure is the result of lack of endogenous growth hormone secretion.

3. **Menotropins** are used to induce ovulation and pregnancy in anovulatory infertile women whose anovulation is not the result of primary ovarian failure. In men, menotropins are used to induce spermatogenesis.

4. **Vasopressin** is used to treat neurogenic diabetes insipidus and to treat postoperative abdominal distention.

5. **Oxytocin** is used to promote delivery by initiating and improving uterine contractions and to control postpartum bleeding or hemorrhage.

D. Adverse effects

1. **Corticotropin** is only rarely associated with adverse effects, which include hypersensitivity reactions or corticosteroid excess.

2. **Growth hormone** is associated with adverse effects primarily related to the development of antibodies to growth hormone. The antibodies are nonbinding in most cases and do not interfere with continued growth hormone treatment.

3. **Menotropins** are associated with:
   a. **Hypersensitivity,** arterial thromboembolism, febrile reactions, ovarian enlargement hyperstimulation syndrome, hemoperitoneum, and (rarely) birth defects in women
   b. **Gynecomastia** in men

4. **Vasopressin** is associated with:
   a. Gastrointestinal (GI) effects, such as abdominal cramps, flatulence, nausea, and vomiting
   b. Central nervous system (CNS) effects, such as tremor, sweating, vertigo, and headache
   c. Other effects, such as urticaria, bronchoconstriction, and anaphylaxis

5. **Oxytocin** is associated with:
   a. Severe water intoxication with convulsions and coma after slow (24-hr) infusion
   b. Uterine hypertonicity, with spasm, tetanic contraction, or uterine rupture
   c. Postpartum hemorrhage
   d. Nausea, vomiting, and anaphylaxis
   e. Fetal effects, such as bradycardia, neonatal jaundice, cardiac dysrhythmias, and premature ventricular contractions

Figure 16-1. Structural formula of cyclopentanoperhydrophenanthrene, from which the gonadal hormones are derived. *A–D,* rings, which may be modified during subsequent conversions; *1–17,* carbon atom positions on the rings.

III. GONADAL HORMONES.
Most natural and synthetic gonadal hormones are derivatives of cyclopentanoperhydrophenanthrene (Figure 16-1). All hormones having this fused reduced 17-carbon-atom ring system are classified as steroids.

A. Estrogen

1. **Natural and semisynthetic estrogens.** The basic nucleus of the natural estrogens has a methyl group designated as C-18 on position C-13 of cyclopentanoperhydrophenanthrene. This basic nucleus is known as **estrane.** Unlike other steroid hormones, all estrogens have an aromatic A ring (Figure 16-2).

   a. **Estradiol,** the principal estrogenic hormone, exists in the body in equilibrium with estrone, which is converted to estriol before excretion (Figure 16-2).

   b. The various routes of administration for estradiol include oral, vaginal (creams, rings, tablets), transdermal patch, and topical emulsion or gel. Estradiol is only weakly active when administered orally owing to metabolism.

   c. Several synthetic estradiol esters, such as **estradiol cypionate (Depo-Estradiol)** and **estradiol valerate (Delestrogen)** (Figure 16-3), are prepared as intramuscular injections in oil, to prolong their action. These estradiol esters are slowly hydrolyzed in muscle tissues to estradiol before absorption and thus are considered to be prodrugs. Another prodrug, **estradiol acetate,** is available for oral and vaginal administration.

   d. Several 17α-ethinyl estradiols increase resistance to first-pass metabolism and enhance oral effectiveness. The estradiol derivatives, **ethinyl estradiol** and its 3-methyl ether **mestranol,** are used principally as the estrogenic components of serial-type oral contraceptives (Figure 16-4). Mestranol is a prodrug and is metabolized to ethinyl estradiol after its oral administration.

   e. **Conjugated estrogens** are a mixture of estrogen metabolites, most often estrogen sulfates, that can be administered orally. Included in this class are **Premarin, Cenestin, Menest, Enjuvia,** and **estropipate.**

2. **Pharmacology.** The specificity of estrogen actions is the result of the presence of estrogen receptors in estrogen-responsive tissues (e.g., vagina, uterus, mammary glands, anterior pituitary, hypothalamus). The receptors are located in the nucleus. When the estrogen is bound to the estrogen receptor, the receptor undergoes a conformational change that activates the estrogen-receptor complex, increases its affinity for DNA, and alters the production of messenger RNA (mRNA). This ultimately leads to either an increase or decrease in enzyme or protein synthesis.

3. **Therapeutic indications**
   a. **Estrogens**

Estradiol   Estrone   Estriol

Figure 16-2. Structural formula of estradiol, which exists in the body in equilibrium with estrone, which in turn is converted to estriol before excretion.

Estradiol acetate

Figure 16-3. Structural formulas of estradiol cypionate (Depo-Estradiol), estradiol valerate (Delestrogen), and estradiol acetate.

    (1) Oral contraceptives (in combination with progestins)
    (2) Treatment of menopausal symptoms
        (a) Vasomotor disorder
        (b) Urogenital atrophy
        (c) Psychological disorder
    (3) Acne
    (4) Osteoporosis, both senile and postmenopausal osteoporosis
    (5) Prostate cancer
    (6) It is not recommended to use estrogens, with or without progestins, for the prevention of cardiovascular disease or dementia.

  4. Adverse effects of estrogens
    a. GI effects, such as GI distress, nausea, vomiting, anorexia, and diarrhea
    b. Cardiovascular effects, such as hypertension and an increased incidence of thromboembolic diseases, stroke, and myocardial infarction
    c. Fluid and electrolyte disturbances, such as increased fluid retention and increased triglyceride level
    d. An increased incidence of endometrial cancer and hepatic adenomas (associated with long-term use)

B. Antiestrogens

  1. The nonsteroidal antiestrogens (estrogen antagonists) **clomiphene, tamoxifen citrate** (Nolvadex), and **toremifene citrate** (Fareston) are triphenylethylene derivatives with an important

R = H, Ethinyl estradiol
R = CH₃, Mestranol

Figure 16-4. Structural formulas of ethinyl estradiol and mestranol.

Figure 16-5. Structural formulas of the antiestrogens tamoxifen, toremifene, clomiphene, and fulvestrant. Clomiphene, tamoxifen, and toremifene are structurally similar, whereas fulvestrant is a larger and more lipid-soluble analog of estradiol.

basic amine side chain (Figure 16-5). These agents are structurally related to nonsteroidal synthetic estrogens with a stilbene structure. **Fulvestrant** (Faslodex) is a potent steroidal antiestrogen (Figure 16-5). These agents have different in vivo binding sites and activities.

2. Pharmacology
   a. Tamoxifen and **toremifene** are predominantly estrogen antagonists and inhibit the action of estrogens by competitively binding to estrogen receptors in breast tissue. These agents have a weak estrogen agonist effect on the endometrium, bone, and lipid levels.
   b. Clomiphene has estrogenic and antiestrogenic activity and induces ovulation by causing an increase in the secretion of the pituitary gonadotropins FSH and LH.
   c. Fulvestrant inhibits the action of estrogens by competitively binding to estrogen receptors and preventing estrogen receptor dimerization in target tissues.

3. Therapeutic indications
   a. Tamoxifen, toremifene, and fulvestrant are used to treat estrogen-dependent breast cancer.
   b. Clomiphene is used to induce ovulation in women who have ovulation failure.

C. Aromatase inhibitors and selective estrogen receptor modulators
   ### a. Pharmacology
   (1) Anastrozole (Arimidex) and **letrozole (Femara)** (Figure 16-6) are potent and selective nonsteroidal **inhibitors of aromatase. Exemestane (Aromasin)** is the only steroidal irreversible inhibitor of aromatase (Figure 16-6), an enzyme responsible for the conversion of androgens (e.g., androstenedione and testosterone) to estrogens (e.g., estrone and estradiol).
   (2) Raloxifene (Evista) is a **selective estrogen receptor modulator** (SERM; Figure 16-6). It reduces bone resorption and decreases bone turnover. Its biological actions, like those of estrogen, are mediated through binding to the estrogen receptor. Clinical data indicate that raloxifene has estrogen-like effects on bone and lipid metabolism but exhibits estrogen antagonist effects on uterine and breast tissue.
   ### b. Therapeutic indications
   (1) Aromatase inhibitors are used to treat advanced breast cancer.
   (2) SERMs are used for the prevention of osteoporosis.

D. Progestins

   1. The **naturally occurring** progestin progesterone is a C-21 steroid. Its basic nucleus is known as pregnane (Figure 16-7). The routes of administration for progesterone include oral, vaginal gel, and intramuscular injection. Progesterone has a half-life of 5–10 min owing to rapid liver metabolism at C-5 and C-20.

   2. Steroidal synthetic progestins have structural features that hinder metabolism at C-5 and C-20. They consist of three types:

Figure 16-6. Structures of the aromatase inhibitors anastrozole, letrozole, and exemestane and the selective estrogen receptor modulator (SERM) raloxifene.

a. The **17α-hydroxyprogesterone derivatives** (e.g., medroxyprogesterone acetate, megestrol acetate) typically introduce a methyl group at position C-6 of progesterone and an acetoxyl group at position C-17. These substitutions increase lipid solubility and decrease first-pass metabolism, enhancing oral activity and the progestin effect (Figure 16-8).

b. The second group of progestins are **19-nortestosterone derivatives** (17α-ethinylandrogens) They are structurally classified as androgens because they lack the 19-methyl group. Although these compounds have progestational and androgenic activity, their primary activity is progestational.

   (1) The absence of the 19-methyl group increases progestational activity.

   (2) The 17α-ethinylandrogens are more liposoluble than progesterone and undergo less first-pass metabolism. The 17α-ethinyl substitutent increases progestational activity relative to androgenic activity in addition to blocking metabolism at C-17.

progesterone

Figure 16-7. Structural formula of progesterone, which is a derivative of pregnane.

Medroxyprogesterone acetate **Megestrol acetate**

Figure 16-8. Structural formulas of medroxyprogesterone acetate (Provera) and megestrol acetate (Megace), synthetic progestins.

(3) These agents, with a 17α-ethinyl group, have potent oral activity and are extensively used as oral contraceptives in combination with ethinyl estradiol (Figure 16-9). Other orally active 17α-ethinylandrogens include the positional isomer of **norethindrone, norethindrone acetate, norethynodrel,** its 18-methyl homolog **norgestrel,** and its 3,17-diacetate analog **ethynodiol diacetate. Norgestimate** is a orally active 3-oxime

R = H   Norethindrone
     COCH₃ Norethindrone acetate   Norethynodrel   Norgestrel

Ethynodiol diacetate   Norgestimate   Desogestrel

Norelgestromin
(Ortho-Evra)   Etonogestrel
(NuvaRing)   Drospirenone
(Yasmin)

Figure 16-9. Structural formulas of norethindrone, norethindrone acetate, norethynodrel, norgestrel, ethynodiol diacetate, norgestimate, desogestrel, norelgestromin, etonogestrel, and drospirenone.

prodrug that is metabolically deacetylated and oxidized to norgestrel. **Desogestrel** is a prodrug that is metabolically oxidized to the 3-ketone.

    (4) Norelgestromin (Ortho-Evra) and Etonogestrel (NuvaRing) are also used as contraceptive agents given in combination with ethinyl estradiol (Figure 16-9). Norelgestromin is administered as a transdermal patch to avoid first-pass metabolism, and etonogestrel is a vaginal ring.

  c. Miscellaneous progestin. Drospirenone (Yasmin), an oral contraceptive agent given in combination with ethinyl estradiol, is structurally different from other progestins (**Figure 16-9**).

3. Pharmacology. The mechanism of action of progestins is similar to estrogen. Progestins bind to progesterone receptors located in the nucleus of progestin-responsive tissues. The formation of the progestin-receptor complex results in the increase in the synthesis of mRNA and specific enzyme or protein synthesis.

4. Therapeutic indications

  a. Progestins are predominately used as oral contraceptive agents. Progestins can be given alone (progestin only) or in combination with estrogens as monophasic, biphasic, and triphasic combinations. Extended oral contraception (**Seasonale**) is also available for a 91-day cycle.

  b. Emergency contraception

    (1) PlanB (levonorgestrel)

    (2) Preven (levonorgestrel in combination with ethinyl estradiol)

  c. Menstrual disorder (dysfunctional uterine bleeding, dysmenorrhea)

  d. Endometriosis

5. Adverse effects

  a. Gynecological effects, such as irregular menses, breakthrough bleeding, and amenorrhea

  b. Weight gain and edema

  c. Exacerbation of breast carcinoma

E. Antiprogestin

1. Mifepristone (Mifeprex) is a steroidal progestin receptor antagonist that can be used to medically terminate pregnancy through 49 days (Figure 16-10). At 2 days after administration of mifepristone, a healthcare provider will administer the prostaglandin E_1 (PGE_1) analog **misoprostol.**

2. Pharmacology. Mifepristone inhibits the action of progestins by competitively binding to progestin receptors. Misoprostol induces uterine contractions.

3. Therapeutic indication. Termination of intrauterine pregnancy.

F. Androgens and anabolic steroids

1. The primary natural androgen is **testosterone,** a C-19 steroid with various routes of administration (oral, gel, buccal, transdermal patch, subcutaneous) (Figure 16-11). Testosterone has two physiological effects: androgenic and anabolic effects.

  a. Compounds used for **androgenic effects**

    (1) Esters of testosterone, such as **testosterone 17-enanthate (Delatestryl)** and **testosterone cypionate (Depo-Testosterone),** are prodrugs and provide increased duration of

Figure 16-10. Structural formula of the antiprogestin mifepristone (Mifeprex).

Figure 16-11. Testosterone is converted to 5α-dihydroxytestosterone (DHT) by the enzyme 5α-reductase.

action when administered intramuscularly owing to slow ester hydrolysis (Figure 16-12).

    (2) Introduction of a 17α-methyl group results in potent, orally active androgens, such as **methyltestosterone** and **fluoxymesterone** (Figure 16-12). The 17α-methyl group decreases first-pass oxidative metabolism to the 17-ketone.

  b. Compounds used for **anabolic effects** include drugs resulting from structural modifications of testosterone. These drugs have a much-enhanced anabolic–androgenic activity ratio (e.g., **oxymetholone, nandrolone decanoate, oxandrolone;** Figure 16-13). Agents with 17α-methyl groups are orally active.

  c. **Miscellaneous androgens. Testolactone (Teslac)** is a weak anabolic steroid that is used primarily to treat breast cancer as a competitive irreversible aromatase inhibitor (Figure 16-14). **Danazol,** a weak androgen, suppresses the pituitary–ovarian axis and is used for treatment of endometriosis and fibrocystic breast disease (Figure 16-14).

2. Pharmacology. The mechanism of action of androgens is similar to that of estrogens. However, the molecule that binds to an androgen receptor is not testosterone. Testosterone is converted to DHT in the cytoplasm of androgen-responsive tissue by the enzyme 5α-reductase (Figure 16-11). DHT binds to an androgen receptor in the nucleus. The formation of androgen-receptor complex results in the increase in the synthesis of mRNA and specific enzyme or protein synthesis.

Figure 16-12. Structural formulas of testosterone enanthate, testosterone cypionate, methyltestosterone, and fluoxymesterone.

Figure 16-13. Structural formulas of the anabolic steroids oxymetholone, nandrolone decanoate, and oxandrolone.

3. Therapeutic indications
a. Androgen-replacement therapy
b. Breast cancer and endometriosis
c. Female hypopituitarism, in combination with estrogen therapy
d. Anabolic therapy, use in patients with negative nitrogen balance
e. Anemia

4. Adverse effects
a. Fluid retention
b. Increased low-density lipoprotein (LDL) and decreased high-density lipoprotein (HDL) cholesterol levels associated with increased risk of atherosclerosis and coronary artery diseases.
c. Psychological changes
d. Liver disorders
e. Development of masculine features in female
f. Decreased fertility in male

G. Antiandrogens

1. Most of the antiandrogens are **nonsteroidal** in nature. They include **flutamide, bicalutamide, and nilutamide** (Figure 16-15).

2. **Pharmacology. Flutamide,** bicalutamide (**Casodex**), and nilutamide (**Nilandron**) inhibit the action of androgens by competitively binding to androgen receptors in the target tissue.

3. **Therapeutic indication.** Antiandrogens are used in the treatment of prostate cancer. Flutamide and bicalutamide are given in combination with luteinizing hormone-releasing hormone (LHRH) agonists.

**Testolactone
(Teslac)**

Danazol

Figure 16-14. Structural formulas of testolactone and danazol.

Figure 16-15. Structures of the antiandrogens flutamide, bicalutamide, and nilutamide.

H. 5α-Reductase inhibitors

1. Available agents include **finasteride (Proscar, Propecia)** and **dutasteride (Avodart;** Figure 16-16).

2. **Pharmacology.** Finasteride and dutasteride are competitive inhibitors of 5α-reductase, an enzyme that converts testosterone to the potent androgen **DHT.**

3. **Therapeutic indications**
   a. Benign prostatic hyperplasia (BPH)
   b. Finasteride (Propecia) is used for androgenic alopecia at one fifth the dose used in BPH.

IV. ADRENOCORTICOSTEROIDS

A. **Chemistry.** The adrenal cortex synthesizes adrenocorticosteroids. Adrenocorticoids are divided into two classes. The first class is **mineralocorticoids,** possessing sodium-retaining and potassium-excreting effects, and the second class is glucocorticoids, possessing anti-inflammatory, protein-catabolic, and immunosuppressant effects. However, most naturally occurring adrenocorticosteroids have some degree of both mineralocorticoid and glucocorticoid activity. All adrenocorticosteroids are derived from the C-21 pregnane steroidal nucleus.

1. **Cortisone** and **hydrocortisone** (cortisol), the prototypical glucocorticoids, are formed in the middle (fascicular) layer of the adrenal cortex (Figure 16-17).
   a. The 17β-ketol side chain (—$COCH_2OH$), the 4-ene, and the 3-ketone structures are found in all clinically useful adrenocorticosteroids (Figure 16-17).
   b. Many natural, semisynthetic, and synthetic glucocorticoids are available. **Modifications** of the prototypes cortisone and hydrocortisone represent attempts to increase glucocorticoid activity while decreasing mineralocorticoid activity.

Finasteride
(Proscar, 5 mg; Propecia, 1 mg)

Dutasteride
(Avodart)

Figure 16-16. Structures of 5α-reductase inhibitors finasteride and dutasteride.

Figure 16-17. Structural formulas of cortisone, hydrocortisone, prednisone, prednisolone, triamcinolone acetonide, betamethasone, and dexamethasone.

(1) The oxygen atom at position C-11 is essential for glucocorticoid activity.

(2) A double bond between positions C-1 and C-2 increases glucocorticoid activity without increasing mineralocorticoid activity as with **prednisone** and **prednisolone** (Figure 16-17).

(3) Fluorination at position C-9 greatly increases both mineralocorticoid and glucocorticoid activity, as with fludrocortisone (Figure 16-18); whereas fluorination at position C-6 increases glucocorticoid activity with less effect on mineralocorticoid activity (Figure 16-17).

(4) A 17α-hydroxyl group in combination with either a 16α-hydroxyl group (as with triamcinolone) or a 16-methyl group (as with betamethasone or dexamethasone) enhances glucocorticoid activity and abolishes mineralocorticoid activity (Figure 16-17).

(5) **Triamcinolone acetonide** a 16α-, 17α-isopropylidenedioxy group, or an acetate ester at C-21, enhances topical absorption (Figure 16-17).

2. **Aldosterone,** which is formed in the outer (glomerular) layer of the adrenal cortex, is the prototypical mineralocorticoid. The clinically useful mineralocorticoid used to treat Addison disease is **fludrocortisone acetate** (Figure 16-18).

Fludrocortisone Acetate

Figure 16-18. Structural formula of fludrocortisone acetate, the clinically useful mineralocorticoid.

B. Pharmacology

1. Therapeutically useful adrenocorticosteroids mimic the activity of the natural glucocorticoids and have metabolic, anti-inflammatory, and immunosuppressive activity.

2. Adrenocorticosteroids require cytoplasmic receptors for transportation to the nuclei of target tissue cells, where they stimulate production of mRNA and ribosomal RNA (rRNA). Adrenocorticosteroids also act in the feedback regulation of pituitary corticotropin.

C. Therapeutic indications

1. Replacement therapy, to treat acute and chronic adrenal insufficiency for Addison disease or Cushing syndrome

2. As the therapy of last resort, to treat severe, disabling arthritis

3. Severe allergic reactions, seasonal allergic rhinitis, or bronchial asthma

4. Chronic ulcerative colitis

5. Rheumatic carditis

6. Renal diseases, including nephrotic syndrome

7. Collagen vascular diseases

8. Cerebral edema

9. Topically used for skin disorders and inflammatory ocular disorders

D. Adverse effects. Adrenocorticosteroids are associated with:

1. Suppression of pituitary–adrenal integrity

2. GI effects, such as peptic ulcer, GI hemorrhage, ulcerative esophagitis, and acute pancreatitis

3. CNS effects, such as headache, vertigo, increased intraocular and intracranial pressures, muscle weakness, and psychological disturbances (euphoria or dysphoria, depression, suicidal tendencies)

4. Cardiovascular effects, such as edema and hypertension

5. Other effects, including weight gain, osteoporosis, hyperglycemia, flushed face and neck, acne, hirsutism, cushingoid "moon face" and "buffalo hump," and increased susceptibility to infection

E. Mineralocorticoids receptor antagonists. **Spironolactone** and **eplerenone (Inspra)** are steroidal aldosterone-receptor antagonists (Figure 16-19). These agents are discussed in detail in Chapters 15, 41, and 42.

Spironolactone   **Eplerenone**
                                    (Inspra)

Figure 16-19. Structural formulas of mineralocorticoid-receptor antagonists spironolactone and eplerenone.

V. THYROID HORMONES AND INHIBITORS

A. Chemistry

1. **Synthesis of thyroid hormones** is a four-step process beginning with the concentration of iodide in the thyroid gland. The enzyme iodoperoxidase then catalyzes steps two and three: iodination of tyrosine residues located on thyroglobulin, a 650,000-mol wt glycoprotein located within the thyroid gland, and coupling of the iodinated tyrosine precursors. Finally, proteolysis of thyroglobulin produces the two naturally occurring thyroid hormones: **thyroxine (levothyroxine; T_4)** and **triiodothyronine (liothyronine; T_3)** in a ratio of 4:1.
   a. Levothyroxine is less potent than liothyronine but possesses a longer duration of action (6–7 days versus 1–2 days).
   b. Peripheral deiodination by **5′-deiodinase** converts T_4 to T_3.
   c. **Regulation** of thyroid hormone production involves a hypothalamic–pituitary–thyroid feedback system. **TRH** is secreted by the hypothalamus and stimulates the release of **TSH (thyrotropin)** from the anterior pituitary. Thyrotropin stimulates the thyroid gland to produce T_4 and T_3. These hormones then regulate their own synthesis by binding to specific sites in the anterior pituitary and inhibiting the release of TSH.

2. **Available thyroid preparations**
   a. The **sodium salts** of T_3 and T_4 are used therapeutically (Figure 16-20). Owing to peripheral conversion, the administration of levothyroxine sodium alone will produce the natural 4:1 ratio of T_4 to T_3.
   b. **Liotrix** (Thyrolar) is a 4:1 mixture of levothyroxine sodium to liothyronine sodium, which is equivalent to, but offers no advantages over, levothyroxine only.
   c. **Thyroid USP** is made from dried, defatted thyroid glands of domestic animals and is standardized based on iodine content.

Sodium Liothyronine   Sodium Levothyroxine

Figure 16-20. Sodium salt forms of the naturally occurring thyroid hormones, liothyronine (T_3) and levothyroxine (T_4).

Figure 16-21. Structures of the thiourylene class of antithyroid hormones.

    d. Thyrotropin (TSH) is a highly purified and lyophilized thyrotropic hormone isolated from bovine anterior pituitary glands.

  3. Inhibitors of thyroid function directly or interfere indirectly with the synthesis of thyroid hormones. These agents include potassium or sodium iodide, radioactive iodine (e.g., $Na^{131}I$), and the thiourylenes (e.g., propylthiouracil, methimazole; Figure 16-21).

B. Pharmacology

  1. Thyroid hormone preparations mimic the activity of endogenous and thyroid hormones. These hormones regulate growth and development, have calorigenic and metabolic activity, and (through sensitization of β-adrenergic receptors) have positive inotropic and chronotropic effects on the myocardium.

  2. Thyroid inhibitors act via several different mechanisms.

    a. Iodides in high concentrations (e.g., Lugol solution) have profound effects in all aspects of thyroid synthesis, release, and metabolism. Iodides limit their own transport, inhibit the synthesis of both iodotyrosine and iodothyronine, and—most important—inhibit the release of thyroid hormones.

    b. Radioactive iodine (^{131}I) is administered as a sodium salt, is rapidly trapped by the thyroid gland, and is incorporated into both tyrosine precursors and mature thyroid hormones. Radioactive β-particle decay produces localized destruction of thyroid cells and the desired therapeutic effect.

    c. Thiourylenes inhibit the enzyme iodoperoxidase, thereby inhibiting two crucial steps in thyroid synthesis: the incorporation of iodine into tyrosine precursor molecules and the coupling of iodinated tyrosines to form T_4 and T_3. In addition, propylthiouracil inhibits the conversion of T_4 to T_3.

C. Therapeutic indications

  1. The major indications for **thyroid hormone preparations** are hypothyroidism (i.e., myxedema), myxedema coma, cretinism, and simple goiter. Other indications include endemic goiter and thyrotropin-dependent carcinoma.

  2. Thyrotropin is used as an adjunct in the detection and treatment of thyroid cancer.

  3. Thyroid inhibitors are used to treat hyperthyroidism. The two most common types of hyperthyroidism are **Graves disease** and **toxic adenoma.** Less common causes are toxic multinodular goiter, thyroiditis, and single hyperfunctioning thyroid nodules.

    a. High concentrations of iodide (Lugol solution) are used before thyroid surgery to make the thyroid gland firmer and reduce its size.

    b. ^{131}I is useful particularly in treating hyperthyroidism in older patients and in patients with heart disease.

    c. Thiourylenes (e.g., propylthiouracil, methimazole) are used to control mild cases of hyperthyroidism, in conjunction with ^{131}I, and to prepare patients before thyroid surgery. They are less effective in producing permanent remission of Graves disease.

D. Adverse effects

  1. Thyroid hormone preparations are only **rarely associated** with adverse effects. Overdosage can cause palpitations, nervousness, insomnia, and weight loss.

2. Thyrotropin is associated with nausea, vomiting, headache, urticaria, anaphylaxis, thyroid gland swelling, transient hypotension, tachycardia, and arrhythmias.

3. Thyroid inhibitors are associated with adverse effects that depend on the agent used.
  a. Iodides are associated with the following adverse effects.
    (1) Iodism, including increased salivation, brassy taste, sore teeth and gums, swollen eyelids, inflamed larynx and pharynx, frontal headache, skin lesions, and skin eruptions
    (2) Hypersensitivity reactions with fever, arthralgia, eosinophilia, and angioedema
    (3) Large doses of iodides given over long periods can cause goiter and hypothyroidism, which can be corrected by the administration of thyroid hormone.
  b. ^{131}I is associated with
    (1) Delayed hypothyroidism (relatively high incidence)
    (2) Possible effects on the future offspring of young adults
  c. Thiourylenes are associated with:
    (1) Dermatological effects such as urticarial papular rash and dermatitis
    (2) Hematological effects, such as agranulocytosis, thrombocytopenia, and granulocytopenia
    (3) GI effects, such as nausea, vomiting, and GI distress
    (4) Pain, stiffness in the joints, headache, and paresthesias
    (5) Other effects, such as drug fever, hepatitis, nephritis, and systemic lupus erythematosus–like syndrome are rare.

E. Drug interactions with thyroid hormones

  1. Bile acid sequestrants (BAS), calcium, ferrous sulfate, sucralfate, iron, and aluminum hydroxide antacids can **decrease the absorption** of thyroid hormones. An appropriate solution to this problem is to adequately space the administration of these agents (e.g., take the thyroid hormone 1 hr before or 4 hr after taking the BAS).

  2. A number of drugs, including phenytoin, carbamazepine, and rifampin, **accelerate thyroid metabolism.** An appropriate solution to this problem is to increase the dose of the thyroid hormone.

VI. ANTIDIABETIC AGENTS

A. Chemistry. Antidiabetic agents include insulin preparations, oral hypoglycemic agents, and peptidic mimetics that can be used to improve glycemic control.

  1. Insulin is an endocrine hormone secreted by the β cells of the pancreas. It is a 51 amino acid protein composed of **two polypeptide chains:** an A chain of 21 amino acids and a B chain of 30 amino acids. Two interchain disulfide bonds connect the A and B chains, and a third intrachain disulfide bond is found between Cys_6 and Cys_{11} of the A chain. Insulin is derived from an 86 amino acid precursor known as proinsulin.
    a. Source. At one time, insulin was available as bovine insulin (which differs from human insulin by 3 amino acids), and porcine insulin (which differs from human insulin only in the terminal amino acid); however, owing to concerns of the transmission of mad cow disease and the limited use of these products, regular insulin is currently available only as recombinant human insulin.
      (1) Human insulins are prepared either by enzymatic conversion of the terminal amino acid of porcine insulin (Novolin) or by means of recombinant DNA technology (Humulin).
      (2) Five synthetic insulin analogs—**lispro insulin** (Humalog), **insulin aspart** (NovoLog), **insulin glulisine** (Apidra), **insulin glargine** (Lantus), and **insulin detemir** (Levemir)—are also available.
    b. Categories. Preparations of insulin are divided into three categories according to their onset, duration, and intensity of action after subcutaneous (SC) administration: short-acting, intermediate-acting, and long-acting. Insulin solubility at the injection site depends on the physical state, the zinc content, the nature of the buffer, and the protein content.
      (1) Short-acting insulins include lispro insulin, insulin aspart, insulin glulisine, and regular insulin.

(a) **Lispro insulin** differs from normal insulin in that the Lys_{29} and Pro_{28} residues of the B chain are reversed. This structural alteration provides for a shorter onset (15–30 min) and duration (3–4 hr) than that of regular insulin.

(b) **Insulin aspart** differs from normal insulin in that the Pro_{28} residue of the B chain is replaced with Asp. This structural change reduces the tendency of insulin to self-associate as hexamers and thus provides for a rapid onset and short duration, similar to that described for lispro insulin.

(c) **Insulin glulisine** differs from normal insulin in two ways. Asn_3 of the B chain is replaced by lysine, and Lys_{29} of the B chain is replaced by Glu. Similar to lispro insulin and insulin aspart, insulin glulisine has a rapid onset and a short duration. All three of these synthetic insulins can be taken from 15 min before to 15 min after the initiation of a meal. Compared to regular insulin, all three of these synthetic analogs have a lower propensity to cause hypoglycemia, thus reducing the need for snacks between meals.

(d) **Regular insulin** (also called insulin injection or crystalline zinc insulin) is a soluble insulin prepared at neutral pH. It can be mixed with most other insulins (with the exceptions of glargine and detemir) and is the only type that can be given intravenously.

(2) **Intermediate-acting** insulins include isophane insulin (neutral protamine Hagedorn; NPH) and combination products of lispro insulin and insulin aspart.

(a) Isophane insulin (NPH) is a complex containing stoichiometric amounts of the protamine, a protein found in certain types of fish, and insulin in a phosphate buffer. The presence of protamine, along with low concentrations of zinc, enhances the aggregation of insulin into dimers and hexamers after subcutaneous injection and prolongs its duration.

(b) Lispro and aspart insulin are available as combination products with their respective protamine complexes, neutral protamine lispro (NPL) and neutral protamine aspart (NPA). Each combination contains 30 U/mL of either lispro or aspart insulin along with 70 U/mL of NPL or NPA, respectively.

(3) **Long-acting** insulins include insulin glargine and insulin detemir.

(a) **Insulin glargine** differs from normal insulin in that Gly replaces the Asn_{21} residue of the A chain and a basic Arg-Arg dipeptide replaces the Thr_{30} of the B chain. These structural alterations cause a decreased solubility at physiological pH, precipitation and delayed absorption after subcutaneous injection, and an increased duration of action. This allows for a once daily administration that produces a constant concentration/time profile that more closely mimics endogenous basal insulin secretion.

(b) **Insulin detemir** differs from normal insulin in two ways. A 14-carbon fatty acid (myristic acid) is covalently bound to Lys_{29} of the B chain, and Thr_{30} of the B chain is removed.

2. **Oral antidiabetic agents** can be classified as either sulfonylureas, biguanides, meglitinides, thiazolidinediones, or β-glucosidase inhibitors.

a. **Sulfonylureas** are acidic compounds and include both first- and second-generation agents (Table 16-1). Second-generation agents (**glyburide, glipizide,** and **glimepiride**) have larger groups attached to the aromatic ring (i.e., larger R_1 substituents), are more lipid soluble, and are more potent than first-generation agents (**tolbutamide, chlorpropamide, tolazamide,** and **acetohexamide**).

b. **Metformin**, a **biguanide,** is a basic compound and is currently the only available agent in its chemical class (Figure 16-22). An additional agent, **phenformin,** was withdrawn from the market in 1977 because of a high incidence of fatal lactic acidosis.

c. **Meglitinides** are acidic compounds. Currently available compounds in this chemical class include **repaglinide** and **nateglinide** (Figure 16-22).

d. **Rosiglitazone** and **pioglitazone** are acidic compounds and can be chemically classified as **thiazolidinediones.** A third agent, **troglitazone,** was withdrawn from the market because of rare but severe hepatic toxicity (Figure 16-22).

e. **Inhibitors of α-glucosidase** are basic analogs of either monosaccharides or polysaccharides. The monosaccharide **miglitol** has better oral absorption than the α-1-4 linked tetrasaccharide **acarbose** (Figure 16-22).

Table 16-1. Oral Hypoglycemic Agents: The Sulfonylureas

General Sulfonylurea Structure

Drug	R₁ Substituent	R₂ Substituent
First-generation agents Tolbutamide (Orinase)	CH_3	$CH_2CH_2CH_2CH_3$
Chlorpropamide (Diabinese)	Cl	$CH_2CH_2CH_3$
Tolazamide (Tolinase)	CH_3	
Acetohexamide (Dymelor)		
Second-generation agents Glyburide (DiaBeta, Micronase)		
Glipizide (Glucotrol)		
Glimepiride (Amaryl)		

3. **Peptide mimetics** include exenatide and pramlintide.
   a. **Exenatide** is an **incretin mimetic.** Incretins are endogenous compounds, such as gluca-gon-like peptide 1 (GLP-1), that improve glycemic control. Exenatide is isolated from the salivary gland venom of the lizard *Heloderma suspectum* (Gila monster).
   b. **Pramlintide** is an **amylinomimetic agent** (i.e., a synthetic analog of human amylin). **Amylin** is a naturally occurring 37 amino acid neuroendocrine peptide that is secreted by pancreatic β cells in response to food intake. Pramlintide contains proline in place of Ala_{25}, Ser_{28}, and Ser_{29} normally present in amylin. This decreases the viscosity, instabil-ity, and aggregation that occur if amylin is placed into solution.

Figure 16-22. Structures of oral hypoglycemic agents: biguanides (metformin), meglitinides (repaglinide and nateglinide), thiazolidinediones (pioglitazone and rosiglitazone) and α-glucosidase inhibitors (miglitol and acarbose).

B. Pharmacology

1. **Insulin preparations** mimic the activity of endogenous insulin, which is required for the proper use of glucose in normal metabolism. Insulin interacts with a specific cell surface receptor to facilitate the transport of glucose and amino acids.

2. **Oral antidiabetic agents** act through a variety of mechanisms.
   a. **Sulfonylureas** block adenosine triphosphate– (ATP-) sensitive potassium channels, which stimulates the release of insulin from pancreatic β cells. Thus sulfonylureas can also be classified as potassium channel blockers (or closers). In addition, sulfonylureas can enhance the peripheral response to a given amount of insulin by increasing the number or affinity of cell surface insulin receptors. The clinical significance of this extrahepatic effect has been questioned.

    b. Biguanides do not stimulate the release of insulin, do not cause hypoglycemia, and thus are best described as antihyperglycemic agents. The reduction in glucose levels seen with these agents is thought to be caused by an increase in insulin action in peripheral tissues as well as an inhibition of gluconeogenesis. It has been proposed that these compounds increase glucose transport across skeletal muscle cell membranes. Biguanides also inhibit hepatic gluconeogenesis.

    c. Meglitinides are similar to the sulfonylureas in that they lower glucose levels by stimulating the release of insulin. They differ from the sulfonylureas in that they have a more rapid onset of action and a shorter duration of action.

    d. Thiazolidinediones do not stimulate insulin secretion, but instead bind to nuclear peroxisome proliferator-activated receptors (PPARs) involved in transcription of insulin-responsive genes and in regulation of adipocyte differentiation and lipid metabolism. Specifically, they enhance the synthesis and translocation of glucose transporter proteins, enhance insulin sensitivity, and cause a favorable redistribution of fat. These effects decrease insulin resistance and improve target cell response to insulin. These compounds are active only when insulin is present.

    e. α-Glucosidase inhibitors inhibit the digestion of carbohydrates in the small intestine and therefore decrease the postprandial rise in glucose levels.

3. Peptide mimetics act through a variety of mechanisms.

    a. Exenatide binds and activates the human GLP-1 receptor. This stimulates glucose-dependent insulin synthesis, enhances insulin secretion by the pancreatic β cells, suppresses inappropriately elevated glucagon secretion, and slows gastric emptying.

    b. Amylin slows gastric emptying; however, it does not alter the overall absorption of nutrients. In addition, it causes a suppression of postprandial glucagon secretion and modulates central processes, resulting in a decreased appetite and caloric intake.

C. Therapeutic indication

1. Insulin preparations are used to treat insulin-dependent diabetes mellitus (IDDM) that cannot be controlled by diet alone. They can also be used in patients with non-insulin-dependent diabetes mellitus (NIDDM) who are not adequately controlled by either diet or oral antidiabetic agents.

2. Oral antidiabetic agents are used as an adjunct to diet in treating NIDDM that cannot be controlled by diet alone. Each class of compounds can be used either as monotherapy or in combination with one another.

3. Peptide mimetics are used as adjunct therapy in combination with either insulin or oral antidiabetic agents. Specifically, **exenatide** is used to improve glycemic control in patients with type 2 diabetes who have not been adequately controlled by oral antidiabetic agents, whereas **pramlintide** is used as an adjunct to mealtime insulin in patients with either type 1 or type 2 diabetes mellitus.

D. Adverse effects

1. Insulin preparations are associated with the following adverse effects:

    a. Hypoglycemia, with sweating, tachycardia, and hunger; possibly progressing to insulin shock with hypoglycemic convulsions

    b. Hypersensitivity reactions

    c. Local irritation at the injection site

2. Oral antidiabetic agents produce a variety of adverse effects, which depend on both the class and the mechanism of the compounds.

    a. Sulfonylureas are associated with the following adverse effects:

        (1) Hypoglycemia, particularly in patients with renal or hepatic insufficiency who are taking longer-acting agents (e.g., chlorpropamide)

        (2) GI effects, such as nausea, vomiting, diarrhea, and constipation

        (3) Hypersensitivity reactions, such as skin rash and photosensitivity. Cross-sensitivity may occur among classes of compounds that also contain the benzene sulfonamide functional group (e.g., **sulfanilamide antibacterials, thiazides, loop diuretics,** and **carbonic anhydrase inhibitors**).

        (4) Blood dyscrasias, such as leukopenia, thrombocytopenia, agranulocytosis, and hemolytic anemia

        (5) Cholestatic jaundice

        (6) Hyponatremia owing to a potentiation of the effects of antidiuretic hormone (seen primarily with chlorpropamide)

   b. Biguanides do not cause hypoglycemia but have been associated with the following adverse effects:

        (1) Fatal lactic acidosis. Phenformin was withdrawn from the U.S. market in 1977 because of a high incidence of this serious adverse effect. The frequency of this effect in metformin is considerably less than that seen with phenformin; and in most if not all reported cases, the lactic acidosis occurred in patients in whom metformin was contraindicated.

        (2) Metallic taste

        (3) GI effects, such as epigastric distress, nausea, vomiting, diarrhea, and anorexia

   c. Repaglinide is associated with the adverse effects listed below. **Nateglinide,** the other commercially available **meglitinide,** is associated only with hypoglycemia.

        (1) Hypoglycemia. Owing to its shorter duration of action, it is not as likely as the sulfonylureas to cause severe hypoglycemia.

        (2) Upper respiratory infection, rhinitis, and bronchitis

        (3) Headache and back pain

   d. Thiazolidinediones used alone, have a low probability of producing hypoglycemia. This probability increases when they are used in combination with either insulin or sulfonylureas. Other adverse effects associated with this class of agents include

        (1) Hepatotoxicity, although rare, can be severe and fatal. To date, this has occurred only with troglitazone, resulting in its removal from the market. As a result, strict monitoring is used during the first year of therapy and then periodically afterward.

        (2) GI effects, such as nausea and vomiting, abdominal fullness, epigastric discomfort, and diarrhea

        (3) An initial and reversible decrease in hemoglobin and white blood count during the first 4–8 weeks of therapy

        (4) Weight gain and **edema**

        (5) Headache

        (6) Upper respiratory infection

   e. α-Glucosidase inhibitors do not cause hypoglycemia but have been associated with **GI distress** as a result of the presence of undigested carbohydrates in the lower GI tract. Smaller compounds such as the monosaccharide **miglitol** are better absorbed and produce fewer GI effects than larger compounds such as **acarbose.**

  3. Peptide mimetics produce a variety of adverse effects. depending on the specific agent.

   a. Exenatide is associated with the following adverse effects:

        (1) CNS effects, such as asthenia, dizziness, restlessness, and jittery effects.

        (2) GI effects, such as nausea, vomiting, diarrhea, dyspepsia, anorexia, and gastroesophageal reflux.

        (3) Metabolic effects, such as hypoglycemia and excessive sweating (hyperhidrosis or diaphoresis).

   b. Pramlintide is associated with the following adverse effects:

        (1) Allergic reaction

        (2) CNS effects, such as dizziness, fatigue, and headache.

        (3) GI effects, such as abdominal pain, anorexia, nausea, and vomiting

        (4) Arthralgia

        (5) Respiratory effects, such as cough and pharyngitis.

E. Drug interactions for oral antidiabetic agents and peptide mimetics can be separated into two major groups: those that alter glucose levels and those that are agent or class specific.

  1. There are a number of compounds that alter glucose levels and thus require changes in drug therapy. These interactions do not specifically interfere with the absorption, distribution, mechanism, or elimination of any specific oral antidiabetic drug and have been referred to as pharmacodynamic drug interactions.

   a. Thiazide diuretics can cause an increase in blood glucose levels by altering carbohydrate metabolism.

   b. β-Blockers can have a variety of effects on glucose levels. They can potentiate hypoglycemia by inhibiting glycogenolysis and glucagon release; however, they can also promote hyperglycemia by inhibiting insulin secretion and decreasing tissue sensitivity to insulin.

In addition, these compounds can mask the signs of hypoglycemia by blunting the reflex tachycardia.

c. **Oral contraceptives and glucocorticoids** can decrease the efficacy of antidiabetic agents by promoting insulin resistance. In addition, glucocorticoids produce metabolic effects that are opposite those of insulin.

d. A number of other drugs can also decrease the glucose-lowering effects of antidiabetic agents. These include **phenytoin, sympathomimetics, corticotropin, ACTH, salicylates,** and **isoniazid.**

e. Some **androgens and anabolic steroids** can cause hypoglycemia in diabetic patients, but not in nondiabetic individuals.

f. **Monoamine oxidase inhibitors** (MAOIs) can stimulate insulin secretion and can contribute to hypoglycemia.

g. **4-Fluoroquinolones** (e.g., ciprofloxacin, ofloxacin) have been reported to cause alterations in blood glucose levels—hypoglycemia in some individuals; hyperglycemia in others.

2. **Drug or drug class specific interactions**
   a. **Sulfonylureas** are highly plasma protein bound; cause the release of insulin by blocking potassium channels in pancreatic cells; and, with the exception of acetohexamide, are oxidatively metabolized by cytochrome P450 enzymes. As a result, drug interactions will occur with:
      (1) Drugs capable of causing **plasma protein displacement** (e.g., fibrates, sulfonamides, phenylbutazone).
      (2) The **potassium channel openers** minoxidil and diazoxide.
      (3) Drugs capable of **inducing or inhibiting** cytochrome P450 enzymes. Glimepiride is metabolized by the cytochrome P2C9 isoform; however, literature references do not provide specific isoform designations for other sulfonylureas.
   b. **Biguanides.** An increased risk of lactic acidosis and acute renal failure can occur if metformin is co-administered with any of the following agents:
      (1) **Cationic drugs** eliminated by renal tubular secretion (e.g., amiloride, cimetidine, dofetilide, midodrine, morphine, procainamide, quinidine, quinine, ranitidine, triamterene, trimethoprim, or vancomycin). These compounds may interfere with the renal tubular secretion of metformin.
      (2) **Iodinated contrast** materials
      (3) **Corticosteroids**
   c. **Meglitinides** have the same drug interaction profile as the sulfonylureas. Nateglinide is oxidatively metabolized by the cytochrome P2C9 and cytochrome P3A4 isozymes, whereas repaglinide is metabolized solely by cytochrome P3A4. Drug interactions involving metabolism would, therefore, be limited to those capable of inducing or inhibiting these two isozymes.
   d. **Thiazolidinediones.** Pioglitazone requires cytochrome P3A4 for oxidative metabolism and, therefore, has possible drug interactions with other compounds that inhibit or induce this isozyme. In addition, pioglitazone can induce cytochrome P3A4 and may decrease the bioavailability of oral contraceptives and other compounds requiring its activity. In contrast, rosiglitazone is metabolized by cytochrome P2C8 and has no clinically significant drug interactions involving cytochrome P450 enzymes.
   e. **α-Glucosidase inhibitors** may impair the oral absorption of digoxin.
   f. **Exenatide and pramlintide** can decrease the rate and/or extent of oral absorption of other drugs owing to their ability to slow gastric emptying. In addition, co-administration of medications that significantly alter gastric motility (i.e., antimuscarinics) should be avoided. Pramlintide and insulin should not be mixed together but rather administered as separate injections.

STUDY QUESTIONS

Directions for questions 1–10: Each of the questions, statements, or incomplete statements in this section can be correctly answered or completed by **one** of the suggested answers or phrases. Choose the **best** answer.

1. The following structure is a hormone. It would be classified best as

(A) an estrogen.
(B) a progestin.
(C) an androgen.
(D) a gonadotropin.
(E) an adrenocorticosteroid.

2. All of the following substances are endogenous tropic hormones secreted by the pituitary gland *except*

(A) somatotropin.
(B) human chorionic gonadotropin (hCG).
(C) follicle-stimulating hormone (FSH).
(D) thyroid-stimulating hormone (TSH).
(E) adrenocorticotropic hormone (ACTH).

3. Which of the following substances when present in urine is the most likely positive sign of pregnancy?

(A) Thyroid-stimulating hormone (TSH)
(B) Adrenocorticotropic hormone (ACTH)
(C) Human chorionic gonadotropin (hCG)
(D) Interstitial cell-stimulating hormone (ICSH)
(E) Isophane insulin (neutral protamine Hagedorn; NPH)

4. All of the following hormonal drugs possess a steroidal nucleus *except*

(A) ethinyl estradiol.
(B) norethindrone.
(C) liothyronine.
(D) prednisolone.
(E) fluoxymesterone.

5. Which of the following glucocorticoids produces the least sodium retention?

(A) Cortisone
(B) Hydrocortisone
(C) Prednisolone
(D) Dexamethasone
(E) Fludrocortisone

6. Which of the following insulins can be administered intravenously?

(A) Regular insulin
(B) Isophane insulin (neutral protamine Hagedorn; NPH)
(C) Insulin aspart
(D) Insulin glargine
(E) Insulin glulisine

7. In comparing levothyroxine to liothyronine, which of the following statements is *not* correct?

(A) Both levothyroxine and liothyronine are naturally occurring thyroid hormones.
(B) Liothyronine can be converted in the peripheral circulation to levothyroxine.
(C) Liothyronine is more potent than levothyroxine.
(D) The plasma concentration of liothyronine is less than that of levothyroxine.
(E) Liothyronine has a shorter duration of action than levothyroxine.

8. Which of the following classes of compounds stimulates the release of insulin from pancreatic β cells?

(A) Progestins
(B) Biguanides
(C) α-Glucosidase inhibitors
(D) Thiourylenes
(E) Sulfonylureas

9. Which of the following compounds is incorrectly matched with its mechanism of action?

(A) Flutamide: competitively blocks the binding of androgens to their receptor
(B) Finasteride: inhibits 5α-reductase
(C) Miglitol: inhibits α-glucosidase
(D) Pioglitazone: competitively blocks the binding of estrogens to their receptor
(E) Anastrazole: inhibits aromatase

10. Which of the following compounds is incorrectly matched with one of its therapeutic uses?

(A) Raloxifene: advanced breast cancer
(B) Metformin: non-insulin-dependent diabetes mellitus (NIDDM)
(C) Finasteride: benign prostatic hyperplasia
(D) Propylthiouracil: hyperthyroidism
(E) Tamoxifen: estrogen-dependent breast cancer

Directions for questions 11–12: The questions and incomplete statements in this section can be correctly answered or completed by **one or more** of the suggested answers. Choose the answer, **A–E.**

A   if **I only** is correct
B   if **III only** is correct
C   if **I and II** are correct
D   if **II and III** are correct
E   if **I, II, and III** are correct

11. Hormones that form lipophilic esters without prior structural modifications include

I. hydrocortisone.
II. testosterone.
III. progesterone.

12. Insulin preparations that contain a modifying protein include

I. insulin glargine.
II. regular insulin.
III. isophane insulin (neutral protamine Hagedorn; NPH).

Directions for questions 13–15: Each statement in this section is most closely related to **one** of the following hormones. The hormones may be used more than once or not at all. Choose the **best** answer, **A–E.**

A   Testosterone
B   Insulin
C   Corticotropin
D   Estradiol
E   Vasopressin

13. Secreted by pancreatic β cells to facilitate glucose and amino acid transport for normal cellular metabolic processes

14. Initiates and controls male sexual development and maintains the integrity of the male reproductive system

15. Promotes the resorption of water at the renal distal convoluted tubule

Directions for questions 16–18: Each statement in this section is most closely related to **one** of the following drug classes. The drug classes may be used more than once or not at all. Choose the **best** answer, **A–E.**

A   Antithyroid agents
B   Sulfonylureas
C   Adrenocorticosteroids
D   Progestins
E   Androgens

16. Peptic ulceration and gastrointestinal hemor-rhage; hyperglycemia, hypertension, and edema; "buffalo hump" and "moon face"; psychological disturbances; and increased susceptibility to infection

17. Agranulocytosis and other blood dyscrasias, cholestatic jaundice, nausea and vomiting, hypoglycemia, and hypersensitivity reactions

18. Hepatotoxicity and jaundice, urinary reten-tion and azoospermia, prostatic hypertrophy and priapism, and paradoxical gynecomastia

ANSWERS AND EXPLANATIONS

1. The answer is A *[see III.A.1; Figure 16-2].*
Ring A is aromatic. Because the only type of steroidal hormone that has an aromatic A ring is an estrogen, this structure represents an estrogen. Other structural characteristics of estrogens include the fact that the structure contains 18 carbon atoms; thus it is an estrane and contains a β-alcohol group in position 17.

2. The answer is B *[see II.A.2.a–b].*
hCG is produced by placental tissue and serves to stimulate the secretion of progesterone during pregnancy. Growth hormone (somatotropin), FSH, TSH, and ACTH are all secreted by the anterior pituitary gland.

3. The answer is C *[see II.A.2.b.(3)].*
hCG is a proteinaceous tropic hormone that is secreted by chorionic (e.g., placental) tissue. Thus hCG is present in the urine only after conception has occurred.

4. The answer is C *[see V.A.1; Figures 16-4, 16-9, 16-12, 16-17, 16-20].*
Liothyronine is a thyroid hormone. Thyroid hormones consist of iodinated aromatic amino acids and are not steroidal in nature. Ethinyl estradiol is a steroidal estrogen, norethindrone is a steroidal 19-norprogestin, prednisolone is an adrenocorticosteroid, and fluoxymesterone is a steroidal androgen.

5. The answer is D *[see IV.A.1.b.(4); Figure 16-17].*
Glucocorticoids have varying degrees of mineralocorticoid activity. This mineralocorticoid activity, which can result in sodium and fluid retention, can be blocked by the introduction of a methyl or hydroxyl group in position 16 of the steroidal nucleus. Dexamethasone has a 16α-methyl substituent.

6. The answer is A *[see VI.A.1.b].*
Most insulin preparations are suspensions; thus they contain particulate matter. Only clear solutions may be administered intravenously. Regular insulin, which consists of water-soluble crystalline zinc insulin is therefore suitable for intravenous administration. All other insulin preparations normally are injected subcutaneously.

7. The answer is B *[see V.A.1.a–b].*
The thyroid gland produces both levothyroxine (T_4) and liothyronine (T_3). The natural ratio of these compounds is 4:1 in favor of levothyroxine; therefore, liothyronine is normally present at a lower concentration than levothyroxine. Liothyronine is more potent than levothyroxine, but has a shorter duration of action. Peripheral conversion involves deiodination, thus levothyroxine is converted to liothyronine. The reverse process is not possible.

8. The answer is E *[see VI.B.2.a–b; VI.B.2.e].*
Of the five classes of compounds listed, only biguanides, α-glucosidase inhibitors, and sulfonylureas are used in the treatment of NIDDM. These classes provide their beneficial effects through different mechanisms of action. Biguanides enhance the peripheral use of insulin, suppress gluconeogenesis, and are often referred to as antihyperglycemic agents. α-Glucosidase inhibitors decrease the absorption of glucose. Sulfonylureas and the structurally unrelated compounds, repaglinide and nateglinide, stimulate the secretion of insulin from pancreatic β cells.

9. The answer is D *[see III.C.a.1; III.G.2; III.H.2; VI.A.2.d–e; VI.B.2.d–e].*
Pioglitazone does not interact with estrogen receptors. It is an oral antidiabetic agent that produces its effects by binding to nuclear PPARs involved in transcription of insulin-responsive genes and in regulation of adipocyte differentiation and lipid metabolism. The other four agents are correctly matched to their mechanisms.

10. The answer is A *[see III.B.3.a; III.C.b.2; III.H.3.a; V.C.3.c; VI.A.2.b; VI.C.2].*
Raloxifene is a SERM and is not used to treat breast cancer. Instead, because of its ability to reduce bone resorption and decrease bone turnover, it is used for the prevention of osteoporosis. All of the other four compounds are correctly matched to their therapeutic use. Finasteride is also used to treat androgenic alopecia.

11. The answer is C (I, II) *[see III.F.1; Figures 16-7, 16-11, 16-17].*
Hydrocortisone has a 21-hydroxyl group, and testosterone has a 17-hydroxyl group; therefore, both of these agents can form esters (e.g., hydrocortisone acetate, testosterone propionate). Progesterone does not have any alcohol groups in its molecule; therefore, it cannot directly form any esters.

12. The answer is B (III) *[see VI.A.1.b].*
Regular insulin, which is a rapid-acting insulin preparation, contains only zinc insulin crystals. Insulin glargine is a synthetic insulin that has been structurally altered at two sites. The structural alterations cause a decreased solubility and an increased duration of action; however, no protein modifiers are added to this preparation. NPH insulin contains protamine, a strongly basic protein. The protamine reduces the water solubility of zinc insulin and lengthens its duration of action. Isophane insulin is classified as an intermediate-acting insulin preparation, having a duration of action of about 24 hr.

13. The answer is B *[see VI.A.1; VI.B.1].*

14. The answer is A *[see III.F.2].*

15. The answer is E *[see II.B.4].*
Insulin is required for the proper use of glucose and the transport of glucose and amino acids across cell membranes. Testosterone, which is produced principally from the Leydig cells of the testes, is responsible for male sexual characteristics. Vasopressin is secreted from the posterior pituitary and is sometimes referred to as an antidiuretic hormone.

16. The answer is C *[see IV.D].*

17. The answer is B *[see VI.D.2.a].*

18. The answer is E *[see III.F.4].*
Exogenously administered adrenocorticosteroids are effective anti-inflammatory agents but give rise to a wide range of metabolic and immunosuppressive effects that result in severe adverse effects. Sulfonylureas are oral antidiabetic agents and can cause blood dyscrasias, impaired liver function, nausea/vomiting, hypoglycemia, and hypersensitivity reactions. Exogenously administered androgens suppress sperm formation and cause paradoxical gynecomastia. Most significant is the hepatotoxicity produced by alkyl-substituted androgen compounds.

17
Drug Metabolism, Prodrugs, and Pharmacogenetics

Marc W. Harrold

I. INTRODUCTION TO DRUG METABOLISM. Drug metabolism (also called **biotransformation**) refers to the biochemical changes that drugs and other foreign chemicals **(xenobiotics)** undergo in the body, leading to the formation of different metabolites with different effects. Xenobiotics can undergo a variety of biotransformation pathways, resulting in the production of a mixture of intermediate metabolites and excreted products, including unchanged parent drug. Rarely is only one metabolite produced from a single drug.

   A. Inactive metabolites. Some metabolites are inactive (i.e., their pharmacologically active parent compounds become inactivated or detoxified).

   1. The hydrolysis of **procaine** to *p*-aminobenzoic acid and diethylethanolamine results in a loss of anesthetic activity.

   2. The oxidation of **6-mercaptopurine** to 6-mercapturic acid results in a loss of anticancer activity.

   B. Metabolites that retain similar activity. Certain metabolites retain the pharmacological activity of their parent compounds to a greater or lesser degree.

   1. Imipramine is demethylated to the essentially equiactive antidepressant, **desipramine.**

   2. Acetohexamide is reduced to the more active hypoglycemic, **l-hydroxyhexamide.**

   3. Codeine is demethylated to the more active analgesic, **morphine.**

   C. Metabolites with altered activity. Some metabolites develop activity different from that of their parent drugs.

   1. The antidepressant **iproniazid** is dealkylated to the antitubercular, **isoniazid.**

   2. The vitamin **retinoic acid** (vitamin A) is isomerized to the anti-acne agent, **isoretinoic acid.**

   D. Bioactivated metabolites. Some pharmacologically inactive parent compounds are converted to active species within the body. These parent compounds are known as **prodrugs.**

   1. The prodrug **enalapril** is hydrolyzed to **enalaprilat,** a potent antihypertensive.

   2. The prodrug **sulindac,** a sulfoxide, is reduced to the active sulfide.

   3. The antiparkinsonian **levodopa (L-dopa)** is decarboxylated in the neuron to active **dopamine.**

II. BIOTRANSFORMATION PATHWAYS

   A. Phase I reactions are those in which polar functional groups are introduced into the molecule or unmasked by oxidation, reduction, or hydrolysis.

   1. Oxidation is the most common phase I biotransformation.
      a. The majority of oxidations occur in the **liver;** however, extrahepatic tissues, such as the **intestinal mucosa, lungs,** and **kidney,** can also serve as metabolic sites.
      b. The vast majority of oxidations are catalyzed by a group of mixed-function oxidases known as **cytochrome P_{450} (CYP450).** These oxidases are bound to the smooth endoplastic reticulum of the liver and require both NADPH and a porphyrin prosthetic group. Unlike most enzymes, CYP450 uses a variety of oxidative biotransformations to metabolize a diverse group of substrates.

   c. CYP450 exists in **multiple isoforms** or families. The presence of these different isoforms is responsible for the large substrate variation seen with CYP450.

     (1) CYP450 isoforms are named using the root "CYP" followed by an arabic number designating the family, a letter designating the subfamily, and a second arabic number indicating the individual gene (e.g., CYP3A4).

     (2) Six mammalian families are involved in steroid and bile acid metabolism: CYP7, CYP11, CYP17, CYP19, CYP21, and CYP27.

     (3) Four mammalian families are involved in xenobiotic, or drug, metabolism: CYP1, CYP2, CYP3, and CYP4. Examples of drugs metabolized by these families and subfamilies are shown in Table 17-1. Note that a number of drugs (e.g., tricyclic antidepressants, diazepam, ondansetron, theophylline) are metabolized by multiple isoforms.

   d. Additional oxidations (e.g., ethanol to acetaldehyde) are catalyzed by nonmicrosomal oxidases located in cytosol and mitochondria of extrahepatic tissues.

   e. CYP450 and nonmicrosomal oxidases catalyze aromatic, aliphatic, olefinic, benzylic, allylic, and α-hydroxylations; N-, O-, and S-dealkylations; oxidative deamination; N- and S-oxidations; desulfuration; dehalogenation; and oxidations of alcohols and aldehydes (Table 17-2).

   f. The **increased polarity** of the oxidized products (metabolites) enhances their water solubility and reduces their tubular reabsorption to some extent, thus favoring their excretion in the urine. These metabolites are somewhat **more polar** than their parent compounds and very commonly undergo further biotransformation by phase II pathways (see II B).

2. Reduction is less commonly encountered than oxidation; however, the overall goal is the same: to create polar functional groups that can be eliminated in the urine. There is evidence suggesting that the CYP450 system might be involved in some reductions. Additionally, bacteria resident in the GI tract are known to be involved in azo and nitro reductions. Reactions catalyzed by reductases are shown in Table 17-3.

3. Enzymatic hydrolysis, the addition of water across a bond, also results in more polar metabolites (see Table 17-3).

   a. Esterase enzymes, usually present in plasma and various tissues, are nonspecific and catalyze de-esterification, hydrolyzing relatively nonpolar esters into two polar, more water-soluble compounds: an alcohol and an acid. Esterases are responsible for converting many prodrugs into their active forms.

   b. Amidase enzymes hydrolyze amides into amines and acids (deamidation). Deamidation occurs primarily in the liver.

   c. Ester drugs susceptible to plasma esterases (e.g., procaine) are usually shorter acting than structurally similar **amide drugs** (e.g., procainamide), which are not significantly hydrolyzed until they reach the liver.

   d. Lactones and **lactams** are cyclic esters and amides, respectively, and are thus also susceptible to hydrolytic metabolism.

B. Phase II reactions are those in which the functional groups of the original drug (or metabolite formed in a phase I reaction) are masked by a **conjugation reaction.** Most phase II conjugates are very polar, resulting in rapid drug elimination from the body.

1. Conjugation reactions combine the **parent drug** (or its metabolites) with certain **natural endogenous constituents,** such as glucuronic acid, glycine, glutamine, sulfate, glutathione, the two-carbon acetyl fragment, or the one-carbon methyl fragment. These reactions generally require both a **high-energy molecule** and an **enzyme.**

   a. The **high-energy molecule** consists of a **coenzyme** bound to the endogenous substrate, the parent drug, or the drug's phase I metabolite.

   b. The **enzymes** (called **transferases**) that catalyze conjugation reactions are found mainly in the liver and, to a lesser extent, in the intestines and other tissues.

   c. Most conjugates are **highly polar** and **unable to cross cell membranes,** making them almost always **pharmacologically inactive** and of little or no toxicity. Exceptions to this are acetylated and methylated conjugates. These conjugates do not possess increased polarity; however, they are usually pharmacologically inactive.

2. There are **six conjugation pathways** (Table 17-4).

   a. Glucuronidation is the **most common** conjugation pathway because of a readily available supply of glucuronic acid as well as a large variety of functional groups, which can enzymatically react with this sugar derivative.

Table 17-1. Examples of Drugs Metabolized by Specific Cytochrome P450 (CYP) Isoforms

CYP1A2
Acetaminophen
Amitriptyline and
   other TCAs
Diazepam
Methadone
Olanzapine
Propranolol
Riluzole
Tacrine
Theophylline

CYP2B1
Chlorpheniramine

CYP2B6
Bupropion
Cyclophosphamide
   and ifosfamide

CYP2C8
Diazepam
Diclofenac
Mephobarbital
Omeprazole
Paclitaxel
Retinoids
Tolbutamide

CYP2C9
Amitriptyline and
   other TCAs
Chlorpheniramine
Carvedilol
Dapsone
Diazepam
Glimepiride
Hexobarbital
Losartan
NSAIDs
Phenytoin
Tolbutamide
Torsemide
Verapamil
Warfarin
Zafirlukast

CYP2D6
Amitriptyline and
   other TCAs
β-blockers
Benztropine
Captopril
Chlorpheniramine
Chlorpromazine
Clemastine
Clozapine
Codeine
Delavirdine
Dextromethorphan
Diphenhydramine
Dolasetron and
   Ondansetron
Donepezil
Encainide
Fenfluramine
Fentanyl
Flecainide
Fluphenazine
Hydrocodone
Hydroxyzine
Imipramine
Lidocaine
Loratadine
Meperidine
Methadone
Methamphetamine
Mexiletine
Morphine
Ondansetron
Oxycodone
Risperidone
Selegiline
SSRIs
Tamoxifen
Thioridazine
Tolterodine
Tramadol
Trazodone

CYP2E1
Acetaminophen
Ethanol
Felbamate
General anesthetics
Isoniazid
Ondansetron
Tamoxifen
Theophylline

CYP3A4
Acetaminophen
Alfentanil
Benzodiazepines
Amitriptyline and
   other TCAs
Amiodarone
Anastrazole
Azole antifungals
Buspirone
Busulfan
Carbamazepine
Chlorpromazine
Cimetidine
Clozapine
Codeine
Cyclophosphamide
   and ifosfamide
Cyclosporin
Dapsone
Darifenacin
Delavirdine
Dexamethasone
Dextromethorphan
Dihydroergotamine
Dihydropyridines
   (*i.e.,* nifedipine)
Diltiazem
Disopyramide
Docetaxel and
   paclitaxel
Dolasetron and
   ondansetron
Donepezil
Doxorubicin
Efavirenz
Enalapril
Ergot alkaloids
Erlotinib
Estrogens
Ethosuximide
Etoposide
Erythromycin and
   clarithromycin
Felbamate
Fentanyl
Fexofenadine
Finasteride
Flutamide
Glyburide
Granisetron

CYP3A4 (cont.)
Haloperidol
HIV protease
   inhibitors
HMG-CoA reductase
   inhibitors
Hydrocodone
Hydrocortisone
Irinotecan
Lansoprazole
Lidocaine
Loperamide
Loratadine
Losartan
Midazolam
Mifepristone
Navelbine
Nefazodone
Nevirapine
Norethisterone
Omeprazole
Ondansetron
Oral contraceptives
Oxybutynin
Pimozide
Prednisone and
   prednisolone
Quinidine
Repaglinide
Rifampin and
   analogs
Risperidone
Salmeterol
Sildenafil
SSRIs
Sulfamethoxazole
Tacrolimus
Tadalafil
Tamoxifen
Teniposide
Testosterone
Theophylline
Tolterodine
Tretinoin
Valproic acid
Vardenafil
Verapamil
Vinca alkaloids
Warfarin

HMG CoA, β-hydroxy-β-methylglutaryl-coenzyme A; *NSAIDs,* nonsteroidal anti-inflammatory drugs; *SSRIs,* selective serotonin reuptake inhibitors; *TCAs,* tricyclic antidepressants.

Table 17-2. Phase I Metabolism: Oxidative Pathways

Type of Reaction (Examples)	Reaction Pathway
1. Aromatic Hydroxylation (phenytoin, phenylbutazone)	1. $R\text{-}C_6H_5 \longrightarrow R\text{-}C_6H_4\text{-}OH$
2. Aliphatic Hydroxylation (pentobarbital, meprobamate)	2. $R\text{-}CH_2\text{-}CH_3 \longrightarrow R\text{-}CH(OH)\text{-}CH_3$
3. Olefinic Hydroxylation (carbamazepine, cyproheptadine)	3. $R\text{-}CH=CH\text{-}R \longrightarrow R\text{-}CH(OH)\text{-}CH(OH)\text{-}R$
4. Benzylic Hydroxylation (tolbutamide, imipramine)	4. $R\text{-}C_6H_4\text{-}CH_3 \longrightarrow R\text{-}C_6H_4\text{-}CH_2OH$
5. Allylic Hydroxylation (pentazocine, hexobarbital)	5. $R\text{-}CH=CH\text{-}CH_3 \longrightarrow R\text{-}CH=CH\text{-}CH_2OH$
6. Hydroxylation-α to a Carbonyl (diazepam, ketamine)	6. $R_1\text{-}NH\text{-}C(=O)\text{-}CH_2\text{-}R_2 \longrightarrow R_1\text{-}NH\text{-}C(=O)\text{-}CH(OH)\text{-}R_2$
7. Oxidative Deamination (amphetamine, dopamine)	7. $R\text{-}CH(NH_2)\text{-}CH_3 \longrightarrow R\text{-}CH_2\text{-}C(=O)\text{-}CH_3$
8. N-Dealkylation (morphine, ephedrine)	8. $R\text{-}NH\text{-}CH_3 \longrightarrow R\text{-}NH_2$
9. N-Oxidation (acetaminophen, guanethidine)	9. $Ar\text{-}NH\text{-}CH_3 \longrightarrow Ar\text{-}N(OH)\text{-}CH_3$
10. O-Dealkylation (codeine, papaverine)	10. $R\text{-}O\text{-}CH_3 \longrightarrow R\text{-}OH$
11. S-Dealkylation (6-methylmercaptopurine)	11. $R\text{-}S\text{-}CH_3 \longrightarrow R\text{-}SH$
12. S-Oxidation (chlorpromazine, mesoridazine)	12. $Ar\text{-}S\text{-}R \longrightarrow Ar\text{-}S(=O)\text{-}R$
13. Desulfuration (thiopental)	13. $R_1\text{-}C(=S)\text{-}R_2 \longrightarrow R_1\text{-}C(=O)\text{-}R_2$
14. Dehalogenation (halothane, chloramphenicol)	14. $CF_3\text{-}CHClBr \longrightarrow CF_3\text{-}CHO$
15. Oxidation of Alcohols (ethanol, estradiol)	15. $R\text{-}CH_2OH \longrightarrow R\text{-}CHO$
16. Oxidation of Aldehydes (acetaldehyde, PGE_2)	16. $R\text{-}CHO \longrightarrow R\text{-}CO_2H$

Table 17-3. Phase I Metabolism: Reductive and Hydrolytic Pathways

Type of Reaction (Examples)	Reaction Pathway
Reduction	
1. Carbonyl Reduction (acetohexamide)	1. $R_1\text{-CO-}R_2 \longrightarrow R_1\text{-CH(OH)-}R_2$
2. Azoreduction (sulfasalazine, olsalazine)	2. $R_1\text{-C}_6H_4\text{-N=N-C}_6H_4\text{-}R_2 \longrightarrow R_1\text{-C}_6H_4\text{-NH}_2 + H_2N\text{-C}_6H_4\text{-}R_2$
3. Nitroreduction (chloramphenicol, clonazepam)	3. $O_2N\text{-C}_6H_4\text{-}R \longrightarrow H_2N\text{-C}_6H_4\text{-}R$
Hydrolysis	
4. Ester Hydrolysis (procaine, meperidine)	4. $R_1\text{-CO-O-}R_2 \longrightarrow R_1\text{-COOH} + HO\text{-}R_2$
5. Amide Hydrolysis (lidocaine, indomethacin)	5. $R_1\text{-CO-NH-}R_2 \longrightarrow R_1\text{-COOH} + H_2N\text{-}R_2$

(1) The high-energy form of glucuronic acid, **uridine diphosphate glucuronic acid,** reacts with a variety of functional groups under the influence of glucuronyl transferase.

(2) Drugs that possess **hydroxyl** or **carboxyl** functional groups readily undergo glucuronidation to form ethers and esters, respectively. In addition, *N*-, *S*-, and *C*-glucuronides are also possible.

(3) As shown in Table 17-4, the addition of glucuronic acid to a drug molecule adds three hydroxyl groups and one carboxyl group. This addition greatly increases the **hydrophilicity** of the drug molecule. As a result, it is unlikely to penetrate cell membranes and elicit pharmacological activity. It is also poorly reabsorbed by the renal tubules and, thus, is readily excreted.

(4) Glucuronides with **high molecular weight** (more than 500) are often excreted into the bile and, eventually, into the intestines. The intestinal enzyme β-glucuronidase can then hydrolyze the conjugate, releasing the unaltered drug (or its primary metabolite) for reabsorption by the intestine.

    b. **Sulfate conjugation** is much less common than glucuronide conjugation because there is no available pool of endogenous sulfate. Additionally, there are fewer functional groups capable of forming sulfate conjugates. The high-energy form of sulfate, **3′-phosphoadenosine-5′-phosphosulfate (PAPS),** reacts with phenols, alcohols, arylamines, and *N*-hydroxyl compounds under the influence of **sulfotransferase** to form highly polar metabolites.

    c. **Amino acid conjugation** involves the reaction of either glycine or glutamine with aliphatic or aromatic acids to form amides. A drug molecule is first converted to an acyl coenzyme A intermediate. An *N*-acyltransferase enzyme then catalyzes the conjugation of the activated drug molecule with the amino acid.

    d. **Glutathione conjugation** is extremely important in preventing toxicity from a variety of harmful electrophilic agents. Glutathione, a tripeptide containing a nucleophilic sulfhydryl group, is present in almost all mammalian tissues. Under the influence of **glutathione S-transferase,** glutathione can react with halides, epoxides, and other electrophilic compounds to form harmless inactive products. When glutathione has reacted with an electrophile, it undergoes a series of reactions to produce a mercapturic acid derivative, which is eliminated.

Table 17-4. Phase II Metabolism: Conjugation Pathways

Type of Conjugate	Reaction Pathway R = Drug Molecule; X = Functional Group
1. Glucuronide (X = OH, NR_2, CO_2H, SH, acidic carbon atoms)	**1.** (structure of UDP-glucuronic acid) + R–X ⟶ (glucuronide conjugate)
2. Sulfate (X = OH, arylamines, NH—OH)	**2.** (structure of PAPS with Adenine, H_2O_3PO, OH) + R–X ⟶ $HO-\overset{O}{\underset{O}{S}}-X\diagdown R$
3. Amino Acid (Occurs only with acid functional groups)	**3.** $R\overset{O}{\underset{S}{\diagdown}}$–CoA + $H_2N\overset{H\ \ Y}{\underset{CO_2H}{\diagup}}$ ⟶ $R\overset{O}{\diagdown}N\overset{H\ \ Y}{\underset{H\ \ CO_2H}{}}$ Y = H or $CH_2CH_2CO_2H$
4. Glutathione (X = electrophilic center such as halide, epoxide, or Michael acceptor)	**4.** (glutathione with SH) + R–X ⟶ (glutathione with S—R)
5. Methyl (X = OH, NH_2, SH)	**5.** (structure of SAM with CH_3, Adenine, HO_2C, NH_2, H_2O_3PO, OH) + R–X ⟶ $R-X-CH_3$
6. Acetylation (X = NH_2, $NHNH_2$, SO_2NH_2, CO—NH_2)	**6.** $H_3C\overset{O}{\underset{S}{\diagdown}}$–CoA + R–X ⟶ $H_3C\overset{O}{\diagdown}X\diagdown R$

    e. Methylation of oxygen-, nitrogen-, and sulfur-containing functional groups results in metabolites that are usually less polar than the unaltered drugs. Methylation can inactivate certain compounds [e.g., catechol O-methyl transferase (COMT) methylates a number of catecholamine neurotransmitters], but overall it plays a minor role in the elimination of drugs. Its major role is in the biosynthesis of endogenous compounds (e.g., epinephrine). The high-energy form required for methyltransferase enzymes is *S*-adenosylmethionine (SAM).

    f. Acetylation can occur with primary amines, hydrazides, sulfonamides, and, occasionally, amides. It leads to the formation of *N*-acetylated products. These products are usually less polar than the unaltered drug and can retain pharmacological activity.

        (1) *N*-acetylated metabolites can accumulate in tissue or in the kidneys, as in the case of certain antibacterial sulfonamides. Crystalluria and subsequent tissue damage may result.

        (2) The high-energy molecule for acetylation is acetyl-CoA. The reaction is catalyzed by *N*-acetyltransferase.

III. FACTORS INFLUENCING DRUG METABOLISM

A. Chemical structure specifically influences a drug's metabolic pathway. The presence or absence of certain functional groups will determine the necessity, route, and extent of metabolism.

B. Species differences

1. **Qualitative differences** in the actual metabolic pathway. Such a variation can result from a genetic deficiency of a particular enzyme or a difference in a particular endogenous substrate. In general, qualitative differences occur primarily with **phase II reactions.**

2. **Quantitative differences** are differences in the extent to which the same type of metabolic reaction occurs. Such a variation can result from a difference in the enzyme level, the presence of species specific isozymes, a difference in the amount of endogenous inhibitor or inducer, or a difference in the extent of competing reactions. In general, quantitative differences occur primarily with **phase I reactions.**

C. Physiological or disease state

1. Because the liver is the major organ involved in biotransformation, **pathological factors** that **alter liver function** can affect a drug's hepatic clearance.

2. **Congestive heart failure** decreases hepatic blood flow by reducing cardiac output, which alters the extent of drug metabolism.

3. An **alteration in albumin production** (the plasma's major drug-binding protein) can alter the fraction of bound to unbound drug. Thus, a decrease in plasma albumin can increase the fraction of unbound (free) drug, which then becomes available to exert a more intense pharmacological effect. The reverse is true when plasma albumin increases.

D. Genetic variations

1. The **acetylation rate** depends on the amount of N-acetyltransferase present, which is determined by genetic factors. The general population can be divided into **fast acetylators** and **slow acetylators.** For example, fast acetylators are more prone to **hepatotoxicity** from the antitubercular agent isoniazid than slow acetylators, whereas slow acetylators are more prone to isoniazid's other toxic effects (see VII.B.4.d).

2. The discovery of isoforms and families of CYP450 enzymes has shown that genetic variations exist in isoforms that oxidize **debrisoquine.** Individuals who are poor metabolizers of this compound **(PM phenotype)** also exhibit impaired metabolism of more than 20 other therapeutic agents, including β-blockers, antiarrhythmics, opioids, and antidepressants. Approximately 5%–10% of whites, 2% of Asians, and 1% of Arabs express the PM phenotype and are at risk for adverse drug reactions.

E. Drug dosage

1. An **increase** in drug dosage results in increased drug concentrations and can saturate certain metabolic enzymes. As drug concentration exceeds 50% saturation for a particular enzyme, drug elimination via this path no longer follows solely first-order kinetics, but rather is a mix of zero- and first-order kinetics. At 100% saturation, metabolism via this enzyme follows zero-order kinetics.

2. **When the metabolic pathway is saturated** (either because of an exceedingly high drug level or because the supply of an endogenous conjugated agent is exhausted), an alternative pathway may be pursued. For example, at normal doses, 98% of a dose of acetaminophen undergoes conjugation with either glucuronic acid or sulfate; however, at toxic doses, conjugation pathways become saturated and acetaminophen undergoes extensive N-hydroxylation, which can lead to hepatotoxicity.

F. Nutritional status

1. The levels of some **conjugating agents** (or endogenous substrates), such as sulfate, glutathione, and (rarely) glucuronic acid, are sensitive to body nutrient levels. For example, a **low-protein diet** can lead to a deficiency of certain amino acids, such as glycine. Low-protein diets also decrease oxidative drug metabolism capacity.

2. Diets **deficient in essential fatty** acids (particularly linoleic acid) reduce the metabolism of ethyl-morphine and hexobarbital by decreasing synthesis of certain drug-metabolizing enzymes.

3. A **deficiency of certain dietary minerals** also affects drug metabolism. Calcium, magnesium, and zinc deficiencies decrease drug-metabolizing capacity, whereas iron deficiency appears to increase it. A copper deficiency leads to variable effects.

4. **Deficiencies of vitamins** (particularly vitamins A, C, E, and the B group) affect drug-metabolizing capacity. For example, a vitamin C deficiency can result in a decrease in oxidative pathways, whereas a vitamin E deficiency can retard dealkylation and hydroxylation.

G. Age

1. Metabolizing enzyme systems are not fully developed at birth; thus, **infants** and **young children** need to receive smaller doses of drugs than adults to avoid toxic side effects. This is particularly true of drugs that require glucuronide conjugation.

2. In **older children,** some drugs may be less active than in adults, particularly if the dosage is based on weight. The liver develops faster than the increase in general body weight and, thus, represents a greater fraction of total body weight.

3. In the **elderly,** metabolizing enzyme systems decline. The lowered level of enzyme activity slows the rate of drug elimination, causing higher plasma drug levels per dose than in young adults.

H. Gender. Metabolic differences between the sexes have been observed for a number of compounds, suggesting that androgen, estrogen, and/or adrenocorticoid activity might affect the activity of certain CYP450 enzyme isozymes.

1. Metabolism of diazepam, prednisolone, caffeine, and acetaminophen is **slightly faster in women.**

2. Oxidative metabolism of propranolol, chlordiazepoxide, lidocaine, and some steroids occurs **faster in men** than in women.

I. Circadian rhythms. The **nocturnal plasma levels** of drugs, such as theophylline and diazepam, are lower than the **diurnal plasma levels.**

J. Drug administration route

1. **Oral administration.** The drug is absorbed from the GI tract and transported to the liver through the hepatic portal vein before entering the systemic circulation. Thus, the drug is subject to hepatic metabolism before it reaches its site of action. This is an effect known as the **first-pass effect, or presystemic elimination** (Table 17-5).
   a. The first-pass effect can cause **significant clinical problems.** Because drugs are metabolized in the liver from their active forms to inactive forms, this effect must be counteracted to achieve the desired plasma or tissue drug level.
   b. A common approach is to **increase the oral dose,** offsetting the loss of drug activity from the first-pass effect.

Table 17-5. Examples of Drugs That Undergo First-Pass Metabolism

Acetaminophen	Fluorouracil	Oxprenolol
Albuterol	Imipramine	Pentazocine
Alprenolol	Isoproterenol	Progesterone
Aspirin	Lidocaine	Propoxyphene
Cortisone	Meperidine	Propranolol
Cyclosporin	Methyltestosterone	Salbutamol
Desipramine	Metoprolol	Terbutaline
Dihydropyridines	Nortriptyline	Testosterone
Estradiol	Organic Nitrates	Verapamil

Table 17-6. Examples of Common CYP3A4 Inhibitors and Inducers

Potent Inhibitors	Moderate Inhibitors	Inducers
Amiodarone	Amprenavir	Carbamazepine
Atazanavir	Ciprofloxacin	Efavirenz
Clarithromycin	Diltiazem	Nevirapine
Indinavir	Erythromycin	Phenytoin
Itraconazole	Fluconazole	Phenobarbital
Ketoconazole	Fluvoxamine	Rifabutin
Nefazodone	Grapefruit juice	Rifapentine
Nelfinavir	Norfloxacin	Rifampin
Ritonavir	Verapamil	St. John's Wort
Telithromycin		
Troleandomycin		
Voriconazole		

2. **Intravenous administration** bypasses the first-pass effect because the drug is delivered directly to the bloodstream without being metabolized in the liver. Thus, intravenous doses of drugs undergoing considerable first-pass effects are much smaller than oral doses.

3. **Sublingual administration** and **rectal administration** also bypass first-pass effects, although rectal administration can produce variable effects.

K. **Concurrent drug therapy.** The co-administration of drugs that are capable of either inhibiting or inducing specific CYP450 isozymes can increase or decrease, respectively, the plasma levels of other drugs that require these isozymes for normal drug metabolism.

1. As indicated on Table 17-1, most drugs are metabolized by the following three isozymes: CYP2C9, CYP2D6, and CYP3A4. The potential for drug interactions due to enzyme inhibition or induction is therefore greater with these compounds.

2. Drugs that alter the activity of CYP450 isozymes are usually substrates of these same isozymes. This can be observed by comparing Tables 17-1 and 17-6.

3. The clinical outcome of these types of drug interactions depends upon three factors:
   a. The potency of the inhibitor or inducer (Table 17-6)
   b. The availability of alternate elimination pathways
   c. The extent to which the higher or lower plasma concentrations of the drug causes symptoms and/or undesirable effects.

IV. EXTRAHEPATIC METABOLISM

A. **Definition.** Extrahepatic metabolism refers to drug biotransformation that takes place in **tissues other than the liver.** The most common sites include the **portals of entry** (e.g., GI mucosa, nasal passages, lungs) and the **portals of excretion** (e.g., kidneys). However, metabolism can occur throughout the body.

B. **Metabolism sites**

1. **Plasma** contains **esterases,** which are responsible primarily for hydrolysis of esters. **Simple esters** (e.g., procaine, succinylcholine) are rapidly hydrolyzed in the blood. Additionally, plasma esterases can activate a variety of ester prodrugs.

2. Metabolizing enzymes in the **intestinal mucosa** are especially important for drugs undergoing microsomal oxidation, glucuronide conjugation, and sulfate conjugation.
   a. As a lipid-soluble drug passes through the intestinal mucosa during drug absorption, it can be metabolized into polar or inactive metabolites before entering the blood. The result is **comparable to a first-pass effect.**

   b. The intestinal mucosa's drug-metabolizing capacity compares to that of the liver. However, it shows much greater individual variation because of its greater exposure to the environment.

3. Intestinal bacterial flora secrete a number of enzymes capable of metabolizing drugs and other xenobiotics.

   a. Any factor that **modifies the intestinal flora** may also **modify drug activity.** Age, diet, disease state, and exposure to environmental chemicals or drugs may all be important.

      (1) Certain **diseases,** particularly **intestinal disease,** affect intestinal flora. Ulcerative colitis, for example, promotes bacterial growth. Diarrhea reduces the number of bacteria.

      (2) Certain **environmental chemicals** and **drugs** also act on intestinal flora. Antibiotics, for example, decrease the number of bacteria.

   b. Bacterial flora **secrete** β-glucuronidase, which hydrolyzes the polar glucuronide conjugates of bile and allows the free, nonpolar bile acids to be reabsorbed. This **enterohepatic circulation** partially maintains the pool of bile acids. This same principle applies to certain glucuronide conjugates of drugs.

   c. Certain bacterial flora **convert** vitamin precursors to their **active forms,** as with vitamin K.

   d. Bacterial flora can also **convert** certain substances to their **toxic forms,** as with the conversion of the artificial sweetener cyclamate to cyclohexylamine, a suspected carcinogen.

   e. Intestinal bacteria produce **azoreductase,** which reduces the prodrug sulfasalazine to the active anti-inflammatory aminosalicylic acid and the active antibacterial sulfapyridine. Sulfasalazine is one of the few agents effective in the treatment of ulcerative colitis.

4. The **acidic environment** of the **stomach** produces nonenzymatic degradation of a number of drug molecules, including penicillin G, carbenicillin, erythromycin, and tetracycline. Additionally, gastric acid assists in the degradation of proteins and peptides (e.g., insulin).

5. The **nasal mucosa** provides a high level of CYP450 activity, which can significantly alter the amount of drug that reaches the systemic circulation. Nasal decongestants, anesthetics, nicotine, cocaine, and other compounds have been shown to undergo nasal metabolism.

6. The **lung** is responsible for first-pass metabolism of drugs administered intravenously, intramuscularly, transdermally, or subcutaneously.

   a. The **total amount** of **metabolizing enzymes** present in the lungs is less than that in the liver; however, the specific activities of the enzymes are comparable to those in the liver.

   b. The lungs provide **second-pass metabolism** for drugs leaving the liver.

C. Placental and fetal metabolism

1. Placenta. In general, if a drug or other xenobiotic is lipid soluble enough to be absorbed into the circulation when administered to a pregnant woman, it will likely also pass through the placenta.

   a. The placenta is not a physical or metabolic barrier to xenobiotics. Very little xenobiotic-metabolizing enzyme activity has been demonstrated in the placenta.

   b. Drugs present in their **active form** in the maternal circulation likely pass **unchanged** into the fetal circulation.

   c. An exception to this lack of enzyme activity in the placenta is the presence of a small amount of **aryl aromatic hydroxylase,** which is **inducible in pregnant women who smoke cigarettes.** A potential consequence is an increase in the production of penultimate carcinogens from the action of this enzyme on the polycyclic aromatic hydrocarbons present in cigarette smoke and other environmental sources.

2. Fetus. In terms of fetal metabolism, there are varying degrees of drug-metabolizing activity dependent upon a number of factors including fetal age.

   a. A **major deficiency** is that of **glucuronic acid conjugating activity** both in the **fetus and the neonate.**

   b. Two consequences of this are the **gray baby syndrome,** resulting from decreased chloramphenicol glucuronidation, and **neonatal hyperbilirubinemia,** resulting from a decrease in bilirubin glucuronide formation.

V. STRATEGIES TO MANAGE DRUG METABOLISM. A variety of methods have been used to circumvent the rapid metabolism of certain drugs. These methods seek to improve drug therapy by decreasing the overall extent of metabolism and increasing the duration of action. In some instances, these methods have provided increased site specificity.

A. Pharmaceutical strategies involve the use of different **dosage forms** to either avoid or compensate for rapid metabolism.

1. **Sublingual tablets** are useful for delivering drugs directly into the systemic circulation and bypassing hepatic first-pass metabolism. **Nitroglycerin,** a rapidly acting antianginal agent, is essentially ineffective when administered orally due to an extremely high first-pass effect but is very effective in treating acute attacks of angina if given sublingually.

2. **Transdermal patches** and **ointment formulations** provide a continuous supply of drug over an extended period of time and are useful for rapidly metabolized compounds such as nitroglycerin. These delivery systems, while not suited to treat acute anginal symptoms, are effective in providing prophylactic concentrations of nitroglycerin.

3. **Intramuscular depot injections** also provide a continuous supply of drug over an extended period of time. Highly lipid soluble esters of **estradiol** and **testosterone** (e.g., estradiol benzoate, testosterone enanthate) are slowly absorbed from their administration site. Hydrolysis of these prodrugs (see VI) produces a steady supply of these rapidly metabolized hormones.

4. **Enteric-coated formulations** can protect acid-sensitive drugs as they pass through the acidic environment of the stomach. **Methenamine, erythromycin,** and **omeprazole** are examples of acid-sensitive agents that are available as enteric-coated preparations.

5. **Nasal administration** allows for the delivery of peptides, such as **calcitonin salmon,** which have very low (if any) oral bioavailability. Characteristics of the lung make it ideal for the administration of peptides. Aerosolized drugs only need to penetrate a thin epithelial layer to reach abundant capillary beds. Additionally, the lungs contain protease inhibitors, which allow for greater stability of the peptides.

B. Pharmacological strategies involve the concurrent use of enzyme inhibitors to decrease drug metabolism. In some instances, the concurrent use of an additional agent does not prevent metabolism but rather prevents the toxicity caused by metabolites of the therapeutic agent.

1. **Levodopa (L-dopa),** the amino acid precursor of dopamine, is used in the treatment of parkinsonism. Unlike dopamine, L-dopa can penetrate the blood–brain barrier and reach the central nervous system (CNS). When in the brain, it is decarboxylated to dopamine. To ensure that adequate concentrations of L-dopa reach the CNS, peripheral metabolism of the drug must be blocked. The concurrent administration of **carbidopa,** a dopa decarboxylase inhibitor that cannot penetrate the blood–brain barrier, prevents peripheral formation of dopamine and allows site-specific delivery of dopamine to the CNS.

2. **β-Lactam antibiotics.** The antibacterial activity of a number of β-lactam antibiotics is reduced by microorganisms capable of secreting the enzyme β-lactamase. This enzyme hydrolyzes the β-lactam ring and inactivates the antibiotic. To counter this resistance mechanism, a β-lactamase inhibitor, such as **clavulanic acid,** is used in conjunction with a penicillin, such as **amoxicillin,** to successfully treat infections caused by β-lactamase–producing bacteria.

3. **Ifosfamide** is an alkylating agent that must undergo in vivo metabolism to produce an active nitrogen mustard. In the process of this metabolic activation, significant concentrations of **acrolein** are produced. These acrolein molecules react with nucleophiles on renal proteins and produce hemorrhagic cystitis. To prevent this toxicity, ifosfamide is always coadministered with **mesna,** a sulfhydryl-containing compound that reacts with and neutralizes any acrolein that is present in the kidney.

4. **HIV protease inhibitors** are extensively metabolized by CYP3A isozymes. In addition, compounds within this class can inhibit these same isozymes. This latter action has been used to optimize therapy. **Ritonavir** is an HIV protease inhibitor that is known to cause hepatoxicity at therapeutic doses. **Lopinavir** is an HIV protease inhibitor that is ineffective if used alone due to rapid CYP3A oxidation. A new strategy combines a low dose of ritonavir with

Testosterone

Methyltestosterone

Tolbutamide

Chlorpropamide

Figure 17-1. Selected examples of chemical modification that eliminate metabolic transformations. Methylation of testosterone blocks the rapid oxidation of the 17-hydroxyl group and allows oral activity, whereas replacement of the metabolically labile *para*-methyl group on tolbutamide with a chloro group allows for a much longer duration of action.

a therapeutic dose of lopinavir. This results in an inhibition of CYP3A, the establishment of adequate plasma levels of lopinavir, and therapeutic efficacy without hepatotoxicity.

C. **Chemical strategies** involve the addition, deletion, or isosteric modification of key functional groups. These molecular modifications hinder or completely eliminate metabolic transformations (Figure 17-1).

1. **Testosterone** is not orally active due to rapid oxidation of its 17-hydroxyl group to a ketone. Addition of a 17α-methyl group converts the labile secondary alcohol to a stable tertiary alcohol. The resulting compound, **methyltestosterone,** is only half as potent as testosterone; however, it is not subject to rapid first-pass metabolism and can be used orally. A similar strategy has been used to make orally active estradiol analogues.

2. **Tolbutamide** is an oral hypoglycemic with a short duration of action. This sulfonylurea rapidly undergoes oxidation of its para-methyl group. A structurally similar compound, **chlorpropamide,** has a nonmetabolizable para-chloro group and, as a result, has a much longer duration of action.

3. **Isoproterenol** is a potent β-adrenergic agonist used for the relief of bronchospasm associated with bronchial asthma. Because it is a catechol (i.e., 3,4-dihydroxy–substituted benzene ring), isoproterenol is subject to rapid metabolism by catechol O-methyl transferase (COMT) and, thus, has poor oral activity. Alteration of the 3,4-dihydroxy substitution to a 3,5-dihydroxy substitution produces **metaproterenol,** a bronchodilator that is not susceptible to COMT, is orally active, and has a longer duration of action than isoproterenol.

4. **Octreotide** is a synthetic octapeptide used to suppress or inhibit severe diarrhea associated with certain tumors. Octreotide mimics the actions of **somatostatin,** a naturally occurring, 14–amino acid peptide. Somatostatin undergoes rapid proteolysis, has a half-life of 1–3 minutes, and must be administered as a continuous intravenous infusion. Octreotide contains the amino acids essential for clinical efficacy but replaces two of the amino acids with their D-enantiomers. These unnatural D–amino acids are more resistant to hydrolysis. As a result, octreotide has an increased half-life and can be administered as a subcutaneous injection.

VI. **PRODRUGS.** These drugs are molecules that are either inactive or very weakly active and require in vivo biotransformation to produce the physiologically active drug. The phase I metabolic processes discussed previously are used to activate prodrugs. A variety of **advantages** can be gained by using a prodrug instead of the active form of the drug.

A. An **increase in water solubility** is useful for the preparation of ophthalmic and parenteral formulations. **Sodium succinate esters** and **sodium phosphate esters** have been used to make a number of water-soluble steroid prodrugs.

B. An **increase in lipid solubility** is useful for a variety of reasons.

1. **Increased duration of action.** Lipid-soluble esters of estradiol, such as benzoate, valerate, and cypionate, are used to prolong estrogenic activity. IM injections of these esters in oil result in a deposit of drug that is slowly hydrolyzed, thereby releasing free estradiol over a prolonged period of time (see V.A.3).

2. **Increased oral absorption** is obtained by converting carboxylic acid groups to esters. These esters can then be rapidly converted to the active acids by plasma esterases. **Enalaprilat** is a potent angiotensin-converting enzyme (ACE) inhibitor that is used for parenteral administration, but, due to its high polarity, it is orally inactive. Its monomethyl ester, **enalapril,** is considerably more lipophilic and, thus, provides good oral absorption. This strategy has been successfully used for a variety of other compounds, including additional ACE inhibitors, fibric acid derivatives, ampicillin, and several cephalosporins.

3. **Increased topical absorption** of steroids is obtained by masking hydroxyl groups as esters or acetonides. These prodrugs are much less polar than the parent compounds and allow increased dermal permeability for the treatment of inflammatory, allergic, and pruritic skin conditions. Examples include **triamcinolone acetonide, diflorasone diacetate,** and beta**methasone valerate.**

4. **Increased palatability.** Antibiotics such as **sulfisoxazole** have a bitter taste and are not suitable for administration to young children who cannot yet swallow tablets or capsules. Esterification to produce **sulfisoxazole acetyl** decreases the water solubility of the antibiotic and, thus, decreases its interaction with bitter taste receptors on the tongue. This compound is marketed as a flavored suspension. Similar strategies have been used to mask the bitter taste of **chloramphenicol** and other antibiotics.

C. **A decrease in GI irritation.** Nonsteroidal anti-inflammatory agents (NSAIDs) produce gastric irritation and ulceration via two mechanisms: a direct irritant effect of the acidic molecule and inhibition of gastroprotective prostaglandin production. The prodrugs **sulindac** and **nabumetone** produce less GI irritation because the gastric and intestinal mucosa are not exposed to high concentrations of active drug during oral administration. Additionally, nabumetone is a ketone, not an acid, and lacks any direct irritant effects.

D. **Site specificity** is useful for increasing the concentration of drug at the active site and for decreasing side effects.

1. **Methyldopa** is a prodrug that is structurally similar to L-dopa. As a result, methyldopa is transported into the CNS and metabolized to the active compound, α**-methyldopamine,** via the same path used for the synthesis of dopamine. This allows a significant amount of α-methyldopamine to reach the CNS and bind to central α_2-adrenergic receptors.

2. **Omeprazole** is used to treat gastric ulcers and other hypersecretory disorders. After oral absorption, it is selectively activated at the acidic pH levels (pH less than 1) seen in gastric parietal cells. This allows the active form of the drug to be produced in close proximity to the enzyme H^+/K^+-ATPase (proton pump), resulting in irreversible inhibition of the enzyme and a decrease in gastric acid secretion. Activation in the stomach prior to absorption can be prevented by the use of enteric-coated formulations (see V.A.4).

3. **Formaldehyde** is an effective urinary tract antiseptic; however, oral administration results in significant toxicity. To avoid this problem, the prodrug **methenamine** is administered instead. Methenamine is stable and nontoxic at normal physiological pH, but is selectively hydrolyzed to formaldehyde and ammonium ions in the acidic urine (pH less than 5.5). As with omeprazole, activation before absorption can be prevented by the use of enteric-coated formulations (see V.A.4).

4. **Olsalazine** is a highly polar dimer of 5-aminosalicylic acid that is poorly absorbed after oral administration. On reaching the large intestine, colonic bacteria cleave the azo bond and liberate the active anti-inflammatory agent. Olsalazine and a related compound, **sulfasalazine,** are useful in treating inflammatory bowel disease.

5. **Diethylstilbestrol** is a synthetic estrogen that can produce undesirable, feminizing side effects when used in the treatment of prostate cancer. These side effects can be avoided by the use of the ester prodrug, **diethylstilbestrol diphosphate.** This prodrug is inactive until dephosphorylated by acid phosphatase, an enzyme that is highly active in prostate tumor cells. This allows for a localized release of active compound and a decrease in systemic side effects.

E. Increased shelf life of both solids and parenteral admixtures can be obtained by the use of prodrugs.

1. **Cefamandole** is a second-generation cephalosporin that is unstable in solid dosage forms. Esterification of the α-hydroxyl group with formic acid produces **cefamandole nafate,** a stable prodrug that is hydrolyzed by plasma esterases to produce the parent antibiotic.

2. **Cyclophosphamide** is a prodrug that requires in vivo oxidation, followed by nonenzymatic decomposition, to produce the active phosphoramide mustard. As a result, aqueous solutions of cyclophosphamide are much more stable than those of other nitrogen mustards (i.e., mechlorethamine). **Mechlorethamine** is highly reactive, does not require in vivo activation, and can rapidly decompose in aqueous environments before administration.

VII. PHARMACOGENETICS

A. **Genes and their involvement in drug response and toxicity**

1. **Genes** can be defined as discrete segments of DNA that are capable of reproduction during cell replication and that are responsible for guiding the biosynthesis of specific proteins and enzymes.

2. Genes encode proteins involved in the **absorption, transport, metabolism, and elimination** of drug molecules. Additionally, they encode proteins that serve as **drug receptors.** It is obvious then that a genetic disposition that would result in either an **over- or an under-expression of these genes** could significantly alter drug response and toxicity.

3. Assuming that a patient has been prescribed a medication that is indicated for his or her condition or disease state, there are several reasons why a patient may not respond or may suffer severe adverse effects:
   a. **Inappropriate dosing**
   b. **Drug–drug interactions**
   c. **Drug allergies**
   d. **Medication errors**
   e. **Genetic predisposition**

4. In its most simplistic form, **pharmacogenetics** can be defined as the use of genetic information to select the "right drug for the right patient." This area of study primarily seeks to identify the individual genetic differences and predispositions that influence drug response and safety.

B. **Genetic variation** in the DNA sequence can cause certain populations of individuals to be **more likely to develop specific disease states,** to be **more likely to follow a specific path of disease progression,** to be **more likely to respond to specific drug therapy,** and/or to be **more likely to develop certain adverse drug effects.**

1. The genetic variation between any two unrelated individuals is approximately one base pair change in every 1000 base pairs.

2. These changes are referred to as **single nucleotide polymorphisms (SNPs)** and are the most common form of genetic variation.

3. **The effects of SNPs vary** based upon the **type and location** of the variation.
   a. **An SNP located within the coding region** of a gene could produce no discernable

effects, negligible effects, or a significant alteration in effects depending upon how the SNP affected the amino acid coding.

(1) An SNP that **did not alter** the amino acid sequence in a protein would produce **no discernable effects.**

(2) An SNP that resulted in one amino acid being replaced by a **similar amino acid** would have a **negligible effect** (e.g., changing a portion of the genetic code from AUU to GUU would result in isoleucine being replaced by valine, a similar hydrophobic amino acid).

(3) An SNP that resulted in one amino acid being replaced by one with **significantly different chemical properties** would cause **a significant alteration of effects** (e.g., changing a portion of the genetic code from GUU to GAU would result in valine being replaced with the acidic, and more hydrophilic, aspartic acid).

b. **An SNP in a splicing control region** could result in the formation of a novel protein that is either larger or smaller in size than that which is naturally occurring.

c. **An SNP in a promoter region** could alter the transcription rate, resulting in either an increase or a decrease in the production of the target protein.

d. An SNP residing outside of any of the above locations is **genetically silent** and does not produce any observable effects.

4. Examples of known genetic variations and their effects on drug efficacy and safety

a. **Warfarin.** Patients with specific variations in the gene for the metabolizing enzyme CYP2C9 require lower doses and are at an increased risk of bleeding.

b. **Salmeterol and albuterol.** Genetic variations in the gene coding for the β_2-adrenergic receptor (ADBR2) can result in a decreased efficacy.

c. **6-Mercaptopurine.** Genetic variations affecting the enzyme thiopurine methyltransferase are known to produce increased toxicity.

d. **Procainamide, hydralazine, and isoniazid.** Genetic variations affecting the rate of *N*-acetylation affect both the efficacy and adverse effect profiles of these agents. The identification of fast and slow acetylators is one of the best known examples of how genetic variation can affect therapeutic safety and efficacy.

e. **Quinidine, cisapride, and clarithromycin.** Genetic variations in the gene coding for potassium channels can result in increased risk and prevalence of QT-syndrome and arrhythmias.

f. **Zileuton.** Patients with genetic variations in the gene coding for the enzyme 5-lipoxygenase do not respond to this drug.

C. Clinical pharmacogenetic assays

1. The **goal** of a clinical pharmacogenetic assay is to place patients into one of four categories.

a. Individuals who are most likely to respond and are at a low risk for adverse effects

b. Individuals who are most likely to respond and are at a high risk for adverse effects

c. Individuals who are less likely to respond and are at a low risk for adverse effects

d. Individuals who are less likely to respond and are at a high risk for adverse effects

2. Issues in the development of pharmacogenetic assays include:

a. Improvement in a medically important response (i.e., the assay should allow healthcare providers to make a better decision than would otherwise be possible).

b. **False positives for efficacy-based assays should be kept at a minimum** in order to prevent nonresponders from being prescribed drugs that will not provide the desired therapeutic outcomes. False negatives (i.e., responders identified as nonresponders) are not as crucial since they would be prescribed appropriate alternative therapy.

c. **False negatives for safety-based assays should be kept at a minimum** in order to prevent at-risk patients from being exposed to potential serious adverse effects. A higher rate of false positives (i.e., patients identified as "at risk") is acceptable. Excluding a certain percentage of patients in order to avoid serious adverse effects has been proposed to be a reasonable trade-off.

d. The results for the assays must be both interpretable and provide clinically useful results. The assays should be simple to use in a clinical setting and should provide results that are easily understood by the patient, physician, pharmacist, and other health-care providers.

e. Analytical and clinical validation of the assay must meet FDA approval standards.

Figure 17-2. Hypothetical single nucleotide polymorphism (SNP) maps. At the top is a composite SNP profile developed by using genetic information from a large database of patients/volunteers. This overall SNP can then be compared to individual SNP maps (i.e., **Patients A–D**) to help determine the overall benefit/risk for the given drug in each of these four patients.

3. As defined here, pharmacogenetic assays do not test for the presence or absence of a disease-specific mutation, nor do they provide any information that could be used to predict disease states in an individual or his or her family. As such, it has been suggested that legal and ethical issues surrounding disease-specific gene tests should not apply to predictions of safety and efficacy of drugs (i.e., the primary focus of pharmacogenetics).

D. SNP maps and their potential use

1. An SNP map for an individual contains the specific number and locations of base pair variations. Such a map could be used to predict patient response and susceptibility to serious adverse reactions.

2. **A simplified example of this is shown in Figure 17-2.** A large database would initially be used to identify SNPs that could be used as predictors of efficacy and safety. At the top of Figure 17-2, the two outside, shaded regions in this **hypothetical model** should be regarded as SNPs that would predict that a patient would favorably respond to the drug. Similarly, the two inner, black regions should be regarded as SNPs that would indicate that a patient was more prone to the development of serious adverse effects. Other SNPs (i.e., the nonhighlighted rectangles shown for the four patients) should be regarded as irrelevant here (i.e., they do not predict either efficacy or safety for the drug in question).

   a. Patient A would be predicted to respond to treatment without the development of any serious adverse effects.

   b. Patient B would be predicted to respond to treatment but would also be expected to develop serious adverse effects.

   c. Patient C would be predicted to be a nonresponder to treatment but would be unlikely to experience any serious adverse effects.

   d. Patient D would be predicted to be a nonresponder to treatment but would be expected to develop serious adverse effects.

STUDY QUESTIONS

Directions: Each of the numbered items or incomplete statements in this section is followed by answers or by completions of the statement. Select the one lettered answer or completion that is **best** in each case.

1. Which of the following statements concerning drug metabolism is true?

(A) Generally, a single metabolite is excreted for each drug administered.
(B) Often, a drug may undergo a phase II reaction followed by a phase I reaction.
(C) Drug-metabolizing enzymes are found only in the liver.
(D) All metabolites are less active pharmacologically than their parent drugs.
(E) Phase I metabolites more likely are able to cross cellular membranes than phase II metabolites.

2. Which of the following metabolites would be the least likely excretion product of orally administered aspirin (see structure below)?

(A) Glycine conjugate
(B) Ester glucuronide
(C) Unchanged drug
(D) Ether glucuronide
(E) Hydroxylated metabolite

3. Sulfasalazine (see structure below) is a prodrug that is activated in the intestine by bacterial enzymes. The enzyme most likely responsible is

(A) azoreductase
(B) pseudocholinesterase
(C) *N*-acetyltransferase
(D) β-glucuronidase
(E) methyltransferase

4. Chloramphenicol (see structure below) is considered to be toxic in infants (gray baby syndrome). This is due to tissue accumulation of unchanged chloramphenicol, resulting from an immature metabolic pathway. Which of the following enzymes would most likely be deficient?

(A) Pseudocholinesterase
(B) Glucuronyl transferase
(C) *N*-Acetyltransferase
(D) Azoreductase
(E) Methyltransferase

5. Which of the following therapeutic advantages cannot be obtained by the use of prodrugs? Increased

(A) oral absorption
(B) water solubility
(C) duration of action
(D) potency
(E) palatability

6. Which of the following statements regarding pharmacogenetics is INCORRECT?

(A) Single nucleotide polymorphisms (SNPs) in a promoter region can result in a decreased production of a target protein.
(B) It is crucial that false positives for safety-based assays be kept at a minimum.
(C) The area of pharmacogenetics focuses primarily on the genetic variations that affect drug efficacy and safety.
(D) The effects of SNPs vary based upon the type and location of the variation.
(E) Genetic variation occurs whenever there is a change in the DNA nucleotide base pair sequence.

Directions: Each question below contains three suggested answers, of which **one or more** is correct. Choose the answer

A	if **I only** is correct
B	if **III only** is correct
C	if **I and II** are correct
D	if **II and III** are correct
E	if **I, II, and III** are correct

7. Terms that may be used to describe the following metabolic reaction include

I. *N*-dealkylation
II. oxidative deamination
III. phase I metabolism

8. Which of the following reactions can be classified as phase II metabolism?

I.

II.

III.

9. Conditions that tend to increase the action of an orally administered drug that undergoes phase II metabolism include

   I. enterohepatic circulation
   II. enzyme saturation
   III. first-pass effect

10. Which of the following statements concerning CYP450 are correct?

   I. The CYP7, CYP11, and CYP27 subfamilies are involved in cholesterol metabolism.
   II. A single drug may be metabolized by multiple isoforms of CYP450.
   III. The majority of xenobiotics, or drugs, are metabolized by the CYP4B and CYP1A subfamilies.

11. Metabolic reactions likely to be affected by a protein-deficient diet include

   I. glycine conjugation
   II. hydrolysis
   III. glucuronidation

Directions: The group of items in this section consists of lettered options followed by a set of numbered items. For each item, select the **one** lettered option that is most closely associated with it. Each lettered option may be selected once, more than once, or not at all.

Questions 12–15

For each drug, select its most likely metabolic pathway.

(A) Ether glucuronidation
(B) Ester glucuronidation
(C) Nitroreduction
(D) Oxidative deamination
(E) Ester hydrolysis

12. Benzoic acid

13. Procaine

14. Acetaminophen

15. Amphetamine

ANSWERS AND EXPLANATIONS

1. The answer is E *[I; II.A.1, B].*
Phase I metabolites are often somewhat more polar than their parents. With the exception of acetylated and methylated metabolites, phase II metabolites are always much more polar than their parents. Thus, phase I metabolites are more likely to retain some liposolubility and are more likely to cross cellular membranes.

It is unusual for a single metabolite to be excreted for a given drug. Most drugs yield a mixture of metabolites. Because of the high polarity and subsequent high excretion of phase II metabolites, they are not likely to undergo further metabolism. Phase I metabolites, on the other hand, are less polar and are very likely to undergo further phase II metabolic reactions.

Whereas the major site of metabolism is the liver, there are many extrahepatic sites that secrete drug-metabolizing enzymes. Although many metabolites are less pharmacologically active than their parents, there are many drugs whose metabolites have equal or greater pharmacological activity and sometimes greater toxicity as well. Prodrugs (i.e., drugs inactive in the form administered) always form at least one active metabolite.

2. The answer is C *[II.A.1.e, 3.a, B.2.a.(2), c; Tables 17-2, 17-3, and 17-4].*
Because of the types of functional groups present, aspirin may undergo a number of different metabolic reactions. These include hydroxylation of the aromatic nucleus, conjugation of the carboxyl group with glycine, conjugation of the carboxyl group with glucuronic acid with the formation of an ester glucuronide, hydrolysis of the acetate ester, and conjugation of the phenol group (resulting from hydrolysis of the acetate ester) with glucuronic acid to form an ether glucuronide.

Because the acetate ester is a simple ester, aspirin is susceptible to hydrolysis in the acid media of the stomach before absorption takes place. In addition, any acetylated molecules that are absorbed are subjected to hydrolysis and are catalyzed by the many esterases present in the circulation. Any acetylated molecules not hydrolyzed in the circulation are subject to hydrolysis in the liver. All of these processes occur before the drug reaches the glomerular filtrate; therefore, excretion of the unchanged acetylated drug is highly unlikely.

3. The answer is A *[II.A.2; Table 17-3].*
Sulfasalazine has both anti-inflammatory and antibacterial activity when converted to aminosalicylic acid and sulfapyridine in the body. This reaction occurs by reductive cleavage of the "azo" linkage contained in the sulfasalazine molecule and is catalyzed in the intestine by bacterial azoreductase. This is a form of site-specific delivery because the intact drug is not absorbed from the stomach or upper intestine and reaches the colon, where it is metabolized. Sulfasalazine is one of a few drugs that is effective for the treatment of ulcerative colitis.

4. The answer is B *[II.B.2.a.(2); III.G.1; Tables 17-2, 17-3, and 17-4].*
The chloramphenicol molecule contains an aromatic nucleus, which would be subject to hydroxylation, a nitro group that is subject to reduction, an amide group that is subject to liver hydrolysis, and alcohol groups that are subject to glucuronidation. Of all the enzyme systems responsible for these reactions, the system responsible for glucuronidation is developed poorly in premature infants and infants up to approximately 6–8 weeks of age.

5. The answer is D *[VI.A, B.1–4].*
By definition, prodrugs are inactive or very weakly active molecules that require in vivo activation to the parent molecule. Thus, conversion of a drug molecule to a prodrug does not increase potency because the original molecule, with whatever potency it contains, is produced after administration. A variety of advantages, including increased water solubility, duration of action, oral absorption, and palatability, can be obtained through the use of prodrugs, but none of these advantages results in an increase in potency of the parent molecule.

6. The answer is B *[VII.A.4, B.1–3, C.2.c].*
While keeping false positives and false negatives at a minimum is always desirable, it is most crucial that false negatives be kept at a minimum for safety-based assays in order to prevent at-risk patients from being exposed to potential serious side effects. A higher rate of false positives is acceptable since preventing serious adverse effects is perceived to be more important than excluding some patients from therapy.

Genetic variation occurs whenever there are base pair changes in the DNA nucleotide sequence. The most common form of genetic variation is a single nucleotide polymorphism (SNP). The cumulative effects of these variations vary based on the types and locations of the SNPs. Variations in coding regions can alter protein function, while those in splicing and promoter regions can alter protein size and protein production, respectively. Some SNPs produce no discernable changes and are therefore genetically silent. Pharmacogenetics primarily seeks to use SNPs and other genetic information to predict predispositions that influence drug response and safety in individual patients.

7. The answer is D (II, III) *[II.A; Table 17-2].*
The reaction shown in the question involves the conversion of one functional group to another (amine to carbonyl); thus, it is classified as a phase I reaction. The introduction of oxygen into the molecule indicates oxidation, and the loss of the amino group signifies deamination; thus, the reaction also can be classified as oxidative deamination. *N*-Dealkylation implies the removal of an alkyl group from a nitrogen. The nitrogen in the parent molecule does not have an alkyl group attached to it.

8. The answer is C (I, II) *[II.A, B; Table 17-4].*
Phase II metabolic reactions involve masking an existing functional group with a natural endogenous constituent. The formulas shown in choices I and II represent this type of reaction, with choice I being an acetylation reaction and choice II, a glycine conjugation reaction. Choice III represents a change in an existing functional group and, thus, represents a phase I reaction. It is an oxidative deamination reaction.

9. The answer is C (I, II) *[II.B.2.a.(4), III.E.1, 2; IV.B.3.b].*
Enterohepatic circulation refers to the process by which glucuronides, which are secreted into the intestine with the bile, are hydrolyzed by intestinal bacterial β-glucuronidase. The hydrolyzed free drug, which is no longer polar, becomes available for intestinal reabsorption into the system and subsequent penetration to its active site.

If an enzyme system becomes saturated, then the active drug cannot be inactivated by that pathway. If the drug cannot undergo an alternative pathway, the increased plasma levels of an unchanged active drug can result in increased activity or toxicity.

The first-pass effect results in metabolism of a drug by the liver before the drug reaches its site of action, resulting in an overall decrease in its activity. Drugs that undergo first-pass metabolism generally are effective in much smaller intravenous doses as compared to oral doses.

10. The answer is C (I, II) *[II.A.1.c; Table 17-1]*
There are six mammalian families involved in steroid and bile acid metabolism. These are CYP7, CYP11, CYP17, CYP19, CYP21, and CYP27. Since cholesterol is the common intermediate for the biosynthesis of all endogenous steroids, some of these enzymes are directly involved in cholesterol metabolism. The families listed, CYP7, CYP11, and CYP27, all metabolize cholesterol, while the other three families catalyze additional oxidations of the initial metabolites.

As is evident from Table 17-1, multiple isoforms of CYP450 can metabolize a single drug. An example of this is seen with imipramine, an antidepressant that is metabolized by CYP1A, CYP2C, and CYP2D isoforms. Additionally, Table 17-1 indicates that the subfamilies CYP2C, CYP2D, and CYP3A metabolize the majority of drugs, or xenobiotics.

11. The answer is A (I) *[III.F.1].*
Phase II metabolic reactions require natural endogenous substrates, which normally are supplied in the diet. A deficiency of these substances results in a decrease in the biotransformation of drugs that use these pathways. Glycine conjugation is a phase II reaction. Glycine is an amino acid that requires dietary protein. A diet deficient in protein, therefore, could lead to a deficiency of glycine and, thus, a decrease in glycine conjugation. Glucuronidation is also a phase II reaction that requires endogenous glucuronic acid, but this substance is supplied by dietary carbohydrates. Hydroxylation is a phase I metabolic reaction and does not require dietary protein.

12–15. The answers are: 12-B *[II.B.2.a.(2)],* **13-E** *[II.A.3.a],* **14-A** *[II.B.2.a.(2)],* **15-D** *[II.A.1.e].*
Benzoic acid contains a carboxylic acid, a functional group that commonly undergoes conjugation with glucuronic acid. The resulting conjugation produces an ester. Carboxylic acids can also undergo conjugation with the amino acids glycine and glutamine. Additionally, benzoic acid can undergo aromatic hydroxylation, a common phase I pathway for drugs containing unsubstituted aromatic rings. Of these options, ester glucuronidation is the only answer available here.

Procaine is an ester-containing local anesthetic. Due to the wide physiological distribution of esterase enzymes, it is extremely susceptible to in vivo hydrolysis. This susceptibility to hydrolysis is the major reason why ester-containing local anesthetics have shorter durations of action as compared to those in other chemical classes.

One of the principal functional groups in acetaminophen is the phenol group. Similar to the carboxylic acid in benzoic acid, the phenol commonly undergoes glucuronide conjugation. The one difference is that a phenol (or an alcohol) produces an **ether** glucuronide, while a carboxylic acid produces an **ester** glucuronide. Phenols also commonly undergo sulfate conjugation reactions and occasionally undergo O-methylation reactions.

The principal functional group in amphetamine is its primary amine. Oxidative deamination is a very common metabolic path for primary amines. Occasionally, primary amines undergo phase II acetylation; however, this is a less common pathway. Aromatic hydroxylation, similar to that discussed above for benzoic acid, is also possible for amphetamine.

18
Drug–Drug and Drug–Nutrient Interactions

Alice C. Engelbrecht

Leon Shargel

I. INTRODUCTION

A. Definition of drug interaction

1. **Drug interaction** refers to an **adverse** drug response produced by the administration of a drug or co-exposure of the drug with another substance, which modifies the patient's response to the drug. Some drug interactions are intentional to provide improved therapeutic response or to decrease adverse drug effects. A **precipitant** drug is the drug, chemical, or food element causing the interaction. An **object** drug is the drug affected by the interaction.

2. Drug interactions include
   a. **Drug–drug** interactions
   b. **Drug–herbal** interactions
   c. **Food–drug** interactions
   d. **Pharmacogenetic** interactions
   e. **Chemical–drug** interactions, such as the interaction of a drug with alcohol or tobacco
   f. **Drug–laboratory test** interactions, such as chemical interactions.

B. Classification of drug interactions. Drug interactions that occur in vivo are generally classified as **pharmacokinetic** or **pharmacodynamic** interactions.

1. **Pharmacokinetic** or **biopharmaceutical** interactions occur when the absorption, distribution (protein and tissue binding), or elimination (excretion and/or metabolism) of the drug is affected by another drug, chemical, or food element.

2. **Pharmacodynamic** interactions occur when the pharmacodynamic effect of the drug is altered by another drug, chemical, or food element, producing an antagonistic, synergistic, or additive effect.

3. **Pharmacogenetic** interactions occur when the pharmacokinetic effect of the drug is altered by genetic factors that affect processes of metabolism.

4. **Pharmaceutical** interactions are caused by a chemical or physical incompatibility when two or more drugs are mixed together. Pharmaceutical interactions can occur during the extemporaneous compounding of drugs, including the preparation of intravenous (IV) solutions. For example, an IV solution of aminophylline has an alkaline pH and should not be mixed with such drugs as epinephrine, erythromycin gluceptate, or cephalothin sodium, which decompose in alkaline pH. Phenytoin sodium will precipitate from a solution that has an acid pH, such as dextrose 5%. Pharmaceutical interactions are usually considered during the development, manufacturing, and marketing of the drug product. Only drug interactions involving pharmacokinetic, pharmacodynamic, and pharmacogenetic processes are considered in this chapter.

II. PHARMACOKINETIC INTERACTIONS

A. Absorption

1. Drug interactions can affect the **rate** and the **extent** of systemic drug absorption (bioavailability) from the absorption site, resulting in increased or decreased drug bioavailability (Table 18-1).

Table 18-1. Drug Interactions That Affect the Bioavailability of the Drug from the Gastrointestinal (GI) Tract

Drug Interaction	Examples (Precipitant Drugs)	Effect (Object Drugs)
Complexation/ chelation	Calcium, magnesium, or aluminum and iron salts	Levofloxacin complexes with divalent cations, causing decreased bioavailability
	Sodium polystyrene sulfonate	Cations in antacids bind to sodium polystyrene sulfonate, causing reduced renal clearance of bicarbonate, resulting in systemic acidosis
Adsorption	Cholestyramine	Decreased bioavailability of digoxin, levothyroxine
	Kaolin	Decreased bioavailability of digoxin
	Activated charcoal	Decreased bioavailability of many drugs
	Acarbose	Decreased bioavailability of digoxin
Increased GI motility	Laxatives, cathartics	Increases GI motility, decreases bioavailability for drugs that are absorbed slowly; decreases bioavailability of drugs from controlled-release products
Decreased GI motility	Anticholinergic agents	Propantheline decreases gastric emptying of acetaminophen, delaying acetaminophen's absorption from small intestine
Alteration of gastric pH	H_2-blockers, antacids, and proton pump inhibitors	Increase gastric pH; dissolution of ketoconazole is reduced at basic pH, causing decreased drug absorption and therapeutic failure
Alteration of intestinal flora	Antibiotics	Digoxin has better bioavailability taken after erythromycin; erythromycin administration reduces bacterial inactivation of digoxin
		Estrogen/progestin birth control requires intestinal flora to facilitate enterohepatic circulation; antibiotics reduce intestinal flora and reduce estrogen/progestin levels, resulting in failure of ovulation suppression and menstrual changes
Inhibition of drug metabolism in intestinal cells	Monoamine oxidase inhibitors (e.g., tranylcypromine, phenelzine)	Inhibit metabolism of albuterol and levalbuterol, leading to hypertension

2. The most common drug absorption **site** is in the **gastrointestinal (GI) tract.** However, drug bioavailability from other absorption sites, such as the skin, can be affected by drug interactions. For example, epinephrine, a vasoconstrictor, will decrease the percutaneous absorption of transdermal lidocaine or transdermal fentanyl.

3. Other **potential** drug interactions that affect bioavailability in the GI tract could be the result of:
   a. **Competition** for carrier-mediated drug absorption in which the participant drug (e.g., purine, pyrimidine) competes for the same carrier as the object drug (e.g., purine or pyrimidine antimetabolite).
   b. **Alteration** of intestinal blood flow caused by the precipitant drug. In congestive heart disease, the blood flow to the GI tract is poor, and an orally administered drug can have a slower rate of absorption. After digoxin therapy, the perfusion of the GI tract is improved along with bioavailability of the object drug.

B. **Distribution.** The distribution of the drug may be affected by plasma protein binding and displacement interactions or tissue and cellular interactions.

1. Plasma protein binding and displacement on albumin and α_1-acid glycoprotein carrier proteins.
   a. **Valproic acid** displaces phenytoin from plasma albumin protein binding sites and reduces hepatic phenytoin clearance by inhibiting the liver's metabolism of phenytoin.
   b. **Aspirin** decreases protein binding and inhibits the metabolism of valproate.

2. **Tissue and cellular interactions.** Digoxin toxicity can be enhanced by concurrent administration of quinidine. Quinidine reduces digoxin clearance and displaces digoxin from both α_1-glycoprotein and albumin tissue-binding sites, leading to a higher plasma digoxin concentration.

C. Drug elimination and clearance

1. **Drug metabolism and hepatic clearance**
   a. Drug metabolism (hepatic clearance) can be affected by enzyme induction, enzyme inhibition, substrate competition for the same enzyme, and changes in hepatic blood flow (Table 18-2).
   b. Many drugs that share the same drug-metabolizing enzymes have a potential for a drug interaction. For example, fluconazole inhibits the hepatic metabolism of warfarin, causing increased risk of bleeding. Carbamazepine is both a substrate and an inducer of the cytochrome P450 3A4 (CYP34A) isoenzyme, thereby inducing its own metabolism and taking 3–5 weeks to reach stable blood levels. (Table 18-3).
   c. Over-the-counter (OTC) drugs and herbal preparations can also be involved in CYP450 isoenzyme metabolism and can cause serious drug–herbal interactions. For example, St. John's Wort may induce CYP3A4 isoenzymes and decrease cyclosporin to subtherapeutic levels. Tobacco use (smoking) can induce the CYP1A2 isoenzyme and decrease clozapine levels, increasing the risk of therapeutic failure in treating obsessive–compulsive disorder (OCD).
   d. Foods may also interfere with hepatic drug metabolism. For example, grapefruit juice is a powerful inhibitor of the CYP3A4 isoenzyme, and will increase blood levels of saquinavir if taken together.
   e. Nonhepatic enzymes can be involved in drug interactions. For example, serotonin syndrome has been reported in patients receiving antidepressants similar to citalopram in combination with a monamine oxidase (MOA) inhibitor. A considerable portion of the 3A4 isoenzymes are found not only in the liver but also in the GI tract, where some of these substrates are metabolized.
   f. A decrease in the hepatic blood flow can decrease the hepatic clearance for high-extraction drugs, such as propranolol and morphine.

Table 18-2. Drug Interactions That Affect Drug Metabolism

Drug Interaction	Examples (Precipitant drugs)	Effect (Objective Drugs)
Enzyme induction		
	Smoking (polycyclic aromatic hydrocarbons)	Increases theophylline metabolism and decreases theophylline levels
	Phenytoin	Decreased tacrolimus levels because of increased metabolism
Enzyme inhibition		
Mixed-function oxidase	Cimetidine	Decreased atorvastatin clearance; increased drug levels
Other enzymes	Monoamine oxidase inhibitors (e.g., pargyline, tranylcypromine)	Serious hypertensive crisis can occur after ingestion of foods with a high content of tyramine or other pressor substances (e.g., Cheddar cheese, red wines, avocado), and catecholamines

Table 18-3. Drug, Herb, and Food Actions with Cytochrome P450 Isoenzymes

Isoenzyme	Inhibitor	Inducer	Substrate
CYP1A2	Ciprofloxacin	Phenytoin	Naproxen
	Levofloxacin	Carbamazepine	Amitriptyline
	Ticlopidine	Charbroiled foods	Verapamil
	Fluvoxamine	Tobacco	Propranolol
			Clozapine
CYP2C9	Cimetidine	Rifampin	Tamoxifen
	Fluoxetine	Carbamazepine	Losartan
	Voriconazole	Phenytoin	Warfarin
	Fluconazole		Celecoxib
	Amiodarone		Phenytoin
CYP2C8	Gemfibrozil	Phenobarbital	Paclitaxel
		Rifampin	Repaglinide
CYP2C19	Ketoconazole	Rifampin	Diazepam
	Omeprazole	Carbamazepine	Phenytoin
	Ticlopidine		Lansoprazole
	Fluoxetine		Clomipramine
	Fluvoxamine		Diphenhydramine
CYP2D6	Methadone	Carbamazepine	Amitriptyline
	Cimetidine	Phenytoin	Metoprolol
	Fluoxetine	Ethanol	Paroxetine
	Ritonavir	St. John's Wort	Codeine
	Haloperidol		Haloperidol
	Diphenhydramine		Venlafaxine
CYP2E1	Cimetidine	Ritonavir	Acetaminophen
	Disulfiram	Isoniazid	Caffeine
		Ethanol	Venlafaxine
CYP3A family	Erythromycin	Carbamazepine	Atorvastatin
	Ketoconazole	Phenobarbital	Warfarin
	Saquinavir	St. John's wort	Lidocaine
	Verapamil	Efavirenz	Ethyl estradiol
	Metronidazole	Garlic supplements	Cyclosporin
		Grapefruit	Doxorubicin
		Seville oranges	Amitriptyline
		Bitter orange	Methadone
			Cyclosporin
			Amlodipine
			Indinavir
			Cyclosporin
			Paclitaxel
			Ritonavir

2. **Renal drug clearance** can be affected by changes in glomerular filtration, tubular reabsorption, active drug secretion, and renal blood flow and nephrotoxicity (Table 18-4).

III. PHARMACODYNAMIC INTERACTIONS

A. Drugs that have similar pharmacodynamic actions may produce an excessive pharmacological or **toxic response.** For example, central nervous system (CNS) depressants, such as the combination of narcotics and antihistamines (e.g., diphenhydramine, chlorpheniramine) can produce increased drowsiness in the patient. Drugs that have anticholinergic effects, such as

Table 18-4. Drug Interactions That Affect Renal Clearance

Drug Interaction	Examples	Effect
Glomerular filtration rate (GFR) and renal blood flow	Methylxanthines (e.g., caffeine, theobromine)	Increased renal blood flow and GFR decrease time for reabsorption of various drugs, leading to more rapid urinary drug excretion
Active tubular secretion	Probenecid	Probenecid blocks the active tubular secretion of penicillin and some cephalosporin antibiotics
Tubular reabsorption and urine pH	Antacids, sodium bicarbonate	Alkalinization of the urine increases the reabsorption of amphetamine and decreases its clearance
		Alkalinization of urine pH increases the ionization of salicylates, decreases reabsorption, and increases its clearance

promethazine and OTC antihistamines, can cause excessive dryness of the mouth, blurred vision, and urinary retention.

B. The pharmacodynamic effect of one drug can be antagonized by the opposite pharmacodynamic effect of a second drug. For example, the antihypertensive effect of β-blockers can be overcome by the use of vasopressors. Obviously, this can have a deleterious effect, be a therapeutic failure, or be a therapeutic strategy in clinical treatment, depending on the situation.

C. Drug therapy can produce an adverse effect that results in an **increased sensitivity** or **toxicity** when another drug is given. For example, the alteration of electrolyte concentrations produced by a diuretic, such as a thiazide derivative, will deplete potassium, resulting in sensitization of the heart to digoxin therapy. Depletion of sodium by a diuretic can also result in lithium toxicity.

D. Therapies that have **intrinsically opposite effects** on the same target system, can result in therapeutic failure. For example, naloxone competes with narcotics at the narcotic receptor site, resulting in therapeutic failure of narcotic-based analgesia therapy.

E. **Pharmacodynamic** drug interactions also can occur with drug–herbal interactions and drug–food interactions. For example, by ingesting large amounts of vitamin K in the diet, the effect of anticoagulation by warfarin is **antagonized.**

IV. DRUG–HERBAL INTERACTIONS

A. Herbal preparations contain combinations of herbs or a single herb. Some herbal preparations represent a single herb containing a variety of alkaloids or constituents that may exhibit a variety of pharmacological activities.

    1. Some herbs contain a number of different pharmacologically active constituents. For example, St. John's wort has at least six different constituents: hyperforin, biapigenin, hypericin, quercitin, chlorogenic acid, and pseudohypericin. Each constituent has its own metabolism, binding, and pharmacologic action. The predominant effect or interaction depends on the relative potency of each constituent in the herb. For example, the constituents of St. John's wort have inhibitory effects on the cytochrome P450 isoenzymes 3A4, 2C9, 1A2, 2D6, and 2D9, but none of these effects is considered clinically significant. St. John's wort appears overall to be an inducer of CYP3A4, and its constituents have many additional effects on metabolism and binding sites (Table 18-5).

    2. Many herbal drugs interact at the same transport, metabolism, and receptor sites as traditional prescription drugs (Table 18-6).

Table 18-5. Pharmacokinetic Activity of the Constituents of St. John's Wort

Activity	Site
Metabolized by	Cytochrome P450, most notably 3A4 isoenzyme
Transported by	Intestinal P-glycoprotein
Active at	γ-Aminobutyric acid, norepinephrine, dopamine, L-glutamate receptor sites
	Serotonin reuptake, norepinephrine reuptake sites
Inhibits	Monoamine oxidase, possibly cellular phosphodiesterase sites
	β-Adrenergic and muscarinic receptor sites
Binding site competition at	DNA sites in human leukemia cells

Table 18-6. St. John's Wort Drug Interactions

Pharmacokinetic Process	Site	Action	Results in	Drug
Metabolism	CYP3A4	Induces	Lower levels of	NNRTI Protease inhibitors Benzodiazepines Calcium channel blockers Carbamazepine Cyclosporin Irinotecan Digoxin
	CYP2C9	Induces	Lower levels of	Warfarin
	CYP1A2	Induces	Lower levels of	Warfarin
Transporter proteins	Intestinal P-glycoprotein transporter proteins	Increases catalyzed efflux of substrate drug	Lower levels of	Digoxin Calcium channel blockers Simvastatin
Pharmacodynamic toxicity	Serotonin reuptake receptor sites	Inhibits serotonin reuptake	Additive SSRI activity	SSRIs
		Serotonin agonist activity	Additive serotonin toxicity	Serotonin agonists (e.g. fenfluramine) and "triptans"
	MAO receptor sites	Increases MAOI and serotonin activity	Additive serotonin toxicity	MAOIs
Pharmacokinetic	Serotonin and norepinephrine reuptake sites	Inhibits reuptake	Norepinephrine and serotonin toxicity	Nefazodone
	DNA binding sites in human leukemia cells	Distorts DNA binding sites	Reversed etoposide-stabilized cleavage complexes	Antagonizes chemotherapy effect of etoposide (in vitro)

CYP, cytochrome P450; *NNRTI*, nonnucleoside reverse transcriptase inhibitor; *MAO*, monoamine oxidase; *MAOI*, monoamine oxidase inhibitor; *SSRI*, selective serotonin reuptake inhibitor.

3. Traditional Chinese medicine (TCM) may contain a combination of herbs. Some imported TCM products have been found to contain unlisted legend drugs. An example is a TCM medication advertised to treat diabetes that was found to contain the pharmaceuticals glyburide and phenformin.

4. Some herbal preparations may contain unrecognized contaminants such as heavy metals, or a similar-appearing herb that is mistakenly harvested. These are quality-control issues that are to a large extent unregulated by government agencies.

B. **Drug-herbal interactions** can occur as pharmacokinetic or pharmacodynamic interactions (Table 18-7).

C. Drugs with narrow therapeutic windows are at greater risk for drug–herbal interactions. For example, important drug–herbal interactions occur with patients taking warfarin:

1. Coenzyme Q10 has a chemical structure related to vitamin K. The combination of warfarin and coenzyme Q10 results in antagonized warfarin activity and inadequate anticoagulation.

2. Ginger, garlic, and feverfew also increase bleeding in patients taking warfarin by directly inhibiting platelets and causing increased risk of bleeding.

3. Wheat grass actually contains high levels of vitamin K, which directly antagonizes warfarin, causing inadequate anticoagulation and therapeutic failure.

D. **Potency of herbal preparations** is influenced by a variety of factors:

1. The stage of growth during which the herb was harvested

2. The drying time

3. The solvents used in extraction of the herb

4. The shelf life and storage conditions of the herbal extract

V. FOOD–DRUG INTERACTIONS

A. **Food can increase, decrease, or not effect the absorption of drugs** (Table 18-8).

B. **Food can influence the bioavailability of a drug** from a modified-release dosage form—for example, controlled release and delayed release (enteric coated)—rather than from an immediate-release dosage form. For example, opening the capsule of enteric-coated omeprazole beads and giving it in an acidic food such as applesauce or with orange juice, eases administration of the drug while maintaining the enteric coating on the omeprazole beads until the drug reaches the basic pH of the duodenum.

C. **Complexation and adsorption** of the drug in the GI tract with another food element is a common drug interaction that reduces the extent of drug absorption. For example, quinolone antibiotics complex with calcium (found in milk products).

D. **Food can be metabolized by the same liver enzymes that metabolize drugs,** causing enzyme inhibition or induction, and resulting in toxic or subtherapeutic drug levels. For example, grapefruit and Valencia oranges inhibit the CYP3A4 isoenzyme system, causing increased levels of substrate drugs such as saquinavir, indinavir, midazolam, nimodipine, nifedipine, lovastatin, cyclosporin, carbamazepine, and verapamil.

E. **Food can pharmacodynamically antagonize the effect of some drugs.** For example, spinach and broccoli provide dietary sources of vitamin K, which antagonizes the effect of warfarin. Garlic can cause additive antiplatelet effect in combination with warfarin, heparin, and low molecular weight heparin (LMWH), and cause increased risk of bleeding.

F. **Foods can contain pharmacologically active compounds** that interact with drugs meant to inhibit endogenous compounds. Monoamine oxidase inhibitors (MAOIs) prevent normal metabolism of catecholamines. They also inhibit the metabolism of tyramine from tyramine-containing foods such as red wine and cheese. The increased levels of tyramine cause hypertensive crisis.

Table 18-7. Common Herbs and Potential Drug Interactions

Herb	Drug/Drug Class	Interaction	Effect
Black cohosh	Antihypertensives	Pharmacodynamic potentiation	Increased effect of antihypertensives (hypotension)
Coenzyme Q10	Warfarin	Pharmacodynamic antagonism	Vitamin K antagonism (increased INR and risk of bleed)
Dong quai	β-Blockers	Inhibition of cytochrome P450 isoenzyme	Increased level (increased hypotension)
	Benzodiazepines		Increased levels (increased drowsiness; CNS depression)
Echinacea	Immunosuppressants; monoclonal antibodies	Pharmacodynamic antagonism	Decreased immunosuppression (flair of autoimmune disease, transplant graft rejection)
Ephedrine; ma huang	β-Blockers	Pharmacodynamic antagonism	Sympathomimetic effect (hypertension)
	MAOIs	Blocked metabolism	Increased and prolonged sympathomimetic effect (hypertensive crisis)
	Corticosteroids	Increased metabolism; induced hepatic metabolism	Decreased corticosteroid levels (decreased steroid effectiveness)
Evening primrose oil	Antiplatelets	Pharmacodynamic potentiation	Decreased platelet aggregation (increased risk of bleed)
	Phenothiazines	Additive toxicity	Reduced seizure threshold (seizures)
Ginkgo biloba	Warfarin, LMWH	Pharmacodynamic potentiation	Increased inhibition of platelet aggregation (increased risk of bleed)
Ginseng	MAOIs	Pharmacodynamic effect	Increased GABA metabolism; increased dopamine levels (mania symptoms)
Kava kava	Acetaminophen; azole antifungals; statins	Additive toxicity	Increased potential for hepatic toxicity (elevated LFTs; hepatic failure)
	Barbiturates; benzodiazepines	Synergy	Increased GABA receptor binding affinity (increased drowsiness; CNS depression)
	Levodopa	Antagonism	Dopamine blockade (decreased effectiveness of levodopa)
Soy	Levothyroxine	Impaired absorption	Decreased levels (hypothyroid symptoms)
St. John's wort	Irinotecan	Induced cytochrome P450 3A4 metabolism	Reduced levels of active irinotecan metabolite for chemotherapy (decreased myelosuppression)
Valerian	Sedatives	Pharmacodynamic	Increased CNS depression (drowsiness; sedation)
	Benzodiazepines	Displacement from binding sites	Displaced drug but additive CNS depression (possible increased drowsiness)

CNS, central nervous system; *GABA,* γ-aminobutyric acid; *INR,* international normalized ratio; *LFTs,* liver function tests; *LMWH,* low molecular weight heparin; *MAOI,* monoamine oxidase inhibitor.

Table 18-8. Affect of Food on Drug Bioavailability

Reduced or Delayed	Increased	No Effect
Nonsteroidal anti-inflammatory drugs, naproxen, naproxen sodium	Griseofulvin	Theophylline[a]
	Metoprolol	Metronidazole
Aspirin	Phenytoin	
Acetaminophen	Propoxyphene	
Antibiotics (tetracycline and penicillin)	Dicumarol	
Ethanol	Morphine	

[a]Food does not significantly affect drug absorption of theophylline in an immediate-release dosage form. However, food may affect theophylline absorption from a controlled-release formulation.

VI. CHEMICAL–DRUG INTERACTIONS

A. **Smoking** by inhaling aromatic polycyclic hydrocarbons can induce CYP1A2 isoenzyme metabolism and decrease levels of substrate drugs, such as theophylline, diazepam, and tricyclic antidepressants.

B. **Ethanol** can increase or decrease the activity of hepatic drug metabolizing enzymes.

1. Chronic alcoholism can increase the rate of metabolism of tolbutamide, warfarin, and phenytoin.

2. Acute alcohol intoxication can inhibit hepatic enzymes in nonalcoholic individuals.

3. Ethanol induces metabolism in CYP1A2 and CYP2E1 isoenzymes. Levels of the CYP1A2 substrates clozapine, cyclobenzaprine, imipramine, and naproxen are decreased. Levels of the CYP2E1 substrate acetaminophen are reduced.

4. Disulfiram inhibits alcohol dehydrogenase, resulting in limited metabolism of ethanol and causing severe ethanol intolerance.

VII. PHARMACOGENETICS AND DRUG INTERACTIONS

A. **Genetic differences** in drug metabolism are the result of variations in **alleles** for genes that code for enzymes responsible for the metabolism of drugs.

1. In normal enzyme function, the gene encoding for the enzyme is composed of two normal alleles. In **polymorphisms,** the genes contain abnormal pairs or multiples of abnormal alleles, leading to altered enzyme function.

2. Polymorphisms can occur in any enzyme system, including the cytochrome P450 hepatic enzymes and the mixed oxidase and *N*-acetyltransferase systems. The CYP2D6, CYP2C9, and CYP2C19 polymorphisms are the most extensively studied.

3. Differences in enzyme activity occur at different rates in different racial groups (Table 18-9).

4. **Polymorphisms** (differences in the alleles) can also vary within a racial group by geographic distribution, as seen with the CYP2D6 alleles in western Europe: There are 10 times as many ultra-metabolizers (UMs) in Greek populations as there are in Austrian populations.

5. The extent of the drug interaction is predicted based on the baseline activity of the enzyme in an individual. Baseline enzyme efficiency varies greatly among individuals, depending on the type and extent of polymorphic changes to the enzyme.

Table 18-9. Ethnic Differences in Cytochrome P450 2D6 Isoenzyme Activity

Ethnicity	Percent of the Population
White	7–10% PM; 1% UM
African American	8% PM
Asian	> 50% PM ; 1% UM

PM, poor metabolizer; *UM,* ultrarapid metabolizer. Reprinted with permission from Zagaria MAE. The promise of pharmacogenomics. US Parm [online] 2004;29(1).

B. **Single nucleotide polymorphisms (SNPs)** are single changes in an allele of a gene responsible for a variety of metabolic processes, including enzymatic metabolism.

1. SNPs can be of several different kinds, resulting in many different variants of an enzyme. For example, more than 70 variant alleles are known for CYP2D6.

2. The combination of alleles encoding the gene determines the activity of the enzyme. The combinations can include missing alleles, defective alleles, duplicated alleles, and multiple alleles. In addition, alleles can demonstrate amplification, substitution, or defective splicing. Errors in transcription and splicing and changes in start and stop codons and amino acids can result in null (abolished) enzyme activity.

3. The combination of alleles for a particular gene can affect the effectiveness of the enzyme or gene product. The overall function of an enzyme is an aspect of the **phenotype** of a particular combination of alleles.
   a. Poor metabolizers (PMs) carry two defective alleles—for example, CYP2D6*4/*5 and CYP2D6*4/*4. Or PMs may possess an allele that codes for a nonfunctioning enzyme or may be missing one allele—for example CYP2D6*5 and CYP2D6*4/deletion.
   b. Normal metabolizers (NMs) carry what are referred to as wild-type alleles—for example, CYP2D6*1/*33. Wild-type alleles encode enzymes with normal function.
   c. Intermediate metabolizers (IMs) are heterozygous—that is, they have one wild-type allele and one defective allele.
   d. Extensive metabolizers (EMs) carry one wild-type and one amplified allele—for example CYP2D6*2/*2, CYP2D6*A/*1a, and CYP2D6*1A/*5.
   e. Ultrarapid metabolizers (UMs) carry two or more copies of an amplified allele, for example CYP2D6*2/*2.

4. Some genetic changes inactivate or reduce enzymatic activity (resulting in PMs), leading to increases in the substrate drug.

5. Gene duplication may increase enzymatic activity (resulting in UMs), leading to lower levels of the substrate drug.

6. In the case of the CYP2D6 isoenzyme, genetic variation among patients accounts for a 10-fold to 30-fold difference in the levels of drugs metabolized by that enzyme. Table 18-10 lists a few CYP2D6 variants and their effects on the drug metabolism activity of the enzyme.

C. **Effect on inhibitors and inducers.** Some polymorphisms affect drug interactions by altering the effect of inhibitors and inducers on the enzymes. The result is an exaggerated effect or a minimal effect on the substrate.

1. In an **EM,** the level of substrate drug is normally low because of the rapid metabolism by the enzyme. An **inhibitor** to the enzyme will substantially inhibit the extensive metabolism, causing significant elevations in the substrate drug. The substrate levels rise dramatically because the effect of the inhibitor is much greater than normal in an EM (Table 18-11).

2. In a **PM,** the level of substrate drug remains high because the metabolism of the substrate is much less than normal. When an **inhibitor** is added to the regimen, the additional inhibition of metabolism is not much greater than what is already occurring in a PM.

Table 18-10. Enzyme Activity and Phenotypes of CYP2D6 Isoenzyme Alleles

Gene	Allele	Enzyme activity	Phenotype
CYP2D6*1	Wild type	Normal	EM or normal
CYP2D6*2	Same as 2D6*1, but possible duplication or amplification	Increased	EM/UM
CYP2D6*4	Defective splicing	Inactive	PM
CYP2D6*5	Gene depletion	No enzyme	PM
CYP2D6*10	Single amino acid substitution; predominant variant in people of Asian descent	Reduced	PM
CYP2D6*17	Single amino acid substitution; predominant variant in people of African descent	Reduced	PM

PM, poor metabolizer; *UM,* ultrarapid metabolizer.
Data from Zagaria MAE. The promise of pharmacogenomics. US Parm [online] 2004;29(1); Ingelman-Sundberg M. Genetic polymorphisms of cytochrome P4502D6 (CYP2D6): clinical consequences, evolutionary aspects and functional diversity. Pharmacogenomics J [online] 2005;5; Lee LS, Nafziger AN, Bertino JS Jr. Evaluation of inhibitory drug interactions during drug development: Genetic polymorphisms must be considered. Clin Pharmacol Ther 2005; 78:1–6.

Therefore, the effect of an inhibitor on a PM is less than it would be for a normal metabolizer. The drug interaction may not occur.

3. In an **EM,** the level of substrate drug is again lower than what would be expected in a normal metabolizer because of the rapid metabolism. The addition of an **inducer** does not cause a great difference in the level of substrate because the metabolism is already increased greatly. The drug interaction may not occur.

4. In a **PM,** the level of substrate drug is again higher than what would be expected in a normal metabolizer because of the lower metabolism of the substrate. The addition of an **inducer** will cause a significant increase in the metabolism of the substrate and cause a much lower level of substrate than what would be expected in a normal metabolizer. The drug interaction may occur to a greater extent than in a normal metabolizers, or the drug interaction may result in substrate levels similar to those of a normal metabolizer.

5. As a general rule, the effect of inhibitors is greater in EMs than in PMs. The effect of inducers is greater in PMs than in EMs.

6. The difference between EMs and UMs can be explained by the difference in their genotypes (allele combinations). EMs are heterozygotes, with one wild-type allele and one amplified allele; UMs are homozygotes, with two amplified alleles (or may carry a gene duplication). The addition of an inhibitor to an UM would be expected to show an even greater drug reaction than would be seen in an EM.

7. Complex drug interactions can be seen when a substrate is metabolized through more than one enzyme system, when one or more enzymes are affected by polymorphism. In

Table 18-11. The Effect of Inhibition of Extensive/Poor Metabolism (EM/UM) and Poor Metabolism (PM) on CYP2D6 Substrates

Isoenzyme	Inhibitor	Substrate	Effect of EM/UM on the Substrate	Effect of PM on the Substrate
CYP2D6	Diphenhydramine	Metoprolol	Increased 61%	Little change
CYP2D6	Quinidine	S-venlafaxine	Increased 4 times	Little change
CYP2D6		R-venlafaxine	Increased 12 times	No change
CYP2D6	Diphenhydramine	Venlafaxine	Increased 2 times	Little change
CYP2D6	Fluoxetine	Risperidone	Increased 4 times	Increase 1.3 times

Reprinted with permission from Lee LS, Nafziger AN, Bertino JS Jr. Evaluation of inhibitory drug interactions during drug development: Genetic polymorphisms must be considered. Clin Pharmacol Ther 2005;78:1–6.

these cases, the substrate is metabolized through a polymorphic enzyme and becomes an active metabolite and an inhibitor or inducer in a second system. Polymorphism in the first enzyme can cause the level of the inhibitor or inducer to be greater or less than expected, thus significantly changing the extent of the inhibition or induction of the second enzyme.

D. Specific pharmacogenomic drug interactions reported in the literature

1. **Omeprazole.** In one study of omeprazole activity on the inhibition of moclobemide in EMs and PMs of CYP2C19, the effect of inhibition varied according to the degree of genetic polymorphism. One would expect inhibition of the metabolism of the substrate moclobemide by the inhibitor omeprazole. But in EMs, the area under the curve (AUC) of the substrate moclobemide almost doubled, reflecting a greater effect of inhibition on moclobemide than was originally extensively metabolized. In comparison, because PMs, by definition, are already poor metabolizers of moclobemide, inhibition of the 2C19 enzyme by omeprazole did not extensively change the AUC levels of moclobemide. [SOURCE: Yu KS, Yim DS, Cho JY et al. Effect of omeprazole on the pharmacokinetics of moclobemide according to the genetic polymorphism of CYP2C19. Clin Pharmacol Ther 2001;69: 266–273.]

2. **Fluvoxamine.** Fluvoxamine inhibits the metabolism of diphenhydramine by the CYP2C19 isoenzyme. When EMs who take diphenhydramine were given the CYP2C19 inhibitor fluvoxamine, the AUC and maximal drug concentration (C_{max}) levels of diphenhydramine increased significantly over placebo. When PMs who take diphenhydramine were given the inhibitor fluvoxamine, the AUC and C_{max} of diphenhydramine did not change significantly. The effect of inhibition on the substrate in EMs of CYP2C19 was greater than it would have been in normal metabolizers. The effect of inhibition on the substrate in PMs of CYP2C19 is not significant. In addition, those EMs who were homozygous showed greater inhibition (reduction in enzyme activity) than those who were heterozygous. This demonstrates that the degree of inhibition varies by genotype. In the same way, EMs show greater inhibition than PMs because PMs already have reduced enzyme activity and thus do not show a great change in C_{max} or AUC, even with inhibition. [SOURCE: Yasui-Furukori N, Saito M, Uno T, et al. Effects of fluvoxamine on lansoprazole pharmacokinetics in relation to CYP2C19 genotypes. J Clin Pharmacol 2004;44:1223–1229.]

3. **Diphenhydramine**
   a. Diphenhydramine inhibits the metabolism of metoprolol. In EMs of CYP2D6, the C_{max} and AUC of diphenhydramine increased by 16% and 61%, respectively, compared to nonpolymorphisms. The inhibitor diphenhydramine decreased conversion of metoprolol to its metabolite by a factor of 3. In PMs, the change in metoprolol conversion was insignificant. Again, the effect of inhibition on the substrate in EMs was greater than that in PMs. [SOURCE: Hamelin BA, Bouayad A, Methot J, et al. Significant interaction between the nonprescription antihistamine diphenhydramine and the CYP2D6 substrate metoprolol in healthy men with high or low CYP2D6 activity. Clin Pharmacol Ther 2000;67:466–477.]
   b. Diphenhydramine inhibits the metabolism of venlafaxine by the CYP2D6 isoenzyme. When diphenhydramine is given to EMs who are taking venlafaxine, the levels of venlafaxine rise twofold. Diphenhydramine given to PMs who are taking venlafaxine causes insignificant change in the levels of venlafaxine. Similar to the interaction with metoprolol (see VII.D.3.a), the extent of inhibition in EMs is much greater than in PMs. [SOURCE: Lessard E, Yessine MA, Hamelin BA, et al. Diphenhydramine alters the disposition of venlafaxine through inhibition of CYP2D6 activity in humans. J Clin Psychopharmacol 2001;21:175–184.]

E. The effect of polymorphism on drug development and drug safety

1. During drug development most drug companies do not determine the genotypes of their test subjects for heterozygosity of the polychrome P450 isoenzymes. In small studies and in studies in which the test subjects are genetically homogenous, the pharmacokinetics described for the drug may be skewed toward the genotypes prevalent in the subject population. The results could be affected, for example, when the study population consists primarily of individuals of Asian descent and the focus drug is metabolized by the CYP2C19 isoenzyme. Varient CYP2C19 alleles occur in 20–25% of the Asian population.

2. When the effects of genotype on pharmacogenomics are not considered during drug development, the potential for toxicity in some populations may be missed. Some drugs have been withdrawn from the market as a result—for example, troglitazone (Rezulin) and mibefradil.

3. Pharmacogenomics testing during drug development could identify the dosing variables by genotype, leading to greater safety in the use of the drug.

4. The identification of the interaction of genotype during drug development may limit the clinical use of that drug to particular pharmacogenomic populations.

VIII. CLINICAL SIGNIFICANCE AND MANAGEMENT OF DRUG INTERACTIONS

A. Potential drug interactions

1. **Multiple-drug therapy,** including both **prescription** and **nonprescription** (OTC) medication, can potentially lead to drug interactions. The more drugs used by a patient, the greater the potential for a drug interaction.

2. **Multiple prescribers.** Patients can be seen by different prescribers who prescribe interacting medication.

3. **Patient compliance.** Patients need to follow proper instructions for taking medications. For example, a patient might take tetracycline with food rather than before meals.

4. **Patient risk factors**
   a. Older patients are at more risk for drug interactions than are younger patients.
      (1) Changes in physiological and pathophysiological conditions in older patients may lead to altered body composition, altered GI transit time and drug absorption, decreased protein binding, altered distribution, and decreased drug clearance. These changes can exacerbate or increase the risk of a drug interaction.
      (2) Older patients generally take more drugs than younger patients, which leads to a greater probability of a drug–drug interaction.
      (3) Older patients may not fully understand the appropriate directions for use of their medications and become unintentionally noncompliant.
   b. Patients with predisposing illness (diabetes, asthma, AIDS, and alcoholism) and patients who are clinically hypersensitive (atopic) are more at risk for drug interactions than nonatopic patients.
   c. Pharmacogenetic variations in enzyme function can occur at different rates in different ethnic populations and, to a lesser extent, in different geographical areas. Such pharmacogenetic factors can lead to a wide variation in the potential for a drug interaction.

B. Clinical significance

1. Not all drug interactions are clinically significant or cause an adverse effect. In some cases, interacting drugs can be prescribed for patients as long as the patient is given proper instructions and is compliant. For example, cimetidine and an antacid might be prescribed to the patient, but the patient should be instructed not to take both medications at the same time.

2. Combination drug therapy can have beneficial effects. Drug combinations are used to improve the therapeutic objective or to decrease adverse events. Some examples are the following:
   a. Trimethoprim and sulfamethoxazole—combination antibiotic for increased efficacy in urinary tract infections
   b. Amoxicillin and clavulanate potassium—combination containing a β-lactamase inhibitor (clavulanate) to inhibit the breakdown of amoxicillin
   c. Hydrochlorothiazide and triamterene—combination diuretic and antihypertensive to minimize potassium excretion

3. Some drug–food and drug–drug interactions are used for their beneficial effects.
   a. Phenytoin is given with dietary fats to increase its bioavailability through enhanced absorption.

    b. Probenecid inhibits renal tubular secretion of penicillin, thereby prolonging the plasma half-life of the antibiotic.

  4. The determination of the clinical significance of a potential drug interaction should be documented in the literature. The likelihood of a drug interaction can be classified as follows:
    a. Established—a drug interaction supported by well-proven clinical studies
    b. Probable—a drug interaction that is very likely but might not be proven clinically
    c. Suspected—a drug interaction that might occur; some data might be available
    d. Possible—a drug interaction that could occur; limited data are available
    e. Unlikely—a drug interaction that is doubtful; no good evidence of an altered clinical effect is available

  5. The clinical relevance of a potential drug interaction should also consider the following:
    a. Size of the dose and the duration of therapy
    b. Onset (rapid, delayed) and **severity** (major, moderate, minor) of the potential interaction
    c. Extrapolation to related drugs

  6. Genetic polymorphisms may affect the toxicity and the clinical efficacy of certain drugs in certain populations. Known inhibitors may pose significant risks to EMs of particular enzyme systems.

C. Management of drug interactions

  1. Review the patient profile, including drug history and patient risk factors. The patient's past medical history can reveal a tendency for noncompliance, past therapeutic failures, and evidence for pharmacogenetic considerations.

  2. Avoid complex therapeutic drug regimens.

  3. Determine the probability of a clinically significant drug interaction.

  4. Suggest a different drug if there is a high probability for a clinically significant drug interaction. For example, acetaminophen can be used for headache instead of aspirin for a patient on anticoagulant therapy.

  5. Carefully instruct the patient as to the timing of the medication. For example, an antacid and H_2-blocker should not be taken at the same time. The patient should use maximum spacing between drugs. Inform the patient about the timing of medications to be taken "on an empty stomach."

  6. Monitor the patient for adverse events. Sulfonamides, such as sulfisoxazole and sulfamethoxazole, can prolong prothrombin time in patients given warfarin therapy. The prothrombin times should be monitored in these patients.

  7. Reevaluate the patient profile and drug history when changing drug therapy. For example, when discontinuing the diuretic of a congestive heart failure patient on digoxin, a review of the profile may reveal a potassium supplement that should be discontinued as well.

  8. Evaluate the risks of drug therapy with respect to the patient's possible genotype and the status of drug metabolism. Consider risks identified with ethnic groups and geographical distribution. Test for enzyme phenotype when feasible. Select drugs and adjust doses as indicated by genetic factors and according to clinical response. Consider determining the patient's genotype when unexpected variations in clinical response are noted. Commercial DNA diagnostic chips are now available for determining CYP450 isoenzyme genotypes.

IX. REFERENCES. A vast number of drug interactions are reported in the literature. General references that are updated periodically include the following:

  A. Drug Interaction Facts. Facts and Comparisons, St. Louis, MO.

  B. Hansten PD, Horn JR, eds. Drug Interactions and Updates. Applied Therapeutics, Vancouver, WA.

C. Drug evaluations. In: DRUGDEX® System [Internet database]. Thompson Micromedex, Greenwood Village, CO.

D. Natural Medicines Comprehensive Database. www.naturaldatabase.com.

E. Cytochrome P450 drug-interaction table. Indiana University School of Medicine, Division of Clinical Pharmacology. medicine.iupui.edu/flockhart/table.htm.

F. PDR Physician's Desk Reference: PDR Guide to Drug Interactions, Side Effects and Indications. Medical Economics Data, Montvale, NJ.

G. PharmGKB: The Pharmacogenetics and Pharmacogenomics Knowledge Base. www.pharmgkb.org.

H. Zucchero FJ, Hogan MJ, Schultz CD, eds. Evaluations of Drug Interactions. Professional Drug Systems, St. Louis, MO.

STUDY QUESTIONS

Directions for questions 1–2: The questions and incomplete statements in this section can be correctly answered or completed by **one or more** of the suggested answers. Choose the answer, **A–E.**

> A   if **I only** is correct
> B   if **III only** is correct
> C   if **I and II** are correct
> D   if **II and III** are correct
> E   if **I, II, and III** are correct

1. Drug interactions may be classed as

   I. pharmacokinetic interactions.
   II. pharmacodynamic interactions.
   III. pharmaceutical interactions.

2. Situations that can potentially lead to drug interactions include

   I. multiple-drug therapy.
   II. multiple prescribers.
   III. patient compliance.

Directions for questions 3–10: Each of the questions, statements, or incomplete statements in this section can be correctly answered or completed by **one** of the suggested answers or phrases. Choose the **best** answer.

3. Which of the following statements regarding drug interactions is true?

   (A) All drug interactions can potentially cause an adverse response in the patient.
   (B) The clinical significance for each potential drug interaction must be considered individually.
   (C) A precipitant drug that inhibits the metabolism of the object drug causes a more serious drug interaction than a precipitant drug causing an increase in the bioavailability of the object drug.
   (D) If the patient is prescribed drugs that can potentially interact, the prescriber should be called and a different precipitant drug should be suggested.

4. A patient on indinavir antiretroviral therapy (ART) begins taking St. John's wort for depression and suffers unexpected reduction in CD4 count. This is most likely the result of

   (A) a pharmacodynamic interaction producing additive toxicity.
   (B) a pharmacodynamic interaction producing an antagonistic therapeutic effect.
   (C) an enzyme induction by St. John's wort causing increased metabolism of ART.
   (D) an enzyme inhibition by St. John's wort causing toxic levels of ART.

5. Which of the following is a valid therapeutic use of a drug interaction?

   (A) The use of probenecid with penicillin G to prolong high penicillin levels to treat a sexually transmitted disease.
   (B) Giving aspirin with warfarin to enhance anticoagulation.
   (C) Instructing the patient to take levofloxacin with milk or antacid to decrease GI intolerance to oral therapy.
   (D) The treatment of depression with a combination of citalopram and a monoamine oxidase inhibitor (MAOI).

6. Which of the following is *not* a harmful food–drug interaction?

   (A) Raw green salads for patients on warfarin deep vein thrombosis (DVT) prophylaxis.
   (B) Grapefruit juice and cyclosporin to prevent graft vs host rejection of a transplanted kidney.
   (C) Omeprazole beads in applesauce for a patient with problems swallowing capsules secondary to gastroesophageal reflux disease (GERD).
   (D) Milk with doxycycline to treat *Helicobacter pylori*.

7. Which of the following statements regarding pharmacogenetic polymorphisms is false?

(A) An extensive metabolizer (EM) who takes metoprolol for hypertension begins to regularly take over-the-counter (OTC) Tagamet for heartburn; the patient is at increased risk for bradycardia and cardiac arrhythmias.
(B) An EM who takes methadone begins taking Tegretol for neuropathic pain; the patient is at risk for treatment failure and pain crisis.
(C) A poor metabolizer (PM) who takes atorvastatin for hyperlipidemia is placed on ketoconazole for a fungal infection; the patient is at increased risk for myalgia and rhabdomyolysis.
(D) A PM who takes metoprolol for tachycardia begins taking Benadryl for sleep; the patient is not at risk for significant bradycardia and cardiac block.

8. Asians are at greatest risk of all ethnic groups for genetic polymorphism in which one of the following cytochrome P450 (CYP) isoenzymes?

(A) CYP2D6
(B) CYP3A4
(C) CYP2C19
(D) CYP1A2

9. Which of the following statements regarding pharmacogenetics is false?

(A) Polymorphisms occur only in the CYP450 hepatic enzymes.
(B) Polymorphisms result in many variations of the CYP450 isoenzymes.
(C) The overall expression of the combined alleles makes up the individual's phenotype in regard to the specific enzyme.
(D) Single nucleotide polymorphisms (SNPs) can occur as the result of errors of transcription, defective splicing, changes in the start and stop codons, and amino acid changes.

10. Which of the following statements regarding genetic polymorphisms is false?

(A) Wild-type alleles encode for normal metabolism.
(B) Ultrarapid metabolizers (UMs) have two or more amplified alleles.
(C) Poor metabolizers (PMs) carry one defective allele and one amplified allele.
(D) Extensive metabolizers (EMs) who are heterozygous at an isoenzyme's locus have slower metabolism than individuals who are homozygous at that locus.

ANSWERS AND EXPLANATIONS

1. The answer is E (I, II, III) *[see I.B]*.
Most drug interactions in vivo are caused by pharmacokinetic and pharmacodynamic interactions. Pharmaceutical interactions can occur during extemporaneous compounding, preparation of intravenous admixtures, and improper dosing, as in the case of giving aspirin with acidic juices (e.g., orange, cranberry).

2. The answer is E (I, II, III) *[see IV.A.1–3]*.
Patient profiles might not contain all the drug history information of the patient. Patients who take nonprescription (OTC) medications, go to several different physicians, or purchase drugs at more than one pharmacy may neglect to inform their physician(s) and pharmacist(s) of all the medications they take.

3. The answer is B *[see IV.B]*.
Not all drug interactions are clinically significant. Some potential clinically significant drug interactions can be prevented by proper patient instruction and compliance. The potential for a clinically significant drug interaction should be documented before calling a physician concerning the prescribed medication.

4. The answer is C *[see II.C.1.c; Table 18-3]*.
St. John's wort induces CYP3A4 isoenzymes, increasing the metabolism of the indinavir and resulting in low indinavir levels and therapeutic failure of ART. St. John's wort itself has no direct effect on CD4.

5. The answer is A *[see II.C.2; Table 18-4]*.
Probenecid is given with penicillin and some cephalosporins for the treatment of some sexually transmitted diseases. Probenecid competes with penicillins for renal elimination, prolonging the half-life of the penicillin. Aspirin and warfarin cause additive anticoagulation, leading to bleeding. Levofloxacin taken with milk to decrease GI irritation causes complexation of the levofloxacin with the calcium in the milk, resulting in decreased levofloxacin availability. Concomitant treatment of depression of citalopram and MAOI results in serotonin syndrome, an additive toxicity.

6. The answer is C *[see V.B]*.
Omeprazole beads are enteric coated. Giving an enteric-coated bead with an acidic food, such as applesauce, preserves the enteric coating and allows the drug to pass intact through the acidic stomach environment and into the basic duodenum environment where it is absorbed. The result is improved drug absorption and decreased drug destruction in the acidic stomach.

7. The answer is C *[see VII.C.2]*.
The PM already has inhibited metabolism of atorvastatin; thus additional inhibition will not significantly increase the blood levels of atorvastatin. Therefore dose-related toxicity is unlikely. The EM who takes metoprolol and Tagamet (cimetidine) will show a greater increase in the metoprolol levels owing to the exaggerated effect of the inhibitor. The EM who takes methadone and Tegretol (carbamazepine) will have increased enzyme induction and metabolism of the methadone, lowering methadone levels and putting the patient at risk for treatment failure for the pain. The PM who takes metoprolol and Benadryl (diphenhydramine) will show inhibition of the metabolism of the metoprolol and increased levels of metoprolol, leading to a higher risk of bradycardia and cardiac block.

8. The answer is A *[see VII.A.3]*.
Polymorphism is highest in the CYP2D6 isoenzyme in Asians; the incidence is > 50%.

9. The answer is A *[see VII.A.2]*.
Polymorphisms can occur in any genetic system, including the mixed oxidase and N-acetyltransferase systems as well as the CYP450 hepatic enzyme system.

10. The answer is C *[see VII.B.3]*.
PMs carry one normal allele and one defective or deleted allele.

19
Nuclear Pharmacy

Stephen C. Dragotakes

Jeffrey P. Norenberg

I. INTRODUCTION

A. Overview

1. **Nuclear pharmacy** is defined as a "patient-oriented service that embodies the scientific knowledge and professional judgment required to improve and promote health through the safe and efficacious use of radioactive drugs for diagnosis and therapy."[1]

2. **Radiopharmaceuticals** are drug products that contain a biological moiety and a radioactive element. The biological construct targets a physiological or pathophysiological process of interest, allowing the localization of radiation that, in turn, may be imaged or used to effect therapy. Most radiopharmaceuticals are used in diagnostic medical imaging; however, they are also used in therapeutic applications, such as in the treatment of hyperthyroidism, thyroid cancer, polycythemia vera, and in the alleviation of bone pain.

3. **Nuclear pharmacy practice** entails the:
   a. Procurement of radiopharmaceuticals
   b. Compounding of radiopharmaceuticals
   c. Performance of routine quality control procedures
   d. Dispensing of radiopharmaceuticals
   e. Distribution of radiopharmaceuticals
   f. Implementation of basic radiation protection procedures and practices
   g. Consultation with and/or education of the nuclear medicine community, patients, pharmacists, other health professionals, and the general public regarding
      (1) Physical and chemical properties of radiopharmaceuticals
      (2) Pharmacokinetics and biodistribution of radiopharmaceuticals
      (3) Drug interactions and other factors that alter patterns of distribution
   h. Monitoring of patient outcomes
   i. Research and development of radiopharmaceuticals

B. Properties of radiopharmaceuticals

1. **Pharmacological effects.** Typically, radiopharmaceuticals lack pharmacological effects because the mass quantities range from picogram (pg) to nanogram (ng) per kilogram (kg) of administered dose.

2. **Route of administration.** Most radiopharmaceuticals are prepared as sterile, pyrogen-free intravenous (IV) solutions or suspensions to be administered directly to the patient. Other routes of administration include intradermal, oral, interstitial, and inhalation (e.g., radioactive gases, aerosols).

3. **Radionuclides**
   a. The radioactive component of a radiopharmaceutical is referred to as a radionuclide. Nuclides are identified as atoms having a specific number of protons and neutrons in the nucleus. A nuclide is typically identified by the chemical symbol of the element with a mass number shown as a superscript, indicating the sum of protons and neutrons (e.g., iodide-131 is indicated as ^{131}I). When the atom is radioactive, it is called a radionuclide.
   b. Radionuclides undergo spontaneous radioactive decay accompanied by the release of energy. The distribution, metabolism, and elimination of the radiopharmaceutical can

---

[1]American Pharmaceutical Association. Nuclear Pharmacy Practice Guidelines. Academy of Pharmacy Practice, 1995.

be determined by measuring this energy with imaging equipment. There are four major types of radiation emitted through this process: α-, β-, γ-, and x-rays. α- and β-radiations are not useful in medical imaging and are, therefore, undesirable in diagnostic applications. Most diagnostic radiopharmaceuticals use penetrating γ-radiation, which can be easily detected and converted into imaging data.

4. **Half-lives of radiopharmaceuticals**
   a. The **physical half-life** of a radiopharmaceutical is the amount of time necessary for the radioactive atoms to decay to one half their original number. Each radionuclide is characterized by a specific half-life that is a physical constant.
   b. The **biological half-life** of a radiopharmaceutical is the amount of time required for the body to metabolize or eliminate one half of the administered dose of any substance through biological processes.
   c. The **effective half-life** of a radiopharmaceutical is the time required for an administered radiopharmaceutical dose to be reduced by one half as a result of both physical decay and biological mechanisms. It is defined as:

$$T_e = T_p + (T_b/T_p) \times T_b$$

   where T_e is the effective half-life, T_p is the physical half-life, and T_b is the biological half-life.

C. **Optimal radiopharmaceuticals**

1. **Optimal diagnostic radiopharmaceuticals**
   a. Should contain a radionuclide with a half-life short enough to minimize radiation exposure to the patient, yet long enough to allow for collection of imaging information. The optimal relationship is a physical half-life equal to approximately 67% of the biological process of interest.
   b. Should incorporate a γ-emitting radionuclide, which decays with the emission of a photon energy between 100 and 300 kiloelectron volts (keV), which is efficiently detected with current instrumentation
   c. Should contain a biological component that allows rapid localization in the organ system of interest and be metabolized or excreted from the nontarget tissues to maximize contrast and minimize the radiation absorbed dose to nontarget organs
   d. Should be readily available and cost-effective

2. **Optimal therapeutic radiopharmaceuticals,** in addition to I.C.1.c–d, should contain α- or β-emitting radionuclides that can effectively deliver radiation in quantities sufficient to cause the desired therapeutic effect. Such effects include apoptosis, DNA damage, or irreparable cell damage leading to tissue effects.

II. SODIUM PERTECHNETATE ^{99m}TC GENERATOR

A. **Overview**

1. ^{99m}Tc, the most commonly used radionuclide in diagnostic imaging today, is produced by the radioactive decay of molybdenum-99 (^{99}Mo).
   a. ^{99m}Tc is obtained via commercially supplied, sterile, pyrogen-free generator systems. A generator is a device used to separate a short half-life radionuclide from the longer-lived parent nuclide while retaining the parent to produce more of the daughter nuclide. In this way, short half-life nuclides can be made available continuously at great distances from the sites of generator production.
   b. All of the commercially supplied generators currently use ^{99}Mo obtained from the fission of uranium-235 (^{235}U). This ^{99}Mo parent is absorbed on an alumina ion (Al_2O_3) exchange column, and the ^{99m}Tc formed from its decay is exchanged for the chloride ion (Cl^-) available in the 0.9% saline eluate solution washed through the column, as the sodium pertechnetate $Na^+(^{99m}TcO_4)^-$ form.

2. The chemical valence state of $Na^+(^{99m}TcO_4)^-$ as it is eluted from the column is +7. Typically, it must be reduced to a lower valence state before it is able to react with other compounds. Although many processes can reduce ^{99m}Tc, the stannous ion (Sn^{++}) reduction method is most commonly used in ^{99m}Tc radiopharmaceutical kits.

a. A radiopharmaceutical kit consists of sterile, pyrogen-free vials containing a reducing agent, the biological compound to be labeled, and any additional adjutants necessary to effect the reaction or to stabilize the labeled product.
b. In most cases, they are lyophilized under inert atmospheres, so as to minimize oxidation of the reducing agent (e.g., Sn^{++}).

B. **Sodium pertechnetate ^{99m}Tc** *USP* (*United States Pharmacopeia*; **$Na^{+99m}TcO_4^-$**) as eluted from a generator in 0.9% sodium chloride (NaCl) solution is an isotonic, sterile, nonpyrogenic, diagnostic radiopharmaceutical suitable for IV injection, oral administration, and direct instillation.

1. **Physical properties**
   a. The solution should be clear, colorless, and free of visible foreign material. The pH is 4.5–7.0.
   b. $Na^{+99m}TcO_4^-$ is itself a radiopharmaceutical, or it may be used to radiolabel all other ^{99m}Tc radiopharmaceuticals.

2. **Biodistribution**
   a. $^{99m}TcO_4^-$ is handled by the body in a fashion similar to ^{131}I—that is, it is taken up and released but not organified by the thyroid.
   b. After IV administration, $^{99m}TcO_4^-$ concentrates in the choroid plexus, thyroid gland, salivary gland, and stomach, but remains in the circulation long enough for first-pass blood-pool studies, organ perfusion, and major vessel studies.
   c. It is primarily excreted by the kidneys unchanged and is expressed in the urine 15–50% by 24 hr.
   d. Between 10 and 55% of the administered dose is eliminated via feces within 3 days.

3. **Decay data**
   a. ^{99m}Tc decays by isomeric transition with a physical half-life of 6 hr.
   b. The primary radiation emissions are 140 keV γ energy photons.

4. **Purity**
   a. *USP* radionuclidic purity requires a ^{99}Mo breakthrough limit of < 0.15 μCi/mCi of ^{99m}Tc at the time of patient administration.
   b. *USP* chemical purity requires an aluminum ion (Al^{+3}) test result of less than 10 μg/mL.

5. **Administration and dosage.** All of the following imaging studies are administered via IV, except nasolacrimal imaging, which is instilled into the lacrimal canal.
   a. Brain imaging: 10–20 mCi (370–740 megabecquerels; MBq)
   b. Thyroid imaging: 1–10 mCi (37–370 MBq)
   c. Salivary gland imaging: 1–5 mCi (37–185 MBq)
   d. Placenta localization: 1–3 mCi (37–111 MBq)
   e. Blood-pool imaging: 10–30 mCi (370–740 MBq)
   f. Urinary bladder imaging: 0.5–1 mCi (18–37 MBq)
   g. Nasolacrimal imaging: < 100 μCi (< 3.7 MBq)

III. RADIOPHARMACEUTICALS FOR CARDIOVASCULAR IMAGING

A. **Perfusion agents for cardiac imaging.** Radiopharmaceuticals are useful in cardiac imaging as agents that provide information on the regional myocardial blood perfusion. They typically are administered as part of a cardiac stress test so as to provide information at peak cardiac output. The patient will run on a treadmill to "stress" the heart. IV coronary vessel dilating agents are used in place of the treadmill when the patient is not physically able to exercise. Examples of these pharmacological agents are dipyridamole, adenosine, and dobutamine. The patient will also be imaged when the heart is at "rest."

1. **Thallous chloride thallium-201 (^{201}Tl)** is a radionuclide that is produced by a cyclotron. It is used for myocardial perfusion imaging in the diagnosis of coronary artery disease and localization of myocardial infarction.

a. Biodistribution

   (1) ^{201}Tl is a monovalent cation with distribution analogous to a potassium ion (K^+); myocardial uptake is by active transport via the Na^+/K^+-adenosine triphosphatase (ATPase) pump.

   (2) Biodistribution is generally proportional to organ blood flow at the time of injection, with blood clearance by myocardium, kidneys, thyroid, liver, and stomach. The remainder is distributed uniformly throughout the rest of the body.

   (3) ^{201}Tl is excreted slowly and equally in both urine and feces.

b. Decay data

   (1) Physical half-life: 73 hr

   (2) Effective half-life: 2.4 days

   (3) Biological half-life: 11 days

   (4) Primary radiation emissions: 68–80 keV x-rays and 167 and 135 keV γ energy photons.

c. Administration and dosage. IV, 2–4 mCi (74–148 MBq)

2. ^{99m}Tc sestamibi (^{99m}Tc-MIBI) exists as a sterile, pyrogen-free IV injection after kit reconstitution with $Na^{+99m}TcO_4^-$ and heating at 100°C for 10 min.

a. Biodistribution

   (1) ^{99m}Tc sestamibi is a cation complex that has been found to accumulate in viable myocardium by passive diffusion into the myocyte with subsequent binding to the mitochondria within the cell.

   (2) The major pathway for clearance of ^{99m}Tc sestamibi is the hepatobiliary system. This agent is excreted without any evidence of metabolism via urine and feces.

b. Decay data

   (1) Effective half-life: 3 hr (myocardium)

   (2) Biological half-life: 6 hr (myocardium)

c. Administration and dosage. IV, 10–30 mCi (370–1110 MBq)

3. ^{99m}Tc tetrofosmin exists as a sterile and pyrogen-free IV injection after kit reconstitution with sodium pertechnetate ^{99m}Tc injection *USP*.

a. Description. ^{99m}Tc tetrofosmin is a lipophilic, cationic ^{99m}Tc complex that has been found to accumulate in viable myocardium.

b. Biodistribution. The major pathways for clearance of ^{99m}Tc tetrofosmin are the renal system and the hepatobiliary system with 26% of the administered dose excreted in the feces and 40% excreted in the urine within 48 hr.

c. Physical properties. See II.A; II.B.3.

d. Administration and dosage. IV during exercise, 5–8 mCi (185–296 MBq); during rest, 15–24 mCi (555–1443 MBq)

4. ^{99m}Tc teboroxime. No longer available

5. Rubidium-82 (^{82}Rb) chloride is a generator-produced radiopharmaceutical obtained by the decay of its accelerator-produced parent strontium (^{82}Sr; half-life is 25 days) adsorbed on a stannous oxide column.

a. Biodistribution

   (1) When eluted with 0.9% NaCl at a rate of 50 mL/min, a solution of the short-lived daughter ^{82}Rb is eluted from the generator for direct IV administration.

   (2) After IV administration, ^{82}Rb rapidly clears from the blood and is extracted by the myocardial tissue in a manner analogous to K^+.

   (3) Myocardial activity is visualized within 1 min after administration.

b. Decay data

   (1) Physical half-life: 75 sec.

   (2) The **decay mode** is by positron emission.

   (3) The **primary radiation emissions** are annihilation 511 keV γ energy photons.

   (4) Parent ^{82}Sr and contaminant ^{85}Sr breakthrough must be closely monitored. Acceptable levels of strontium breakthrough are < 0.02 μCi ^{82}Sr/mCi ^{82}Rb and < 0.2 μCi ^{85}Sr/mCi ^{82}Rb.

c. Administration and dosage. IV, 30–60 mCi (1110–2220 MBq)

6. Ammonia ^{13}N exists under a USP monograph as an on site cyclotron produced, sterile IV solution of $^{13}NH_3$, useful as a myocardial perfusion agent.

  a. **Decay data**
    (1) **Physical half-life:** 10 min.
    (2) **Decay mode:** positron emission resulting in the production of two 511 keV annihilation γ photons.
  b. **Biodistribution**
    (1) After IV injection, it circulates as $^{13}NH_3$ but localizes into the myocytes via diffusion as $^{13}NH_3$. It is then metabolized to glutamine and retained by the myocytes.
    (2) After IV injection, it is cleared rapidly from the blood; < 2% of the administered dose remains after 5 min postinjection.
    (3) It is predominantly metabolized to ^{13}N-glutamine by different organs of the body.
    (4) Between 10% and 20% is excreted via the renal system.
  c. **Administration and dosage.** IV, 15–20 mCi (555–740 MBq)

B. Agents used to measure cardiac function. Regional myocardial wall motion

  1. **^{99m}Tc-labeled red blood cells (^{99m}Tc-RBCs)** are used for blood-pool imaging, including cardiac first-pass and gated equilibrium imaging (regional cardiac wall motion).
    a. **Physical properties.** Autologous RBCs can be labeled by a number of techniques that use the Sn^{++} radiolabeling method with three general steps.
      (1) The cells are treated with Sn^{++} to provide an intracellular source of the reducing agent. This step can be carried out with either in vivo or in vitro labeling procedures.
      (2) The next step is the removal of excess Sn^{++} either by chemical oxidation (in vitro method) or by biological clearance (in vivo method).
      (3) All of the methods include the addition of sodium pertechnetate ($^{99m}TcO_4^-$). This ^{99m}Tc, while in the +7 valence state, crosses the intact erythrocyte membrane and binds to intracellular hemoglobin (Hb) after being reduced by the available intracellular Sn^{++}.
    b. **Biodistribution.** After IV injection, the labeling RBCs distribute within the blood pool and are well maintained in the blood pool with a bi-exponential whole body clearance of 2.5–2.7 hr and 75–176 hr (e.g., major route of excretion is via the urine).
    c. **Administration and dosage.** IV, 10–20 mCi (370–740 MBq)

  2. **Pyrophosphate injection *USP* and phosphates *USP*.** The major use for these agents in nuclear medicine is as convenient and stable sources of Sn^{++} for the labeling of autologous RBCs. In this application, the kits are reconstituted with normal saline and injected via IV.

  3. **^{99m}Tc albumin (^{99m}Tc-HSA) injection**
    a. **Biodistribution**
      (1) ^{99m}Tc albumin distributes initially within the intravascular space and leaves this space at a rate slow enough to permit imaging of the blood pool.
      (2) Plasma clearance is bi-exponential: a fast component clearing with a half-life of 2 hr and a slow component clearing with a half-life of 10–16 hr.
      (3) The major route of elimination is via the urine.
    b. **Administration and dosage.** IV, 20 mCi (740 MBq)

C. Agents for imaging myocardial infarction include pyrophosphate injection *USP* and phosphates *USP*.

  1. **Mechanism of localization.** The skeletal localizing radiopharmaceutical pyrophosphate has been shown to accumulate also in zones of myocardial infarction. This localization is thought to be the result of binding of the pyrophosphate to microcalcification with hydroxyapatite crystals found in infarcted tissue.

  2. **Biodistribution** of labeled pyrophosphate depends on the ability of phosphates to become involved with calcium ion (Ca^{++}) deposition in necrotic cardiac tissue.

IV. SKELETAL IMAGING

A. Skeletal-imaging agents

  1. **Overview.** ^{99m}Tc-labeled bone agents are useful in the detection of bone lesions that are associated with metastatic neoplasms, metabolic disorders, and infections of the bone. The imaging advantages of ^{99m}Tc, coupled with the sensitivity of bone agent localization in

skeletal bone hydroxyapatite, allows for detection of bone pathology before evidence is shown by conventional x-rays.

2. **^{99m}Tc bone agents.** There are many different forms of ^{99m}Tc bone agents, with minor differences in their individual chemical structure. Currently used bone-imaging agents are based on either the P—C—P diphosphonate structure, including ^{99m}medronate disodium and ^{99m}Tc oxidronate, or the inorganic P—O—P phosphate structure, such as ^{99m}Tc pyrophosphate. These bone agents are S^{++} reduction method kits, which exist as sterile, pyrogen-free IV radiopharmaceuticals after reconstitution with $Na^{+99m}TcO_4^-$.

   a. **Physical properties**
      (1) All of the ^{99m}Tc bone-imaging agents are susceptible to radiological decomposition with reoxidation of the ^{99m}Tc to a higher valence state. These agents sometimes include antioxidants (e.g., ascorbic or gentisic acid) in their formulation to improve their in vitro stability.
      (2) They should be stored at room temperature before and after reconstitution.
   b. **Biodistribution**
      (1) It is believed that the localization of the diphosphonates occurs by chemisorption onto the hydroxyapatite mineral matrix of skeletal bone with uptake related to bone metabolic activity and bone blood flow.
      (2) For ^{99m}Tc medronate disodium and ^{99m}Tc oxidronate, approximately 50% of the administered dose localizes in the skeleton, and 50% is excreted by the kidneys within the first 4–6 hr after IV injection.
   c. **Administration and dosage.** IV, 10–20 mCi (370–740 MBq)

B. **Bone marrow imaging.** See VI.A.1; VI.A.3; VI.B.

V. **LUNG IMAGING.** Radiopharmaceuticals are used to evaluate both pulmonary perfusion and pulmonary ventilation, to detect pulmonary embolism and to assess pulmonary function before pneumonectomy.

A. **Pulmonary perfusion imaging**

   1. **^{99m}Tc albumin (^{99m}Tc-MAA)**
      a. **Physical properties**
         (1) The ^{99m}Tc albumin aggregated kit contains HSA albumin that has been aggregated by heat denaturation.
         (2) This Sn^{++} reduction method kit exists as a sterile, pyrogen-free suspension of radiolabeled aggregated particles after reconstitution with $Na^{+99m}TcO_4^-$.
         (3) It should be stored at 2°–8°C after reconstitution.
      b. **Biodistribution**
         (1) After IV administration of ^{99m}Tc albumin aggregated, 80% of the radiolabeled albumin particles become trapped by capillary blockade in the pulmonary circulation.
         (2) After trapping, the particles are cleared from the lungs mainly by mechanical breakup. These smaller particles are ultimately cleared from the circulation by the reticuloendothelial system.
         (3) Particle size should be controlled—that is, 90% of the particles should be between 10 and 90 μm, and none should be > 150 μm, to ensure adequate trapping by the lung capillary bed but no occlusion of the large-bore vessels.
         (4) Particle number should be between 200,000 and 700,000 particles per adult dose to obtain uniform imaging data without compromising capillary blood flow. Neonates should receive < 125,000 particles.
      c. **Decay data.** Biological half-life in the lung: 2–3 hr
      d. **Administration and dosage.** IV, 1–4 mCi (37–148 MBq)

B. **Pulmonary ventilation imaging** with radioactive gases is a routine nuclear medicine procedure that can provide valuable information about regional lung ventilation. Radiopharmaceuticals used are either radioactive gases or radioaerosols.

   1. **Xenon-133 (^{133}Xe)** is supplied as a radioactive gas contained in glass septum vials to be administered by inhalation through a closed respiratory system or a spirometer. It is a byproduct of ^{235}U fission.

   a. Biodistribution
   (1) ^{133}Xe is a readily diffusible gas, which is neither used nor produced by the body. It passes through membranes and freely exchanges between blood and tissue, tending to concentrate more in body fat.
   (2) Inhaled ^{133}Xe distributes within the alveoli and enters the pulmonary venous circulation via the capillaries; most of the absorbed ^{133}Xe ia returned and exhaled from the lungs after a single pass through the peripheral circulation.
   (3) In concentrations used for diagnosis, the gas is physiologically inactive.
   b. Decay data
   (1) Effective half-life in the lung: 2 min
   (2) Physical half-life: 5.2 days.
   (3) Decay mode: β minus and γ decay.
   (4) Primary radiation emissions: 100 keV β energy and 81 keV γ energy photons.
   c. Administration and dosage. Inhalation, 2–30 mCi (74–1110 MBq)

2. **Xenon-127 (^{127}Xe)** is supplied as a radioactive gas contained in glass septum vials to be administered by inhalation through a closed respiratory system or a spirometer. It is produced by a cyclotron.
   a. Biodistribution. Localization is the same as ^{133}Xe.
   b. Decay data
   (1) Physical half-life: 36.4 days
   (2) Decay mode: by electron capture
   (3) Primary radiation emissions: 203 keV, 190 keV, 172 keV, and 375 keV γ energy photons.
   c. Administration and dosage. Inhalation, 5–10 mCi (185–370 MBq)

3. **Radioaerosols** have become increasingly used with the advent of nebulizers that produce particles of a consistent size necessary for uniform lung distribution.
   a. Biodistribution
   (1) ^{99m}Tc pentetate (DTPA) radioaerosols of approximately 0.25 μm mass median aerodynamic diameter are useful in determining lung ventilation.
   (2) After deposition of the nebulized droplets within the airways, the ^{99m}Tc pentetate is absorbed into the pulmonary circulation.
   (3) The material is subsequently excreted by the kidneys. Clearance from the lungs is sufficiently slow to allow for imaging of the lungs in multiple projections from a single administration.
   b. Physical properties. See II.B.3.
   c. Administration and dosage. Inhalation, 30 μCi (1110 MBq)

VI. HEPATIC IMAGING

A. **Overview.** Hepatic imaging requires the use of two different classes of radiopharmaceuticals to evaluate the two cell types responsible for hepatic function.

1. **Reticuloendothelial system imaging.** The liver, spleen, and bone marrow are evaluated with radiolabeled colloidal material, ranging in size from 0.1 to 3.0 μm. These particles are rapidly cleared from the blood by phagocytosis by the Kupffer cells or trapped in the space of Disse, which is found between the polygonal hepatocytes and the Kupffer cells.

2. **Liver spleen imaging.** Radiopharmaceuticals are useful in imaging space-occupying primary tumors and metastatic neoplasms as well as hepatic defects caused by abscesses, cysts, and trauma.

3. **Bone marrow imaging.** Images that localize in the bone marrow are useful in the evaluation of pathologies that affect bone marrow.

4. **Hepatobiliary imaging.** Hepatocyte function can be evaluated by substances meeting requirements of molecular weight, lipophilicity, and chemical structure, to be excreted by the polygonal cells into the hepatobiliary system. Hepatobiliary-imaging radiopharmaceuticals are useful in the diagnosis of cystic duct obstruction in acute cholecystitis as well as defining postcholecystectomy anatomy and physiology.

B. Reticuloendothelial-imaging agents

1. **^{99m}Tc sulfur colloid (^{99m}Tc$_2$S$_7$)** is a sterile, pyrogen-free IV radiopharmaceutical formed via a chemical reaction between ^{99m}TcO$_4^-$ and an acidified solution of sodium thiosulfate at 100°C.

   a. **Physical properties**

      (1) Tc$_2$S$_7$ is thought to remain in the +7 valence state as the heptasulfide coprecipitate of elemental sulfur that occurs during the reaction.

      (2) The use of Na^{+99m}TcO$_4^-$ with Al^{+3} levels > 10 μg/mL can lead to the formation of particles > 5 μm, which can result in lung uptake.

      (3) Heating times should be controlled to preclude large particle formation.

   b. **Biodistribution.** After administration, 80%–90% of the dose is phagocytized by the Kupffer cells of the liver or trapped in the space of Disse, 5%–10% by the spleen, and the balance by the bone marrow. The blood clearance half-life is approximately 2.5 min. Particles are not metabolized and reside in the reticuloendothelial system for a prolonged period.

   c. **Administration and dosage.** IV, liver/spleen: 1–8 mCi (37–296 MBq); bone marrow: 3–12 mCi (111–444 MBq)

C. Hepatobiliary-imaging agents

1. **Overview**

   a. **Iminodiacetic acid (IDA) derivatives,** which are lidocaine analogs, are useful as hepatobiliary-imaging agents because of their lipophilicity, which allows them to be selectively cleared by carrier-mediated hepatocyte metabolic pathways. Because these agents share the same excretion pathway as bilirubin, patients who have increased bilirubin levels exhibit decreased hepatic clearance and an increased renal clearance. Lack of gallbladder visualization is an abnormal finding, suggesting acute cholecystitis.

   b. **Cholecystokinetic agents,** such as sincalide and cholecystokinin, may be used to empty the contents of the gallbladder in fasting patients before injection of IDA compounds in an attempt to promote gallbladder filling and visualization. These agents can also be injected after the injection of the IDA compound to cause a visualized gallbladder to empty. Cholecystokinetic agents are used to increase the specificity and sensitivity of the imaging procedure.

   c. **Narcotic analgesics,** such as morphine, have been used to constrict the sphincter of Oddi to produce increased intraductal pressures to promote retrograde gallbladder filling.

2. **^{99m}Tc disofenin (^{99m}Tc-DISIDA)**

   a. **Physical properties.** See II.B.3.

   b. **Biodistribution**

      (1) ^{99m}Tc-DISIDA is rapidly cleared from the blood; 8% remains in the blood after 30 min.

      (2) Approximately 9% of the administered activity is excreted in the urine during the first 2 hr. The remainder of the activity is cleared through the hepatobiliary system.

      (3) Peak liver uptake is within 10 min; peak gallbladder uptake is by 30–40 min.

      (4) Gallbladder and intestinal visualization occurs within 60 min postadministration.

   c. **Administration and dosage.** IV, nonjaundiced patient: 1–5 mCi (37–185 MBq); IV, jaundiced patient: 3–8 mCi (111–296 MBq)

3. **^{99m}Tc lidofenin (^{99m}Tc-HIDA).** No longer commercially available

4. **^{99m}Tc mebrofenin**

   a. **Physical properties.** See II.B.3.

   b. **Biodistribution**

      (1) ^{99m}Tc mebrofenin is rapidly cleared from the blood; 17% remains after 10 min. Only 1% of the administered activity is excreted in the urine within the first hours; the remainder of the activity clears through the hepatobiliary system.

      (2) Peak liver uptake occurs within 10 min; visualization of the hepatic duct and gallbladder, within 10–15 min; then intestinal activity, within 30–60 min.

   c. **Administration and dosage.** IV, nonjaundiced patient: 2–5 mCi (74–185 MBq); IV, jaundiced patient: 3–10 mCi (111–370 MBq)

VII. RENAL IMAGING

A. Overview

1. Radiopharmaceuticals are used in renal imaging to determine renal function, renal vascular flow, and renal morphology. They are also useful for the evaluation of renal function in posttransplant patients for complications such as obstruction, infarction, leakage, tubular necrosis, and rejection.

2. The use of radiopharmaceuticals to determine renal function or renal morphology is based on the two physiological mechanisms responsible for excretion: glomerular filtration and tubular secretion.

B. Agents cleared by glomerular filtration are useful in determining the glomerular filtration rate (GFR), renal artery perfusion, and the visualization of the collecting system.

1. **^{99m}Tc pentetate (^{99m}Tc-DTPA)**
   a. **Physical properties.** See II.B.3.
   b. **Biodistribution**
      (1) After administration, ^{99m}Tc pentetate rapidly distributes throughout extracellular fluid space, from which it is rapidly cleared by glomerular filtration only.
      (2) Up to 10% may be protein bound, leading to a decrease in measured GFR.
      (3) After administration, 50% of the dose is cleared by the kidneys within 2 hr, and up to 95% is cleared by 24 hr.
   c. **Administration and dosage.** IV, 10–20 mCi (370–740 MBq)

2. **Sodium iothalamate iodine-125 (^{125}I) injection** is a commercially supplied, sterile, pyrogen-free injection containing 1 mg sodium iothalamate per milliliter.
   a. **Biodistribution**
      (1) Sodium iothalamate ^{125}I is used for determination of the GFR but not for imaging because of poor imaging emissions of ^{125}I.
      (2) Thyroid blockade with oral potassium iodide (KI) is suggested.
   b. **Decay data**
      (1) **Physical half-life:** 59 days
      (2) **Decay mode:** by electron capture
      (3) **Primary radiation emissions:** 35 keV γ energy photons and x-rays.
   c. **Administration and dosage.** IV, 10–50 μCi (3.7–18.5 MBq)

C. Tubular secretion agents are used to evaluate renal tubular function and measure effective renal plasma flow.

1. **Iodohippurate iodine-131 (^{131}I) hippuran.** No longer commercially available

2. **^{99m}Tc mertiatide (^{99m}Tc-MAG3)**
   a. **Description**
      (1) Supplied as a sterile, pyrogen-free, lyophilized kit containing betiatide, precursor of mertiatide, and chelation adjutants.
      (2) After the sodium pertechnetate is added to the kit, it must be heated in a hot water bath or heating block at 100°C for 10 min to form ^{99m}Tc mertiatide from the betiatide precursor.
   b. **Biodistribution**
      (1) Mertiatide is renally excreted, 90% of the administered dose is excreted within 3 hr postinjection.
      (2) It is primarily cleared via active tubular secretion and to a small extent via glomerular filtration.
   c. **Physical properties.** See II.B.3.
   d. **Administration and dosage.** IV, 5–10 mCi (185–370 MBq)

D. Renal cortical imaging agents are used to evaluate renal anatomy because of their ability to accumulate in the kidney and provide anatomical imaging data.

1. **^{99m}Tc gluceptate (^{99m}Tc-GLH)**
   a. **Physical properties.** See II.B.3.
   b. **Biodistribution**

(1) ^{99m}Tc-GLH rapidly distributes throughout the body, with rapid blood clearance via glomerular filtration and tubular secretion and reabsorption.

(2) Approximately 25% of the administered dose is excreted within the first hour; 65%, within 6 hr; and 70%, within 24 hr.

(3) After 3–6 hr, a maximum of 5%–15% of the dose administered is concentrated in the proximal renal tubular cells of the renal cortex.

c. **Administration and dosage.** IV, 10–20 mCi (370–740 MBq)

2. ^{99m}**Tc succimer (^{99m}Tc-DMSA)**

a. **Physical properties**

(1) See II.B.3.

(2) ^{99m}Tc succimer complex must be allowed to incubate for 10 min postreconstitution and must be used within 4 hr postincubation.

b. **Biodistribution**

(1) Within 3–6 hr postadministration, 40%–50% of the dose localizes in the renal cortex, where it is taken up by the tubular cells.

(2) Excretion into the urine is slow; 5%–20% is excreted within the first 2 hr, 10%–30% by 6 hr, and < 40% by 24 hr.

c. **Administration and dosage.** IV, 2–6 mCi (74–222 MBq)

VIII. THYROID IMAGING

A. Overview

1. The basic function of the thyroid gland is the production of thyroid hormone for the regulation of metabolism. The thyroid hormones are produced within the gland through the organification of iodine obtained from the oxidation of available iodide circulating in the blood. The inability of the body to distinguish between the isotopes of iodine provides a perfect metabolic tracer for the thyroid biochemical system.

2. The function of the thyroid gland can be evaluated by the uptake of ^{131}I or ^{123}I, allowing the detection of hypothyroidism with decreased uptake and hyperthyroidism with increased uptake.

3. ^{99m}TcO$_4$$^-$ is a monovalent anion with an ionic radius similar to iodide. As a result, the pertechnetate ion is trapped by the thyroid gland in a fashion similar to iodide. The two species are sufficiently different in that ^{99m}TcO$_4$$^-$ is not organified no incorporated into thyroid hormone, and it is subsequently released unchanged.

B. Thyroid imaging agents

1. **Sodium iodide iodine-123 (^{123}I)** is a radiopharmaceutical available in either solution or capsule form for oral administration. It is produced by a cyclotron.

a. **Biodistribution**

(1) Orally administered iodine is rapidly absorbed from the gastrointestinal (GI) tract; thyroid gland uptake is evident within minutes.

(2) Sodium iodide ^{123}I is considered an ideal radiopharmaceutical for iodine uptake and imaging studies because of its short half-life and useful 159 keV primary γ emissions.

b. **Decay data**

(1) **Physical half-life:** 13.2 hr

(2) **Biological half-life:** 3.5 days

(3) **Decay mode:** by electron capture

(4) **Primary radiation emissions:** 159 keV, 27 keV, and 529 keV γ energy photons

c. **Administration and dosage.** Oral thyroid uptake: 100–200 μCi (3.7–7.4 MBq); thyroid image: 100–500 μCi (3.7–18.5 MBq)

2. **Sodium iodide ^{131}I** is used for thyroid uptake and imaging studies; however, it is now used less often because of the high radiation dose absorbed.

a. **Biodistribution**

(1) Orally administered iodine is rapidly absorbed from the GI tract; with thyroid gland uptake is within minutes.

(2) Sodium iodide ^{131}I is not considered an ideal radioiodine radiopharmaceutical for iodine uptake and imaging studies because of its long half-life, poor imaging properties, and the high radiation dose to the thyroid from its β decay component.
(3) The radiation dose from the high-energy β particle with the imaging potential of its γ emissions make this radionuclide the agent of choice for therapeutic treatment of hyperthyroidism and thyroid cancer.
b. Decay data
  (1) Physical half-life: 8.08 days
  (2) Decay mode: by β decay
  (3) Primary radiation emissions: 606 keV and 333 keV β energy; 364 keV, 637 keV, and 284 keV γ energy photons.
c. Administration and dosage. ^{131}I is available as either a capsule or in solution for oral administration.
  (1) Diagnostics
    (a) Thyroid uptake: 2–15 μCi (0.074–0.555 MBq)
    (b) Thyroid image: 30–50 μCi (1.11–1.85 MBq)
    (c) Whole body image: 1–5 mCi (37–185 MBq)
  (2) Therapeutics
    (a) Hyperthyroidism: 10–30 mCi (370–1110 MBq)
    (b) Thyroid carcinoma: 50–200 mCi (1850–7400 MBq)

3. Na^{+99m}TcO$_4$$^-$. See II.B.

4. ^{201}Tl. Parathyroid imaging
  a. Biodistribution. ^{201}Tl concentrates in the thyroid and also in parathyroid adenomas, which can be detected by a dual isotope subtraction technique of subtracting thyroid uptake counts from Na^{+99m}TcO$_4$$^-$ to unmask nonthyroid thallium uptake counts (see III.A.1).
  b. Administration and dosage. IV, 2 mCi (74 MBq)

IX. BRAIN IMAGING

A. Cerebral perfusion brain-imaging agents. Radiopharmaceuticals for evaluating brain perfusion must possess a lipophilic partition coefficient sufficient to diffuse passively across the blood–brain barrier (BBB) almost completely within one pass of the cerebral circulation, as well as being sufficiently retained to permit data collection. The regional uptake of these agents is proportional to cerebral blood flow. This class of radiopharmaceuticals is useful in the diagnosis of altered regional blood perfusion in stroke.

1. ^{99m}Tc exametazime (^{99m}Tc-HMPAO) exists as a sterile, pyrogen-free IV injection after reconstitution with sodium pertechnetate *USP,* which may be stabilized with the addition of a methylene blue/phosphate buffer stabilizing solution.
  a. Description
    (1) ^{99m}Tc exametazime is a neutral, lipid-soluble complex that freely crosses the BBB. This is a relatively unstable complex, which rapidly converts to a secondary, less lipophilic complex incapable of penetrating into the brain. The in vitro addition of a methylene blue/phosphate buffer stabilizing solution after preparing the ^{99m}Tc exametazime will stabilize the lipid-soluble complex for 4 hr.
    (2) Additional limitations on kit preparation parameters require the use of high mole fraction technetium generator eluates of < 2 hr postelution from a generator previously eluted within 24 hr.
  b. Biodistribution
    (1) ^{99m}Tc exametazime rapidly clears from the blood, with a maximum brain uptake of 3.5%–7%, and up to 2.5% remaining after 24 hr.
    (2) The activity is widely distributed throughout the body; 30% distributes to the GI tract.
    (3) Within 48 hr, 40% of the dose is excreted through the urine and 15% is eliminated via the feces.
  c. Physical properties. See II.B.3.
  d. Administration and dosage. IV, 10–20 mCi (370–740 MBq)

2. **^{99m}Tc bicisate (^{99m}Tc-ECD)**
   a. **Description**
      (1) ^{99m}Tc bicisate exists as a sterile, pyrogen-free IV injection after reconstitution with sodium pertechnetate ^{99m}Tc *USP* and the addition of a phosphate buffer.
      (2) After reconstitution, a stable lipophilic ^{99m}Tc bicisate complex is formed, which is able to cross the BBB by passive diffusion.
   b. **Biodistribution**
      (1) ^{99m}Tc bicisate is rapidly cleared from blood; a maximum of 6.5% of the administered dose is localized in the brain, and 5% is left in the blood after 1 hr.
      (2) Once located in the brain cells, ^{99m}Tc bicisate is metabolized by endogenous enzymes to a polar compound that is unable to diffuse out of the brain cells.
      (3) ^{99m}Tc bicisate is primarily eliminated via the kidneys; 50% is excreted within 2 hr, and 74% in 24 hr. Hepatobiliary excretion accounts for approximately 12.5% of the administered dose after 48 hr.
   c. **Radionuclide properties.** See II.B.3.
   d. **Administration and dosage.** IV, 10–30 mCi (370–1110 MBq)

3. **Iofetamine hydrochloride ^{123}I.** Not commercially available

B. **Carrier-mediated transport (cerebral metabolism) mechanisms.** These are responsible for transporting glucose across the BBB. Agents such as ^{18}F fludeoxyglucose aid in the evaluation of cerebral function by mapping the distribution of glucose metabolism. ^{18}F fludeoxyglucose is produced by a cyclotron.

1. **Biodistribution.** Currently, there is a *USP* monograph for on-site cyclotron-produced ^{18}F fludeoxyglucose, which is a glucose analog. ^{18}F fludeoxyglucose concentrates in the brain, where it is phosphorylated but does not undergo subsequent metabolism because of the replacement of the hydroxyl group in the 2 position with a fluorine atom. It is then metabolically trapped for a sufficient time to allow imaging.

2. **Decay data**
   a. **Physical half-life:** 109.7 min
   b. **Decay mode:** by positron emission
   c. **Primary radiation emissions:** 633 keV energy positrons and 511 keV γ energy photons.

3. **Administration and dosage.** IV, 5–10 mCi (185–370 MBq)

C. **Cerebral neurotransmitter imaging: Fluorodopa fluorine-18 (^{18}F) injection**

1. **Description**
   a. Cerebral neurotransmitter synthesis can be studied with fluorodopa ^{18}F injection. The intracerebral distribution of this neurotransmitter tracer can be used in the assessment of neurodegenerative diseases such as parkinsonism.
   b. Fluorodopa ^{18}F injection exists under a *USP* monograph as an on-site-produced sterile IV solution of a levodopa analog in which a portion of the molecule has been replaced with ^{18}F, a positron-emitting radionuclide.

2. **Biodistribution**
   a. After IV injection, plasma activity decreases to 10% of the administered dose within 5 min after injection.
   b. Fluorodopa ^{18}F injection is predominantly metabolized in periphery via dopa decarboxylase, and catechol-*O*-methyl transferase. To maximize brain uptake, carbidopa may be used to decrease peripheral metabolism.
   c. Rapid excretion via renal system as dopamine metabolites

3. **Radionuclide data.** See IX.B.2.

4. **Administration and dosage.** IV, 10–20 mCi (370–740 MBq)

D. **Cerebrospinal fluid (CSF) dynamics.** Radionuclide cisternography is useful in the evaluation of hydrocephalus and in detecting CSF leaks. In CSF imaging, the radiopharmaceutical **indium-111 pentetate (^{111}In-DTPA)** is introduced intrathecally into the spinal subarachnoid space, ascends through the basal cisterns, proceeds over the cerebral hemispheres, and eventually drains into the superior sagittal sinus. ^{111}In pentetate is commercially supplied as a sterile, pyrogen-free unit dose injection. It is produced by a cyclotron.

1. **Biodistribution**
   a. After intrathecal injection, this radiopharmaceutical normally ascends to the parasagittal region within 24 hr.
   b. After absorption into the bloodstream via the arachnoid villi, the major route of elimination is by kidney; 65% of the dose is excreted within 48 hr; and 85%, within 72 hr.

2. **Decay data**
   a. **Physical half-life:** 67 hr
   b. **CSF biological half-life:** 12 hr
   c. **Effective half-life:** 10 hr
   d. **Decay mode:** by electron capture
   e. **Primary radiation emissions:** 171 keV and 245 keV γ energy photons

3. **Administration and dosage.** Intrathecal, 500 μCi (18.5 MBq)

X. **INFECTION AND INFLAMMATION.** Evaluation of sites of infection include the use of agents that can associate with components of the natural defense mechanisms and can accumulate where they localize.

A. **Gallium (^{67}Ga) citrate**

1. **Description**
   a. It is supplied as a sterile, pyrogen-free radiopharmaceutical with preservatives.
   b. The mechanism of localization is thought to depend on the formation of a gallium transferrin complex in the blood and on binding to transferrin receptors associated with infection and inflammation.
   c. It accumulates in areas of white blood cell (WBC) localization.

2. **Biodistribution**
   a. After administration, the highest concentration of ^{67}Ga citrate, other than at the site of infection, is in the renal cortex. After 24 hr, the maximum concentration shifts to bone and lymph nodes; but after 1 week, it is mainly concentrated in the liver and spleen.
   b. ^{67}Ga citrate is excreted slowly from the body; 26% is via urine, and 9% is via feces. Whole body retention is 65% after 7 days.

3. **Radionuclide data**
   a. **Mode of production:** by cyclotron
   b. **Decay mode:** by electron capture
   c. **Physical half-life:** 78 hr
   d. **Decay emissions:** 93 keV, 185 keV, 300 keV, and 393 keV γ photons

4. **Administration and dosage.** IV, for infection, 3–8 mCi (111–300 MBq). A daily laxative or an enema should be used by the patient after the injection and before the images to cleanse the bowel of radioactivity that may interfere with the images and possibly lead to a false positive result.

B. **WBC labeling agents.** Radiolabeled WBCs are used in the detection of a wide variety of infectious and inflammatory processes. Current use includes the diagnosis of intra-abdominal abscesses, inflammatory bowel disease, appendicitis, fever of unknown origin, and osteomyelitis. WBCs can be radiolabeled with ^{111}In oxine or ^{99m}Tc-exametazime.

1. **^{111}In oxyquinoline solution (^{111}In oxine)**
   a. **Description**
      (1) ^{111}In oxyquinoline is supplied as a sterile preservative-free, pyrogen-free, radiopharmaceutical solution for use in the radiolabeling of autologous leukocytes.
      (2) ^{111}In forms a saturated neutral lipophilic complex with oxyquinoline (1:3 ratio), which enables it to penetrate a cell membrane.
      (3) After incubation of ^{111}In oxyquinoline with a population of autologous leukocytes, the ^{111}In is thought to become firmly bound to cytoplasmic components, thereby allowing the free oxine to be released by the cell.
   b. **Biodistribution**
      (1) After radiolabeling, the autologous leukocytes are reinjected; 30% is taken up by the spleen, and 30% is taken up by the liver, reaching a peak at 2–4 hr postinjection.

(2) Pulmonary uptake is immediately evident postinjection, but it clears, with minimal visible activity, after 4 hr.

(3) There is a biexponential blood clearance; 9%–24% clears with a biological half-life of 2–5 hr, and the remaining 13%–18% clears with a biological half-life of 64–116 hr.

(4) Elimination is mainly through radioactive decay; < 1% is excreted in feces and urine during the first 24 hr.

c. Radionuclide data

(1) Mode of production: by cyclotron

(2) Decay mode: by electron capture

(3) Physical half-life: 67 hr

(4) Decay emissions: 245 keV and 171 keV

d. Administration and dosage. IV, 200–500 μCi (7.4–8.5 MBq)

2. ^{99m}Tc-HMPAO. As a sterile and pyrogen-free IV injection after reconstitution with sodium pertechnetate, ^{99m}Tc-HMPAO may be used to radiolabel leukocytes.

a. Description

(1) ^{99m}Tc-HMPAO is a neutral, lipid-soluble complex that is able to penetrate the WBC membrane. This lipophilic complex is relatively unstable and rapidly converts to a secondary complex incapable of penetrating the WBCs.

(2) The methylene blue/phosphate buffer stabilized solution is not able to radiolabel cells and should not be used.

(3) Additional limitations on kit preparation parameters require the use of high mole fraction technetium generator elutes of < 2 hr postelution from a generator previously eluted within 24 hr.

b. Biodistribution

(1) After IV injection, the radiolabeled cells localize in the lungs, liver, spleen, blood pool, bone marrow, and bladder.

(2) Elimination is primarily via the liver.

c. Radionuclide data. See II.B.1.b; II.B.3.a–b.

d. Administration and dosage. IV, for infection, 7–25 mCi (260–925 MBq)

XI. BREAST IMAGING

A. ^{99m}Tc-MIBI

1. Description

a. ^{99m}Tc-MIBI is used for both breast and cardiac imaging.

b. ^{99m}Tc-MIBI is indicated for planar imaging as a second line of evaluating breast lesions in patients with an abnormal mammogram or a palpable breast mass.

c. ^{99m}Tc-MIBI may not be used to screen for breast cancer, to confirm the presence or absence of malignancy, or to replace a biopsy.

2. Biodistribution. ^{99m}Tc-MIBI is primarily excreted by the hepatobiliary system.

3. Physical properties. See II.B.3.

4. Administration and dosage. IV, 20–30 mCi (740–1110 MBq)

XII. DEEP VEIN THROMBOSIS (DVT) IMAGING

A. ^{99m}Tc apcitide injection. No longer commercially available

XIII. TUMORS

A. The usefulness of radiopharmaceuticals in the detection of tumors varies in sensitivity and specificity, with differences in tumor location and type.

1. **^{67}Ga**
   a. **Description**
      (1) ^{67}Ga is supplied as a sterile, pyrogen-free radiopharmaceutical with preservatives.
      (2) The mechanism of localization is thought to depend on the formation of a gallium transferrin complex or binding to transferrin receptors on tumor cells.
      (3) It accumulates in primary metastatic tumor sites and may detect the presence of Hodgkin disease, lymphoma, and bronchogenic carcinoma.
   b. **Biodistribution.** See X.A.2.
   c. **Radionuclide data.** See X.A.3.
   d. **Administration and dosage.** IV, for tumor, 10 mCi (370 MBq)

2. **^{111}In pentetreotide**
   a. **Description**
      (1) It is supplied as a sterile, pyrogen-free kit for the preparation of ^{111}In pentetreotide. The two-component kit consists of a reaction vial containing a lyophilized mixture of pentetreotide with stabilizer adjutants and a second vial containing an indium ^{111}In chloride/ferric chloride solution.
         (a) The pentetreotide molecule is a conjugate of pentetate (diethylenetriamine pentaacetic acid; DTPA) and octreotide, which is a somatostatin analog.
         (b) ^{111}In pentetreotide is prepared by adding the ^{111}In/Fe chloride solution to the vial containing the pentetreotide. The pentetate portion of the molecule acts as a bifunctional chelate, linking the ^{111}In radionuclide to the biological active octreotide portion of the agent.
      (2) ^{111}In pentetreotide is indicated for localization of primary and metastatic neuroendocrine tumors expressing somatostatin receptors.
   b. **Biodistribution**
      (1) Within 1 hr after IV injection, ^{111}In pentetreotide distributes from the plasma to extravascular space; less than one third of the administered dose remains in the plasma 10 min postinjection.
      (2) ^{111}In pentetreotide localizes as a function of somatostatin receptor density, with accumulation in normal pituitary, thyroid, liver, spleen, and the urinary bladder.
      (3) Elimination is primarily renal; 50% of the administered dose is excreted within 6 hr postinjection; 85%, after 24 hr, and < 90% after 48 hr. Less than 2% of the administered dose is cleared via the feces within 72 hr post-injection.
   c. **Radionuclide data**
      (1) Mode of production: iby cyclotron
      (2) Decay mode: by electron capture
      (3) Physical half-life: 67 hr
      (4) Decay emissions: 245 keV and 171 keV
   d. **Administration and dosage.** IV, 3–6 mCi (111–222 MBq)

3. **Iobenguane ^{131}I injection (^{131}I-MIBG)**
   a. **Description**
      (1) It is supplied as a sterile, pyrogen-free radiopharmaceutical for use as an adjunctive diagnostic agent for the localization of primary and metastatic pheochromocytomas and neuroblastomas.
      (2) Iobenguane (meta-iodobenzylguanidine) labeled with ^{131}I acts as a physiological analog of norepinephrine and is transported and accumulated in the adrenal medulla. This allows for the detection of neuroendocrine tumors via the specific uptake of labeled iobenguane.
      (3) Because of its physiological similarities to norepinephrine, many classes of drugs that interfere with catecholamine transport and function may affect the uptake and localization of labeled iobenguane.
   b. **Biodistribution**
      (1) After IV injection, there is rapid uptake in the liver, with lesser amounts accumulating in the lungs, heart, and spleen.
      (2) Normal adrenal gland uptake is low; but for tumors such as pheochromocytomas and neuroblastomas, the uptake is relatively higher.
      (3) Elimination is renal; most of the drug is excreted mainly unchanged. Between 40% and 50% of the administered dose is excreted within 24 hr, and 70%–90% is excreted within 4 days postinjection.

(4) Administration of potassium iodide 1 day before and for 10 days after administration is suggested to reduce thyroid uptake of potential radioiodide contaminants.

c. Physical data. See VIII.B.2.b.

d. Administration and dosage. IV, 0.5–1 mCi (18.5–37 MBq)

4. ^{201}**Tl.** This agent has utility as a tumor-imaging agent because of its accumulation in the rapidly metabolizing cells of certain tumors in accordance with its mechanism of localization (see III.A.1).

a. Administration and dosage. IV, 1.5–3 mCi (55–111 MBq)

5. ^{18}**F fludeoxyglucose *USP*.** Currently, there is a *USP* monograph for on-site cyclotron-produced ^{18}F fludeoxyglucose, which is a glucose analog. This agent has utility as a tumor-imaging agent because of an increased demand for glucose by tumors with an advanced state of malignancy. Not only can ^{18}F fludeoxyglucose locate and differentiate tumors but it can also help distinguish between recurrent brain tumor and radiation necrosis in patients receiving radiation therapy (see IX.B).

a. Biodistribution. ^{18}F fludeoxyglucose concentrates in metabolically active cells, where it is phosphorylated but does not undergo subsequent metabolism because of the replacement of the hydroxyl group in the 2 position with a fluorine atom. It is then metabolically trapped for a sufficient time to allow imaging.

b. Administration and dosage. IV, 5–25 mCi (185–370 MBq)

6. ^{99m}**Tc depreotide**

a. Description

(1) ^{99m}Tc depreotide is based on a synthetic peptide with a high binding affinity for somatostatin receptors in normal and abnormal tissues. ^{99m}Tc depreotide is used to identify somatostatin-receptor-bearing pulmonary masses in patients presenting with pulmonary lesions and who are known to have had a malignancy or have a history highly suspect for malignancy.

(2) ^{99m}Tc depreotide is supplied as a vial containing a sterile, nonpyrogenic, freeze-dried mixture of depreotide, stannous chloride dihydrate, sodium glucoheptonate dihydrate, and edetate disodium dihydrate.

(3) ^{99m}Tc depreotide exists as a sterile, pyrogen-free IV injection after kit reconstitution with $Na^{+99m}TcO_4^-$ and heating at 100°C for 10 min.

(4) Caution should be exercised when giving this drug to patients with insulinomas because depreotide exists as a somatostatin analog that can produce severe hypoglycemia in patients with insulinomas.

b. Biodistribution. Approximately 12% of the administered dose is excreted through the urine within 4 hr.

c. Radionuclide data. See II.B.3.

d. Administration and Dosage. Peripheral IV injection, 15–20 mCi (555–740 MBq)

B. Antibodies

1. ^{99m}**Tc arcitumomab**

a. Description

(1) ^{99m}Tc arcitumomab is a murine monoclonal antibody Fab fragment.

(2) It is indicated in conjunction with standard diagnostic evaluations for the detection of recurrent and/or metastatic colorectal cancer involving the liver, extrahepatic abdomen, and pelvis in patients with confirmed colorectal cancer.

(3) The use of a Fab fragment helps reduce the human antimouse antibody (HAMA) reaction.

b. Biodistribution

(1) Approximately 28% of the dose is excreted in the urine over the first 24 hr.

(2) Approximately 93% of the dose is eliminated from the blood after 24 hr.

(3) The Fab fragment minimizes liver metabolism and facilitates rapid blood clearance.

c. Radionuclide data. See II.B.3.

d. Administration and dosage. IV, 1 mg arcitumomab with 20–30 mCi of ^{99m}Tc (740–1110 MBq)

XIV. THERAPEUTIC AGENTS. The therapeutic use of radiopharmaceuticals is based on the concept of selective localization of radiopharmaceuticals coupled with the lethality of the same because of the tissue damage resulting from highly ionizing particulate emissions such as β particles.

A. Chromic phosphate phosphorus-32 (^{32}P) suspension

1. **Description.** Available as a sterile, pyrogen-free aqueous suspension used in the treatment of peritoneal or pleural effusions caused by metastatic disease. Also used in the treatment of ovarian and prostate cancer.

2. **Biodistribution**
   a. Colloidal suspension of ^{32}P is rapidly taken up by macrophages adhering to the cavity wall, thereby concentrating and localizing the irradiation effect of the ^{32}P radionuclide β particulate emission.
   b. After infusion, the suspension rapidly distributes from within the cavity and may localize in the lungs, adrenal glands, kidneys, lymph nodes, liver, spleen, bone marrow, plasma, erythrocytes, and leukocytes, depending on colloidal particle size.
   c. Elimination is primarily renal.

3. **Radionuclide data**
   a. **Mode of production:** by reactor
   b. **Decay mode:** β
   c. **Physical half-life:** 14.3 days
   d. **Decay emissions:** 695 keV mean energy β, 100% abundance

4. **Administration and dosage**
   a. Intraperitoneal instillation: 10–20 mCi (370–740 MBq)
   b. Intrapleural instillation: 6–12 mCi (222–444 MBq)
   c. Carcinoma interstitial: 0.1–0.5 mCi (3.7–18.5 MBq)
   d. Caution is advised for visual inspection to prevent misadministration of the sodium phosphate form (clear, colorless), which is designated for intravascular use only.

B. Sodium phosphate ^{32}P solution

1. **Description**
   a. It is available as a commercially supplied, sterile, pyrogen-free radiopharmaceutical.
   b. It is primarily used as an antineoplastic for the treatment of polycythemia rubra vera and is selectively used for the palliative treatment of metastatic bone pain.
   c. Its therapeutic effect is owing to cell damage resulting from irradiation produced by beta particulate emission.

2. **Biodistribution**
   a. It concentrates as phosphate within the DNA of rapidly dividing hematopoietic cells in the treatment of polycythemia rubra vera and as phosphate in areas of increased bone formation.
   b. After IV administration, it diffuses rapidly into extracellular and intracellular space, concentrating in the bone marrow, spleen, and liver.
   c. Elimination is primarily renal; 5%–10% is excreted within 24 hr, and 20% within 1 week.
   d. Whole body biological half-life is approximately 39 days.

3. **Radionuclide data**
   a. **Mode of production:** by reactor
   b. **Decay mode:** by β
   c. **Physical half-life:** 14.3 days
   d. **Decay emissions:** 695 keV mean energy β, 100% abundance

4. **Administration and dosage**
   a. Polycythemia rubra vera: IV, 3–5 mCi (111–185 MBq)
   b. Metastatic bone lesions: IV, 10–21 mCi (370–777 MBq)
   c. Caution is advised for visual inspection to prevent misadministration of the chromic phosphate form (green, cloudy), which is designated for interstitial use only.

C. Sodium iodide ^{131}I (therapeutic)

1. **Description**
   a. It is indicated for treatment of hyperthyroidism and thyroid carcinoma.
   b. Its therapeutic action is owing to the accumulation and retention of iodine and its isotope ^{131}I.

2. Biodistribution
   a. See VIII.A; VIII.B.2.
   b. **Biological half-life in the thyroid:** euthyroid patient, 80 days; hyperthyroid patient, 5–40 days

3. Radionuclide data. See VIII.B.2.b.

4. Administration and dosage. Oral capsule or oral solution
   a. Hyperthyroidism: 10–30 mCi (370–1110 MBq)
   b. Thyroid carcinoma: 30–200 mCi (1110–7400 MBq)

D. Strontium-89 (^{89}Sr) chloride

1. Description
   a. It is indicated for the alleviation of bone pain arising from metastatic bone disease.
   b. As a metabolic analog of calcium, ^{89}Sr concentrates selectively in areas of increased osteogenesis, thus delivering a radiation dose sufficient to provide a palliative effect.
   c. Pain relief begins 7–21 days after administration, with maximum relief by 6 weeks and an average duration of 6 months.
   d. Reduction in patient analgesic usage occurs in up to 75% of patients treated; complete pain relief is seen in 20% of treated patients, and no pain relief in 20%–25% of treated patients.
   e. Bone marrow suppression effects limit ^{89}Sr use to patients with initial WBC counts > 2,400 and platelet counts > 60,000.

2. Biodistribution
   a. After administration, ^{89}Sr clears rapidly from blood and localizes in the bone hydroxy-apatite.
   b. Initial biological half-life in normal bone is 14 days; longer retention is seen in metastatic bone lesions. Between 12% and 90% of the administered dose is retained for up to 3 months after administration.
   c. Elimination is primarily renal; 66% of the administered dose clears via GFR within the first 2 days, and 33% is excreted via feces.

3. Radionuclide data
   a. **Mode of production:** by accelerator
   b. **Decay mode:** by β
   c. **Emission data:** 1.46 MeV maximum β energy, 100% abundance
   d. **Physical half-life:** 50.5 days

4. Administration and dosage. IV, 4 mCi (148 MBq), 40–60 μCi/kg (1.5–2.2 MBq/kg)

E. Samarium-153 (^{153}Sm) lexidronam

1. Description
   a. ^{153}Sm is indicated for the relief of pain in patients who have confirmed metastatic cancer of the bone.
   b. ^{153}Sm concentrates in areas of high bone turnover and accumulates more in osteoblastic lesions than in the normal bone.
   c. The goal of ^{153}Sm therapy is for patients to be able to reduce the amount of narcotic analgesics needed to control their pain.

2. Biodistribution
   a. The lesion to normal bone ratio is 5:1.
   b. The percentage of uptake of ^{153}Sm is directly proportional to the number of lesions the patient has.
   c. Less than 1% of the dose remains in the blood 5 hr postinjection.
   d. ^{153}Sm is 100% renally excreted over 12 hr.
   e. The onset is approximately 1 week.

3. Radionuclide data
   a. **Mode of production:** by cyclotron
   b. **Decay mode:** by β and γ decay

    c. Physical half-life: 46.3 hr

    d. Decay emissions: 640 keV, 710 keV, and 840 keV β energy and 103 keV γ energy photons

4. Precautions. [153]Sm may cause bone marrow suppression, which should return to baseline within 8 weeks postinjection.

5. Administration and dosage. IV, 1 mCi/kg (37 MBq/kg)

F. Yttrium-90 (^{90}Y) ibritumomab tiuxetan and ^{111}In ibritumomab tiuxetan

1. Overview

    a. [111]In ibritumomab tiuxetan and ^{90}Y ibritumomab tiuxetan are part of a therapeutic regimen used in the treatment of non–Hodgkin lymphoma (NHL) patients with relapsed refractory low-grade, follicular, or transformed B cell NHL and patients with rituximab refractory NHL.

    b. Ibritumomab tiuxetan is an immunoconjugate consisting of a monoclonal antibody ibritumomab, which is linked to the chelator tiuxetan.

    c. The ibritumomab antibody is a murine immunoglobulin G1 (IgG1) κ monoclonal antibody produced in Chinese hamster ovary (CHO) cells. The ibritumomab antibody is directed against the CD20 antigen, which is expressed on the surface of normal and malignant B lymphocytes.

    d. The linker chelator tiuxetan provides a high-affinity chelation site for ^{111}In in the case of the imaging dose and for ^{90}Y in the case of the therapeutic dose.

    e. The therapeutic regimen is administered in two separate doses. This allows for the qualitative evaluation of the biodistribution to avoid potential toxicities such as abnormally high bone marrow localization or prolonged renal excretion. In each administration, patients must be premedicated with diphenhydramine 50 mg and acetaminophen 650 mg 0.5 hr before receiving the rituximab infusion required before administering the radiolabeled antibody.

        (1) Step 1 is the administration of rituximab followed by the ^{111}In ibritumomab tiuxetan diagnostic imaging dose.

        (2) Step 2 follows step 1 by 7–9 days and consists of a second rituximab infusion followed by the ^{90}Y ibritumomab therapy dose.

2. Description

    a. Supplied as two separate kits to produce a single dose of ^{111}In ibritumomab tiuxetan and a single dose of ^{90}Y ibritumomab tiuxetan

    b. Each kit consists of four vials containing:

        (1) Ibritumomab tiuxetan in saline, 3.2 mg

        (2) Sodium acetate, 50 mM

        (3) Formulation buffer (contains human serum albumin)

        (4) One empty reaction vial

    c. Exists as a sterile, nonpyrogenic IV solution after formulation with either ^{111}In or [90]Y

3. Biodistribution

    a. The mean half-life for ^{90}Y ibritumomab tiuxetan in the blood is 30 hr.

    b. Approximately 7.8% of the administered dose is excreted in the urine over 7 days.

    c. The estimated biological half-life is 48 hr.

4. Radionuclide data

    a. [111]In. See XIII.B.1.c.

    b. [90]Y

        (1) Mode of production: by reactor

        (2) Decay mode: by β

        (3) Physical half-life: 64.1 hr

        (4) Decay emission: 935 mean keV, 100% emission

5. Precautions

    a. [90]Y ibritumomab tiuxetan should not be administered to patients with altered biodistributions of the ^{111}In ibritumomab tiuxetan imaging and dosimetry dose.

b. ^{90}Y ibritumomab tiuxetan should not be administered to patients with:
  (1) ≤25% lymphoma marrow involvement
  (2) Platelet counts < 100,000 cell/mm^3
  (3) Neutrophil count < 1,500 cells/mm^3
  (4) Hypocellular bone marrow
  (5) History of failed stem cell collection
c. Ibritumomab tiuxetan is contraindicated in patients with known hypersensitivity or anaphylactic reactions to murine proteins.
d. Patients who have previously received murine-based protein therapy should be screened for human antimouse antibodies.
e. Infusion-related adverse events, including asthenia, chills, and nausea, are common and are usually self-limited. Tumor lysis syndrome has been reported after rituximab infusions, which are part of ^{90}Y ibritumomab tiuxetan therapy. Patients should be monitored closely for this potentially fatal adverse event.

XV. REFERENCES

A. American Pharmaceutical Association. Nuclear Pharmacy Practice Guidelines. Academy of Pharmacy Practice, 1995.

B. Bernier DR, Christian PE, Langan JK. Nuclear Medicine Technology and Techniques. St. Louis, Mosby 1994.

C. Chilton HM, Witcofski R: Nuclear Pharmacy: An Introduction to the Clinical Applications of Radiopharmaceuticals. Philadelphia, Lea & Febiger 1986.

D. Swanson DP, Chilton HM, Thrall JH. Pharmaceuticals in Medical Imaging. New York, Macmillan 1990.

E. United States Pharmacopeia Drug Information (USPDI) 2002.

STUDY QUESTIONS

Directions for questions 1–7: Each of the questions, statements, or incomplete statements in this section can be correctly answered or completed by **one** of the suggested answers or phrases. Choose the **best** answer.

1. Which of the following emissions from the decay of radionuclides is most commonly used in nuclear medicine diagnostic imaging?

(A) x-ray
(B) β
(C) α
(D) γ
(E) Positron

2. Which of the following radionuclides is most commonly used in nuclear pharmacy practice?

(A) gallium-67 (^{67}Ga)
(B) thallium-201 (^{201}Tl)
(C) technetium-99m (^{99m}Tc)
(D) iodine-123 (^{123}I)
(E) xenon-133 (^{133}Xe)

3. Which of the following radionuclides is produced using a generator?

(A) technetium-99m (^{99m}Tc)
(B) thallium-201 (^{201}Tl)
(C) gallium-67 (^{67}Ga)
(D) xenon-133 (^{133}Xe)
(E) iodine-123 (^{123}I)

4. Which of the following radiopharmaceuticals can be used in skeletal imaging?

(A) technetium-99m albumin aggregated
(B) technetium-99m medronate disodium
(C) xenon-133 gas *USP*
(D) thallous chloride (^{201}Tl) *USP*
(E) technetium-99m disofenin

5. Which of the following radiopharmaceuticals is used in the diagnosis of acute cholecystitis?

(A) technetium-99m sulfur colloid
(B) technetium-99m medronate disodium
(C) technetium-99m albumin
(D) technetium-99m exametazime
(E) technetium-99m disofenin

6. Which of the following cyclotron-produced radiopharmaceuticals is used for assessing regional myocardial perfusion as part of an exercise stress test?

(A) thallous chloride ^{201}Tl *USP*
(B) sodium iodide ^{123}I
(C) gallium citrate ^{67}Ga *USP*
(D) indium-111 pentetate
(E) cobalt-57 cyanocobalamin

7. Glomerular filtration and the urinary collection system can best be evaluated using which of the following agents?

(A) technetium-99m sulfur colloid
(B) technetium-99m albumin
(C) technetium-99m sestamibi
(D) technetium-99m disofenin
(E) technetium-99m pentetate'

Directions for questions 8–11: The questions and incomplete statements in this section can be correctly answered or completed by **one or more** of the suggested answers. Choose the answer, **A–E.**

A	if **I only** is correct
B	if **III only** is correct
C	if **I and II** are correct
D	if **II and III** are correct
E	if **I, II, and III** are correct

8. The definition of the optimal radiopharmaceutical includes which of the following attributes?

I. short half-life
II. γ photon with a 100–300 keV energy
III. rapid localization in target tissue and quick clearance from nontarget tissue

9. Which of the following statements are true for sodium pertechnetate technetium-99m (^{99m}Tc) *USP*?

I. It is used to radiolabel all other ^{99m}Tc radiopharmaceuticals.
II. The molybdenum-99 (^{99}Mo) breakthrough limit is < 0.15 μCi ^{99}Mo/mCi ^{99m}Tc (< 0.15 kBq/MBq).
III. It has a physical half-life of 16 hr.

10. Which of the following organs can be imaged with technetium-99m (^{99m}Tc) sulfur colloid?

 I. liver
 II. spleen
 III. bone marrow

11. Which of the following radiopharmaceuticals may be used to image the thyroid gland?

 I. sodium iodide ^{131}I
 II. sodium pertechnetate technetium-99m *USP*
 III. sodium iodide ^{123}I

Directions for questions 12–16: Each of the following mechanisms of localization is most closely related to one of the following radiopharmaceuticals. The mechanisms may be used more than once or not at all. Choose the **best** answer, **A–E.**

A	metabolic trapping
B	phagocytosis
C	capillary blockade
D	active transport
E	passive diffusion

12. thallous chloride ^{201}Tl USP

13. technetium-99m albumin aggregated USP

14. technetium-99m sulfur colloid

15. technetium-99m exametazime

16. fluorine-18 fludeoxyglucose

ANSWERS AND EXPLANATIONS

1. The answer is D *[see I.B.3.b]*.
Current camera technology most efficiently detects γ radiation. α and β emissions are not useful in nuclear medicine imaging because of their harmful particulate emissions and low tissue penetration. Although x-ray emissions can be used as in the case of the mercury daughter of the thallous chloride ^{201}Tl parent, they are not efficiently detected. Annihilation radiation associated with positron decay can be imaged, but this technology is currently limited to a few specialized centers.

2. The answer is C *[see II.A.1]*.
^{99m}Tc has become the radionuclide of choice in current nuclear pharmacy practice since its introduction in the mid-1960s. ^{99m}Tc fulfills all of the requirements of the optimal radiopharmaceutical, with its physical half-life of 6 hr, 140 keV γ energy emission, ready availability, cost, and ability to be radio-labeled to a wide variety of biologically active compounds.

3. The answer is A *[see II.A.1.a]*.
^{99m}Tc is obtained via commercially supplied, sterile, pyrogen-free generator systems. A generator is a device used to separate a short half-life radionuclide from the longer-lived parent nuclide, while retaining the parent to produce more of the daughter nuclide. In this way, short–half-life nuclides can be made available on a continuous basis at great distances from the sites of generator production.

4. The answer is B *[see IV.A.2]*.
The ^{99m}Tc diphosphonate compounds are the most popular bone-imaging agents currently used in nuclear medicine imaging. They are rapidly taken up by skeletal bone; 50% of the administered dose is adsorbed onto bone hydroxyapatite and the remainder is excreted by the kidneys. The imaging advantages of the ^{99m}Tc, coupled with the sensitivity of bone agent localization in skeletal bone hydroxy-apatite, allow for detection of bone pathology before evidence of pathology can be shown by conventional x-ray.

5. The answer is E *[see VI.C.1–2]*.
^{99m}Tc disofenin is an iminodiacetic acid derivative, which is useful for hepatobiliary imaging due to its ability to be selectively cleared by a carrier-mediated hepatocyte pathway. Lack of gallbladder visualization is an abnormal finding suggestive of acute cholecystitis.

6. The answer is A *[see III.A.1]*.
Regional uptake of thallous chloride ^{201}Tl *USP* is proportional to myocardial blood supply. The injection of ^{201}Tl in concert with a treadmill exercise stress test determines myocardial perfusion at maximum cardiac output when cardiac demand outstrips supply and the distribution of ^{201}Tl is less after affected by collateral blood supply within the myocardium. Regions that do not take up ^{201}Tl are interpreted as areas of infarct or ischemia. If these focal areas of decreased uptake subsequently fill in with redistributed ^{201}Tl, they are interpreted to be areas of ischemia, in contrast with areas of infarct, which remain as diminished areas of activity.

7. The answer is E *[see VII.B.1]*.
^{99m}Tc pentetate is cleared through glomerular filtration in the same manner as inulin and can be used to determine the GFR as well as in the evaluation of obstruction of vascular supply and renal morphology.

8. The answer is E (I, II, III) *[see I.C]*.
The optimal radiopharmaceutical has a half-life short enough to minimize radiation exposure to the patient yet long enough to allow for collection of imaging information. It should incorporate a γ- emitting radionuclide, which decays with the emission of a photon energy between 100 and 300 keV, which is efficiently detected with current instrumentation. The radiopharmaceutical should localize rapidly in the organ system of interest and be metabolized, excreted, or both from the nontarget tissues to maximize contrast and minimize radiation-absorbed dose.

9. The answer is C (I, II) *[see II.A–B]*.
Sodium pertechnetate ^{99m}Tc *USP* decays by isomeric transition and has a physical half-life of 6 hr. The emission of a γ photon has the energy of 140 keV.

10. The answer is E (I, II, III) *[see VI.B.1].*
^{99m}Tc sulfur colloid localizes within the reticuloendothelial system; 80%–90% of the dose is phagocytized by the Kupffer cells of the liver; 5%–10%, by the spleen; and the balance, by the bone marrow.

11. The answer is E (I, II, III) *[see VIII.B].*
Although all of the listed agents accumulate in the thyroid gland, only sodium iodide ^{123}I possesses ideal imaging characteristics and organification into thyroid hormone. While the imaging properties of sodium pertechnetate ^{99m}Tc *USP* are good, the pertechnetate ion is trapped only by the thyroid and not organified, thus limiting the information provided by the image.

12. The answer is D *[see III.A.1].*
Thallous chloride ^{201}Tl *USP* is a monovalent cation with distribution analogous to potassium ion (K^+). Myocardial uptake is by active transport via the Na^+/K^+-ATPase pump.

13. The answer is C *[see V.A.1]*
After IV administration of ^{99m}Tc albumin aggregated *USP*, 80% of the radiolabeled albumin particles become trapped by capillary blockade in the pulmonary circulation.

14. The answer is B *[see VI.B.1].*
After the administration of ^{99m}Tc sulfur colloid, 80%–90% of the dose is phagocytized by the Kupffer cells of the liver; 5%–10%, by the spleen; and the balance, by the bone marrow.

15. The answer is E *[see IX.A.1].*
^{99m}Tc exametazime is used for evaluating brain perfusion. It possesses a lipophilic partition coefficient that is sufficient to diffuse passively across the BBB almost completely within one pass of the cerebral circulation, and that is sufficiently retained to permit data collection.

16. The answer is A *[see IX.B.1].*
^{18}F fludeoxyglucose is used in evaluating cerebral function by mapping the distribution of cerebral glucose metabolism. As an analog of glucose, ^{18}F fludeoxyglucose is transported into the brain by carrier-mediated transport mechanisms responsible for transporting glucose across the BBB. Because the presence of the flourine atom in the 2 position prevents metabolism beyond the phosphorylation step, ^{18}F fludeoxyglucose becomes metabolically trapped within the brain.

PART II

PHARMACY PRACTICE

20
Pharmaceutical Care and Disease State Management

Peggy C. Yarborough

I. INTRODUCTION

A. **Practice of pharmacy.** The practice of pharmacy embraces a variety of settings, patient populations, and specialist and generalist pharmacists. Central to the practice of pharmacy, however, is the provision of clinical services directly to, and for the benefit of, **patients.**

B. **Definition.** The term **pharmaceutical care** (sometimes called **pharmacist care**) describes specific activities and services through which an individual pharmacist "cooperates with a patient and other professionals in designing, implementing and monitoring a therapeutic plan that will produce specific therapeutic outcomes for the patient."[1]

C. Pharmaceutical care is increasingly being augmented by activities that may be described as **focused areas of practice,** wherein the pharmacist is engaged in:

1. **Drug monitoring,** for a specific drug or for therapy for a specific disease state

2. **Disease monitoring,** for a specific disease state

3. **Drug therapy and disease management/collaborative practice,** by protocol

4. A pharmacist may incorporate one or more areas of focused practice into a general practice of pharmacy or may specialize within a narrow field of practice. Examples of highly specialized practice include pharmacist-directed diabetes management clinics, hypertension clinics, anticoagulation clinics, and hospital-based infectious disease services.

II. SCOPE OF PRACTICE WITHIN PHARMACEUTICAL CARE

A. **Role.** Pharmaceutical care has evolved from an emphasis on prevention of drug-related problems (basically **drug management**) to the expanded roles of pharmacists in the **triage of patients, treatment of routine acute illnesses, management of chronic diseases,** and **primary disease prevention.**

B. **Function.** The provision of pharmaceutical care does not imply that the pharmacist is no longer responsible for dispensing functions. In many instances, however, implementation of pharmaceutical care services necessitates a redesign of the professional work flow, with assignment of technical functions to technical personnel under the direct supervision and responsibility of the pharmacist.

---

[1]Hepler CD, Strand LM. Opportunities and responsibilities in pharmaceutical care. Am J Hosp Pharm 1990;47: 533–543.

Table 20-1. Uniqueness of Pharmaceutical Care

Characteristic	Traditional Pharmacy	Clinical Pharmacy	Pharmaceutical Care
Primary focus	Prescription order or OTC request	Physicians or other health professionals	Patient
Continuity	On demand	Discontinuous	Continuous
Strategy	Obey	Find fault or prevention	Anticipate or improve
Orientation	Drug product	Process	Outcomes

OTC, over the counter.

III. UNIQUENESS OF PHARMACEUTICAL CARE. Provision of pharmaceutical care overlaps somewhat with other aspects of pharmacy practice (Table 20-1). However, pharmaceutical care is not the same as these other areas, which include

A. Clinical pharmacy

B. Patient counseling

C. Pharmaceutical services; when the activities of a pharmacy or pharmacy department are performed for "faceless" patients or charts, the activity is one of pharmacy service, not pharmaceutical care (i.e., chart or drug profile reviews without input from the patient or caregiver is not pharmaceutical care).

IV. ESSENTIAL COMPONENTS OF PHARMACEUTICAL CARE

A. Pharmacist–patient relationship. The importance of putting a face and personality with the clinical picture is a key component of pharmaceutical care. A pharmacist can have a caring relationship with a patient but not with a chart or drug profile. A pharmacist cannot have empathy for words on a page or on a computer screen. Pharmaceutical care is based on a collaborative effort between pharmacist and patient.

B. Pharmacist's workup of drug therapy (PWDT). The provision of pharmaceutical care is often centered around a process described as the PWDT.[2] The PWDT contains the *thought processes* necessary for pharmaceutical care. The PWDT is too lengthy to be used as the chart note for pharmacist interventions; an abbreviated format known as a FARM (findings, assessment, resolutions/recommendation, and monitoring) note or a SOAP (subjective, objective, assessment, and plan) note is more appropriate for a chart notation (Table 20-2). Nonetheless, it is helpful to the pharmacy student, or to a pharmacist entering a new field of pharmacy practice, to write out complete PWDTs for a variety of patients as training or orientation exercises. Although the forms and methods used for the PWDT may vary, the components are essentially the same.

1. **Data collection.** Collect, synthesize, and interpret relevant information, such as:
   a. Patient demographic data: age, race, sex
   b. Pertinent medical information
      (1) Current and past medical history
      (2) Family history
      (3) Social history
      (4) Dietary history
      (5) Medication history (prescription, OTC, social drugs; allergies)
      (6) Physical findings (e.g., weight, height, blood pressure, edema)
      (7) Laboratory or other test results (e.g., serum drug levels, potassium level, serum creatinine as relevant to drug therapy)
   c. Patient complaints, symptoms, signs

[2]Strand LM, Morley PC, Cipolle RJ, et al. Drug-related problems: Their structure and function. Ann Pharmacother 1990;24:1093–1097.

Table 20-2. Components of a FARM Note and a SOAP Note

PWDT Component	FARM Note	SOAP Note
Findings	The identified or suggestive patient-specific information that gives a basis for or leads to the recognition of a pharmacotherapy problem or indication for pharmacist intervention	
	Findings (F) Subjective and objective data incorporated into same section	**Subjective data (S)** separated from **objective data (O)**
Desired outcomes	**Assessment (A)** *The pharmacist's clinical judgment based on his or her findings*—thus it is no better than the database (the findings); the assessment forms the basis for the intervention plan	
Desired end points		
Drug-related problems		
Therapeutic selection	**Resolutions/ Recommendation (R)**	**Plan (P)**
Monitoring parameters	**Monitoring (M)**	
Follow-up		

2. Develop or identify the **CORE pharmacotherapy plan**[3]
   a. **C = condition** or patient need. Note that this may include nonmedical conditions or needs and is thus not a reiteration of the current medical problems.
   b. **O = outcome(s)** desired for the conditions or needs.
      (1) **Patient outcomes** (POEMS: patient-oriented evidence that matters). There are generally five categories of patient outcomes:.
         (a) Mortality
         (b) Morbidity
            (i) Related to disease process
            (ii) Related to medication/treatment plan
         (c) Behavior
         (d) Economic
         (e) Quality of life
      (2) **Therapeutic end points** (surrogate markers; DOES: disease-oriented evidence)
         (a) A therapeutic end point represents the pharmacological or therapeutic effect that is expected, ultimately, to achieve the desired outcome(s).
         (b) More than one end point is usually needed to achieve an outcome—for example, both near-normal glycemic control and normalization of blood pressure are necessary to significantly reduce the risk of end-stage renal disease.
   c. **R = regimen** to achieve the desired outcome(s)
      (1) **Therapeutic regimens**
         (a) **Existing therapy.** For example, a pharmacist is asked to work with a patient for whom one or more agents are already prescribed for the disease process or problem.
            (i) Evaluate the current drug regimen for its potential to achieve desired end points and to meet the patient's individual needs.
            (ii) Revise the regimen as appropriate.
         (b) **Initial therapy.** A pharmacist is asked to work with a patient whose condition was newly diagnosed or is asked to develop an initial treatment plan.
            (i) List the therapeutic options (drug and regimen) most likely to achieve the desired end points.
            (ii) Select the option best suited for the patient's medical, physical (e.g., handicap), psychosocial (e.g., support system), mental (motivation, denial, fear), and financial well-being.

[3]Canaday BR, Yarborough PC. Documenting pharmaceutical care: Creating a standard. Ann Pharmacother 1994; 28:1292–1296.

    (2) Goal setting and behavior regimens. The patient is an essential partner for setting and achieving intermediate- and short-term goals and the behavior changes necessary to achieve those goals. To construct effective behavior regimens, the pharmacist practitioner must incorporate the following concepts:

      (a) Identify the **type of goal** being set, such as the following:

        (i) Start a new positive action—for example, start an exercise program.

        (ii) Increase the frequency or intensity of a positive action—for example, drink two more cups of water daily.

        (iii) Stop or decrease the frequency or intensity of a destructive action—for example, stop smoking.

        (iv) Continue an action that is "perfect"—for example, continue to exercise 30 min a day, every day.

      (b) State the behavior goal in terms that are **clear, specific,** and **reasonable.**

        (i) Set **time limits**—for example, "Over the next 3 weeks."

        (ii) Target a **specific action**—for example, "I will walk."

        (iii) Set **measures and frequency**—for example, "six blocks, three days a week."

        (iv) Divide a big task into several small ones, making each change small relative to the current patient behavior. The old saying "It's hard by the yard, but a cinch by the inch" is true.

  d. E = evaluation parameters to assess outcome achievement.

    (1) Efficacy parameters. What should be monitored, how often, and by whom to ensure that therapeutic end points or patient outcomes are being achieved.

    (2) Toxicity parameters. What should be monitored, how often, and by whom to ensure that adverse effects, allergic reactions, or toxicity is not occurring.

3. Identify the PRIME pharmacotherapy problems or indications for pharmacist interventions, [4] sometimes referred to as drug-related problems.[5] The goal is to identify actual or potential problems that could compromise the desired patient outcomes (Table 20-3).

  a. P = pharmaceutical-based problems

    (1) Patient not receiving a prescribed drug, device, or intervention

    (2) Routine monitoring (labs, screenings, exams) missing

Table 20-3. PRIME Pharmacotherapy Problem Types

P = Pharmaceutical-based problems
- Patient not receiving a prescribed drug, device, or intervention
- Routine monitoring (labs, screenings, exams) missing

R = Risks to patient
- Adverse drug reaction/drug allergy
- Potential for overlap of adverse effects (must be kept in mind as part of the workup or evaluation of any new complaint or problem reported by patient)

I = Interactions
- Drug–drug, drug–disease, drug–food interactions

M = Mismatch between medications and condition or patient needs
- No indication for a current drug, device, or intervention
- Indication for a drug, device, or intervention but none prescribed

E = Efficacy issues
- Too much of the correct drug
- Too little of the correct drug
- Wrong drug, device, intervention, or regimen prescribed; more efficacious choice possible

Adapted with permission from Canaday BR, Yarborough PC. Documenting pharmaceutical care: Creating a standard. Ann Pharmacother 1994;28:1292–1296.

---

[4]Canaday BR, Yarborough PC. Documenting pharmaceutical care: Creating a standard. Ann Pharmacother 1994; 28:1292–1296.

[5]Foppe van Mil JW, Westerlund LT, Hersberger KE, et al. Drug-related problem classification systems. Ann Pharmacother 2004;38:859–867.

b. R = risks to patient
  (1) Adverse drug reaction/drug allergy
  (2) Potential for overlap of adverse effects; must be kept in mind as part of the workup or evaluation of any new complaint or problem reported by patient

c. I = interactions
  (1) Drug–drug, drug–disease, drug–food, drug–lab interactions

d. M = mismatch between medications and condition or patient needs
  (1) No indication for a current drug, device, or intervention
  (2) Indication for a drug, device, or intervention but none prescribed
  (3) Perceived or actual barriers to implementation of medication or behavior regimen, such as financial constraints; lifestyle issues; and intellectual, physical, or emotional limitations.

e. E = efficacy issues
  (1) Too much of the correct drug
  (2) Too little of the correct drug
  (3) Wrong drug, device, intervention, or regimen prescribed or more efficacious choice possible

C. Documentation of pharmaceutical care. Formulate a **FARM note** or **SOAP note** to describe and document the interventions intended or provided by the pharmacist.[6] Some healthcare facilities may specify one format over the other; pharmacists need to become proficient in each.

1. Format of a FARM note
  a. F = findings. The patient-specific information that gives a basis for, or leads to, the recognition of a pharmacotherapy problem or indication for pharmacist intervention. Within the FARM format, findings include subjective and objective information about the patient.
  b. A = assessment. The pharmacist's evaluation of the findings, including statements of:
    (1) Any additional information that is needed to best assess the problem to make recommendations
    (2) The severity, priority, or urgency of the problem
    (3) The short-term and long-term goals of the intervention proposed or provided.
      (a) Examples of **short-term goals:** eliminate symptoms, lower blood pressure (BP) to 140/90 mm Hg within 6 weeks, manage acute asthma flareup without requiring hospitalization
      (b) Examples of **long-term goals:** prevent recurrence, maintain BP at <130/80 mm Hg, prevent progression of diabetic nerve disease
  c. R = resolution (including prevention). The intervention plan includes actual or proposed actions by the pharmacist or recommendations to other healthcare professionals. The rationale for choosing a specific intervention should be stated. Intervention options may include the following:
    (1) Observing, reassessing, or following—no intervention necessary at this time. If no action was taken or recommended, the FARM note serves as a record of the event and should constitute part of the patient's pharmacy chart or database.
    (2) Counseling or educating the patient or caregiver
    (3) Making recommendations to the patient or caregiver
    (4) Informing the prescriber
    (5) Making recommendations to the prescriber
    (6) Withholding medication or advising against use
  d. M = monitoring and follow-up. The parameters and timing of follow-up monitoring to assess the efficacy, safety, and outcome of the intervention. This portion of the FARM note should include the following:
    (1) The parameter to be followed (e.g., pain, depressed mood, serum potassium level)
    (2) The intent of the monitoring (e.g., efficacy, toxicity, adverse event)
    (3) How the parameter will be monitored (e.g., patient interview, serum drug level, physical examination)

[6]Canaday BR, Yarborough PC. Documenting pharmaceutical care: Creating a standard. Ann Pharmacother 1994; 28:1292–1296.

(4) Frequency of monitoring (e.g., weekly, monthly)

(5) Duration of monitoring (e.g., until resolved, while on antibiotic, until resolved then monthly for 1 year)

(6) Anticipated or desired finding (e.g., no pain, euglycemia, healing of lesion)

(7) Decision point to alter therapy when or if outcome is not achieved (e.g., pain still present after 3 days, mild hypoglycemia more than two times a week)

2. Format of a SOAP note. The SOAP format is the one used most often by medical practitioners; however, when used within the pharmaceutical care context, the content of the sections must be revised to match the pharmacist's legal scope of practice.

    a. S = subjective findings. The patient-specific *subjective* information that gives a basis for, or leads to, the recognition of a pharmacotherapy problem or indication for pharmacist intervention. Within the SOAP format, patient findings are delineated into subjective and objective data.

        (1) Subjective data are open to individual interpretation, whereas objective data are easily duplicated or quantified. Examples of subjective findings include the patient's statement of complaint (the chief complaint; cc) and duration or severity of symptoms.

        (2) Sometimes, the data to be noted are not clearly delineated as subjective or objective or there may be a preponderance of one type of data. In these instances, the subjective and objective data may be combined as a single section, labeled "S/O Findings."

    b. O = objective findings. The patient-specific *objective* information that gives a basis for, or leads to, the recognition of a pharmacotherapy problem or indication for pharmacist intervention. Examples of objective information include laboratory data, weight, height, blood pressure, and pulse.

    c. A = assessment. In the medical model, the assessment states the physician's working diagnosis and/or possible explanations for the patient's medical problem(s). In the pharmaceutical care model, however, diagnosis is not normally within the pharmacist's scope of practice. Instead, the assessment section includes the pharmacist's evaluation of the subjective and objective findings in a manner similar to the description of the assessment in the FARM format (see IV.C.1.b).

    d. P = plan. In the medical model, the plan states the physician's intended drug regimen(s), surgical procedures, and/or diagnostic tests. In the pharmaceutical care model, pharmacists may not have the authority to initiate or alter drug therapy regimens or order laboratory tests. Laboratory or prescriptive authority may be granted on a state-by-state basis, under collaborative protocol with specific physician(s) or within a specific healthcare facility or system. Actions included within the plan section should be identified as *recommended* actions when appropriate. In the pharmaceutical care model, the plan is usually expanded to describe information included in the monitoring and follow-up section of the FARM note (see IV.C.1.d).

V. FOCUSED AREAS OF PRACTICE. This phrase refers to areas of speciality practice in which pharmacists are increasingly being recognized for their therapeutic or management expertise. As such, pharmaceutical care provided by the pharmacist is augmented by activities not normally provided within the generalist pharmacist role. Categories of focused practice may best be described by the type and extent of specialty activities. *Activities for each descriptive level are additive to, or augment, the previous level*—that is, focused drug monitoring incorporates and expands the activities of pharmaceutical care; focused disease monitoring incorporates the activities of pharmaceutical care plus focused drug monitoring, and so on.

    A. Drug monitoring. Specialized monitoring for a specific drug or drug therapy for a specific disease state. Examples are the following:

        1. Extensive patient education concerning the drug, the drug monitoring process, and the pharmacist's and patient's responsibilities for focused drug monitoring. It must be stressed to the patient that for the focused drug monitoring program to be effective, the pharmacist must have access to information concerning *all* the medications being taken by, or prescribed for, the patient.

2. Each time the patient returns for a refill of the monitored medication (e.g., for hypertension, diabetes, hyperlipidemia, circulation, cardiovascular disease, glaucoma):
   a. Perform a **compliance check** (expected versus actual refill date) and determine *why* the needed medication or supplies are not being refilled. Physical, financial, intellectual, mental, or emotional issues may be involved, requiring referral to other healthcare providers or requiring other innovative solutions. Take the responsibility and appropriate action to resolve these issues.
   b. Ask about the occurrence and frequency of **side effects,** especially those related to quality of life—such as orthostatic hypotension, changes in sexual function, energy level, exercise tolerance, hypoglycemia, hyperglycemia, and ability to concentrate. Counsel the patient about strategies to minimize these effects or contact the prescriber to offer options to resolve the patient's reported problems.

3. With each new **prescription or over-the-counter (OTC) medication** added to the monitored drug regimen, observe and counsel the patient concerning the following:
   a. Drugs that may affect the efficacy of the monitored drug (drug–disease and drug–drug interactions). For example, with diabetes medications:
      (1) Certain drugs may directly change blood glucose levels.
      (2) Certain drugs may indirectly change blood glucose levels by interacting with the hypoglycemic agent.
   b. Drugs that may affect the course of the disease for the monitored drug. For example, certain drugs added to a diabetes regimen may affect the complications of diabetes by aggravating neuropathy and nephropathy as a result of decreased circulation.
   c. Drugs that may affect comorbidity conditions of the disease for the monitored drug. For example, certain drugs added to a diabetes regimen may affect concurrent hypertension, lipid abnormalities, and other conditions that occur more frequently in the diabetic population.

4. Remind and encourage patients to adhere to schedules for recommended **laboratory tests** during the course of the drug therapy. Examples include prothrombin time tests, liver function tests, eye examinations, and renal function tests. Adherence to such monitoring parameters will allow prevention or early detection and treatment of certain adverse drug effects.

B. **Disease monitoring.** Specialized monitoring for a specific disease state. Disease-monitoring activities are optimally performed at regular intervals (e.g., at set appointment times), but should at least be performed each time the patient returns for refill of a disease-related medication or supply.

1. A focused disease-monitoring program is extensive in time, effort, and patient education. At this level, however, the pharmacist does not initiate changes in pharmacological therapies. Recommendations for changes are relayed to the medical provider, who then directs the pharmacist concerning specific regimen adjustments.

2. Examples of focused disease-monitoring activities are the following:
   a. **Extensive patient education** concerning the disease and its treatment, the disease-monitoring process, and the pharmacist's and patient's responsibilities for focused disease monitoring. Education will likely be needed initially and periodically during the monitoring program.
   b. Focused monitoring of a *chronic* disease would include patient education to establish the patient's desired *targets or goals* and strategies to attain them.
      (1) Encourage and assist patients to set long-term goals—for example, lose 30 lb or quit smoking.
      (2) Encourage and assist patients to set short-term goals that are directed toward meeting the long-term goals—for example, lose 1 lb in 1–2 weeks or decrease smoking by one cigarette per day.
   c. Assessment for **subjective evidence** of *improvement or worsening of disease symptoms.*
      (1) The frequent or consistent occurrence of certain symptoms (such as asthma attacks, hypoglycemia, chest pain, diarrhea from ulcerative colitis) should be brought to the attention of the medical provider.

        (2) Lack of subjective evidence of efficacy (failure of pain control, minimal or no improvement of nocturia) should also be reported to the prescriber.

        (3) The patient's report of days of work or school missed owing to exacerbation of disease symptoms is a valuable assessment of disease control or treatment.

    d. Assessment for **objective evidence** or *certain indices of disease control or treatment.* For example, a pharmacist may review and guide a diabetic patient in interpretation of self-monitored blood glucose (SMBG) records. Using these data, the pharmacist can then advise the patient concerning the application of a prescribed insulin adjustment algorithm.

        (1) Some data may be patient derived, such as SMBG, weight, measurement of calf circumference, and readings from a peak-flow meter.

        (2) Some data may be pharmacist initiated, such as a pharmacy-based lipid-monitoring program, blood glucose testing, and blood pressure measurements. It should be noted that a pharmacy may need to be **Clinical Laboratories Improvement Act** (CLIA) certified before performing certain waived or moderately complex laboratory procedures.

        (3) Some data may be obtained through the physician's office; a copy is forwarded to the pharmacist or brought in by the patient.

C. Drug/disease management by protocol. The components of this focused practice include the following:

    1. Disease and drug monitoring, including a significant component of patient education

    2. Disease and quality-of-life outcomes identified and agreed on by patient, medical provider, and pharmacist

    3. Application of a drug-disease-management protocol, developed as a collaborative work relationship between pharmacist and medical provider, which elaborates specific authorizations or limitations for the pharmacist's activities. Components of a drug-disease-management protocol may include the following:

        a. Process by which the physician refers the patient to the pharmacist

        b. Drugs, devices, medical treatment, tests and procedures that may be prescribed, administered, or ordered, as appropriate for the treatment of the health problem addressed by the protocol

            (1) Drug initiation, dosage adjustment and/or discontinuation

            (2) Specific laboratory orders and interpretation

        c. Limited physical assessment

        d. Integration of the pharmaceutical care plan into the total medical care plan for the patient

        e. Predetermined plan for emergency services

        f. Written communication/documentation to/from medical provider (e.g., chart access and note entry)

VI. CLINICAL SKILLS AND PHARMACIST'S ROLES IN PHARMACEUTICAL CARE. The skills, activities, and services inherent in the provision of pharmaceutical care include the following:

A. Patient assessment

    1. Physical assessment

    2. Barriers to adherence

    3. Psychosocial issues

B. Patient education and counseling

    1. Interview skills

    2. Communication skills (e.g., empathy, listening, speaking or writing at the patient's level of understanding)

    3. Ability to motivate, inspire

    4. Develop and implement a patient education plan based on an initial education assessment

    5. Identification and resolution of compliance barriers

C. Patient-specific pharmacist care plans

    1. Recognition, prevention, and management of drug interactions

    2. Pharmacology and therapeutics (innovative and conventional)

    3. Interpretation of laboratory tests

    4. Knowledge of community resources, professional referrals

    5. Communication and rapport with community medical providers

D. Drug-treatment protocols

    1. Develop and maintain (update) protocols.

    2. Follow protocols as a pharmacist clinician.

    3. Monitor aggregate adherence to treatment protocols (e.g., drug-use evaluations; DUEs), especially for a managed-care or health-system facility.

E. Dosage adjustment

    1. Identify patients at risk for exaggerated or subtherapeutic response.

    2. Apply pharmacokinetic principles to determine patient-specific dosing.

    3. Order and interpret relevant tests at correct time intervals to assess dosage adjustment (e.g., plasma drug concentrations, blood glucose levels, blood pressure measurements).

F. Selection of therapeutic alternatives

    1. Use drug information resources effectively.

    2. Review and critique drug literature.

    3. Construct comparative analyses to support therapeutic decisions.

G. Prescriptive authority in designated practice sites or positions

H. Preventive services

    1. Immunizations

    2. Screenings

    3. Health and wellness education

I. Managerial skills

    1. Plan, direct, and implement pharmaceutical-care activities within a variety of practice environments, such as community pharmacy, ambulatory-care settings, managed or contractual care, home-health services, long-term-care facilities, inpatient hospital practice, and others.

    2. Allocate resources.

VII. PHARMACEUTICAL CARE AS THE MODEL FOR PHARMACY PRACTICE. The concepts, activities, and services of pharmaceutical care form the basis for provision of clinical services directly to, and for the benefit of, patients in all pharmacy practice settings. These settings include home-health, hospital, ambulatory-care, primary-care, consultation, long-term-care, and community pharmacy practice. Work flow, staffing patterns, processes, and pharmacy programs might differ, but the core approach to patient care remains pharmaceutical care in all settings.

VIII. DOCUMENTATION OF PHARMACEUTICAL CARE. "If it isn't documented, it isn't done!" Documentation of pharmaceutical care is integral to continuity of care, demonstration of clinician competence, communication among health-care providers, evidence of contributions to patient care, and reimbursement of professional services.

A. **Pharmaceutical care,** including the pharmaceutical care plan process (CORE, PRIME, FARM, or SOAP), is a systematic method for recording the pharmacist's examination of a patient's pharmacotherapy and subsequent identification of medication-related problems.

B. **Computer software programs,** in most practice settings, maintain patient data and drug-profile records. Thus after documentation of the initial pharmaceutical care plan, patient data or drug regimens are included in subsequent FARM (or SOAP) notes only if a change occurs that is relevant to the therapeutic issue being addressed in the note.

C. Forms that summarize pharmacists' interventions using a **unified coding system** are useful for processing reimbursement or billing forms, but these forms are not adequate documentation of pharmaceutical care. These forms do not communicate to other health professionals the depth and quality of pharmacist interventions or the pharmacist's plan for ongoing pharmaceutical care.

IX. PHARMACEUTICAL CARE: AN ONGOING PROCESS. The **patient profile** (database) is revised and reassessed each time a new drug is added to or deleted from the medication regimen, a new disease or condition is diagnosed, or the patient undergoes other clinical intervention, such as surgery. When the patient returns to the pharmacy or is readmitted to the health system facility, the pharmacist uses the patient profile, PWDT, and FARM (or SOAP) notes (maintained in the patient pharmacy chart or in the medical chart) as the basis for ongoing pharmacist–patient interactions.

X. IMPORTANCE OF PHARMACEUTICAL CARE IN TODAY'S PHARMACY PRACTICE

A. The potential for **medication errors** is growing, and one professional group must assume a primary role in addressing this issue, rather than various groups or individuals making fragmented efforts. The pharmacist is trained specifically to address these therapeutic issues.

B. The use of prescription and nonprescription medications is growing and now constitutes the primary therapeutic modality available to healthcare practitioners and patients.

C. The number, complexity, and potency of prescription and nonprescription drug products are increasing.

D. The need for pharmaceutical care secures an enduring role for the pharmacist in the U.S. healthcare system. Every encounter with patients, regardless of practice setting, provides pharmaceutical care.

E. Pharmaceutical-care activities integrate pharmacists into the healthcare system of the future.

STUDY QUESTIONS

Directions: Each of the questions, statements, or incomplete statements can be correctly answered or completed by **one** of the suggested answers or phrases. Choose the **best** answer.

1. Which of the following statements best describes FARM?

(A) cultivation of a pharmacist's knowledge to better serve the public
(B) findings, assessment, resolution, monitoring
(C) findings, assessment, recognition, management
(D) the process by which an individual pharmacist interacts with a specific patient to attain pertinent medical information

2. An example of an expanded role of the pharmacist is

(A) community leader.
(B) preparation of compounded prescriptions.
(C) maintaining adequate inventory of orphan drugs.
(D) triage of patients.

3. What is the most important focus of pharmaceutical care?

(A) pharmacist
(B) patient
(C) prescription
(D) patient chart

4. Which of the following statements regarding pharmaceutical care is true? Pharmaceutical care

(A) usually does not overlap into other areas of heath care.
(B) and clinical pharmacy are synonymous.
(C) implies that the pharmacist is no longer responsible for dispensing functions.
(D) is based on strategies to provide continuous patient care to attain desired outcomes.

5. Essential components of pharmaceutical care include

(A) patient–pharmacist relationship, legible physician orders, and accurate data collection.
(B) pharmacist–patient relationship and workup of drug therapy.
(C) a software program that accesses medication history and prompts the pharmacist concerning questions to ask the patient.
(D) maintenance of patient medication history for at least 2 years and a focus on acute illness.

6. In the CORE pharmacotherapy plan, what does the *E* stand for?

(A) education of patient or caregiver
(B) efficacy issues
(C) elaboration
(D) evaluation parameters

7. The most important reason for using the FARM note is to

(A) collect information for the physician.
(B) document problem-solving and/or interventions performed by the pharmacist.
(C) keep a log of all drug interactions.
(D) create a uniform method of recording patient information.

8. Which of the following topics would *not* be included in the assessment portion of the FARM note?

(A) recommendations made to the patient or caregiver
(B) severity, priority, or urgency of the problem
(C) short-term and long-term goals of the intervention
(D) additional information that is needed to best assess the problem

9. Immunizations, screenings, and wellness education are examples of which clinical skill?

(A) community health overview
(B) patient medication education and counseling
(C) preventive services
(D) managerial services

10. The pharmacist's role in the selection of therapeutic alternatives requires which of the following clinical skills?

(A) review and critique drug literature
(B) motivate and inspire patients
(C) perform drug-use evaluations (DUEs)
(D) knowledge of community resources

ANSWERS AND EXPLANATIONS

1. The answer is B *[see IV.C]*
A FARM progress note is used to describe and document the interventions intended or provided by the pharmacist. The acronym FARM stands for findings, assessment, resolution, and monitoring and follow-up.

2. The answer is D *[see II.A]*.
Pharmaceutical care has evolved from an emphasis on prevention of drug-related problems to the expanded roles of triage of patients, treatment of routine acute illnesses, management of chronic diseases, and primary disease prevention.

3. The answer is B *[see IV.A]*.
Pharmaceutical care is based on a collaborative effort between pharmacist and patient.

4. The answer is D *[see I.B; IX]*.
The term *pharmaceutical care* describes specific activities and services through which an individual pharmacist cooperates with a patient and other professionals in designing, implementing, and monitoring a therapeutic plan that will produce specific therapeutic outcomes for the patient. The patient profile (database) is revised and the potential for drug-related problems is reassessed each time a new drug is added to or deleted from the medication regimen, a new disease or condition is diagnosed, or the patient undergoes other clinical intervention (e.g., surgery).

5. The answer is B *[see IV.A–B]*.
The essential components of pharmaceutical care are the pharmacist–patient relationship and the pharmacist's workup of drug therapy.

6. The answer is D *[see IV.B.2]*.
The acronym CORE refers to the components of the pharmacotherapy plan, which is part of the pharmacist's workup of drug therapy. CORE stands for condition (or patient need), outcome (desired for that condition), regimen (selected to achieve that outcome), and evaluation parameters (to assess outcome achievement).

7. The answer is B *[see IV.C; VIII; IX]*.
The FARM note is the pharmacist's progress note, describing and documenting the interventions intended or provided by the pharmacist. This constitutes the progress note in the medical chart (in health-system facilities) or in the pharmacy patient chart (in community pharmacy or sites without ready access to the medical chart).

8. The answer is A *[see IV.C]*.
The assessment portion of the FARM note states the pharmacist's evaluation of the findings. Recommendations are made to the patient or caregiver to resolve or prevent an actual or potential problem identified by the pharmacist. Thus such recommendations would be included in the resolution portion of the FARM note.

9. The answer is C *[see VI.H]*.
Immunizations, screenings, and health and wellness education are examples of clinical skills used in a pharmacist's provision of preventive services.

10. The answer is A *[see VI.F]*.
For effective selection of therapeutic alternatives, a pharmacist would use certain clinical skills, including use of drug information resources, comparative analyses, and review and critique of drug literature.

21

Drug Information Resources

Paul F. Souney

Connie Lee Barnes

I. **DEFINITION.** Drug information is current, critically examined, relevant data about drugs and drug use in a given patient or situation.

A. **Current information** uses the most recent, up-to-date sources possible.

B. **Critically examined information** should meet the following criteria:

1. More than one source should be used when appropriate.

2. The extent of agreement of sources should be determined; if sources do not agree, good judgment should be used.

3. The plausibility of information, based on clinical circumstances, should be determined.

C. **Relevant information** must be presented in a manner that applies directly to the circumstances under consideration (e.g., patient parameters, therapeutic objectives, alternative approaches).

II. **DRUG INFORMATION RESOURCES.** There are three sources of drug information: journals (primary sources), indexing and abstracting services (secondary sources), and textbooks (tertiary sources).

A. **Primary sources**

1. **Benefits.** Journal articles provide the most current information about drugs and, ideally, should be the source for answering therapeutic questions. Journals enable pharmacists to:
   a. Keep abreast of professional news
   b. Learn how another clinician handled a particular problem
   c. Keep up with new developments in pathophysiology, diagnostic agents, and therapeutic regimens
   d. Distinguish useful from useless or even harmful therapy
   e. Enhance communication with other healthcare professionals and consumers
   f. Obtain continuing education credits
   g. Share opinions with other healthcare professionals through letters to the editor
   h. Prepare for the board certification examination in pharmacotherapy, nutrition support, and so on.

2. **Limitations.** Although publication of an article in a well-known, respected journal enhances the credibility of information contained in an article, this does not guarantee that the article is accurate. Many articles possess inadequacies that become apparent as the ability to evaluate drug information improves.

B. **Secondary sources**

1. **Benefits.** Indexing and abstracting services are valuable tools for quick and selective screening of the primary literature for specific information, data, citation, and articles (Table

Table 21-1. Examples of Abstracting and Indexing Services

Secondary References	Journals Indexed	Lag Time
CINAHL	1200	—
ClinAlert	150	1–6 weeks
Current Contents Connect	8000	1–6 weeks
Embase	4550	20 days
Medline/PubMed	4500	1 week
Inpharma	1800	3 weeks–6 months
International Pharmaceutical Abstracts	500	6–14 months
Iowa Drug Information System	200	3–12 months
Pharmaceutical News Index	—	2–8 weeks
Reactions	1800	3 weeks–6 months
Science Citation Index	3700	3–12 months

Cumulative Index to Nursing and Allied Health Literature

21-1). In some cases, the sources provide sufficient information to serve as references for answering drug information requests.

2. **Limitations.** Each indexing or abstracting service reviews a finite number of journals. Therefore, relying on only one service can greatly hinder the thoroughness of a literature search. Another important fact to remember is the substantial difference in lag time (i.e., the interval between the publication of an article and the citation of that article in an index) among the available services. Several examples are given in Table 21-1.
   a. Secondary sources usually **describe** only articles and clinical studies from journals. Frequently, readers respond to, criticize, and add new information to published articles and studies through letters. Services such as Medline/PubMed or the Iowa Drug Information Service generally do include pertinent letters to the editor within the scope of coverage.
   b. Indexing and abstracting services are primarily used to **locate** journal articles. In general, abstracts should not be used as primary sources of information because they are generally interpretations of a study and may be a misinterpretation of important information. Pharmacists should obtain and evaluate the original article because abstracts might not tell the whole story.

C. Tertiary sources

1. **Benefits.** General-reference textbooks can provide easy and convenient access to a broad spectrum of related topics. Background information on drugs and diseases is often available. Although a textbook might answer many drug-related questions, the limitations of these sources should not be overlooked.
   a. It could take several years to publish a text, so information available in textbooks might not include the most recent developments in the field. Other resources should be used to update or supplement information obtained from textbooks.
   b. The author of a textbook might not have done a thorough search of the literature, so pertinent data could have been omitted. An author also might have misinterpreted the primary or secondary literature. Reference citations should be available to verify the validity and accuracy of the data.

2. **General considerations** when examining and using textbooks as sources of drug information include the following:
   a. The author, publisher, or both: What are the author's and publisher's track records?
   b. The year of publication (copyright date)
   c. The edition of the text: Is it the most current edition?
   d. The presence of a bibliography: If a bibliography is included, are important statements accurately referenced? When were the references published?
   e. The scope of the textbook: How accessible is the information?
   f. Alternative resources that are available (e.g., primary and secondary sources, other relevant texts)

III. INTERNET

A. Benefits. The Internet expands the ability to search therapies that have been recently published or discussed in the media. An Internet search may be required for the following: company-specific information, issues currently in the news, alternative medicine, or U.S. government information. The most popular Web browsers are Mozilla Firefox and Microsoft Internet Explorer. A variety of search engines, software tools for searching the Internet, have been developed. General search engines (AltaVista, Google, Yahoo, About, HotBot, Lycos) attempt to index as much of the Internet as possible.

B. Limitations

1. Unlike information published in journals and textbooks, information obtained from the Internet may not be peer reviewed or edited before release.

2. Information received from the Internet may be only as reliable as the person who posted it and the users who read and comment on its content. A Web site should be evaluated by its source (author) of information. The name, location, and sponsorship should be disclosed. Also, a reputable site will provide easy access to information and the ability to give feedback. Pharmacists should use traditional literature evaluation skills to determine whether information on Web site is clear, concise, unbiased, relevant, and referenced.

C. Use. To obtain information from the Internet, the user must have an address (referred to as a URL, or uniform resource locator) to type into the browser, which will then find the site automatically. Many associations and organizations have Web sites that are linked to other Web pages. Table 21-2 provides a selection of Web sites.

Table 21-2. Selected Web Sites

Site	URL (Web Address)
Agency for Healthcare Research and Quality	www.ahrq.gov
American Association of Colleges of Pharmacy	www.aacp.org
American Cancer Society	www.cancer.org
American Diabetes Association	www.diabetes.org
American Heart Association	www.americanheart.org
American Society of Health-System Pharmacists	www.ashp.org
Centers for Disease Control and Prevention	www.cdc.gov
Clinical Trial Results	www.clinicaltrialresults.org
Clincal Trials	www.clinicaltrials.gov
Drug Infonet	www.druginfonet.com
eMedicine	www.emedicine.com
Healthfinder	www.healthfinder.gov
Health on the Net Foundation	www.hon.ch
Mayo Clinic College of Medicine	www.mayo.edu
Medscape	www.medscape.com
MedWatch	www.fda.gov/medwatch
National Cancer Institute	www.cancer.gov
National Guideline Clearinghouse	www.guideline.gov
National Heart, Lung, and Blood Institute	www.nhlbi.nih.gov
National Institutes of Health	www.nih.gov
National Library of Medicine	www.nlm.nih.gov
Pharmaceutical Research and Manufacturers of America	www.phrma.org
PharmacyOneSource	www.pharmacyonesource.com
Pharmscope	www.pharmscope.com
RxList	www.rxlist.com
RxMed	www.rxmed.com
U.S. Department of Health and Human Services	www.os.dhhs.gov
U.S. Food and Drug Administration	www.fda.gov
WebMD	www.webmd.com

IV. STRATEGIES FOR EVALUATING INFORMATION REQUESTS. It is important to obtain as many clues as possible about drug information requests before beginning a literature search. Both time and money can be wasted doing a vast search. Below are important questions to ask the inquirer or to evaluate before a manual or computerized search.

   A. Talk with the inquirer. Before spending time searching for information, talk to the person who is requesting the information and acquire any necessary additional information.

      1. Determine the reason for the inquiry. Find out where the inquirer heard or read about the drug. Is he or she taking the medication? If so, why? Because the search can be done by the drug or disease name, determine if the inquirer has a medical condition. Ascertaining the reason for the inquiry helps determine what additional information should be provided. For example, if the inquiry concerns a foreign drug, the inquirer might ask for a domestic equivalent.

      2. Clarify the drug's identification and availability. Make sure that the drug in question is available and double-check information about the drug, such as:
        a. The **correct spelling** of the drug's name
        b. Whether it is a **generic** or **brand name drug**
        c. What **pharmaceutical company** manufactures the drug and in what **country** the drug is manufactured
        d. Whether the drug is **prescription** or **nonprescription**
        e. Whether the drug is still **under investigation** and, if it is on the market, **the length of time on the market**
        f. The **dosage form** of the drug
        g. The **purpose** of the drug (i.e., what medical condition or symptom the drug is intended to alleviate; this information helps narrow the search if products with similar names are found)

   B. To **identify** or **assess product availability,** consider using the following resources (see also Appendix E). Some of these resources are available in an electronic format or in an Internet/intranet version.

      1. For drugs manufactured in the **United States,** the following resources are available:
        a. *The American Drug Index,* updated annually
        b. *Drug Facts and Comparisons,* updated monthly and bound annually
        c. *Drug Topics Red Book,* periodically supplemented and updated annually
        d. *Physician's Desk Reference (PDR),* updated annually
        e. *American Hospital Formulary Service (AHFS) Drug Information,* supplemented quarterly and updated annually
        f. *Martindale: The Complete Drug Reference,* updated every 3 years

      2. For drugs manufactured in **foreign countries,** the following resources are available:
        a. *Martindale: The Complete Drug Reference*
        b. *Index Nominum*
        c. *United States Adopted Names (USAN)* and the *United States Pharmacopoeia (USP) Dictionary of United States Adopted Names (USAN)*

      3. For **investigational drugs,** the following resources are available:
        a. *Martindale: The Complete Drug Reference*
        b. *Drug Facts and Comparisons*
        c. F-D-C Reports, including "The Pink Sheet"
        d. *The NDA Pipeline* published by FDC Reports

      4. For **orphan drugs**—that is, drugs that are used to prevent or treat a rare disease (affects < 200,000 people in the United States, so the cost of development is not likely to be offset by sales) and for which the U.S. Food and Drug Administration (FDA) offers assistance and financial incentives to sponsors undertaking the development of the drugs—the following resources are available:
        a. *Drug Facts and Comparisons*
        b. *The National Information Center for Orphan Drugs and Rare Diseases (NICODARD),* maintained by the FDA Office of Orphan Products Development
        c. The National Institutes of Health (NIH) Office of Rare Diseases
        d. National Organization for Rare Disorders

5. For an **unknown drug** (i.e., one that is in hand but not identified), chemical analysis can be performed or the drug can be identified by physical characteristics, such as color, special markings, and shape. Consult the following sources for help:
   a. *PDR's Drug Facts and Comparisons (eFacts), Drug Topics Red Book, Ident-A-Drug Reference*
   b. *Identidex (Micromedex)*
   c. The manufacturer
   d. A laboratory
   e. *Lexi-Comp (Lexi-Drug ID)*
   f. *Clinical Pharmacology Product Identification*

V. SEARCH STRATEGIES.
To develop an effective search strategy for locating drug information literature, the following tactics should be followed after determining whether primary or secondary sources are desired.

   A. Determine whether the question at hand is **clinical** or **research related. Define the question** as specifically as possible. Also, identify appropriate index terms (also called keywords or descriptors) with which to search for the information.

   B. Determine the **type of information** and **how much** is needed (i.e., only one fact, the most recent journal articles, review articles, or a comprehensive database search).

   C. Ascertain as much information as possible about the drug being questioned and the **inquirer's association** with it. Remember that data on adverse drug effects or drug interactions are often fragmented and inadequately documented. See IV.A.2 for the specific drug information that should be acquired. Determine the answers to the following questions:
   1. What is the indication for the prescribed drug?
   2. Is the drug's use approved or unapproved? This information can be found in the following resources (remember to check how often these resources are updated to ensure having the latest information).
      a. **Approved uses** of drugs can be checked in:
         (1) *AHFS Drug Information* for the current year and in the year's supplements
         (2) *Drug Facts and Comparisons (eFacts)*
         (3) *PDR*
         (4) *USP Drug Information*
         (5) *Drugdex (Micromedex)*
         (6) *Clinical Pharmacology*
         (7) *Drug Information Handbook (Lexi-Comp)*
      b. **Unapproved uses** of drugs can be found in:
         (1) *AHFS Drug Information*
         (2) *Drug Facts and Comparisons*
         (3) *Martindale: The Complete Drug Reference*
         (4) Medline
         (5) *Drugdex*
         (6) *Inpharma*
         (7) *USP Drug Information*
   3. What are the age, sex, and weight of the patient in question?
   4. Does the patient have any other medical conditions or renal or hepatic disease?
   5. Is the patient taking any other medications?
   6. What drugs has the patient taken during the past 6 months, and what were the dosages?
   7. Did the patient experience any signs or symptoms of a possible adverse drug reaction? If so:
      a. How severe was the reaction?
      b. When did the reaction appear?
      c. Has the patient (or any member of the patient's family) experienced any allergic or adverse reactions to medications in the past?

 d. Consult the following resources for more information:
   (1) Meyler's *Side Effects of Drugs* (SEDBASE online)
   (2) A general drug reference
   (3) *Reactions* (Ovid)
   (4) Medline
 e. The manufacturer of the drug may be a useful source for missing information. In exchange for information, most companies expect to receive an adverse drug reaction form.

8. Did the patient experience any signs or symptoms of a drug interaction? If so:
 a. What were the specific drugs in question?
 b. What were the respective dosages of the drugs?
 c. What was the duration of therapy?
 d. What was the length of the course of administration?
 e. What are the details of the events secondary to the suspected reaction?
 f. Consult the following resources for more information:
   (1) A drug interactions reference—for example, *Drug Interaction Facts,* Hansten's *Drug Interaction Analysis and Management, Evaluations of Drug Interactions (EDI)*
   (2) A general drug reference (e.g., *PDR*)
   (3) *Reactions*
   (4) Medline

9. What is the patient's current medication status?

10. Does the patient have any underlying diseases?

11. How has the patient been managed so far?

12. What is the stability of the drug? How is compatibility of the drug with other drugs? What are the administration technique and the equipment that holds it? Resources to check for this information include
 a. Trissel's *Handbook on Injectable Drugs*
 b. King's *Guide to Parenteral Admixtures*
 c. Trissel's *Stability of Compounded Formulations*

D. Explore other possible information resources if necessary. For example, it may be useful to find background material in textbooks (tertiary references), and then go to the journal literature (primary references) for more current information.

VI. EVALUATING A CLINICAL STUDY. Resource identification is followed by a critical assessment of the available information. This step is critical in developing an appropriate response for the inquirer.

A. Evaluate the objective of the study. Determine the aim of the research that was performed.

 1. What did the researchers intend to examine?

 2. Is this goal stated clearly (i.e., is the objective specific)?

 3. Was the research limited to a single objective, or were there multiple drugs or effects being tested?

B. Evaluate the subjects of the study. Determine the profile of the study population by looking for the following information:

 1. Were healthy subjects or affected patients used in the study?

 2. Were the subjects volunteers?

 3. What were the criteria for selecting the subjects?

 4. How many subjects were included, and what is the breakdown of age, sex, and race?

 5. If a disease was being treated, did any of the subjects have diseases other than that initially being treated? Were any additional treatments given? Were there any contraindications to the therapy?

6. What was the patient selection method and who was excluded from the study?

7. A patient selection review should be done. You will find that most groups of subjects are homogeneous (i.e., they all have comparable characteristics). If a disease state is studied, patients should exhibit similar severity of symptoms. Researchers wish to eliminate interpatient variability. By selecting patients with similar characteristics, researchers can avoid results that are caused by individual differences among patients. Strong individual differences can obscure the results of the experiment. If studying a group of patients who exhibit significant interpatient variability is necessary, researchers may divide the patients into groups according to the variables likely to be associated with responsiveness to therapy. This is known as stratification.

C. Evaluate the administration of the drug treatment. For each drug being investigated, determine the following information:

    1. Details of treatment with the agent being studied:
        a. Daily dose
        b. Frequency of administration
        c. Hours of day when administered
        d. Route of administration
        e. Source of drug (i.e., the supplier)
        f. Dosage form
        g. Timing of drug administration in relation to factors affecting drug absorption
        h. Methods of ensuring compliance
        i. Total duration of treatment

    2. Other therapeutic measures in addition to the agent being studied

D. Evaluate the setting of the study. Try to determine the environment of the study and the dates on which the trial began and ended. Look for the following information:

    1. People who made the observations; various professionals who offer different and unique perspectives based on their backgrounds and interests (Were the same people making observations throughout the study?)

    2. Whether the study was done on an inpatient or outpatient basis

    3. Description of physical setting (e.g., hospital, clinic, ward)

    4. Length of the study (i.e., dates on which the trial began and ended)

E. Evaluate the methods and design of the study. The method section of the research paper explains how the research was conducted. The study design (i.e., retrospective, prospective, blind, crossover) and the methods used to complete the study are important in judging whether the study and the results are reliable and valid. From the study, try to determine answers to the following questions:

    1. Are the methods of assessing the therapeutic effects clearly described?

    2. Were the methods standardized?
        a. Retrospective versus prospective
            (1) Retrospective studies look at events that have already occurred to find some common link among them, require reliance on patient memories and accurate medical records, and are unable to show cause and effect. Retrospective studies are useful for studying rare diseases (or effects) and can help a healthcare professional decide if enough information exists to warrant prospective examination of a problem.
            (2) Prospective studies look forward in time at a question the study seeks to answer. They can be observational or experimental (i.e., clinical trials).
        b. Treatment allocation
            (1) Parallel study design is a protocol in which two or more patient groups are studied concurrently. The groups are treated identically except for one variable, such as a drug therapy (Figure 21-1).
            (2) Crossover design may be used as an additional control for interpatient and intrapatient variability (Figure 21-2). In this type of design, each patient group undergoes each type of treatment. However, the sequence in which the subjects undergo treat-

Figure 21-1. Parallel study design.

ment is reversed for one group. Crossover design reduces the possibility that the results were strongly influenced by the order in which therapy was given. And because both groups of patients receive both types of treatment, any differences in responsiveness between the groups as a result of patient selection will be uncovered.

3. Were **control measures** used to reduce variation that might influence the results? Examples of such control methods include
   a. Concurrent controls
   b. Stratification or matched subgroups
   c. A run-in period
   d. The patient as his or her own control (i.e., crossover design)
   e. Identical ancillary treatment

4. Were controls used to reduce bias? Examples of such controls include
   a. **Blind assessment,** which means that the people observing the patients do not know who is a subject and who is a control
   b. **Blind patients,** which means that the patients do not know whether they received the substance being studied or a placebo (**double-blind** combines this point with point a above [VI.E.4.a]) (Table 21-3)
   c. **Random allocation,** which means that patients involved in the study have an even chance of being assigned to either the group of subjects receiving the active drug or the group receiving a placebo
   d. **Matching dummies,** which are placebos that are physically identical to the active agent being studied
   e. **Comparison** of a placebo or a therapy to a recognized standard practice

F. **Evaluate the analysis of the study.** After looking at specific areas of the study separately, gather the information together to determine whether the trial is acceptable and the conclusions are justified by determining answers to the following questions (Figure 21-3):

1. Were the subjects suitably selected in relation to the aim(s) of the study?

2. Were the methods of measurement valid in relation to the aim(s) of the study?

3. Were the methods adequately standardized?

4. Were the methods sufficiently sensitive?

5. Was the design appropriate?

6. Were there enough subjects?

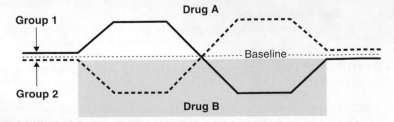

Figure 21-2. Crossover study design.

Table 21-3. Types of Blind Studies

Types of Blinds	Patient Aware of Treatment	Physician Aware of Treatment
Open label (nonblind)	X	X
Single-blind	—	X
Double-blind	—	—

7. Was the dosage appropriate?

8. Was the duration of treatment adequate?

9. Were carryover effects avoided, or were compensations made for them?

10. If no controls were used, were they unnecessary or overlooked?

11. If controls were used, were they adequate?

12. Was the comparability of treatment groups examined?

13. Are the data adequate for assessment?

14. If statistical tests were not done, were they unnecessary or overlooked?

15. If statistical tests are reported, assess the following:
    a. Is it clear how the statistical tests were done?
    b. Were the tests appropriately used?
    c. If results show no significant difference between test groups, were there enough patients (i.e., statistical power)?

VII. GENERAL GUIDELINES FOR RESPONSES TO DRUG INFORMATION REQUESTS

A. **Do not guess!**

B. Responses to a member of the public must take several ethical issues into account.

1. Patient privacy must be protected.

2. Professional ethics must be maintained.

3. The patient–physician relationship cannot be breached.

4. Response is not necessary if the inquirer intends to misuse or abuse information that is provided. The inquirer often admits intent or offers clues to potential abuse, such as in the following examples:
    a. A patient asks how a certain drug is dosed (i.e., how much the drug can be increased, when it can be increased, what the maximum daily dose is). This kind of inquiry signals that the patient might be adjusting his or her own therapy.
    b. A patient asks a pharmacist to identify a tablet that is a prescription product known for a high rate of abuse.

C. Organize information before attempting to communicate the response to the inquirer. Anticipate additional questions.

D. Tailor the response to the inquirer's background. Also, consider the environment of the practice, institutional policy and procedure, and formulary.

E. Tell the inquirer where the information was found. Exercise caution when making statements such as, "There are no reports in the literature."

F. Use *extreme* caution when making statements such as, "I recommend . . ." Do not hesitate to refer consumers to their physicians.

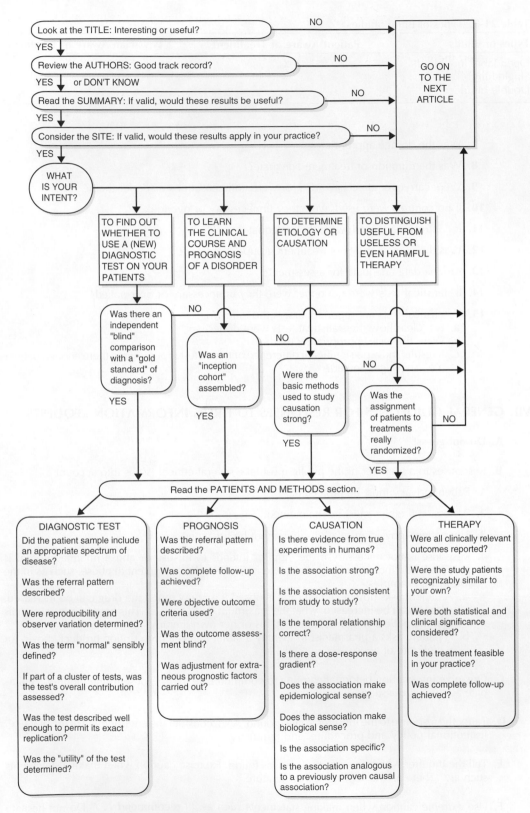

Figure 21-3. Evaluation of study analysis.

G. Use more than abstracts to answer drug information questions because they might be taken out of context and do not include all of the data available in the original article.

H. Alert the inquirer of a possible delay when it takes longer than anticipated to answer the question.

I. Ask if the information that is provided answers the inquirer's questions.

J. Ask if the inquirer wishes to have reprints of articles or a written response.

22
Adverse Drug Reaction Reporting
Barbara Szymusiak-Mutnick

I. INTRODUCTION. Adverse drug reactions (ADRs) are a cause of significant morbidity and mortality in patients in all areas of health care today. There is wide variation in the current healthcare literature, but it has been estimated that from one third to as high as one half of ADRs are believed to be preventable. The Institute of Medicine reported in January 2000 that an estimated 7000 deaths occur each year as a result of medication errors. Other studies estimate significantly higher numbers of deaths. The cost of morbidity and mortality owing to drug-related adverse events in the ambulatory population was recently estimated to be $75 billion annually. There are an estimated 3 million hospital admissions each year caused by the misuse of pharmaceuticals. The suffering that patients experience because of drug-related events cannot be quantified.

II. DEFINITIONS. The terms *adverse drug reaction, adverse drug event, untoward drug reaction, drug misadventure, side effect, medication errors, misuse of pharmaceuticals,* and *drug-related problem* are many times used interchangeably but do not always describe the same situation.

A. The National Coordinating Council for Medication Error Reporting and Prevention defines a **medication error** as "any event that may cause or lead to inappropriate medication use or patient harm while medication is in the control of the health care professional, patient, or consumer."[1]

B. The U.S. Food and Drug Administration's (FDA) definition of an **adverse drug** event is "any adverse event associated with the use of a drug in humans, whether or not considered drug related, including the following: an adverse event occurring in the course of the use of a drug in professional practice; an adverse event occurring from a drug overdose, whether accidental or intentional; an adverse event occurring from drug abuse; an adverse event occurring from drug withdrawal; and any significant failure of expected pharmacological action."[2]

C. Adverse drug reaction is defined by the World Health Organization (WHO) as "one which is noxious and unintended, and which occurs at doses normally used in man for the prophylaxis, diagnosis, or therapy of disease, or for the modification of physiological function."[3]

III. TYPES OF ADVERSE DRUG REACTIONS

A. Type A

1. Type A reactions are extensions of the drug's known pharmacology and are responsible for the majority of ADRs.

2. Type A reactions are usually dose dependent and predictable but can be the result of concomitant disease states, drug–drug interactions, or drug–food interactions.

3. Ways to minimize type A reactions include understanding the pharmacology of the drug being prescribed, monitoring drugs with a narrow therapeutic index, and avoiding polypharmacy when possible.

---

[1]http://www.nccmerp.org/aboutMedErrors.html
[2]http://a257.g.akamaitech.net/7/257/2422/04nov20031500/edocket.access.gpo.gov/cfr_2001/aprqtr/pdf/21cfr314.80. pdf#search=%2221%20CFR%20314.80(a)%22
[3]http://www.who.int/patientsafety/highlights/COE_patient_and_medication_safety_gl.pdf

B. Type B

1. Type B reactions include idiosyncratic reactions, immunological or allergic reactions, and carcinogenic/teratogenic reactions.

2. Type B reactions are usually not the result of a known pharmacology of the drug but seem to be a function of patient susceptibility. They are rarely predictable, are usually not dose dependent, and seem to concentrate in certain body systems such as the liver, blood, skin, kidney, and nervous system.

3. Type B reactions are uncommon but are generally serious and can be life threatening.

4. Except for immediate hypersensitivity reactions, type B reactions usually take 5 days before the patient demonstrates hypersensitivity to a drug. There is no maximum time for the occurrence of a reaction, but most occur within 12 weeks of initiation of therapy.

IV. RECOGNITION

A. Drugs must always be considered as a possible cause of disease or symptoms that are among a patient's list of complaints. Complete drug histories, including nonprescription drugs, must also be carried out.

B. Recognition is often subjective, and it is not always possible to demonstrate strong causality between the drug and the occurrence.

1. Several factors may help in assessing the determination of causality.
   a. Did the patient actually ingest the drug in question?
   b. Did the onset of symptoms occur after the drug was taken?
   c. What is the time interval between taking the drug and the onset of symptoms?
   d. Did the symptoms resolve or improve after the drug was stopped or the dose decreased?
   e. Did the symptoms reoccur after the drug was reintroduced?
   f. Did drug–drug interactions contribute to the symptoms?
   g. Were the drugs measured in "toxic levels" in the patient's serum?
   h. Has this reaction been previously seen with use of the drug?
   i. What is the personal experience of the clinician with previous use of the drug and reactions secondary to the drug?

2. Nomograms have been developed to aid in the assessment of causality.

V. SURVEILLANCE PROGRAMS. Pharmacists as well as all healthcare professionals should take an active role in monitoring, reporting, and trending ADR information. Some of the activities involved in a concurrent and ongoing ADR surveillance program at an institutional level include the following components:

A. Pharmacy departments should take the lead in the collection of information and should submit all reviews and reports to the pharmacy and therapeutics committees for review and evaluation.

1. Encourage all healthcare professionals to be involved in reporting.

2. Monitor patients who are using high-risk agents.

3. Review patients who have received "antidote"-type drugs.

4. Notify prescribers of suspected ADRs, and encourage thorough documentation of the description of the reaction as well as the outcome in patients' medical records.

5. Report appropriately identified ADRs to the FDA.

6. Develop the use of pharmacy computer systems to track ADRs.

B. Evaluation of the causes of ADRs should be carried out. ADR report information should be used for educational purposes and identification of drug use and medication use processes to prevent further occurrences of such reactions. ADR reporting information should be incorporated into institutional risk management programs.

VI. REPORTING TO THE FDA. Three of the five major centers at the FDA are involved with evaluating the safety and efficacy of drugs. The largest center is the Center for Drug Evaluationand Research (CDER), which oversees both prescription and nonprescription—over-the-counter (OTC)—drugs. In 2002, CDER established the Adverse Events Reporting System (AERS), a computerized data base designed to support the FDA's postmarketing safety program for drugs and therapeutic biologic products. Annually, the AERS receives about 400,000 reports of adverse experiences possibly associated with drugs. The Center for Biological Evaluation and Research (CBER) ensures the safety and efficacy of blood products, vaccines, allergenics, biological therapeutics, gene therapy, medical devices and tests, xenotransplantation products, and banked human tissue and cellular products. The Center for Food Safety and Applied Nutrition (CFSAN) established the CFSAN Adverse Events Reporting System (CAERS) in 2002. The CAERS provides a monitoring system to identify potentially serious problems secondary to non-FDA-approved herbs, minerals, vitamins, dietary supplements, and other substances.

A. The national **Vaccine Adverse Event Reporting System** (VAERS) is coadministered by the CBER and the Centers for Disease Control and Prevention (CDC). More than 10 million vaccines are given to children and many million more doses to adults each year. Although vaccines protect many people from dangerous diseases, they do have the potential to cause adverse effects.

    1. The National Childhood Vaccine Injury Act (NCVIA) requires health professionals to report
        a. Adverse events after the administration of vaccines specified in the act, as described in the "Reportable Events Table," within the specified time period (available at www.vaers.hhs.gov/reportable.htm or 1-800-822-7967)
        b. Any event listed in the manufacturer's package insert as a contraindication to subsequent doses of the vaccine

    2. In 1990, VAERS was set up to receive all reports of suspected adverse events caused by any U.S. licensed vaccine (Figure 22-1).

    3. The VAERS depends on voluntary reporting by health professionals to:
        a. Identify rare adverse reactions not detected in prelicensing studies
        b. Monitor for increases in already known reactions
        c. Identify risk factors or preexisting conditions that promote reactions
        d. Identify particular vaccine lots with unusually high rates or unusual types of events

B. MedWatch, the FDA's Medical Products Reporting Program established in 1993, is a voluntary system for healthcare providers(Figure 22-2). However, manufacturers and distributors of FDA-approved drugs, biologics, radiation-emitting devices, special nutritional products, dietary supplements, infant formulas, and devices are mandated to report problems to the FDA. The goals of the program are to increase awareness of reporting of medical-product–induced diseases and the importance of reporting, to clarify what should be reported, to make reporting as easy as possible, and to provide feedback to health professionals.

    1. Importance of reporting
        a. The incidence of ADRs occurs at a high rate in health care today.
            (1) Generally, it is reported that 3%–11% of all hospital admissions can be attributable to ADRs, although some studies report the figure to be as high as 29%.
            (2) The likelihood that a patient will experience an ADR while hospitalized is reported in the literature to be in a range from 1% to 44%.
        b. Prevention of ADRs is an important strategy in health care. It has been estimated that at least one third of all ADRs may be preventable. It has been further noted that preventable ADRs tend to be the most costly to treat and cause the greatest degree of patient morbidity.
            (1) Future ADRs can be prevented in individual patients by careful and consistent documentation in patient records.
            (2) A program that tracks ADRs can help discover previously unidentified trends. These trends can be used within the institution to develop programs of prospective intervention to prevent reoccurrence of the reaction in the patient populations that are at similar risk.
        c. Recognition of previously undiscovered ADRs attributable to a drug is particularly true in the case of newly marketed products.
            (1) Although clinical trials are generally effective in assessing efficacy and risk to benefit ratio, inherent limitations exist in premarketing trials.

VAERS

VACCINE ADVERSE EVENT REPORTING SYSTEM
24 Hour Toll Free Information 1-800-822-7967
P.O. Box 1100, Rockville, MD 20849-1100
PATIENT IDENTITY KEPT CONFIDENTIAL

For CDC/FDA Use Only

VAERS Number _____

Date Received _____

Patient Name:

_____

Last _____ First _____ M.I.

Address

_____

_____

_____

City _____ State _____ Zip

Telephone no. (____) _____

Vaccine administered by (Name):

_____

Responsible
Physician _____
Facility Name/Address
_____
_____
_____

City _____ State _____ Zip

Telephone no. (____) _____

Form completed by (Name):

_____

Relation ☐ Vaccine Provider ☐ Patient/Parent
to Patient ☐ Manufacturer ☐ Other
Address *(if different from patient or provider)*
_____
_____
_____

City _____ State _____ Zip

Telephone no. (____) _____

| 1. State | 2. County where administered | 3. Date of birth / / mm dd yy | 4. Patient age | 5. Sex ☐M ☐F | 6. Date form completed / / mm dd yy |

7. Describe adverse events(s) (symptoms, signs, time course) and treatment, if any

8. Check all appropriate:
☐ Patient died (date ___/___/___ mm dd yy)
☐ Life threatening illness
☐ Required emergency room/doctor visit
☐ Required hospitalization (_____ days)
☐ Resulted in prolongation of hospitalization
☐ Resulted in permanent disability
☐ None of the above

9. Patient recovered ☐ YES ☐ NO ☐ UNKNOWN

12. Relevant diagnostic tests/laboratory data

10. Date of vaccination / / mm dd yy
Time _____ AM PM

11. Adverse event onset / / mm dd yy
Time _____ AM PM

13. Enter all vaccines given on date listed in no. 10

Vaccine (type)	Manufacturer	Lot number	Route/Site	No. Previous Doses
a.				
b.				
c.				
d.				

14. Any other vaccinations within 4 weeks prior to the date listed in no. 10

Vaccine (type)	Manufacturer	Lot number	Route/Site	No. Previous doses	Date given
a.					
b.					

15. Vaccinated at:
☐ Private doctor's office/hospital ☐ Military clinic/hospital
☐ Public health clinic/hospital ☐ Other/unknown

16. Vaccine purchased with:
☐ Private funds ☐ Military funds
☐ Public funds ☐ Other/unknown

17. Other medications

18. Illness at time of vaccination (specify)

19. Pre-existing physician-diagnosed allergies, birth defects, medial conditions(specify)

20. Have you reported this adverse event previously?
☐ No ☐ To health department
☐ To doctor ☐ To manufacturer

Only for children 5 and under

22. Birth weight _____ lb. _____ oz.

23. No. of brothers and sisters

21. Adverse event following prior vaccination (check all applicable, specify)

	Adverse Event	Onset Age	Type Vaccine	Dose no. in series
☐ In patient				
☐ In brother or sister				

Only for reports submitted by manufacturer/Immunization project

24. Mfr./imm. proj. report no.

25. Date received by mfr./imm.proj.

26. 15 day report? ☐ Yes ☐ No

27. Report type ☐ Initial ☐ Follow-Up

Health care providers and manufacturers are required by law (42 USC 300aa-25) to report reactions to vaccines listed in the Table of Reportable Events Following Immunization Reports for reactions to other vaccines are voluntary except when required as a condition of immunization grant awards.

Form VAERS-1(FDA)

Figure 22-1. VAERS form for reporting possible adverse drug reactions.

Figure 22-2. Form for reporting possible adverse drug reactions to the FDA Medical Products Reporting Program.

(a) The trials are usually relatively short in duration and do not effectively mimic the exposure patients would experience if using the drug as a chronically administered agent.

(b) Drug–drug interactions and use in patients with concomitant disease states may not be tested for in these trials.

(c) The small size of the trials (usually 1000–3500 individuals) is insufficient to detect rarely occurring adverse reactions.

(d) Racial and ethnic groups may not be participating in the same numbers as represented in the general population.

    d. Prompt recall in cases of product problems are accomplished when the MedWatch Program is used to report product problems or device defects.

  2. What should be reported?

    a. ADRs that are serious, even if causality is not proven, including

      (1) A patient's death that is suspected of being a direct outcome of an ADR

      (2) A life-threatening event

      (3) An initial or prolonged hospitalization

      (4) A significant, persistent, or permanent change or disability/incapacity

      (5) A congenital anomaly (including those occurring in a fetus)

      (6) Other problems that aren't listed in the manufacturer's package insert as a known side effect

    b. Malfunctioning medical devices such as heart valves, latex gloves, dialysis machines, and ventilators and problems with nutritional products

    c. Product problems that can result in compromised safety or quality, including product contamination, mislabeling, unclear labeling, poor packaging, potency problems, and questionable stability

    d. Counterfeit or suspected counterfeit drugs

    e. Adverse events with food, herbs, vitamins, cosmetics, or dietary supplements, although CAERS is the prefered reporting system

    f. Adverse events owing to blood products, allergenics, gene therapy, human tissue and cellular products, and xenotransplantation products

    g. Medication errors

  3. Confidentiality of both the reporter and the patients whose cases are reported are substantially protected by the FDA.

  4. Reporting of problems with OTC medications are required when the product has been marketed with a new drug application (NDA), including drugs formerly marketed as prescription-only drugs. OTC products marketed without an NDA do not require reporting, but reporting is strongly encouraged. Approval of the FDA is not required for the marketing of nonprescription herbs, minerals, vitamins, dietary supplements, and other substances. Because the FDA does not approve these substances, efficacy and safety do not have to be demonstrated, nor is it mandated to report problems to the FDA.

  5. Reporting to manufacturers is not described in the FDA's guidelines, although a section of the MedWatch form can be checked off to inform the FDA that a copy of the report has been forwarded to the manufacturer by the reporter.

C. Information on previously reported events

  1. The FDA Web site provides on-line safety information at www.fda.gov/medwatch/safety.htm gathered from approximately 25,000 reports that are submitted each year.

  2. Clinically important product safety alerts are available via an automated e-mail message-delivery system from www.fda.gov/medwatch/elist.htm.

  3. FDA alerts also appear on www.Pharmacist.com, a joint venture of the American Pharmacist Association and the National Association of Boards of Pharmacy.

VII. American Society of Health-Systems Pharmacists (ASHP) Guidelines define criteria for classifying an ADR as significant. They encourage reporting of serious or unexpected ADRs to the FDA, the manufacturer, or both.

VIII. Joint Commission on Accreditation of Healthcare Organizations (JCAHO) requirements for accreditation describe the need for each healthcare organization to monitor for adverse events involving drugs and devices in a continual, collaborative fashion.

IX. *United States Pharmacopeia (USP).* Medication Errors Reporting Program at www.usp.org/ patientSafety/mer/ and the USP-Institute for Safe Medication Practices (ISMP) Medication Errors

Reporting Program at https://www.ismp.org/orderforms/reporterrortoISMP.asp are two programs involved in collection of medication error data.

X. FURTHER INFORMATION

A. Information about the MedWatch program can be obtained by phone at 1-800-FDA-1088 and at www.fda.gov/Medwatch/.

B. Information about VAERS can be obtained by phone at 1-800-822-7967 and at www.fda.gov/cber/vaers/vaers.htm.

C. Information about reporting to the CFSAN program can be obtained by phone at 301-436-2405 or at www.cfsan.fda.gov.

D. Further information about the FDA's reporting systems and programs, such as CDER, can be found on the FDA's Web site (www.fda.gov).

STUDY QUESTIONS

Directions: Each of the questions, statements, or incomplete statements can be correctly answered or completed by **one** of the suggested answers or phrases. Choose the **best** answer.

1. The phrase "one which is noxious and unintended, and which occurs at doses normally used in man for the prophylaxis, diagnosis, or therapy of disease, or for the modification of physiological function," describes

(A) a side effect.
(B) an adverse drug reaction.
(C) an adverse drug event.
(D) a medication error.

2. Type A reactions are characterized by which of the following?

(A) idiosyncratic reactions
(B) a function of patient susceptibility
(C) caused by drug–drug interactions
(D) All of the above
(E) None of the above

3. The MedWatch form is *not* the appropriate form to report which of the following events?

(A) a vaccine event described in the Vaccine Adverse Event Reporting System (VAERS) "Reportable Events Table"
(B) a suspected counterfeit drug
(C) a malfunctioning ventilator
(D) a drug that is contained in a package with unclear labeling
(E) None of the above

4. Preventable adverse drug reactions (ADRs)

(A) generally display mild symptoms.
(B) are always easily recognized.
(C) are problems that are easily medically managed.
(D) All of the above
(E) None of the above

5. Reporting problems with vitamins to the FDA is required by law in which of the following situations?

(A) when the problem is discovered by the consumer
(B) when safety and efficacy have been proven by manufacturers to the FDA
(C) when a healthcare professional discovers the problem
(D) All of the above
(E) None of the above

ANSWERS AND EXPLANATIONS

1. The answer is B *[see II.C].*
This is the definition from the WHO.

2. The answer is C *[see III.A.2].*
Type A reactions can be caused by drug–drug interactions. Idiosyncratic reactions and reactions caused by patient susceptibility are generally in the classification of Type B reactions.

3. The answer is A *[see VI.A.1].*
All the others are reportable on the MedWatch form. The National Childhood Vaccine Injury Act requires the use of a VAERS form to report vaccine-related injuries.

4. The answer is E *[see VI.B.1].*
Preventable ADRs can be the cause of serious medical problems that require intensive medical care. Although some preventable ADRs may appear obvious on review of a patient's medication history, this is not always the case.

5. The answer is E *[see VI.B.4].*
Marketing of these products does not depend on the manufacturers proving efficacy and safety of the products. No law requires reporting of subsequent problems. These products do not require an NDA. Although it is not required for healthcare professionals to report problems, it is essential that voluntary reporting takes place.

23
Medication Errors
Robert Cisneros

I. MEDICATION ERROR PROBLEM

  A. The 2000 Institute of Medicine (IOM) report *To Err Is Human* brought the problem of errors in medicine to national attention.[1]

   1. An estimated 44,000–98,000 **deaths per year** are caused by medical errors. **Of those deaths,** approximately 7,000 are the result of medication errors.

   2. A call to action was given to improve patient safety.

  B. In recent years, tragic medication errors have focused attention on concerns regarding patient safety.

   1. A chemotherapy mix up at a major cancer center resulted in the death of a patient from a **fourfold overdose** daily for 4 days.

   2. A child accidentally received an **intravenous rather than intramuscular** dose of long-acting penicillin and died.

   3. A compounding error resulted in death of a child who received a tricyclic antidepressant at a dose **10 times greater than the dose prescribed** by physician.

II. ERROR DEFINITION.
The National Coordinating Council for Medication Error Reporting and Prevention (NCCMERP) defines a medication error as follows: "A medication error is any preventable event that may cause or lead to inappropriate medication use or patient harm while the medication is in the control of the health care professional, patient, or consumer. Such events may be related to professional practice, health care products, procedures, and systems, including prescribing; order communication; product labeling, packaging, and nomenclature; compounding; dispensing; distribution; administration; education; monitoring; and use."[2]

III. TYPES OF ERRORS.
The following categories of errors have been used in numerous research studies.[3]

  A. **Wrong drug error.** A drug that was not ordered for a patient was administered—for example, a patient accidentally received furosemide 40 mg orally. Possible causes: The pharmacist accidentally filled the patient's prescription for an antibiotic with furosemide; the pharmacist reached for the wrong bottle on the shelf and did not check the label carefully enough.

  B. **Extra dose error.** A patient receives more doses of a drug than were ordered—for example, a patient was supposed to receive a medication with breakfast for 3 days but received it for 5 days. Possible cause: The patient's nurse was confused by the medication directions.

  C. **Omission error.** A dose of a drug was not administered as ordered but was skipped—for example, a patient was supposed to receive digoxin 0.25 mg orally in the morning but did not receive the dose. Possible cause: The patient's nurse was so busy that he or she forgot to administer the dose.

---

[1]Kohn LT, Corrigan JM, Donaldson MD, et al., eds. To Err Is Human: Building a Safer Health System. Washington, DC, National Academy Press, 2000.
[2]NCCMERP, "What Is a Medication Error," available at www.nccmerp.org/aboutMedErrors.html.
[3]Cohen MR, ed. Medication Errors. Washington, DC, American Pharmaceutical Association, 1999.

D. Wrong dose or wrong strength error. Either the wrong dose of a medicine or the wrong strength is administered—for example, the patient was supposed to receive warfarin 0.5 mg but received warfarin 5 mg instead. Possible causes: The pharmacist misread the label; the physician wrote the order as "warfarin .5 mg." Another example: a patient was supposed to receive timolol 0.25% but was given timolol 0.5%. Possible cause: The pharmacist took the wrong product off of the shelf, confused by the concentrations.

E. Wrong route error. A patient receives a dose of a medication by a route that was not ordered by the physician—for example, a patient was supposed to receive prochlorperazine 10 mg intramuscularly but the drug was administered intravenously. Possible causes: The nurse misread the orders; the physician mistakenly wrote "IV" instead of "IM".

F. Wrong time error. A patient does not receive a dose of medication at the time at which it was to be administered—for example, a hospitalized patient with diabetes is scheduled to receive a dose of insulin immediately before breakfast (at 7:00 A.M.) but the dose is given 2 hr after breakfast. Possible cause: The nurse was busy and could not give dose on time.

G. Wrong dosage form error. A patient receives a dose of medicine in a dosage form that was not intended—for example, nicotinic acid 500 mg tablets were ordered for a patient who instead receives nicotinic acid 500 mg slow-release capsules. Possible cause: The pharmacist did not carefully check the product or was confused by the label.

H. Other. Errors that do not fit into any of the into any of the other categories.

IV. COMMON ERROR HAZARDS

A. Dangerous abbreviations. Numerous common abbreviations and symbols have been associated with errors. Detailed lists are available from the Institute for Safe Medication Practices (ISMP) at www.ismp.org/Tools/abbreviationslist.pdf and the Joint Commission on Accreditation of Healthcare Organizations (JCAHO) at http://www.jointcommission.org/PatientSafety/DoNot UseList/. JCAHO's accredited organizations are required to avoid using the potentially confusing abbreviations on its "Do Not Use" list.

  1. **U, IU: unit(s).** The letter *U* can easily be misinterpreted as a number (e.g., 0 or 4), and serious harm has occurred with insulin and heparin as a result of this confusion. For example, a patient received 66 units of insulin instead of 6 units. The order, which was written for "6U" of regular insulin was misread as 66. The word *units* should be written out in full.

  2. **QD, Q.D., qd, q.d. (daily).** These common abbreviations have been misinterpreted as "QID" or "qid" (four times daily) resulting in overdoses. The word *daily* should be written out in full.

  3. **Q.O.D, QOD, qod (every other day).** These common abbreviations have been misinterpreted as QID (four times daily), resulting in overdoses. The words *every other day* should be written out completely.

  4. **Trailing zero.** When a dose is ordered and followed with a decimal point and a zero, such as 2.0 mg or 25.0 mg, errors can occur. The decimal point may be missed and an overdose can occur. For example, warfarin 2.0 mg may be misinterpreted as 20 mg. Trailing zeros should be avoided, and the dose written without the additional zero—for example, warfarin 2 mg (instead of 2.0 mg).

  5. **Lack of leading zero.** A drug's dose may be less than 1 mg, such as for digoxin. Often the dose is written without a leading zero: digoxin .25 mg instead of digoxin 0.25 mg. Errors have occurred because the decimal point is missed—for example, warfarin .5 mg may be interpreted as warfarin 5 mg. Leading zeroes should be included, so the dose is written as digoxin 0.25 mg or warfarin 0.5 mg.

  6. **MS, MSO$_4$ (morphine sulfate), MgSO$_4$ (magnesium sulfate).** The abbreviations for morphine sulfate and magnesium sulfate are quite similar and can be confused. It is recommend that *morphine sulfate* and *magnesium sulfate* be written in out in full.

B. **Other confusing symbols, abbreviations.** There are numerous other hazardous symbols and abbreviations that should be used with caution when writing prescription orders and carefully examined when filling prescriptions. Examples include the following:

   1. **cc.** Stands for cubic centimeters and is often used instead of mL. This has been misinterpreted as a 0 (zero); use mL.

   2. **μg.** Used for micrograms—for example, levothyroxine 250 μg daily. The abbreviation has been mistaken for mg, and overdoses have occurred; better to use mcg or to write out the word *micrograms.*

   3. **<, >.** Symbols for less than (<) and greater than (>) have been mistaken for each other or misinterpreted as numbers. Better to write out the words *less than* or *greater than.*

   4. **HCT.** This abbreviation for "hydrocortisone" has been misinterpreted as hydrochlorothiazide. Better to write the word out completely.

   5. **HCl.** The abbreviation for "hydrochloric acid" has been misinterpreted as KCl (potassium chloride). Better to write out the words completely.

C. **Sound-a-like or look-a-like drug names.** A detailed list of confusing drug names can be found in the 2004 *United States Pharmacopeia* publication "USP Quality Review" (www.usp.org/pdf/EN/patientSafety/qr792004-04-01.pdf). Another list is available from ISMP (www.ismp.org/Tools/confuseddrugnames.pdf).

   1. Examples include the following:
      a. Amitriptyline and aminophylline
      b. Cisplatin and carboplatin
      c. K-Dur and Cardura

   2. To avoid these problems, the ISMP offers several suggestions, including the use of computerized reminders, name-alert stickers, and independent checks; opening the bottle in front of the patient, who can confirm the appearance; and reporting errors.

D. **High-risk drugs.** Certain **potent drugs** have been implicated in many serious and tragic medication errors. These have been called high-risk or high-alert drugs. A list of such medications can be found at www.ismp.org/Tools/highalertmedications.pdf. Examples include the following:

   1. **Blood-modifying agents such as heparin and warfarin.** Errors have resulted in serious injury or death from hemorrhaging as a result of overdose (patient receiving 10 mg instead of 1 mg) or from blood clots as a result of underdose (patient receiving 0.5 mg instead of 5 mg).

   2. **Narcotics and sedatives.** Central nervous system depression and respiratory arrest have resulted from errors with these drugs, such as diazepam 25 mg given intravenously instead of 2.5 mg.

   3. **Neuromuscular paralyzing agents such as succinylcholine and vecuronium.** Accidental use or inadvertent use before adequate ventilation procedures were started have resulted in respiratory arrest and death.

   4. **Chemotherapy drugs.** These drugs are associated with potent adverse effects, affecting numerous body systems, such as the immune, neurologic, and clotting systems. Deaths have occurred as a result of errors with these products. For example, vincristine was accidentally given to a child instead of vinblastine, resulting in death. Confusion over the dosing of cyclophosphamide resulted in a fatal fourfold overdose

V. SEVERAL SAFETY TECHNIQUES OBSERVED IN COMMUNITY PHARMACIES[4]

A. Keep work procedures organized and simplified.

B. Don't work on several prescriptions at once, just one at a time.

---

[4]Flynn EA, Barker KN, Carnahan BJ. National observation study of prescription dispensing accuracy and safety in 50 pharmacies. J Am Pharm Assoc 2003;43:191–200.

C. Manage interruptions, don't be pressured to rush.

D. Smell check.

E. Bar code check.

F. Use a magnifying glass when needed.

G. Enhance the design of the facility.

VI. ROOT CAUSE ANALYSIS (RCA). This is a structured process for identifying direct and indirect factors that contributed to a medication error. A framework for conducting an RCA is available at http://www.jointcommission.org/SentinelEvents/. See "Framework For Conducting a Root Cause Analysis."

A. Important questions to ask:

1. What happened and why?

2. What were the contributing factors?
    a. Age? Hours worked? Staffing?
    b. Workload? Stress? Confusing names? Location on shelf?
    c. Inadequate information? Communication?
    d. Inadequate equipment?
    e. Workplace atmosphere conducive to safety?
    f. Inadequate training of pharmacist or technician?

B. Latent defect. A **weakness in a system** that does not immediately result in an error but, under the right set of circumstances, can contribute to a mistake. For example:

1. Stocking look-alike or sound-alike drugs next to each other, contributing to a pharmacist incorrectly filling a prescription.

2. Inadequate training of employees, contributing to an error in which an automated dispensing machine was used improperly and a patient received the wrong medication.

VII. NATIONAL SAFETY EFFORTS

A. JCAHO's National Patient Safety Goals for Accredited Organizations can be found at http://www.jointcommission.org/PatientSafety/NationalPatientSafetyGoals/. Hospital goals include:

1. Improve the accuracy of patient identification. Have two means of identifying the patient other than room number.

2. Improve communication among caregivers. Verify and read back telephone and oral orders.

3. Create a list of "do not use" abbreviations. Standardize the abbreviations used, and prohibit the use of those that are prone to confusion and misinterpretation.

4. Improve the safe use of medicines.
    a. Limit the number of different concentrations available per drug product; standardize.
    b. Develop methods of identifying and reviewing sound-alike and look-alike drugs, preventing errors with them.
    c. All medications and containers should be properly labeled.

5. Reduce the risk of infections.
    a. Comply with all Centers for Disease Control and Prevention (CDC) recommendations for hand washing and hygiene.
    b. Thoroughly investigate all serious adverse events and deaths associated with infection acquired in a healthcare setting.

6. Keep accurate patient medication records and histories throughout the continuum of care.
    a. Ensure that a patient's medication records are complete and accurate when he or she is referred or transferred within or between organizations.

USP MEDICATION ERRORS REPORTING PROGRAM
Presented in cooperation with the Institute for Safe Medication Practices
USP is an FDA **medWatch** partner

MEDI-CATION ERRORS REPORTING PROGRAM

Date and time of event:

Please describe the error. Include description/sequence of events, type of staff involved, and work environment (e.g., code situation, change of shift, short staffing, no 24-hr. pharmacy, floor stock). If more space is needed, please attach a separate page.

Did the error reach the patient?   ❏ Yes ❏ No

Was the incorrect medication, dose, or dosage form administered to or taken by the patient?   ❏ Yes ❏ No

Circle the appropriate Error Outcome Category (select one—see back for details): A B C D E F G H I

Describe the direct result of the error to the patient (e.g., death, type of harm, additional patient monitoring).

Indicate the possible error cause(s) and contributing factor(s) (e.g., abbreviation, similar names, distractions, etc.).

Indicate the location of the error (e.g., hospital, outpatient or community pharmacy, clinic, nursing home, patient's home, etc.).

What type of staff or health care practitioner made the initial error?

Indicate if other practitioner(s) were also involved in the error (type of staff perpetuating error).

What type of staff or health care practitioner discovered the error or recognized the potential for error?

How was the error (or potential for error) discovered/intercepted?

If available, provide patient age, gender, diagnosis. Patient identification not required.

Please complete the following for the product(s) involved. (If more space is needed for additional products, please attach a separate page.)

	Product #1	Product #2
Brand Name		
Generic Name		
Manufacturer		
Labeler		
Dosage Form		
Strength/Concentration		
Type and Size of Container		

Reports are most useful when relevant materials such as product label, copy of prescription/order, etc., can be reviewed. Can these materials be provided? ❏ Yes ❏ No   Please specify:

Suggest any recommendations to prevent recurrence of this error, or describe policies or procedures you instituted or plan to institute to prevent future similar errors.

Name and Title

Telephone Number

E-mail

Facility Name, Address, and Zip

Your name and a copy of this report are routinely shared with the Institute for Safe Medication Practices (ISMP). Copies of reports will be sent to third parties such as the manufacturer/labeler, and to the Food and Drug Administration (FDA). You have the option of including your name on these copies.

In addition to releasing my name to ISMP, USP may release my identity to these third parties as follows (check boxes that apply):
❏ The manufacturer and/or labeler as listed above ❏ FDA ❏ Other persons requesting a copy of this report ❏ Anonymous to all third parties

Signature

Date

Return to:
USP PRN
12601 Twinbrook Parkway
Rockville, MD 20852-1790

Submit via the Web at www.usp.org/mer
Call Toll Free: **800-23-ERROR** (800-233-7767)
or FAX: 301-816-8532

Date Received by USP

File Access Number

PPE049G

©USPC 2001

Figure 23-1. The medication error form used by the *United States Pharmacopeia*. [Reprinted with permission of the *United States Pharmacopeia*.]

b. Proper communication of accurate patient medication information is critical for everyone involved in the patient's care.

B. The 100,000 Lives Campaign from the Institute for Healthcare Improvement can be found at www.ihi.org/IHI/Programs/Campaign/.

1. Use **evidence-based therapeutic measures** to prevent deaths from **acute myocardial infarction.**

2. **Prevent adverse drug events** (ADEs) by implementing medication reconciliation and ensuring accurate and up-to-date medication records throughout the patient's hospital stay.

3. **Prevent central line infections** by implementing appropriate procedures.

4. **Prevent surgical site infections** by appropriate care and antibiotic use.

5. **Prevent ventilator-associated pneumonia** by following appropriate proven steps.

C. The IOM in July 2006 released its report "Preventing Medication Errors." Several recommendations were made to improve patient safety including: enhancing role of patient in medication management, improving patient education, and increasing the use of technology, such as e-prescribing. This report can be accessed at www.iom.edu.

D. Medication error reporting. The reporting of medication errors provides critical safety feedback. Figure 23-1 shows the form used in the *United States Pharmacopeia's* error reporting program. Errors can be submitted anonymously via the Internet, by telephone, or by mail.

STUDY QUESTIONS

Directions: Each of the questions, statements, or incomplete statements can be correctly answered or completed by **one** of the suggested answers or phrases. Choose the **best** answer.

1. A major result in the 2000 Institute of Medicine (IOM) report is that

   (A) pharmacists are not blamed for the majority of medical errors.
   (B) surgeons make more mistakes than any other health professional.
   (C) pharmacists make more mistakes than any other health professional.
   (D) there is now more emphasis on error prevention.

2. A pharmacist is presented a prescription for 250 mcg of levothyroxine. Which of the following dosages would be equivalent to that amount?

   (A) 2.5 mg
   (B) 0.25 gm
   (C) 0.25 mg
   (D) 25 gm

3. A prescription is written for warfarin 1.0 mg. The community pharmacist accidentally dispenses 10 mg. The patient develops severe bleeding within 3 days and nearly dies. Which of the following is the most accurate assessment of this prescription?

   (A) A trailing zero is present in this prescription and could have contributed to the pharmacist's error.
   (B) This is an example of a leading zero, which contributed to the error and the patient tragedy.
   (C) Sound-alike medications contributed to this error.
   (D) This does not qualify as an error based on the National Coordinating Council for Medication Error Reporting and Prevention (NCCMERP) definition.

4. A hospital pharmacy begins stocking new intravenous mini-bags of a neuromuscular-blocking agent. The packaging is similar to a commonly used intravenous antibiotic. The addition of the new mini-bags was not widely communicated to all personnel. One weekend, several doses of this new product were accidentally dispensed in place of the intended doses of antibiotic. Several patients suffered respiratory arrest and one of the patients eventually died. What would a root cause analysis of this error find?

   (A) The only cause of this error was a pharmacist who was not paying attention. The pharmacist should be dismissed.
   (B) Poor communication practices is a latent defect in this pharmacy system and significantly contributed to the error.
   (C) The pharmacy technicians are to blame for this error, not the pharmacist, because the technicians obtained the mini-bags from stock and placed the labels on the bags. The pharmacist checked only the technician's work. The technician should be dismissed.
   (D) This is an example of an extra dose error.

5. What do the following abbreviations MS, MSO_4 and $MgSO_4$ have in common?

   (A) common abbreviations for morphine sulfate
   (B) common abbreviations for magnesium sulfate
   (C) should not be used in JCAHO-accredited institutions
   (D) approved abbreviations in most hospitals

6. A major error in a hospital pharmacy resulted in a total parenteral nutrition solution being mistaken for a cardioplegic solution for coronary bypass surgery. Which of the following is true regarding the root cause analysis that was done at the hospital after the error?

   (A) The primary objective is to find out which pharmacist made the mistake that allowed this to take place.
   (B) The result of the analysis would be the admission that an error had taken place.
   (C) All factors that could have contributed to this error would be identified and analyzed.
   (D) A root cause analysis would be inappropriate in this case.

ANSWERS AND EXPLANATIONS

1. The correct answer is D *[see I.A.2]*.
The IOM report revealed alarming data on deaths related to medical errors. The report contributed to increased efforts to improve patient safety.

2. The correct answer is C *[see III.D]*
Although this may seem to be an elementary question and answer, a wrong dose error such as this could easily lead to a serious injury or death to a patient.

3. The correct answer is A *[see IV.A.4]*
Warfarin 1.0 mg. is an example of a trailing zero. JCAHO has included this in its "Do Not Use" list of abbreviations. However, in the community setting, it is a practice that can still be frequently seen on prescriptions. When a trailing zero is observed, much caution should be exercised in interpreting the prescription.

4. The correct answer is B *[see VI.A.2]*
Poor communication was a major contributing factor to this tragic series of errors. The drug was a high-risk drug and had similar packaging as another commonly used drug. These are two major ingredients for the serious error that took place. This does not absolve the technician and pharmacist totally from any blame but emphasizes the significant role that failure of communication played within this pharmacy system. The system was as much or more to blame than any individuals. Firing the individuals does not repair the problem of poor communication in the system but only sets the stage for a similar mistake to occur again.

5. The correct answer is C *[see IV.A.6]*
These abbreviations are included in JCAHO's "Do Not Use" list. Errors resulting in serious harm have occurred after mix ups with morphine and magnesium.

6. The correct answer is C *[see VI.A.2]*
A root cause analysis is not intended to focus on blame but on all factors that could have been related to this error. Factors might have included training of pharmacist and technicians, the actual drug order, and the label. The contribution of such factors might not be discovered if the focus is on only identifying which pharmacist, technician, or other professional is to blame.

24
Clinical Toxicology
John J. Ponzillo

I. OVERVIEW

A. This chapter is intended to provide the reader with an overview of the management of various toxic exposures. Emergency medical services (EMS) should be immediately contacted to provide advanced life support for patients with unstable vital signs resulting from a poisoning exposure. In addition, these patients should be referred to a hospital for follow-up. A nationwide toll-free poison center number became available. This number, 800-222-1222 is available 24 hr/day and should be used by healthcare professionals and the general public when dealing with exposures to potentially toxic substances.

B. Definitions

1. **Clinical toxicology.** Focuses on the effects of substances in patients caused by accidental poisonings or intentional overdoses of medications, drugs of abuse, household products, or various other chemicals

2. **Intoxication.** Toxicity associated with any chemical substance

3. **Poisoning.** A clinical toxicity secondary to accidental exposure

4. **Overdose.** An intentional exposure with the intent of causing self-injury or death

C. Epidemiology. In 2004, more than 2.4 million accidental and intentional poisonings were reported to the American Association of Poison Control Centers (AAPCC). The majority of poison exposures (84.1%) were accidental. However, 1183 of these exposures resulted in death. More information can be found at the AAPCC's Web site (www.aapcc.org).

D. Information resources

1. **Computerized databases**
   a. ***Poisindex*** is a computerized CD-ROM database that is updated quarterly and is a primary resource for poison control centers.

2. **Printed publications.** Textbooks and manuals provide useful information regarding the assessment and treatment of patients exposed to various substances, although their usefulness is limited by the lag time of information published in the primary literature reaching updated editions.
   a. Ellenhorn MJ, ed. Medical Toxicology: Diagnosis and Treatment of Human Poisonings, 2nd ed. New York, Elsevier Science, 1997.
   b. Fraunfelder FT, Fraunfelder FW. Drug-Induced Ocular Side Effects, 5th ed. Little Rock: Butterworth-Heinemann, 2001.
   c. Goldfrank L, ed. Toxicologic Emergencies. 7th ed. Norwalk, CT: Appleton & Lange, 2002.
   d. Grant WM. Toxicology of the Eye, 4th ed. Springfield, IL: Charles C Thomas, 1995.
   e. Haddad LM, Shannon MW, Winchester JF, eds. Clinical Management of Poisoning and Drug Overdose, 3rd ed. Philadelphia: Saunders, 1998.
   f. Hedges JR, Henderson RG, eds. Terrorism and critical care: chemical, biological, radiologic, and nuclear weapons. Crit Care Clin 2005;21(4).
   g. Holstege CP, Rusyniak DE, eds. Medical Toxicology. Med Clin North Am 2005;8(6).
   h. Leikin JB, Paloucek FP. Poisoning and Toxicology Compendium, 3rd ed. Hudson, OH: Lexi-Comp, 2002.
   i. Olson KR, ed., with, Anderson IB, Benowitz NL, Blanc PD, et al. Poisoning and Drug Overdose, 4th ed. Stamford, CT, Appleton & Lange, 2004.

3. **Internet**[1]
   a. Centers for Disease Control and Prevention (CDC) at www.cdc.gov
   b. U.S. Food and Drug Administration (FDA) at www.fda.gov
   c. National Library of Medicine at www.nlm.nih.gov
   d. National Institute for Occupational Safety and Health (NIOSH) at www.cdc.gov/niosh
   e. American Society of Health-System Pharmacists at www.ashp.org
   f. Material Safety Data Sheets at www.msdssearch.com
   g. U.S. Environmental Protection Agency (EPA) at www.epa.gov
   h. Chemical Abstracts Service at www.cas.org

4. **Poison control centers** accredited by the AAPCC provide information to the general public and healthcare providers. These centers are the most reliable and up-to-date sources of information; thus the AAPCC's phone number (800-222-1222) should be readily available.

II. GENERAL MANAGEMENT

A. **Supportive care and ABCs.** Evaluating and supporting the vital functions (airway, breathing, and circulation [ABCs]) are the mandatory first steps in the initial management of drug ingestions. After the patient is stabilized, the specific issue(s) of poison management should be addressed.[2]

B. **Treatment** for patients with depressed mental status includes the following:

   1. To rule out or treat hypoglycemia, 50 mL of 50% dextrose in adults and 1 mL/kg in children, intravenously (IV)

   2. Thiamine 100 mg IV push (glucose can precipitate the Wernicke-Korsakoff syndrome in thiamine-deficient patients)

   3. Naloxone (Narcan) 0.4–2 mg IV push, if opiate ingestion is suspected

C. **Obtaining a history of exposure**

   1. **Identify** the substance(s) ingested, the route of exposure, the quantity ingested, the amount of time since ingestion, signs and symptoms of overdose, and any associated illness or injury. **Corroborate** history and other physical evidence (e.g., pill containers) from prehospital providers.

   2. **Neurological examination** evaluates any seizures, alterations in consciousness, confusion, ataxia, slurred speech, tremor, headache, or syncope.

   3. **Cardiopulmonary examination** evaluates any syncope, palpitations, cough, chest pain, shortness of breath, or burning or irritation of the upper airway.

   4. **Gastrointestinal (GI) examination** evaluates any abdominal pain, nausea, vomiting, diarrhea, or difficulty in swallowing.

   5. **Past medical history** should include
      a. Medications, including nonprescription (over-the-counter [OTC]) substances
      b. Use of herbal medications
      c. Alcohol or drug abuse
      d. Psychiatric history
      e. Allergies
      f. Occupational or hobby exposures
      g. Travel
      h. Prior ingestions
      i. Social history with potential for domestic violence or neglect
      j. Last normal menstrual period or pregnancy

---

[1] Since the terrorist attacks of September 11, 2001, there has been an increased awareness regarding bioterrorism. Although this chapter is not intended to review the management of biological or chemical warfare, the Web sites in this section contain specific and updated links regarding the treatment of these exposures. The reader is encouraged to review this information.

[2] American College of Emergency Physicians. Clinical policy for the initial approach to patients presenting with altered mental status. Ann Emerg Med 1999;33:251–281.

D. Routine laboratory assessment

    1. Complete blood cell (CBC) count

    2. Serum electrolytes

    3. Blood urea nitrogen (BUN); serum creatinine (SCr)

    4. Blood glucose

    5. Urinalysis

    6. Electrocardiogram (ECG)

    7. Chest roentgenogram and/or kidneys, ureters, and bladder (**KUB**) x-ray

E. Toxicology laboratory tests

    1. Advantages
        a. Confirm or **determine** the presence of a particular agent
        b. Predict the anticipated toxic effects or severity of exposure to some poisons
        c. Confirm or **distinguish** differential or contributing diagnosis
        d. Occasionally help **guide therapy**

    2. Disadvantages
        a. These tests cannot provide a specific diagnosis for all patients.
        b. All possible intoxicating agents cannot be screened.
        c. In critically ill patients, supportive treatment is needed before laboratory results of the toxicology screen are available.
        d. Laboratory drug-detection abilities differ.
        e. In general, only a **qualitative determination** of a substance or substances is necessary; however, **quantitative levels** of the following drugs are necessary to guide therapy:
            (1) Acetaminophen
            (2) Arsenic
            (3) Carbamazepine (Tegretol)
            (4) Carboxyhemoglobin
            (5) Digoxin (Lanoxin)
            (6) Ethanol
            (7) Ethylene glycol
            (8) Iron
            (9) Lead
            (10) Lithium (Eskalith)
            (11) Mercury
            (12) Methanol
            (13) Methemoglobin
            (14) Phenobarbital
            (15) Phenytoin (Dilantin)
            (16) Salicylates
            (17) Theophylline
            (18) Valproic acid (Depakene)

F. Skin decontamination should be performed when percutaneous absorption of a substance may result in systemic toxicity or when the contaminating substance may produce local toxic effects (e.g., acid burns). The patient's clothing is removed, and the areas are irrigated with copious quantities of water. **Neutralization should not be attempted.** For example, neutralizing acid burns with sodium bicarbonate will produce an exothermic chemical reaction, thereby exacerbating the patient's condition.

G. Gastric decontamination may be attempted when supportive care is begun. GI decontamination involves removal of the ingestant with emesis or lavage, the use of activated charcoal potentially to bind any ingestants, and the use of cathartics to hasten excretion and thereby limit absorption.

1. **Emesis**
   a. **Contraindications**
      (1) Children younger than 6 months of age
      (2) Patients with central nervous system (CNS) depression or seizures
      (3) Patients who have ingested a strong acid, alkali, or a sharp object
      (4) Patients with compromised airway protective reflexes (including coma and convulsions)
      (5) Patients who have ingested some types of hydrocarbons or petroleum distillates
      (6) Patients who have ingested substances with an extremely rapid onset of action
      (7) Patients with emesis after the ingestion
   b. **Syrup of ipecac.** Owing to concerns of safety, efficacy and the delay of antidote administration, syrup of ipecac is no longer recommended for general use. Ipecac may be administered within 30 min of an ingestion and **only on the advice of a poison control center.**[3]
      (1) Mechanism of action. The onset of emesis usually occurs within 30 min after syrup of ipecac. The effects last for approximately 2 hr and produce approximately three episodes of emesis in 60 min.
      (2) Dosages. Patients 6–12 months of age, 5–10 mL; patients 1–12 years of age, 15 mL; patients older than age 12 years, 30 mL. Each dose of syrup of ipecac should be followed with 120–240 mL of water. The patient should be upright to avoid accidental aspiration and should be supervised.
      (3) Adverse effects. Diarrhea, lethargy/drowsiness, and prolonged (> 1 hr) emesis

2. **Gastric lavage**
   a. **Use.** Gastric lavage is infrequently used in patients who are not alert or have a diminished gag reflex. This procedure should also be considered in patients who are seen early after massive ingestions. This procedure is **contraindicated in patients who have ingested acids, alkalis, or hydrocarbons.** In addition, **patients should not receive gastric lavage if they are at risk for GI perforation or if they are combative.**
   b. **Procedure.** Patients are placed in the left lateral decubitus position. Lavage is performed after a cuffed endotracheal tube is in place to protect the airway. After aspiration of the gastric contents, 250–300 mL of tap water or saline is instilled and then aspirated. The sequence should be repeated until the return is continuously clear for at least 2 L.

3. **Activated charcoal** adsorbs almost all commonly ingested drugs and chemicals and is usually administered to most overdose patients as quickly as possible. Commonly ingested substances not adsorbed include **ethanol, iron, lithium, cyanide, ethylene glycol, lead, mercury, methanol, organic solvents, potassium, strong acids,** and **strong alkalis.**
   a. **Dosage.** Activated charcoal (Actidose with sorbitol) is available as a colloidal dispersion with water or sorbitol. In **adults,** the dose of activated charcoal is 25–100 g; the dose in **children** 1–12 years of age is 25–50 g; the dose in children up to 1 year of age is 1 g/kg. Constipation has not been observed after the administration of a single dose of activated charcoal. **Multiple doses** of any cathartics should be avoided because they can cause electrolyte imbalances and/or dehydration. Toxic ingestions with drugs having an enterohepatic circulation (e.g., carbamazepine, theophylline, phenobarbital, tricyclic antidepressants, phenothiazines, digitalis) generally require that the charcoal be readministered every 6 hr to prevent reabsorption during recirculation.
   b. **Adverse effects.** Charcoal aspiration and empyema have been reported in the literature. As such, charcoal should be withheld if patients are vomiting. Bowel obstruction may occur with multiple doses of activated charcoal and/or patients who are receiving concomitant therapy with neuromuscular-blocking drugs.[4]

H. **Whole-bowel irrigation** has been shown to be effective under certain conditions, particularly when activated charcoal lacks efficacy. An isosmotic cathartic solution such as polyethylene glycol (GoLYTELY, Colyte) is used. The dosage is 1–2 L/hr given orally or by nasogastric tube until the rectal effluent is clear.

---

[3] American Academy of Clinical Toxicology and European Association of Poisons Centres and Clinical Toxicologists. Position statement: Syrup of ipecac. Clin Toxicol 1997;35:699–709.
[4] American Academy of Clinical Toxicology and European Association of Poisons Centres and Clinical Toxicologists. Position statement: Single-dose activated charcoal. Clin Toxicol 1997;35:721–741.

I. **Forced diuresis** and **urinary pH manipulation** may be used to enhance the elimination of substances, whose elimination is primarily renal, if the substance has a relatively small volume of distribution with little protein binding. However, the use of these methods is associated with fluid and electrolyte disturbances.

   1. **Alkaline diuresis** promotes the ionization of weak acids, thereby preventing their reabsorption by the kidney, which facilitates the excretion of such weak acids. This procedure has been used in the management of patients who have ingested long-acting barbiturates such as phenobarbital or salicylic acid. Patients are given 50–100 mEq of sodium bicarbonate IV push, followed by a continuous infusion of 50–100 mEq of sodium bicarbonate in 1 L of 0.25%–0.45% normal saline, maintaining a urine pH of 7.3–8.5. Urine output should be 5–7 mL/kg/hr. **Complications** include metabolic alkalosis, hypernatremia, hyperosmolarity, and fluid overload.

J. **Dialysis.** In patients who fail to respond to the measures of decontamination already outlined, hemodialysis, and to a lesser extent peritoneal dialysis, may enhance drug elimination. Substances that are removed by hemodialysis generally are water soluble, have a small volume of distribution (< 0.5 L/kg), have a low molecular weight (< 500 daltons), and are not significantly bound to plasma proteins. Hemodialysis usually is indicated for life-threatening ingestions of ethylene glycol, methanol, or paraquat. This technique also has been used to enhance the elimination of ethanol, theophylline, lithium, salicylates, and long-acting barbiturates.

K. **Hemoperfusion** is a technique in which anticoagulated blood is passed through (perfused) a column containing activated charcoal or resin particles. This method of elimination clears substances from the blood more rapidly than hemodialysis, but it does not correct fluid and electrolyte abnormalities, as does hemodialysis. Hemoperfusion, although more effective in removing phenobarbital, phenytoin, carbamazepine, methotrexate, and theophylline than hemodialysis, is less effective in removing ethanol or methanol. **Complications** of hemoperfusion include thrombocytopenia, leukopenia, hypocalcemia, hypoglycemia, and hypotension.

III. MANAGEMENT OF SPECIFIC INGESTIONS

A. **Acetaminophen (Tylenol)** is an antipyretic-analgesic that can produce fatal hepatotoxicity in untreated patients through the generation of a toxic metabolite.

   1. **Available dosage forms.** Acetaminophen is available in a variety of OTC and prescription drug products.

   2. **Toxicokinetics.** Acetaminophen is well absorbed from the GI tract and has a half-life between 2 and 3 hr. Less than 5% is excreted unchanged in the urine; the remainder is metabolized in the liver by the cytochrome P450 system.

   3. **Clinical presentation**
      a. **Phase I** (12–24 hr postingestion). Nausea, vomiting, anorexia, and diaphoresis
      b. **Phase II** (1–4 days postingestion). Asymptomatic
      c. **Phase III** (2–3 days in untreated patients). Nausea, abdominal pain, progressive evidence of hepatic failure, coma, and death

   4. **Laboratory data**
      a. **Serum acetaminophen levels.** Patients with levels greater than 150, 70, or 40 mg/mL at 4, 8, or 12 hr after ingestion require antidotal therapy with *N*-acetyl-L-cysteine (NAC) according to the Rumack-Matthews nomogram.
      b. Baseline liver function tests should be done in all patients.
      c. Renal function tests, including a BUN and SCr, should be done.
      d. Coagulation studies include prothrombin time (PT), partial thromboplastin time (PTT), and bleeding time.

   5. **Treatment**
      a. Adult patients who have ingested > 10 g or children who have ingested > 200 mg/kg require treatment. Elderly and alcoholic patients have an increased susceptibility to acetaminophen hepatotoxicity.
      b. The recommended treatment is GI decontamination with activated charcoal.

c. Antidotal therapy with NAC is indicated for patients with toxic blood levels of acetaminophen.

   (1) NAC dosage is 140 mg/kg as a loading dose followed by 70 mg/kg every 4 hr for a total of 17 doses. NAC is administered either orally or via a nasogastric tube. NAC (Mucomyst) 20% contains 200 mg/mL. Each dose must be diluted 1:3 in either cola or fruit juice to mask the unpleasant taste and smell. The dose of NAC should be repeated if the patient vomits within 30 min of administration. Patients with severe nausea secondary to NAC may be pretreated with IV metoclopramide (Reglan) 10 mg every 6 hr. Metoclopramide acts as an antiemetic while increasing the rate of NAC absorption.

   (2) IV NAC (Acetadote)
      (a) Loading dose: 150 mg/kg over 60 min
      (b) Maintenance dose: 50 mg/kg over 4 hr followed by 100 mg/kg over 16 hr
      (c) Anaphylactoid reactions are observed in approximately 20% of patients. **Caution** should be exercised in patients with a history of **asthma.**

B. Alcohols[5]

1. Ethylene glycol
   a. Available forms. Ethylene glycol commonly is used in antifreeze and windshield deicing solutions. This form is sometimes colorless and has a sweet taste.
   b. Toxicokinetics. Ethylene glycol is hepatically metabolized by alcohol dehydrogenase to glycolaldehyde, which is metabolized by aldehyde dehydrogenase to glycolic acid. Glycolic acid is converted to glyoxylic acid, whose most toxic metabolite is oxalic acid.
   c. Clinical presentation
      (1) Stage I (0.5–12 hr postingestion). Ataxia, nystagmus, nausea and vomiting, decreased deep tendon reflexes, and severe acidosis (more severe overdoses: hypocalcemic tetany and seizures, cerebral edema, coma, and death)
      (2) Stage II (12–24 hr postingestion). Tachypnea, cyanosis, tachycardia, pulmonary edema, and pneumonitis
      (3) Stage III (24–72 hrspostingestion). Flank pain and costovertebral angle tenderness; oliguric renal failure
   d. Laboratory data may reveal severe metabolic acidosis, hypocalcemia, and calcium oxalate crystals in the urinalysis.
   e. Treatment
      (1) Gastric lavage is performed within 30 min of ingestion.
      (2) IV ethanol (EtOH) is used in situations in which fomepizole is not available.
         (a) Indications include an ethylene glycol level > 20 mg/dL, suspicion of ingestion pending level, or an anion gap metabolic acidosis with a history of ingestion, regardless of the level.
         (b) EtOH dosage
            (i) An EtOH level of at least 100 mg/dL should be maintained.
            (ii) Loading dose is 7.5–10 mL/kg of a 10% ethanol in dextrose 5% in water (D_5W) over 1 hr, followed by a maintenance infusion of 1.4 mL/kg/hr.
            (iii) Infusion rates may need to be increased in patients receiving hemodialysis.
      (3) Fomepizole (Antizol) is a potent inhibitor of alcohol dehydrogenase that can prevent the formation of the toxic metabolites of either methanol or ethylene glycol.
         (a) Administer a **loading dose** of 15 mg/kg (up to 1 g) in 100 mL of D_5W or 0.9% sodium chloride (NaCl) infused over 30 min.
         (b) Maintenance doses: 10 mg/kg every 14 hr for 4 doses, then increase to 15 mg/kg (to offset autoinduction phenomenon) until methanol or ethylene glycol levels are < 20 mg/dL.
      (4) Pyridoxine (100 mg IV every day) and **thiamine** (100 mg IV every day) are cofactors that may convert glyoxylic acid to nonoxalate metabolites.
      (5) Sodium bicarbonate is used as needed to correct the acidosis.
      (6) Hemodialysis. EtOH infusion must be continued, and the rate of administration may need to be increased. **Indications** include ethylene glycol level > 50 mg/dL, congestive heart failure, renal failure, and severe acidosis.

[5] Megarbane B, Borron SW, Baud FJ. Current recommendations for the treatment of severe toxic alcohol poisonings. Intensive Care Med 2005;31:189–195.

2. **Methanol**
   a. **Available forms** include gas-line antifreeze, windshield washer, and some sterno.
   b. **Toxicokinetics.** Alcohol dehydrogenase converts methanol to formaldehyde, which is then converted to formic acid.
   c. **Clinical presentation**
      (1) **Stage I.** Euphoria, gregariousness, and muscle weakness for 6–36 hr, depending on the rate of formation of formic acid
      (2) **Stage II.** Vomiting, upper abdominal pain, diarrhea, dizziness, headache, restlessness, dyspnea, blurred vision, photophobia, blindness, coma, cerebral edema, cardiac and respiratory depression, seizures, and death
   d. **Laboratory data** include severe metabolic acidosis, hyperglycemia, and hyperamylasemia.
   e. **Treatment**
      (1) **Gastric lavage.** Charcoal has not been shown to absorb alcohols.
      (2) **IV EtOH (used in situations in which fomepizole is not available)**
         (a) **Indications** include any peak methanol level > 20 mg/dL, a suspicious ingestion with a positive history, or any symptomatic patient with an anion gap acidosis.
         (b) **Administration** is the same as per ethylene glycol (see III.B.1).
      (3) **Folic acid** administered at 1 mg/kg (maximum 50 mg) IV every 4 hr for 6 doses increases the metabolism of formate.
      (4) **Fomepizole (Antizol)** (see III.B.1.e.(3))
      (5) **Sodium bicarbonate** is used for severe acidosis.
      (6) **Hemodialysis** is used for methanol levels > 50 mg/dL, severe and resistant acidosis, renal failure, or visual symptoms.

C. **Anticoagulants**[6]

   1. **Heparin/ Low Molecular Weight Heparin (LMWH)**
      a. **Available dosage forms** include parenteral dosage forms for IV and subcutaneous administration.
      b. **Toxicokinetics.** Heparin has a half-life of 1–1.5 hr and is primarily metabolized in the liver. The newer LMWHs—enoxaparin (Lovenox), dalteparin (Fragmin), tinzaparin (Innohep)—have a longer half-life, especially in patients with renal failure.
      c. **Clinical presentation.** Look for any signs or symptoms of bleeding or bruising.
      d. **Laboratory data.** Obtain PTT, bleeding time, and platelet counts.
      e. **Treatment**
         (1) **Stopping heparin administration for 1–2 hr and restarting therapy at a reduced dose can reverse mild over-anticoagulation.**
         (2) **Severe overdoses** may require the administration of **protamine.**
            (a) Protamine combines with heparin and neutralizes it: **1 mg protamine neutralizes 100 U heparin.**
            (b) Protamine should be administered slowly, intravenously over 10 min. The maximum dose of protamine is 50 mg in any 10-min period.
            (c) Considerable controversy exists about the method of reversing the over-anticoagulation with LMWHs. Some sources recommend the administration of protamine to neutralize part of the effects of these anticoagulants, whereas case reports reported successes with recombinant factor VII (NovoSeven).
            (d) These overdoses should be referred to a hematologist and/or the poison control center.

   2. **Warfarin (Coumadin)**
      a. **Available dosage forms** include oral tablets and a solution for parenteral administration.
      b. **Toxicokinetics.** Warfarin is well absorbed after oral administration. Its mean half-life is 35 hr; protein binding is 99%, with a 5-day duration of activity. Vitamin K–dependent

[6] Ansell J, Hirsh J, Poller L, et al. The pharmacology and management of the vitamin K antagonists. [Paper presented at the 7th ACCP Conference on Antithrombotic and Thrombolytic Therapy.] Chest 2004;126:204s–233s. Hirsh J, Raschke R. Heparin and low-molecular-weight heparin. [Paper presented at the 7th ACCP Conference on Antithrombotic and Thrombolytic Therapy.] Chest 2004;126:188s–203s. Levine MN, Raskob G, Beyth S, et al. Hemorrhagic complications of anticoagulant treatment. [Paper presented at the 7th ACCP Conference on Antithrombotic and Thrombolytic Therapy.] Chest 2004;126:287s–310s.

clotting factors begin to decline 6 hr after administration, but therapeutic anticoagulation may require several days.

c. **Clinical presentation** includes minor bleeding, bruising, hematuria, epistaxis, and conjunctival hemorrhage. More serious bleeding includes GI, intracranial, retroperitoneal, and wound site.

d. **Laboratory data** include PT, international normalized ratio (INR), and bleeding time.

e. **Treatment**

   (1) If **PT** or **INR** is **slightly elevated,** withhold warfarin for 24–48 hr; then reinstitute therapy with a reduced dosage.

   (2) If **PT** or **INR** is **elevated** and **bleeding,** administer 10 mg of phytonadione (vitamin K) over 30 min. Patients who are bleeding may require the administration of blood products that contain clotting factors.

   (3) For mild over-anticoagulation, follow American College of Clinical Pharmacy (ACCP) guidelines.

D. Antidepressants

1. Tricyclic antidepressants (TCAs)

   a. **Available forms** include amitriptyline (Elavil), nortriptyline (Aventyl), imipramine (Tofranil), desipramine (Norpramin), doxepin (Sinequan), protriptyline (Vivactil), and clomipramine (Anafranil).

   b. **Toxicokinetics.** The compounds are hepatically metabolized, undergo enterohepatic recirculation, are highly bound to plasma proteins, and have an elimination half-life of approximately 24 hr.

   c. **Clinical presentation.** Anticholinergic effects include mydriasis, ileus, urinary retention, and hyperpyrexia. **Cardiopulmonary toxicity** exhibits tachycardias, conduction blocks, hypotension, and pulmonary edema. **CNS manifestations** range from agitation and confusion to hallucinations, seizures, and coma.

   d. **Laboratory data.** Blood level monitoring does not correlate well with clinical signs and symptoms of toxicity. Some authors suggest that electrocardiographic monitoring is a better guide to assessing the severity of ingestion.

   e. **Treatment**

      (1) **GI decontamination.** Syrup of ipecac is not recommended because patients may quickly become comatose, increasing the risk of aspiration. **Activated charcoal** is given every 6 hr.

      (2) **Alkalinization** with sodium bicarbonate 1–2 mEq/kg to maintain an arterial pH of 7.45–7.55 decreases the free fraction of the absorbed toxins, while reversing some of the cardiac abnormalities.

      (3) **Phenytoin (Dilantin)** and/or **benzodiazepines** may be required to control seizures. Phenytoin must be administered at a rate not exceeding 25 mg/min because of hypotensive side effects. **(Fosphenytoin [Cerebyx]** may be used because it has a lower incidence of hypotension than phenytoin.)

      (4) **Physostigmine** 2 mg IV over 1 min may be used to reverse **severe** anticholinergic toxicity owing to these drugs. **Because this antidote may cause asystole, the use of this antidote for TCA overdoses is declining.**

2. Selective serotonin reuptake inhibitors (SSRIs)

   a. **Available forms** (nontricyclic agents) include fluoxetine (Prozac), sertraline (Zoloft), and paroxetine (Paxil).

   b. **Toxicokinetics.** SSRIs are well absorbed after oral administration. Peak levels occur within 2–6 hs. SSRIs are hepatically metabolized with a half-life between 8 and 30 hr.

   c. **Clinical presentation** includes mild symptomatology. Patients may become agitated, drowsy, or confused. Seizures and cardiovascular toxicity are rare.

   d. **Laboratory data.** ECG monitoring is recommended. Blood level monitoring is not recommended.

   e. **Treatment** includes gastric lavage and supportive treatment. Some toxicologists may recommend the use of cyproheptadine (Periactin) to manage the serotonin syndrome, which may manifest as a result of these ingestions.

E. Benzodiazepines

1. **Available forms** include chlordiazepoxide (Librium), diazepam (Valium), flurazepam (Dalmane), midazolam (Versed), lorazepam (Ativan), alprazolam (Xanax), and triazolam (Halcion).

2. **Toxicokinetics.** These drugs are hepatically metabolized.

3. **Clinical presentation** includes drowsiness, ataxia, and confusion. Fatalities are rare.

4. **Laboratory data.** Drug level monitoring is not indicated.

5. **Treatment**
   a. **Supportive** treatment includes gastric emptying, activated charcoal, and a cathartic.
   b. **Flumazenil** (Romazicon) is given 0.2 mg IV over 30 sec; repeat doses of 0.5 mg over 30 sec at 1-min intervals for a maximum cumulative dose of 5 mg.
      (1) Flumazenil has a short elimination half-life.
      (2) **Careful observation** for **resedation** is necessary, especially for ingestions of long-acting benzodiazepines.
      (3) **Flumazenil is contraindicated in mixed overdose patients (particularly involving tricyclic antidepressants) in whom seizures are likely.**

F. **β-adrenergic antagonists**

   1. **Available dosage forms.** Class examples include propranolol (Inderal), metoprolol (Lopressor), and atenolol (Tenormin). Oral and parenteral dosage forms are available.

   2. **Toxicokinetics.** All of the members within this class differ in regard to renal versus hepatic elimination, lipid solubility, and protein binding. Patients may become toxic owing to changes in organ function.

   3. **Clinical presentation** includes hypotension, bradycardia, and atrioventricular block. Bronchospasm may occur, particularly with noncardioselective agents.

   4. **Laboratory data** include serum electrolytes and blood glucose (patients may become hypoglycemic).

   5. **Treatment**
      a. **GI decontamination** includes gastric lavage and activated charcoal.
      b. **Glucagon** is given 50–150 μg/kg as a loading dose over 1 min, followed by a continuous infusion of 1–5 mg/hr.
      c. **Epinephrine** should be used cautiously in β-blocker overdoses. Unopposed α-receptor stimulation in the face of complete β-receptor block may lead to profound hypertension.

G. **Calcium channel antagonists**

   1. **Available forms** include verapamil (Calan), diltiazem (Cardizem), and the dihydropyridine class (nifedipine derivatives [Procardia]).

   2. **Toxicokinetics.** Onset of action is approximately 30 min, whereas the duration is 6–8 hr. Several compounds are available as sustained-release dosage forms, which may contribute to prolonged toxicity.

   3. **Clinical presentation.** Hypotension is common to all classes. Bradycardia and atrioventricular block are more commonly seen with ingestions of verapamil or diltiazem. Pulmonary edema and seizures (verapamil) have been reported.

   4. **Laboratory data** include ECG and serum electrolytes.

   5. **Treatment**
      a. **GI decontamination** includes gastric lavage, activated charcoal, and whole-bowel irrigation (especially for ingestions with sustained-release products).
      b. **Calcium.** Calcium chloride 10% (10–20 mL) IV push is given for the management of hypotension, bradycardia, or heart block.
      c. **Glucagon** dosage is the same as for β-blocker overdose.
      d. **Combined insulin and dextrose administration** has been used in selected cases. This should be **used only in consultation with a poison control center.**

H. **Cocaine**

   1. **Available forms** include alkaloid obtained from *Erythroxylon coca*.

   2. **Toxicokinetics.** Cocaine is well absorbed after oral, inhalational, intranasal, and IV administration. Cocaine is metabolized in the liver and excreted in the urine.

3. **Clinical presentation** includes CNS and sympathetic stimulation (e.g., hypertension, tachypnea, tachycardia, nausea, vomiting, seizures). Death may result from respiratory failure, myocardial infarction, or cardiac arrest.

4. **Laboratory data** include cocaine and cocaine metabolite urine screens.

5. **Treatment** is **supportive**: benzodiazepines for seizures, labetalol (Normodyne) for hypertension, and neuroleptics for psychosis.

I. Corrosives

1. **Available forms** include strong acids or alkalis.

2. **Toxicokinetics.** Corrosives are well absorbed after oral and inhalational administration.

3. **Clinical presentation.** These compounds produce burns on contact.

4. **Laboratory data.** Arterial blood gases (ABGs), chest radiographs, and at least 6 hr of observation are required for inhalation exposure.

5. **Treatment** is **decontamination.** Exposed skin must be irrigated with water. **Neutralization** should be **avoided** because these reactions are exothermic and will produce further tissue damage.

J. Cyanide

1. **Available forms** include industrial chemicals and some nail-polish removers.

2. **Toxicokinetics.** The drug is rapidly absorbed after oral or inhalation exposure.

3. **Clinical presentation** includes headache, dyspnea, nausea, vomiting, ataxia, coma, seizures, and death.

4. **Laboratory data** include cyanide levels, ABGs, electrolytes, and an ECG.

5. **Treatment.** A cyanide antidote kit is used. It contains the following:
   a. **Amyl nitrite'** Pearls are crushed and held under the patient's nostrils.
   b. **Sodium nitrite** 10 mL IV push. Converts hemoglobin to methemoglobin, which binds the cyanide ion.
   c. **Sodium thiosulfate** 50 mL of a 25% solution IV push. May be repeated if there is no response.
   d. **Oxygen**
   e. **Sodium bicarbonate.** As needed for severe acidosis
   f. **Hyperbaric oxygen.** For patients not responding to already outlined treatment

K. Digoxin (Lanoxin)

1. **Available dosage forms** include oral and parenteral.

2. **Toxicokinetics.** Digoxin is well absorbed, is primarily renally eliminated, and has a half-life of 36–48 hr. Its volume of distribution is 7–10 L/kg. Equilibration between serum level and myocardial binding requires 6–8 hr.

3. **Clinical presentation** includes confusion, anorexia, nausea, and vomiting in mild cases. In more severe cases, cardiac dysrhythmias are seen.

4. **Laboratory data** include serum digoxin levels, electrolytes, particularly serum potassium levels, and an ECG.

5. **Treatment**
   a. **Decontamination** with activated charcoal is recommended.
   b. **Supportive therapy** includes managing hyperkalemia or hypokalemia and inotropic support as needed.
   c. **Digoxin-specific Fab antibodies (Digibind).** To determine the dosage, use the following formula

$$\text{Dose (vials)} = \frac{[\text{ingested digoxin (mg)} \times 0.8]}{0.6}$$

Each vial contains 40 mg of digoxin antibodies (Digibind) and should be reconstituted with 4 mL of sterile water.

L. Electrolytes

1. Magnesium

a. **Available dosage forms** include oral, rectal, and parenteral. Magnesium-containing cathartics (e.g., magnesium citrate) have been reported to produce hypermagnesemia in patients receiving repetitive doses with activated charcoal.

b. **Toxicokinetics.** Magnesium is found intracellularly and is renally eliminated.

c. **Clinical presentation**
   (1) **Mild:** Deep tendon reflexes may be depressed; lethargy and weakness
   (2) **Severe:** Respiratory paralysis and heart block; prolonged PR, QRS, and QT intervals

d. **Laboratory data**
   (1) **Mild:** > 4 mEq/L
   (2) **Severe:** > 10 mEq/L

e. **Treatment** is **10% calcium chloride** 10–20 mL to temporarily antagonize the cardiac effects of magnesium. In severe cases, **hemodialysis** may be required.

2. Potassium

a. **Available dosage forms** are oral and parenteral.

b. **Toxicokinetics.** Potassium is primarily an intracellular cation. Changes in acid–base balance produce shifts in serum potassium values (e.g., a 0.1-U increase in serum pH produces a 0.1–0.7 mEq/L decrease in serum potassium values).

c. **Clinical presentation** includes cardiac irritability and peripheral weakness with minor increases. Cardiac dysrhythmias, including bradycardia, may progress to asystole.

d. **Laboratory data.** ECG data include **peaked T waves** and prolongation of the QRS complex.

e. **Treatment**
   (1) **Calcium.** Administer calcium chloride 10% 10–20 mL to antagonize the cardiac effects of hyperkalemia.
   (2) **Sodium bicarbonate.** 1–2 mEq/kg IV increases serum pH and causes an intracellular shift of potassium.
   (3) **Glucose and insulin.** 50 mL of 50% dextrose and 5–10 U of regular insulin are administered via IV push to shift potassium from the extracellular fluid into the cells.
   (4) **Cation exchange resins** bind potassium in exchange for another cation (sodium). **Sodium polystyrene sulfonate** (Kayexalate) is given 15 g/60 mL with 23.5% sorbitol in doses 15–30 g by mouth every 3–4 hr as needed until the hyperkalemia resolves. Alternatively, 50 g of sodium polystyrene sulfonate can be given rectally in 200 mL of sodium chloride as a retention enema.
   (5) **Hemodialysis** is reserved for life-threatening hyperkalemia that does not respond to the above measures.

M. Iron (Fe)

1. **Available dosage forms.** Numerous OTC products are available. Toxicity is based on the amount of elemental iron ingested: sulfate salt 20% elemental Fe; fumarate salt 33% elemental Fe; and gluconate salt 12% elemental Fe.

2. **Toxicokinetics.** Iron is absorbed in the duodenum and jejunum.

3. **Clinical presentation**
   a. **Phase I.** Nausea, vomiting, diarrhea, GI bleeding, hypotension
   b. **Phase II.** Clinical improvement seen 6–24 hr postingestion
   c. **Phase III.** Metabolic acidosis, renal and hepatic failure, sepsis, pulmonary edema, and death

4. **Laboratory data** include serum Fe levels, total iron-binding capacity (TIBC; **is controversial**), ABGs, liver function tests (LFTs), hemoglobin, and hematocrit. Radiological evaluation of the abdomen notes the presence of radiopaque pills.

5. **Treatment**
   a. **Decontamination.** For ingestions > 40 mg/kg. Gastric lavage using sodium bicarbonate is of questionable efficacy. Whole-bowel irrigation is used for large ingestions.

b. **Supportive treatment**

c. **Deferoxamine** (Desferal) is used to chelate iron. Administer 25–50 mg/kg up to a dose of 1 g, and observe for a red color in the urine. Then administer at a rate of 15 mg/kg/hr up to a maximum dose of 6 g/day. Continue until serum iron is within the therapeutic range.

N. **Isoniazid (INH)**

1. **Available dosage forms** include oral and parenteral.

2. **Toxicokinetics.** INH is well absorbed orally. Peak levels are within 1–2 hr postingestion. Isoniazid is hepatically metabolized.

3. **Clinical presentation** includes nausea, vomiting, slurred speech, ataxia, generalized tonic–clonic seizures, and coma.

4. **Laboratory data** include severe lactic acidosis, hypoglycemia, mild hyperkalemia, and leukocytosis.

5. **Treatment**

a. **Decontamination.** Avoid emesis because patients are at high risk for developing seizures; for severe ingestions use activated charcoal gastric lavage.

b. **Pyridoxine,** which reverses INH-induced seizures, is given in gram doses equivalent to the amount of isoniazid ingested. Pyridoxine is mixed as a 10% solution in D_5W and infused over 30–60 min.

c. **Sodium bicarbonate** corrects the acidosis.

O. **Lead**

1. **Available forms** include lead-containing paint or gasoline fume inhalation.

2. **Toxicokinetics.** Lead has slow distribution, with a half-life of approximately 2 months.

3. **Clinical presentation** includes nausea, vomiting, abdominal pain, peripheral neuropathies, convulsions, and coma.

4. **Laboratory data** include anemia and an elevated blood-lead level.

5. **Treatment**

a. **Edetate calcium disodium (calcium disodium Versenate)** is given 50–75 mg/kg/day intramuscularly (IM) or via slow IV in 4 divided doses.

b. **Dimercaprol (BAL)** is given 4 mg/kg IM every 4 hr for 3–5 days.

P. **Lithium (Eskalith)**

1. **Available dosage forms** include liquid, capsules, and tablets (immediate and sustained release).

2. **Toxicokinetics.** Lithium is well absorbed after oral administration. It is not appreciably bound to plasma proteins and has a small volume of distribution (V_d) of 0.5 L/kg. Elimination is renal, with a half-life of 14–24 hr.

3. **Clinical presentation**

a. **Mild:** Polyuria, blurred vision, weakness, slurred speech, ataxia tremor, and myoclonic jerks

b. **Severe:** Delirium, coma, seizures, and hyperthermia

4. **Laboratory data**

a. Therapeutic range: 0.6–1.2 mEq/L

b. Mild toxicity: 1.5–2.5 mEq/L

c. Moderate toxicity: 2.5–3 mEq/L

d. Severe toxicity: > 3 mEq/L

5. **Treatment**

a. **Supportive** care, including basic life support and fluid and electrolyte replacement

b. **Decontamination**

(1) **Syrup of ipecac not recommended**
(2) **Activated charcoal** ineffective
(3) **Sodium polystyrene sulfonate** has been effective in experimental models. Need to monitor potassium levels.
(4) **Whole-bowel irrigation** for large ingestions, especially those involving sustained-release products
(5) **Hemodialysis** for severely symptomatic patients with acute exposure levels > 2.5 mEq/L or chronic levels > 1.5 mEq/L. **Note:** Lithium levels may rise after dialysis owing to a rebound effect.

Q. Opiates

1. **Available dosage forms** include oral immediate-release and sustained-release preparations as well as parenteral agents.

2. **Toxicokinetics.** Some agents have prolonged elimination half-lives (e.g., heroin, methadone).

3. **Clinical presentation** includes respiratory depression and a decreased level of consciousness. Rare effects include hypotension, bradycardia, and pulmonary edema. Seizures have been reported in patients with renal dysfunction in individuals who are receiving meperidine owing to the accumulation of the metabolite normeperidine.

4. **Laboratory data** include baseline ABGs and toxicology screens.

5. **Treatment**
   a. **Naloxone** is given 0.4–2 mg every 5 min up to 10 mg and 0.03–0.1 mg/kg in pediatric patients. Naloxone has a very short half-life, and resedation is a concern in patients overdosing on long-acting opioids or sustained-release dosage forms.
   b. **Nalmefene (Revex)** has a half-life of 4–8 hr. Initial dosages are 0.5 mg/70 kg. A follow-up dose 2–5 min later is 1 mg/70 kg.

R. Organophosphates

1. **There are a variety of available forms;** they are usually pesticides or chemical warfare agents.

2. **Toxicokinetics.** Organophosphates are absorbed through the lungs, skin, GI tract, and conjunctiva.

3. **Clinical presentation** includes excessive cholinergic stimulation.

4. **Laboratory data** include red blood cell acetylcholinesterase activity.

5. **Treatment**
   a. **Decontamination**
   b. **Atropine** is given 0.5–2 mg IV to reverse the peripheral muscarinic effects.
   c. **Pralidoxime (2-PAM; Protopam)** is given 1 g IV over 2 min and repeated in 20 min as needed.

S. Salicylates

1. **Available dosage forms** include a variety of OTC products: oral, rectal, and topical.

2. **Toxicokinetics.** Salicylates are well absorbed after oral administration. The half-life is 6–12 hr at lower doses. In overdose situations, the half-life may be prolonged to more than 20 hr.

3. **Clinical presentation** includes nausea, vomiting, tinnitus, and malaise (mild toxicity). Lethargy, convulsions, coma, and metabolic acidosis appear in more severe overdoses. Potential **complications** from therapeutic and toxic doses include GI bleeding, increased PT, hepatic toxicity, pancreatitis, and proteinuria.

4. **Laboratory data** for the following 6-hr postingestion levels are:
   a. 40–60 mg/dL: tinnitus
   b. 60–95 mg/dL: moderate toxicity
   c. More than 95 mg/dL: severe toxicity
   d. With the presence of acidemia and aciduria, evaluate ABGs.

    e. In addition, laboratory evaluation may show leukocytosis, thrombocytopenia, increased or decreased serum glucose and sodium, hypokalemia, and increased serum BUN, creatinine, and ketones.

  5. Treatment
    a. Decontamination. Repetitive doses of activated charcoal every 6 hr, with 1 dose of cathartic for patients who ingested > 150 mg/kg. Whole-bowel irrigation for large ingestions.
    b. Alkaline diuresis is given as noted in decontamination section to enhance salicylate excretion. This is indicated for levels> 40 mg/dL.
    c. Hemodialysis is used for severe intoxications when serum levels are > 100 mg/dL. This method of decontamination is much better than repetitive doses of activated charcoal.
    d. Fluid and **electrolyte** replacement is administered as needed.
    e. Vitamin K (Aquamephyton) and **fresh frozen plasma** are used to correct any coagulopathy.

T. Snake bites

  1. Types. There are numerous species of snakes found worldwide. The venomous snakes found in North America include the following: rattlesnake, cottonmouth, copperhead, and coral. Because patients may be exposed to more exotic snakes, a herpetologist should be consulted for a more definitive identification.

  2. Toxicokinetics. Onset of symptomatology depends on the species of snake and the patient's underlying medical condition.

  3. Clinical presentation includes nausea; vomiting; diarrhea; syncope; tachycardia; and cold, clammy skin. Local findings include pain, edema, and erythema. More severe envenomations can lead to severe tissue injury, compartment syndrome, and shock.

  4. Laboratory data
    a. CBC and platelet count
    b. Coagulation profile
    c. Fibrin degradation products
    d. Electrolytes
    e. BUN, SCr, and urinalysis

  5. Treatment
    a. Supportive. Move the patient away from striking distance of the snake. Ideally, the patient should be transported to a medical facility as soon as possible. Constrictive clothing, rings, watches, etc. should be removed. Tetanus immunization should be assessed, and surgical intervention may be necessary for severe cases.
    b. Antivenoms
      (1) Antivenin (Crotalidae) polyvalent is a horse-derived product that has been reported to produce allergic reactions. For mild bites, the recommended dose is 5–10 vials; moderate, 10–20; and severe envenomations may require 20 or more vials.
      (2) Crotalidae polyvalent immune Fab is a polyvalent antivenin made from sheep sources. The initial dose is 4–6 vials diluted in 250 mL of 0.9% normal saline (NS) administered over 1 hr. Additional doses may be required for severe envenomations.

U. Theophylline

  1. Available dosage forms include liquid, sustained-release tablets and capsules as well as parenteral forms.

  2. Toxicokinetics. Well absorbed orally with a V_d of approximately 0.5 L/kg. Theophylline is hepatically metabolized and has a half-life of 4–8 hr. Theophylline clearance depends highly on age, concomitant disease states, and interacting drugs.

  3. Clinical presentation includes nausea, vomiting, seizures, and cardiac dysrhythmias. Chronic toxicity carries a poorer prognosis than acute toxicity.

4. **Laboratory data.** Therapeutic theophylline levels are 5–20 µg/mL. Hyperglycemia and hypokalemia are seen with acute ingestions. Other useful laboratory tests include serum electrolytes, BUN, creatinine, hepatic function, and ECG monitoring.

5. **Treatment**
   a. **Supportive** therapy includes maintaining an airway and treating seizures and dysrhythmias as they occur.
   b. **Decontamination. Syrup of ipecac not recommended.**
   c. **Activated charcoal** (repetitive doses) to enhance elimination. **Whole-bowel irrigation** for massive ingestions (especially with sustained-release products). **Charcoal hemoperfusion** is used in unstable patients who are in status epilepticus. **Hemodialysis** is used when hemoperfusion is unavailable.
   d. **β-adrenergic antagonists** (e.g., esmolol, Brevibloc) are used to treat the hypotension, tachycardia, and dysrhythmias caused by elevated cyclic adenosine monophosphate levels.

IV. REFERENCES

A. American Academy of Clinical Toxicology and European Association of Poisons Centres and Clinical Toxicologists. Position statement: Single-dose activated charcoal. Clin Toxicol 1997; 35:721–741.

B. American Academy of Clinical Toxicology and European Association of Poisons Centres and Clinical Toxicologists. Position statement: Syrup of ipecac. Clin Toxicol 1997;35:699–709.

C. American College of Emergency Physicians. Clinical policy for the initial approach to patients presenting with acute toxic ingestion or dermal or inhalation exposure. Ann Emerg Med 1999; 33:735–762.

D. American College of Emergency Physicians. Clinical policy for the initial approach to patients presenting with altered mental status. Ann Emerg Med 1999;33:251–281.

E. American Heart Association. Toxicology in ECC. Circulation [Special issue] 2005;112: IV126–IV132. Available at www.circulationaha.org.

F. Ansell J, Hirsh J, Poller L, et al. The pharmacology and management of the vitamin K antagonists. [Paper presented at the 7th ACCP Conference on Antithrombotic and Thrombolytic Therapy.] Chest 2004;126:204s–233s.

G. Bond RC. The role of activated charcoal and gastric emptying in gastrointestinal decontamination: A state-of-the-art review. Ann Emerg Med 2002;39:273–285.

H. Gold BS, Dart RC, Barish RA. Bites of venomous snakes. New Engl J Med 2002;347:347–356.

I. Hirsh J, Raschke R. Heparin and low-molecular-weight heparin. [Paper presented at the 7th ACCP Conference on Antithrombotic and Thrombolytic Therapy.] Chest 2004;126:188s–203s.

J. Levine MN, Raskob G, Beyth S, et al. Hemorrhagic complications of anticoagulant treatment. [Paper presented at the 7th ACCP Conference on Antithrombotic and Thrombolytic Therapy.] Chest 2004;126:287s–310s.

K. Litovitz TL, Klein-Schwartz, Rodgers GC, et al. 2001 annual report of the American Association of Poison Control Centers Toxic Exposure Surveillance System. Am J Emerg Med 2002;20:1–62.

L. Megarbane B, Borron SW, Baud FJ. Current recommendations for the treatment of severe toxic alcohol poisonings. Intensive Care Med 2005;31:189–195.

M. Mokhlesi B, Leiken JB, Murray P, et al. Adult toxicology in critical care part 1: General approach to the intoxicated patient. Chest 2003;123:577–592.

N. Mokhlesi B, Leiken JB, Murray P, et al. Adult toxicology in critical care part 2: General approach to the intoxicated patient. Chest 2003;123:897–922.

O. Paloucek F. Antidotal flumazenil use—The protamine of the 90s. Crit Care Med 1999; 27: 10–11.

STUDY QUESTIONS

Directions: Each of the questions, statements, or incomplete statements can be correctly answered or completed by **one** of the suggested answers or phrases. Choose the **best** answer.

1. A physician receives a call from the parent of a 2-year-old child who has ingested an unknown quantity of morphine controlled-release tablets and is now unconscious. The physician's initial recommendation is to

   (A) call emergency medical services (EMS) and have the child taken to the hospital emergency department.
   (B) administer 1 g/kg of activated charcoal with sorbitol.
   (C) administer syrup of ipecac 15 mL by mouth to induce vomiting.
   (D) suggest that the child receive emergency hemodialysis.
   (E) suggest that the child receive acid diuresis with ammonium chloride.

2. A grandfather arrives at your pharmacy asking to purchase a bottle of syrup of ipecac to keep in his home in the event of a poisoning when grandchildren are visiting. What should you tell him?

   (A) Administer 15 mL of syrup of ipecac at the first sign of an ingestion.
   (B) Syrup of ipecac is no longer recommended by the American Association of Poison Control Centers and the American Academy of Pediatrics.
   (C) Provide him with the toll-free number for the poison control center.
   (D) Both B and C.

3. An unconscious patient is brought into the emergency department. The patient is given 50 mL of 50% dextrose in water, thiamine 100 mg IV, followed by naloxone 1 mg, at which point he awakens. This patient most likely has overdosed on which of the following substances?

   (A) methanol
   (B) amitriptyline
   (C) cocaine
   (D) haloperidol
   (E) heroin

4. Contraindications to the administration of syrup of ipecac include which of the following?

   (A) an unconscious patient
   (B) a patient who is experiencing a generalized tonic clonic seizure
   (C) a patient who has ingested a caustic substance
   (D) All of the above
   (E) None of the above

5. An unconscious patient is brought to the emergency department with a history of an unknown drug overdose. Which of the following actions should the physician perform?

   (A) administer 50 mL of 50% dextrose, thiamine 100 mg IV push, and naloxone 0.4 mg IV push
   (B) protect the patient's airway and ensure that vital signs are stable
   (C) order the following laboratory tests: complete blood count (CBC), electrolytes, and a toxicology screen
   (D) All of the above

6. A patient who overdoses on acetaminophen is admitted to the hospital for antidotal therapy with N-acetyl-L-cysteine (NAC). The patient has the following medication orders: NAC 140 mg/kg loading dose followed by 70 mg/kg for a total of 17 doses, ranitidine 50 mg IV every 8 hr, prochlorperazine 10 mg IM every 6 hr as needed for nausea, thiamine 100 mg IV every day for 3 doses, and Darvocet N-100 1–2 tablets every 4 hr as needed for headache. What is the best course of action?

   (A) Call the physician to increase the dosage of ranitidine to 50 mg IV every 6 hr.
   (B) Call the physician to have the Darvocet N-100 discontinued.
   (C) Call the physician to initiate hemodialysis therapy.
   (D) Have the patient prophylactically intubated to protect the airway.
   (E) Administer ethanol 10% at a loading dose of 7.5 mL/kg over 1 hr, followed by a continuous infusion of 1.4 mL/kg/hr for 48 hr.

7. Ethyl alcohol (EtOH) is administered to patients who have ingested either ethylene glycol or methanol because EtOH

(A) helps sedate patients.
(B) increases the metabolism of ethylene glycol and methanol.
(C) blocks the formation of the toxic metabolites of ethylene glycol and methanol.
(D) increases the renal clearance of ethylene glycol and methanol.
(E) is not an antidote for ethylene glycol or methanol overdoses.

8. A patient with renal failure is inadvertently given 3 doses of potassium chloride 40 mEq IV in 100 mL of 0.9% sodium chloride over a 3-hr period. This error is immediately discovered and a STAT serum potassium level is 8.0 mEq/L. The patient is bradycardic with a markedly prolonged QRS complex. The patient should receive which of the following?

(A) calcium chloride 10% 10 mL IV push
(B) sodium bicarbonate 50 mEq IV push
(C) insulin 10 U and 50% dextrose 50 mL IV push
(D) sodium polystyrene sulfonate 30 g by mouth every 3 hr for 4 doses
(E) None of the above

9. Parenteral calcium is used as an antidote for which of the following situations?

(A) verapamil overdoses
(B) hyperkalemia
(C) cocaine intoxication
(D) verapamil overdoses and hyperkalemia

10. A 65-year-old woman with normal renal function is administered a 0.25 mg dose of digoxin IV push. A serum level obtained 1 hr after drug administration is 5 ng/mL. Your recommendation to the physician is which of the following?

(A) Administer 2 vials of digoxin immune antibodies STAT.
(B) Administer repetitive doses of activated charcoal.
(C) Call a nephrologist, and put the patient on hemodialysis.
(D) Repeat the serum digoxin level 6–8 hr after the dose, and reassess the patient.

11. A 16-year-old woman is reported to have overdosed on 40 sustained-release theophylline tablets. She is transported to the emergency department, where gastric lavage was performed and she was given one dose of activated charcoal. An initial theophylline level is 42 μg/mL, but a follow-up level in the intensive care unit (ICU) is 95 μg/mL. What is the most appropriate course of therapy?

(A) charcoal hemoperfusion and multiple-dose activated charcoal
(B) syrup of ipecac administration
(C) forced alkaline diuresis
(D) nasogastric administration of sodium-polystyrene sulfonate

12. A 23-year-old man is admitted to the intensive care unit (ICU) after ingesting 20 acetaminophen tablets 500 mg with a six-pack of beer. He was initially awake and alert in the emergency department and was given one dose of activated charcoal. His initial acetaminophen level taken approximately 2 hr after ingestion is 90 μg/mL. What would be the most appropriate course of action?

(A) Administer repeated doses of activated charcoal and sorbitol.
(B) Administer syrup of ipecac.
(C) Administer a loading dose of N-acetyl-L-cysteine (NAC), and repeat the acetaminophen level in 4 hr.
(D) Discharge the patient to home.

13. An overdose victim presents to the emergency department with an elevated heart rate, decreased blood pressure, dilated pupils, and lethargy. Upon arrival to the intensive care unit (ICU), she has a generalized tonic–clonic seizure that is treated with IV diazepam and fosphenytoin. Which of the following is the most likely intoxicant?

(A) ethyl alcohol
(B) methanol
(C) acetaminophen
(D) oxycodone
(E) amitriptyline

ANSWERS AND EXPLANATIONS

1. The answer is A *[see I.A]*.
Patients with unstable vital signs should be taken to an emergency department for immediate treatment.

2. The answer is D *[see II.G.1.a]*.
Induced vomiting is no longer an acceptable option of managing poisonings at home because it is a relatively ineffective method of removing toxins and results in a delay in administering antidotal therapy. It is important to council patients on poison prevention and to give parents and other friends and relatives the toll-free number for the poison control center. Parents should also know basic first aid and cardiopulmonary resuscitation (CPR).

3. The answer is E *[see III.Q.5]*.
Naloxone reverses the effects of opioid receptor agonists, such as heroin, morphine, and propoxyphene.

4. The answer is D *[see II.G.1]*.
Contraindications to ipecac include the three Cs: caustics, conscious, and convulsions; see also the answer to question 2. The use of syrup of ipecac is reserved for rare circumstances and only under the direction of the poison control center and/or a physician. These are new recommendations and many parents, relatives, and friends may have this product in their medicine cabinets.

5. The answer is D *[see II]*.
The management of unconscious overdose patients involves aggressive support of vital signs and the administration of empiric antidotal therapy, while obtaining various laboratory tests to determine the nature of the overdose.

6. The answer is B *[see III.A]*.
Darvocet N-100 is an acetaminophen-containing product that should not be given to a patient with documented acetaminophen toxicity. Be aware particularly of OTC products containing acetaminophen.

7. The answer is C *[see III.B]*.
Ethanol saturates alcohol dehydrogenase and prevents the formation of the toxic metabolites of either ethylene glycol or methanol, however this antidote is falling out of favor owing to its adverse metabolic and central nervous system effects. Fomepizole (Antizol), a specific inhibitor of alcohol dehydrogenase, is becoming the preferred antidote for methanol or ethylene glycol overdoses. Ethanol may be used in situations in which fomepizole is not available.

8. The answer is A *[see III.L.2]*.
All of the selections are used to manage hyperkalemia. Although, in an unstable patient, the cardiac effects of hyperkalemia must first be reversed with intravenous calcium.

9. The answer is D *[see III.G; III.L.2]*.
Parenteral calcium is used to reverse the cardiac effects of calcium channel blocker overuse and hyperkalemia.

10. The answer is D *[see III.K]*.
The plasma–tissue distribution phase for digoxin is 6–8 hr postadministration. Sampling digoxin levels sooner may give a falsely elevated level. Only symptomatic patients should receive digoxin immune antibodies. Hemodialysis is of no value in managing digoxin overdoses.

11. The answer is A *[see III.T]*.
Large ingestions of sustained-release products may act as drug reservoirs, necessitating aggressive measures to remove the toxin.

12. The answer is C *[see III.A].*
Large acetaminophen ingestions (> 140 mg/kg) may be fatal if unrecognized. The Rumack-Matthew nomogram requires a 4-hr level to accurately assess the potential for toxicity. If the 4-hr level is in the toxic range, the full course of NAC therapy should be administered.

13. The answer is E *[see III.D].*
Tricyclic antidepressant overdoses will produce seizures, hypotension, mydriasis, hypotension, and ventricular dysrhythmias. The cardiac and CNS effects of tricyclic antidepressant toxicity will respond to bicarbonate therapy. Opiates such as oxycodone will produce miosis.

25
Federal Pharmacy Law

Robert C. Pavlan, Jr.

I. FEDERAL CONTROLLED SUBSTANCES ACT

A. Schedules of controlled substances. Certain drugs have a potential for abuse that leads to physical or psychological dependence. As a result, the U.S. federal government has placed these drugs into schedules (I, II, III, IV, and V) and refers to them as controlled substances. The Attorney General of the United States has the authority to add or remove a drug or substance from one of the federal schedules, or to transfer a drug from one federal schedule to another. The federal schedules are updated and published annually by the federal government.

1. Schedule I (CI; C-I) Schedule I drugs may not be kept in a pharmacy nor dispensed pursuant to a prescription (except for properly registered facilities for investigative or research purposes). A controlled substance analogue of a drug in any federal schedule, commonly referred to as a "designer drug," is considered a schedule I substance to the extent intended for human consumption. Required findings by the government for placement of a drug into schedule I include:
   a. The drug or other substance has a high potential for abuse.
   b. The drug or other substance has no currently accepted medical use in treatment in the United States.
   c. There is a lack of accepted safety for use of the drug or other substance under medical supervision.

2. Schedule II (CII; C-II). Required findings for placement of a drug into schedule II include:
   a. The drug or other substance has a high potential for abuse.
   b. The drug or other substance has a currently accepted medical use in treatment in the United States or a currently accepted medical use with severe restrictions.
   c. Abuse of the drug or other substance may lead to severe psychological or physical dependence.

3. Schedule III (CIII; C-III). Required findings for placement of a drug into schedule III include:
   a. The drug or other substance has a potential for abuse less than the drugs or other substances in schedules I and II.
   b. The drug or other substance has a currently accepted medical use in treatment in the United States.
   c. Abuse of the drug or other substance may lead to moderate or low physical dependence or high psychological dependence.

4. Schedule IV (CIV; C-IV). Required findings for placement of a drug into schedule IV include:
   a. The drug or other substance has a low potential for abuse relative to the drugs or other substances in schedule III.
   b. The drug or other substance has a currently accepted medical use in treatment in the United States.
   c. Abuse of the drug or other substance may lead to limited physical dependence or psychological dependence relative to the drugs or other substances in schedule III.

5. Schedule V (CV; C-V). Required findings for placement of a drug into schedule V include:
   a. The drug or other substance has a low potential for abuse relative to the drugs or other substances in schedule IV.
   b. The drug or other substance has a currently accepted medical use in treatment in the United States.
   c. Abuse of the drug or other substance may lead to limited physical dependence or psychological dependence relative to the drugs or other substances in schedule IV.

B. Registration requirements. This Act regulates the use of controlled substances by requiring all entities that lawfully handle them to register with the federal government, specifically, the Drug Enforcement Administration (DEA).

1. **Entities that must register**
   a. **Manufacturers** and **wholesalers** of controlled substances must register with the DEA initially and reregister every year thereafter.
   b. **Dispensers** (practitioners and pharmacies) of controlled substances must register with the DEA initially and reregister every 3 years thereafter. Pharmacists, pharmacy interns, pharmacy technicians, and all other employees or agents of a pharmacy do not have to register, providing the pharmacy is properly registered and the employee or agent is acting in the usual course of employment or business.
   c. All other entities that lawfully handle any controlled substance must register with the DEA, including researchers, clinics and laboratories, and teaching institutions.

2. **Separate registration for separate activities.** Every entity that engages in one of the following activities must register with the DEA. A separate registration is required for each activity, with certain exceptions (e.g., a manufacturer of a schedule of a controlled substance is allowed to distribute that schedule without being registered as a distributor).
   a. Manufacturing controlled substances
   b. Distributing controlled substances
   c. Dispensing controlled substances listed in schedules II–V (e.g., practitioners, pharmacies)
   d. Conducting research with controlled substances listed in schedules II–V
   e. Conducting instructional activities with controlled substances listed in schedules II–V
   f. Conducting a narcotic treatment program using any narcotic drug listed in schedules II, III, IV, or V
   g. Conducting research and instructional activities with controlled substances listed in schedule I
   h. Conducting chemical analysis with controlled substances listed in any schedule
   i. Importing controlled substances
   j. Exporting controlled substances
   k. Participating in maintenance or detoxification treatment and mixing, preparing, packaging, or changing the dosage form of a narcotic drug listed in schedules II, III, IV, or V for use in maintenance or detoxification treatment by another narcotic treatment program.

3. **Separate registrations for separate locations.** Each principal place of business of a registrant having more than one location must have its own registration certificate. Each pharmacy, chain pharmacy, and hospital that dispenses controlled substances must have its own registration certificate. Registration is not required for an office that is used by a registrant where controlled substances are neither stored nor dispensed.
   a. **Warehouses.** A warehouse where controlled substances are stored by or on behalf of a registrant is not required to register unless one of the following occurs:
      (1) Controlled substances are directly distributed from the warehouse to a registered location different than the location from which the substances were shipped.
      (2) Controlled substances are directly distributed from the warehouse to a person or entity not required to register under the Act.

4. **Registration procedure.** Applications to become registered must be submitted to the DEA on the appropriate form with the required fee, information, and signature of one of the following:
   a. The individual who owns and operates the entity, if doing business as an individual
   b. A partner of the applicant, if a partnership
   c. An officer of the applicant, if a corporation, corporate division, association, trust, or other entity
   d. One or more individuals who have been granted a power of attorney by an applicant. A **power of attorney** allows one to lawfully act in place of another. The power of attorney must be signed by one of the individuals listed above in a–c and by the individual receiving the power of attorney. The power of attorney remains valid until revoked by the applicant.

5. **Registration action by the DEA.** If an application is complete, it will be accepted for filing. If it is defective, the DEA will return the application with a statement indicating the reason for its nonacceptance. The application may be corrected and resubmitted at any time.
   a. **Issuance of certificate of registration.** A certificate of registration will be issued by the DEA when it determines that the registration is required by law in order to conduct

such activity (e.g., manufacturing, distributing, or dispensing a controlled substance). The certificate must be conspicuously maintained and readily retrievable at the registered location.

    b. Denial of registration. If the DEA determines that a registration is not required by law, it will issue an Order To Show Cause why the registration should not be denied. The applicant may request a hearing and explain why the certificate of registration should be issued. After the hearing, the DEA may deny the application or issue the certificate.

6. Modification of registration. A registrant may submit a letter of request to the DEA seeking to modify its registration. A modification may be sought when there is a change in the name or address that appears on the certificate, or when the pharmacy seeks DEA approval to dispense additional controlled substances [if initially authorized to only dispense a particular schedule(s) of controlled substances].

7. Transfer of registration. A registration to dispense controlled substances may not be transferred to any other person or entity except when the ownership of a pharmacy is being transferred from one entity to another. In such a case, controlled substances in schedules II–V must be properly disposed of or transferred to the new entity.

8. Suspension or revocation of registration. The DEA may suspend or revoke any registration. The DEA must first issue an Order To Show Cause (upon the registrant) why the registration should not be revoked or suspended. The registrant may request a hearing to explain why the registration should not be suspended or revoked. After a hearing, the DEA may suspend, revoke, or take no action on the registration.

    a. Order of suspension or revocation. After a registrant has received an order suspending or revoking its registration, it must take the following action:

        (1) Immediately deliver its certificate of registration and any DEA 222 order forms in its possession to the nearest office of the DEA

        (2) As instructed by the DEA, either:

            (a) deliver all controlled substances in its possession to the nearest office of the DEA or to authorized agents of the DEA or

            (b) place all controlled substances in its possession under seal.

    b. Imminent danger to public health or safety. The DEA may serve on a registrant an order of immediate suspension when it finds that there is an **imminent danger** to the **public health** or **safety.** The immediate suspension remains in effect until the conclusion of all proceedings, either administrative proceedings by the DEA or judicial proceedings. After receiving an order of immediate suspension, the registrant must take the same action as outlined above under I B 8 a.

9. Exemptions from registration. Certain individuals are exempt from registration under the Act. The following are exempt:

    a. Military officials. Military officials, including Public Health Service and Bureau of Prisons officials, who are authorized to prescribe, dispense, or administer, but not to procure or purchase, controlled substances in the course of their official duties, are exempt from registering with the DEA. The individual must, however, obtain a registration for such activities conducted during any separate private practice.

    b. Law-enforcement officials. Federal and state law-enforcement personnel acting in the course of enforcing any law relating to controlled substances are exempt from registration.

    c. Civil defense officials. Civil defense and disaster-relief organization officials are exempt from registration in order to maintain and dispense controlled substances during times of proclaimed emergencies or disasters.

    d. Agents and employees of registrants. Agents and employees, while acting lawfully in the usual course of their business or employment, are exempt from registration when the business or employment is conducted on behalf of a person (or business) who is registered under the Act. Delivery personnel (e.g., United Parcel Service, Federal Express) are therefore not required to register. Likewise, pharmacists working for a registered pharmacy are not required to register.

10. Termination of registration. The registration of any person or entity will terminate when the person dies, ceases legal existence (e.g., corporate dissolution, partnership dissolution), or discontinues business or professional practice. The DEA must be notified promptly when any of these occurs. In such a case, all controlled substances in schedules II–V must be properly disposed of.

C. Required inventories. The Act requires all pharmacies and hospitals (every separately registered location) to conduct an initial inventory and biennial inventory of all controlled substances in schedules II, III, IV, and V.

1. **Initial inventory.** The initial inventory must be taken on the date the entity commences business and begins dispensing controlled substances. If the entity has no controlled substances on hand, a record of this fact must be maintained as its initial inventory.

2. **Biennial inventory.** The biennial inventory must be taken at least every 2 years from the date of the initial inventory.
   a. **Biennial date.** The biennial date may be **any** date that is within 2 years of the previous biennial (or initial) date. This date does **not** have to be reported to the DEA if it is different than the biennial date that would otherwise apply (i.e., on the exact day 2 years after the previous inventory).

3. **Inventory procedures**
   a. All inventories must be maintained in a **written, typewritten,** or **printed form** and be conducted at either the opening of business or the close of business on the inventory date (which must be noted on the inventory).
   b. **Separate inventory record for schedule II controlled substances.** Because all records for schedule II controlled substances must be maintained separately from other records, schedule II inventories must be maintained separately from other controlled-substance inventories.

4. **Inventory content.** All inventory records must contain the following:
   a. Date the inventory is taken
   b. Each finished form of the substance (dosage form and strength)
   c. Number of units or volume of each finished form in each commercial container (e.g., 100-tablet bottle). For opened commercial containers, inventory must be taken as follows:
      (1) For schedule II controlled substances, an exact count or measure must be taken.
      (2) For schedule III, IV, and V controlled substances, an estimated count or measure may be taken, except that an exact count must be taken if the container holds more than 1000 tablets or capsules.
   d. For each controlled substance maintained for extemporaneous compounding, or for substances that are damaged, defective, or impure and awaiting disposal:
      (1) Name of the substance
      (2) Total quantity to the nearest metric unit weight or the total number of units of finished form
      (3) Reason the substance is being maintained and whether it is capable of use in the manufacture of any controlled substance in finished form

5. **Inventory record maintenance.** Every inventory record must be maintained at the registered location (e.g., pharmacy, hospital) for at least 2 years from the date of the inventory.
   a. Schedule II inventories must be maintained separately from all other records of the pharmacy.
   b. Schedule III–V inventory records must be maintained either separately from all other records of the pharmacy or in such a manner that the required information is readily retrievable from ordinary business records of the pharmacy. "Readily retrievable" means that the inventory records can be separated out from all other records in a reasonable time.

6. **Perpetual inventories.** The Act does not require a dispenser registrant (e.g., pharmacy, hospital) to maintain a perpetual inventory of any controlled substance.

7. **Newly controlled substances or changes in scheduling of a substance.** An inventory of a substance must be taken when, by order of the DEA, it becomes a newly controlled substance or it shifts into another schedule. The inventory of that particular controlled substance must be taken on the effective date of the change. A complete inventory of all controlled substances is not required, nor is an inventory required when a substance moves from a controlled-substance schedule to a nonfederal schedule.

8. **Transfer of business activity.** An inventory of controlled substances II–V must be taken at the time a pharmacy or hospital undergoes a change in ownership. The inventory must

be taken on the date of transfer and serves as the final inventory of the transferor and the initial inventory of the transferee.

9. **Inventory record submission.** The Act does not require the submission of inventory records to anyone, including the DEA. The records must be maintained at the registered location for inspection and copying by authorized agents of the DEA.

D. **Obtaining controlled substances.** Schedule II controlled substances must be obtained from a supplier (wholesaler, manufacturer) by using DEA Form 222. The Act does not require the use of any special form to obtain controlled substances in schedules III–V.

1. **DEA Form 222.** Only entities that are registered to dispense or handle schedule II controlled substances may obtain Form 222. The forms are serially numbered and issued by the DEA with the name, address, registration number, authorized activity, and schedules of the registrant. Each form contains an original, duplicate, and triplicate copy (Copy 1, Copy 2, and Copy 3, respectively).

   a. **Execution of Form 222.** Form 222 may be executed only on behalf of the registrant named on the form and only if the registration has not expired nor been revoked or suspended. The form must be prepared in triplicate as provided by the DEA by use of a typewriter, pen, or indelible pencil in the following manner:

      (1) Only one item may be ordered on each of the 10 numbered lines on the form. The total number of items ordered must be noted on the form in the space provided.

      (2) One item may consist of one or more commercial or bulk containers of a product. A separate item must be made for different commercial or bulk containers of a product. For each item, the form must contain the following information:

         (a) Name of the article ordered

         (b) Finished or bulk form of the product (dosage form and strength)

         (c) Number of units or volume in each commercial or bulk container (e.g., 100-tablet bottle)

         (d) Number of commercial or bulk containers ordered

         (e) If the article is not in pure form, the name and quantity per unit of the controlled substances contained in the article.

      (3) The supplier's name and address must be included on the form. Only one supplier may be listed on any one form.

      (4) Each form must include the date of the order, and no form is valid more than 60 days after its execution by the purchaser.

      (5) The form must be signed either by the person who signed the most recent application for registration or reregistration, or by a person authorized to obtain and execute order forms by a **power of attorney.**

         (a) Any purchaser may authorize one or more individuals (does not have to be an attorney-at-law), whether or not located at the registered location, to obtain and execute 222 Forms by executing a power of attorney for the individual(s).

         (b) The power of attorney must be signed by the person who signed the most recent application for registration or reregistration and by the individual(s) receiving the power of attorney. This form must be similar or identical to the DEA's "Power of Attorney for DEA Order Forms."

         (c) Once properly executed, the individual receiving the power of attorney may obtain and sign DEA Form 222 to the same extent as the individual who signed the most recent application for registration or reregistration.

         (d) The power of attorney must be filed with the executed 222 Forms of the purchaser and be retained for the same period as any order form bearing the signature of the attorney [see I.D.1.a (8)]. The power of attorney does not have to be submitted to the DEA.

      (6) Copies 1 and 2 must be submitted to the supplier. Copy 3 must be retained by the purchaser.

      (7) When the ordered schedule II controlled substances are received by the pharmacy, the following information must be recorded on the retained Copy 3:

         (a) Number of commercial or bulk containers furnished on each item (or line)

         (b) Date on which the containers are received by the pharmacy

      (8) DEA 222 Forms must be maintained at the registered location (pharmacy or hospital) for at least 2 years from their execution. The time of execution would be the date the last entry was made on Copy 3.

    b. Cancellation by purchaser. A purchaser may cancel all or part of an order by notifying the supplier in writing. The supplier must indicate the cancellation on Copies 1 and 2 by drawing a line through the canceled items and printing the word "canceled" in the space provided for number of items shipped. Likewise, a supplier may void all or part of an order by notifying the purchaser in writing and printing the word "canceled" in the space provided for number of items shipped.

    c. Maintenance of DEA Form 222. Executed Copy 3 forms and Copies 1 and 2 of each unaccepted or defective form and the statement of refusal from the supplier must be maintained by the purchaser. They must be kept separate from all other records and be available for inspection for at least 2 years. All forms must be maintained at the registered location preprinted on the form, and not at a central location.

    d. Loss or theft of DEA Form 222. Any used or unused form stolen from or lost by a purchaser or supplier must be reported immediately to the DEA. Such notification must include the serial number of each form lost or stolen.

2. Obtaining schedule III–V controlled substances. There is no special form for obtaining schedule III–V controlled substances. Each registrant must, however, maintain a complete and accurate record of receipt for each such substance. The record must be maintained at either the registered location of the pharmacy or hospital, or at a central location, for 2 years. If a central location is used, the pharmacy must first notify the DEA, indicating its intention to keep central records. Central records may then be maintained unless the DEA denies the request to keep such records. An invoice or packing slip will suffice as a record of receipt, providing the following information is included:

    a. Name of the controlled substance

    b. Finished form of the substance (dosage form and strength)

    c. Number of units or volume of the finished form in each commercial container (e.g., 100-tablet bottle)

    d. Number of commercial containers of each such finished form received from other persons

    e. Date of actual receipt of each commercial container

    f. Name, address, and registration number of the person from whom the containers were received

E. Storage of controlled substances. All controlled substances in schedules II–V must be stored in one of the following ways:

1. In a securely locked, substantially constructed cabinet

2. Dispersed throughout the stock of unscheduled prescription medication to prevent any theft or diversion

F. Theft or significant loss of schedule II–V controlled substances. Every registrant must promptly notify the regional office of the DEA of the theft or significant loss of any controlled substance in schedules II–V. This report must be done using DEA **Form 106.**

G. Disposal of controlled substances. Every disposal of a controlled substance must be accomplished by submitting DEA **Form 41** to the DEA (except for disposals pursuant to a valid prescription, discussed below). The form must list the controlled substances earmarked for disposal. The DEA will authorize the disposal and instruct the registrant to dispose of the controlled substances in one of the following ways:

1. By the transfer to a person or entity registered with the DEA and authorized to possess the substance. Schedule II controlled substances must be transferred by use of the transferee's (another pharmacy or hospital, or the wholesaler or manufacturer) DEA Form 222. A written record of the transfer of schedule III–V controlled substances must be kept for at least 2 years and include the following information:

    a. Name of the controlled substance

    b. Finished form of the substance (dosage form and strength)

    c. Number of units or volume of the finished form in each commercial container (e.g., 100-tablet bottle)

    d. Number of commercial containers of each finished form transferred

    e. Date of the transfer

    f. Name, address, and registration number of the transferee

2. By the delivery to an agent of the DEA or to the nearest office of the DEA

3. By the destruction in the presence of an agent of the DEA or other authorized person

4. By any other means that the DEA determines to ensure that the substance does not become available to unauthorized persons or entities

H. Regular disposals of controlled substances. If a registrant (usually a hospital) regularly disposes of controlled substances in schedules II–V the DEA may authorize disposals without prior approval in each instance. If the DEA grants this authority, the registrant must keep records of each disposal and file periodic reports to the regional office of the DEA summarizing the disposals. The DEA may place additional conditions on such disposal, including the method of disposal and the frequency and detail of reports.

I. Disposal of controlled substances pursuant to a valid prescription

1. Persons who may issue prescriptions for controlled substances. A controlled-substance prescription may be issued only by a practitioner who is granted such authority by the state in which that practitioner is licensed. Although the Act is federal legislation, each state determines who will be authorized to dispense controlled substances. Most states allow the following individuals to prescribe: physicians, dentists, podiatrists, and veterinarians. Some states allow the following individuals, referred to as midlevel practitioners, to prescribe (usually with certain restrictions): physician's assistants, nurse practitioners, certified nurse midwives, psychiatric nurses, mental health clinical specialists. All prescribers must be registered with the DEA or exempted from registration (see I.B.9).

    a. DEA numbers and authenticity. After registering with the DEA, all registrants are assigned a DEA number by the DEA. A practitioner's DEA number consists of nine characters. The first two characters are letters. The first letter will be either A or B. The second letter will be the first letter of the practitioner's last name. The next six characters are randomly chosen numbers. The last character is a number often referred to as the "check digit." For example, Dr. Henry Jones may have a DEA number of AJ 4357782.

        (1) Authentication of DEA number. The DEA assigns DEA numbers with a quick method of verification built into the number. This allows a dispensing pharmacist to make a cursory review of the number for authenticity. For example, using the above DEA number, the practitioner's last name must start with a J. Also, the following quick calculation can be made to verify that the "check digit" is correct:

            (a) The digits in positions 1, 3, and 5 are added together to reach a number. In the above example, that would be $4 + 5 + 7 = 16$.

            (b) The digits in positions 2, 4, and 6 are added together, then multiplied by 2. In the above example, that would be $(3 + 7 + 8) \times 2 = 36$.

            (c) These numbers above are added together: $16 + 36 = 52$. The far-right digit becomes the check digit. The check digit must therefore be a 2. If the check digit is anything other than a 2, the number may not be a valid DEA number. In such a case, the DEA should be notified in order to verify the number.

        (2) Midlevel practitioner DEA numbers. Midlevel practitioner DEA numbers are similar to practitioner DEA numbers except for the first character. Instead of the letter A or B, midlevel practitioners have the letter M as the first character in their DEA number. The mathematical method for verifying the authenticity of the number is the same.

        (3) DEA numbers for practitioners and midlevel practitioners who are employees of institutions. Practitioners and midlevel practitioners who issue prescriptions in the course of their employment with an institution may issue prescriptions for all controlled substances under the institution's DEA registration. The practitioner's or mid-level practitioner's "DEA number" will be a specific internal code number issued by the institution. The code number must consist of numbers, letters, or a combination of numbers and letters and must be a suffix to the institution's DEA number, preceded by a hyphen (e.g., AP0123456-10 or AP0123456-A12).

2. Purpose of issuance of controlled-substance prescriptions. A controlled-substance prescription may be issued only in good faith for a legitimate medical purpose by a practitioner acting in the usual course of his or her professional practice. The practitioner and the dispensing pharmacist have the responsibility to ensure that a prescription is properly issued and dispensed (referred to as corresponding responsibility of the pharmacist).

    a. Legitimate medical purpose. Legitimate medical purpose and good faith are prerequisites for all controlled-substance prescriptions. With respect to a pharmacist, these requirements will be apparent from an objective point of view. As a general rule, if, from all the surrounding facts and circumstances, a reasonably prudent pharmacist would form the opinion that a prescription was issued for a legitimate medical purpose, then the pharmacist has fulfilled his or her responsibility under the Act, and the prescription may be legally dispensed.

    b. Usual course of professional practice. A **practitioner–patient relationship** for the purpose of treating and caring for the patient must be present. Usually, such a relationship includes the taking and recording of an appropriate medical history, and an appropriate physical exam. This limits a practitioner's ability to prescribe outside his or her course of professional practice (e.g., a veterinarian may not prescribe a controlled substance for a human). The notion of "usual course of practice" becomes more unclear with respect to medical doctors who specialize. Such specialists often issue prescriptions "outside" their specialty. Generally, all controlled-substance prescriptions from medical doctors are deemed to be "in the usual course of professional practice" as long as it is issued for a human, regardless of whether the problem being treated is within the doctor's specialty.

    c. Restrictions on issuance of a controlled-substance prescription

        (1) A prescription may not be issued by a practitioner in order for that practitioner to obtain controlled substances for the purpose of **general dispensing** to his or her patients.

        (2) A prescription may not be issued for the dispensing of controlled substances for **detoxification** or maintenance treatment. Administration and direct dispensing of controlled substances are allowed only when conducted in properly registered treatment programs. A prescription for **methadone** is valid only when issued as an analgesic in cases of severe pain. Methadone may be dispensed in a hospital to maintain a patient's addiction as long as the patient is admitted and being treated for some other medical condition and is not administered methadone solely for detoxification purposes.

3. Manner of issuance of a controlled-substance prescription. Schedule II controlled-substance prescriptions must be written with ink or indelible pencil or typewritten (except in cases of oral emergency schedule II prescriptions). Schedule III–V controlled-substance prescriptions may be orally ordered by the practitioner. Prescriptions may be prepared by either the practitioner or an agent of the practitioner, and communicated to the pharmacy by the practitioner or the agent. Authorization for the prescription (or refill) must, however, originate with the practitioner. Both the practitioner and dispensing pharmacist are responsible for the completeness of the prescription. All prescriptions for controlled substances must include the following information:

    a. Full name and address of the patient

    b. Date the prescription is issued and signed (one and the same)

    c. Drug name, dosage form and strength

    d. Quantity of drug prescribed

    e. Directions for use

    f. Name, address, and DEA registration number of the practitioner

    g. The signature of the practitioner (no preprinted or stamped signatures) as he or she would sign any legal document (all schedule II controlled-substance prescriptions must be manually signed by the practitioner)

4. Emergency dispensing of schedule II controlled substances

    a. An oral schedule II controlled-substance prescription may be received from a practitioner in an emergency situation. An emergency prescription must include all of the information required for any controlled-substance prescription. An emergency situation exists when **all three** of the following factors are present:

        (1) The immediate administration of the controlled substance is necessary for proper treatment of the patient.

        (2) No appropriate alternative treatment is available, including administration of a controlled substance that is not in schedule II.

        (3) It is not reasonably possible for the practitioner to provide a written prescription to be presented to the person dispensing the controlled substance before the dispensing.

b. Proper dispensing. The quantity prescribed and dispensed must be limited to the amount necessary to adequately treat the patient during the emergency period. If the practitioner is not known to the pharmacist, the pharmacist must make a reasonable good-faith effort to determine that the oral authorization came from a registered practitioner.

   (1) Delivery of written prescription. The practitioner who authorizes the emergency prescription must, within 7 days of the oral authorization, deliver a written prescription to the dispensing pharmacist. The prescription must contain the information required of all controlled-substance prescriptions, have written on its face the words "Authorization for Emergency Dispensing," and the date of the oral authorization. The prescription may be delivered in person or by mail; if delivered by mail, it must be postmarked within the 7-day period. Upon receipt, the dispensing pharmacist must attach it to the oral emergency prescription, which was previously reduced to writing.

   (2) Failure to deliver a written prescription. If a practitioner fails to deliver the written prescription as required, the dispensing pharmacist must notify the regional office of the DEA. Failure by the pharmacist to notify the DEA serves to void the pharmacist's authority to dispense an oral emergency schedule II prescription. The pharmacist will be deemed to have unlawfully dispensed a schedule II controlled substance.

5. Facsimile prescriptions. Prescriptions for controlled substances III, IV and V (and non-federal controlled substances such as penicillin and furosemide) may be delivered to the dispensing pharmacy via facsimile machine. A facsimile prescription is deemed to be the written, signed prescription from the prescriber so long as it contains the information required of all prescriptions under federal law. The prescription must be sent directly from the prescriber or his authorized agent to the pharmacy.

   a. Schedule II controlled substances. Prescriptions for schedule II controlled substances may be sent via facsimile to a dispensing pharmacy to facilitate dispensing of the prescription. **No drug may be released** to the patient until the original, signed prescription is presented to the dispensing pharmacist. A schedule II controlled-substance facsimile prescription **will serve** as the original, signed prescription in the following situations:

   (1) Injectable home-health prescriptions. A facsimile schedule II narcotic prescription calling for the compounding of a solution for direct administration to a patient in a private residence, long-term–care facility, or hospice setting may serve as the original prescription. The exception applies so long as the solution will be administered by means of parenteral, intravenous, intramuscular, subcutaneous, or intraspinal infusion.

   (2) Long-term–care facility prescriptions. Any facsimile schedule II prescription issued for a resident of a long-term–care facility may serve as the original, signed prescription.

   (3) Hospice patient prescriptions. Any facsimile schedule II narcotic prescription issued for a patient enrolled in a hospice-care program certified and/or paid for by Medicare under Title XVIII or licensed by state law may serve as the original prescription. The prescriber, or his agent, **must** note on the prescription that the patient is a hospice patient.

6. Electronic data transmission prescriptions. Prescription information that is transmitted directly from a practitioner to a pharmacy by electronic means such as the Internet is referred to as electronic data transmission prescriptions. Electronic signatures are recognized as legally acceptable signatures of practitioners and legend drugs, except for controlled substances, may be transmitted to pharmacies via the Internet if allowed by state law. A state may allow a practitioner and pharmacy to maintain the prescription information in electronic form without reducing it to writing, so long as they comply with state-mandated safeguards.

   a. Controlled-substance prescriptions. The DEA does not yet recognize electronic data transmission prescriptions as a means of communicating prescription information for any controlled substance. Therefore, prescription information for controlled substances may not be communicated from a practitioner to a pharmacy by electronic means.

7. Persons who may dispense controlled-substance prescriptions. A **pharmacist** acting in the usual course of his or her professional practice in a DEA-registered pharmacy (or hospital or other registered facility) may dispense a controlled substance pursuant to a prescription.

A **pharmacy intern** acting under the direct supervision of his preceptor in a DEA-registered facility may also dispense a controlled substance pursuant to a prescription.

8. **Dispensing procedures of controlled substances pursuant to a prescription.** Once a controlled-substance prescription has been lawfully issued by a practitioner and presented to a pharmacist, it may be dispensed in accordance with the following:
   a. **Presentation to the pharmacist.** Schedules III and IV controlled-substance prescriptions are valid for 6 months from the date of issuance by the practitioner. Schedule II controlled-substance prescriptions have no time limit for presentation under the Act, although they are often recognized to be valid for up to 6 months. Schedule V controlled-substance prescriptions also have no set time limit for presentation under the Act. Regardless of which schedule of controlled substance is involved, the good-faith and "legitimate medical purpose" limitation will always apply and may serve to otherwise limit the validity of a prescription.
   b. **Information that must be recorded on the prescription by the dispensing pharmacist.** Under the Act, a filled prescription is considered to be a lawful record of disposition for a controlled substance. As a result, every prescription for a controlled substance must contain certain information. Some of the information will already be contained in the prescription, although the dispensing pharmacist is responsible for ensuring that all of the following information is recorded (usually on the face of the prescription):
      (1) Name of the controlled substance
      (2) Finished form of the controlled substance (dosage form and strength)
      (3) Name and address of the person to whom it was dispensed
      (4) Date of dispensing
      (5) Number of units or volume dispensed (quantity)
      (6) Written or typewritten name or initials of the individual who dispensed the controlled substance
      (7) Serial number of the prescription
   c. **Required information on prescription labels.** Every prescription label for a controlled substance must include the following information:
      (1) Name and address of the pharmacy
      (2) Serial number assigned to the prescription
      (3) Date of the initial filling of the prescription (for refills, the date originally filled)
      (4) Name of the patient
      (5) Name of the prescribing practitioner
      (6) Directions for use, and cautionary statements, if any
      (7) For schedule II, III, and IV controlled substances, the federal crime transfer warning must appear on the container: "Caution: Federal law prohibits the transfer of this drug to any person other than the patient for whom it was prescribed."
   d. **Allowable quantities that may be dispensed.** The Act contains no limitation concerning the quantity of a controlled substance that may be dispensed pursuant to a prescription. All quantities are, of course, limited to the good-faith and "legitimate medical purpose" standards.
   e. **Filing controlled substance prescriptions.** Written controlled-substance prescriptions must be maintained at the pharmacy for a period of 2 years from the date of the original dispensing or last refill, whichever is later. They must be available for inspection and copying by employees and agents of the DEA and be filed **segregated** from all other records in one of the following ways (state law usually dictates the method to be used):
      (1) Using **three separate files** as follows:
         (a) One file for schedule II controlled-substance prescriptions
         (b) One file for schedule III, IV, and V controlled-substance prescriptions
         (c) One file for unscheduled prescription drugs
      (2) Using **two separate files** as follows:
         (a) One file for all controlled-substance prescriptions (II–V), as long as schedule III, IV, and V prescriptions have the letter "C" stamped in red ink in the lower-right corner no less than 1 inch high
         (b) One file for unscheduled prescription drugs
      (3) Using **two separate files** as follows:
         (a) One file for schedule II controlled-substance prescriptions
         (b) One file for all other controlled substances (III–V) and unscheduled prescription drugs, as long as schedule III, IV, and V prescriptions have the letter "C" stamped in red ink in the lower-right corner no less than 1 inch high

(4) In either **(2)** or **(3)** above, if a pharmacy utilizes an electronic record-keeping system for prescriptions (i.e., computerized records), which permits identification by prescription number and retrieval of original documents by prescriber's name, patient's name, drug dispensed, and date filled, then the requirement to mark the hard copy prescription with a red "C" is waived.

f. Refill dispensing of controlled substances. Prescriptions for schedule II controlled substances may not be refilled. Prescriptions for schedules III and IV controlled substances may be refilled up to five times within 6 months from the date of issue of the prescription. Schedule V controlled-substance prescriptions have no limitations for refilling under the Act; however, once again, the good-faith and "legitimate medical purpose" limitations apply here, as well as to all controlled-substance refills.

(1) Refill information may be maintained either manually or by use of a computer. The Act requires that the information be maintained one way or the other, but not both ways. If **computerized refill records** are maintained, the system must have certain capabilities and the dispensing pharmacist must follow certain procedures.

(a) The computer must be able to provide on-line retrieval of the original prescription information, provide on-line retrieval of the refill history, a refill-by-refill audit trail, and an auxiliary procedure in those cases where the system experiences downtime.

(b) The system must also allow the pharmacist who refills a prescription to document that the information he or she entered into the computer is correct.

(2) When dispensing a refill, the pharmacist must record, on the back of the original prescription or by computer, the following information:

(a) Date of the refill

(b) Name or initials of the refilling pharmacist

(c) Amount of the medication dispensed (if the amount is omitted, the refill will be deemed to have been for the full face amount prescribed by the practitioner)

g. Partial dispensing of controlled substances. The Act does not prohibit the partial dispensing of controlled substances in schedules III and IV, provided that each partial filling is recorded in the same manner as refills, the total quantity dispensed in all partial fillings does not exceed the total quantity prescribed, and no partial filling occurs after 6 months from the date of issuance of the prescription. Likewise, all partial fillings of a schedule V prescription must not exceed the total quantity prescribed.

(1) Partial dispensing of a schedule II controlled substance. The partial dispensing of a schedule II prescription is allowed if the pharmacist is unable to supply the full quantity or the prescription is for a terminally ill patient or a patient in a long-term–care facility (LTCF). Under no other circumstance may a schedule II prescription be partially dispensed.

(a) Inadequate supply. In cases of an inadequate supply, the dispensing pharmacist must note on the face of the prescription the amount dispensed. The remaining balance of the schedule II prescription must be dispensed within 72 hours of the first partial filling. If, for any reason, the balance is not dispensed within the 72-hour period, the pharmacist must notify the prescribing practitioner of this fact. The pharmacist may not dispense any further amounts pursuant to this prescription beyond the 72-hour period.

(b) Terminally ill and patients in LTCFs. It is the pharmacist's responsibility to ensure that a patient has a medical diagnosis documenting a terminal illness or that the patient is in an LTCF. Before any partial dispensing, the pharmacist must record on the prescription whether the patient is "terminally ill" or an "LTCF patient." Any partial dispensing without one of these notations shall be deemed to be a dispensing in violation of the Act. The total amount of the schedule II substance dispensed in all partial fillings must not exceed the total quantity prescribed. Schedule II prescriptions for a terminally ill patient or a patient in an LTCF are valid up to 60 days from the date of issuance of the prescription by the practitioner. All of the following information must be recorded, either manually on the back of the prescription or via computer (with similar capabilities required for computerized refill record keeping), when partially dispensing a schedule II prescription for a terminally ill patient or a patient in an LTCF:

(i) Date of the partial filling

(ii) Quantity of drug dispensed

(iii) Remaining quantity authorized to be dispensed

(iv) Identification of the dispensing pharmacist

h. Transfer of refill information for a controlled-substance prescription. Refill information concerning schedules III, IV, and V controlled substances may be transferred to another pharmacy only once (if allowed by state law). Pharmacies electronically sharing a real-time, on-line database (such as chain pharmacies) may transfer refill information for these controlled substances up to the maximum number of refills permitted by law and the prescriber's authorization. The communication must be made directly between two licensed pharmacists. Both the original prescription and the transferred prescription must be maintained for 2 years from the date of the last refill. Certain information must be recorded as follows:

(1) The **transferring pharmacist** must:

(a) Write the word "void" on the face of the original prescription

(b) On the back of the prescription, record the name, address, and DEA registration number of the pharmacy to which it was transferred and the name of the pharmacist receiving the information

(c) Record the date of the transfer and the name of the transferring pharmacist

(2) The **receiving pharmacist** must:

(a) Write the word "transfer" on the face of the transferred prescription

(b) Record all of the information required for any controlled-substance prescription (see I I 3), and include the following:

(i) Date of issuance of the original prescription

(ii) Original number of refills authorized on the original prescription

(iii) Date the prescription was initially dispensed

(iv) Number of valid refills remaining and the date of the last refill

(v) Pharmacy's name, address, DEA registration number, and original prescription number from which the prescription information was transferred

(vi) Name of the transferring pharmacist

J. Disposal of controlled substances to a patient without a prescription. Controlled substances that are not prescription (or legend) drugs under federal law may be dispensed to a patient at retail without a prescription. These drugs do not have on the manufacturer's label the federal statement: "Caution: Federal law prohibits dispensing without a prescription." The substances may be dispensed without a prescription in accordance with the following:

1. The dispensing must be made only by a licensed pharmacist. The actual cash transfer or delivery may be made by a nonpharmacist.

2. Not more than 8 oz of any substance containing opium, 4 oz of any other controlled substance, 48 dosage units of any substance containing opium, or 24 dosage units of any other controlled substance may be dispensed to the same purchaser in any 48-hour period.

3. The purchaser is at least 18 years old.

4. Any purchaser not known to the pharmacist must furnish suitable identification.

5. A bound record book must be maintained for 2 years from the date of the last entry. The following information must be recorded for each purchase:

a. Name and address of the purchaser

b. Name and quantity of controlled substance purchased

c. Date of each purchase

d. Name or initials of the pharmacist who dispensed the substance to the purchaser

6. All dispensing of a controlled substance without a prescription must be done in good faith and not to evade the provisions of the Act.

K. Security considerations

1. Controlled-substance seals. Manufacturers must package certain controlled substances in a container with a securely affixed seal to reveal any tampering. Every bottle, multiple-dose vial, or other commercial container of any controlled substance listed in schedule

II, or of any narcotic controlled substance listed in schedule III or IV, must be packaged with such a seal.

2. **Felony convictions.** No DEA registrant may employ an individual who has access to controlled substances if that individual had previously been convicted of a felony offense related to controlled substances.

3. **Manufacturer's label.** Every commercial container of a controlled substance must have on its label the symbol designating the schedule in which the controlled substance is listed. The symbol must appear in the upper-right corner of the label or be overprinted on the label.

L. **Record maintenance.** All records required to be maintained under the Act must be kept by the registrant for 2 years. The records may be maintained at a central location (e.g., at a chain pharmacy's regional office) after notifying the DEA. However, executed DEA 222 Forms (Copy 3), all controlled-substance prescriptions, and all inventories must be maintained at the pharmacy, not centrally. All schedule II controlled-substance records must be maintained separately and readily retrievable from all other records.

M. **DEA inspections.** Inspections by the DEA of any registered facility may be conducted only in a reasonable manner and during regular business hours. Inspection may be conducted after obtaining consent of the registrant or after the DEA has obtained an administrative warrant from a judge. An application for an administrative warrant must state with specificity the nature, extent, and authority to conduct the requested inspection. The scope of an administrative inspection extends to any records required under the Act, equipment and containers used in the handling of controlled substances, and the verification of compliance with any requirement of the Act. If records are removed from the registrant by the DEA, a receipt given to the registrant will list the items taken.

N. **Long-term–care facilities (LTCFs).** An LTCF is defined as a nursing home, retirement care, mental care, or other facility or institution that provides extended health care to resident patients. LTCFs are not normally registered with the DEA, although they often maintain controlled substances that are dispensed to a patient by prescription from a pharmacy. They are not required to be registered with the DEA because the controlled substance is dispensed to the ultimate user (the patient) and is not issued by or through the LTCF. When disposing of controlled substances, LTCFs must contact the nearest DEA Diversion Field Office for disposal instructions.

1. **Emergency kits for LTCFs.** An LTCF may maintain controlled substances in emergency kits so long as state law specifically approves of such use and the state sets forth procedures that require the following:
   a. **Source of supply:** The LTCF must obtain controlled substances for the emergency kits from a DEA-registered hospital/clinic, pharmacy, or practitioner.
   b. **Security safeguards:** Access to each emergency kit in the LTCF must be restricted, and the type and quantity of controlled substances that may be placed in the emergency kit must be specifically limited.
   c. **Proper control, accountability, and record keeping:** The LTCF and the providing DEA-registered hospital/clinic, pharmacy, or practitioner must maintain complete and accurate records of the controlled substances placed in the emergency kit, including the disposition of these controlled substances, as well as take periodic physical inventories of the drugs.
   d. **Administration of controlled substances.** In emergency medical situations when medication is needed from the emergency kit, only LTCF personnel who are authorized by an individual practitioner can administer the controlled substances.
   e. **Prohibited activities:** Prohibited activities can result in the state revocation, denial, or suspension of having emergency kits containing controlled substances in an LTCF.

O. **Violations under the Act.** Penalties for violations of the Federal Controlled Substances Act depend on the schedule of controlled substance involved, the unlawful act, **and the knowledge and intent of the violator.** It will also depend on whether it is a first offense or a subsequent offense.

1. **Civil penalty.** Generally, each violation of the Act may subject an individual to a civil penalty (fine) of up to $10,000. The government must prove that the violator was negligent with respect to compliance under the Act, as opposed to mere mistake or inadvertence.

2. **Imprisonment.** If an individual knowingly and intentionally violates the Act, he or she may be sentenced to a term of years, in addition to a civil penalty.

II. FEDERAL FOOD, DRUG, AND COSMETIC ACT (FDCA).
In 1937, sulfanilamide elixir containing deadly diethylene glycol (automobile antifreeze) was manufactured without any safety data. There were numerous deaths associated with its use, which prompted the federal government to pass the 1938 FDCA. The FDCA requires that all new drug products intended for use as labeled by the manufacturer in the United States must be proven to the federal government to be safe and effective. Such proof is submitted to the Food and Drug Administration (FDA) by use of a New Drug Application (NDA).

A. **Definition.** Under the FDCA, the term "drug" is defined as including all of the following:

1. Articles recognized in the official *United States Pharmacopeia (USP),* official *Homeopathic Pharmacopoeia of the United States,* or official *National Formulary,* or any supplement to these

2. Articles intended for use in the diagnosis, cure, mitigation, treatment, or prevention of disease in man or other animals

3. Articles (other than food) intended to affect the structure or any function of the body of man or other animals

4. Articles intended for use as a component of any article specified in 1, 2, or 3 above

B. **Legend drugs.** Legend drugs are those medications that have on their label from the manufacturer the following federally required statement: "**Rx** only." Such medications may be dispensed directly to the patient by means of a valid written or oral prescription from a practitioner or by a valid refill authorization of either. By law, these medications must bear a label with adequate directions for use, which can only be given by a licensed practitioner and, therefore, the requirement of a prescription. A drug, intended for use by humans, is considered a legend drug (and have the above caution on its label) if any of the following apply:

1. Because of the drug's toxicity or other potential for a harmful effect, or its method of use, or collateral measures necessary to its use, it is **not safe** for use **except under the supervision** of a practitioner licensed by law to administer such drug.

2. The drug is a **new drug** for which an approved NDA limits its use to the professional supervision of a practitioner licensed by law to administer such drug. A new drug is broadly defined as being one that generally is not recognized among experts as safe and effective for use under the conditions prescribed, recommended, or suggested in the labeling. It is also defined as being a drug that, as a result of investigations to determine its safety and effectiveness for use under such conditions, has become so recognized but that has not, other than in the investigations, been used to a material extent or for a material time under such conditions. Finally, a new drug may result from a change in the dosage form, labeling, indications, or any other change in a drug product that is already being marketed. The ultimate decision of whether a drug is a new drug lies with the FDA because of its expertise in resolving technical and scientific questions.

   a. **NDA.** Every new drug marketed in the United States must be safe and effective for its intended use as labeled by the manufacturer. Proof of safety and effectiveness must be submitted to the FDA by the manufacturer via the NDA. When a new chemical entity (NCE) is identified by a manufacturer, the manufacturer must obtain an Investigational New Drug Application (IND) before conducting preclinical animal tests and clinical human investigations.

   b. **IND.** Because an NCE has not yet been approved by the FDA as a safe and effective drug, a manufacturer is required to file an IND with the FDA. The IND allows a manufacturer to conduct research with the NCE and exempts the drug from certain prohibitions of the FDCA in order to facilitate clinical investigations; thus, INDs are sometimes referred to as an Investigational New Drug Exemption. Generally, clinical investigation of an NCE is divided into three phases, with each phase involving a greater number of human subjects.

   (1) **Phase 1.** A phase 1 investigation is the initial introduction of an investigational new drug into humans to determine the metabolism, pharmacology, side effects, mechanism of action, and early evidence on effectiveness.

   (2) **Phase 2.** A phase 2 investigation includes the well-controlled, closely monitored clinical studies in order to evaluate the effectiveness of the drug for a particular indication and to further determine side effects and risks.

   (3) **Phase 3.** A phase 3 investigation includes expanded clinical trials to gather additional information concerning safety, effectiveness, and the overall benefit–risk relationship associated with the drug's use. This phase also includes gathering information to provide an adequate basis for physician labeling.

   c. **Treatment INDs (or treatment protocols).** The FDA may allow a treatment IND, which allows a researcher (physician) to use an investigational drug as treatment in serious and life-threatening diseases where no comparable or satisfactory alternative drug or other therapy is available.

C. **Over-the-counter (OTC) medications.** Certain medications may be dispensed OTC at retail distributors without a prescription. The federal government has determined that these medications may be safely and properly self-administered without the supervision of a practitioner licensed by law to administer (or prescribe) such a drug. Generally, these medications are not habit-forming and have a low toxicity or other potential for a harmful effect. These medications do not have the federal statement "**Rx** only" on their label (see II.B).

   1. OTC preparations must have **adequate directions** for use on their label, and the product must comply with the applicable FDA monograph. The FDCA requires all drugs marketed in the United States to be generally recognized as safe and effective. As a result, it convened review panels to review OTC drug effectiveness and create monographs for each therapeutic class of OTC drugs. This review is referred to as the Drug-Efficacy (or Effectiveness) Study Implementation (DESI). All OTC drugs must comply with the applicable drug monograph or be considered misbranded (see II.I) and subject to FDA regulatory action.

   2. OTC preparations must have the following information on its label:
      a. Identity, in bold face, of the OTC product on the principal display panel
      b. Adequate directions for use
      c. Ingredients (including inert or inactive ingredients) in the product
      d. Net quantity of contents
      e. Expiration date of the product
      f. Lot number of the product
      g. Name and place of business of the manufacturer, packer, or distributor
      h. Disclosure of certain contents and the declaration of certain warnings, including habit-forming ingredients and warnings, pregnancy/nursing warnings, and aspirin warnings

   3. **Prescription drug conversion to OTC.** A legend drug will convert to an OTC drug when the FDA finds that the prescription-only limitation is not necessary for the protection of the public health by reason of the drug's toxicity or other potential for harmful effect, the method of its use, or the collateral measures necessary to its use. The FDA must also find that the drug is safe and effective for use in self-medication as directed in proposed labeling.

   4. **Miscellaneous regulations for OTCs.**
      a. **Ipecac syrup.** Although ipecac syrup can only be dispensed pursuant to a prescription, the FDA believes that it should be readily available OTC as an emergency treatment emetic for use in poisonings. The FDA allows the OTC sale of ipecac syrup in 1 fluid ounce containers so that it will be readily available in the household for emergency treatment of poisonings, under medical supervision, and that the drug be appropriately packaged and labeled for this purpose.
      b. **Pregnancy-nursing warning.** All OTC drugs intended for systemic absorption must contain a warning that if the user is pregnant or nursing a baby, she should first seek the advice of a health professional before using the product. Exceptions to this labeling requirement exist when an OTC is intended to benefit the fetus or nursing infant, and for OTC drugs that are labeled exclusively for pediatric use.
      c. **Aspirin warnings.** All OTC aspirin containing preparations must have a warning to keep out of children's reach and to contact a physician immediately in case of accidental

overdose. Oral or rectal OTC aspirin containing preparations must also have a warning concerning Reye's syndrome in children and teenagers.

    d. Chemicals and precursors. It was discovered that combination drug products containing ephedrine, pseudoephedrine, or phenylpropanolamine are the precursor materials used by illegal methamphetamine laboratories. The Comprehensive Methamphetamine Control Act of 1996 requires all retail distributors of these OTC products to fulfill certain obligations. A retail distributor includes a grocery store, general merchandise store, a pharmacy, or any other entity or person who sells these items to customers for personal use. For regulated transactions, a retailer must maintain a record of these transactions for a period of 2 years, must obtain proof of identity from customers, and must report suspicious regulated sales immediately to the DEA. The record must be maintained separately from other records of controlled substances, and the DEA suggests that the record be made in a bound log book similar to the record kept for the sale of OTC controlled substances (see IJ). The following single transactions of these products in the amounts stated are considered to be "regulated transactions."

        (1) Phenylpropanolamine (PPA). PPA is no longer in any OTC drug product.

        (2) Pseudoephedrine. Sales of combination products containing more than 24 g of pseudoephedrine. Blister-pack sales of these products exceeding 24 g are **not** regulated sales.

        (3) Ephedrine. Sales of combination products containing more than 24 g of ephedrine **and all** single-entity ephedrine products regardless of the amount of ephedrine (more than zero grams).

D. Generic drugs

    1. Definition. The *generic name* of a drug has been defined as its chemical name, a common name, or an official name used in an official compendium. A manufacturer seeking approval from the FDA for a drug that has already been proven to be safe and effective may file an Abbreviated New Drug Application (ANDA).

    2. ANDA. A filing of an ANDA allows the approval of a drug for which exhaustive safety and efficacy studies have already been performed. A drug is considered to be the same as an approved drug when the two are identical in active ingredient(s), dosage form, strength, route of administration, indications, and conditions of use. Rigorous animal and human data to determine safety and effectiveness are not required in the ANDA. However, information showing that the generic version of the drug is bioavailable and bioequivalent to the pioneer (original) drug is necessary. Such approved drugs are listed by the FDA in the "Approved Drug Products with Therapeutic Equivalence Evaluations," commonly referred to as the FDA Orange Book (because it comes from the FDA in an orange binder).

E. Proprietary drugs. The *proprietary name* of a drug is the name given by the manufacturer to designate the drug's source of manufacture and to differentiate it from the same or chemically similar drugs from other manufacturers. Another name for the proprietary name of a drug is its trade name.

F. Established names for drugs. The FDCA authorizes the Commissioner of the FDA to designate an official name for any drug if he determines that such action is necessary or desirable in the interest of usefulness and simplicity. The FDCA also requires that a drug's established name appear on the label and labeling of the drug. A drug's *established name* is defined as follows:

    1. It may be an **official name** designated by the Commissioner of Food and Drugs. For NCEs, the name should be simple and useful. In this regard, the FDA recognizes the U.S. Adopted Names Council (USAN) in deriving names for NCEs. The USAN name is considered to be an official name recognized in an official compendium. The FDA may use another name if the USAN or common or usual name is unduly complex, misleading, or is not useful for any other reason.

    2. If no official name has been designated for the drug and the drug is an article recognized in an official compendium, then the **official title** contained in the compendium may be the established name.

    3. If neither of the above two apply, then the **common** or **usual name** of the drug may be its established name.

G. Dispensing a prescription drug. A prescription drug may be dispensed only by a practitioner or by a pharmacist pursuant to a written or oral prescription of a practitioner, or a refill of either. The prescription label on the container dispensed to the patient must contain certain information, or it will be considered misbranded and dispensed in violation of the FDCA. This information is minimal under the FDCA and is usually supplemented by state laws, which require more information. So long as this information is in English, the dispensing pharmacist will be in compliance with the FDCA. If any of the required information is in another language, then all of the required information must be in that language. The prescription must also be packaged in a child-resistant container as required under the Poison Prevention Packaging Act (see III). The following information must appear on every prescription label:

1. Name and address of the pharmacy

2. Serial number of the prescription

3. Date the prescription is filled or the date of the prescription

4. Name of the prescriber

5. Name of the patient (if stated in the prescription)

6. Directions for use and any cautionary statements contained in the prescription

H. Drug recall. The FDCA allows the FDA to initiate regulatory actions to ensure that unsafe, unfit, or ineffective products do not reach the market, or to promptly remove those products that do reach the marketplace. The enforcement actions that may be initiated include the release of information to the general public and/or professional groups; administrative actions and inspections; the institution of recall; or seizure, injunction, or criminal prosecution.

1. **Voluntary action of the manufacturer.** After several unsuccessful attempts by the FDA to receive court-ordered recalls, the FDA recognizes that recalls are voluntary actions of the manufacturers and distributors. As a result, a recall may be undertaken at any time, or upon request of the FDA. If the FDA is unsuccessful in persuading a company to recall a product, or when the FDA determines that a recall is or will be ineffective, it may seek a court order condemning the product and allowing the product's seizure.

2. **Drug recall classification.** After the FDA has evaluated the problem(s) associated with the product and after the degree of health hazard has been determined, the FDA will assign the recall one of the following classifications:
   a. **Class I**—a situation in which there is a reasonable probability that the use of or exposure to a violative product will cause serious adverse health consequences or death
   b. **Class II**—a situation in which use of or exposure to a violative product may cause temporary or medically reversible adverse health consequences or where the probability of serious health consequences is remote
   c. **Class III**—a situation in which use of or exposure to a violative product is not likely to cause adverse health consequences

3. **Recall procedure.** A recall strategy will be developed that will consider the depth of the recall (consumer level, retail level, wholesale level), the need for public warnings, and the extent of effectiveness checks for the recall. Every recalling company is responsible for notifying each of its affected direct accounts by first-class mail, mailgram, or telegram. Public notification is made by the FDA via the weekly *FDA Enforcement Report,* which publishes each recall according to its classification.

I. Adulteration and misbranding. A misbranding or adulteration of a drug is prohibited by the FDCA. Although the misbranding and adulteration provisions are mainly concerned with the manufacturing of a drug, a pharmacist may also misbrand or adulterate a drug. The purpose of the misbranding and adulteration statutes is to protect the public health of consumers who are largely unable to protect themselves where drugs are involved. The adulteration and misbranding statutes are criminal in nature and may subject a pharmacist to criminal proceedings in federal court, in addition to administrative proceedings.

1. **Adulteration.** In general, the term *adulteration* refers to a change or variation from official formulary standards or from the manufacturer's standards. A drug is considered adulterated if any of the following conditions occur:

a. If the drug consists in whole or in part of any filthy, putrid, or decomposed substance
b. If the drug has been prepared, packed, or held under unsanitary conditions where it may have been contaminated with filth or rendered injurious to health
c. If the drug's container is composed, in whole or in part, of any poisonous or deleterious substance that may render the contents injurious to health
d. If the drug contains, for purposes of coloring only, a color additive that is unsafe within the meaning of the FDCA
e. If the drug is a new animal drug, or an animal feed containing a new animal drug, that is unsafe within the meaning of the FDCA
f. If the drug is purported to be a drug that is recognized in an official compendium, and its strength differs from, or its quality or purity falls below, the standard set forth in the compendium, unless the deviation is plainly and specifically stated on its label
g. If the drug is not a compound recognized by name in an official compendium; if its strength differs from, or its purity or quality falls below, that which it purports or is represented to possess
h. If the drug has been mixed or packed with another substance so as to reduce the drug's quality or strength
i. If the drug has been substituted, wholly or partially, with another substance
j. If the drug is an OTC drug and it is not packaged in the required tamper-resistant packaging or properly labeled in conformity with the tamper-resistant regulations (see IV)
k. If the drug (or medical device) is an ophthalmic preparation offered or intended for ophthalmic use that is not sterile

2. **Misbranding.** In general, the term *misbranding* means that a drug is sold or dispensed with a label or labeling that is in violation of the FDCA. *Label* is defined as being a display of written, printed, or graphic matter upon the immediate container of any article (or drug). *Labeling* is more broadly defined to include the label as well as other written, printed, or graphic matter upon any article or any of its containers or wrappers, or accompanying the article (or drug). A drug is considered misbranded if any of the following conditions occur:
a. If the labeling is false or misleading in any particular
b. If the drug is an imitation of another drug, or if it is offered for sale under the name of another drug
c. If the drug is composed wholly or partly of insulin and it is not properly batch certified under the FDCA
d. If the drug is composed wholly or partly of an antibiotic and it is not properly batch certified under the FDCA
e. If the drug is dispensed by a name that is recognized in an official compendium and it is either not packaged or not labeled in conformity with the official compendium
f. If the drug is determined by the federal government to be liable to deterioration and it is not packaged in a proper form and manner, and the label fails to bear a statement of proper precautions
g. If the drug is dispensed in a non–child-resistant container, when a child-resistant container is otherwise required (see III)
h. If the manufacturer fails to place on the label any of the following:
   (1) Fact that certain drugs may be habit forming
   (2) Name of each active ingredient
   (3) Name and place of business of the manufacturer, packer, or distributor
i. If a pharmacist fails to place on a prescription container label any of the following:
   (1) Name and address of the pharmacy
   (2) Serial number of the prescription
   (3) Date of filling the prescription or the date of the prescription
   (4) Name of the prescriber
   (5) Name of the patient
   (6) Directions for use and any cautionary statements contained in the prescription
j. If an oral contraceptive is dispensed without the required patient package insert
k. If an intrauterine device that must be dispensed with a patient package insert is dispensed without the insert
l. If an estrogen product is dispensed without the required patient package insert
m. If a progestogen-containing product is dispensed without the required patient package insert

n. If a legend drug is dispensed (or refilled) without a prescription (or refill authorization) of a licensed practitioner, it is deemed to be misbranded by the dispensing pharmacist.

o. If the drug is an OTC drug and it is not packaged in tamper-resistant packaging or properly labeled in conformity with the tamper-resistant regulations (see IV)

p. If the drug is an OTC drug and it is not properly labeled in conformity with the labeling requirements of the FDCA

q. If the drug (or medical device) is an ophthalmic preparation offered or intended for ophthalmic use that is not sterile

3. **Violations under the Act.** Any misbranding or adulteration of a drug may subject the individual (e.g., a pharmacist) to imprisonment, a fine, or both. A pharmacy and pharmacist will be exempt from criminal sanctions in either of the following cases:

   a. **Certain cases of good faith.** When adulterated or misbranded products are received from a manufacturer or wholesaler in good faith by the pharmacy, the pharmacy may not be held responsible in certain situations. This exemption applies only if it is a first violation and, if requested, the pharmacy or pharmacist furnishes to the government the name and address of the person from whom the drug was received and copies of all documents pertaining to its delivery.

   b. **Receipt of drug with a signed, written guaranty.** A pharmacy and pharmacist will be exempt from misbranding and adulteration violations when a signed, written guaranty is received from the wholesaler or manufacturer. The guaranty must contain the name and address of the person residing in the United States from whom the drug was received in good faith and a statement that the drug is not adulterated or misbranded.

4. **Seizures.** Any adulterated or misbranded drug will be subject to condemnation and seizure by the U.S. government after a hearing in any district court of the United States (or territory) with proper jurisdiction. A seizure may be done without a hearing if the federal government has probable cause to believe that the violation would be dangerous to health or that the labeling of the misbranded article is fraudulent or would be materially misleading to the injury or damage of the purchaser or consumer.

5. **Investigations and inspections**

   a. The U.S. Secretary of Health and Human Services has the authority to conduct examinations and inspections through federal employees and by officers and employees of any state, territory, or political subdivision duly commissioned by the U.S. Secretary of Health and Human Services as an officer of the U.S. Department of Health and Human Services.

   b. **Scope of investigation.** An investigator may enter a pharmacy or other establishment where adulterated or misbranded drugs are held and inspect all drugs, materials, containers, and labeling. The inspection does not extend to financial data, sales data other than shipment data, pricing data, personnel data, and other records that have no bearing on adulteration and misbranding. The investigator must present appropriate credentials and a written notice to the owner, operator, or agent in charge that he or she is authorized to conduct an investigation. The inspection must be done at reasonable times, within reasonable limits, and in a reasonable manner.

6. **Current Good Manufacturing Practice (cGMP).** Under the FDCA, a drug is considered adulterated if it is not manufactured "in conformity with current Good Manufacturing Practice." FDA regulations state with particularity the minimum cGMPs for methods to be used in, and the facilities or controls to be used for, the manufacture, processing, packing, or holding of a drug. The cGMPs ensure that a drug meets the requirements of the FDCA as to safety and has the identity and strength and meets the quality and purity characteristics that it purports.

J. Registration of producers of drugs

1. Manufacturers and businesses that distribute a drug manufactured by another but sold under their own label or trade name must register their establishment with the FDA. They also must submit a list of every drug (prescription and OTC) in commercial distribution, with updates every June and December.

2. Pharmacies properly licensed by state law that do not manufacture or possess drugs for sale other than in the regular course of the practice of pharmacy are not required to register with the FDA. A pharmacy engaged in manufacturing or processing activities that are

considered beyond the normal practice of pharmacy must register with the FDA and supply a list of every drug in commercial distribution.

   a. Scope of pharmacy practice. A pharmacy or pharmacist may not manufacture drug products. They may only compound drug preparations pursuant to a valid prescription of a practitioner for a particular patient. Large-scale manufacturing of drug products by a pharmacy or pharmacist is outside the scope of pharmacy practice and requires proper registration with the FDA and compliance with cGMPs.

K. Package inserts. The federal government has determined that prescription medication information needs to be disseminated to health professionals and, in the case of certain drugs, to the patient.

   1. Manufacturer's insert. An amendment to the FDCA required that all manufacturers provide "full disclosure" concerning prescription medication that they market. Full disclosure is accomplished by means of a package insert that is enclosed with every commercial container of a drug product. The insert should contain essential scientific information needed for the safe and effective use of the drug and should be informative and accurate. It must not be promotional in tone, false, or misleading.

   2. Patient package insert. The FDA has determined that, because of certain side effects associated with the use of particular drug products, patient package inserts must be dispensed to the patient at the time of dispensing the medications. The following products must be dispensed with a patient package insert, which is supplied with the product from the manufacturer:

   a. Oral contraceptives. Hospital inpatients or LTCF patients may receive the insert before administration of the first oral contraceptive and every 30 days thereafter, as long as the therapy continues.

   b. Intrauterine devices for human use in contraception. Every practitioner dispensing such a device must provide the patient with an informative insert.

   c. Estrogen and estrogen-containing products. Hospital inpatients or LTCF patients may receive the insert before administration of the first estrogen dose and every 30 days thereafter, as long as the therapy continues.

   d. Progestational drug products. Hospital inpatients or LTCF patients may receive the insert before administration of the first progestational drug product and every 30 days thereafter, as long as the therapy continues.

   e. Isoproterenol inhalation products require the following warning statement on the immediate container label of such a product: "Warning: Do not exceed the dose prescribed by your physician. If difficulty persists, contact your physician immediately."

   f. Miscellaneous drug products. Certain drug products were approved by the FDA with the provision that they must be dispensed along with a patient package insert that includes a particular warning or statement of benefits and risks associated with the use of the drug. For example, isotretinoin was approved for dispensing with an insert warning about serious fetal harm when administered to pregnant women.

L. Prescription drug samples

   1. An **amendment** to the FDCA (Prescription Drug Marketing Act) severely restricted the distribution of drug samples by manufacturers. Under the FDCA, no person may sell, purchase, or trade, or offer to sell, purchase, or trade any drug sample. Samples may only be distributed upon written request of a practitioner. Manufacturers must maintain records of every sample distribution for a period of three years. Pharmacies may not receive samples from a manufacturer except in certain situations in which a practitioner requests storage of his or her samples in the pharmacy.

   2. Importation under the FDCA. The Prescription Drug Marketing Act prohibits the import of prescription drugs once exported. Importation is allowed after notification and approval of the FDA and in cases of an emergency.

M. Medical devices. An amendment to the FDCA in 1976 (Medical Device Amendments) required a device manufacturer to provide reasonable assurance of the safety and effectiveness of the device. The amendment required the FDA to categorize each device on the market in 1976 into one of three classes: Class I, Class II, or Class III, depending on each device's safety and effectiveness. Generally, **Class I** devices are those that have a reasonable assurance of safety and effectiveness. **Class II** devices are those that do not have the reasonable assurance of safety and effectiveness, but there is sufficient information about the device to establish special controls to ensure its safety and effectiveness (and may be marketed with such controls). **Class III** devices are those for which information is not sufficient to provide reasonable assurance of their safety and effectiveness. Class III devices may be marketed only if they are proven to be substantially equivalent to a device on the market before 1976, by approval of a premarket application, or by reclassification into Class I or II.

1. **Medical device tracking.** Manufacturers of medical devices whose failure would be reasonably likely to have a serious adverse health consequence must track the device down the chain of distribution to the patient. Such tracking allows the manufacturer to take appropriate action with respect to recalls, defects, or other relevant information concerning the device. Every final distributor such as a pharmacy, hospital, or home health-care company must report certain information to the manufacturer. Tracking information must be maintained by the manufacturer and distributor for the useful life of the device and be available for inspection by FDA personnel.

2. **Manufacturer's reports.** Every device manufacturer must report to the FDA information, when received or made aware of, that reasonably suggests that one of its marketed devices may have caused or contributed to a death or serious injury. Likewise, hospitals and other medical service facilities must provide reports on adverse reactions to, or malfunctioning of, medical devices.

3. **Adulteration and misbranding.** Medical devices may be adulterated or misbranded in the same way that drugs are adulterated or misbranded (see II.I).

III. **POISON PREVENTION PACKAGING ACT (PPPA).** The PPPA of 1970 requires that drugs for human use in an oral dosage form must be packaged for the consumer in special packaging. All such federal controlled substances and drugs dispensed pursuant to a prescription must be dispensed to the consumer in special packaging. *Special packaging,* referred to as **child-resistant** containers, is defined as a container that is designed to be significantly difficult for children under 5 years of age to gain access to within a reasonable time. The container must not be too difficult for normal adults (ones with no overt physical or mental handicaps) to use properly and does not include packaging that all such children cannot gain access within a reasonable time. The Consumer Products Safety Commission is responsible for interpreting, establishing rules and regulations for, and enforcing the provisions of the PPPA.

A. **Exceptions.** The following medications are exempt from the special packaging requirements:

1. Sublingual dosage forms of nitroglycerin; other dosage forms intended for oral administration, such as nitroglycerin sustained-release preparations, must be packaged in child-resistant containers

2. Sublingual and chewable forms of isosorbide dinitrate in dosage strengths of 10 mg or less

3. Erythromycin ethylsuccinate granules for oral suspension and oral suspensions in packages containing not more than 8 g of the equivalent of erythromycin

4. Cyclically administered oral contraceptives in manufacturers' mnemonic (memory-aid) dispenser packages that rely solely on the activity of one or more progestogen or estrogen substances

5. Anhydrous cholestyramine in powder form

6. All unit-dose forms of potassium supplements, including individually wrapped effervescent tablets, unit-dose vials of liquid potassium, and powdered potassium in unit-dose packages, containing not more than 50 mEq of potassium per unit dose

7. Sodium fluoride drug preparations, including liquid and tablet forms, containing no more than 264 mg of sodium fluoride per package and containing no other prescription medication

8. Betamethasone tablets packaged in manufacturers' dispenser packages, containing no more than 12.6 mg betamethasone

9. Pancrelipase preparations in tablet, capsule, or powder form and containing no other prescription medication

10. Prednisone in tablet form, when dispensed in packages containing no more than 105 mg of the drug, and containing no other prescription medication

11. Mebendazole in tablet form in packages containing not more than 600 mg of the drug and no other prescription medication

12. Methylprednisolone in tablet form in packages containing not more than 84 mg of the drug and no other prescription medication

13. Colestipol in powder form in packages containing not more than 5 g of the drug and no other prescription medication

14. Erythromycin ethylsuccinate tablets in packages containing no more than the equivalent of 16 g erythromycin

15. Conjugated estrogen tablets USP, when dispensed in mnemonic packages containing not more than 32 mg of the drug and no other prescription medication

16. Norethindrone acetate tablets USP, when dispensed in mnemonic packages containing not more than 50 mg of the drug and no other prescription medication

17. Medroxyprogesterone acetate tablets

B. **Requests for a non–child-resistant container.** A prescribing practitioner may make a request in the prescription that the medication be dispensed in a non–child-resistant container. A practitioner may not, however, make a blanket request that all prescriptions issued by him or her be dispensed in non–child-resistant containers. The purchaser, or patient, may also make a request that the medication be dispensed in a non–child-resistant container. The request of the purchaser, or patient, does not (under the PPPA) have to be in writing. The purchaser, or patient, may make a blanket request that none of his or her medications be dispensed in a child-resistant container. A dispensing pharmacist may never make the decision to use non–child-resistant containers.

C. **Reuse of child-resistant containers.** Reuse of child-resistant containers are prohibited by regulation of the federal Consumer Products Safety Commission. However, the Commission has indicated that glass containers may be reused as long as a new safety closure is used.

D. **Manufacturer's packaging.** Packaging from the manufacturer that is intended to be dispensed directly to the patient must be in child-resistant packaging. Bulk packaging intended to be repackaged by the pharmacist for each prescription does not have to be in special packaging from the manufacturer. Unit packaging from the manufacturer that will be dispensed directly to the consumer, or patient, must comply with the child-resistant requirements of the PPPA (unless specifically exempted; see III.A).

E. **Exemptions for easy access.** Special packaging is not required in cases where OTC medication needs to be readily available to the elderly or handicapped persons. A manufacturer may supply a single size of a drug product in non–child-resistant packaging, as long as it also supplies the medication in packages that use the special packaging. Additionally, the package must be conspicuously labeled with the statement: "This package for households without young children." For those packages too small for this statement, the statement "Package not child-resistant" may be used.

F. **Hospitals and institutions.** The special packaging requirements of the PPPA apply to household substances. *Household substance* is defined as "any substance which is customarily produced or distributed for sale for consumption or use, or customarily stored, by individuals in or about the household. . . ." As long as the medication is administered by institutional personnel and is not directly dispensed to the consumer (patient), child-resistant containers are not required.

G. **Miscellaneous products requiring special packaging.** The PPPA requires that certain household substances be distributed to the consumer in special packaging. Examples of these substances include furniture polish containing petroleum distillates, drain pipe cleaners, turpentine, paint solvents, and lighter fluid.

IV. ANTI-TAMPERING ACT. The U.S. Congress passed the Anti-Tampering Act in 1984 due to a number of deaths that occurred in the early 1980s from OTC medication capsules contaminated with cyanide.

   A. Violations. Unlawful acts involving a consumer product can be broken down into one of the following listed violations. The term *consumer product* includes any food, drug, device, or cosmetic, as well as any article, product, or commodity that is customarily used by individuals for purposes of personal care or to perform services ordinarily done within a household.

   1. Tampering. Any individual who tampers or attempts to tamper with any consumer product that affects interstate or foreign commerce, or its labeling or container, may be in violation of the statute. A violation occurs when the individual acts (or threatens to act) with reckless disregard for the risk that another person will be placed in danger of death or bodily injury. Any individual who taints any consumer product or causes its labeling or container to be materially false or misleading is in violation of the statute if done with intent to cause serious injury to the business of another.

   2. False communications. Knowingly communicating false information that a consumer product has been tainted may be a violation. If such tainting, had it occurred, would create a risk of death or bodily injury to another person, then the false communication is deemed a violation.

   3. Conspiracy. An agreement between two or more persons to do (or further) either of the above acts is considered a violation.

   B. OTC tamper-resistant packaging. Certain OTC products must be packaged, by FDA regulation, in tamper-resistant packaging. Examples include contact lens solutions and other ophthalmic solutions. A **tamper-resistant package** is one having one or more indicators or barriers to entry that, if breached or missing, can reasonably be expected to provide visible evidence to consumers that tampering has occurred. To reduce tampering, the package must have **one** of the following characteristics:

   1. Be distinctive by design so that the product cannot be duplicated by commonly available materials or processes or

   2. Use one or more indicators or barriers to entry that employ an identifying characteristic

   C. OTC tamper-resistant labeling. The OTC product must be labeled with a prominently placed statement alerting consumers to the specific tamper-resistant feature of the package. The statement must be placed so that it will be unaffected if the tamper-resistant feature is breached or missing.

   D. Medical devices and cosmetics. Certain medical devices and cosmetics must be packaged in tamper-resistant packaging. The packaging requirements are similar to the requirements outlined above for OTC drug products.

V. MAILING PRESCRIPTION MEDICATION

   A. All prescription medication, including controlled substances and narcotics in schedules II–V, may be mailed from a physician, or pharmacist pursuant to a prescription, to the patient. Flammable substances (e.g., acetone) and alcoholic beverages may not be sent to a patient through the U.S. mail.

   B. The medication must be placed in a plain outer container or be securely overwrapped in plain paper. There must be no markings of any kind on the outside wrapper or container that would indicate the nature of the contents.

VI. OMNIBUS BUDGET RECONCILIATION ACT OF 1990 (OBRA '90). Under the Constitution of the United States, the federal government has no power or authority to directly regulate the practice of pharmacy. Such power rests with each state. The federal government can, however, indirectly regulate, or affect, the practice of pharmacy by attaching conditions of participation and reimbursement for federally funded programs.

A. **Medicaid prescriptions.** With respect to prescriptions dispensed to Medicaid patients (paid in part by the federal government along with the state government), the federal government has attached certain conditions for reimbursement. Such conditions were deemed necessary to stem the always increasing cost of the Medicaid programs. It was believed that improved medication compliance by Medicaid recipients would, in the long run, reduce the cost of the programs by reducing subsequent hospitalizations and other subsequent utilization of health care. As a result, pharmacists are required to do the following in the course of dispensing a Medicaid prescription:

1. Make a reasonable good-faith effort to obtain and maintain a history of the patient, including a medication history

2. Conduct a review of every prescription for appropriateness and to screen for potential drug therapy problems

3. Make an offer to counsel each Medicaid recipient concerning the drug (if the offer is accepted, the counseling must include the drug's proper administration, common adverse or severe side effects, techniques for self-monitoring, and proper storage)

B. **Manufacturer's best price.** OBRA '90 requires manufacturers that wish to participate in the Medicaid program to offer the federal government their best price for prescription drugs. *Best price* is defined as the lowest price at which any purchaser is purchasing that drug product.

VII. HEALTH INSURANCE PORTABILITY AND ACCOUNTABILITY ACT OF 1996 (HIPAA).
HIPAA is federal legislation that requires all health-care providers, including pharmacies, to protect patient information from unauthorized use and disclosures. This is referred to as the Privacy Rule and was established as a result of the government's recognition that individually identifiable health information is readily available due to health-care plans, health-care clearinghouses, third-party billing practices, clinical research trials, and the transmission of health information in electronic form. Protected health information (PHI) must be confidentially maintained by a health-care provider to prevent any unauthorized use or disclosure. Other covered entities, such as Organized Health Care Arrangements, HMO's and insurance plans, must also follow the Privacy Rule.

A. **Definitions.** Under the Privacy Rule, certain terms have specific meanings.

1. **"Covered entity"** means:
   a. a health plan (e.g., group health insurance, Medicaid, Medicare).
   b. a health-care clearinghouse (e.g., billing service companies and companies that process health information received from another entity).
   c. a health-care provider who transmits any health information in electronic form in connection with a transaction covered by HIPAA. "Health care" is defined as including the sale or dispensing of a drug, device, equipment, or other item in accordance with a prescription.

2. **"Individually identifiable health information"** is information created or received by a covered entity that relates to the past, present, or future physical or mental health or condition of an individual; the provision of health care to an individual; or any payment for any provision of any health care, **and** that identifies the individual **or** that provides a reasonable basis to identify the individual. The items listed below are deemed sufficient to identify an individual:
   a. Name
   b. Address, including all geographic subdivisions smaller than a state (e.g., street address, city, county, zip code)
   c. Dates (except year), including birth dates, admission dates, discharge dates, dates of death
   d. Telephone numbers
   e. Fax numbers
   f. E-mail addresses

    g. Social Security numbers
    h. Medical record numbers
    i. Health plan beneficiary numbers
    j. Account numbers
    k. Certificate/license numbers
    l. Vehicle identifiers and serial numbers, including license plate numbers
    m. Device identifiers
    n. Web universal resource locaters (URLs)
    o. Internet protocol (IP) address numbers
    p. Biometric identifiers, including fingerprints and voice prints
    q. Full face photographic images and any comparable images
    r. Any other unique identifying number, charactistic, or code, except for codes assigned to reidentify information that has been de-identified
    s. Names of any relative, employer, or household member of the individual

3. **"Protected health information" (PHI)** is all individually identifiable health information that is transmitted or maintained in **any** form or medium, electronically or otherwise.

4. **"Notice of privacy practices for protected health information."** An individual has the right to adequate notice of the uses and disclosures of PHI that may be made by the covered entity, and of the individual's rights and the covered entity's legal duties with respect to PHI. Generally, the notice must contain information describing the individual's rights under the Privacy Rule and the covered entity's responsibilities.
    a. **Header.** Every notice must contain the following statement as a header or be otherwise prominently displayed: "THIS NOTICE DESCRIBES HOW MEDICAL INFORMATION ABOUT YOU MAY BE USED AND DISCLOSED AND HOW YOU CAN GET ACCESS TO THIS INFORMATION. PLEASE REVIEW IT CAREFULLY."
    b. **Individual's rights.** An individual has the right to request restrictions on certain uses and disclosures of PHI, the right to receive confidential communications of PHI by alternative means or at alternative locations, the right to inspect and copy his PHI, the right to amend his PHI, the right to receive an accounting of disclosures of PHI, and the right to obtain a paper copy of the notice from the covered entity.
    c. **Covered entity's responsibilities.** The notice must include a statement that the covered entity is required by law to maintain the privacy of PHI, a statement of its legal duties and privacy practices with respect to PHI, a statement that it must abide by the notice currently in effect, and a statement that it reserves the right to change the terms of its notice and how it will provide individuals with a revised notice.
    d. **Miscellaneous contents of notice.** The notice must contain a statement that individuals may complain to the covered entity and to the U.S. Department of Health and Human Services if they believe their privacy rights have been violated. The notice must state a date on which it becomes effective. The effective date must be no later than the date of the first service delivery.
    e. **Posting of notice.** A pharmacy must post the notice in a clear and prominent location where it is reasonable to expect individuals to be able to read the notice.
    f. **Written acknowledgment of notice.** Every covered entity must obtain a written acknowledgment of receipt of the notice by the individual. If one is not obtained, the covered entity must document its good-faith efforts to obtain the acknowledgment and the reason why it was not obtained.
    g. **Exceptions for inmates.** A person incarcerated in or otherwise confined to a correctional institution does not have a right to notice under the Privacy Rule, and the notice requirements do not apply to a correctional institution that is a covered entity.

5. **"Authorization"** for a covered entity to use or disclose PHI: a patient must give written authorization before a covered entity, including pharmacies and pharmacists, may use or disclose PHI. **No patient consent or authorization** is necessary when PHI use and disclosure is for **treatment, payment, or health-care operations.** This allows a health-care provider to consult with other covered entities (i.e., other health-care providers) to provide proper patient care without being unduly hindered by the Privacy Rule. For uses and disclosures that require an authorization, the **written authorization** must be written in plain language, and a **signed copy** must be provided to the individual. The signed authorization must be maintained by the covered entity for **6 years** from the date of its creation or the date when it was last in effect, whichever is later. The written authorization must at least contain the following core elements and statements:

    a. A description of the information to be used or disclosed that identifies the information in a specific and meaningful fashion.

    b. The name or other specific identification of the person(s), or class of persons, authorized to make the requested use or disclosure.

    c. The name or other specific identification of the person(s), or class of persons, to whom the covered entity may make the requested use or disclosure.

    d. A description of each purpose of the requested use or disclosure.

    e. An expiration date or an expiration event that relates to the individual or the purpose of the use or disclosure.

    f. Signature of the individual and date. If signed by a personal representative, it must also include a description of such representative's authority to act for the individual.

    g. The written authorization must contain the following statements:

        (1) The individual's right to revoke the authorization in writing along with the exceptions to the right to revoke and a description of how the individual may revoke the authorization.

        (2) The ability or inability to condition treatment, payment, enrollment, or eligibility for benefits on the authorization, by stating either that the covered entity cannot require authorization, or that if the covered entity can require authorization, the consequences to the individual of his or her refusal to sign the authorization.

        (3) The potential for the disclosed information to be redisclosed by the recipient and no longer be protected by the Privacy Rule.

  6. "Minimum necessary." When using or disclosing PHI or when requesting PHI from another covered entity, a covered entity must make reasonable efforts to limit PHI to the **minimum necessary** to accomplish the intended purpose of the use, disclosure, or request. The minimum necessary rule **does not apply** to disclosures or requests by a health-care provider for treatment, uses or disclosures made pursuant to an authorization, and uses or disclosures that are required by law. "Required by law" means a mandate in a law that compels an entity to make a use or disclosure of PHI. It includes a covered entity's compliance with state and federal laws and regulations that require the production of information; court orders and court-ordered warrants, subpoenas or summons issued by a court, a governmental or tribal inspector general, or an administrative body authorized to require the production of information and Medicare conditions of participation with respect to health-care providers participating in the program.

  7. "Business associates." A business associate of a covered entity is a person or business that performs a function or activity on behalf of the covered entity, such as claims processing, billing, utilization review, quality assurance, etc., **and** that requires the use or disclosure of individually identifiable health information. A business associate would also include persons who provide services to the covered entity, **and** the service involves disclosure of individually identifiable health information, such as legal, actuarial, accounting, consulting, data aggregation, management, administrative, accreditation, or financial services. **Excluded** from the definition of business associates are members of the workforce of the covered entity, and functions or services that do not require disclosure of individually identifiable health information.

    a. Business associate contracts. Every business associate must enter into an agreement with the covered entity to ensure compliance with the Privacy Rule. Generally, the agreement must establish the required uses and disclosures of PHI by the business associate and require the return or destruction of PHI at termination of the contract.

B. Additional responsibilities of covered entities. Every covered entity must create policies and procedures for compliance with the Privacy Rule, must designate a privacy official responsible for creating such policies and procedures, must designate a contact person or office that is responsible for receiving complaints and that is able to provide further information about matters covered by the notice, and must train all members of its workforce with respect to the Privacy Rule. Every designation must be maintained by the covered entity for 6 years from the date it last was in effect. Lastly, every covered entity must have and apply appropriate sanctions against members of its workforce who fail to comply with the Privacy Rule.

C. State law privacy rules. The federal Privacy Rule is intended as the minimum requirement for privacy standards. If a state law is more stringent, then a covered entity must follow that state's privacy standards. If a state privacy law is not as stringent, the federal Privacy Rule preempts any contrary state law and a covered entity must abide by the federal Privacy Rule.

D. Penalties for violation of the Privacy Rule. Any person who violates the Privacy Rule may not be fined more than $100 for each violation up to a total of $25,000 per calendar year for all violations of an identical requirement. Additional penalties may be imposed for the following **wrongful disclosure** of individually identifiable health information:

1. Wrongful obtainment or disclosure of PHI: fined not more than $50,000, imprisoned not more than 1 year, or both.

2. Wrongful obtainment or disclosure of PHI under false pretenses: fined not more than $100,000, imprisoned not more than 5 years, or both.

3. Wrongful obtainment or disclosure of PHI committed with intent to sell, transfer, or use same for commercial advantage, personal gain, or malicious harm: fined not more than $250,000, imprisoned not more than 10 years, or both.

VIII. NARCOTIC TREATMENT PROGRAMS. Methadone use is currently allowed as part of a total treatment program for narcotic addiction. Regulations concerning methadone treatment programs have been jointly established by the DEA and FDA. Narcotic-dependent individuals are those who physiologically need heroin or a morphine-like drug to prevent the onset of signs of withdrawal.

A. Definition. A narcotic treatment program is an organization that administers or dispenses a narcotic drug to a narcotic addict for maintenance or detoxification treatment, and provides, when appropriate or necessary, a comprehensive range of medical and rehabilitative services. The program must be:

1. Approved by the FDA

2. Approved by the appropriate state agency, usually the state's Department of Public Health or equivalent

3. Registered under the Federal Controlled Substances Act with the DEA to use a narcotic drug for the treatment of narcotic addiction

B. Detoxification treatment is defined as dispensing of narcotic drugs in decreasing doses to an individual to alleviate adverse physiological or psychological effects incident to withdrawal of narcotic drug use. Detoxification is for a period not in excess of 180 days.

C. Maintenance treatment is the dispensing of a narcotic drug, at relatively stable dosage levels, in the treatment of an individual for dependence on heroin or other morphine-like drug.

D. Requirements to admit patients into a program. In general, for a patient to be admitted into a comprehensive maintenance program, the following requirements must be met:

1. A program physician must determine that the person is currently physiologically dependent on a narcotic drug and became physiologically dependent at least 1 year before admission to the program.

2. The patient must have voluntarily chosen to participate in the program and must sign a "Consent to Methadone Treatment" (provided by the FDA) after being clearly and adequately informed about the use of methadone.

E. Take-home methadone. Take-home methadone may be given only to patients who, in the clinical judgment of the program physician, are responsible in handling narcotic drugs. The patient must come to the clinic for observation daily or at least 6 days a week. Over time, the program physician may reduce clinical observations to once weekly. Methadone for take-home use must be dispensed similarly to the dispensing of any schedule II controlled substance and include the treatment center's name, address, and telephone number on its label

STUDY QUESTIONS

Directions: Each of the numbered items or incomplete statements in this section is followed by answers or by completions of the statement. Select the **one** lettered answer or completion that is **best** in each case.

1. All of the following prescription medications may be delivered by mail to the patient via the U.S. Postal Service EXCEPT

(A) procainamide
(B) ampicillin
(C) hydromorphone
(D) diazepam
(E) all of the above may be delivered by mail

2. Which of the following narcotic drugs has been approved by the FDA for use in the treatment of narcotic addiction?

(A) Morphine
(B) Codeine
(C) Methadone
(D) Hydrocodone
(E) None of the above

3. For the U.S. government to place a drug into schedule III, which of the following findings must be made concerning the drug?

(A) The drug or other substance has a high potential for abuse.
(B) Abuse of the drug or other substance may lead to limited physical dependence or psychological dependence relative to the drugs or other substances in schedule IV.
(C) The drug or other substance has no currently accepted medical use in treatment in the United States.
(D) Abuse of the drug or other substance may lead to moderate or low physical dependence or high psychological dependence.
(E) There is a lack of accepted safety for use of the drug or other substance under medical supervision.

4. Under the Federal Controlled Substances Act, all of the following items must appear on a controlled-substance prescription label EXCEPT the

(A) name, address, and DEA number of the pharmacy
(B) name of the patient
(C) name of the prescribing practitioner
(D) serial number assigned to the prescription
(E) date of the initial filling of the prescription

5. Under the Federal Controlled Substances Act, all of the following entities must register with the DEA EXCEPT

(A) prescribers of controlled substances
(B) pharmacists who dispense controlled substances
(C) distributors of controlled substances
(D) importers of controlled substances
(E) universities conducting instructional activities with controlled substances listed in schedules II–V

6. Under the Federal Controlled Substances Act, which of the following statements concerning the emergency dispensing of a schedule II controlled substance is true?

(A) The practitioner who authorizes the oral prescription must, within 7 days, deliver a written prescription to the dispensing pharmacist.
(B) The quantity prescribed and dispensed must be limited to the amount necessary to adequately treat the patient during the emergency period.
(C) It is not reasonably possible for the practitioner to provide a written prescription to be presented to the person dispensing the controlled substance before the dispensing.
(D) No appropriate alternative treatment is available, including administration of a controlled substance that is not in schedule II.
(E) All of the above statements are true.

7. Under the Federal Controlled Substances Act, the crime transfer warning, "Caution: Federal law prohibits the transfer of this drug to any person other than the patient for whom it was prescribed," must appear on the prescription container label of all controlled substances EXCEPT

(A) schedule II controlled substances
(B) schedule III controlled substances
(C) schedule IV controlled substances
(D) schedule V controlled substances

8. Which of the following statements concerning drug recall classification is true?

(A) A Class I recall is a situation in which use of, or exposure to, a violative product is not likely to cause adverse health consequences.

(B) A Class I recall is a situation in which use of, or exposure to, a violative product may cause temporary or medically reversible adverse health consequences or in which the probability of serious health consequences is remote.

(C) A Class I recall is a situation in which there is a reasonable probability that the use of, or exposure to, a violative product will cause serious adverse health consequences or death.

(D) A Class II recall is a situation in which use of, or exposure to, a violative product is not likely to cause adverse health consequences.

(E) A Class III recall is a situation in which there is a reasonable probability that the use of, or exposure to, a violative product will cause serious adverse health consequences or death.

9. Under the Federal Food, Drug, and Cosmetic Act, all of the following statements are considered a misbranding of a drug EXCEPT if

(A) the labeling is false or misleading in any particular.

(B) an oral contraceptive is dispensed without the required patient package insert.

(C) the drug is an imitation of another drug, or if it is offered for sale under the name of another drug.

(D) the drug consists in whole or in part of any filthy, putrid, or decomposed substance.

10. All of the following oral medications are exempt from child-resistant packaging EXCEPT

(A) anhydrous cholestyramine in powder form

(B) nitroglycerin preparations in sustained release form

(C) cyclically administered oral contraceptives in manufacturers' mnemonic (memory-aid) dispenser packages that rely solely upon the activity of one or more progestogen or estrogen substances

(D) pancrelipase preparations in tablet, capsule, or powder form that contain no other prescription medication

ANSWERS AND EXPLANATIONS

1. The answer is E *[V]*.
Narcotics and controlled substances in schedules II–V may be delivered to the patient by mail. The U.S. Postal Service no longer prohibits the mailing of narcotics by a physician or pharmacist (pursuant to a prescription) to the patient.

2. The answer is C *[VIII; VIII.A; I.I.2.c.(2)]*.
Methadone is approved by the FDA for use in the treatment of narcotic addiction. Only a properly registered narcotic treatment program may dispense methadone for maintenance or detoxification treatment. Pharmacies that are not so registered may only dispense methadone for severe pain.

3. The answer is D *[I.A.3]*.
To place a drug into schedule III, the U.S. government must make the following findings concerning the drug: (1) it has a potential for abuse less than the drugs or other substances in schedules I and II; (2) it has a currently accepted medical use in treatment in the United States; and (3) abuse of the drug may lead to moderate or low physical dependence or high psychological dependence.

4. The answer is A *[I.I.8.c.(1)–(7)]*.
A pharmacy's DEA number is not required to appear on the medication container label dispensed to the patient.

5. The answer is B *[I.B.2.a–k; I.B.9.d]*.
Agents and employees of DEA registrants, such as pharmacists, are exempt from registering with the DEA. Pharmacies, not the individual pharmacists, must register with the DEA.

6. The answer is E *[I.I.4.a, b]*.
Emergency dispensing of an oral schedule II controlled-substance prescription must be done in strict compliance with the law. Before dispensing such a prescription, the pharmacist must make the threshold determination that ALL three factors that define an emergency situation (see I.I.4.a) are present. If any one of the three factors is absent, the prescription is not for an emergency situation, and a written prescription must be presented to the pharmacist.

7. The answer is D *[I.I.8.c.(7)]*.
The federal crime transfer warning label is not required to appear on the prescription container label of schedule V controlled substances.

8. The answer is C *[II.H.2.a–c]*.
A Class I recall is a situation in which there is a reasonable probability that the use of, or exposure to, a violative product will cause serious adverse health consequences or death.

9. The answer is D *[II.I.1, 2]*.
The Federal Food, Drug, and Cosmetic Act states that a drug is considered adulterated if it consists in whole or in part of any filthy, putrid, or decomposed substance. The terms "misbranding" and "adulteration" are often referred to in literature and case law as being the same or similar violations under the law. However, the Act sets forth specific instances of adulteration and specific instances of misbranding.

10. The answer is B *[III.A.1]*.
Only sublingual dosage forms of nitroglycerin are exempt from child-resistant packaging.

26
Reviewing and Dispensing Prescription and Medication Orders

Todd A. Brown

I. DEFINITIONS

A. Prescriptions are orders for medications, nondrug products, and services that are written by a licensed practitioner or midlevel practitioner who is authorized by state law to prescribe (see Appendix A). Pharmacists are increasingly being given prescribing privileges by enactment of state **collaborative drug therapy management** (CDTM) legislation. This allows pharmacists to change the dose of existing medications or order new medication under established protocols or guidelines agreed on by the pharmacist and physician. Practitioners may prescribe only medications that are within their scope of practice. Prescriptions may be written, presented orally (by telephone), or presented electronically (i.e., via fax or computer network) to the pharmacist. The requirements of the prescription form may vary with state regulations. The prescription serves as a vehicle for communication from the prescriber to the pharmacist about the needs of the patient. The following information should be included on a prescription:

1. **Patient information,** including full name and address

2. **Date** on which the prescription was issued

3. **Name and dosage form of the product.** The name can be any of the following:
   a. Proprietary (brand)
   b. Nonproprietary (generic)
   c. Chemical

4. **Product strength.** The strength of the product is not required if only one strength is commercially available or if the product contains a combination of active ingredients. It is advisable to include the strength to reduce the chance of misinterpreting the prescription. If the dose is to be calculated by the pharmacist, then the pharmacist can decide the strength of the product dispensed after calculating the patient's dose.

5. **Quantity to be dispensed.** This should include the amount and the units of measure (e.g., grams, ounces, tablets). If the amount is not specified, the directions should specify the dose to be taken and the duration of therapy so that the pharmacist can calculate the quantity required for the patient.

6. **Directions for the pharmacist.** Directions may be required for:
   a. Preparation (e.g., compounding)
   b. Labeling (i.e., information to be put on the prescription label)

7. **Directions for the patient.** These should include explicit instructions on the quantity, schedule, and duration for proper use. "As Directed" should be avoided. If the directions vary, a minimum and maximum dose can be used.

8. **Refill information.** If refill information is not supplied, it is generally assumed that no refills are authorized. "As needed" (pro re nata [prn]) refills are usually interpreted as allowing for refills for 1 year unless laws or regulations restrict the amount or time period in which a prescription is valid.

9. **Prescriber information.** This should include the name, office address, signature of the prescriber, and the Drug Enforcement Administration (DEA) number (for controlled substances only). In some circumstances, prescriptions may be written by a midlevel practitioner (not licensed to prescribe alone) under the supervision of a licensed prescriber. In these cases, both the midlevel practitioner writing the prescription and the supervising licensed prescriber's name should be included.

B. Medication orders are orders for medications by an individual authorized to prescribe and are intended for use by patients while in an institutional setting. They may be written, presented orally (by telephone), or presented electronically (i.e., via fax or computer network) to the pharmacist. The medication order generally includes

1. **Patient information** (e.g., full name, identification number)

2. **Date and time** the order was written

3. **Name of the product.** The name can be any of the following:
   a. Proprietary (brand)
   b. Nonproprietary (generic)
   c. Chemical

4. **Product strength, dosage, and route of administration.** The strength of the product is not required if only one strength is commercially available or if the product contains a combination of active ingredients. It is advisable to include the strength to reduce the chance of misinterpreting the order. The pharmacist may decide the strength of the product dispensed after calculating the patient's dose. The dosage and route of administration should be included to reduce the chance of misinterpreting the order and to allow for correct administration to the patient.

5. **Prescriber's signature.** If the order was taken verbally, the name of the person transcribing the order should be included.

6. **Directions for the pharmacist.** These can be used for:
   a. Preparation (e.g., compounding)
   b. Labeling (i.e., information to be put on the label)

7. **Instructions for administration,** including quantity, route of administration, schedule, and duration of use

II. UNDERSTANDING THE PRESCRIPTION OR MEDICATION ORDER AND EVALUATING ITS APPROPRIATENESS

A. Understanding the order. A complete understanding of all information contained in a prescription or medication order is required. Each piece of information should be appropriate and consistent with the remaining information (i.e., the instructions for use should be appropriate for the medication being ordered). The pharmacist should read the entire prescription or medication order carefully to determine the prescriber's intent by interpreting the following information:

1. The name and address of both the patient and the prescriber

2. The patient's disease or condition requiring treatment

3. The reason the order is indicated, relative to the medical need of the patient (e.g., an antibacterial for an infection)

4. The name of the product, the quantity prescribed, and instructions for use

5. All terminology, including units of measure (apothecary, metric, or English) and Latin abbreviations (see Appendix A for common abbreviations)

B. Evaluating the appropriateness. Complete information is required on the prescription or medication order to provide the necessary information to allow the pharmacist to evaluate the appropriateness of the order. When the order is incomplete, the pharmacist must obtain the required information from either the patient or the prescriber. The following should be considered during an evaluation:

1. The patient's disease or condition requiring treatment

2. The patient's allergies or hypersensitivities

3. The pharmacological or biological action of the prescribed product

4. The prescribed route of administration

5. Whether the prescribed product might result in a drug–drug, drug–disease, or drug–food interaction

6. Whether the dose, dosage form, and dosage regimen are safe and likely to meet the needs of the patient

7. Whether the patient will have any difficulties adhering to the regimen and the potential impact on the therapeutic outcome desired

8. Whether the total quantity of medication prescribed is sufficient to allow proper completion of a course of therapy

9. Whether a physical or chemical incompatibility might result (i.e., if the product requires extemporaneous compounding)

10. Whether a licensed practitioner, acting in the course and scope of practice, issued the prescription in good faith, for a legitimate medical purpose

C. **Discovering inappropriate prescriptions or medication orders.** Pharmacists are required to review medication profiles to ensure the appropriateness of prescriptions or medication orders. This is commonly called drug utilization review (DUR). Pharmacists should not fill prescriptions or medication orders that they have concerns with or that are considered inappropriate but, rather, should contact the prescriber. The process of calling a prescriber to discuss concerns identified during a DUR is commonly called **therapeutic intervention.**

1. When performing a therapeutic intervention, the following information should be provided:
   a. A brief description of the problem
   b. A reference source that documents the problem
   c. A description of the clinical significance of the problem
   d. A suggestion of a solution to the problem

2. The following resolutions are possible to solve the problem or concern:
   a. The prescription or medication order will be dispensed as written.
   b. The prescription or medication order will not be dispensed.
   c. The prescription or medication order will be altered and dispensed.

3. Documentation of the results of a therapeutic intervention are required if the prescription or medication order is changed. The name of the prescriber, date of communication, issues discussed, and resolution should be included in the documentation. This information should be kept for the same time period as the prescription or medication order.

4. If the pharmacist feels that, in his or her professional judgment, an order is inappropriate and could harm the patient, the pharmacist should not process the order. The pharmacist may also be required to explain the situation to the patient. If, after a therapeutic intervention, the pharmacist believes the order is still inappropriate, the guidelines of the institution and professional judgment should be followed.

III. **PROCESSING PRESCRIPTIONS AND MEDICATION ORDERS** requires that the pharmacist follow appropriate guidelines. An environment that limits distractions and disruptions during these activities will assist in increasing the accuracy of this process. Automation and the use of pharmacy technicians allow the pharmacist to oversee these functions but spend less time performing these activities. The time saved allows the pharmacist greater time for patient-focused activities, such as counseling and patient education.

A. **The following** information should be recorded on the prescription:

1. The prescription number (for initial filling)

2. The original date of filling

3. The product and quantity dispensed

4. The pharmacist's initials

B. **Product selection.** Generic substitution statutes, as well as formulary and therapeutic substitution policies, might provide direction in product selection.

C. Product preparation for use by the patient. The following might be necessary for preparation:

1. Obtaining the proper amount of medication to be dispensed

2. Reconstitution (the addition of liquid to make a solution or suspension)

3. Extemporaneous compounding (see Chapter 5)

4. Assembly of the medication delivery unit

D. Selection of the proper package or container is required to ensure product stability, to promote patient compliance, and to comply with legal requirements. This information is commonly found in the *United States Pharmacopeia* (*USP*).

E. Labeling the prescribed product

1. The **prescription label** must contain the following information:
   a. Name and address of the pharmacy
   b. Patient's name
   c. Original date of filling
   d. Prescription number
   e. Directions for use
   f. Product's brand name or generic name and manufacturer
   g. Product strength (if available in more than one strength)
   h. Quantity of medication dispensed
   i. Prescriber's name
   j. Expiration date of the medication
   k. Pharmacist's initials

2. **Unit-dose packages** contain one dose or one unit of medication. For a medication order that is dispensed in **unit-dose packages,** the label should identify the product's brand or generic name, strength, lot number, and expiration date.

3. **Auxiliary and cautionary labels.** To ensure proper medication use, storage, and compliance with applicable statutes, and to reinforce information provided during counseling, auxiliary and/or cautionary labels should be affixed when appropriate (see Appendix A).

4. For medication in schedules II–IV (see Chapter 25), a federal transfer warning is required.

F. Record keeping and confidentiality. The pharmacist is required to maintain **prescription files** and **records** in accordance with standards of sound practice and statutory requirements. The implementation of the **Healthcare Insurance Portability and Accountability Act** (HIPAA) has put additional requirements on all health professionals who have access to health information (see Chapter 25). The records include a **patient profile,** containing patient demographic information and a complete chronological record of all medication use and services provided in the delivery of pharmaceutical care.

1. The patient profile should contain the following **patient information:**
   a. Patient's name
   b. Patient's address (or room number in institutional settings)
   c. Any known allergies, sensitivities, or history of idiosyncratic reactions to previous medications
   d. Birth date (i.e., to assess the appropriateness of the dose)
   e. Clinical condition(s) (to help assess the appropriateness of the medication and to prevent drug–disease interactions)
   f. Weight (to assess the appropriateness of the dose)
   g. Occupation (to detect conditions associated with a particular occupation and to help determine if the patient will be able to comply with the regimen)
   h. Nonprescription medication use (to prevent drug–drug and drug–disease interactions, to assess medication effectiveness, and to detect possible adverse effects)

2. In addition, the patient profile should contain the following information from each prescription or medication order:
   a. Name of the medication
   b. Medication strength
   c. Dosage form

    d. Quantity dispensed
    e. Directions for use
    f. Prescription number
    g. Dispensing date
    h. Number of refills authorized and remaining
    i. Prescriber's name
    j. Pharmacist's initials

IV. DISPENSING MEDICATION AND COUNSELING. The dispensing of medication requires that the pharmacist verify that patients have the necessary knowledge and ability to adhere to the prescribed treatment. This will increase the likelihood of obtaining the desired outcomes.

  A. Counseling patients. The pharmacist should evaluate the patient's understanding of each medication and supply additional information when the patient's information is incorrect or insufficient. The pharmacist might need to advise patients regarding the proper dosage, appearance, and name of the medication. Information about the route of administration, instructions for use, duration of use, and the reason the product was prescribed may also be needed. In addition, the following topics might also be appropriate during the counseling session:

    1. Special procedures. As appropriate, the pharmacist should advise patients on how to take the medication (e.g., on an empty stomach, with plenty of water) and instruct them on foods to avoid while taking the medication (e.g., alcoholic beverages, dairy products).

    2. Potential adverse effects. The pharmacist should ensure that patients are aware of the possible adverse effects associated with the medication. Patients should understand the following:
      a. The **frequency** of an adverse effect. This will help patients recognize common adverse effects and not be overly concerned with those that are rare.
      b. The **severity** of an adverse effect. This will help patients focus on those adverse effects that are severe and not those that are inconsequential.
      c. What action should be taken to **manage** or **minimize** the adverse effect. This will help patients deal with possible adverse effects in the appropriate manner.

    3. Proper storage. The pharmacist should counsel patients on how to store medications properly to ensure stability and potency.

    4. Over-the-counter (OTC) products. The pharmacist should instruct patients about the use of OTC products that might or might not be appropriate when taking a prescribed product.

  B. Counseling health professionals. Health professionals (i.e., in an institutional setting) may administer medications to patients. In these cases, the pharmacist should ensure that the health professional has sufficient knowledge to administer the product. Information that health professionals would need to administer medications safely and effectively include the following:

    1. The choice of a particular product

    2. The proper dosage, dosage regimen, and route of administration

    3. The cost of the prescribed product and the costs associated with its use (i.e., administration costs and costs of treating possible adverse effects)

    4. The availability of commercially made products

    5. Potential adverse effects

    6. Drug interactions

    7. Physical incompatibilities

    8. Safe handling and disposal procedures

    9. Nutritional interactions or requirements

    10. Drug interference with laboratory tests

V. PATIENT MONITORING. The provision of pharmaceutical care requires a **pharmaceutical care plan** (see Chapter 20). Monitoring a patients' need for medication and the effect of the medication on the patient maximizes the effectiveness of the medications being taken. Undesired outcomes associated with drug therapy are frequently called **drug-related problems.**

A. **Pharmaceutical care plan.** To increase the frequency and benefits of desired outcomes, a pharmaceutical care plan should include the following:

1. **Assessment.** A review of the medical conditions and symptoms to determine the need for medication

2. **Plan.** A decision of an appropriate drug therapy based on the assessment of the patient

3. **Monitoring.** A review of the outcomes of drug therapy (i.e., goals and end points) to determine if the patient is obtaining the desired outcomes

B. **Drug-related problems** are evidence of less-than-optimal drug therapy. Detection of drug-related problems requires an assessment of the need for a change in drug therapy. Possible problems include

1. **Unnecessary drug therapy.** The medication cannot be associated with a medical condition or the presence of a condition in which nondrug therapy is more appropriate.

2. **Wrong drug.** The drug is not indicated for the condition or is not delivering the desired outcomes, or a more effective drug is available.

3. **Dose too low.** Incorrect dose, frequency, administration, or duration of therapy results in an insufficient dose of drug to the patient.

4. **Adverse drug reaction.** An allergic reaction, drug interaction, or an undesirable effect occurs from a medication.

5. **Dose too high.** Incorrect dose, frequency, or duration, results in more medication than is required.

6. **Inappropriate compliance.** The patient is not taking the optimal amount of medication owing to cost, administration difficulties, alternative health beliefs, or a lack of understanding of the need for the medication.

7. **Need additional drug therapy.** Owing to an undertreated condition, synergism with concurrent drug therapy or prophylactic therapy is required.

STUDY QUESTIONS

Directions: Each of the questions, statements, or incomplete statements can be correctly answered or completed by **one** of the suggested answers or phrases. Choose the **best** answer.

1. Medication orders differ from prescriptions in which of the following ways? They

(A) are intended for ambulatory use.
(B) contain only the generic name of the medication.
(C) are intended for institutional use.
(D) may be transmitted electronically.
(E) contain the quantity of medication to be dispensed.

2. If a therapeutic intervention is necessary, all of the following information should be communicated to the prescriber *except*

(A) a declaration that "a mistake was made."
(B) a brief description of the problem.
(C) a reference source that documents the problem.
(D) an alternative or suggestion to resolve the problem.
(E) a description of the clinical significance of the problem.

3. The following information should be recorded on a prescription *except* the

(A) prescription number.
(B) date of filling.
(C) expiration date.
(D) product and quantity dispensed.
(E) pharmacist's initials.

4. A prescription label should contain all of the following *except* the

(A) quantity dispensed.
(B) lot number.
(C) patient's diagnosis.
(D) expiration date.
(E) prescriber's name.

5. Auxiliary and cautionary labels should be used for all of the following purposes *except* to

(A) substitute for verbal consultation.
(B) ensure proper usage.
(C) inform of storage requirements.
(D) comply with regulatory requirements.
(E) warn against the concomitant use of certain drugs or foods.

6. The following items are essential for a patient profile system *except*

(A) the patient's name.
(B) the prescriber's Drug Enforcement Administration (DEA) registration number.
(C) the patient's allergies.
(D) the patient's birth date.
(E) instructions for medication use.

7. The following are drug-related problems *except*

(A) an adverse effect from a medication.
(B) symptoms caused by undertreatment.
(C) a drug–drug interaction.
(D) an undiagnosed condition.
(E) an allergic reaction to a medication.

ANSWERS AND EXPLANATIONS

1. The answer is C *[see I.B].*
Medication orders are written for the care of inpatients. Both medication orders and prescriptions may contain the brand or generic name of the drug and may be transmitted electronically. Only prescriptions contain the quantity of medication to be dispensed.

2. The answer is A *[see II.C.1].*
Information provided to the prescriber during a therapeutic intervention should include a description of the problem, reference source, description of the clinical significance, and an alternative. Informing the prescriber that a mistake was made does not encourage cooperation and resolution of the problem.

3. The answer is C *[see III.A].*
The prescription number, date of filling, product and quantity dispensed, and pharmacist's initials should be recorded on the prescription. The expiration date of the product being dispensed is not required.

4. The answer is C *[see III.E.1].*
The quantity of medication dispensed, lot number, expiration date of the product, and prescriber's name should be included on the label. The patient's diagnosis, although listed in the patient's profile, is not included on the prescription label.

5. The answer is A *[see III.E.3; IV.A.1].*
Auxiliary and cautionary labels are an adjunct to, not a replacement for, verbal consultation. Appropriate uses for such labels include ensuring proper use, storage requirements, and compliance with statutory requirements, and warning against food and drug interactions.

6. The answer is B *[see III.F.1–2].*
The patient's name is required to identify each patient. Often, the address or room number is required to identify patients with similar names. The patient's allergies, birth date, and instructions for use are required to prevent drug allergies and to assess the appropriateness of the prescription or medication order.

7. The answer is D *[see V.B].*
Adverse effects, undertreated conditions, allergic reactions, and drug–drug interactions are all drug-related problems. An undiagnosed condition may lead to a drug-related problem once diagnosed; however, diagnosis is required before the need for medication can be assessed.

27
Sterile Products
John Fanikos

I. INTRODUCTION. The *United States Pharmacopeia* (*USP*) and the *National Formulary* (*NF*) published practice standards for compounding sterile preparations after case reports of patient harm and fatality. The procedures and requirements outlined in *USP* Chapter 797 are intended to prevent patient harm resulting from ingredient errors and microbial contamination. The chapter includes the responsibilities of personnel performing compounding, training and evaluation requirements, verification of sterility and accuracy of medication preparations, classification of microbial contamination risk, and equipment and environmental quality and control. Although these standards apply to all facilities (hospitals, nursing homes, pharmacies) and all practitioners (physicians, nurses, technicians), they are especially important for pharmacists, who are most often involved with sterile medication preparation. Because the standards require substantial investment in labor, equipment, and supplies, regulatory agencies (the U.S. Food and Drug Administration [FDA], Joint Commission on Accreditation of Healthcare Organizations [JCAHO], and U.S. state boards of pharmacy) expected implementation by January 2006, with evidence of long-term compliance and routine monitoring thereafter.

II. DEFINITIONS

A. Sterility, an absolute term, means the absence of living microorganisms.

   1. A **microbe** is a microscopic organism, such as a bacterium, fungus, protozoan, or virus.

   2. **Pyrogens** are metabolic by-products of living or dead microorganisms that cause a pyretic response (i.e., a fever) on injection.

   3. **Sterile products** are pharmaceutical dosage forms that are sterile. This includes products such as parenteral preparations, irrigating solutions, and ophthalmic preparations (see Chapter 29). Sterile product compounding requires not only clean facilities but personnel who have received training in and have been tested on the principals and practices of sterilization and stability.

   4. **Aseptic manipulation** refers to the techniques and procedures used during compounding that maintain the sterility of pharmaceutical dosage forms.

   5. **Compounded sterile preparations** (CSPs) include the following:
      a. Preparations that, when prepared according to manufacturer instructions, expose a sterile agent to potential microbial contamination.
      b. Preparations made from nonsterile ingredients that must be sterilized before patient administration.
      c. Sterile or nonsterile biologicals (vaccines, immunoglobulins), diagnostic products, medications, nutritional products, and radiopharmaceuticals that must be sterilized before being administered to a patient or used for irrigation, in a bath, as an implant, for inhalation, for an injection, in the eye, or in the ear.

   6. **Microbial contamination risk levels** are assigned according to the probability of contaminating a preparation with microbial organisms, endotoxins, or foreign chemical or physical particulate matter.
      a. **Low-risk CSPs** are compounded by aseptically transferring a single sterile dosage form from a sterile ampule, vial, bottle, or bag using sterile needles and syringes to a final sterile container or device for patient administration.
      b. **Medium-risk CSPs** are compounded by aseptically transferring multiple sterile dosage forms from sterile ampules, vials, bottles, or bags using sterile needles and syringes to a single final sterile container or device for patient administration.
      c. **High-risk CSPs** are compounded from nonsterile ingredients and terminally sterilized before patient administration or are compounded from sterile ingredients that are compounded under inferior air quality conditions.

7. **Compounded parenteral preparations** are pharmaceutical dosage forms that are injected through one or more layers of skin. Because the parenteral route bypasses the protective barriers of the body, parenteral preparations must be sterile. The pH of a solution may markedly influence the stability and compatibility of parenteral preparations (see VII.B).

B. **Design and function of sterile compounding areas**

1. **Clean rooms** are areas specially constructed and maintained to reduce the probability of environmental contamination of sterile products during the manufacturing process. Engineering controls to reduce the potential for airborne contamination include airflow through high-efficiency particulate-air (HEPA) filters, use of horizontal flow clean benches, vertical flow clean benches, biological safety cabinets, and barrier isolators. Clean rooms are traditionally designed with multiple compartments or partitioned work areas for aseptic processing (Figure 27-1).

   a. The **anteroom** provides a clean area for personal cleaning and hygiene and for donning personal protective equipment such as hair covers, gloves, gowns, or full clean room attire (Figure 27-2). Supplies are removed from shipping cartons in this area and decontaminated with a disinfecting agent.

   b. **Buffer area** contains the work surfaces in which sterile products are prepared and should provide at least an International Organization for Standardization (ISO) class 8 work environment. The buffer area should contain no sinks or drains and be free of objects that shed particles (e.g., cardboard, paper, cotton). Traffic flow in and out is minimized and restricted to qualified compounding personnel.

   c. **HEPA filters** are used to cleanse the air entering the room. These filters remove all airborne particles 0.3 mm or larger, with an efficiency of 99.97%. The reference standards for HEPA-filtered rooms are now on a metric-based system (Table 27-1). HEPA-filtered rooms are classified as ISO class 3–8. An ISO class 8 room contains no more than 3,520,000 particles of 0.5 mm or larger per cubic meter of air.

   d. **Positive-pressure airflow** is used to prevent contaminated air from flowing into the clean room. To achieve this, the air pressure inside the clean room must be greater than the pressure outside the room, so that when a door or window to the clean room is opened, the airflow is outward.

   e. **Counters** in the clean room are made of stainless steel or other nonporous, easily cleaned material.

Figure 27-1. Clean room design.

Figure 27-2. Clean room attire. [Photograph by William Salkin.]

    f. Walls, floors, and ceilings do not have cracks or crevices and have rounded corners. All surfaces should also be nonporous and washable to enable regular disinfection. If walls or floors are painted, an epoxy paint is used.

    g. Airflow. As with the HEPA filters used in clean rooms, the airflow moves with a uniform velocity along parallel lines. The velocity of the airflow is 27 m/min (90 ft/min).

    h. A **critical site** is any opening providing a direct path between a sterile product and the environment or any surface coming in direct contact with the sterile product and the environment. Laminar flow workbenches (LFWBs) are used to provide an adequate critical site environment. *USP* Chapter 797 requires sterile preparation compounding be performed in an air environment of at least an ISO class 5 rating.

2. Laminar flow workbenches are generally used in conjunction with clean rooms and are specially designed to create an aseptic environment for the preparation of sterile products. An ISO class 5 environment exists inside a certified horizontal or vertical LFWB.

    a. HEPA filter requirement. Like clean rooms, laminar flow workbenches use HEPA filters, but the benches use a higher-efficiency air filter than do clean rooms.

Table 27-1. International Organization of Standardization (ISO) Classification of Particulate Matter in Room Air

Class		Particle Size	
ISO	U.S. Federal Standard[a]	ISO (per cubic meter)	U.S. Federal Standard[a] (per cubic foot)
3	Class 1	35.2	1
4	Class 10	352	10
5	Class 100	3520	100
6	Class 1000	35,200	1,000
7	Class 10,000	352,000	10,000
8	Class 100,000	3,520,000	100,000

[a]Federal Standard No. 209E, General Services Administration.

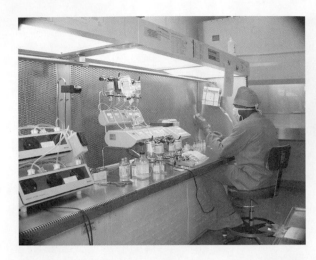

Figure 27-3. Horizontal laminar flow hood. [Photograph by William Salkin.]

b. Types of laminar flow workbenches
   (1) Horizontal laminar flow hoods were the first hoods used in pharmacies for the preparation of sterile products (Figure 27-3). Airflow in horizontal hoods moves across the surface of the work area, flowing first through a prefilter and then through the HEPA filter. The major disadvantage of the horizontal hood is that it offers no protection to the operator, which can be significant when hazardous compounds or antineoplastic agents are being prepared (see VII.D.2).
   (2) Vertical laminar flow hoods provide two major **advantages** over horizontal flow hoods (Figure 27-4).
      (a) The airflow is vertical, flowing down on the work space. This airflow pattern protects the operator against potential hazards from the products being prepared.
      (b) A portion of the HEPA-filtered air is recirculated a second time through the HEPA filter. The remainder of the filtered air is removed through an exhaust filter, which may be vented to the outside to protect the operator from chronic, concentrated exposure to hazardous materials.

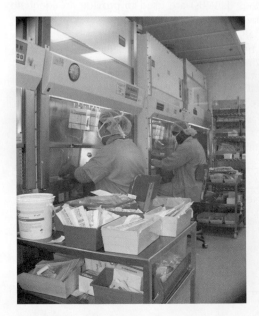

Figure 27-4. Vertical laminar flow hood. [Photograph by William Salkin.]

3. **Biological safety cabinets** (BSCs) are vertical laminar flow hoods; four major types are available. They are differentiated by the amount of air recirculated in the cabinet, whether this air is vented into the room or outside, and whether contaminated ducts are under positive or negative pressure.

   a. **Type A cabinets** recirculate 70% of cabinet air through HEPA filters back into the cabinet; the remainder is discharged through a HEPA filter into the clean room. Contaminated ducts are under positive pressure.

   b. **Type B1 cabinets** recirculate 30% of cabinet air through HEPA filters back into the cabinet; the remainder is discharged through HEPA filters to the outside environment. Contaminated ducts are under negative pressure.

   c. **Type B2 cabinets** discharged all cabinet air through HEPA filters to the outside environment. Contaminated ducts are under negative pressure.

   d. **Type B3 cabinets** recirculate 70% of cabinet air through HEPA filters back into the cabinet; 30% is discharged through HEPA filters to the outside. Contaminated ducts are under negative pressure.

4. **Barrier isolators** provide a ISO class 5 environment for product preparation; aseptic manipulations occur inside a closed, pressurized environment accessible only via sealed gloves that reach into the work area. (Figure 27-5). Isolators use unidirectional or turbulent airflow to remove contaminants from the unit. It uses positive air pressure to keep external airborne particles out of the isolator. This technology represents an acceptable alternative to LFWBs in a clean room for aseptic processing.

5. **Inspection and certification.** Clean rooms, LFWBs, BSCs, and barrier isolators are inspected and certified when they are first installed and at least every 6 months thereafter. Inspection and certification are also required when LFWB, BSCs, and isolators are moved to a new location.

   a. **Inspections** should be conducted by National Sanitation Foundation (NSF) accredited and certified technicians with expertise and training in contamination control technologies. Equipment used for testing has appropriate tolerance for the specified testing and is calibrated to National Institute of Standards and Technology (NIST) traceable standards.

Figure 27-5. Barrier isolator. [Photograph courtesy of Innovative Technology.]

b. Testing is performed per relevant industry standards, and at minimum includes
 (1) HEPA filter integrity testing
 (2) Airflow testing: down flow and inflow where appropriate
 (3) Particulate monitoring
 (4) Pressurization monitoring (clean rooms and barrier isolators) ensures that no particle > 0.3 mm passes through the HEPA filter. In addition, an anemometer is used to determine airflow velocity, and a particle counter is used to determine the particle count.

III. QUALITY CONTROL AND QUALITY ASSURANCE

A. Definitions

1. **Quality control** is the day-to-day assessment of all sterile compounding operations. This includes receipt of raw materials, preparation, storage, distribution, patient administration, and includes analytic testing of the finished product.

2. **Quality assurance,** an oversight function, involves the auditing of quality control procedures and systems, with suggestions for changes as needed.

B. Testing procedures. Various types of tests are used to ensure that all sterile products are free of microbial contamination, pyrogens, and particulate matter.

1. **Clarity testing** is used to check sterile products for particulate matter and leaks. Before dispensing a parenteral solution, compounding personnel should check for particulates by swirling the solution and looking at it against both light and dark backgrounds, using a clarity testing lamp or other standard light source.

2. **Compound accuracy checking** is a double-check of the used drug products and supplies by a person other than the compounder. This includes an inspection of the label and syringes used to measure the additives.

3. **Beyond-use dating** represents the date and time beyond which a product should not be administered because of potency, sterility, or storage concerns. Beyond-use dating should be assigned in accordance with the manufacturer's product labeling and *USP* Chapter 797 requirements.
 a. High-risk CSPs should not be used beyond 24 hr when stored at room temperature, 3 days when stored under refrigeration, and 45 days when stored in a freezer ($\leq 20°C$).
 b. Medium-risk CSPs should not be used beyond 30 hr when stored at room temperature, 7 days when stored under refrigeration, and 45 days when stored in a freezer ($\leq 20°C$).
 c. Low Risk Level CSPs should not be used beyond 48 hours when stored at room temperature, 14 days when stored under refrigeration, and 45 days when stored in a freezer ($\leq 20°C$).

4. **End product testing** is sterility and pyrogen testing, which should be performed on all high-risk CSPs that are prepared in batches of 25 units or more, multidose vials, or preparations that are exposed > 6–12 hr before sterilization.
 a. **Sterility testing** ensures that the process used to sterilize the product was successful. The **membrane sterilization method** is often used to conduct sterility testing. Test samples are passed through membrane filters, and a nutrient medium is then added to promote microbial growth. After an incubation period, microbial growth is determined.
 b. **Pyrogen testing** can be accomplished by means of qualitative fever response testing in rabbits or by in vitro limulus lysate testing. Commercial laboratories are available to perform these tests. Personnel handling sterile products can attempt to avoid problems with pyrogens by purchasing pyrogen-free water and sodium chloride for injection from reputable manufacturers and by using proper handling and storage procedures.

C. Environmental testing includes air and surface sampling to measure microbiology conditions of the clean room and assesses the effectiveness of cleaning and sanitizing procedures.

1. **Air sampling** evaluates airborne organisms by exposing sterile nutrient plates containing trypticase soy broth (TSB) or trypticase soy agar (TSA) to the compounding environment for a suitable time frame.

2. Surface sampling uses TSA plates called replicate organism detection and counting (RODAC) plates to capture microorganism.

Both air- and surface-sampling plates are collected and incubated. The number of discrete colonies of organisms, colony-forming units (CFUs), are counted and reported.

D. Practical quality assurance programs for noncommercial sterile products include training, monitoring the manufacturing process, quality control checks, and documentation.

    1. Training of pharmacists and technicians in proper aseptic techniques and practices is the single most important aspect of an effective quality assurance program. Training should impart a thorough understanding of compounding policies and procedures.

    2. By **monitoring the manufacturing process,** a supervisor can check adherence to established policies and procedures and take corrective action as necessary.

E. Process validation provides a mechanism for ensuring processes consistently result in sterile products of acceptable quality. This should include a written procedure to follow as well as evaluation of aseptic technique through process simulation.

F. Process simulation testing or personnel evaluation duplicates sterile compounding of low-, medium-, and high-risk CSPs under most stressful conditions, except that an appropriate growth media (soybean–casein digest medium) is used in place of the drug products. After preparation and incubation of the final product, no growth indicates that proper aseptic techniques were followed. *USP* Chapter 797 requires compounding personnel complete process-simulation testing annually for those manufacturing low- and medium-risk CSPs and semi-annually for those producing high-risk CSPs.

G. Quality control checking includes monitoring the sterility of a sample of manufactured products. The membrane sterilization method is practically employed using a commercially available filter and TSB media.

H. Documentation of training procedures, quality control results, laminar flow hood certification, and production records are required by various agencies and organizations.

IV. STERILIZATION METHODS AND EQUIPMENT.
Sterilization is performed to destroy or remove all microorganisms in or on a product. Sterilization can be achieved through thermal, chemical, radioactive, or mechanical methods.

A. Thermal sterilization involves the use of either moist or dry heat.

    1. Moist-heat sterilization is the **most widely used** and reliable sterilization method.
        a. Microorganisms are destroyed by **cellular protein coagulation.**
        b. The objects to be sterilized are exposed to saturated steam under 1 atm pressure at a minimum temperature of **121°C** for at least 20–60 min.
        c. An **autoclave** is commonly used for moist-heat sterilization.
        d. Because it does not require as high a temperature, moist-heat sterilization causes **less product and equipment damage** compared to dry-heat sterilization.

    2. Dry-heat sterilization is appropriate for materials that cannot withstand moist-heat sterilization. Objects are subjected to a temperature of at least **160°C** for **120 min** (if higher temperatures can be used, less exposure time is required).

B. Chemical (gas) sterilization is used to sterilize surfaces and porous materials (e.g., surgical dressings) that other sterilization methods may damage.

    1. In this method, **ethylene oxide** is used generally in combination with heat and moisture.

    2. Residual gas must be allowed to dissipate after sterilization and before use of the sterile product.

C. Radioactive sterilization is suitable for the industrial sterilization of contents in sealed packages that cannot be exposed to heat (e.g., prepackaged surgical components, some ophthalmic ointments, and powders).

    1. This technique involves either **electromagnetic** or **particulate radiation.**

    2. Accelerated drug decomposition sometimes results.

D. Mechanical sterilization (filtration) removes but does not destroy microorganisms and clarifies solutions by eliminating particulate matter. For solutions rendered unstable by thermal, chemical, or radiation sterilization, filtration is the preferred method. A depth filter or screen filter may be used. Personnel should ensure the filter used either during compounding or administration is chemically and physically compatible with the CSP at the temperature and pressure conditions used.

    1. Depth filters usually consist of fritted glass or unglazed porcelain (i.e., substances that trap particles in channels).

    2. Screen (membrane) filters are films measuring 1–200 mm thick made of cellulose esters, microfilaments, polycarbonate, synthetic polymers, silver, or stainless steel.

        a. A **mesh** of millions of microcapillary pores of identical size filter the solution by a process of physical sieving.

        b. Flow rate. Because pores make up 70%–85% of the surface, screen filters have a higher flow rate than depth filters.

        c. Types of screen filters

            (1) Particulate filters remove particles of glass, plastic, rubber, and other contaminants.

                (a) Other uses. These filters also are used to reduce the risk of phlebitis associated with administration of reconstituted powders. Filtration removes any undissolved powder particles that may cause venous inflammation.

                (b) The **pore size** of standard particulate filters ranges from 0.45 to 5 mm. Special particulate filters are required to filter blood, emulsions (e.g., fat emulsions), or colloidal dispersions or suspensions because these preparations have a larger particle size.

            (2) Microbial filters, with a pore size of 0.22 μm or smaller, ensure complete microbial removal and sterilization. This is referred to as cold sterilization.

            (3) Final filters, which may be either particulate or microbial, are often included as part of the tubing used in drug administration. They are referred to as in-line filters and are used to remove particulates or microorganisms from an intravenous (IV) solution during infusion.

V. PACKAGING OF PARENTERAL PRODUCTS.
Parenteral preparations and other sterile products must be packaged in a way that maintains product sterility until the time of use and prevents contamination of contents during opening.

A. Types of containers

    1. Ampules, the oldest type of parenteral product containers, are made entirely of **glass.**

        a. Intended for **single use only,** ampules are opened by breaking the glass at a score line on the neck.

        b. Disadvantages. Because glass particles may become dislodged during ampule opening, the product must be filtered before it is administered. Their unsuitability for multiple-dose use, the need to filter solutions before use, and other safety considerations have markedly reduced the ampule as a package form.

    2. Vials are glass or plastic containers closed with a rubber stopper and sealed with an aluminum crimp (Figure 27-6).

        a. Vials have several **advantages** over ampules.

            (1) Vials can be designed to hold multiple doses (if prepared with a bacteriostatic agent).

            (2) The drug product is easier to remove from vials than from ampules.

            (3) Vials eliminate the risk of glass particle contamination during opening.

Figure 27-6. Syringes and vials. [Photograph by William Salkin.]

b. However, vials also have certain **disadvantages.**
  (1) The rubber stopper can become **cored,** causing a small bit of rubber to enter the solution.
  (2) Multiple withdrawals (as with multiple-dose vials) can result in microbial contamination.
c. Some drugs that are unstable in solution are packaged in vials unreconstituted and must be **reconstituted** with a diluent before use. Sterile water or sterile sodium chloride for injection are the most commonly used drug diluents.
  (1) To accelerate the dissolution rate and permit rapid reconstitution, many powders are lyophilized (freeze dried).
  (2) Some of these drugs come in vials that contain a double chamber.
     (a) The top chamber, containing sterile water for injection, is separated from the unreconstituted drug by a rubber closure.
     (b) To dislodge the inner closure and mix the contents of the compartments, external pressure is applied to the outer rubber closure. This system eliminates the need to enter the vial twice, thereby reducing the risk of microbial contamination.

3. Some drugs come in vials that may be attached to an diluent containing bag for reconstitution and administration (**ADD-Vantage,** Abbott; Figure 27-7).

Figure 27-7. *Left,* prefilled antibiotic piggyback dose. *Right,* Abbott ADD-Vantage system. [Photograph by William Salkin.]

    a. The ADD-Vantage vial is screwed into the top of an ADD-Vantage diluent bag, and the rubber diaphragm is dislodged from the vial, allowing the diluent solution to dissolve the drug.

    b. The reconstituted ADD-Vantage vial and IV bag are ready for administration when hung.

4. Prefilled syringes and **cartridges** are designed for maximum convenience (Figure 27-6).

    a. Prefilled syringes. Drugs administered in an emergency (e.g., atropine, epinephrine) are available for immediate injection when packaged in prefilled syringes.

    b. Prefilled cartridges are ready-to-use parenteral packages that offer improved sterility and accuracy. They consist of a plastic cartridge holder and a prefilled medication cartridge with a needle attached. The medication is premixed and premeasured. Narcotics such as meperidine (Demerol) and hydromorphone (Dilaudid) are commonly available in prefilled cartridges.

5. Infusion solutions are divided into two categories: **small-volume parenterals** (SVPs), those having a volume < 100 mL; and **large-volume parenterals** (LVPs), those having a volume of ≥ 100 mL. Infusion solutions are used for the intermittent or continuous infusion of fluids or drugs (see X.B).

B. Packaging materials. Materials used to package parenteral products include glass and plastic polymers.

1. Glass, the original parenteral packaging material, has superior clarity, facilitating inspection for particulate matter. Compared to plastic, glass less frequently interacts with the preparation it contains.

2. Plastic polymers used for parenteral packaging include polyvinyl chloride (PVC) and polyolefin.

    a. PVC is flexible and nonrigid.

    b. Polyolefin is semirigid; unlike PVC, it can be stored upright.

    c. Both types of plastic offer several **advantages** over glass, including durability, easier storage and disposal, reduced weight, and improved safety.

VI. PARENTERAL ADMINISTRATION ROUTES.
Parenteral preparations may be given by a variety of administration routes.

A. Subcutaneous (SC or SQ) administration refers to injection into the subcutaneous tissue beneath the skin layers, usually of the abdomen, arm, or thigh. Insulin is an example of a subcutaneously administered drug.

B. Intramuscular (IM) administration means injection into a muscle mass. The mid-deltoid area and gluteus medius are common injection sites.

1. No more than 5 mL of a solution should be injected by this route.

2. Drugs intended for prolonged or delayed absorption such as medroxyprogesterone (Depo-Provera) and methylprednisolone (Depo-Medrol) are commonly administered intramuscularly.

C. Intravenous (IV) administration is the most important and most common parenteral administration route. It allows an immediate therapeutic effect by delivering the drug directly into the circulation. However, this route precludes recall of an inadvertent drug overdose. Antibiotics, cardiac medications, and many other drugs are given intravenously.

D. Intradermal (ID) administration involves injection into the most superficial skin layer. Because this route can deliver only a limited drug volume, its use is generally restricted to skin tests and certain vaccines.

E. Intra-arterial (IA) administration is injection directly into an artery. It delivers a high drug concentration to the target site with little dilution by the circulation. Generally, this route is used only for radiopaque materials, thrombolytic agents, and some antineoplastic agents.

F. Intracardiac (IC) administration is injection of a drug directly into the heart.

G. Hypodermoclysis refers to injection of large volumes of a solution into subcutaneous tissue to provide a continuous, abundant drug supply. This route occasionally is used for antibiotic administration in children.

H. Intraspinal administration refers to injection into the spinal column. Local anesthetics (e.g., lidocaine, bupivacaine) are frequently administered via this route before and after surgical procedures.

I. Intra-articular administration means injection into a joint space. Corticosteroids (e.g., methyl-prednisolone, hydrocortisone) are administered via this route for the treatment of arthritis.

J. Intrasynovial administration refers to injection into the joint fluid.

K. Intrathecal (IT) administration is injection into the spinal fluid; it sometimes is used for antibiotics and cancer chemotherapy.

L. Epidural (ED) administration refers to the injection of medications, usually local anesthetics and/or narcotics near or outside the dura mater of the central nervous system. This route is frequently used during childbirth.

VII. PARENTERAL PREPARATIONS

A. IV admixtures. These preparations consist of one or more sterile drug products added to an IV fluid, generally dextrose or sodium chloride solution alone or in combination. IV admixtures are used for drugs intended for continuous infusion. Drugs that may cause irritation or toxicity when given as a rapid direct IV injection are also prepared as IV admixtures.

    1. Hypotonic solutions exert a lower osmotic pressure than blood or sodium chloride 0.9% solution.

    2. Isotonic solutions have the same osmotic pressure as blood or sodium chloride 0.9% solution.

    3. Hypertonic solutions exert a greater osmotic pressure than blood or sodium chloride 0.9% solution. To avoid phlebitis and tissue damage, these solutions are administered through a large vein, either the subclavian vein or the internal jugular vein.

B. IV fluids and electrolytes

    1. Fluids used in the preparation and administration of parenteral products include sterile water and sodium chloride, dextrose, and Ringer solutions, all of which have multiple uses. These fluids serve as vehicles in IV admixtures, providing a means for reconstituting sterile powders. They serve as the basis for correcting body fluid and electrolyte disturbances and provide a caloric source in parenteral nutrition.

      a. Dextrose (D-glucose) solutions are the most frequently used glucose solutions in parenteral preparations.

        (1) Uses. Generally, a solution of dextrose 5% in water (D_5W) is used as a vehicle in IV admixtures. D_5W may also serve as a hydrating solution. In higher concentrations (e.g., a 10% solution in water), dextrose provides a source of carbohydrates in parenteral nutrition solutions.

        (2) Considerations. Because the pH of D_5W ranges from 3.5 to 6.5, instability may result if it is combined with an acid-sensitive drug.

          (a) Dextrose concentrations > 15% must be administered through a central vein.

          (b) Dextrose solutions should be used cautiously in patients with diabetes mellitus.

      b. Sodium chloride usually is given as a 0.9% solution. Because it is isotonic with blood, this solution is called normal saline solution (NSS). A solution of 0.45% sodium chloride is termed half-normal saline. A solution of 0.225% sodium chloride is termed quarter-normal saline.

(1) **Sodium chloride for injection,** which is a solution of 0.9% sodium chloride, is used as a vehicle in IV admixtures and for fluid and electrolyte replacement. In smaller volumes, it is suitable for the reconstitution of various medications.

(2) **Bacteriostatic sodium chloride for injection,** which is also a 0.9% solution, is intended solely for multiple reconstitutions. It contains an agent that inhibits bacterial growth (e.g., benzyl alcohol, propylparaben, methylparaben), which allows for its use in multiple-dose preparations.

c. **Waters** are used for reconstitution and for dilution of such IV solutions as dextrose and sodium chloride. Waters suitable for parenteral preparations include sterile water for injection and bacteriostatic water for injection.

d. **Ringer solutions,** which are appropriate for fluid and electrolyte replacement, are commonly administered to postsurgical patients.

(1) **Lactated Ringer injection** (i.e., Hartmann solution, Ringer lactate solution) contains sodium lactate, sodium chloride, potassium chloride, and calcium chloride. Frequently, it is combined with dextrose (e.g., as 5% dextrose in lactated Ringer injection).

(2) **Ringer injection** differs from lactated Ringer injection in that it does not contain sodium lactate and has slightly different concentrations of sodium chloride and calcium chloride. Like lactated Ringer injection, it may be combined in solution with dextrose.

2. **Electrolyte preparations.** With ions present in both intracellular and extracellular fluid, electrolytes are crucial for various biological processes. Surgical and medical patients who cannot take food by mouth or who need nutritional supplementation require the addition of electrolytes in hydrating solutions or parenteral nutrition solutions.

a. **Cations** are positively charged electrolytes.

(1) **Sodium** is the chief extracellular cation.

(a) **Importance.** Sodium plays a key role in interstitial osmotic pressure, tissue hydration, acid–base balance, nerve-impulse transmission, and muscle contraction.

(b) **Parenteral sodium preparations** include sodium chloride, sodium acetate, and sodium phosphate.

(2) **Potassium** is the chief intracellular cation.

(a) **Importance.** Potassium participates in carbohydrate metabolism, protein synthesis, muscle contraction (especially of cardiac muscle), and neuromuscular excitability.

(b) **Parenteral potassium preparations** include potassium acetate, potassium chloride, and potassium phosphate.

(3) **Calcium**

(a) **Importance.** Calcium is essential to nerve-impulse transmission, muscle contraction, cardiac function, bone formation, and capillary and cell membrane permeability.

(b) **Parenteral calcium preparations** include calcium chloride, calcium gluconate, and calcium gluceptate.

(4) **Magnesium**

(a) **Importance.** Magnesium plays a vital part in enzyme activities, neuromuscular transmission, and muscle excitability.

(b) **Parenteral preparation.** Magnesium is given parenterally as magnesium sulfate.

b. **Anions** are negatively charged electrolytes.

(1) **Chloride** is the major extracellular anion.

(a) **Importance.** Along with sodium, it regulates interstitial osmotic pressure and helps control blood pH.

(b) **Parenteral chloride preparations** include calcium chloride, potassium chloride, and sodium chloride.

(2) **Phosphate** is the major intracellular anion.

(a) **Importance.** Phosphate is critical to various enzyme activities. It also influences calcium levels and acts as a buffer to prevent marked changes in acid–base balance.

(b) **Parenteral phosphate preparations** include potassium phosphate and sodium phosphate.

(3) Acetate
  (a) Importance. Acetate is a bicarbonate precursor that may be used to provide alkali to assist in the preservation of plasma pH.
  (b) Parenteral acetate preparations include potassium acetate and sodium acetate.

C. Parenteral antibiotic preparations are available as sterile unreconstituted powders—which must be reconstituted with sterile water, normal saline, or D_5W—or as a sterile, ready-to-use liquid parenteral.

  1. Administration methods. Parenteral antibiotics may be given intermittently by direct IV injection, short-term infusion, intramuscular injection, or intrathecal injection.

  2. Uses. Parenteral antibiotics are used to treat infections that are serious and require high antibiotic blood levels or when the gastrointestinal tract is contraindicated, such as in ileus.

  3. Dosing frequencies of parenteral antibiotics vary from once daily to as often as every 2 hr, depending on the kinetics of the drug, seriousness of the infection, the site of infection, and the patient's disease or organ status (e.g., renal disease).

D. Parenteral antineoplastic agents. Studies suggest that these medications may be toxic to the personnel who prepare and administer them. The evidence is not conclusive, which necessitates special precautions to ensure safety and minimize risks. In response to concerns, the Occupational Safety and Health Administration (OSHA) published the technical manual *Controlling Occupational Exposure to Hazardous Drugs.* Every facility must have a written plan that includes drug preparation precautions, storage, transport, personal protective equipment (gloves, gowns, masks), work equipment, waste disposal, spill management, and personnel medical surveillance.

  1. Administration methods. Parenteral antineoplastics may be given by direct IV injection, short-term infusion, or long-term infusion. Some are administered by a non-IV route, such as the subcutaneous, intramuscular, intra-arterial, or intrathecal route.

  2. Safe antineoplastic handling guidelines. All compounding personnel who prepare or practitioners who administer antineoplastics should receive special training in the following guidelines to reduce the risk of exposure to these drugs.
   a. A **vertical laminar flow hood** should be used during drug preparation, with exhaust directed to the outside.
   b. All syringes and IV tubing should have **Luer-Lok fittings** (see IX.B.1; IX.B.4).
   c. Clothing. Personnel should wear personal protective equipment, including closed-front cuffed surgical gowns and double-layered latex surgeon's gloves.
   d. Negative-pressure technique should be used during withdrawal of medication from vials. This will prevent pressure from building up inside the vial and causing the drug to spray around the needle.
   e. Final dosage adjustment should be made into the vial, ampule, or directly into an absorbent gauze pad.
   f. Priming equipment. Special care should be taken when IV administration sets are primed. The IV tubing should be primed before adding the drug, or the tubing can be primed with drug-free fluid before connecting it to the chemotherapy drug container. If these are not available, prime the tubing into sterile gauze in a sealable plastic bag.
   g. Proper procedures should be followed for **disposal** of materials used in the preparation and administration of antineoplastics.
    (1) Needles should not be clipped or recapped.
    (2) Preparations should be discarded in containers that are puncture-proof, leak-proof, and properly labeled.
    (3) Hazardous waste. There is no completely acceptable method for disposing of hazardous waste. High-temperature incineration may be the preferred method. These materials may also be buried in an EPA-licensed hazardous waste dump or chemically deactivated.
   h. After removal of gloves, personnel should **wash hands** thoroughly.
   i. Personnel and equipment involved in the preparation and administration of antineoplastic agents should be **monitored** routinely.

  3. Patient problems. Infusion phlebitis and extravasation are the most serious problems that may occur during the administration of parenteral antineoplastics.

a. **Infusion phlebitis** (inflammation of a vein) is characterized by pain, swelling, heat sensation, and redness at the infusion site. Drug dilution and filtration can eliminate or minimize the risk of phlebitis.

b. **Extravasation** (infiltration of a drug into subcutaneous tissues surrounding the vein) is especially harmful when antineoplastics with vesicant properties are administered. Measures must be taken immediately if extravasation occurs.

   (1) Depending on the drug involved, emergency measures may include stopping the infusion, injecting hydrocortisone or another anti-inflammatory agent directly into the affected area, injecting an antidote (if available), and applying a cold compress (to facilitate a drug–antidote reaction).

   (2) A warm compress may then be applied to increase the flow of blood, and thus the vesicant, away from damaged tissue.

E. **Parenteral biotechnology products** are created by the application of recombinant technology to generate therapeutic agents, such as monoclonal antibodies, various vaccines, and colony-stimulating factors.

1. **Uses** of these agents include cancer therapy, infections, transplant rejection, rheumatoid arthritis, inflammatory bowel disease, respiratory diseases, and malaria as well as vaccines against cancer, HIV infection, and hepatitis B.

2. **Characteristics.** Protein and peptide biotechnology drugs have a shorter half-life, often require special storage such as refrigeration or freezing, and must not be shaken vigorously to avoid destroying the protein molecules.

3. **Administration.** Many biotechnology products require reconstitution with sterile water or normal saline and may be parenterally administered by direct IV injection or infusion, or by intramuscular or subcutaneous injection.

VIII. IRRIGATING SOLUTIONS.

Although these sterile products are manufactured by the same standards used to process IV preparations, they are **not intended for infusion into the venous system.** Labeling differences between irrigation solutions and injections are specified in the *USP* and reflect differences in acceptable particulate matter levels, volume of solution available for use, and the container design.

A. **Topical administration.** Irrigating solutions for topical use are packaged in pour bottles so that they can be poured directly onto the desired area. These solutions are intended for such purposes as irrigating wounds, moistening dressings, and cleaning surgical instruments.

B. **Infusion of irrigating solutions.** This procedure, using an administration set attached to a Foley catheter, is commonly used for many surgical patients. Surgeons performing urological procedures often use irrigating solutions to perfuse tissues, to maintain the integrity of the surgical field, remove blood, and provide a clear field of view. To decrease the risk of infection, 1 mL Neosporin G.U. Irrigant, an antibiotic preparation, is often added to these solutions.

C. **Dialysis.** Dialysates are irrigating solutions used in the dialysis of patients with such disorders as renal failure, poisoning, and electrolyte disturbances. These products remove waste materials, serum electrolytes, and toxic products from the body.

1. In **peritoneal dialysis,** a hypertonic dialysate is infused directly into the peritoneal cavity via a surgically implanted catheter. The dialysate, which contains dextrose and electrolytes, removes harmful substances by osmosis and diffusion. After a specified period of time, the solution is drained. Antibiotics and heparin may be added to the dialysate.

2. In **hemodialysis,** the patient's blood is transfused through a dialyzing membrane unit that removes the harmful substances from the patient's vascular system. After passing through the dialyzer, the blood reenters the body through a vein.

IX. NEEDLES AND SYRINGES

A. **Hypodermic needles** are stainless-steel or aluminum devices that penetrate the skin for the purpose of administering or transferring a parenteral product (Figure 27-8).

1. **Needle gauge** is the outside diameter of the needle shaft; the larger the number, the smaller the diameter. Gauges in common use range from 13 (largest diameter) to 27. Subcutaneous injections usually require a 24-gauge or 25-gauge needle. Intramuscular injections require a needle with a gauge between 19 and 22. Needles between 18 gauge and 20 gauge are commonly used for compounding parenterals.

2. **Bevels** are slanting edges cut into needle tips to facilitate injection through tissue or rubber vial closures.
   a. **Regular-bevel needles** are the most commonly used type, and they are suitable for subcutaneous and intramuscular injections and hypodermoclysis.
   b. **Short-bevel needles** are used when only shallow penetration is required (as in IV injections).
   c. **Intradermal-bevel needles** are designed for intradermal injections and have the most beveled edges.

3. **Needle lengths** range from 1/4 to 6 inches. Choice of needle length depends on the desired penetration.
   a. For **compounding parenteral preparations,** 1 1/2-inch-long needles are commonly used.
   b. **Intradermal and subcutaneous injections** necessitate a short needle length, usually 1/4 to 5/8 inch.
   c. **Intraspinal injection** requires a needle length of 3 1/2 inches.
   d. **IV infusion** requires needles that range in length from 1 1/4 to 2 1/2 inches.

B. **Syringes** are devices for injecting, withdrawing, or instilling fluids. Syringes consist of a glass or plastic barrel with a tight-fitting plunger at one end; a small opening at the other end accommodates the head of a needle (Figure 27-9).

1. The **Luer syringe,** the first syringe developed, has a universal needle attachment accommodating all needle sizes.

2. **Syringe volumes** range from 0.3 to 60 mL. Insulin syringes have unit gradations (100 units/mL) rather than volume gradations.

3. **Calibrations** are in the metric system, and vary in specificity, depending on syringe size. The smaller the syringe, the smaller the measurement scale.

4. **Syringe tips** come in several types.
   a. **Luer-Lok tips** are threaded to ensure the needle fits tightly in the syringe. Antineoplastic agents should be administered with syringes of this type (see VII.D.2).

Figure 27-8. Needles. *Top,* 20 gauge, 3 1/2 inch. *Bottom, left to right,* 18 gauge, 1 1/2 inch; 20 gauge, 1 inch; 23 gauge, 1 inch; 25 gauge, 5/8 inch; 27 gauge, 1/2 inch. [Photograph by William Salkin.]

Figure 27-9. Syringes. *Left to right,* 60 mL catheter tip, 60 ml, 30 mL, 10 mL, 5 mL, 3 mL, 1 mL. [Photograph by William Salkin.]

    b. Luer-slip tips are unthreaded so that the syringe and needle do not lock into place. Because of this, the needle may become dislodged.

    c. Eccentric tips, which are set off center, allow the needle to remain parallel to the injection site and minimize venous irritation.

    d. Catheter tips are used for wound irrigation and administration of enteral feedings. They are not intended for injections.

X. INTRAVENOUS DRUG DELIVERY

  A. Injection sites

    1. Peripheral vein injection is preferred for drugs that do not irritate the veins, administration of isotonic solutions, and patients who require only short-term IV therapy. Generally, the dorsal forearm surface is chosen for venipuncture.

    2. Central vein injection is preferred for administration of irritating drugs or hypertonic solutions, patients requiring long-term IV therapy, and situations in which a peripheral line cannot be maintained. Large veins in the thoracic cavity, such as the subclavian vein, are used.

  B. Infusion methods

    1. Continuous-drip infusion is the slow, primary-line infusion of an IV preparation to maintain a therapeutic drug level or provide fluid and electrolyte replacement.

      a. Flow rates must be carefully monitored. Generally, these rates are expressed as volume per unit of time (e.g., mL/hr, drops/min) and sometimes as milligrams per minute (mg/min) for certain drugs.

      b. Administration. Drugs with a narrow therapeutic index such as oxytocin (Pitocin), heparin, and pressor agents such as norepinephrine (Levophed) and phenylephrine (Neo-Synephrine) typically are administered by this method.

    2. Intermittent infusion allows drug administration at specific intervals (e.g., every 4 hr) and is most often used for antibiotics.

      a. Three different techniques may be used.

        (1) Direct (bolus) injection rapidly delivers small volumes of an undiluted drug. This method is used to:

          (a) Achieve an immediate effect (as in an emergency)

          (b) Administer drugs that cannot be diluted

          (c) Achieve a therapeutic serum drug level quickly

        (2) Additive set infusion, using a volume-control device, is appropriate for the intermittent delivery of small amounts of IV solutions or diluted medications. The fluid chamber is attached to an independent fluid supply or placed directly under the established primary IV line.

(3) The **piggyback method** is used when a drug cannot be mixed with the primary solution. A special coupling for the primary IV tubing permits infusion of a supplementary secondary solution through the primary system.

   (a) This method eliminates the need for a second venipuncture or further dilution of the supplementary preparation.

   (b) **Admixtures** in which the vehicle is added to the drug are known as manufacturers' piggybacks. Admixtures in which a special drug vial is attached to a special IV bag are available in the ADD-Vantage system (Figure 27-7).

b. In some cases, **intermittent infusion injection devices** are used. Also called scalp-vein, heparin-lock, or butterfly infusion sets, these devices permit intermittent delivery while eliminating the need for multiple venipunctures or prolonged venous access with a continuous infusion. To prevent clotting in the cannula, dilute heparin solution or sodium chloride 0.9% may be added. Benefits of intermittent infusion injection devices include the following:

   (1) This method is especially suitable for patients who do not require, or would be jeopardized by, administration of large amounts of IV fluids (e.g., those with congestive heart failure).

   (2) Because intermittent infusion injection devices do not require continuous attachment to an IV bottle or bag and pole, they permit greater patient ambulation.

C. **Pumps** and **controllers** are the electronic devices used to administer parenteral infusions when the use of gravity flow alone might lead to inaccurate dosing or risk patient safety. Pumps and controllers are used to administer parenteral nutrition, chemotherapy, cardiac medications, and blood products.

1. **Pumps** are used to deliver IV infusions with accuracy and safety.

   a. Two **types of mechanisms** are used in infusion pumps.

      (1) **Piston-cylinder mechanisms** use a piston in a cylinder or a syringe-like apparatus to pump the desired volume of fluid.

      (2) **Linear peristaltic mechanisms** use external pressure to expel the fluid out of the pumping chamber.

   b. **Types of pumps**

      (1) **Volumetric pumps** are used for intermittent infusion of medications such as antibiotics. They are also used for continuous infusion of IV fluid, parenteral nutrition, anticoagulants, and antiasthma medications.

      (2) **Syringe pumps** are used to administer intermittent or continuous infusions of medications (e.g., antibiotics, opiates) in concentrated form.

      (3) **Mobile infusion pumps** are small infusion devices designed for ambulatory and home patients and used for administering chemotherapy and opiate medications.

      (4) **Implantable pumps** are infusion devices surgically placed under the skin to provide a continuous release of medication, typically an opiate. The reservoir in the pump is refilled by injecting the medication through a latex diaphragm in the pump.

      (3) **Patient-controlled analgesic pumps** are used to administer narcotics intermittently or on demand by the patient within the patient-specific parameters, which are ordered by the physician and programmed into the pump.

   c. **Benefits.** Despite their extra costs and the training required by personnel, pumps provide a number of important benefits. They maintain a constant, accurate flow rate and can detect infiltrations, occlusions, and air. Pumps also may decrease the amount of time a nurse spends dispensing medication. Newer devices are equipped with "drug libraries" that have prespecified high and low dose infusion limits which may facilitate medication administration and reduce errors.

2. **Controllers,** unlike pumps, exert no pumping pressure on the IV fluid. Rather, they rely on gravity and control the infusion by counting drops electronically, or they infuse the fluid mechanically and electronically (e.g., volumetric controllers). In **comparison to pumps,** the following are characteristics of controllers:

   a. They are less complex and generally less expensive.

   b. They achieve reasonable accuracy.

   c. They are very useful for uncomplicated infusion therapy but cannot be used for arterial drug infusion or for infusion into small veins.

D. IV incompatibilities. When two or more drugs must be administered through a single IV line or given in a single solution, an undesirable reaction can occur. Although such incompatibilities are relatively rare, their consequences can be deadly. A patient who receives a preparation in which an incompatibility has occurred could experience toxicity or an incomplete therapeutic effect.

1. Types of incompatibilities

a. A **physical incompatibility** occurs when a drug combination produces a visible change in the appearance of a solution. The solution should never be administered to a patient.

(1) An **example** of physical incompatibility is the evolution of carbon dioxide when sodium bicarbonate and hydrochloric acid are admixed.

(2) Various **types** of physical incompatibilities may occur:

(a) Visible color change or darkening

(b) Formation of precipitate, which may result from the combination of phosphate and calcium

b. A **chemical incompatibility** reflects the chemical degradation of one or more of the admixed drugs, resulting in toxicity or therapeutic inactivity.

(1) The degradation is not always visible. **Nonvisible chemical incompatibility** may be detected only by analytical methods.

(2) Chemical incompatibility occurs in several **varieties.**

(a) **Complexation** is a reaction between products that inactivates them. For example, the combination of calcium and tetracycline leads to formation of a complex that inactivates tetracycline.

(b) **Oxidation** occurs when one drug loses electrons to the other, resulting in a color change and therapeutic inactivity.

(c) **Reduction** takes place when one drug gains electrons from the other.

(d) **Photolysis** (chemical decomposition caused by light) can lead to hydrolysis or oxidation, with resulting discoloration.

c. A **therapeutic incompatibility** occurs when two or more drugs, IV fluids, or both are combined and the result is a response other than that intended. An example of a therapeutic incompatibility is the reduced bactericidal activity of penicillin G (Pfizerpen) when given after tetracycline (Sumycin). Because tetracycline is a bacteriostatic agent, it slows bacterial growth; penicillin, on the other hand, is most effective against rapidly proliferating bacteria.

2. Factors affecting IV compatibility

a. pH. Incompatibility is more likely to occur when the components of an IV solution differ significantly in pH. This increased risk is explained by the chemical reaction between an acid and a base, which yields a salt and water; the salt may be an insoluble precipitate.

b. Temperature. Generally, increased storage temperature speeds drug degradation. To preserve drug stability, drugs should be stored in a refrigerator or freezer, as appropriate.

c. Degree of dilution. Generally, the more diluted the drugs are in a solution, the less chance there is for an ion interaction leading to incompatibility.

d. Length of time in solution. The chance for a reaction resulting in incompatibility increases with the length of time that drugs are in contact with each other.

e. Order of mixing. Drugs that are incompatible in combination, such as calcium and phosphate, should not be added consecutively when an IV admixture is being prepared. This keeps these substances from pooling, or forming a layer on the top of the IV fluid, and, therefore, decreases the chance of an incompatibility. Thorough mixing after each addition is also essential.

3. Preventing or minimizing incompatibilities. To reduce the chance for an incompatibility, the following steps should be taken:

a. Each drug should be mixed thoroughly after it is added to the preparation.

b. Solutions should be administered promptly after they are mixed to minimize the time available for a potential reaction to occur.

c. The number of drugs mixed together in an IV solution should be kept to a minimum.

d. If a prescription calls for unfamiliar drugs or IV fluids, compatibility references should be consulted.

E. Hazards of parenteral drug therapy. A wide range of problems can occur with parenteral drug administration.

1. **Physical hazards**
   a. **Phlebitis,** which is generally a minor complication, may result from vein injury or irritation. Phlebitis can be minimized or prevented through proper IV insertion technique, dilution of irritating drugs, and a decreased infusion rate.
   b. **Thrombosis,** the formation of a blood clot in a vein or artery.
   c. **Extravasation** may occur with administration of drugs with vesicant properties (see VII.D.3.b).
   d. **Irritation** at the injection site can be reduced by varying the injection site and applying a moisturizing lotion to the area.
   e. **Pain** from infusion is most common with peripheral IV administration of a highly concentrated preparation. Switching to central vein infusion and/or diluting the drug might alleviate the problem.
   f. **Air embolism,** potentially fatal, can result from entry of air into the IV tubing.
   g. **Infection,** a particular danger with central IV lines, may stem from contamination during IV line insertion or tubing changes. Infection may be local or generalized (septicemia). The infection risk can be minimized by following established protocols for the care of central lines.
   h. **Allergic reactions** can result from hypersensitivity to an IV solution or additive.
   i. **Central catheter misplacement** may lead to air embolism or pneumothorax. To ensure that the catheter has passed into the subclavian vein and advanced to the level of the vena cava, the placement should always be verified radiologically.
   j. **Hypothermia,** possibly resulting in shock and cardiac arrest, might stem from administration of a cold IV solution. This problem can be prevented by allowing parenteral products to reach room temperature.
   k. **Neurotoxicity** may be a serious complication of intrathecal or intraspinal administration of drugs containing preservatives. Preservative-free drugs should be used in these circumstances.

2. **Mechanical hazards**
   a. **Infusion pump** or **controller failure** can lead to runaway infusion, fluid overload, or incorrect dosages.
   b. **IV tubing** can become kinked, split, or cracked. It also may produce particulates, allow contamination, or interfere with the infusion.
   c. **Particulate matter** may be present in a parenteral product and can cause embolism.
   d. **Glass containers** may break, causing injury.
   e. **Rubber vial closures** may interact with the enclosed product.

3. **Therapeutic hazards**
   a. **Drug instability** may lead to therapeutic ineffectiveness.
   b. **Incompatibility** may result in toxicity or reduced therapeutic effectiveness.
   c. **Labeling errors** can cause administration of an incorrect drug or improper dosage.
   d. **Drug overdose** can be caused by runaway IV infusion, failure of an infusion pump or controller, or nursing or pharmacy errors.
   e. **Preservative and solubilizing agent toxicity** can be a serious complication, especially in children. For example, premature infants receiving parenteral products containing benzyl alcohol can develop a fatal acidotic toxic syndrome, which is referred to as the gasping syndrome. Rapid administration of phenytoin (Dilantin) and diazepam (Valium), both of which use propylene glycol as a solubilizing agent, has been associated with cardiovascular collapse.

STUDY QUESTIONS

Directions: Each of the questions, statements, or incomplete statements can be correctly answered or completed by **one** of the suggested answers or phrases. Choose the **best** answer.

1. Parenteral products with an osmotic pressure less than that of blood or 0.9% sodium chloride are referred to as

(A) isotonic solutions.
(B) hypertonic solutions.
(C) hypotonic solutions.
(D) iso-osmotic solutions.
(E) neutral solutions.

2. Aseptic technique should be used in the preparation of all of the following medications with the exception of

(A) a neomycin irrigation solution.
(B) a ganciclovir (Cytovene) intraocular injection.
(C) a phytonadione (AquaMEPHYTON) subcutaneous injection.
(D) an ampicillin (Principen) intravenous (IV) admixture piggyback.
(E) bacitracin ointment.

3. Which needle has the smallest diameter?

(A) 25 gauge, 3 3/4 inches
(B) 24 gauge, 3 1/2 inches
(C) 22 gauge, 3 1/2 inches
(D) 20 gauge, 3 3/8 inches
(E) 26 gauge, 3 5/8 inches

4. Intra-articular injection refers to injection into the

(A) muscle mass.
(B) subcutaneous tissue.
(C) spinal fluid.
(D) superficial skin layer.
(E) joint space.

5. Advantages of the intravenous route include

(A) ease of removal of the dose.
(B) a depot effect.
(C) low incidence of phlebitis.
(D) rapid onset of action.
(E) a localized effect.

6. A central vein, either subclavian or internal jugular, may be considered a suitable route for intravenous (IV) administration in which of the following situations?

(A) when an irritating drug is given
(B) when hypertonic drugs are given
(C) for long-term therapy
(D) for administering dextrose 35% as parenteral nutrition
(E) All of the above

7. To prepare a total parenteral nutrition (TPN) that requires 10 mEq calcium gluconate and 15 mM potassium phosphate, the appropriate action to take would be which of the following?

(A) Add the calcium first, add the other additives, then add the phosphate last, thoroughly mixing the solution after addition.
(B) Add the calcium gluconate and potassium phosphate consecutively.
(C) Do not combine the agents but give them as separate infusions.
(D) None of the above.

8. Which needle gauge would be most likely used for the subcutaneous injection of epoetin?

(A) 25 gauge, 5/8 inch
(B) 16 gauge, 1 inch
(C) 18 gauge, 1 1/2 inches
(D) 22 gauge, 1 1/2 inches
(E) None of the above

9. Which of the following drugs should *not* be prepared in a horizontal laminar flow hood?

(A) ampicillin
(B) dopamine
(C) cisplatin (Platinol)
(D) nitroglycerin
(E) bretylium tosylate (Bentylol)

10. All of the following statements about D_5W are true *except* which one?

(A) Its pH range is 3.5–6.5.
(B) It is hypertonic.
(C) It is a 5% solution of D-glucose.
(D) It should be used with caution in diabetic patients.
(E) It is often used in IV admixtures.

11. All of the following are potential hazards of parenteral therapy *except* which one?

(A) hypothermia
(B) phlebitis
(C) extravasation
(D) allergic reactions
(E) ileus

12. Procedures for the safe handling of antineoplastic agents include all of the following *except* the

(A) use of Luer-Lok syringe fittings.
(B) wearing of double-layered latex gloves.
(C) use of a negative-pressure technique when medication is being withdrawn from vials.
(D) wearing of closed-front, surgical-type gowns with cuffs.
(E) use of a horizontal laminar flow hood.

13. In preparing an intraspinal dose of bupivacaine, the best pore size filter for cold sterilization would be a(n)

(A) 8-mm filter.
(B) 5-μm filter.
(C) 0.45-μm filter.
(D) 0.22-μm filter.
(E) None of the above

14. Process simulation

(A) is a method of quality assurance.
(B) evaluates the adequacy of a practitioner's aseptic technique.
(C) requires the use of a microbial growth medium.
(D) is carried out in a manner identical to normal sterile admixture production under routine operating conditions.
(E) All of the above.

For questions 15–18: The pharmacist receives a prescription for hydromorphone (Dilaudid) injection to be compounded to a solution of 15 mg/mL. Dilaudid is commercially available in an ampule but the concentration is 10 mg/mL. The physician would like a more concentrated solution prepared so that 50 mL can be instilled into the titanium reservoir of a Medtronic infusion pump. The hydromorphone solution will be continuously infused, intrathecally, over approximately 30 days, for a patient with chronic back pain uncontrolled with oral narcotics. The pharmacist checks the inventory and finds a bottle of hydromorphone powder *USP*. The pharmacists proceeds to weigh out enough powder for a 60-mL preparation. The weighing step is checked by a colleague pharmacist.

15. According to *USP* Chapter 797 this sterile preparation would be considered a

(A) high-risk CSP.
(B) medium-risk CSP.
(C) low-risk CSP.
(D) None of the above

16. What would be an appropriate environment for the aseptic manipulations required for this preparation?

(A) pharmacy workbench or counter in ambient room air
(B) inside an anteroom, with ISO class 8 quality air
(C) inside a barrier isolator with ISO class 5 quality air
(D) a horizontal laminar flow workbench bench, newly installed, with no certification, but manufacturer guaranteed to be ISO class 5 air quality.

17. The pharmacist begins to gather the supplies for this preparation, which include

(A) Millipore 0.45-μ HV filter with sterile water for injection.
(B) Millipore 0.22-μ GS filter with sodium chloride 0.9%.
(C) Becton-Dickinson 16-gauge, 5 -μ filter needle with sodium chloride 0.9%.
(D) Millipore 0.8-μ AA filter with dextrose 5% in water.

18. After the solution was prepared, the appropriate quality control or double-check by another pharmacist would include

(A) inspection of the powder and the label to ensure hydromorphone was the prepared ingredient and that the label contained a beyond-use date and the 15 mg/mL concentration.
(B) sending a solution sample or aliquot to a microbiology laboratory to test for the presence of bacteria and pyrogens before dispensing.
(C) a check to ensure the correct sterilizing filter was used.
(D) a visual inspection to ensure the final aqueous solution had no visible participates.
(E) All of the above.

ANSWERS AND EXPLANATIONS

1. The answer is C *[see VII.A.1–3].*
Hypotonic solutions have an osmotic pressure less than that of blood (or 0.9% saline), whereas hypertonic solutions have an osmotic pressure greater than that of blood, and isotonic or iso-osmotic solutions have an osmotic pressure equal to that of blood.

2. The answer is E *[see II.A.7].*
Irrigation solutions, ophthalmic preparations, parenteral products, and subcutaneous and IV medications should be prepared using aseptic technique. Since Bacitracin ointment is applied to the skin and does not bypass the body's protective barriers, its preparation would not be held to the same requirements.

3. The answer is E *[see IX.A.1].*
The gauge size refers to the outer diameter of the needle. The lower the gauge size number, the larger the needle.

4. The answer is E *[see VI.I].*
Intra-articular injection refers to an injection into the joint space. This administration route generally is used for certain types of corticosteroids to reduce inflammation associated with injury or rheumatoid arthritis.

5. The answer is D *[see VI.C].*
The IV route of drug administration allows for rapid onset of action and, therefore, immediate therapeutic effect. There can be no recall of the administered dose, and phlebitis, or inflammation of a vein, can occur. In addition, a depot effect (i.e., accumulation and storage of the drug for distribution) cannot be achieved by administering a drug intravenously. Delivering a drug intravenously results in a systemic rather than a localized effect.

6. The answer is E *[see VII.B.1.a; X.A.2].*
Irritating drugs, hypertonic drugs, long-term therapy, and dextrose 35% are best given by central IV administration. Peripheral vein injection is used for postoperative hydration, administration of nonirritating drugs, or isotonic solutions and for short-term IV therapy.

7. The answer is A *[see X.D.1.a].*
Physical incompatibilities occur when two or more products are combined and produce a change in the appearance of the solution, such as the formation of a precipitate. Calcium and phosphate solutions when directly combined or added consecutively to a solution will form a white precipitate. By altering the order of mixing, they can be safely added to TPN solutions.

8. The answer is A *[see IX.A.1; IX.A.3.b].*
Since subcutaneous injection does not require penetration through several skin layers or muscle tissue, a short needle with a narrow diameter is used. A 16- or 18-gauge needle is most commonly used in the pharmacy for preparing parenteral solutions. A 22-gauge needle would be used for intramuscular injection.

9. The answer is C *[see II.B.2.b.(2)(a)].*
Cisplatin is an antineoplastic agent and, consequently, should be prepared only in a vertical laminar flow hood because of the potential hazard of these toxic agents to the operator.

10. The answer is B *[see VII.B.1.a].*
D_5W is acidic, its pH ranges from 3.5 to 6.5, and it is isotonic. It is often used in IV admixtures and should be used with caution in diabetic patients.

11. The answer is E *[see X.E.1].*
Parenteral therapy is often a treatment for ileus. Hypothermia, phlebitis, extravasation, and allergic reactions can be hazards of parenteral therapy.

12. The answer is E *[see VII.D].*
To prevent drug exposure, a vertical flow laminar hood (not horizontal) should be used when an antineoplastic agent is prepared. The other precautions mentioned in the question are important safety measures for handling parenteral antineoplastics. All pharmacy and nursing personnel who handle these toxic substances should receive special training.

13. The answer is D *[see IV.D.2; IV.C.2.(a)].*
Because intraspinal and epidural doses of bupivacaine are frequently prepared from nonsterile powders, cold sterilization, accomplished by filtration, is a simple method of ensuring complete microbial removal. Filters listed 8 mm to 0.45 μm will remove only particulate matter. A 0.22-μm filter ensures the removal of microorganisms.

14. The answer is E *[see III.F].*
Process simulation is one part of an overall quality assurance program. It requires duplicating sterile product preparation using a growth medium in place of actual products. It serves to evaluate the aseptic technique of the individual performing all the necessary steps of sterile product preparation.

15. The answer is A *[see II.6.c].*
The hydromorphone preparation is a high-risk CSP because it is made from nonsterile powder.

16. The answer is C *[see II.B.4].*
USP Chapter 797 requires an ISO class 5 air quality environment for this preparation. A barrier isolator within a clean room creates an ISO class 5 environment. Ambient room air is unacceptable for any preparation. An anteroom is generally an area of relatively high personnel and supply traffic. Although air quality may be acceptable, it does not provide an acceptable critical site for aseptic manipulations. All new laminar flow work benches should be tested for air velocity and filter integrity before use.

17. The answer is B *[see IV.D.2.c(2)].*
The hydromorphone requires sterilization before intrathecal administration. This is best achieved with a 0.22-μ filter. Sodium chloride 0.9% is the solution most similar to the CNS fluid and would be a better choice over sterile water or dextrose 5% injection.

18. The answer is E *[see III].*
Each step in sterile compounding should have an associated quality assurance double-check. Inspection of the initial ingredients, review of supplies, monitoring of aseptic technique, and examination of the final product create multiple opportunities to intercept an error and make necessary corrections. High-risk CSPs should be used within 24 hr in the absence of sterility testing. Given that this product will be administered over 30 days, a sterility and pyrogen test would be appropriate.

28
Parapharmaceuticals, Home Diagnostics, and Medical Devices

Jenny A. Van Amburgh

Todd A. Brown

I. AMBULATORY AIDS

A. Canes. These simple ambulatory aids provide balance and allow for the transfer of weight off a weakened leg.

1. **Height.** The height of the cane must be adjusted to the individual patient. A cane that is correctly fitted allows for maximum weight transfer without allowing the patient to lock the elbow. The correct height should provide a 25° angle at the elbow, or the top of the cane should come to the crease of the wrist while the patient is standing erect.

2. **Types of canes.** Canes may be made of wood or metal.
   a. **Wooden canes** come in varying thicknesses. The thicker ones are intended for males, and the thinner ones are for females. They may be cut to the correct height for the patient.
   b. **Metal canes** are usually adjustable in height to fit the individual patient.
   c. **Folding canes** will fold to allow for easy transport or storage when not in use.
   d. A **quad cane** is a metal cane that has a quadrangular base with four legs. This allows for greater weight transfer. The base of the quad cane comes in two sizes. The larger base provides greater stability but is more difficult to manipulate because of the size and weight.
   e. **Seat canes** contain an area that can be folded down and used to sit on. They are useful for individuals who cannot walk long distances without resting.

B. Crutches may be used by patients with temporary disabilities (e.g., sprains, fractures) or by those with chronic conditions.

1. **Use.** Crutches are used to take all the weight off an injured or weakened leg. The crutches are used in place of the leg. Crutch sizes range from toddler to adult. Accessories that are used with a crutch include a tip to prevent slipping, handgrip cushion, and arm pad (for axillary crutch).

2. **Types of crutches**
   a. An **axillary crutch,** the **most commonly used** crutch, is typically used for temporary disabilities. The top of the crutch should be 2 inches below the axilla to prevent "crutch paralysis" (i.e., injury to the axillary nerves, blood vessels, and lymph nodes). The height of the handgrip should be set so that the elbow forms a 25° angle.
   b. A **forearm crutch** (also called a **Canadian** or **Lofstrand** crutch) remains in position by attaching to the forearm by a collar or cuff. It is commonly used by patients who need crutches on a long-term basis.
   c. A **quad crutch** is a forearm crutch with a quadrangular base that has four legs. The base is attached to the crutch with a flexible rubber mount. This allows for more stability and constant contact with the ground.
   d. A **platform crutch** contains a rectangular area in which to place the forearm. The crutch may be held by a handgrip or secured by a belt that wraps around the forearm. It is commonly used by patients who do not have enough hand strength and control for a forearm crutch.

C. Seat lift chairs are electric-powered chairs that raise the patient from a sitting to a standing position.

D. Walkers are lightweight rectangular-shaped devices that are made of metal tubing and have four widely placed legs.

1. **Use.** Walkers are used by patients who need more **support** than a cane or crutch or who have trouble with balance during ambulation. The use requires reasonably good arm, hand, and wrist function. The patient holds on to the walker and takes a step, then moves the walker and takes another step.

2. **Types of walkers.** Walkers come in two sizes: **adult** and **child.** Walkers may be adjustable in height. Some walkers will fold to make storage or transporting easier. Walkers can have wheels on the front legs to allow the user to move the walker by raising the back legs and rolling it instead of having to pick it up. Patients with loss of arm, wrist, or hand function on one side might use a **hemiwalker** or a **side walker.**
    a. A **hemiwalker** is similar to a standard walker except that it has one handle in the center of the walker for manipulation.
    b. A **side walker** is placed to the side of the patient instead of in front of the patient.
    c. A **reciprocal walker** contains two hinges, one on each side of the walker. This allows the user to swing each side alternately during ambulation.
    d. A **rollator** is a walker with wheels on all four legs. The movement is controlled by hand brakes.

E. Wheelchairs. Many different types of wheelchairs are available. The patient's disabilities, size, weight, and activities are the main considerations in wheelchair selection. The following options should be considered when selecting a wheelchair.

1. **Seat size.** The standard chair is 18 inches wide and 16 inches deep. A narrow wheelchair is 16 inches wide. Wheelchairs are available in widths up to 48 inches. The chair should be 2 inches wider than the widest part of the patient's body (usually around the buttocks or thighs).

2. **Arms** can be fixed or detachable to allow the patient to transfer on and off the chair. Half-length arms (as opposed to full length) allow the use to get closer to a table or work surface. Various types of padding and adjustments in the arm position can assist the patient in obtaining a position that is comfortable and keeping the arms on the arm rests.

3. **Tires** can be hard rubber or pneumatic (i.e., air filled) which allows the chair to transverse rougher surfaces.

4. **Wheels** can be reinforced with spokes or can be composite based.

5. **Leg rests** can be of different sizes and are available with padding. Some have adjustable elevation to aid in healing an acute injury.

6. **Footrests** can be of different sizes and are available with or without heel loops to keep the foot on the footrest.

7. **Casters** (i.e., **front wheels**) can be hard rubber or pneumatic.

8. **Calf rests** can be of different sizes and are available with padding.

9. **Seat upholstery** holds the patient in the chair. Seats come in a variety of materials to accommodate patients' needs.

10. **Back upholstery** supports the patient's back while he or she is sitting in the chair. The material in the seat and back are usually the same.

11. **Cross braces** add stability and durability to the chair.

12. **Weight.** Standard wheelchairs weigh 35–50 lb. Lightweight wheelchairs (25–35 lb.) are available for those who are unable to manipulate a standard chair and for ease of transport.

F. Sports chairs are wheelchairs that are lightweight and durable. They are designed for people who are very active.

G. Powered wheelchairs are designed for people who cannot wheel themselves. This type of wheelchair is powered by an electric motor and battery.

II. BATHROOM EQUIPMENT. This equipment is used for patients who cannot get to the bathroom or for patients who need assistance using the toilet or bathtub.

   A. Elevated toilet seats are used to increase the height at which the patient sits over the toilet. This assists patients with limited mobility in getting on and off the toilet. Additional support can be provided with **toilet safety rails.** These rails allow the patient to transfer weight from the feet to the hands, and they help prevent the patient from falling when getting on or off the toilet.

   B. Commodes are portable toilets that are used by patients who cannot get to the bathroom. Commodes contain a frame (with or without a backrest), a seat, and a bucket. Some are adjustable in height and have arms that drop to facilitate transfer to and from the commode. Folding commodes are available to make storage easier.

   C. Three-in-one commodes function as combination commode, elevated toilet seat, and toilet safety rails. These are beneficial for patients requiring varying assistance during recuperation.

   D. Bath benches are seats with or without a back that fit in the bathtub and allow the patient to sit while taking a shower.

   E. Transfer benches are placed over the outside of the bathtub. They are available with or without a back. A transfer bench assists the patient in getting into the bathtub and serves as a bath bench while the patient takes a shower.

   F. Grab bars are bars that either attach to the wall around the bathtub or to the bathtub itself to assist patients in getting on and out of the bathtub.

III. BLOOD PRESSURE MONITORS. Patients with hypertension use this equipment to monitor blood pressure so that appropriate therapeutic decisions can be made. A patient's blood pressure measured at home is typically 5 mm Hg lower than when measured at the office.[1] The type of monitor that is recommended should be determined by the patient's ability to use the product correctly. Items to consider when assisting a patient in the selection of a blood pressure monitor: ease of use (e.g. automatic inflation), use of the monitor with one hand (has D-ring cuff), the size of the display monitor (visually impaired patients), blood pressure cuff size, and the capability to store readings. Types of monitors include the following:

   A. Mercury sphygmomanometer. This type of monitor is the **most accurate** and does not need calibration. Mercury in a graduated column rises in response to pressure applied to the cuff. The blood pressure is determined by measuring the length of the mercury column while listening for the Korotkoff sounds in the stethoscope. Mercury monitors are usually not used as a home device because of their large size, the need for use of a stethoscope, and the potential for mercury spill. Owing to the risk of mercury exposure, this type of sphygmomanometer is being phased out of healthcare facilities.

   B. Finger monitors. These detect blood pressure by compressing the finger and converting blood vessel movement into blood pressure by oscillometric technology. Many environmental conditions and medications can interfere with the results of these monitors. Finger blood pressure monitors are **least accurate** and not recommended for home monitoring.

   C. Aneroid sphygmomanometer. This is similar to a mercury sphygmomanometer, except that instead of a column of mercury, it has a dial to be read. Aneroid models have the advantage of being **less expensive** than mercury models; however, they do require regular calibration in a healthcare provider's office with a mercury sphygmomanometer to ensure proper results. These types of monitors are portable and lightweight, however. Most require manual inflation of the cuff, but a separate stethoscope is not required.

---

[1] National Heart, Lung, and Blood Institute. The seventh report of the Joint National Committee on Prevention, Detection, Evaluation, and Treatment of High Blood Pressure. August 2004. Available at www.nhlbi.nih.gov/guidelines/hypertension/jnc7full.htm.

D. Electronic or digital monitor. This type of monitor detects blood pressure by using a microphone or by oscillometric technology, which converts movement of vessels into blood pressure. This type is easier to use than a mercury or aneroid sphygmomanometer as most offer automatic inflation and deflation and there is not a need for a separate stethoscope. These models are more **expensive,** can provide inaccurate readings if the patient moves while the blood pressure is being performed, and requires frequent calibration against a mercury sphygmomanometer; but they represent an alternative for patients who cannot use a sphygmomanometer. Some of these monitors come with a wrist cuff which may be useful in overweight or obese patients for whom the regular size arm blood pressure cuff is too small.

IV. HEAT AND COLD THERAPY. For musculoskeletal disorders (e.g., sprains, strains, arthritis), treatment may include the application of heat or cold to specific areas of the body.

A. Heat can be applied in a dry or moist form. **Dry** heat is less effective than moist heat but is tolerated better; thus its clinical effectiveness is similar. **Moist** heat has an advantage of not causing as much perspiration and is often recommended. The application of heat produces vasodilation and muscle relaxation. This facilitates pain relief and healing. Products that can deliver heat include the following:

1. A **hot water bottle,** a rubber container, should be half filled with hot water. The remaining air is squeezed out of the container, which is then capped. This results in a flexible container that can be shaped to the area of the body for which it is being used to provide dry heat.

2. A **heating pad** is an electrically powered pad that can produce moist or dry heat. Moist heat is supplied by inserting a wet sponge in a pocket that is next to the pad. Patients should be instructed to place the pad on top of the body instead of lying on the pad to prevent burning.

3. A **moist-heat pack** (also called a hydrocollator) contains silica beads, which absorb heat when placed in boiling water. The heated pack is wrapped in a towel and applied to the body to provide moist heat. A moist-heat pack must be kept moist to retain its absorbent properties. The pack should be wrapped in plastic and stored in the refrigerator if use is anticipated or in the freezer if long-term storage is required.

4. A **gel pack** provides dry heat after it is heated in boiling water or in the microwave. It is reusable by repeating the heating process.

5. **Chemical hot packs** provide dry heat by mixing chemicals from two compartments. The chemicals undergo an exothermic reaction. Some packs are reusable by reheating in boiling water or in the microwave.

6. **Paraffin baths** provide moist heat by covering the body with heated paraffin. Once the wax cools and hardens, it is removed. This method is commonly used for patients with arthritis in the hands and fingers.

B. Cold application is indicated mainly as acute therapy to decrease circulation to a local area and to provide pain relief. Cold is contraindicated in patients with circulatory stasis or lacerated tissue. Products that can deliver cold include the following:

1. An **ice bag** is a flexible plastic container designed to hold ice. The bag is then applied to the body.

2. A **gel pack** can be used to apply cold by freezing and then applying to the body.

3. **Chemical packs** can be used to apply cold. Chemicals from two compartments are mixed together, resulting in a chemical reaction that produces cold. These packs are used once and then disposed of.

V. HOME DIAGNOSTIC AIDS

A. Self-care tests or **kits** are used as screening tests or for monitoring. Many factors can affect the accuracy of the tests. The most common factors are patients not following directions and patients having poor technique. Pharmacists should be prepared to counsel patients on the selection of a test, on the proper use, and on interpretation of results. Pharmacists should refer patients to the appropriate healthcare provider if necessary.

B. Types of self-care tests

1. **Urine tests**
   a. The **urine glucose test** detects sugar in the urine. Patients with diabetes can use this to evaluate glucose control. Blood glucose monitoring is preferred, however, because it is more accurate and gives a better description of current glycemia.
   b. The **ketone test** detects the presence of ketones in the urine. This is used by patients with diabetes as an indicator of severely uncontrolled diabetes.
   c. **Ovulation prediction tests** predict when ovulation occurs to increase the chance of conception.
      (1) These tests detect the presence of **luteinizing hormone (LH)** in the urine. Its presence means that ovulation should occur within 20–48 hr.
      (2) The test is performed daily until a positive result is obtained. Many kits recommend not using the first morning urine as the LH surge typically starts in the morning and may not be detectable until later in the day. Therefore, it is recommended to test between 10 A.M. and 8 P.M.
      (3) The day on which the patient begins testing depends on the length and regularity of her menstrual cycle. Patients with menstrual cycles of consistent length may need to test only for 4 days, whereas those with menstrual cycles that change in length may need to test for 8 or 9 days.
      (4) False-positive results can occur if the patient is taking fertility medications (e.g., clomiphene), oral contraceptives, or hormone-replacement therapy or if the patient has polycystic ovary syndrome or impaired liver or kidney function.
   d. **Pregnancy tests** detect pregnancy by the presence in the urine of **human chorionic gonadotropin (hCG),** which is secreted after fertilization. Many pregnancy test kits can detect hCG 1 day after missed menses.
      (1) False-positive results can occur if the patient takes the test too early, is taking fertility medications (e.g., hCG), or has ovarian cysts.
      (2) If a patient uses a household container or a waxed cup to collect urine, it may affect the test results.
      (3) Patients should be referred to the appropriate healthcare provider if they receive a positive result or two negative results 7 days apart and have not had menses.
   e. The **urinary bacteria test** detects the presence of nitrite in the urine. The presence of nitrite is used as an indicator of a **urinary tract infection (UTI)** because the most common bacteria associated with UTIs are gram-negative bacteria, which convert nitrate to nitrite.
      (1) Because this test is not specific for bacteria, false results can occur.
      (2) This test is used by patients who have recurrent or chronic UTIs or many risk factors. Risk factors include previous UTIs, diabetes, urinary tract abnormalities, enlarged prostrate, and behavioral risk factors (e.g., frequent sexual activity, delayed urination, the use of spermicides or diaphragms).
      (3) False positives can result from medications (e.g., phenazopyridine) the patient may be taking or from menstrual blood in the urine, depending on the test used. In addition, a false negative may be detected if the patient is taking high doses of vitamin C, adheres to a strict vegetarian diet, or has frequent urination.

2. **Blood tests**
   a. The **cholesterol test** determines a patient's total cholesterol (TC), low-density lipoprotein (LDL), high-density lipoprotein (HDL) and/or triglycerides.
      (1) Some tests provide the patient only with a TC level, whereas others provide a full lipid profile (TC, LDL, HDL, and/or triglycerides).
      (2) Some cholesterol kits are a single-use test in which patient applies a blood sample onto a collecting card, which is mailed to a laboratory for evaluation. Other single-use tests can be performed and evaluated by the patient at home. The measurement of the amount of cholesterol is determined by a color chart, which is provided with the test.
      (3) Reusable cholesterol monitors are available. They use reflectance photometer technology to convert the color change produced into a reading on a liquid crystal display screen.

(4) Regardless of the test used, the patient places a large drop of blood onto the test card or cassette. Some of the tests require the patient to fast—meaning nothing to eat or drink except water for 12–14 hr before collecting the blood.

(5) These tests can be useful for patients who want to monitor their therapy. They are also useful as screening tests. Patients who test borderline or higher for high cholesterol should be referred to the appropriate healthcare provider.

b. The **blood glucose test** measures the concentration of glucose in the blood. Patients with diabetes use this information, along with diet, exercise, and medication, to keep glucose levels within a target range.

(1) Some blood glucose test kits are read by comparing the color change to a chart provided with the test. Visually read tests give an approximation of the blood glucose.

(2) Other tests are designed to be used with **blood glucose meters,** which read the test and display the actual blood glucose value. Some blood glucose meters contain optical units that measure the color change caused by glucose; others measure the electric charge produced by glucose. The result is then calibrated to provide whole blood or plasma glucose concentration. Whole blood is approximately 15% lower than plasma glucose, which is what is measured in the standard laboratory tests. Many of the new glucometers provide results as the "plasma equivalent," meaning they test whole blood but use an internal algorithm to calculate the plasma glucose.

(3) Patients using blood glucose tests must perform the tests properly and understand the appropriate actions to take when the resulting values are outside the desired range.

3. Fecal occult blood tests detect the presence of blood in the stool as a screening test for colorectal cancer. Patients drop a pad into the toilet after defecation. The pad will change color if blood is present. Patients should eat high-fiber foods during the testing period and are instructed to test three consecutive stool samples. Patients with a positive result should be referred to the appropriate healthcare provider. Certain conditions (gastrointestinal bleed, nosebleed, menstruation), foods (red meat), medications (nonsteroidal anti-inflammatory drugs [NSAIDs]), and toilet-bowl cleaners can produce false-positive results.

4. Home specimen collection kits allow for collection of a specimen at home, which is then sent to a laboratory for testing. Blood-collection devices are available so that patients can test themselves for the presence of HIV or hepatitis C virus (HCV) or the concentration of glycosylated hemoglobin A_{1c} (for patients with diabetes). A screening test for illicit drug use is also available. These tests require a urine or hair sample for analysis.

(1) The HIV, HCV, and illicit drug use tests allow the patient to test anonymously by using an identification number included with the kit. The results can be obtained by calling a toll-free number.

(2) There are two glycosylated hemoglobin A_{1c} tests available; one requires the patient to mail in the blood sample, and the other is a single-use monitor by which the patient obtains the results at home within minutes of taking a blood sample. The single-use monitor uses a series of proprietary microoptic procedures, miniaturized digital electronics, and dry reagent chemistries. Results obtained from this kit are comparable to those from laboratory tests. The patient should be encouraged to communicate the results with the appropriate healthcare provider.

5. Fertility microscopes allow women to determine their most fertile time of the month. A woman places saliva on a viewing slide or plate, allows the saliva to dry for 5–7 min, and then views it under a microscope. The appearance of a ferning pattern means ovulation has occurred. Estrogen levels rise and peak with ovulation, causing an increase in salt levels in the saliva, resulting in a fernlike pattern in dried saliva. Simple dots or a bubble-like appearance is found during a nonfertile period. A woman should be advised to avoid smoking, eating, or drinking for 2 hr before testing. Polycystic ovary syndrome and perimenopause can cause false-positive results.

VI. HOSPITAL BEDS AND ACCESSORIES. Hospital beds are used by patients who are confined to bed for long periods of time or who require elevation of the head or feet as part of their treatment. Hospital beds may be manually or electrically operated.

A. Types of hospital beds

1. A **manual** hospital bed has no electrically powered motors; the head, foot, and bed height are adjusted manually.

2. A **semielectric** hospital bed contains two electric motors that raise the head and foot of the bed. The patient can usually adjust the head and foot position with a handheld control. The height of the bed is adjusted manually. The semielectric bed can usually be adjusted manually in case of loss of electricity.

3. A **fully electric** hospital bed contains three motors that can change the height of the bed as well as raise the head and foot via electrically powered motors. The fully electric hospital bed can usually be adjusted manually in case of loss of electricity.

B. Accessories

1. **Bed rails** keep the patient in the bed and allow the patient to change positions.

2. A **trapeze** is a triangular-shaped object that hangs above the patient and is used to change the patient's position.

3. **Alternating pressure pads** are used by patients to prevent decubitus ulcers (i.e., bed sores). As a preventive measure, these pads inflate, thus changing the areas of the body that receive pressure.

VII. INCONTINENCE AND INCONTINENCE PRODUCTS

A. **Urinary incontinence** is a condition in which involuntary urine loss is a social or hygienic problem and is objectively demonstrable. Incontinence is a common problem in the elderly. Types of incontinence include

1. **Urge** incontinence, which is uncontrolled contractions of the bladder

2. **Stress** incontinence, a weakness of the sphincter that causes leakage when intra-abdominal pressure increases (e.g., while laughing, coughing, sneezing) and is common in pregnancy

3. **Overflow** incontinence, which is caused by obstruction of urine flow from the bladder and is common in elderly men as a result of prostate enlargement

4. **Functional incontinence,** which is related to physical or psychological problems that impair the patient's ability to get to the bathroom

5. **Iatrogenic incontinence,** which is caused by drugs or surgery

6. **Mixed incontinence,** which is a combination of more than one type of incontinence

B. **Incontinence products**

1. **Shields** are disposable, absorbent pads that are placed in the underwear and held with an adhesive strip on the back of the pad. These pads are used for light incontinence problems.

2. **Undergarments** are disposable absorbent garments that are worn under the underwear and held in place with elastic straps that go around the hips. They are designed for moderate incontinence problems.

3. **Briefs** look like adult-size diapers that are kept in place with adhesive strips. They are designed for heavy incontinence problems.

4. **Pull-up pants** are absorbant disposable garments that look like underwear and are used for heavy incontinence problems.

5. **Underpads** are absorbent pads to be placed on the bed underneath a patient with incontinence. These pads contain a barrier to protect the bedding.

6. **Waterproof sheets** are plastic or vinyl sheets that protect the mattress. They may be lined with a soft material to prevent friction against the skin.

7. **Incontinence systems** are garments that look like underwear but have a pouch or pocket designed for a disposable or reusable pad.

VIII. ORTHOPEDIC BRACES AND SURGICAL FITTINGS. These products promote proper body alignment and support injured areas. Pharmacists should have additional training before attempting to fit an orthopedic device.

A. Abdominal supports are elastic and are used to support and hold surgical dressings in place. Abdominal supports come in different widths.

B. Arm slings are used to provide comfort and support during recuperation from fractures, sprains, and surgery. The elbow should form a 90° angle in an arm sling to allow for proper circulation.

C. Back supports are worn by patients to provide support or promote proper alignment. Such supports are named after the area of the spine on which it is worn.

   1. A **sacral belt** (also called **sacral cinch** or **sacroiliac belt**) supports the lower back.

   2. A **lumbosacral support** supports the lower and middle back.

   3. A **thoracolumbar support** supports the middle and higher areas of the back.

D. Cervical collars support or limit the range of motion of the neck. Cervical collars should be of sufficient length so that the patient can adjust the degree of compression. The width of the cervical collar should equal the measurement from the chin to the sternum when the patient is standing straight, looking ahead.

   1. **Soft** or **foam** cervical collars provide mild support and remind the wearer to keep the neck straight.

   2. **Hard** or **rigid** cervical collars provide more support and limit movement to a greater degree.

   3. A **Philadelphia** or **extrication** collar is used to immobilize the neck and is commonly used in emergency situations.

E. Clavicle supports are used as aids for the reduction and stabilization of the clavicle (i.e., collarbone). These supports are sometimes called **figure-eight straps** because of their appearance.

F. Knee braces (also called **knee cages**) are used to support the knee. Some braces have metal stays on the side to prevent the lateral movement of the knee. Those with metal stays may also have hinges to allow for movement of the knee. Some knee braces have a cut-out hole and padding around the patella (i.e., knee cap) to prevent its movement.

G. Knee immobilizers prevent any motion of the knee and are used for severe injuries and fractures. They are available in different lengths and are adjustable in size.

H. Nighttime ankle brace keeps the ankle at a 90° angle while sleeping. It can be used in the treatment of Achilles tendon injuries or plantar fasciitis.

I. Shoulder immobilizers prevent movement of the shoulder and arm. The elbow should be at a 90° angle to allow for healing without affecting circulation.

J. Tennis elbow supports apply pressure to the forearm to provide pain relief and decrease inflammation from tennis elbow (i.e., epicondylitis).

K. Wrist braces prevent movement of the wrist to allow healing. The brace may be shaped to have the wrist flexed so that the tendons in the hand remain stretched during the period of inactivity.

IX. OSTOMY APPLIANCES AND ACCESSORIES

A. Definitions. An **ostomy** is a surgical procedure in which an artificial opening is created in the abdominal wall for the purpose of eliminating urine or fecal waste. The opening is called a **stoma.** Ostomies can be temporary to allow for repair or healing of the digestive tract or can be permanent. Each procedure is named to describe the anatomical location involved.

1. In a **colostomy,** part of the colon is cut and attached to the abdominal wall. This procedure is done mainly in patients with colon or rectal cancer, lower-bowel obstruction, or diverticulitis. A colostomy may be temporary or permanent, the discharge may be liquid or semisolid (as with an **ascending** colostomy), or it may be solid (as with a **descending** or **sigmoid** colostomy). Patients with an ascending colostomy and some patients with a transverse colostomy have gastric enzymes present in the discharge. These patients must take extra care to ensure that the discharge does not come into contact with the skin.

2. In an **ileostomy,** the ileum is attached to the abdominal wall. This procedure is performed in patients with ulcerative colitis or Crohn disease.

3. A **urostomy** is performed in patients with bladder cancer. In this procedure, an **ileal conduit** is created by attaching the ureters to the ileum and the distal end of the ileum to the abdominal wall.

B. **Ostomy appliances.** The ostomy appliance contains a **skin barrier** that attaches to the skin around the stoma. The skin barrier protects the skin and allows for the collection device or **pouch** to be worn on the body. The selection of an ostomy appliance depends on the type of discharge produced. In addition to size, color, and flexibility, appliances may have detachable pouches and be able to be drained by releasing a clip at the bottom of the appliance.

C. **Ostomy accessories**

1. **Washers, powder paste,** and **ointments** are designed to be used with a skin barrier and provide additional protection of the skin around a stoma.

2. **Cement, elastic belts,** and **tape** are used to hold the appliance in place.

3. **Deodorizers** help control fecal odor. **External** deodorizers can be placed into the appliance; systemic deodorizers (e.g., bismuth subgallate, chlorophyll, charcoal) can be ingested as **internal** deodorizers.

4. **Moisturizers** and **disinfectants** can be used to treat the skin and prevent complications.

5. **Irrigation devices** are used by patients who have control over the elimination of waste to facilitate removal of the accumulated waste. The devices are used to instill water into the intestine, which produces peristalsis.

D. **Special considerations for ostomy patients.** Drug therapy can present unique problems for ostomates. Absorption of enteric-coated or sustained-release products may not be possible. Antibiotics, sulfa drugs, laxatives, and diuretics are some of the common problem medications in these patients.

X. RESPIRATORY EQUIPMENT

A. **Continuous positive airway pressure** (CPAP) is used in patients with sleep apnea. The pressure supplied from this machine keeps the airway open. It is typically worn while sleeping to allow the patient to sleep without disturbance.

B. A **humidifier** puts moisture into the air by breaking water into small particles and blowing them into the air to be evaporated. Humidifiers are sometimes referred to as called "cool-mist vaporizers."

1. **Vaporizers** are similar to humidifiers in that they are used to deliver moisture to the air. However, a vaporizer produces a steam to increase humidity, whereas a humidifier produces a nonheated mist.

2. An **ultrasonic humidifier** contains a transducer, which produces a finer mist. It is commonly used to promote expectoration in patients with upper-respiratory infections.

3. Both types of humidifiers and vaporizers need to be cleaned regularly to prevent the growth of mold or bacteria.

C. A **nebulizer** is used to deliver medication to the mouth or throat. Patients with a sore throat may use a nebulizer to deliver a topical anesthetic to the throat. An **ultrasonic nebulizer** is used to deliver medication into the lungs. The medication is diluted with normal saline and then inhaled. An ultrasonic nebulizer is used by patients with respiratory infections, asthma, or chronic obstructive pulmonary disease (COPD).

D. Oxygen is administered for a variety of conditions. Oxygen can be stored as a gas or a liquid or can be extracted from the air via a **concentrator.** The amount of oxygen required by the patient is measured in liters per minute (L/min). A **registered respiratory therapist** can be consulted for information on the correct procedures, cautions, and laws regarding oxygen use.

E. A **peak flow meter** is used by patients with asthma to detect constriction of the airways before symptoms appear. Early detection of an upcoming attack allows for therapy designed to stop or minimize the severity of the disease. Patients exhale as much as possible into a peak flow meter to obtain the expiratory flow rate. If this rate is below a predetermined baseline, patients might be instructed to change therapy.

XI. THERMOMETERS. These instruments measure body temperature and are **most commonly used** to detect or evaluate the treatment of infections.

A. A glass **thermometer** has a sealed glass constriction chamber that contains liquid mercury, red- or blue-colored fluid, or Galinstan (a mixture of gallium, indium, and tin). Responding to temperature changes, the mercury, red- or blue-colored fluid, or Galinstan expands or contracts. It remains at the maximum temperature registered until shaken back into the reservoir at the bottom. Glass fever thermometers are graduated from 96°F to 106°F in two-tenths-of-a-degree increments. These types of thermometers should be cleaned and sterilized with alcohol after each use. The American Academy of Pediatrics recommends against the use of mercury-containing thermometers because of the risk of mercury exposure if it breaks. However, more research is needed to assess the accuracy of the newer glass thermometers (red- or blue-colored fluid or Galinstan).[2]

1. The **oral** thermometer has a long slender reservoir. It is placed under the tongue, and the lips are sealed around the thermometer for 3–4 min. Invalid results may occur if the patient eats, drinks, or chews gum before the temperature is taken; incorrectly places the thermometer in the mouth; talks or breathes rapidly through mouth or nose while the temperature is being taken; or has oral abscess or dentures.

2. The **rectal** thermometer has a blunt, pear-shaped bulb to prevent breakage and aid in retention. It is inserted 1 inch into the rectum and left for at least 2 min. A lubricant should be used to aid insertion. Rectal temperature is 1°F higher than oral temperature. Rectal temperatures have been found to lag behind the core temperature. So if a patient has a rapid change in core temperature, the rectal temperature will not immediately reflect it.

3. The **stubby** thermometer has a short, stubby bulb to prevent it from breaking. It can be used as an oral or a rectal thermometer.

4. Any of the three types of glass thermometers can be used to take the **axillary temperature** if an oral or rectal temperature cannot be taken. An axillary temperature is taken by holding the thermometer snugly under the arm for 3–4 min. Axillary temperature is 1°F lower than oral temperature. However, there is controversy about the accuracy of axillary temperature. Using this temperature location can be clinically useful as long as the site is recorded and used consistently.[3]

B. The basal thermometer is used to measure basal body temperature. Basal thermometers are available as a glass or digital thermometer. A digital thermometer may lower the potential for user error as it offers more accuracy. The basal body temperature is used to predict ovulation to increase or decrease the chance of conception. Basal body temperature can be taken orally, rectally, or vaginally, but the route should be consistent.

[2] Smith LS. Using low-tech thermometers to measure body temperatures in older adults: A pilot study. J Gerontol Nurs 2003;29:26–33.
[3] Carroll M, Dip HE. An evaluation of temperature measurement. Nurs Stand 2000;14:39–43.

C. **Digital thermometers** register temperature quickly. Heat alters the current running through a resistor, and the temperature is displayed via a digital readout. The current is supplied by a battery, some of which are rechargeable. Digital thermometers can be used orally or rectally and generally require placing a plastic sheath over the tip of the thermometer before using. Digital thermometers have been integrated into pacifiers to assist in taking an infant's temperature.

D. **Tympanic thermometers** use infrared technology to detect the temperature of the tympanic membrane. The temperature is determined within seconds and is less invasive than other thermometers. These thermometers use disposable tips that are inserted into the ear. The American Academy of Pediatrics recommends that this type of thermometer be used in older babies and children because the probe needs to accurately fit into the ear. Inappropriate placement and too much earwax can cause inaccurate readings.[4]

E. **Skin thermometers** are placed directly on the skin (usually the forehead) to calculate body temperature. This type of thermometer is a liquid-crystal strip that changes colors based on temperature. Environment factors such as sweating and ambient temperature will affect the skin temperature. This method is not as accurate as the others and should be reserved for situations in which other methods are not possible.

XII. **URINARY CATHETERS.** These devices allow for the **collection** and **removal of urine** from the bladder.

A. **External** catheters are used for **heavy incontinence** problems or complete loss of urine control. They are attached to a stationary collection device or a leg bag to allow for ambulation. Types of external catheters include the following:

1. The **male** external catheter is placed around the penis. Some have adhesive to assist in keeping the catheter secure.

2. The **female** external catheter, which is a contoured device that fits snugly in the vagina.

B. **Internal** catheters are used during **surgery** or when external catheters are inappropriate. Internal catheters can be used at home, but the patient must be taught proper insertion techniques to prevent infection. The catheter is inserted through the urethra into the bladder and is attached to a stationary collection device or leg bag. Catheters are sized by the **French scale:** the larger the number, the larger the diameter of the catheter. Types of catheters include the following:

1. The **straight** catheter is used for **intermittent catheterization** to drain the bladder. It consists of a rubber tube; urine drains from one end and the other end connects to the collection device.

2. The **Foley** catheter, an indwelling catheter, can be used for **up to 30 days before changing.** The end inserted into the bladder contains a balloon, which is inflated with sterile water or saline to hold the catheter in place. The balloon is deflated before removal.

---

[4] American Academy of Pediatrics. Fever—How to take a temperature. 2002. Available at: www.aap.org/pubed/ZZZQEB7R25D.htm?&sub_cat=1.

STUDY QUESTIONS

Directions: Each of the numbered items or incomplete statements in this section is followed by answers or by completions of the statement. Select the **one** lettered answer or completion that is **best** in each case.

1. When a patient is fitted with an axillary crutch, how far below the underarm should the top of the crutch rest?

(A) 0.5 inch
(B) 1 inch
(C) 2 inches
(D) 3 inches
(E) 4 inches

2. What angle should the elbow form when a cane is the correct height?

(A) 10°
(B) 25°
(C) 45°
(D) 60°
(E) 90°

3. A product that delivers moisture to the air by heating water to produce steam is called a

(A) nebulizer.
(B) humidifier.
(C) ventilator.
(D) peak flow meter.
(E) vaporizer.

4. An absorbent product designed for patients with light incontinence problems is a

(A) brief.
(B) shield.
(C) undergarment.
(D) underpad.
(E) catheter.

5. When an oral temperature is taken, the thermometer should be placed into the mouth for

(A) 1–2 min.
(B) 3–4 min.
(C) 5–6 min.
(D) 7–8 min.
(E) > 9 min.

6. The diameter of urinary catheters is measured by which of the following scales?

(A) Leur
(B) English
(C) French
(D) gauge
(E) metric

7. A cervical collar that immobilizes the neck is called a

(A) soft cervical collar.
(B) hard cervical collar.
(C) foam cervical collar.
(D) extrication collar.
(E) rigid cervical collar.

8. Incontinence that is caused by an obstruction of the bladder is called

(A) overflow incontinence
(B) urge incontinence
(C) stress incontinence
(D) functional incontinence
(E) iatrogenic incontinence

9. A colostomy or ileostomy could be performed for all of the following conditions *except*

(A) lower bowel obstruction.
(B) malignancy of the colon or rectum.
(C) ulcerative colitis.
(D) duodenal ulcer.
(E) Crohn disease.

10. Pregnancy test kits are designed to detect which substance?

(A) luteinizing hormone (LH)
(B) progesterone
(C) human chorionic gonadotropin (hCG)
(D) estrogen
(E) follicle-stimulating hormone

ANSWERS AND EXPLANATIONS

1. The answer is C *[see I.B.2.a].*
When a patient is fitted for an axillary crutch, the top of the crutch should be 2 inches below the axilla (underarm).

2. The answer is B *[see I.A.1].*
When a patient is properly fitted for a cane, the elbow should form a 25° angle. This allows for maximum weight transfer.

3. The answer is E *[see X.B].*
A vaporizer produces moisture by heating water to produce steam. A humidifier also produces moisture; however, it works by mechanically creating small water particles. A nebulizer is used to deliver liquid to the mouth and throat. A ventilator is used to assist in breathing. A peak flow meter is used to detect airway constriction.

4. The answer is B *[see VII.B.1].*
Shields are pads that are placed in the underwear and held with adhesive strips. They are used for patients with light incontinence problems.

5. The answer is B *[see XI.A.1].*
Oral temperature is taken by inserting the bulb of the thermometer under the tongue and sealing the lips around the thermometer for 3–4 min.

6. The answer is C *[see XII.B].*
The French scale is used to measure the diameter of a urinary catheter. The Leur scale is used to measure syringe tip size. The gauge scale is used to measure needle diameter. The metric scale is a general system of measurement.

7. The answer is D *[see VIII.D.3].*
An extrication collar (also known as a Philadelphia collar) is used to immobilize the neck. It is commonly used in emergency situations. Soft or foam cervical collars provide mild support and remind the patient to keep the neck straight. Hard or rigid cervical collars provide moderate support but allow some movement.

8. The answer is A *[see VII.A.3].*
Overflow incontinence is caused by obstruction of the bladder. Urge incontinence is caused by uncontrolled bladder contractions. Stress incontinence is caused by increases in intra-abdominal pressure. Functional incontinence is related to physical or psychological problems. Iatrogenic incontinence is caused by drugs or surgery.

9. The answer is D *[see IX.A.1–2].*
Lower-bowel obstruction, malignancy of the colon or rectum, and diverticulitis may all require a colostomy. Ulcerative colitis and Crohn disease may require an ileostomy. The treatment of a duodenal ulcer would not include a colostomy or an ileostomy.

10. The answer is C *[see V.B.1.d].*
Pregnancy tests detect hCG in the urine. This is secreted after the embryo has implanted in the uterus. Ovulation-prediction tests detect LH. Progesterone, estrogen, and follicle-stimulating hormone are all involved in controlling the menstrual cycle.

29
OTC Otic, Dental, and Ophthalmic Agents

Jennifer D. Smith

Connie Lee Barnes

I. OTIC OVER-THE-COUNTER (OTC) PRODUCTS

A. The ear can be divided into three distinct parts: the external ear, the middle ear, and the inner ear.

1. The external ear is typically thought of as the part of the ear one can see. However, being made up of the auricle, the external auditory canal, and the outer surface of the tympanic membrane, the external ear extends much farther.
   a. The **auricle,** also referred to as the **pinna,** functions to collect sound and channel it toward the middle ear.
   b. The **external auditory canal,** also known as the **ear canal,** is about 1 inch in length, leading directly to the eardrum. The ear canal contains small glands that are responsible for secreting cerumen, better known as earwax.
   c. The outer surface of the tympanic membrane is known as the **eardrum.** The eardrum separates the external auditory canal from the middle ear.

2. The **middle ear** is an air-filled chamber that provides direct access to the inner ear and indirect access to the nose and throat by way of the eustachian tube. The middle ear houses three small bones (malleus, incus, and stapes) known as the ossicles. When sound strikes the eardrum, it vibrates, transmitting the sound vibrations to the ossicles, which in turn transmit the sound to the inner ear.

3. The **inner ear** is a delicate structure composed of auditory and vestibular components.
   a. The auditory component of the inner ear (the cochlea) is responsible for hearing. The cochlea, a snail-shaped structure filled with fluid, is attached to one of the ossicles (the stapes) in the middle ear. When the stapes moves, it creates waves within the cochlea. Depending on the wave produced, neural impulses are created and transmitted to the brain for interpretation.
   b. The vestibular component of the inner ear (the semicircular canals and the vestibule) is responsible for maintaining balance and equilibrium.

B. **Common ear disorders**

1. **Excessive/impacted cerumen** (earwax). Contrary to current social beliefs, earwax does not need to be removed with objects such as fingers, towels, and cotton-tipped applicators because these objects typically cause impaction of the earwax, rather than its removal. Instead, the external ear has a unique self-cleansing mechanism. Ear canal skin is constantly shed and removed via lateral migration from the tympanic membrane (at a rate of 2–3 mm per day) to the external canal, where cerumen adheres to the shed skin and other debris. Movement such as chewing moves the cerumen outward where it is removed by drying, flaking, or simply falling out. The use of hearing aids or earplugs can block this outward migration, developing earwax impaction and leading to hearing loss.
   a. The **functions** of cerumen include
      (1) Lubrication of the lining of the ear canal
      (2) Temporarily repelling water
      (3) Resistance to infection owing to its acidic nature (pH = 4–5), which creates an unfavorable environment for organism survival
      (2) Trapping dust, debris, and foreign objects
   b. **Epidemiology.** Aside from impaction caused by manipulation, some patient populations are more prone to experience impacted cerumen, including patients with an overproduc-

tion of cerumen, patients with narrowed ear canals, the elderly, and patients with mental retardation.

   c. Symptoms of impacted cerumen include earache, itching of the ear, reflex cough, dizziness, vertigo, tinnitus, and compromised hearing.

   d. Earwax-softening agents may be used alone or followed by the use of an otic syringe (see I.C).

      (1) Carbamide peroxide 6.5% in anhydrous glycerin is the **only U.S. Food and Drug Administration (FDA) approved agent for cerumen removal.** When carbamide peroxide makes contact with tissue enzymes, oxygen is released, producing a foaming action. This **foaming action softens impacted cerumen.**

         (a) Available agents. Murine, Debrox, Dent's Ear Wax

         (b) Instructions for use. Patients **aged 12 and older** should tilt the head sideways and instill 5–10 drops into the ear. The applicator tip should not be inserted into the ear canal. Patients should keep the head tilted to the side (or insert cotton) for several minutes to increase contact time with the cerumen. Repeat the process **twice daily for up to 4 days.** For children < 12 with suspected cerumen impaction, a medical provider should be consulted.

      (2) Olive oil (sweet oil) is used to soften earwax and alleviate itching.

      (3) Mineral oil, recommended as 2 drops in the affected ear(s) once per week, has been used to liquefy the cerumen, thus aiding in its removal.

      (4) Docusate sodium given 15 min before provider in-office irrigation has shown efficacy, but no data exist to support the superiority of docusate sodium over carbamide peroxide.

      (5) Hydrogen peroxide is a component of carbamide peroxide and has weak antibacterial properties. As an otic solution, hydrogen peroxide may be diluted 1:1 with warm water and instilled in the ear to aid in cerumen softening and removal.

      (6) Ear candles, also known as coning candles, are made of paraffin-coated fabric wound into a foot-long cone. Patients are instructed to place the cone in the ear canal and light the distal end with a match. Allegedly, the cerumen is liquefied and negative pressure draws out the wax. In one study of ear candles, more candle wax was deposited into the ears of patients than earwax was removed. However, no data support this dangerous process for efficacy. Furthermore, complications may include external otitis, temporary hearing loss, and burns.

   e. Patients with perforated tympanic membrane, ear drainage, ear pain, or a rash in the ear should be referred to a healthcare provider. In the office, providers may use various devices or irrigating systems to remove impacted cerumen.

2. Vertigo is a loss of equilibrium, in which one might describe a room as spinning. As described in I.A.2.B, the vestibular compartment of the inner ear is responsible for maintaining balance and equilibrium. The autonomic system may become involved if the vertigo is severe, producing dizziness, pallor, sweating, and nausea. Patients expressing symptoms of vertigo (aside from motion sickness) should be referred to a medical provider.

3. Tinnitus may be described by patients as a ringing, buzzing, hissing, whistling, or humming noise lasting from seconds to minutes. Tinnitus has been linked to a variety of causes, including Ménière disease, head injuries, otitis media, syphilis, temporomandibular-joint (TMJ) dysfunction, and certain medications (salicylates, nonsteroidal anti-inflammatory drugs, aminoglycosides, loop diuretics, and chemotherapeutic agents). If tinnitus is constant or severe, a medical consult is advised. Currently, there are no FDA-approved treatments for tinnitus.

4. External otitis, also referred to as otitis externa, is **inflammation of the external auditory canal** secondary to a bacterial or fungal infection.

   a. Cause. External otitis, frequently referred to as swimmer's ear, is thought to be most commonly the result of **local trauma** to the external canal (e.g. cotton-tipped applicators, fingers, sharp objects) or **prolonged exposure to moisture.** Prolonged exposure to moisture (e.g., humid environment, underwater swimming, diving) promotes maceration of the thin skin lining the ear canal, allowing bacteria to penetrate and grow. Trauma to the external canal lends itself to susceptibility to damage and thus easier infiltration of microorganisms. The predominant microorganisms isolated from patients with swimmer's ear are ***Pseudomonas aeruginosa*** and ***Staphylococcus aureus.***

b. Symptoms. Initial symptoms include **itching** and a sensation of **pressure/fullness in the ear,** followed by **pain,** an **otic discharge,** and a possible **decrease in hearing.** The pain may become quite intense, especially if the outer ear is touched or with movement of the jaw, such as chewing.

c. Treatment is with a **prescription otic antibiotic** and **corticosteroid** if bacterial in origin and otic antibiotic alone if fungal in origin, as well as discontinuation of mechanical trauma and/or swimming (until resolution of infection). Oral antibiotics are not necessary unless the infection is unresponsive to otic treatment, the patient is immunocompromised, or a middle ear infection coexists. **External otitis should not be self-treated.**

d. Prevention of external otitis is the key. Mechanical trauma to the ear, by way of cotton-tipped applicators, and fingers should cease immediately. Water should be removed as gently and effectively as possible after swimming or showering/bathing using a towel around the edges of the ear or a hair dryer set on low heat. It may also be beneficial to tilt the head to the side to help expel water. If reoccurrence is frequent, one might consider using molded ear plugs, but consideration should be given to the risk of impacted cerumen with the use of such devices.

5. Water-clogged ear may be a contributing factor to external otitis owing to tissue maceration from prolonged periods of exposure to water; however, water-clogged ear is a separate disorder. Therefore, labeling of products approved by the FDA for the treatment of water-clogged ear may not allude to its use for prevention of external otitis. The only agent FDA approved as safe and effective as an ear-drying agent is isopropyl alcohol 95% in anhydrous glycerin 5%, approved for use in patients 12 years of age and older. A home solution of 50/50 isopropyl alcohol and white vinegar may also be used to dry the ear. Caution must be taken not to recommend self-treatment for water-clogged ear for patients with signs of infection, discharge or bleeding from the ear, ear surgery within the previous 6 weeks, or tympanostomy tubes.

6. Furuncles, also known as boils, are small abscesses surrounding the base of a hair follicle in the outer portion of the external ear canal. *Staphylococcus aureus* is typically the offending organism. Furuncles are usually self-limiting and may be managed with warm compresses and a topical antibiotic.

7. Otitis media is a bacterial infection that is most prevalent between the ages of 3 months and 3 years, owing to the length, angle, and function of the eustachian tube in children. Symptoms include ear pain, fever, fluid discharge from the ear, and possible decreased hearing. All patients with suspected otitis media must be referred to a medical provider for evaluation and treatment.

C. Administration of otic agents

1. Instructions for use of otic drops
   a. Warm the solution by holding the bottle in the hand for a few moments.
   b. Tilt the head sideways with the affected ear upward.
   c. Pull the earlobe up and back to straighten the canal for adults and down and back to straighten in children.
   d. Use the other hand to squeeze the bottle of drops, carefully delivering the number of recommended drops into the ear canal. Caution should be taken not to insert the applicator into the ear canal.
   e. Keep the head tilted sideways for several minutes or place cotton in the ear to prevent the medication from draining out. If cotton is used, it must be large enough, so as not to become lodged in the ear, and should not be left in the ear for longer than 1 hr.
   f. Repeat the procedure on the opposite ear, if necessary.

2. Instructions for use of an otic syringe
   a. Prepare a *warm* solution of plain water. Fill the otic syringe with the warm water solution.
   b. Straighten the ear canal using the appropriate method, as noted above. Tilt the head over a sink or basin to catch the outflow solution.
   c. Insert the tip of the otic syringe into ear, with the tip pointed slightly upward.
   d. Gently squeeze the bulb of the otic syringe to allow the solution to enter the ear. Allow the solution to drain from the ear into the sink or basin. If pain or dizziness occurs, remove the syringe and consult a medical provider.
   e. Repeat on opposite ear, if necessary.

II. DENTAL OTC PRODUCTS

A. Dental anatomy. Anatomically, the teeth are divided into two parts: the **crown** (above the gingival line) and the root (below the gingival line).

1. **Enamel** is the crystalline calcium salts (hydroxyapatite) that cover the crown to protect the underlying tooth structure.

2. **Dentin** is the largest part of the tooth structure, located beneath the enamel. It protects the dental pulp.

3. **Cementum** is a bone-like structure that covers the root and provides the attachment of the tooth with the periodontal ligaments.

4. **Pulp** consists of free nerve endings.

B. Common dental problems and OTC products

1. **Dental caries** (i.e., **cavities**) are formed by the growth and implantation of cariogenic microorganisms.
   a. **Causes**
      (1) **Bacteria** (primarily *Streptococcus mutans* and *Lactobacillaceae*) produce acids (e.g., lactic acid) that demineralize enamel. Initially, demineralized enamel appears as a white, chalky area and becomes bluish white and eventually brown or yellow.
      (2) **Diet** is another factor in the development of dental caries. Foods with a high concentration of refined sugar (i.e., sucrose) increase the risk of dental caries. Sucrose is converted by bacterial plaque into volatile acids that destroy the hydroxyapatite.
         (a) **Fructose** and **lactose** are less cariogenic than sucrose.
         (b) **Noncariogenic sugar substitutes** are xylitol, sorbitol, and aspartame.
   b. **OTC products** for dental caries include products that can alleviate the pain and sensitivity until the patient can get to the dentist. Examples of ingredients that are beneficial in this regard include lidocaine, benzocaine (e.g., Anbesol, Orajel), or an oral analgesic (e.g., aspirin, acetaminophen).

2. **Plaque and calculus**
   a. **Causes**
      (1) **Plaque** is a sticky substance formed by the attachment of bacteria to the pellicle, which is a thin, acellular, glycoprotein (a mucoprotein coating that adheres to the enamel within minutes after cleaning a tooth).
      (2) **Calculus** (or **tartar**) is the substance formed when plaque is not removed within 24 hr. The plaque begins to calcify into calculus when calcium salt precipitates from the saliva. Calculus can be removed only by a professional dental cleaning.
   b. **OTC products**
      (1) **Toothbrushes.** Soft, rounded, nylon bristles are preferred by dentists because hard bristles can irritate the gingival margins and cause the gums to recede. Some toothbrushes have specially designed bristles that reach deep between teeth and along the gumline to remove stains and polish teeth and massage gums. Examples include Colgate Whitening and Colgate Massager toothbrushes. Electric toothbrushes can benefit patients who require someone to clean their teeth for them or patients who have orthodontic appliances. Toothbrushes should be replaced when they begin to show wear or every 3 months, whichever comes first. Patients should replace their toothbrush after having an upper-respiratory infection.
      (2) **Irrigating devices** direct a high-pressure stream of water through a nozzle to the hard-to-clean areas by gently lifting the free gingiva to rinse out crevices. Two types are available: **pulsating** (i.e., intermittent low- and high-pressure water streams) and **steady** (i.e., constant and consistent water pressure), neither of which has shown superior irrigating ability.
         (a) Irrigating devices should serve as adjuncts in maintaining oral hygiene.
         (b) **Examples** include Interplak Water Jet, Hydro-Pik, and the Waterpik oral irrigator.
   c. **Dental floss** is available waxed, unwaxed, thick, thin, flavored, or unflavored. Some dental flosses are impregnated or coated with additives such as baking soda and fluoride. Also, several manufacturers are marketing floss made of materials with superior anti-shredding properties (e.g., Glide, Colgate Precision). There are no differences among

dental flosses in terms of plaque removal and prevention of gingivitis. There is no evidence of a residual wax film with the use of waxed dental floss.

(1) The selection of dental floss depends on the characteristics of the patient, such as tooth roughness or tightness of tooth contacts (e.g., waxed floss is recommended for tight-fitting teeth because it can pass easily between the teeth without shredding).

(2) The American Dental Association (ADA) recognizes the following brands as safe and effective: Butler, Johnson & Johnson, and Oral-B.

d. Dentifrices are products that enhance the removal of stains and dental plaque by the toothbrush. These include toothpastes, antiplaque and anticalculous mouthwashes, cosmetic whiteners, desensitizing agents, disclosing agents, and dental gums.

(1) Toothpastes are beneficial in decreasing the incidence of dental caries, reducing mouth odors, and enhancing personal appearance. Some toothpastes may contain the antioxidant coenzyme Q_{10} (CoQ_{10}; e.g., Perfect Smile Q_{10}). **Ingredients** include the following:

(a) Abrasives are responsible for physically removing plaque and debris. Examples include silicates, sodium bicarbonate, dicalcium phosphate, sodium metaphosphate, calcium pyrophosphate, calcium carbonate, magnesium carbonate, and aluminum oxides. Mentadent contains sodium bicarbonate, whereas PeroxiCare and Colgate baking soda and peroxide whitening contain sodium bicarbonate and peroxide. High-abrasive formulations are not advised for long-term use or for use by patients with exposed root surfaces.

(b) Surfactants are foaming agents that are incorporated into most dentifrices because their detergent action aids in removing debris. The **most frequently used** surfactants are **sodium lauryl sulfate** and **sodium dodecyl benzene sulfonate.** Sodium lauryl sulfate–containing dentifrices have been associated with an increase in the occurrence of canker sores. Dentifrices such as Rembrandt Natural, Sensodyne, and Biotene do not contain sodium lauryl sulfate.

(c) Humectants prevent the preparation from drying. Examples include sorbitol, glycerin, and propylene glycol.

(d) Suspending agents add thickness to the product. Examples include methylcellulose, tragacanth, and karaya gum.

(e) Flavoring agents include sorbitol or saccharin.

(f) Pyrophosphates are found in tartar-control toothpastes. These products retard tartar formation; however, they form an alkaline solution that may irritate the skin. Some patients might experience a rash around the outside of the mouth. These patients should use regular toothpaste and only occasionally brush with tartar-control toothpaste (e.g., Colgate Tartar Control Whitening). Tartar-control toothpastes do not penetrate below the gumline, where tartar does the most damage.

(g) Fluoride is anticariogenic because it replaces the hydroxyl ion in hydroxyapatite with the fluoride ion to form fluorapatite on the outer surface of the enamel. Fluorapatite hardens the enamel and makes it more acid resistant. Fluoride also has demonstrated antibacterial activity.

(i) Fluoride is **most beneficial** if used from birth through **age 12 or 13** because unerupted permanent teeth are mineralizing during that time. Whether or not a patient receives fluoride depends on the concentration in his or her local drinking water (Table 29-1).

Table 29-1. Daily Fluoride Supplement Requirements for Infants and Children, Based on Concentration of Fluoride in Drinking Water

Fluoride Concentration (ppm)	Age	Fluoride Supplement Required (mg/day)
> 0.6	6 months to 3 years	0
	3–6 years	0
0.3–0.6	6 months to 3 years	0
	3–6 years	0.25
	6–16 years	0.50
< 0.3	6 months to 3 years	0.25
	3–6 years	0.50
	6–16 years	1.00

    (ii) Common fluoride compounds in toothpaste include 0.24% sodium fluoride and 0.76% or 0.80% sodium monofluorophosphate (e.g., Aim, Crest, Aquafresh, Colgate). Crest Gum Care contains a reformulated version of stannous fluoride (0.454%), which might reduce gingivitis and bleeding of the gums by an average of 20% and 33%. However, it can also stain the teeth brown.

    (iii) A fluoride warning label, which recommends contacting a poison control center or seeking professional assistance if more than a brushful of fluoride toothpaste is ingested, is required by the FDA on fluoride-containing dentifrices because the federal agency lists fluoride as a toxic substance.

    (iv) The estimated toxic dose of fluoride is 5–10 mg/kg.

    (v) Acute fluoride toxicity causes nausea, vomiting, and diarrhea. The ADA limits the maximum amount of fluoride in ADA-accepted toothpaste to 260 mg per container.

(2) Agents with **antiplaque** potential for inclusion in dentifrices include plant extracts (sanguinarine), metal salts (zinc and stannous), phenolic compounds (triclosan), and essential oils (thymol and eucalyptol).

    (a) Triclosan is an antimicrobial agent that has been demonstrated clinically to help prevent gingivitis, plaque, cavities, and tartar.

        (i) Colgate Total contains 0.24% sodium fluoride and 0.30% triclosan and is formulated with the polymer **Gantrez,** which works to prolong the contact of triclosan with oral structures.

        (ii) Therefore, Colgate Total continues to work in between brushings.

    (b) Colgate Total has been accepted by the ADA as efficacious.

(3) Anticalculous dentifrices include the ingredients zinc chloride, zinc citrate, and 33% pyrophosphate to prevent calculus formation.

    (a) The ADA does not evaluate anticalculous claims because it regards the inhibition of supragingival calculus as a nontherapeutic use.

    (b) The ADA has directed that the following statement appear on all package and container labeling for accepted fluoride dentifrice products with calculus-control activity: "[*Product name*] has been shown to reduce the formation of tartar above the gumline, but has not been shown to have a therapeutic effect on periodontal diseases."

(4) Cosmetic whitening agents. The **most common ingredient** in these products that is responsible for whitening the teeth is **10% carbamide peroxide** (i.e., in Gly-Oxide, Simply White, or Proxigel) and hydrogen peroxide (i.e., in Crest Whitestrips).

    (a) Carbamide peroxide is a white crystal that reacts with water to release hydrogen peroxide, which in turn liberates free oxides.

    (b) Some cosmetic whiteners may contain hydrogen peroxide or perhydrol urea in gel or liquid form.

    (c) Products specifically marketed to dentists include Colgate Platinum Professional Tooth Whitening System and Rembrandt Lighten Gel.

        (i) Patients should perform tooth bleaching only with a dentist's supervision.

        (ii) Crest Extra Whitening uses a patented soft-silica technology. Owing to this technology, the product contains 50% more silica, which greatly enhances the removal of extrinsic stains without increasing abrasiveness.

        (iii) Colgate Luminous also contains a silica whitening technology and fluoride.

    (d) Possible risks associated with using whitening products include alteration of normal flora, tissue damage, tooth sensitivity, gingivitis, and potentiation of carcinogenic effects of other agents.

    (e) Antiseptics have been used as whiteners (e.g., Gly-Oxide, Proxigel).

(5) Desensitizing agents reduce the pain in sensitive teeth caused by cold, heat, acids, sweets, or touch. These products should be nonabrasive and should not be used on a permanent basis unless directed by a dentist.

    (a) Examples of **5% potassium nitrate compounds** include Colgate Sensitive, Sensodyne, Aquafresh Sensitive, and Crest Sensitivity.

    (b) Dibasic sodium citrate in Pluronic gel and 10% strontium chloride were classified as class III pending further evidence of effectiveness.

(6) Disclosing agents aid in visualizing where dental plaque has formed. These products are for occasional use only and should not be swallowed. The FDA-approved product is a vegetable dye, Food, Drug, and Cosmetic (FD&C) Red No 3. Following use, the consumer should rinse the mouth with water and then expectorate.

(7) **Mouthwashes** may contain astringents, demulcents, detergents, flavors, germicidal agents, and fluoride. They can be used for cosmetic purposes, reducing plaque, or supplementing fluoride consumption.

   (a) **Cosmetic mouthwashes** freshen the breath. They are nontherapeutic and are not effective as an antiseptic agent. These mouthwashes are classified by their active ingredients, alcohol content, and appearance. The most popular products are those that contain medicinal phenol and mint. The higher the percent of alcohol, the higher the effect of the flavor within the mouth.

   (b) **Antiplaque mouth rinses.** Mouth rinses claiming anticalculous or tartar-control activity contain the same active ingredients as anticalculus dentifrices. Cool Mint Listerine has received the ADA seal of approval.

      (i) Cetylpyridinium chloride (CPC), a mouthwash ingredient, has been approved for class I for plaque and gingivitis treatment. Examples of products in this class include Cepacol, Scope, Oral-B Anti-Plaque Rinse, and Crest Pro-Health Rinse.

      (ii) Chlorhexidine is an active ingredient in some mouthwashes. An example is Colgate PerioGard.

      (iii) Staining is associated with the overuse of CPC and chlorhexidine.

      (iv) **Fluoridated mouthwashes** are used after cleaning the teeth and should be expectorated. Nothing should be put into the mouth for 30 min after using these mouthwashes. The ADA has approved the following products: ACT Anti-Cavity Dental Rinse, ACT for Kids, Fluorigard Anti-Cavity Dental Rinse, and Reach Fluoride Dental Rinse, Oral-B Rinse Therapy and Anti-Cavity Treatment, and Colgate Phos-Flur.

(8) **Dental gums** are promoted to reduce plaque, whiten teeth, possibly reduce the risk of tooth decay, and freshen breath. Chewing gum is associated with increased salivary flow, which apparently produces a beneficial buffering effect against acids in the oral cavity.

   (a) Some contain baking soda as a mild abrasive cleaner and to neutralize acid.

   (b) Calcium may be added to help remineralize the teeth and prevent cavities.

   (c) These gums also contain xylitol, a sweetener that is less likely to cause cavities than sugar or sorbitol. Examples are Trident Advantage, Arm & Hammer Dental Care, BreathAsure, Dental Care, Advance Breath Care, Aquafresh Whitening, and Biotene. BreathAsure Dental Gum contains an ingredient called PXT-20, which is an emulsion of polydimethylsiloxane and poloxamer 407. It forms a thin coating on the tooth that is supposed to reduce plaque buildup.

   (d) These gums are not a substitute for good oral hygiene, including brushing and flossing, but may be useful for people who are unable to brush after lunch.

   (e) It is not known if these products have any advantage over regular sugarless gum.

3. **Gingivitis** is inflammation of the gingiva. The gingiva may appear larger in size with a bluish hue caused by engorged gingival capillaries and a slow venous return.

   a. **Cause.** Gingivitis is caused by microorganisms that eventually damage cellular and intercellular tissues. **Chronic gingivitis** may be localized or generalized. The gums readily bleed when probed or brushed, and the patient should seek dental assistance.

   b. **OTC products** include anesthetics containing eugenol or benzocaine (e.g., Orajel) to relieve the pain. Mouthwashes may freshen the breath; however, it is important to consider the potential of these products to disguise and delay treatment of pathological conditions (e.g., gingivitis) before use. Also, acetaminophen (Tylenol) can be recommended. The patient should seek the advice of a dentist.

4. **Periodontal disease** is the result of chronic gingivitis left untreated.

   a. The periodontal ligament attachment and alveolar bone support of the tooth deteriorate.

   b. **Risk factors** include gender (men affected more than women), age (> 35 years old), smoking, lack of oral care and regular dentist visits, diabetes, hypertension, rheumatoid arthritis, and loss of anterior teeth.

   c. Periodontitis may be treated with prescription products:

      (1) Periostat (doxycycline hyclate, 20-mg capsules)

      (2) Atridox (doxycycline hyclate 10%) in the Atrigel Delivery System.

         (a) Atridox provides local antibacterial effects.

         (b) Low-dose doxycycline inhibits collagenase, an enzyme that destroys connective tissue in the gums, leading to tooth loss.

5. **Acute necrotizing ulcerative gingivitis (ANUG)** (also called **trench mouth**) is characterized by necrosis and ulceration of the gingival surface with underlying inflammation. This condition is usually seen in teens and young adults.
   a. **Signs** and **symptoms** of ANUG include severe pain, halitosis, bleeding, foul taste, and increased salivation.
   b. The **cause** of ANUG is unknown. It is postulated that it might be associated with the overgrowth of spirochete and fusiform organisms.
   c. **Risk factors** include anxiety, stress, smoking, malnutrition, and poor oral hygiene.
   d. **Treatment** consists of local débridement. Also, penicillin VK (penicillin V is a derivative of penicillin G; however, it is more stable in an acidic medium and, therefore, is better absorbed from the gastrointestinal tract; K stands for potassium) or metronidazole may be used in certain cases (e.g., widespread lesions).
   e. **OTC products** include acetaminophen and products with benzocaine (not eugenol because it may cause soft tissue damage). The patient should be advised to see a dentist. The use of salicylates is not recommended if the patient is predisposed to bleeding. Also, adequate nutrition, high fluid intake, and rest are essential. Rinsing the mouth with warm normal saline or 1.5% peroxide solution might be helpful for the first few days.

6. **Temporomandibular joint syndrome** is caused by an improper working relationship between the chewing muscles and the TMJ.
   a. **Signs** and **symptoms** include a dull, aching pain around the ear, headaches, neck aches, limited opening of the mouth, and a clicking or popping noise upon opening the mouth.
   b. **Risk factors** include bruxism (i.e., grinding the teeth) and occlusal (i.e., bite) abnormalities.
   c. **Treatment** consists of moist heat applied to the jaw, muscle relaxants, bite plates or occlusal splints, a diet of soft foods, correcting the occlusion, or surgery.
   d. **OTC products** that can help relieve the pain include oral analgesics (e.g., acetaminophen, ibuprofen).

7. **Teething pain.** The ADA has not accepted any product for teething pain. A **frozen teething ring** can provide symptomatic relief. Persisting pain may be treated with a local anesthetic such as benzocaine (found in Anbesol Baby and Orajel Baby). If a teething child presents with a fever, a physician should be contacted.

8. **Xerostomia** (i.e., dry mouth) is caused by improper functioning of the salivary glands (as in Sjögren syndrome and diabetes mellitus). **Artificial saliva** is available as an OTC product. The ADA has approved the following artificial saliva products: Moi-Stir, Salivart, Xero-Lube, and OralBalance Gel.

C. **Common oral lesions and OTC products**

1. **Canker sores** (also called **recurrent aphthous ulcers or recurrent aphthous stomatitis**)
   a. The **cause** of canker sores is unknown. Studies suggest that the sores may be caused by hypersensitivity to bacteria found in the mouth or dysfunction of the immune system initiated by minor trauma or stress. This is why physicians or dentists may use prednisone or a topical steroid to reduce allergic reaction or have the patient rinse with a tetracycline suspension. Peridex and Listerine appear to help decrease bacteria in the mouth.
   b. **Lesions** can occur on any nonkeratinized mucosal surface in the mouth (i.e., tongue, lips) and usually appear gray to yellow with an erythematous halo of inflamed tissue surrounding the ulcer. Most lesions persist 7–14 days and heal without scarring.
   c. **OTC products** can control the pain of canker sores, shorten the duration of current lesions, and prevent new lesions. Products include **protectants, local anesthetics,** and **débriding and wound-cleansing agents.**
      (1) **Protectants** include Orabase, denture adhesives (see II.F.2), and benzoin tincture. Denture adhesives are not approved for this use by the FDA.
      (2) **Local anesthetics,** such as benzocaine or butacaine, are the **most common anesthetics** found in these OTC products.
         (a) The FDA has approved the following ingredients:
            (i) Benzocaine (5%–20%)
            (ii) Benzyl alcohol (0.05%–0.1%)
            (iii) Dyclonine (0.05%–0.1%)
            (iv) Hexylresorcinol (0.05%–0.1%)
            (v) Menthol (0.04%–2%)
            (vi) Phenol (0.5%–1.5%)

        (vii) Phenolate sodium (0.5%–1.5%)

        (viii) Salicyl alcohol (1%–6%)

    (b) Examples of OTC local anesthetics for oral use include Anbesol, Blistex, Campho-Phenique, Orajel, Orajel CoverMed, Zilactin-B, Zilactin-L, Benzodent, and Rembrandt Canker Pain Relief Kit.

    (c) The use of products containing substantial amounts of menthol, phenol, camphor, and eugenol should be discouraged owing to their ability to irritate tissue.

    (d) Aspirin should not be retained in the mouth or placed on an oral lesion in an attempt to provide relief.

    (e) Prescription products. Amlexanox (Aphthasol) has been approved for the treatment of canker sores.

        (i) It is applied 4 times daily after meals and at bedtime.

        (ii) Advise patients to start using the product as soon as they notice symptoms and to continue until the ulcer is healed, approximately 10 days.

    (f) Gelclair is indicated for local management and relief of oral pain associated with aphthous ulcers. It provides oral pain relief by acting as a protective adherent barrier over the surface of the mouth and throat.

        (i) Patient should use one packet at least 3 times a day or as needed.

        (ii) Advise patients to mix 1 packet with 3 tablespoons of water, swish for a minute, then expectorate. Do not eat or drink for approximately 1 hr after treatment.

    (g) Investigational **products. Thalidomide** is being studied for the treatment of AIDS-associated oral canker sores.

  (3) Débriding and wound-cleansing agents include 10%–15% carbamide peroxide, 3% hydrogen peroxide, 1.2 g sodium perborate monohydrate, and sodium bicarbonate. The FDA considers these four active ingredients to be safe and effective for débriding or wound-cleansing agents for oral healthcare.

2. Cold sores/fever blisters (also called **herpes simplex labialis**) are caused primarily by the herpes simplex virus type 1 (HSV-1). HSV-1 is contagious and is thought to be transmitted by direct contact. An outbreak may be provoked by stress, minor infection, fever, or sunlight. Cold sores usually occur on the lips and are recurrent, often arising in the same location.

  a. Presentation. An outbreak is preceded by burning, itching, or numbness. Red papules of fluid-containing vesicles then appear, and these eventually burst and form a crust. These sores are typically self-limited and heal in 10–14 days without scarring.

  b. OTC products for cold sores include products that contain softening compounds (e.g., emollient creams, petrolatum, protectants), which keep the cold sore moist to prevent it from drying and fissuring. Local anesthetics in nondrying bases (e.g., Orabase, with benzocaine) decrease pain. Highly astringent bases should be avoided. The ADA contraindicates caustic agents (e.g., phenol, silver nitrate), camphor and other counterirritants, and hydrocortisone for the treatment of cold sores. Lesions should be kept clean by gently washing with mild soap.

        (i) Docosanol 10% cream (**Abreva**) is indicated for the treatment of cold sores. It prevents the cold sore infection from entering healthy cells. It is approved by the FDA to shorten healing time and duration of symptoms. Patients should apply the cream at the first sign of an outbreak and continue to apply the cream five times a day until the lesion is healed.

        (ii) Viractin gel (2% tetracaine) is used for the temporary relief of pain and itching associated with cold sores.

  (1) If a **secondary infection** develops, bacitracin or Neosporin antibiotic ointments should be recommended. If necessary, the patient should consult a physician for a systemic antibiotic prescription.

  (2) A lip **sunscreen** should be used for patients whose cold sores appear to be caused by sun exposure.

  (3) The essential amino acid l-lysine has been used in oral doses of 300–1200 mg daily to accelerate recovery or suppress recurrence of cold sores. However, studies have produced conflicting data regarding l-lysine and its effect on the duration, severity, and recurrence rate of cold sores.

  c. Prescription products

    (1) Valacyclovir (Valtrex) is indicated for the treatment of herpes labialis.

    (2) Acyclovir cream 5% (Zovirax) is indicated for the treatment of cold sores in adults and adolescents > 12 years of age. Therapy should be initiated at the onset of sign and symptoms and applied 5 times per day for 4 days.

(3) **Penciclovir cream 1% (Denavir)** is an antiviral medication for the treatment of cold sores in adults and children 12 years of age and older. Patients should apply the cream every 2 hr while awake for 4 days, beginning at the first sign of tingling or swelling.

D. Common oral infections and OTC products

1. **Candidiasis** (also called **thrush**) is caused by the fungus *Candida albicans,* which is the most common opportunistic pathogen associated with oral infections. Thrush has a milky curd appearance, and affected patients should contact a physician.

2. **Oral cancer.** The most common oral cancer is **squamous cell carcinoma,** which can appear as red or white lesions, ulcerations, or tumors.
   a. **Signs** and **symptoms** include a color change in the tongue, a sore throat that does not heal, and persistent or unexplained bleeding. Patients with any of these signs should contact a physician or a dentist.
   b. **Risk factors** include smoked and smokeless tobacco as well as alcohol.
   c. **Treatment** consists of eliminating use of tobacco and alcohol in any form (e.g., alcoholic beverages, mouth rinses with alcohol). Also, treatment generally includes **wide local excision** for small lesions and **en bloc excisions** for larger lesions (in continuity with radical neck dissection if lymph nodes are involved). Radiation, alone or combined with surgery, may be appropriate. Chemotherapy may be used as palliation or as an adjunct to surgery and radiation.
   d. **OTC medications** should not be administered until after checking with a physician. For example, OTC medications used for inflammation can increase the effects of methotrexate. Chemotherapeutic agents can produce many possible side effects that require immediate medical attention (e.g., chest pain, inflammation, unusual bleeding). Some examples of side effects that usually do not require medical attention include nausea, vomiting, loss of appetite or hair, and trouble sleeping. OTC medications can be useful in these cases; however, nausea and vomiting are treated by prescription medications such as ondansetron or metoclopramide. Nonpharmacological measures, such as avoiding disturbing environmental odors and vestibular disturbances, might be helpful in minimizing nausea and vomiting.

E. Recommended standard prophylaxis for prevention of endocarditis

1. **Amoxicillin** 2.0 g orally 1 hr before the procedure for adults, and 50 mg/kg orally for children, is the recommended standard prophylactic regimen for all dental, oral, upper-respiratory tract, and esophageal procedures.

2. For patients who are **allergic to penicillin,** the recommended **alternative oral regimens** include the following:
   a. **Clindamycin,** 600 mg for adults; 20 mg/kg for children
   b. **Cephalexin** or **cefadroxil,** 2.0 g for adults; 50 mg/kg for children
   c. **Azithromycin** or **clarithromycin,** 500 mg for adults; 15 mg/kg for children, 1 hr before the procedure

F. OTC denture products

1. **Denture cleansers** are either **chemical** or **abrasive** in respect to their cleansing ability.
   a. **Chemical** denture cleansers include alkaline peroxide, alkaline hypochlorite, or dilute acids.
      (1) **Alkaline peroxide** is the **most commonly used** chemical denture cleanser and is available as tablets or powders. It causes oxygen to be released, which creates a cleansing effect. Alkaline peroxide does not damage the surface of acrylic resins; however, it may bleach them.
      (2) **Alkaline hypochlorite** (i.e., bleach) dissolves the matrix of plaque but has no effect on calculus. It is both bactericidal and fungicidal. A **disadvantage** of alkaline hypochlorite is that it **corrodes metal denture components.** It can also bleach acrylic resin. Therefore, it should not be used more than once a week.
   b. **Abrasive** denture cleansers are available as gel, paste, or powder (e.g., silicates, sodium bicarbonate, dicalcium phosphate, calcium carbonate).

      (1) Dentures should not be soaked in hot water because the heat could distort or warp the appliances.

      (2) The ADA accepts the following denture cleansers as safe and effective: Denture-Brite, Efferdent, and Polident.

  2. Denture adherents contain materials (e.g., karaya gum, pectin, methylcellulose) that swell, gel, and become viscous to promote adhesion, which increases the denture attachment to underlying soft tissues.

    a. Disadvantages. As the use of denture adherents increases, the soft tissue deteriorates. Denture adherents can also provide a medium for bacterial and fungal growth. Daily use of denture adherents is not recommended.

    b. The ADA accepts the following denture adherents as safe and effective: Fixodent, ORAfix, Sea-Bond, Super Poli-Grip, and Effergrip.

G. Pharmacists' responsibilities to the patient using OTC oral products

  1. Refer a patient to a dentist if the oral complaint involves an abscess with fever, swelling, malaise, lymphadenopathy, or purulent exudate.

  2. Remind patients that cold and canker sores, with appropriate treatment, are usually a self-limiting problem.

  3. Patients should be informed about **how to use recommended products,** the duration of use, the expectations of using the product, and the procedure to follow if the product is ineffective.

  4. If a nonprescription product does not improve a condition, or if the condition worsens, use of the product should be discontinued and a physician or dentist should be contacted.

III. OPHTHALMIC OTC PRODUCTS

A. Anatomy of the eye

  1. The **sclera,** also known as the white of the eye, functions to protect intraocular contents and maintain the shape of the eye.

  2. The **cornea** is the main refracting surface of the eye.

  3. The anterior chamber of the eye houses a continuous supply of **aqueous humor,** which is produced in relation to the intraocular pressure. The aqueous humor is responsible for nourishing the cornea.

  4. The **iris** is the colored part of the eye that regulates the entrance of light through the pupil.

  5. The **pupil** is the contractile opening at the center of the iris that dilates and constricts in response to light.

  6. The **lens** is found directly behind the iris and pupil and is responsible for enabling the eye to accommodate, focusing for near and distance vision. The lens continues to grow throughout life, gradually becoming thicker over time. The lens is, therefore, susceptible to the degenerative effects of aging, most noticeably evident in the 5th decade of life as the inability to focus and refocus for near and distance vision.

  7. Approximately two thirds of the volume of the eye is occupied by the **vitreous humor.** As one ages, the gel-like characteristics of the vitreous humor is lost and shadows are cast by various cells, giving the illusion of "floaters."

  8. The **retina** is composed of the optic disc, the retinal vessels, and the macula. The optic nerve enters the retina through the optic disc. The macula is responsible for central vision and the remaining parts of the retina are responsible for peripheral and color vision.

  9. The **optic nerve,** also known as the second cranial nerve (CN II), transmits impulses from the retina to the brain.

B. Ophthalmic Formulations

1. **Vehicles** provide increased viscosity, thereby enhancing contact time of the product. Vehicles commonly found in ophthalmic products include carboxymethylcellulose (CMC), povidone, polyvinyl alcohol (PVA), and hydroxypropyl methylcellulose (HPMC).

2. **Preservatives** provide antimicrobial activity for ophthalmic preparations and include benzalkonium chloride (BAK), chlorhexidine, methylparaben, propylparaben, ethylenediaminetetraacetic acid (EDTA), and sorbic acid.

3. **Antioxidants** prevent product deterioration. Common antioxidants found in ophthalmic preparations include edetic acid, sodium bisulfite, sodium metabisulfite, sodium thiosulfate, and thiourea.

4. **Wetting agents** reduce surface tension of the lens and include polysorbate 20, polysorbate 80, poloxamer 282, and tyloxapol.

5. **Buffers** are used in ophthalmic preparations to maintain a pH between 6.0 and 8.0. Buffers include acetic acid, boric acid, hydrochloric acid, phosphoric acid, potassium bicarbonate, potassium borate, potassium citrate, sodium acetate, sodium bicarbonate, sodium bisphosphate, sodium borate, sodium carbonate, sodium citrate, sodium hydroxide, and sodium phosphate.

6. **Tonicity adjusters** ensure an isotonic agent, equal to 0.9%–60.2% sodium chloride. These agents include dextrose, glycerin, potassium chloride, propylene glycol, and sodium chloride.

C. Nonprescription ophthalmic agents

1. **Artificial tears** are used to **hydrate and lubricate the eye** by stimulating tear production and decreasing tear evaporation. Initial dosing is recommended as 2 times daily, up to 4 times daily, as needed. However, solutions may be used hourly, if clinically indicated. To reduce ocular irritation, preservative-free artificial tears should be recommended to patients who will need to use the medication frequently.

2. **Lubricating ointments** include white petrolatum, mineral oil, and lanolin, which act to lubricate and hydrate the eye. As an ointment, these agents are able to **provide increased contact time with the ocular surface but may result in blurred vision.** If possible, blurred vision may be minimized (or less noticeable) by decreasing the amount of ointment instilled into the eye or by administering the ointment at bedtime. Initial dosing is recommended as 2 times daily, but may be used as often as every few hours, or only occasionally, depending on patient response. Preservative-free ophthalmic ointments may reduce ocular irritation in patients requiring frequent dosing. When using eye drops and ointment, **drops should be instilled into the eye before applying ointment.**

3. **Vasoconstrictors** (decongestants) work by producing a **temporary constriction of the conjunctival blood vessels,** thereby reducing eye redness. Available ophthalmic vasoconstrictors include naphazoline, phenylephrine, tetrahydrozoline, and oxymetazoline. These agents **may have a rebound effect (congestion) if used in excess** or for extended durations and should be avoided in patients with narrow-angle glaucoma.

4. **Antihistamines** may be used for the treatment of ophthalmic conditions associated with allergic rhinitis, though their use has been classified by the FDA as less than effective because of the lack of data demonstrating clinical effectiveness. Only two nonprescription ocular antihistamines are available (e.g., pheniramine and antazoline), but only in combination with the ophthalmic decongestant naphazoline.
   a. Typical dosing of ophthalmic antihistamines is 1–2 drops in each eye 3–4 times daily.
   b. Ophthalmic antihistamines should not be recommended in patients with glaucoma or patients at high risk of developing narrow-angle glaucoma, as pupil dilation associated with the use of these agents may cause this disorder.
   c. Side effects of these agents may include burning, stinging, itching, foreign body sensation, dry eye, lid edema, and pupil dilation.

5. **Astringents decrease ocular inflammation.** The only FDA-recommended astringent is **zinc sulfate,** recommended as 1–2 drops four times daily.

6. **Irrigant solutions** work to **rinse and remove debris and contaminants** from the eye, while maintaining ocular moisture.

7. **Hyperosmotic agents** increase the tonicity of the tear film, eventually eliminating excess fluid from the cornea.

D. **Eye disorders**

1. **Dry eye,** also known as keratoconjunctivitis sicca, is a common condition in which patients complain of a foreign body sensation, ophthalmic itching, decreased tear production, redness, pain, and difficulty moving the eyelids. Symptoms are the result of a deficiency to produce aqueous, mucin, or lipid tear film components, which may be attributable to certain disease states (e.g., thyroid disease, Parkinson disease), infection, or medications (e.g., antihistamines, oral contraceptives). Nonprescription treatment for dry eye includes the use of **artificial tears during the day and ophthalmic ointment at** night.

2. **Conjunctivitis** is inflammation of the conjunctiva which may be caused by bacterial or viral infection, allergy, or environmental factors.
   a. **Allergic conjunctivitis** symptoms affect both eyes and include redness, mild edema of the eyelid, excessive tearing, extreme itching, string-like mucoid discharge, and chemosis. Nonprescription treatment recommendations avoidance of the allergen if feasible, cold compresses, vasoconstrictors, and antihistamines. Nonprescription ophthalmic products containing a combination of a vasoconstrictor and an antihistamine are available (e.g., Naphcon A, Opcon A, Visine-A).
   b. The causes of **bacterial conjunctivitis** depend on patient's age. Approximately one quarter of patients presenting with bacterial conjunctivitis will have **concomitant otitis media.** Therefore it is prudent for all children presenting with a purulent ocular discharge on waking in the morning and abrupt onset of redness to have their ears examined for otitis media. **Treatment for bacterial conjunctivitis is prescription only.**
   c. **Viral conjunctivitis** is most often attributable to the **adenovirus** and is **highly contagious.** More commonly known as **"pink eye,"** individuals often experience an upper-respiratory infection or are exposed to another individual with viral conjunctivitis before the onset of symptoms (e.g., pink eye, thick ocular discharge, extreme tearing, foreign body sensation). **Treatment is supportive** and may include cold compresses, artificial tears, and topical vasoconstrictors.

3. **Chemical burns** can result from medications, chlorinated swimming pools, or exposure to toxic fumes or irritants (e.g., hairsprays, battery acid, vinegar, oven cleaners, lye). **Treatment includes immediate and continued irrigation** of the eye(s) with saline or sterile water and emergency attention from a physician or eye care specialist.

4. **Corneal edema** is characterized by **halos or star bursts** around lights, which are the result of an underlying disorder (e.g. damage to the eye). Once diagnosed by a physician, **hyperosmotic agents** such as Muro solution or ointment may be used to **draw the fluid away from the cornea.** Dosing should begin with a 2% solution used 4 times daily with the addition of a 5% ointment used at nighttime if needed. If unresolved, the 2% solution may be changed to a 5% solution with continued use of the ointment.

5. A **hordeolum,** more commonly known as a **sty,** is an infection of the glands of the eyelids caused by *Staphylococcus aureus.* Sties present as painful, red, and edematous but may be relieved by the application of **warm compresses** for 10–15 min 3–4 times daily. Topical antibiotics may be required.

6. A **chalazion,** simply a **granuloma,** may involve the glands of the eyelids or the surrounding area but is **not infectious.** When in its early stages, the inflammation may be relieved by **warm compresses** applied for 10–15 min 3–4 times daily. If not resolved within 1 week, provider consultation is appropriate, and surgical excision may be necessary.

7. **Blepharitis** is a **bilateral inflammation of the eyelid margins,** attributable to *Staphylococcus,* seborrheic dermatitis, or a combination of the two. Blepharitis may be identified by red,

scaly, thickened eyelids with possible loss of the eyelashes. Staphylococcal blepharitis requires antibiotic treatment, but seborrheic blepharitis may respond to lid hygiene with warm compresses for 15-20 min 2–4 times daily, followed by lid scrubs with a mild detergent.

E. Antioxidants

1. The antioxidant vitamins include vitamin A (retinol and β-carotene), vitamin C, and vitamin E. **β-Carotene 50 mg** every other day may prevent the development of cataracts, especially in smokers. However, the **use of antioxidants in patients who smoke increases the risk of lung cancer and should, therefore, not be recommended. Vitamin C** has been studied for the prevention of cataracts. However, insufficient data in published trials limits the recommendation of this supplement for this purpose.

2. **Lutein,** an antioxidant pigment that functions to filter and protect the visual apparatus and its vascular supply, may be beneficial for improvement in vision in patients with dry age-related macular degeneration and prevention of cataracts. However, more data by way of large randomized controlled trials are necessary to assess safety and efficacy of this supplement.

3. Patients with moderate and advanced age-related macular degeneration (ARMD) have shown a reduction in the progression of the disease and its associated vision loss with antioxidants plus zinc, as well as a combination of the following supplements: vitamin C 500 mg, vitamin E 400 IU, β-carotene 15 mg, zinc oxide 80 mg, and copper 2 mg. Ocuvite PreserVision, a formulation of the above antioxidants, zinc, and copper, is a dietary supplement currently under patent based on the promising results of the National Eye Institute's (NEI's) landmark Age-Related Eye Disease Study (AREDS). Studies of patients with mild or borderline ARMD have not shown benefit from antioxidant plus zinc supplementation. Therefore, this formulation should be **recommended only to patients who are nonsmokers** (owing to an increased risk of lung cancer) **with a diagnosis of moderate or advanced ARMD.**

F. Contact Lenses

1. **Types of contact lenses**
   (a) **Hard contact lenses** were the first "original" contact lens, which were made of polymethylmethacrylate (PMMA). Because of the hydrophobic nature of PMMA, the permeability of oxygen is limited, thus restricting the once-common use of hard contact lenses.
   (1) A **spectacle blur,** the inability to see well with glasses after removal of the contact lens, may occur with the use of hard lenses. The small diameter of the lens may also contribute to loss of the lens from the eye.
   (2) Care of hard contact lenses includes cleaning between the fingertips, soaking, and wetting with each removal of the lens from the eye. Furthermore, care must be taken to avoid scratching and chipping the surface of the contact lens.
   b. **Rigid gas-permeable (RGP) lenses** infuse oxygen permeability of soft contact lenses with the features of the hard contact lenses. RGP lenses are generally thicker than soft lenses, but more oxygen is delivered to the cornea by these agents.
   (1) The RGP lenses are available in daily- and extended-wear versions, approved for up to 7 days of wear.
   (2) Care of the RGP lens includes cleaning the lens in the palm of the hand with a surface-active cleaning product and an enzymatic product. The lens should then be soaked for a minimum of 4 hr in a conditioning solution before reinsertion.
   c. **Soft lenses** are more comfortable and easier to remove than other contact lenses, however, the visual improvement noted may not be as significant as that which is seen with RGP or hard lenses. **Soft lenses should not be worn when applying topical ophthalmic products,** except those products specifically formulated for such use (e.g., rewetting solution).
   (1) Extended-wear soft contact lenses are approved for 7 days of continuous wear. However, a relatively new product, Focus Night and Day, is approved for continuous 30-day use, though not all patients will be able to tolerate the lens placement for 30 days.

(2) Daily-wear soft contact lenses are designed to be worn for 1 day, up to 3 months, depending on the lens chosen. Because the lenses will be discarded within a short period of time, an enzymatic solution is generally not necessary for this type of lens, but general cleaning and disinfecting each time they are removed from the eyes is advisable. Sleeping in these lenses is not recommended.

2. Solution ingredients are generally specific to the type of contact lens chosen (e.g., soft, hard, or RPG). Therefore, the patient should ensure the product selected is in accordance with the type of lens worn.

    a. Cleaning solutions act to remove residue (e.g., debris, oils) from the contact lens by nonionic or amphoteric surfactants. If not cleaned regularly, the residue will build and harden, creating an ocular irritant, and possibly an ophthalmic infection. A homemade cleaning solution of baking soda and distilled water may be used, but is not typically recommended owing to the increased risk of ocular infection and difficulty in removing the agent from the lens.

    b. Soaking solutions are used to provide an aseptic environment for the lens once removed from the eye and may also aid in removal of residual contaminant on the lens not removed during cleaning. Soaking solutions generally have a higher concentration of preservative than wetting agents, but the lens should be thoroughly rinsed before insertion.

    c. Wetting solutions are applied directly to the lens before insertion into the eye. The function of the wetting solution is to transition the lens surface from hydrophobic to hydrophilic, provide lubrication, and enhance fingertip adhesion to allow for easier insertion. Wetting solutions are not necessary for insertion if the patient has significant tearing immediately after insertion of the lens. Saliva should not be used in place of a wetting solution because of the potential for infection.

    d. Multipurpose products are generally a solution composed of a cleaning solution, soaking solution, and wetting solution for ease of use with contact lenses. However, a multipurpose product may not be as efficacious in the removal of the residue or providing adequate lubrication as the use of the three individual agents.

    e. Rewetting solutions may be used to clean and moisten the surface of the contact lens while the lens is still in the eye.

    f. Conditioning solution is essentially an enhanced wetting solution, providing improved comfort and wettability of the lens.

G. Instillation of eye medication (Figure 29.1)

    1. Wash hands.

    2. Shake suspensions to evenly distribute ingredients.

    3. Hold the lower eye lid down to form a pouch between the lid and the eyeball.

    4. Always apply eye drops before applying eye ointment. Dispense the recommended number of drops into the pouch for eye drops. Keep the eyelids closed and apply gentle pressure to the inner canthus for 1–2 min. Wait 5–10 min before instilling another eye medication.

    5. Ointments should be applied to the lower conjunctival sac as a 1/2-inch ribbon. To minimize blurred vision, a decreased amount of ointment may be applied to the eye. Blurred vision will be less noticed by the patient if the ointment is administered at bedtime, if feasible.

Guidelines for Instilling Eye Medications:

Follow these general guidelines when instilling eye medication:
- Shake suspensions or "milky" solutions to obtain the desired medication level.
- Wash hands thoroughly before and after the procedure.
- Ensure adequate lighting.
- Read the label of the eye medication to make sure it is the correct medication.
- Assume a comfortable position.
- Do not touch the tip of the medication container to any part of the eye or face.
- Hold the lower lid down; do not press on the eyeball. Apply gentle pressure to the cheek bone to anchor the finger holding the lid.

- Instill eye drops before applying ointments.
- Apply a 1/2-inch ribbon of ointment to the lower conjunctival sac.

- Keep the eyelid closed, and apply gentle pressure on the inner canthus (punctal occlusion) near the bridge of the nose for 1 or 2 minutes immediately after instilling eyedrops.
- Using a clean tissue, gently pat skin to absorb excess eyedrops that run onto cheeks.
- Wait 5 to 10 minutes before instilling another eye medication.

Figure 29-1. Guidelines for instilling eye medication. [Modified with permission from Smeltzer SC, Bare BG. Brunner & Suddarth's Textbook of Medical-Surgical Nursing, 10th ed. Philadelphia: Lippincott Williams & Wilkins, 2004.]

STUDY QUESTIONS

Directions for questions 1–3: The questions and incomplete statements in this section can be correctly answered or completed by **one or more** of the suggested answers. Choose the answer, **A–E.**

1. Which of the following nonprescription products is approved by the U.S. Food and Drug Administration (FDA) for treatment of impacted cerumen?

    I. olive oil
    II. carbamide peroxide
    III. isopropyl alcohol 95% in anhydrous glycerin

A	if **I and II** are correct
B	if **I, II, and III** are correct
C	if **II only** is correct
D	if **III only** is correct
E	if **I only** is correct

2. Which of the following otic conditions can be treated with a nonprescription agent?

    I. vertigo
    II. tinnitus
    III. external otitis
    IV. water-clogged ear

A	if **I, II, and III** are correct
B	if **III and IV** are correct
C	if **I and IV** are correct
D	if **I and II** are correct
E	if **IV only** is correct

3. Which of the following conditions is appropriate for the use of isopropyl alcohol 95% in anhydrous glycerin?

    I. treatment of impacted cerumen
    II. treatment of water-clogged ears
    III. prevention of external otitis
    IV. treatment of external otitis

A	if **I and II** are correct
B	if **II and III** are correct
C	if **III and IV** are correct
D	if **II only** is correct
E	if **III only** is correct

Directions for questions 4–5: Each of the questions, statements, or incomplete statements in this section can be correctly answered or completed by **one** of the suggested answers or phrases. Choose the **best** answer.

4. All of the following are true regarding carbamide peroxide *except* which one?

    (A) Carbamide peroxide softens earwax by the foaming action produced when oxygen is released.
    (B) Carbamide peroxide is safe for pharmacist recommendation in patients age 6 years and older.
    (C) Appropriate dosing for carbamide peroxide is 5–10 drops in the ear 2 times daily.
    (D) Carbamide peroxide should be used for a maximum of 4 days unless otherwise directed.

5. All of the following are true regarding external otitis *except* which one?

    (A) Initial treatment for external otitis is an oral antibiotic and corticosteroid.
    (B) Symptoms of external otitis include otic itching, pressure and fullness in the ear, pain, and otic discharge.
    (C) Mechanical trauma to the ear with cotton-tipped applicators can contribute to increased susceptibility to external otitis.
    (D) External otitis is also referred to as swimmer's ear.

Directions for question 6: The question in this section can be correctly answered by **one or more** of the suggested answers. Choose the answer, **A–E.**

6. Which of the following is an appropriate counseling tip for administration of otic drops?

I. Pull the earlobe up and back to straighten the ear canal for children.

II. Pull the earlobe down and back to straighten the ear canal for adults.

III. Fill the otic syringe with hot water.

IV. If cotton is used to retain medication in the ear, it should not be left in the ear for longer than 1 hr.

A if **III only** is correct
B if **IV only** is correct
C if **I and II** are correct
D if **I, II, and IV** are correct
E if **III and IV** are correct

Directions for questions 7–17: Each of the questions, statements, or incomplete statements in this section can be correctly answered or completed by **one** of the suggested answers or phrases. Choose the **best** answer.

7. All of the following are true regarding ophthalmic formulations *except* which one?

(A) Vehicles enhance contact time of the ophthalmic product.
(B) Antioxidants prevent product deterioration.
(C) Wetting agents reduce surface tension of the lens.
(D) Tonicity adjusters are used to maintain a pH between 6.0 and 8.0.

8. Which of the following is appropriate treatment of diagnosed corneal edema?

(A) hyperosmotic agent
(B) vasoconstrictor
(C) antihistamine
(D) artificial tears

9. Which of the following is also known as "pink eye"?

(A) allergic conjunctivitis
(B) bacterial conjunctivitis
(C) viral conjunctivitis
(D) environmental conjunctivitis

10. All of the following are antioxidants used for the treatment and/or prevention of ophthalmic disorders *except*

(A) vitamin D.
(B) β-carotene.
(C) vitamin C.
(D) lutein.

11. Which of the following solutions may be used to clean and moisten the surface of the contact lens while the lens is still in the eye?

(A) cleaning solution
(B) wetting solution
(C) soaking solution
(D) rewetting solution

12. Which of the following is true regarding ophthalmic antihistamines?

(A) Pheniramine and tetrahydrozoline are the only two nonprescription ophthalmic antihistamines available.
(B) Ophthalmic antihistamines are available only in combination with naphazoline.
(C) Ophthalmic antihistamines should not be recommended in patients with hypertension.
(D) Ophthalmic antihistamines may produce rebound congestion if used in excess or for extended durations.

13. Which of the following is the only astringent used in nonprescription ophthalmic agents that is recommended by the U.S. Food and Drug Administration (FDA)?

(A) edetic acid
(B) benzalkonium chloride
(C) zinc sulfate
(D) povidone

14. The definition of a surfactant (an ingredient in toothpaste) can best be described by which of the following statements?

(A) It prevents drying of the preparation.
(B) It removes debris by its detergent action and causes foaming, which is usually desired by the patient.
(C) It physically removes plaque and debris.
(D) It determines the texture, dispersiveness, and appearance of the product.
(E) It adds flavor to the preparation, which makes it more appealing to the patient.

15. A 16-year-old girl stops by a pharmacy on her way home from school. She says to the pharmacist, "I have been using Proxigel daily to bleach my teeth in preparation for my spring formal. However, my teeth are becoming very sensitive." Each of the following statements is advice that the pharmacist might suggest *except* which one?

(A) There is a possibility that you may damage the gingival tissue and tooth pulp.
(B) Oxidizing agents may have the potential for mutating or enhancing the carcinogenic effects of other agents (e.g., tobacco).
(C) Bleaching teeth is best done under dental supervision.
(D) Proxigel is an antiseptic that contains zinc and should not be used for cosmetic whitening of the teeth.
(E) The most common ingredient in products responsible for teeth whitening is 10% carbamide peroxide, which can cause sensitivity.

16. All of the following products may be recommended by a pharmacist for the treatment of canker sores *except*

(A) benzocaine.
(B) Zilactin-B.
(C) Bayer aspirin placed directly on the oral lesion.
(D) Anbesol.
(E) Orajel.

17. The U.S. Food and Drug Administration (FDA) has approved which ingredient for protection against painful sensitivity of the teeth caused by cold, heat, acids, sweets, or contact?

(A) dicalcium phosphate
(B) sodium lauryl sulfate
(C) 5% potassium nitrate
(D) zinc chloride
(E) calcium carbonate

Directions for questions 18–20: The questions and incomplete statements in this section can be correctly answered or completed by **one or more** of the suggested answers. Choose the answer, **A–E.**

A	if **I only** is correct
B	if **III only** is correct
C	if **I and II** are correct
D	if **II and III** are correct
E	if **I, II, and III** are correct

18. Which of the following compounds is/are considered a suspending agent (an ingredient in dentifrices)?

I. dicalcium phosphate
II. karaya gum
III. methylcellulose

19. Cold-sore treatment might include which of the following ingredients?

I. benzocaine
II. docosanol
III. camphor

20. Pharmacists can recommend over-the-counter (OTC) drug treatment for which of the following ear conditions?

I. treatment of accumulated earwax
II. prevention of blocked ears caused by altitude changes
III. treatment of water-clogged ears

ANSWERS AND EXPLANATIONS

1. The answer is C (II) *[see I.B.1.d.(1)]*.
Carbamide peroxide is the only FDA-approved agent for cerumen removal. Olive oil and mineral oil are used to remove cerumen, but are not FDA approved. Isopropyl alcohol 95% in anhydrous glycerin is FDA approved for water-clogged ears, but not cerumen removal.

2. The answer is E (IV) *[see I.B.1.d; I.B.2–4]*.
Patients exhibiting symptoms of vertigo, aside from motion sickness, should be referred to a medical provider. There is no FDA-approved treatment for tinnitus. External otitis (swimmer's ear) should be treated with a prescription otic antibiotic and corticosteroid. Only impacted cerumen and water-clogged ears may be treated with nonprescription products.

3. The answer is D (II) *[see I.B.5]*.
Isopropyl alcohol 95% in anhydrous glycerin is FDA approved only for treatment of water-clogged ears. Labels on products of isopropyl alcohol 95% in anhydrous glycerin should not claim to be used for treatment or prevention of external otitis (swimmer's ear) because this is a separate disorder from water-clogged ears. Treatment for impacted cerumen is carbamide peroxide.

4. The answer is B *[see I.B.1.d.(1)]*.
Carbamide peroxide softens earwax through its foaming action when oxygen is released. It is labeled for ages 12 and older. Therefore, for children < age 12 with suspected cerumen impaction should be seen by a medical provider. Patients should instill 5–10 drops of carbamide peroxide into the ear 2 times daily for up to 4 days.

5. The answer is A *[see I.B.4.a–c]*.
External otitis is referred to as swimmer's ear. Though prolonged exposure to moisture is the typical cause of external otitis, mechanical trauma, such as the use of cotton-tipped applicators, fingers, or sharp objects in the ear, may cause the external ear canal to be more susceptible to damage and microorganism infiltration. Patients with external otitis may present with otic itching, a sensation of pressure or fullness in the ear, pain, or an otic discharge. Initial treatment is with an otic antibiotic and corticosteroid, not an oral antibiotic. Oral antibiotics are indicated when the infection is unresponsive to otic treatment, the individual is immunocompromised, or a middle ear infection coexists.

6. The answer is B (IV) *[see I.C]*.
The earlobe should be pulled up and back to straighten the canal for adults and down and back to straighten the canal in children. Only warm water should be used in the otic syringe, as cold or hot water may induce dizziness. If cotton is used in the ear to retain the medication, it must be large enough to remove easily and should not be left in the ear for longer than 1 hr.

7. The answer is D *[see III.B]*.
Buffers are used in ophthalmic preparations to maintain a pH between 6.0 and 8.0. Tonicity adjusters ensure the product is isotonic, equal to 0.9%–60.2% sodium chloride.

8. The answer is A *[see III.D]*.
Once diagnosed by a physician, corneal edema is treated with hyperosmotic agents such as Muro solution or ointment to draw the fluid away from the cornea.

9. The answer is C *[see III.D.2]*.
Viral conjunctivitis is most often attributable to the adenovirus and is more commonly known as pink eye.

10. The answer is A *[see III.E]*.
The antioxidant vitamins examined for the prevention and/or treatment of ophthalmic disorders include vitamin A (retinol and β-carotene), vitamin C, and vitamin E. Lutein is an antioxidant pigment that functions to filter and protect the visual apparatus and its vascular supply. Lutein, is therefore, thought to be beneficial for improvement in vision in patients with dry age-related macular degeneration and prevention of cataracts. Vitamin D is not an antioxidant vitamin.

11. The answer is D *[see III.F.2].*
Rewetting solutions are the only contact lens solutions that may be used while the lens is still in the eye.

12. The answer is B *[see III.C.4].*
The only two available nonprescription ophthalmic antihistamines available are pheniramine and antazoline, which are available only in combination with the ophthalmic decongestant naphazoline. Ophthalmic antihistamines should not be recommended in patients with glaucoma or patients at high risk of developing narrow-angle glaucoma but are not contraindicated in patients with hypertension. Vasoconstrictors, not antihistamines, may produce rebound congestion when used in excess or for extended durations.

13. The answer is C *[see III.B].*
Edetic acid is an antioxidant and benzalkonium chloride (BAK) is a preservative used in ophthalmic formulations. Zinc sulfate is the only FDA-recommended astringent. Povidone is a vehicle used in ophthalmic formulations.

14. The answer is B *[see II.B.2.d.(1)].*
Sodium lauryl sulfate is used frequently as a surfactant in most dentifrices. Its detergent action aids in the removal of debris, and the foaming is usually desired by the patient. There is no evidence that surfactants possess anticaries activity or decrease periodontal disease. The FDA considers surfactants an inactive ingredient in dentifrices.

15. The answer is D *[see II.B.2.d.(4)].*
Teeth-whitening agents usually contain 10% carbamide peroxide, which is a white crystal that reacts with water to release hydrogen peroxide and, therefore, liberates free oxides. Cosmetic agents can alter the normal flora or cause tissue irritation, gingivitis, and teeth sensitivity. Antiseptics have been used as cosmetic whiteners (e.g., Gly-Oxide, Proxigel) along with calcium peroxide (e.g., Calprox in EpiSmile). EpiSmile also contains sodium monofluorophosphate.

16. The answer is C *[see II.C.1.c.(2)].*
Local anesthetics can provide relief of canker sore pain. The most common local anesthetics found in OTC products include benzocaine and butacaine. Some examples are Anbesol, Zilactin-B, and Orajel. Aspirin should not be retained in the mouth before swallowing or placed in the area of the oral lesions because of the high risk for chemical burn with necrosis.

17. The answer is C *[see II.B.2.d.(5)].*
Desensitizing agents should not be abrasive or used on a chronic basis unless directed by a dentist. The products approved by the ADA include the ingredients 5% potassium nitrate, 10% strontium chloride, and dibasic sodium citrate 2% in Pluronic gel.

18. The answer is D (II, III) *[see II.B.2.d.(1).D].*
Suspending agents are products that add thickness to the dentifrices. Examples are tragacanth, karaya gum, and methylcellulose. Dicalcium phosphate is categorized as an abrasive product.

19. The answer is C (I, II) *[see II.C.2.a–b].*
Cold-sore treatment involves keeping the lesion moist with emollient creams, petrolatum, or protectants. Local anesthetics (e.g., benzocaine, dyclonine, salicyl alcohol) may be used. In addition, docosanol 10% cream (Abreva) and tetracaine 2% gel (Viractin) are available without a prescription for the treatment of cold sores. Topical counterirritants (e.g., camphor) and caustics or escharotic agents (e.g., phenol, menthol, silver nitrate) are not recommended because they may further irritate the tissue. Cold sores are usually self-limiting and heal within 10–14 days without scarring.

20. The answer is E (I, II, III) *[see I.B].*
OTC drug treatment can be recommended for all of these ear conditions.

30
OTC Dermatological Agents

Larry N. Swanson

I. PEDICULOSIS AND PEDICULICIDES

A. Introduction. Pediculosis is a skin infestation produced by blood-sucking lice. Lice are small, flat, wingless insects with stubby antennae and three pairs of legs that end in sharp, curved claws. Three **types of lice infest humans.**

1. *Pediculus humanus capitis* (i.e., the head louse)

2. *Pediculus humanus corporis* (i.e., the body louse)

3. *Phthirus pubis* (i.e., the pubic, or crab, louse)

B. Life cycles. The lice that infest humans pass through similar life cycles.

1. **Location.** All lice need human warmth to survive.
   a. **Head** and **pubic lice** spend their entire cycle on the skin of the human host.
   b. **Body lice** live in clothing, coming to the skin surface only to feed.

2. **Development**
   a. Each type of louse develops from **eggs (nits)** that incubate for about 1 week. When the small, gray-white, tear-shaped eggs hatch, the nymphs appear.
   b. In about 3 weeks, the **nymphs** mature; then the females start to lay eggs.
   c. Each type of louse survives about 1 month as a **mature adult.** During this time, the female head louse can produce 3–6 eggs a day.

3. **Egg deposit**
   a. **Body lice** deposit their eggs on fibers of clothing, particularly in the seams. These lice can survive without food up to 10 days, and the eggs may remain viable for about 1 month. Daily clothing changes and boiling or ironing infested clothing can eradicate **body lice.**
   b. **Head** and **pubic lice** deposit their eggs on hair strands, about 1/4 inch from the skin. Adult head lice can survive on inanimate objects for about 20 hr; head lice nits may survive up to 10 days off the body.

C. Incidence. The incidence of lice infestations increases each year.

1. More than 10 million cases of head lice occur each year in the United States.

2. The bulk of these cases occur between September and November, when students are back in school.

3. In outbreaks of head lice, 70% of cases occur in children younger than 12 years.

4. Infestations tend to be more common in girls, presumably because of their greater tendency to share grooming items.

5. Unlike the other two forms of lice, body lice are associated with improper hygiene and are often present in homeless people. This infestation is rare in the United States, especially when people follow proper hygiene routines.

D. Medical problems

1. Both adult and nymph lice are blood sucking; they feed on humans by piercing the skin and introducing a small amount of saliva (which contains an **anticoagulant**) into the feeding area. All lice types feed on blood for about 30–45 min every 3–6 hr.
   a. The attachment of lice to the body causes an **erythematous papule,** which may **itch.**
   b. The female louse produces a sticky **cement-like secretion** that holds the eggs in place on the hair shaft so securely that ordinary shampooing does not remove it.

2. Neither head nor crab lice transmit infections, but body lice transmit **typhus, relapsing fever,** and **trench fever.**

3. Lice and humans have a true **parasitic relationship;** lice depend on the human host for shelter, food, and reproductive success. Once hatched, nymphs must have access to the human host within the first 12- to 24-hr period, if they are to survive.

E. Methods of transmission

1. Head lice are most commonly **spread by head-to-head contact** with an infested person through hats, caps, scarves, pillowcases, communal combs and brushes, or clothing that is hung close together (e.g., on a coat rack).

2. Pubic lice are **transmitted primarily through sexual contact,** but also through shared undergarments, towels, or toilet seats.
   a. The lice affect teens and young adults most often through sexual contact.
   b. Lice frequently coexist with other sexually transmitted diseases.
   c. Scratching in the genital areas may transmit pubic lice to other hairy regions, such as the eyelashes, eyebrows, sideburns, and mustaches.

F. Signs and symptoms

1. Head lice
   a. Most patients have fewer than 10 lice.
   b. The most common sign is **head scratching.**
   c. Skin redness around the nape (i.e., back) of the neck and above the ears is usually seen.
   d. The lice can be identified by direct examination using wooden applicator sticks or a comb to part the hair, then looking at the hair through a magnifying glass.
   e. The lice appear as tiny brownish gray spots that are often difficult to see. The shiny, **whitish silver eggs,** which appear almost as grains of sugar, are more likely to be seen than the lice. The nits are initially **deposited** about **1/4 inch from the scalp** on the hair shaft, and they may be **confused with dandruff or hairspray droplets.** Usually, hair grows at a rate of about 1/2 inch per month, so the duration of infestation can be assessed based on this information.

2. Pubic lice. The primary symptom is scratching in the genital area.

3. Body lice. The most common symptoms are bites and itching, which are commonly seen as vertical excoriations on the trunk area.

G. Treatment

1. There are **three steps** in the treatment of **head and body lice.**
   a. Treat the lice and nits with a pediculicide agent.
   b. Control the symptoms of itching to prevent secondary infection.
   c. Clean the environment of potential lice and nits.

2. Itching. Pharmacists should advise patients that even after the causative organism and nits have been killed, itching may persist for several days. This aspect is very important because patients may decide to use pediculicides excessively, thinking that they have been ineffective when the itching continues. **Excessive use of pediculicides may result in excessive drying, which can cause further itching.**

3. Home remedies. Because of the social stigma attached to lice infestation, some individuals may resort to harmful home remedies. Examples of such uncomfortable, ineffective, and potentially dangerous approaches that should not be used include
   a. Shaving the head and pubic area
   b. Applying heat to the infested area with a hair dryer
   c. Soaking the head in hot water for several minutes
   d. Soaking the area of infestation with gasoline or kerosene

4. Over-the-counter (OTC) pediculicide products are considered first-line treatments and include
   a. Pyrethrins 0.17%–0.33% with piperonyl butoxide 2%–4%. This product is safe and effective for the treatment of head and pubic lice. The combination of ingredients is an example of **pharmacological synergism.**

(1) Pyrethrins kill by **disrupting ion-transport mechanisms at the nerve membranes.** These natural insecticides are derived from a mixture of substances obtained **from** the flowers of the **chrysanthemum** plant. Because not all eggs may be killed (it takes about 4 days for the nervous system of the louse to develop) with a single application of this agent or removed with a nit comb, it may be necessary to reapply the pyrethrin product within 7–10 days of the first application (because the usual hatching time of the eggs is 7–10 days).

(2) Piperonyl butoxide enhances the pediculicide effect of pyrethrins by **suppressing the oxidative degradation mechanisms of the lice.** Therefore, the length of time that the pyrethrins contact the lice is increased.

(3) Side effects from either agent are **uncommon.**

    (a) Contact dermatitis (see IV) is the most frequently reported side effect.

    (b) Allergic reactions. Because pyrethrins are derived from a plant (chrysanthemum), they may produce hay fever (i.e., allergic rhinitis) and asthma attacks in susceptible individuals. Thus patients who have known allergies to ragweed or chrysanthemum plants should use this product with caution.

(4) Common **trade names** for this product include Rid Lice Killing Shampoo, Clear Lice Killing Shampoo.

(5) Directions for use (shampoo)

    (a) Apply the product, undiluted, to the dry hair until it is entirely wet.

    (b) Allow the product to **remain on the head for 10 min.**

    (c) Rinse thoroughly with warm water.

    (d) Dry the area, preferably with a disposable cloth.

    (e) Comb hair in the previously infested area **with a fine-toothed comb** to remove dead lice and eggs.

    (f) Do not exceed two applications within 24 hr. It may be necessary to reapply the shampoo in 7–10 days [see I.G.4.a.(1)].

b. Permethrin (Nix) is a pyrethroid (i.e., a synthetic version of a pyrethrin). It is indicated for the treatment of head lice only.

(1) Mechanism of action. Permethrin has a **similar mechanism of action as the pyrethrins.**

(2) Application. Permethrin comes in the form of a 1% **creme rinse** and should be applied like a conventional hair conditioner after the hair has been shampooed (use a shampoo with no conditioner), rinsed, and towel dried. The hair should be thoroughly saturated with undiluted permethrin (25–30 mL), which should **remain on the hair for 10 min. then rinsed.**

(3) Effectiveness. A single application is generally effective in killing lice. Because the agent is retained on the hair shaft, the product provides **continuing activity for up to 14 days.** This residual effect persists regardless of normal shampooing.

    (a) Even with the residual activity, there still may be the need for retreatment in 7–10 days.

    (b) Comb hair in the previously infested area **with a fine-toothed comb** to remove dead lice and eggs.

    (c) There is, at least theoretically, the speculation that because low-level residual amounts of this agent are retained on the hair, it may be possible that when suboptimal levels are present, some lice may survive and give rise to strains that are resistant.

c. OTC pediculicide treatment failure. Treatment failure with the use of the preceding agents has been reported. Speculations as to the cause of this treatment failure include failure to follow product instructions, noncompliance with nit removal, and head-lice drug resistance. Studies support the theory that there are now "super lice" that have survived exposure to pyrethrins and permethrin.

5. Prescription products are included here to put into perspective how the OTC agents fit into therapy.

a. Malathion (Ovide) is an organophosphate cholinesterase inhibitor that has been widely used as a lawn and garden insecticide. Resistance has also become an issue with this agent.

(1) Mechanism of action. Sulfur atoms in the malathion bind with sulfur groups on the hair, giving a residual protective effect against reinfestation.

    (2) Application. Malathion is prepared as a lotion in 78% alcohol; therefore, caution should be used near an open flame or a hair dryer. The product should be sprinkled on dry hair and left for 8–12 hr before rinsing. A fine-toothed comb should be used to remove the dead lice and eggs.

    (3) No systemic **adverse effects** have been reported with topical use of this medication.

      (a) The alcoholic vehicle may produce stinging and possible flammability.

      (b) Although this agent may be effective, its unpleasant odor (owing to sulfhydryl compounds), the required time of 8–12 hr on the scalp, and those points noted in I.G.5.a.(3).(a) represent the main drawbacks.

  b. Lindane, or γ-benzene hexachloride has fallen into disfavor because of the potential for toxicity and the fact that its efficacy is less than the other agents available (both prescription and OTC products). Resistance to this agent is widespread.

    (1) It has **neurotoxicity potential** because of percutaneous absorption; therefore, its use should be avoided in infants, pregnant and nursing women, and anyone with a neurological disorder. Severe **central nervous system (CNS) toxicity** has occurred in infants, with seizures and deaths reported, particularly when the lotion is used or when the agent is ingested. Toxicity has been minimal when the shampoo is used properly to treat head lice.

  6. Adjunctive therapy

    a. Nit removal

      (1) The pediculicide products mentioned vary in their ability to kill the lice nits. To ensure successful therapy, after pediculicide application, the nits should be removed with a **fine-toothed comb.** A sturdy **metal comb** (like the LiceMeister) is recommended by the National Pediculosis Association (NPA). Many schools have a **"no nit" policy**—that is, a child's hair and scalp must be free of nits before he or she is allowed to return to the classroom.

      (2) Although various substances have been used in an effort to dislodge the nits from the hair shafts, most, if not all, have been unsuccessful. A mixture of 50% vinegar and 50% water has been recommended, but its effectiveness has been questioned. A lice egg remover containing various enzymes comes as part of a kit, but challenges have been made to its effectiveness.

    b. Treatment of other household members. Once a lice infestation has been identified in one member of the household, all other members should be examined carefully. Everyone who is infested should be treated at the same time.

    c. Adjunctive methods for controlling lice infestations

      (1) Washable material items such as linens, towels, hats, and clothing should be machine-washed in hot water and dried in a hot dryer to destroy lice and nits.

      (2) Nonwashable material goods should be dry-cleaned or sealed in a plastic bag for 2 weeks.

      (3) Personal items (e.g., comb, brushes) should be soaked in hot water (130°F) for at least 15 min.

      (4) Furniture and household items (e.g., carpets, chairs, couches, pillows) should be vacuumed thoroughly. OTC spray products that contain pyrethrins are no more effective than vacuuming in terms of removing the risk of reinfestation.

    d. Pediculicides should not be used around the eyes. For **eyelash pubic lice infestations, petrolatum** applied five times a day asphyxiates lice, or gentle removal with baby shampoo may be helpful.

H. Head lice myths are numerous. The following additional facts may reassure and inform patients and parents of patients.

  1. No significant difference in incidence occurs among the various socioeconomic classes or races.

  2. Hygiene and hair length are not contributing factors.

  3. Head lice do not fly or jump from person to person.

  4. Head lice do not carry other diseases.

  5. Head lice cannot be contracted from animals, and pets are not susceptible to *Pediculus humanus capitis.*

6. The head does not have to be shaved to get rid of lice.

7. Washing hair with "brown" soap is not effective.

8. Head lice are unrelated to ticks.

9. Hair does not fall out as a consequence of infestation.

10. Head lice infestations can occur at any time of the year.

II. ACNE AND ITS TREATMENT

A. Overview

1. **Definition.** Acne vulgaris is a disorder of the pilosebaceous units, mainly of the face, chest, and back. The lesions usually start as open or closed comedones and evolve into inflammatory papules and pustules that either resolve as macules or become secondary pyoderma, which results in various sequelae.

2. **Incidence**
   a. Acne vulgaris is the **most common** skin disease of adolescence; it affects about 85% of all people between the ages of 12 and 24.
   b. It affects primarily adolescents in junior high and senior high, then decreases in adulthood.

3. **Importance**
   a. Acne vulgaris is usually **self-limiting.**
   b. However, the condition is significant to adolescents because of heightened self-consciousness about appearance.
   c. A great majority of people do not consult a physician for treatment of acne; therefore, a pharmacist can play a significant role.

B. Origins and pathophysiology

1. The **pathogenesis** of acne vulgaris involves **three events.**
   a. **Increased sebum production**
      (1) Sebum secretion is regulated primarily by **androgens,** which are actively secreted in both sexes beginning at puberty.
      (2) One of these androgens, testosterone, is converted to **dihydrotestosterone (DHT).**
      (3) DHT levels induce the sebaceous glands to increase in size and activity, resulting in increased amounts of sebum.
   b. **Abnormal clumping of epithelial horny cells within the pilosebaceous unit**
      (1) Normally, keratinized horny cells are sloughed from the epithelial lining of the pilosebaceous duct in the hair follicles and are carried to the skin surface with a flow of sebum.
      (2) In the patient with acne, the keratinization process is abnormal, characterized by increased adherence and production of follicular epithelial cells. This process is called **retention hyperkeratosis,** and it results in obstruction of the outflow of the pilosebaceous unit.
   c. **Presence of *Propionibacterium acnes*** (a gram-positive anaerobe)
      (1) People with acne have skin colony counts of *P. acnes* that are significantly higher than the counts of those without acne.
      (2) *P. acnes* produces several enzymes, including lipases, that break down sebum triglycerides to short chain free fatty acids (FFAs), which are irritating, cause comedones, and result in inflammation.

2. **Sequence of acne lesion development**
   a. Mechanical blockage of a pilosebaceous duct by clumped horny cells results in a **closed comedo (i.e., a whitehead).**
   b. When a closed comedo develops, it can form either a papule or an **open comedo (i.e., a blackhead).** The **dark color** of the blackhead is attributed to a combination of melanin, oxidized lipid, and keratinocytes, **not** to **dirt.**
   c. The lesion may enlarge and fill with pus, which is then termed a pustule.

    d. In more severe cases of acne, papules may develop into nodules or cysts.

    e. The term *pimple* nonspecifically refers to whiteheads, blackheads, papules, and pustules.

C. Clinical features

    1. Location. Acne vulgaris lesions usually occur on the face, neck, chest, upper back, and shoulders. Any or all types of lesions may be seen on a single patient.

    2. Symptoms. This condition is usually asymptomatic; however, some patients may have pruritus or pain if large, tender lesions are present.

    3. Classification. It is important to differentiate **noninflammatory** from **inflammatory** acne to determine the best treatment approach. There have been many rating or grading scales for acne severity (Table 30-1). **Cystic acne** is present when the follicular wall ruptures occur deeper in the dermis and nodules and cysts are seen. Because of the potential for scarring, cystic acne patients should be referred to a physician for treatment. Scarring occurs with hypertrophic ridges, keloids, or atrophic "ice pick" pits.

D. Complicating factors. Other factors have been implicated in the exacerbation of acne.

    1. Drugs and hormones

        a. Many topical and systemic medications (e.g., bromides, iodides, topical coal tar products, androgens, phenytoin, progestins, lithium, corticosteroids) can be comedogenic and can make acne worse or can induce acne-like eruptions (i.e., acneiform lesions).

        b. Acneiform eruptions differ from true acne lesions in that apparently no comedo forms, eruptions are usually acute, and the lesions usually are all in the same stage of development.

    2. Stress does not cause acne but may exacerbate it.

    3. Diet. There is very little evidence to support a relationship between diet and acne. Many different foods have been blamed for acne, from chocolates and sweets to shellfish to nuts and other fatty foods. Several studies have demonstrated that **chocolate does not affect acne.** The majority of dermatologists today make the following recommendations regarding diet.

        a. The patient should be eating a well-balanced diet. As with most other diseases, and as a matter of good health, excess fats and simple carbohydrates should be avoided.

        b. The patient who insists that certain foods cause exacerbation of acne should probably avoid those foods.

    4. Physical trauma or **irritation** can promote the rupture of plugged follicles, which can produce more inflammatory reactions. Scrubbing the face, wearing headbands, cradling the chin with the hand, and picking at the pimples can contribute to the primary inflammation process. **Gentle** regular **washing** with soap and water can be beneficial.

Table 30-1. Assessment of Acne Severity

Grade of Acne	Qualitative Description	Quantitative Description
I	Comedonal acne	Comedones only, < 10 on face, none on trunk, no scars; noninflammatory lesions only
II	Papular acne	10–25 papules on face and trunk, mild scarring; inflammatory lesions < 5 mm in diameter
III[a]	Pustular acne	More than 25 pustules, moderate scarring; size similar to papules but with visible, purulent core
IV[a]	Severe/persistent pustulocystic acne	Nodules or cysts, extensive scarring, inflammatory lesions > 5 mm in diameter
—	Recalcitrant severe cystic acne	Extensive nodules/cysts

[a]Some overlap with previous grade of acne.
Reprinted with permission from Berardi RR. *Handbook of Nonprescription Drugs: An Interactive Approach to Self-Care,* 14th ed. Washington, DC, American Pharmaceutical Association, 2004:916.

5. **Cosmetics.** Some cosmetic bases and certain cosmetic ingredients are comedogenic (e.g., lanolins, petroleum bases, cocoa butter). Preparations such as cleansing creams, suntan oils, and heavy foundations should be avoided.

6. **Menstrual cycle.** Some women may notice flare-ups of acne during the premenstrual part of the cycle. Fluctuations in the level of progesterone are the probable cause.

7. **Environmental factors.** Very humid environments or heavy sweating lead to keratin hydration, swelling, and a decrease in the size of the pilosebaceous follicle orifice, which results in duct obstruction. The sun, as well as artificial ultraviolet (UV) light, can help acne by drying and peeling the skin, but both also can aggravate acne.

E. **Treatment and care**

1. **General**
   a. Most patients can be treated successfully with either topically or systemically administered medications or both. Acne often improves when patients reach their early 20s.
   b. Even the most effective treatment programs may take several weeks to produce any clinical improvement. This aspect must be emphasized.
   c. People affected with acne should avoid anything that seems to worsen the condition (e.g., cosmetics, clothing, cradling the chin with the hand).
   d. The number and type of lesions should be roughly determined to assess further therapeutic responses.
   e. **Self-treatment with OTC agents** is appropriate only for patients with **noninflammatory grade I acne** of mild to moderate severity.

2. **Cleansing recommendations**
   a. Because many acne patients have oily skin, **gentle cleansing** two to three times daily is recommended for removing excess oil.
   b. Acne lesions cannot be scrubbed away. Compulsive scrubbing may actually worsen the acne by disrupting the follicular walls and thus setting the stage for inflammation.
   c. Mild facial soaps, such as Dove, Neutrogena, and Purpose, should be used to cleanse the skin.
   d. Medicated soaps containing sulfur, resorcinol, or salicylic acid are of little value because the medication rinses away rather than penetrates the follicle.
   e. Patients with mild comedonal acne might find benefit from cleansers containing pumice, polyethylene, or aluminum oxide particles (e.g., Brasivol). However, patients with inflammatory acne or sensitive skin should avoid these products.

3. **Approaches** to treatment depend on the severity of the condition. Although acne cannot be cured, most cases can be managed successfully with topical treatment alone. Based on the pathogenesis of the condition, potential methods include
   a. **Unblocking** the sebaceous duct so that the contents can be easily expelled
   b. **Decreasing** the amount of sebum that is secreted
   c. **Changing** the composition of the **sebum** to make it less irritating by decreasing the population of *P. acnes*

4. **Nonprescription topical medications**
   a. **Benzoyl peroxide** (2.5%–10%)—for example, Clearasil Maximum Strength Acne Treatment Cream, PanOxyl Aqua Gel (U.S. Food and Drug Administration [FDA] category 3)—has traditionally been recognized as the most effective topical OTC agent for acne, and many OTC acne products contain it. However, the latest monograph from the FDA changed the status of benzoyl peroxide from category 1 (generally recognized as safe and effective) to category 3I, indicating that more data are needed to prove its safety in regard to long-term photocarcinogenic effects. Marketing of this agent is permitted pending final evaluation of its tumorigenic potential.
      (1) **Effects.** Benzoyl peroxide has irritant, drying, peeling, comedolytic, and antibacterial effects. The clinical response shows only minimal differences among the 2.5%, 5%, and 10% concentrations.
         (a) A **beneficial effect** should be noticed within about 2 weeks, but the usual length of a therapeutic trial is 6–8 weeks.
         (b) As for **adverse effects,** benzoyl peroxide may cause a burning or stinging sensation, which gradually disappears. Most of the adverse effects from this agent relate to its therapeutic effect of irritating and drying the skin. For this reason,

the lowest concentration available should be chosen initially. About **2.5%** of patients will **develop a contact dermatitis** with its use.

- **(c)** The vehicle for the benzoyl peroxide is also important in its overall activity. The alcohol gel vehicle tends to be more effective than the lotion or cream formulations.
- **(d)** Benzoyl peroxide can discolor certain types of fabric or clothing material and can also bleach hair.

(2) Mechanism of action. Benzoyl peroxide has a dual mode of action, so it is effective against both inflammatory and noninflammatory acne.

- **(a)** Benzoyl peroxide decomposes to release oxygen, which is lethal to the *P. acnes* anaerobe.
- **(b)** As an irritant, it increases the turnover rate of epithelial cells, resulting in increased sloughing and promoting of resolution of comedones.

(3) Application

- **(a)** The affected area should be washed with mild soap and water, then gently patted dry.
- **(b)** The product should be massaged gently into the skin, avoiding the eyes, mouth, lips, and inside of the nose.
- **(c)** The product can be applied at night, left on for 15 or 20 min to test sensitivity, then washed off.
- **(d)** If no excessive irritation develops, apply once daily for the first few days.
- **(e)** If drying, redness, or peeling does not occur in 3 days, increase application to twice daily.
- **(f)** If patients have to use benzoyl peroxide during the day, advise them to use a sunscreen and avoid unnecessary sun exposure.

b. Salicylic acid (0.5%–2%), an irritant keratolytic agent, results in increased turnover of the epithelial lining (category 1). Through this effect, salicylic acid probably promotes the penetration of other acne products.

c. Sulfur (3%–8%), **sulfur** (3%–8%) **combined with resorcinol** (2%), **or resorcinol monoacetate** (3%)—for example, Clearasil Adult Care Acne Treatment Cream, Acnomel (category 1)

- **(1)** Sulfur is a keratolytic agent and has antibacterial actions.
- **(2)** Sulfur traditionally has been recognized as a less desirable product because it may be acnegenic with continued use, and it has an offensive color and odor.

d. Resorcinol (as a single agent) is a keratolytic agent that has been recognized as effective against acne **when the agent is combined with sulfur** (category 2).

F. Prescription medications, both topical and systemic, are included here for completeness and to put into perspective how OTC agents fit into acne therapy.

1. Topical prescription agents

a. Tretinoin (vitamin A acid, *trans*-retinoic acid, Retin-A) increases the turnover rate of nonadhering horny cells in the follicular canal, which results in comedo clearing and inhibits new comedo development.

(1) Effectiveness. Tretinoin is probably the most effective topical agent for acne, especially acne characterized by comedones. It is best used for **noninflammatory** acne. Tretinoin also may be used in combination with antibiotics or benzoyl peroxide for management of inflammatory acne.

(2) Side effects. Because of its irritant properties, tretinoin can cause **excessive irritation, erythema, peeling,** and increased risk for **severe sunburn.** There may be an initial exacerbation of the acne (pustular flare) at 2–4 weeks, but usually by 8 weeks, the patient will see marked improvement. Because this agent may cause photosensitivity, it should generally be applied at night.

(3) Application. The cream formulation of tretinoin, which is less irritating than the gel form should be used initially for patients with dryer skin. The patient with very oily skin may do well initially with the gel form. The retinoids should be applied 30 min after washing because moisture on the skin increases absorption and irritation. To minimize irritation, initially such a product can be applied every other day for 2 weeks, then daily. Other irritating substances, such as strong abrasive cleaners and astringents, should be avoided during treatment with tretinoin. Newer microsize reformulations of this agent (Retin-A Micro, Avita) are less irritating.

b. **Adapalene** (Differin) is a topical retinoid-like compound that is dosed once daily. It can be applied in the morning because of no photodegratdation, and it has less potential for photosensitivity.

(1) **Effectiveness.** It appears to cause less irritation than tretinoin with equivalent efficacy. Therapeutic results should be noticed in 8–12 weeks. It can be used as an alternative to tretinoin in individuals with mild to moderate acne.

(2) **Side effects.** The same precautions that apply to tretinoin apply also for adapalene.

c. **Tazarotene gel and cream** (Tazorac) is a retinoid prodrug for mild to moderately severe facial acne that is applied once daily in the evening. It has similar efficacy and precautions as tretinoin, and the dose-related **adverse effects** include itching, burning, stinging, and erythema (redness). The gel form appears to be more irritating than tretinoin. A pustular flare may occur at about 10–14 days after this product is begun.

d. **Topical antibiotics: erythromycin** (Eryderm), **clindamycin** (Cleocin-1) and **tetracycline.** These topical antibiotics are most effective when used in combination with benzoyl peroxide or topical retinoids. Combination products containing benzoyl peroxide and erythromycin (Benzamycin) and benzoyl peroxide and clindamycin (BenzaClin) are also available. When these antibiotics are used alone, bacterial resistance occurs rapidly. Benzoyl peroxide use in combination with these antibiotics protects against this resistance.

(1) **Mechanism of action.** The mechanism of action apparently involves suppression of the *P. acnes* organism, which in turn minimizes the inflammatory response due to the acne.

(2) **Application.** These antibiotics are applied directly to acne sites, thus minimizing serious side effects from oral administration.

(3) **Side effects.** There are **minimal** side effects to these topically applied antibiotics. **Mild burning** or **irritation** may occur. Although daily topical **Clindamycin** does not produce detectable levels in the urine after 8 weeks of administration, there is a potential risk of **pseudomembranous colitis. Tetracycline** can cause a **yellow staining of the skin.**

e. **Azelaic acid** (Azelex) and **sodium sulfacetamide and sulfur** are additional topical agents that are less effective than the other topical prescription agents. These agents might be used when others are not tolerated or as adjuncts to other therapies.

2. **Systemic prescription agents**

a. **Oral antibiotics/anti-infectives** are the most effective against inflammatory lesions because they suppress *P. acnes.* They may be used when topical combinations are not tolerated or have failed. Oral antibiotics have an onset of action of 3–4 weeks. They are prescribed for daily use over 4–6 months and then tapered and ultimately discontinued with acne improvement. Antibiotics do not affect existing lesions, but prevent future lesions through this effect. *P. acnes* resistance to antibiotic therapy has become an increasing problem; erythromycin resistance is the most commonly reported, and minocycline resistance is reported rarely. As noted previously, concomitant administration of benzoyl peroxide may decrease the incidence of resistance.

(1) **Tetracycline** is the **most frequently used** oral antibiotic for acne. It is preferred because of its effectiveness, low toxicity, and low cost.

(a) **Initial doses** are 250 mg, 2–4 times daily, gradually reduced to a maintenance dose of about 250 mg per day.

(b) **Side effects.** The more common adverse effects include upset stomach, vaginal moniliasis, and photosensitivity.

(2) **Erythromycin** (E-Mycin) may be used as an alternative to tetracycline.

(a) **Initial doses** range from 500 to 2000 mg per day in divided doses. A maintenance dose ranges from 250 to 500 mg per day.

(b) **Side effects.** The primary side effect associated with erythromycin is gastrointestinal distress.

(3) **Minocycline** (Minocin) **or doxycycline** (Vibramycin). Either of these agents can be taken in doses of 50–200 mg per day. Because of greater lipid solubility and enhanced penetration into sebaceous follicles, these agents may be useful for refractory cases. Either can be taken if bacterial resistance is suspected to erythromycin or if intolerable gastric irritation occurs after oral tetracycline. These two agents can be taken with food. Side effects to minocycline, including dizziness or vertigo and headache, discoloration of skin and visceral tissue, and drug-induced lupus erythematosus, limit the use of this agent. Doxycycline may be photosensitizing and should be swallowed with adequate fluids to prevent esophageal ulcerations.

(4) Trimethoprim-sulfamethoxazole (Bactrim, Septra) has been used successfully in patients with acne resistant to erythromycin or tetracyclines. Minocycline and doxycycline are preferred over this agent because of its side-effect profile. **Oral clindamycin** (Cleocin) is used rarely because of the risk of pseudomembranous colitis.

b. Oral isotretinoin (Accutane) is a vitamin A derivative indicated for **severe nodulocystic acne.** A single course of therapy results in a long-term stable remission in > 80% of patients.

    (1) Mechanism of action. Although the exact mechanism is unknown, isotretinoin decreases sebum production and keratinization, and it reduces the population of *P. acnes.*

    (2) Dosage. Treatment is usually begun with a daily dose of 0.5 mg/kg and increased to 1 mg/kg given in two divided doses with food for the usual duration of 20 weeks. A micronized formulation allows for lower once daily dosing with no regard to food intake.

    (3) Side effects include

        (a) Mucocutaneous dryness. Cheilitis (i.e., inflammation of the lips), dryness of the nasal mucosa, and facial dermatitis may occur with isotretinoin use. These effects can be treated with topical lubricants. Dryness of the eyes can also occur, so people using isotretinoin should not wear contact lenses.

        (b) Elevated serum levels. Isotretinoin may elevate serum triglycerides and cholesterol, as well as liver enzymes.

        (c) Birth defects. Isotretinoin is a **potent teratogen** and should not be given to pregnant women. A strict risk management program for isotretinoin use requires physicians to register patients to document negative pregnancy tests before use. Physicians who prescribe this agent and pharmacies that dispense it must be registered in an electronic FDA system.

        (d) Psychiatric effects. There have been reports of depression, suicidal behavior, and suicide. Data are inadequate to establish a causal relationship between isotretinoin administration and depression and suicide. This information must be taken in the context that teenagers with acne may often be depressed related to their appearance.

c. Antiandrogens and hormones

    (1) Estrogens can decrease sebum production through an antiandrogenic effect.

    (2) Some progestin agents in oral contraceptives (e.g., norethindrone, norgestrel) have androgenic activity that can stimulate sebum secretion resulting in acne. One of the progestins, **norgestimate,** is minimally androgenic, and when it is combined with **ethinyl estradiol** as a triphasic combination oral contraceptive agent (Ortho Tri-Cyclen), it is effective in the treatment of moderate acne in some women and is FDA approved for such. **Norethindrone acetate/ethinyl estradiol** (Estrostep) is also FDA approved for acne.

    (3) Spironolactone (Aldactone) is an oral antiandrogen which acts to decrease sebum production and may be used on a limited basis.

    (4) Corticosteroids. Although corticosteroids have been implicated as causing acne, they also can be used to treat severe acne. Intralesional injections of triamcinolone and systemic corticosteroids have been used for severe inflammatory acne and severe cystic acne, respectively. Prednisone (or its equivalent) in doses of 20 mg per day or higher may be used for a short period of time to quickly improve acne for important events like a wedding. Topical corticosteroids are not effective.

III. SUNLIGHT, SUNSCREENS, AND SUNTAN PRODUCTS

A. Introduction. Overexposure to sunlight damages skin. A suntan, which has traditionally been associated with health, is actually a response to injury. Of the three types of solar radiation, only the UV spectrum produces sunburn and suntan.

    1. The **UV spectrum** ranges from 200 to 400 nanometers (nm). Natural and artificial UV light is further subdivided into three bands.

        a. UVA (320–400 nm) can cause the skin to tan, and it tends to be weak in causing the skin to redden. UVA is about 1000 times less potent than a comparable dose of UVB in causing erythema, but it is only slightly blocked out by the ozone layer and reaches the earth's surface in 10–100 times the amount of UVB. Some have proposed that UVA be further subdivided into UVA I (340–400 nm) and UVA II (320–340 nm). UVA I is less erythrogenic and melanogenic than UVA II or UVB. UVA II is similar in effect to UVB.

  (1) **Uses.** UVA is often used in tanning booths and in psoralen plus UVA (PUVA) treatment of psoriasis.

  (2) **Disadvantages.** UVA is responsible for many **photosensitivity** reactions, **photoaging,** and **photodermatoses.** UVA rays can also **penetrate deeply into the dermis** and augment the cancerous effects of UVB rays.

  b. **UVB** (290–320 nm) **causes the usual sunburn reaction** and stimulates tanning. It has long been associated with sunlight skin damage, including the various skin cancers. It is the **most erythrogenic** and **melanogenic** of the three UV radiation bands. Small amounts of this radiation are required for normal **vitamin D synthesis** in the skin.

  c. **UVC** (200–290 nm) does not reach the earth's surface because most of it is absorbed by the ozone layer. Artificial UVC sources (e.g., germicidal and mercury arc lamps) can emit this radiation.

2. The **visible spectrum** (400–770 nm) produces the "brightness" of the sun.

3. The **infrared spectrum** (770–1800 nm) produces the "warmth" of the sun.

B. Sunburn and suntan

1. **Sunburn** is generally a **superficial burn involving the epidermis.** This layer is rapidly repaired while old cells are being sloughed off in a process called **peeling.** The newly formed skin is thicker and offers protection for the lower dermal layers.

  a. **Normal sequence after mild to moderate sunlight UV radiation (UVR) exposure**

    (1) Erythema occurs within 20–30 min as a result of oxidation of bleached melanin and dilation of dermal venules.

    (2) The initial erythema rapidly fades, and true sunburn erythema begins 2–8 hr after initial exposure to the sun.

    (3) Dilation of the arterioles results in increased vascular permeability, localized edema, and pain, which become maximal after 14–20 hr and last 24–72 hr.

  b. **Manifestations** range from mild (a slight reddening of the skin) to severe (formation of blisters and desquamation). If the effect is severe, the patient may experience pain, swelling, and blistering. Fever, chills, and nausea may also develop, as well as prostration, which is related to excessive synthesis and diffusion of prostaglandins.

2. **Suntan** is the result of two processes:

  a. **Oxidation of melanin,** which is already present in the epidermis

  b. **Stimulation of melanocytes** to produce additional melanin, which is subsequently oxidized on further exposure to sunlight

    (1) With increased melanin production, the melanocytes introduce the pigment into keratin-producing cells, which gradually become darkened keratin and a full suntan in 2–10 days.

    (2) Tanning increases tolerance to additional sunlight and reduces the likelihood of subsequent burning. However, dark skin is not totally immune to sunburn.

C. Factors affecting exposure to UVR

1. **Time of day and season.** The greatest exposure to harmful UVB rays occurs between 10 A.M. and 4 P.M. in midsummer. UVA rays are fairly continuous throughout the day and season.

2. **Altitude.** Sunburn is more likely to occur at high altitudes. UVB intensity increases 4% with each 1000-ft. increase in altitude.

3. **Environmental factors.** Atmospheric conditions (e.g., smog, haze, smoke) may affect (i.e., decrease) the amount of UVR reaching the skin. Although direct sunlight greatly reduces the amount of UV exposure needed to produce a burn, sunburn can occur without it. For example, a sunburn can also develop on a cloudy day because there is some UVR penetration through cloud layers (60%–80%). However, the **reflection of light rays** (e.g., by snow, sand, water) greatly **increases** the amount of UV **exposure to sunlight.**

4. **Predisposing factors.** People with fair skin and light hair are at greater risk for developing sunburn and other UVR skin damage than their darker counterparts.

D. Other reactions to sunlight (UVR) exposure

1. **Actinic keratosis** is a precancerous condition and may occur after many years of excessive exposure to sunlight. Typically arising during middle age or later, this disorder manifests as a sharply demarcated, roughened, or hardened growth, which may be flat or raised, and it may progress to **squamous cell carcinoma.**

2. **Skin cancer.** Chronic overexposure to sunlight may lead to **squamous cell carcinoma, basal cell carcinoma,** or **malignant melanoma.**
   a. **Squamous cell carcinoma.** Lesions usually appear as thickened, rough, scaly patches, which can bleed, and most commonly develops from actinic keratosis. It accounts for about 15% of skin cancers.
   b. **Basal cell carcinoma.** This is the most common of all skin cancers and accounts for about 80% of skin cancers. It may appear as pearly or translucent bumps and originates in the basal cells.
   c. **Malignant melanoma.** Malignant melanoma originates from melanocytes and is the deadliest form of skin cancer, and its incidence has been increasing. Moles should be watched for indications of malignancy—the **ABCD**s are
      (1) **A**symmetrical shape
      (2) **B**order irregularity
      (3) **C**olor that is nonuniform
      (4) **D**iameter > 6 mm.
   d. Malignant melanoma formation may be associated with intense, intermittent overexposure to the sun (sunburning).

3. **Drug-induced photosensitivity reactions**
   a. **Types**
      (1) **Photoallergy reactions** occur when light makes a drug become antigenic or act as a hapten (i.e., a photoallergen). These reactions also require previous contact with the offending drug. Photoallergy reactions are relatively **rare** and are associated more frequently with topically applied agents than with oral medications.
         (a) **Occurrence** of these reactions is not dose related. The patient is usually cross-sensitive with chemically related compounds.
         (b) **Rashes** are most prominent on light-exposed sites (i.e., face, neck, forearms, back of hands), and they usually occur, after an incubation period of 24–48 hr of combined drug and sun exposure, as an intensely pruritic eczematous dermatitis (a severe rash).
      (2) **Phototoxic reactions** occur when light alters a drug to a toxic form, which results in tissue damage that is independent of an allergic response.
         (a) **Occurrence.** These reactions are usually dose related, and the patient usually has no cross-sensitivity to other agents.
         (b) **Rashes** often appear as an exaggerated sunburn and are usually confined to areas of combined chemical and light exposure.
   b. **Implicated drugs.** Many drugs have been implicated in causing photoallergy and phototoxic reactions: thiazides, tetracyclines, phenothiazines, sulfonamides, and even sunscreens. Some drugs may produce both types of reactions.
   c. **Prevention.** Standard sunscreens do not always prevent photosensitivity reactions caused by drugs. UV light above 320 nm (i.e., UVA light) has been implicated in inducing photosensitivity reactions, so a chemical or physical sunscreen must cover this spectrum (see III.E.2).

4. **Photodermatoses** are skin conditions that are triggered or worsened by light within specific wavelengths. These conditions include polymorphous light eruption (PMLE), lupus erythematosus, and solar urticaria.

5. **Photoaging** is a skin condition that is not merely an acceleration of normal aging. UVA radiation is thought to be involved. The skin appears dry, scaly, yellow, and deeply wrinkled; it is also thinner and more fragile.

E. Sunscreen agents.
People can protect their skin from harmful UVR by avoiding exposure to sunlight and other sources of UVR, wearing protective clothing, and applying sunscreen.

1. **Application and general information.** All exposed areas should be covered evenly and liberally (2 mg/cm^2, which requires about 1 ounce of sunscreen per one total body application

for an average-size adult in a swimsuit) with sunscreen, optimally 30 min (2 hr for PABA and PABA esters) before sun exposure to allow for penetration and binding to the skin.

   a. **Substantivity.** Perspiration, swimming, sand, towels, and clothing tend to remove sunscreen and may increase the need for reapplication.

   (1) Substantivity is the ability of a sunscreen formulation to adhere to the skin while swimming or perspiring.

   (2) **Water resistant** labeling indicates that the formula retains its sun protection factor (SPF) after 40 min of activity in the water, sweating, or perspiring.

   (3) Labeling a product as **very water resistant** indicates that the product retains SPF after 80 min of activity in the water, sweating, or perspiring.

   b. **Protection.** Sunscreen products vary widely in their ability to protect against sunburn; the SPF and UVA/UVB ray protection should be noted to determine the level of protection. Moreover, baby oil, mineral oil, olive oil, and cocoa butter are not sunscreens (but are often used to attain a tan).

   (1) **SPF** gives the consumer a guide for determining how the product will protect the skin from UV rays, principally UVB rays. An SPF of 30 blocks about 97% of the UVB rays. Scientific evidence shows a point of diminishing returns at levels > 30; any benefits that might be derived from using sunscreens with an SPF > 30 are negligible. The FDA's most recent monograph requires sunscreens with an SPF > 30 to use one collective term "SPF 30 Plus" or "30 +." An SPF of at least 15 for most individuals is recommended by the Skin Cancer Foundation.

   (a) **Definitions.** A **minimal sun protection product** has an SPF of 2 to under 12; a **moderate sun protection product** has an SPF of 12 to under 30; a **high sun protection product** has an SPF of 30 or above.

   (b) **Derivation.** SPF is defined as the **minimal erythema dose (MED)** of protected skin divided by the MED of unprotected skin. MED is the amount of solar radiation needed to produce minimal skin redness.

   (c) **Example.** A person who usually gets red after 20 min in the sun and wants to stay in the sun for 2 hr (120 min) should apply a sunscreen with an SPF of 6 (120 min ÷ 20 min = SPF 6). An SPF 6 product should provide adequate coverage, provided it is not washed off (as from swimming) or dissolved by sweat. An SPF of 15 blocks approximately 93% of the UVB rays.

   (d) There is **no generally accepted comparable term that measures UVA protection,** although a few have been proposed. One major concern is that people may be staying out in the sun longer when they use sunscreen products that have high SPF values. If inadequate UVA protection is provided in that product, these individuals may be exposing themselves to very high amounts of UVA, with the potential for significant overexposure to this form of UV radiation.

   (2) **Skin cancer prevention.** Sunscreen application has been shown to prevent squamous cell carcinoma, but it is not absolutely confirmed that their use prevents melanoma. In fact, some studies have found that individuals who regularly use sunscreen have a higher risk of this cancer (perhaps because they can stay out in the sun longer before burning and thus experience longer periods of sun exposure).

   c. **Sensitivity.** Some people may be hypersensitive to sunscreen agents. Discontinue use if signs of irritation or a rash occur. Contact dermatitis may occur with some of these agents. If sensitive to benzocaine, procaine, sulfonamides, or thiazides, avoid PABA or PABA esters.

   d. **Specific information**

   (1) Do not use these products on infants younger than 6 months of age (there is concern about absorption of these agents).

   (2) Do not use a product with an SPF < 4 on children younger than 2 years of age (there is concern that an SPF < 4 will not provide adequate protection).

   (3) Recommend sunscreen products that are broad-spectrum sunscreens (i.e., that block both UVB and UVA).

2. The two basic **types of sunscreen agents** are physical sun blocks and chemical sunscreens (Table 30-2).

   a. **Physical sun blocks** are opaque formulations that reflect and scatter up to 99% of light in both the UV and visible spectrums (290–700 nm). Examples include **titanium dioxide** and **zinc oxide.** These sun blocks are less cosmetically acceptable than chemical sunscreens because they have a greasy appearance, but they may be useful for protecting

Table 30-2. Sunscreen Ingredients

Type	Sunscreens	UV Spectrum (nm)	Concentrations (%)
Chemical	*Benzophenones* Oxybenzone Dioxybenzone	UVA and UVB 270–350 260–380[a]	 2–6 3
	PABA and PABA esters P-aminobenzoic acid Ethyl dihydroxy propyl PABA Padimate O (octyl dimethyl PABA) Glyceryl PABA	UVB 260–313 280–330 290–315 264–315	 5–15 1–5 1.4–8 2–3
	Cinnamates Cinoxate Ethylhexyl-*p*-methoxycinnamate Octocrylene Octyl methoxycinnamate	UVB[b] 270–328 290–320 250–360 290–320	 1–3 2–7.5 7–10 —
	Salicylates Ethylhexyl salicylate Homosalate Octyl salicylate	UVB[c] 280–320 295–315 280–320	 3–5 4–15 3–5
	Miscellaneous Menthyl anthranilate (meradimate) Digalloyl trioleate Avobenzone (butyl methoxy- dibenzoylmethane; Parsol 1789) Phenylbenzimidazole sulfonic acid	UVB 260–380[d] 270–320 UVA 320–400 290–320	 3.5–5 2–5 3 4
Physical	Titanium dioxide Red petrolatum Zinc oxide	290–700 290–365[e] 290–700	2–25 30–100 —

[a]Values available when used in combination with other screens.
[b]Some UVA spectrum.
[c]Primarily UVB, but has about one third the absorbency of PABA.
[d]Values are concentrations higher than normally found in nonprescription drugs.
[e]At 334 nm, 16% UV radiation is transmitted; at 365 nm, 58% is transmitted.
Reprinted with permission from Drug Facts and Comparisons, 60th ed. St. Louis, MO: Wolters Kluwer, 2005.

small areas (e.g., the nose). These sun blocks are also useful for photosensitization protection. Newer, more dilute versions of titanium dioxide products and microfine, transparent forms of zinc oxide are more cosmetically appealing. Red petrolatum covers a lesser spectrum (290–365 nm).

  b. **Chemical sunscreens** act by absorbing a specific portion of the UV light spectrum to keep it from penetrating the skin. They can be categorized on the basis of their spectra of UVR blockage and basic chemical classification. Five main groups of chemical sunscreens are available.

  (1) **PABA** and **PABA esters** primarily absorb UVB rays. Examples are *p*-aminobenzoic acid, padimate O, and glyceryl PABA.

  (2) **Cinnamates** primarily absorb UVB rays. Examples are cinoxate and octyl methoxycinnamate.

  (3) **Salicylates** primarily absorb UVB rays. Examples are ethylhexyl salicylate and homosalate.

  (4) **Benzophenones** absorb UVB rays and sometimes extend into the UVA range. Examples are oxybenzone and dioxybenzone. Because of their extension into the UVA range, they are somewhat protective against photosensitivity reactions.

(5) Dibenzoylmethane derivatives. Avobenzone (Parsol 1789) or butyl methoxydibenzoylmethane, provides coverage over the entire UVA range although its absorbance decreases dramatically at 370 nm. Photosensitivity reactions from medications may not be completely prevented in the 370–400 nm range. In combination with other agents that cover the UVB range, reasonable protection for both the UVA and UVB ranges can be achieved.

(6) Other chemical sunscreens. Phenylbenzimidazole sulfonic acid does not match up with any of the classes above. It covers just the UVB range 290–320 nm.

(7) A new agent **ecamsule,** incorporated into a combination product (Anthelios SX) with avobenzone and octocrylene was approved by the FDA in July, 2006. The combination protects against both UVA and UVB.

   c. OTC sunscreen products. Most sunscreen products on the market contain combinations of two or more of the classes of chemical sunscreen agents described in preceding sections. To get adequate UVA protection, choose a product with avobenzone or a product with titanium dioxide or zinc oxide.

F. Special agents of interest

   1. **Dihydroxyacetone** (DHA) is a chemical agent that darkens the skin by interacting with keratin in the stratum corneum to produce an **artificial suntan.** It provides **no protection against UV rays** and may not produce a natural-looking tan. This is known as an artificial tan extender. DHA must be applied evenly. If an artificial suntan is achieved with this chemical, it wears off in a few days. In addition, it can discolor hair and clothing.

   2. **Bronzers** are artificial tan products that stain the skin. They are fully washable with soap and water and will not protect against solar radiation.

   3. **β-Carotene,** a vitamin A precursor, may produce skin coloration when ingested orally. Although β-carotene is protective against some forms of abnormal photosensitivity (e.g., erythropoietic protoporphyria), it has not been shown to protect against sunburn in normal individuals.

   4. **Canthaxanthin** is a carotenoid (provitamin A). It has been used as a food-coloring agent but has not been approved by the FDA for use as an oral tanning agent. It **does not produce a true suntan** but is deposited into fatty tissues under the skin. It probably does not protect the skin from sunburn.

   5. **Tyrosine** has been promoted as a **tan accelerator** or **tan promoter.** Because melanin pigment is eventually synthesized from tyrosine, the theory is that topically applied tyrosine will enhance the formation of melanin. However, **studies have not confirmed an enhanced tanning effect from this agent.**

IV. CONTACT DERMATITIS AND ITS TREATMENT

A. Introduction

   1. **Types of contact dermatitis.** Contact dermatitis is one of the **most common** dermatological conditions encountered in clinical practice. It has traditionally been divided into **irritant contact dermatitis** and **allergic contact dermatitis** on the basis of the origin and immunological mechanism.

   a. Irritant contact dermatitis is caused by direct contact with a primary irritant. These irritants can be classified as absolute or relative primary irritants.

   (1) Absolute primary irritants are intrinsically damaging substances that injure, on first contact, any person's skin. Examples include strong acids, alkalis, and other industrial chemicals.

   (2) Relative primary irritants cause most cases of contact dermatitis seen in clinical practice. These irritants are less toxic than absolute primary irritants, and they require repeated or prolonged exposure to provoke a reaction. Examples of relative primary irritants include soaps, detergents, benzoyl peroxide, and certain plant and animal substances.

   b. Allergic contact dermatitis. Many plants, and almost any chemical, can cause allergic contact dermatitis. Poison ivy is a classic example of allergic contact dermatitis, which is classified as a type IV hypersensitivity reaction. This type of allergic reaction is T cell–mediated, and the following **sequence of events** must occur to provoke it:

(1) The epidermis must come in **contact** with the hapten (i.e., the specific allergen).

(2) The **hapten–epidermal protein complex** (i.e., the complete antigen) must form.

(3) The antigen must **enter the lymphatic system.**

(4) Immunologically competent lymphoid cells, which are selective against the antigen, must form.

(5) On **reexposure** to the hapten, the typical, local delayed hypersensitivity reaction (i.e., contact dermatitis) occurs.

(6) The **induction period,** during which sensitivity develops, usually requires 14–21 days but may take as few as 4 days or more than several weeks. **Once sensitivity is fully developed:**

    (a) Reexposure to even minute amounts of the same material elicits an eczematous response, typically with an onset of 12 hr and a peak of 48–72 hr after exposure.

    (b) Sensitivity usually persists for life.

        (i) Most contact allergens produce sensitization in only a small percentage of exposed persons.

        (ii) Allergens or substances such as poison ivy, however, produce sensitization in > 70% of the population (50%–95% are sensitive to the poison ivy plant).

2. General phases of contact dermatitis

  a. Acute stage. Wet lesions, such as blisters or denuded and weeping skin, are evident in well-outlined patches. Also evident are erythema, edema, vesicles, and oozing.

  b. Subacute stage. In this phase, crusts or scabs form over the previously wet lesions. Allergic contact dermatitis and irritant contact dermatitis caused by absolute primary irritants produce both the acute and subacute stages.

  c. Chronic stage. In this phase, the lesions become dry and thickened (i.e., lichenified). Initially, dryness and fissuring are the signs. Later, erythema, lichenification, and excoriations appear. The chronic phase of contact dermatitis usually occurs more often with irritant contact dermatitis caused by relative primary irritants.

B. Toxic plants. Poison ivy and poison oak are the **most common causes** of allergic contact dermatitis in North America. These plants were formerly known as the *Rhus* genus, but they are now properly referred to as the *Toxicodendron* genus.

  1. Poison ivy (*Toxicodendron radicans* and *T. rydbergii*) grows as a vine or as a bush. It is found in most parts of the United States, but is especially prevalent in the northeastern part of the country. Poison ivy is often identified by its characteristic growth pattern, described by the saying "Leaves of three, let it be."

  2. Poison oak (*T. diversilobum*) is found in the western United States and Canada. It grows as an upright shrub or a woody vine. *T. toxicarium* is found in the eastern United States.

  3. Poison sumac (*T. vernix*) grows in woody or swampy areas as a coarse shrub or tree and is prevalent in the eastern United States and southeastern Canada.

C. Toxicodendron dermatitis. For dermatitis to develop, previous sensitization (a 5- to 21-day incubation period) caused by direct contact with a sensitizing agent is required (see IV.A.1.b). An oleoresin, **urushiol oil,** which is a pentadecacatechol, is the active sensitizing agent in poison ivy, poison oak, and poison sumac. There are slight differences in the chemical structures of the sensitizing agent in each of these plants, but the three agents cross-react.

  1. Release of the urushiol oil. The plants must be bruised or injured to release the oleoresin. It is **present in** the **roots, stems, leaves,** and **fruit.** The urushiol oil may remain active on tools, toys, clothes, pets, and under fingernails if those items have had contact with the broken plants.

    a. Urushiol oil does not volatilize, so one cannot get dermatitis from just being near a poison ivy plant; direct contact is necessary. **Burning plants,** however, can cause droplets of oil carried by smoke to enter the respiratory system, which can cause significant respiratory distress.

    b. A cut or damaged poison ivy, poison oak, or poison sumac plant initially yields a **clear fluid** containing the oleoresin, which **turns to a black inky lacquer** on exposure to air within a few minutes. This change can be a means for confirming identification of these plants.

   c. Because the oleoresin can rapidly penetrate the skin, the affected **area must be washed with soap and water within 10 min** after exposure to prevent the dermatitis eruption. Washing up to 30 min after exposure is still useful in removing some of the oleoresin.

2. If an individual has been **previously sensitized,** the lesions usually occur within 6–48 hr after contact with the allergen.

3. Typically, the **initial eruption** exists as small patches of erythematous papules (usually streaks). **Pruritus (itching) is the primary symptom.**
   a. Papules may progress to vesicles, which may then ooze and bleed when they are scratched. Secondary infection may then develop. Often, the inflammation is severe, and a significant amount of edema occurs over the exposed area.
   b. The lesions may last from a few days to several weeks. Left untreated, the condition rarely persists longer than 2–3 weeks.

4. Poison ivy dermatitis does not spread. New lesions, however, may continue to appear for several days despite lack of further contact with the plant. This reaction may be owing to the following facts:
   a. Skin that has been minimally exposed to the antigen begins to react only as the person's sensitivity heightens.
   b. Antigen is absorbed at varying rates through the skin of different parts of the body.
   c. The person inadvertently touches contaminated objects or may have residual oleoresin—for example, underneath the fingernails.

5. Poison ivy is not contagious. The serous fluid from the weeping vesicles are not antigenic. No one can "catch" poison ivy from another person.

D. Treatment. The treatment of irritant and allergic contact dermatitis focuses on therapy for the specific symptomatology.

1. A pharmacist should **refer a patient** with a poison ivy eruption to a physician if:
   a. The eruption involves a large area of the body (about 25%).
   b. The eruption involves the eyes, genital area, mouth, or respiratory tract (some patients may experience respiratory difficulties if they inhale the smoke of burning poison ivy plants).

2. The **severity of the eruption** depends on:
   a. The quantity of allergen that the patient has been exposed to
   b. The individual patient's sensitivity to the allergen

3. For severe eruptions, a patient should consult a physician, who may prescribe **systemic corticosteroids.**
   a. Systemic corticosteroids are the cornerstone of therapy. One should use sufficiently high doses to suppress this inflammation. Generally, it is recommended that prednisone be given in a dose of 60 mg/day for 5 days, then reduced to 40 mg/day for 5 days, then 20 mg/day for 5 days, then discontinued. Prepacked dosage packs of corticosteroids used over 6 days provide too low of a dose over too short a period of time.
   b. Some blisters may be drained at their base. The skin on top of the blister should be kept intact. Draining the blister allows more topical medication to penetrate for an antipruritic effect. Baths and soaks [see IV.D.4.b.(1).(b)] may be beneficial as well.

4. For a less severe eruption, the principal goals are to relieve the itching and inflammation and to protect the integrity of the skin.
   a. Several therapeutic classes of agents can be used **to relieve itching.**
      (1) The application of **local anesthetics**—for example, benzocaine (5%–20%)—may relieve itching. Relief may be of short duration (30–45 min), but application of benzocaine may be especially useful at bedtime, when pruritus is most bothersome. There is some question about the frequency of the sensitizing ability of benzocaine (0.17%–5%). Certainly, treatment should be discontinued if the rash worsens.
      (2) Topical antihistamines—for example, diphenhydramine (Benadryl cream or spray)—may provide relief of mild itching principally through a topical anesthetic effect rather than any antihistamine effect. Many would not recommend their use because they may also have a significant sensitizing potential, and in children with varicella infections (where the integrity of the skin is compromised), systemic absorp-

tion has occurred with symptoms of anticholinergic toxicity produced. Topical and oral diphenhydramine should not be used concurrently.

(3) **Counterirritants** include camphor (0.1%–3%), phenol (0.5%–1.5%), and menthol (0.1%–1%). These agents have an analgesic effect as a result of depression of cutaneous receptors. The exact antipruritic mechanism is not fully known, but a placebo effect may result from the characteristic medicinal odors of these agents.

(4) **Astringents** are mild protein precipitants that result in contraction of tissue, which in turn decreases the local edema and inflammation.

    (a) The principal agent used is **aluminum acetate** (Burow's solution).

    (b) **Calamine** (zinc oxide with ferric oxide, which provides the pink color) is also used sometimes. Calamine contracts tissue and helps dry the area, but the formation of the thick dried paste may not be tolerated by some people.

(5) **Topical hydrocortisone** (e.g., Cortaid), which is available in concentrations up to 1%, is minimally useful for its antipruritic and anti-inflammatory effects.

b. Basic treatment

(1) **Acute (weeping) lesions** (see IV.A.2.a)

    (a) **Wet dressings** work on the principle that water evaporating from the skin cools it and thus relieves itching. Wet dressings have an additional benefit of causing gentle débridement and cleansing of the skin.

    (b) **Burow's solution** (Domeboro) in concentrations of 1:20–1:40 as a wet dressing or a cool bath of 15–30 min 3–6 times per day provides a significant antipruritic effect.

    (c) **Colloidal oatmeal baths** (e.g., Aveeno) may also provide an antipruritic effect.

    (d) **Topical therapy that may hinder treatment**

      (i) **Local anesthetics and topical antihistamines** may sensitize.

      (ii) **Calamine** may make a mess without doing much good!

(2) **Subacute dermatitis** (see IV.A.2.b). **A thin layer of hydrocortisone cream or lotion (0.5%–1%)** may be applied 3–4 times a day to treat subacute dermatitis. Supplemental agents, such as topical anesthetics, may be used as well.

(3) **Chronic dermatitis** (see IV.A.2.c) is best treated with hydrocortisone ointment. This stage is observed more frequently in forms of contact dermatitis that involve continuous exposure to the irritant or allergen.

E. Prevention

1. The best treatment for poison ivy contact dermatitis is to **prevent contact** with the offending cause. This approach involves avoiding the plant and wearing protective clothing.

2. Barrier preparations. Bentoquatam (quaternium-18 bentonite), Ivy Block, an organoclay, is the first poison ivy blocker proven safe and effective. It comes as a lotion that should be applied at least 15 min before contact with the plant and then every 4 hr for continued protection against urushiol. It should be applied to leave a smooth, wet, visible film on the skin. Ivy Block may be removed with soap and water. Because of its alcohol content, patients should be instructed to stay away from flame during application until the product has dried on the skin.

STUDY QUESTIONS

Directions: Each of the questions, statements, or incomplete statements can be correctly answered or completed by **one** of the suggested answers or phrases. Choose the **best** answer.

1. A woman, who has not been in the sun for 4 months, develops redness on her chest after lying in the sun for 20 min. The next day, she applies a suntan lotion and develops the same degree of redness on her back in 2 hr and 20 min. What is the sun protection factor (SPF) of the lotion she is using?

   (A) 14
   (B) 10
   (C) 12
   (D) 9
   (E) 7

2. Which of the following cleansing products would a pharmacist recommend for a patient with inflammatory acne?

   (A) an abrasive facial sponge and soap used 4 times a day
   (B) aluminum oxide particles used 2 times a day
   (C) sulfur 5% soap used 2 times a day
   (D) mild facial soap used 2 times a day

3. If a patient needs a second application of an over-the-counter (OTC) pyrethrin pediculicide shampoo, how many days after the first application should this be done?

   (A) 4–5
   (B) 6
   (C) 7–10
   (D) 14–21
   (E) 15–17

4. All of the following treatments for personal articles infested with head lice would be effective *except*

   (A) placing woolen hats in a plastic bag for 2 weeks.
   (B) using an aerosol of pyrethrins with piperonyl butoxide sprayed in the air of all bathrooms.
   (C) machine-washing clothes in hot water and drying them using the hot setting on the dryer.
   (D) dry-cleaning woolen scarves.
   (E) soaking hair brushes in hot water for 15 min.

5. All of the following sunscreen agents or combinations of agents would likely help prevent a drug-induced photosensitivity reaction *except*

   (A) titanium dioxide,
   (B) octyl methoxycinnamate plus homosalate,
   (C) oxybenzone and padimate O,
   (D) zinc oxide,
   (E) padimate O plus avobenzone,

6. All of the following would be appropriate recommendations for an adult patient in the acute stage (i.e., blistering, weeping) of poison ivy contact dermatitis *except*

   (A) 60 mg per day of prednisone initially, then tapered over 15 days.
   (B) Burow's solution; 1:20 wet dressing to area for 15–30 min, 4 times per day.
   (C) two soaks per day in Aveeno Bath Treatment,
   (D) two applications of Ivy Block,

7. All of the following nonprescription agents have been classified by the U.S. Food and Drug Administration (FDA) as safe and effective (category 1) for acne *except*

   (A) sulfur.
   (B) salicylic acid.
   (C) sulfur-resorcinol combination.
   (D) benzoic acid.

8. Pharmacists educating patients about acne should mention all of the following *except*

   (A) eliminating all chocolate and fried foods from the diet.
   (B) cleansing skin gently 2–3 times daily.
   (C) using water-based noncomedogenic cosmetics.
   (D) not squeezing acne lesions.
   (E) keeping in mind that acne usually resolves by one's early 20s.

9. A 15-year-old male patient has been using benzoyl peroxide 5% cream faithfully every day for the past 2 months with no apparent side effects. All of the following can be said about this patient *except*

(A) he has been using this product for a long enough time to determine if the dose and dosage form are going to have any benefit.

(B) he should use this product no more frequently than every other day because of its irritating properties.

(C) this starting dose and dosage form are useful, especially if he has dry skin or it is wintertime.

(D) his scalp hair may look bleached if the product comes in contact with it.

(E) the product would sting if it got into his eyes.

10. All of the following descriptions match the therapeutic agent for poison ivy *except*

(A) calamine: phenolphthalein gives it the pink color.

(B) Ivy Block: useful in preventing poison ivy dermatitis.

(C) benzocaine: data regarding incidence of hypersensitivity are conflicting.

(D) hydrocortisone: useful for its antipruritic and anti-inflammatory effects.

11. All of the following statements related to sun protection are true *except* which one?

(A) The sun's intensity increases 20% when going from sea level to an altitude of 5000 ft.

(B) Water resistant labeling on a sunscreen product indicates that it will retain its SPF after 40 min of activity in water, sweating, or perspiring.

(C) Baby oil is not a sunscreen, but its application to the skin after tanning causes melanin to rise to the surface.

(D) Per the FDA, a product with an SPF of 50 must now be labeled "SPF 30 Plus."

(E) The SPF is really only a measure of ultraviolet B (UVB) protection.

12. All of the following statements about sunscreens are correct *except* which one?

(A) Malignant melanoma formation may be associated with intense, intermittent overexposure to the sun (sunburning).

(B) Dihydroxyacetone (DHA) will not prevent sunburn.

(C) Sunscreens are best applied immediately before going out in the sun.

(D) Avobenzone provides sunscreen coverage for the UVA spectrum.

(E) Tyrosine has been marketed as a tan accelerator or tan magnifier.

ANSWERS AND EXPLANATIONS

1. The answer is E *[see III.E.1].*
The SPF is the minimal erythema dose (MED) of protected skin divided by the MED of unprotected skin. Thus 2 hr and 20 min (140 min) divided by 20 min equals an SPF of 7.

2. The answer is D *[see II.E.2].*
For patients with inflammatory acne, the best product is a mild facial soap used 2 times a day. The soap should be gently rubbed into the skin with only the fingertips. Cleansing products that irritate already inflamed skin should be avoided.

3. The answer is C *[see I.G.4.a.(1)].*
Reapplication of pyrethrins with piperonyl butoxide should be within 7–10 days of the first application. Any lice nits that were not killed on the first application would have time to hatch and then be killed with the second application.

4. The answer is B *[see I.G.4 a; I.G.6.c].*
Pyrethrins with piperonyl butoxide in an aerosol form can be sprayed directly on inanimate objects (e.g., chairs, headrests) to kill head lice, but the combination should not be sprayed in the air like an aerosol deodorizer. Moreover, vacuuming the furniture would probably be as effective as spraying it. The other selections are appropriate for personal articles infested with head lice.

5. The answer is B *[see III.E.2; III.D.3.c].*
Octyl methoxycinnamate and homosalate protect against only UVB exposure. Because photosensitivity reactions are often associated with UVA radiation exposure, people also need sunscreen protection for this portion of the UV radiation band. The other agents listed cover at least part of both UVA and UVB spectra.

6. The answer is D *[see IV.D.3–4; IV.E.2].*
Ivy Block is used as a barrier protectant for the prevention of poison ivy dermatitis, *not* for the treatment of an acute eruption. The other options are appropriate to recommend to someone suffering from the acute stage of poison ivy dermatitis.

7. The answer is D *[see II.E.4].*
Benzoic acid has not been shown to be effective for acne treatment. The other agents, sulfur, salicylic acid, and a sulfur-resorcinol combination, are all safe and effective products for treating acne.

8. The answer is A *[see II.D.3].*
Evidence does not show that acne worsens from any particular type of food, including chocolate or fried foods. The other choices are pieces of information that the pharmacist should convey to a patient with acne.

9. The answer is B *[see II.E.4.a].*
Although the irritating properties of benzoyl peroxide might dictate applying it only every other day on initiating treatment, this patient has tolerated the agent on a daily basis for 2 months. Thus there would be no need to decrease the application frequency. All of the other choices do apply to this patient's use of benzoyl peroxide.

10. The answer is A *[see IV.D.4.a].*
Ferric oxide provides the pink color of calamine. All of the other descriptions match their associated agents.

11. The answer is C *[see III.C.2; III.E.1.b–c; III.E.2.b].*
Baby oil is not a sunscreen, and it has no effect on melanin. SPF does measure UVB protection, and an SPF higher than 30 must be labeled SPF 30 Plus. Water resistant sunscreen products must retain their SPF value after 40 min of water activity. The intensity of the sun does increase by 4% with each 1000-ft. rise in elevation.

12. The answer is C *[see III.D.2; III.E.1; III.E.2.b; III.F.1; IIIF.4].*
Optimally, sunscreens should be applied 1–2 hr before exposure to the sun. This allows time for the product to bind to the stratum corneum, which provides better protection. The other responses are correct.

31

OTC Weight-Control, Sleep, and Smoking-Cessation Aids

Jennifer D. Smith

I. WEIGHT CONTROL

A. Obesity is a growing epidemic in America, spanning all age groups from childhood to adulthood. Approximately 30.5% of adults were considered obese in the year 2000, and 15.5% of adolescents were considered overweight. This growing epidemic was responsible for 5.7% of total recent U.S. health expenditures.

   1. The U.S. Preventive Services Task Force (USPSTF) determined that the body mass index (BMI) is reliable and valid identifier for **adults** at increased risk for morbidity and mortality owing to overweight and obesity. The BMI is calculated as either weight (in pounds) divided by height (in inches squared) multiplied by 703 or as weight (in kilograms) divided by height (in meters squared). The following guidelines relate BMI to overweight and obesity:
      a. **Morbid obesity** is defined as a **BMI > 40 kg/m^2**.
      b. **Obesity** is defined as a **BMI > 30 kg/m^2**.
      c. **Overweight** is defined as a **BMI between 25 and 30 kg/m^2**.

   2. Trunkal fat accumulation, measured by **waist circumference,** is a **risk factor for cardiovascular disease and other diseases** (e.g., type 2 diabetes, sleep apnea, knee osteoarthritis) regardless if the individual is considered obese. Waist circumference is not a valid measurement in individuals with a BMI > 35 kg/m^2. Individuals with the following waist circumferences are considered at increased risk for cardiovascular and other diseases:
      a. A waist circumference in **men > 40 inches** (102 cm)
      b. A waist circumference in **women > 35 inches** (88 cm)

B. **Management.** Diet and exercise (lifestyle modifications) are the recommended first approach to weight loss, as well as sustained weight control. Though it seems relatively simple to eat a well-balanced diet and exercise regularly, time constraints and ease of access to highly processed foods are hurdles that Americans face in the fight against the bulge.

   1. **Caloric restriction.** To reduce weight (and thus BMI), energy intake should be less than the energy expended.
      a. The approximate adult energy requirements, based on actual weight, may be roughly estimated as follows. A 120 lb. active woman would require approximately 1800 kcal/day to maintain her current weight.
         (1) Bedridden or sedentary individuals: 10–12 kcal/lb.
         (2) Moderately active individuals (walking at regular pace): 13 kcal/lb.
         (3) Active individuals: 15 kcal/lb.
         (4) Very active individuals: 20 kcal/lb.
      b. To lose about 0.5 kg/week, a **deficit of 500–1000 calories (kcal) per day** must be met. A **safe rate of weight loss is considered to be 1–2 lb./week.**
      c. Several commercially available weight loss programs (e.g., Weight Watchers and Jenny Craig) exist today. When compared to self-help weight loss programs, some commercially available programs have shown enhanced and sustained weight loss, which may be attributable to the social support provided.

   2. **Exercise** can decrease the appetite and increase body metabolism. Exercise adds only modestly to initial weight loss but is the key component of **sustained weight loss.**

C. **Dietary supplements.** In 2001, retail sales of weight loss supplements in the United States were estimated to be $>$ **$1.3 billion.** Americans have begun to seek nonprescription weight loss products for a variety of reasons.

   1. Some individuals may view dietary supplements as a quick resolution to the growing epidemic, because the obtainment of desired or reduced body weight with long-term lifestyle

changes is perceived as difficult. Many advertisements of weight loss products give inflated claims, offering rapid results with little to no modification in lifestyle habits. Some people view dietary supplements as natural and, therefore, mistakenly believe they are safe to use.

2. With the implementation of the Dietary Supplement Health and Education Act of 1994, manufacturers are **not required to demonstrate product safety and efficacy before marketing** supplements. In addition, the **adherence to good manufacturing practices is not mandatory** for manufacturers of dietary supplements. The lack of evidence for product safety and efficacy, coupled with potential deviation from good manufacturing practices raises concerns for healthcare providers who attempt to make appropriate recommendations to patients seeking nonprescription weight loss products.

3. The U.S. Food and Drug Administration (FDA) files action against manufactures of supplements determined unsafe, falsely labeled, labeled with misleading claims, adulterated, or misbranded.

4. The Federal Trade Commission (FTC) takes action against manufacturers providing product advertising that is misleading or makes unsubstantiated claims.

5. Numerous single- and multiple-entity products are available on the market today, each under the scrutiny of the FDA and FTC. The most commonly seen ingredients in weight loss products currently marketed, organized by purported mechanisms of action, are the following:
   a. **Increase energy expenditure**
      (1) **Ephedra.** Contains supplements that were **banned by the FDA in April 2004** owing to unreasonable risks of illness or injury when used as labeled. Products formulated with ephedrine alkaloids (ephedra, ma huang, sida cordifolia, Pinellia) were removed immediately, though, unlike other dietary supplements currently available, ephedra-containing supplements did have convincing evidence for short-term weight loss.
      (2) **Bitter orange** is an extract from the peel, flower, leaf, and fruit of the Seville orange. Typical dosage is about 1 g/day, standardized to 1.5%–6.0% synephrine, a stimulating agent that is chemically similar to ephedrine. Currently, there are no data to support its efficacy as an agent for weight loss. If combined with other stimulants such as caffeine, bitter orange may be cardiotoxic.
      (3) **Guarana** seed contains 2.5%–7% caffeine and exerts a diuretic action. Effectiveness has been demonstrated only in combination with ephedrine. Tolerance and dependence can develop with chronic use.
      (4) **Caffeine** is an FDA-approved product, efficacy of this agent for weight loss has been demonstrated only in combination with ephedrine, which has been removed from the market. Tolerance and dependence can develop with chronic use.
   b. **Modulate carbohydrate metabolism**
      (1) **Chromium,** an essential mineral, increases insulin sensitivity, lean body mass, and basal metabolic rate and decreases insulin blood levels and body fat. Chromium is used in weight loss products in the form of chromium picolinate, 200–400 µg/day, with no reported significant adverse effects. Rhabdomyolysis and renal failure have been reported with the use of chromium picolinate in doses exceeding 1000 µg/day. Though widely marketed, there have been no large, well-designed studies for the use of chromium in weight loss. Though its efficacy for weight loss remains uncertain, at least 115 products marketed for weight loss contain chromium.
      (2) **Ginseng,** in the form of Panax ginseng, may improve glucose tolerance, according to preliminary data. Though ginseng is found in at least 20 commercially available weight loss products, it has no demonstrated efficacy for weight loss in humans.
   c. **Enhance satiety**
      (1) **Guar gum,** a fiber derived from the Indian cluster bean, has been deemed relatively safe in doses of 7.5–30.0 g/day, however, it has not demonstrated efficacy for weight loss in at least 20 clinical trials. Adverse effects include abdominal pain, flatulence, and diarrhea.
      (2) **Glucomannan** (*Amorphophallus konjac*) purportedly absorbs water in the gut, contributing to enhanced satiety and thus decreased caloric intake. Preliminary evidence has demonstrated that glucomannan (3–4 g/day) may be well tolerated and efficacious for weight loss. However, this agent can have a laxative effect.
      (3) **Psyllium** forms a fibrous mass with a bulk laxative effect but has not demonstrated efficacy for weight loss. Potential adverse effects are significant, including esophageal obstruction and nephrotoxicity (if seeds are crushed, chewed, or ground, a pigment

may be deposited in the renal tubules). If used, patients should be instructed to not crush, chew, or ground the seeds, and adequate fluids must be consumed.

d. Increase fat oxidation or reduce fat synthesis

(1) L-Carnitine is synthesized in the liver, kidney, and brain. It is fundamentally important for fatty acid transport for energy production. No trials demonstrate efficacy of L-carnitine for weight loss.

(2) Hydroxycitric acid (HCA) is derived from the rind of the brindle berry, a tropical fruit native to India. It is purported to inhibit mitochondrial citrate lyase, thereby suppressing acetyl coenzyme A and fatty acid synthesis. In doses of 300–3,000 mg/day, HCA has been well tolerated, with adverse effects of headache and gastrointestinal symptoms reported. Efficacy of HCA remains questionable.

(3) Green tea contains a polyphenol, epigallocatechin-3-gallate, better known as **EGCG.** Each cup (8 oz) of green tea provides 10–80 mg of caffeine, contributing to the tea's diuretic action and central nervous system (CNS) stimulation (e.g., increased heart rate, increased blood pressure, anxiety). Green tea has demonstrated increased fat oxidation and thermogenesis but lacks data regarding efficacy in weight loss.

(4) Vitamin B$_5$ has been postulated to induce weight loss; however, data are lacking to support this.

(5) Licorice safety and efficacy for weight loss remains unclear. Reported adverse effects of licorice include pseudoaldosteronism, hypertension, and hyperkalemia.

(6) Conjugated linoleic acid (CLA) is a group of *trans*-fatty acids, which is purported to alter body composition by increasing lean tissue deposition and decreasing triglyceride uptake in adipose tissue. In doses of 1.4–6.8 g/day, CLA may have efficacy in weight loss, especially in obese patients. Adverse effects include mild to moderate gastrointestinal symptoms. CLA may increase insulin levels and insulin resistance.

(7) Clinical trials of **pyruvate,** in doses of 6–44 g/day, have demonstrated weak evidence of its effectiveness for weight loss. Reported adverse effects include diarrhea and audible abdominal sounds.

(8) Calcium suppresses parathyroid hormone and 1,25-dihydroxyvitamin D to reduce fat synthesis and increase fat oxidation. Oral doses of calcium obtained through both diet (1.2–1.3 g/day) and supplementation (800 mg/day) have produced positive results in at least one randomized controlled trial ($n = 32$). A larger randomized controlled trial is needed to substantiate current advertising.

e. Block dietary fat absorption. Chitosan, a common ingredient in "fat-trapper" supplements, is derived from the exoskeleton of shellfish. In doses of 2.0–4.5 g/day, chitosan has not demonstrated clinically significant increases in fecal fat excretion or weight loss. Adverse effects include nausea, constipation, and flatulence. Furthermore, it is questionable if chitosan is safe in individuals with shellfish allergies.

f. Increase water elimination

(1) Dandelion (*Taraxacum officinale*) seems to have a diuretic effect, but has not been studied for weight loss in humans. At least 15 dietary supplements for weight loss contain dandelion.

(2) Cascara stimulates peristalsis and evacuation, allowing FDA to approve this agent for use as a stimulant laxative. However, cascara has not been studied in humans for weight loss.

g. Miscellaneous. Spirulina (blue-green algae) contains phenylalanine, an agent theorized to inhibit appetite. Spirulina was declared ineffective for weight loss in 1981 by the FDA, and no published studies have proven otherwise. At least 13 products for weight loss currently on the market contain spirulina.

II. SLEEP AIDS

A. Normal sleep and sleep requirements

1. Sleep requirements vary widely among individuals and change throughout the life cycle. The usual range of sleep time per night is 5–10 hr, with an average of about 7.5 hr. Newborns require a considerable amount of sleep time, up to 18 hr. Adolescents typically do not become sleepy until after midnight and awaken very late in the morning (if allowed), but require a total of 9.5 hr of sleep. The typical adult requires 7–8 hr of sleep to feel adequately restored, but this time may diminish with aging.

2. **Polysomnography** is the predominant tool for characterizing sleep physiology, though guidelines from the American Sleep Disorders Association do not indicate it as useful in the diagnosis and management of patients with insomnia. Using polysomnography, researchers have identified five stages of sleep, subdivided into rapid eye movement (REM) sleep and non-REM sleep.
    a. Non-REM sleep consists of four stages. Each stage is a progression into a deeper sleep; and stages 3 and 4 are considered deep, restorative sleep. If time spent in stages 3 and 4 of sleep is diminished (as seen with aging), then sleep quality is compromised.
    b. REM sleep is considered stage 5 of sleep. Most dreaming occurs during REM sleep. If awoken while in REM sleep, dreams may be described in vivid detail.

B. **Insomnia**
    1. **Definition.** Insomnia is defined as one or more of the following sleep-related complaints: difficulty in sleep initiation (arbitrarily defined as a delay of > 30 min), difficulty in maintenance of sleep, shortened duration of sleep, or quality of sleep that results in adverse daytime consequences.
    2. **Epidemiology.** Insomnia is the most common sleep disorder in the United States, affecting approximately 35% of the adult population. Those affected most include women, the less educated or unemployed, separated or divorced individuals, patients with chronic medical or psychiatric disorders, and substance abusers. Economic costs of insomnia are estimated to be > $46 billion annually in the United States. Direct costs include prescription and nonprescription medications, as well as visits to a healthcare provider. Indirect costs include absenteeism, diminished productivity, fatigue-related automobile crashes, and industrial accidents.
    3. Classification of insomnia by duration.
        a. **Transient insomnia** lasts < **1 week** and is typically the result of acute situational stress or circadian issues such as jet lag or shift work. This type of insomnia is often self-limiting.
        b. **Short-term insomnia** lasts **1–4 weeks** and is attributable to situational stress (e.g., acute personal loss), often related to work and family life or to medical or psychological disorders. If short-term insomnia is not managed appropriately, it may progress to chronic insomnia because individuals become increasingly anxious and frustrated about the inability to sleep. There are no established predictors to determine if short-term insomnia will continue to become chronic insomnia.
        c. **Chronic insomnia** lasts > **1 month.** People with chronic insomnia need further evaluation because the condition is often the result of a medical disorder (e.g., sleep apnea, restless leg syndrome, primary insomnia), psychiatric disorder, or substance abuse. Up to 40% of chronic insomnia cases are correlated with psychiatric disorders, particularly depression.
    4. Classification of insomnia based on cause
        a. **Primary insomnia** is the main pathological condition in which a patient experiences continued insomnia in the absence of a related medical or psychiatric condition. Its pathogenesis is unknown, but the condition is treatable. Idiopathic insomnia is the inability to obtain adequate sleep, possibly stemming from a misaligned circadian rhythm. Psychophysiologic insomnia is increased wakefulness associated with the bed environment.
        b. **Secondary insomnia** is more common than primary and can be attributed to the following:
            (1) Adjustment insomnia is associated with situational stress.
            (2) Inadequate sleep hygiene is associated with lifestyle habits that reduce the amount of quality sleep, such as noise in the bedroom or the use of caffeine.
            (3) Insomnia owing to a psychiatric disorder
            (4) Insomnia owing to a medical condition, which may include restless leg syndrome, chronic pain (arthritis), migraines, or cancer
            (5) Insomnia owing to substance abuse
    5. Treatment
        a. **Nonpharmacologic intervention** is inexpensive and may be effective.
            (1) Maintain a regular schedule and do not nap; avoid sleeping in late after a poor night's sleep.
            (2) Use the bed only for sleep; avoid reading or watching television in bed.
            (3) If unable to initiate sleep (or go back to sleep) within 20 min, engage in a relaxing activity (away from bed) until drowsy, and then return to bed.

(4) Avoid exercise within 3–4 hr of bedtime.
(5) Minimize or avoid caffeine after noon.
(6) Minimize or avoid alcohol, tobacco, or stimulants. Many people believe alcohol to be an agent for sleep induction; however, alcohol can act as a CNS stimulant, thereby increasing nocturnal awakenings.
b. Nonprescription drug therapy: It has been estimated that 40% of patients with insomnia self-medicate with either alcohol or nonprescription medications in an effort to correct the condition. The sales of single-entity nonprescription hypnotics (e.g., diphenhydramine, doxylamine) have increased since that estimate was made, but the sales of nighttime analgesics (nonprescription hypnotic plus an analgesic, typically acetaminophen) have surpassed the single-entity products. Currently, data supporting the safety and efficacy of complementary therapy as sleep aids are lacking.
   (1) Diphenhydramine, an ethanolamine, blocks histamine₁ and muscarinic receptors, thus inducing sedation. Diphenhydramine is marketed as a nighttime sleep aid as Unisom SleepGels, Sleepinal, Compoz, and Simply Sleep.
      (a) Diphenhydramine may be dosed for sleep induction as **25–50 mg/night** in patients aged 13 and older. Doses > **50 mg show no additional benefit,** but increased adverse effects. An initial dose of 25 mg may be recommended for patients over the age of 65 with no contraindications to the agent. A dose of 1 mg/kg/night (not to exceed 50 mg) may be recommended for patients aged 6–12. Diphenhydramine is not recommended for sleep induction in patients younger than age 6.
      (b) Adverse effects of diphenhydramine are **anticholinergic,** including dry mouth, blurred vision, constipation, and urinary retention. Diphenhydramine use should be avoided in patients with glaucoma (narrow-angle), benign prostatic hypertrophy, dementia, or cardiovascular disease.
      (c) The duration of sedation from diphenhydramine is 3–6 hr. However, this may be extended in elderly patients or those with delayed metabolism.
      (d) The use of diphenhydramine for the alleviation of insomnia should be **limited to 7–10 consecutive nights.** If used longer than recommended, decreased efficacy may be noted and REM sleep may be suppressed.
      (e) Diphenhydramine is available in combination with aspirin or acetaminophen as a **nighttime analgesic.** Data are available to support the use of these agents in combination if pain is present. However, in the absence of pain, the addition of an analgesic simply provides increased opportunities for complications and drug-misadventures.
   (2) Doxylamine, like diphenhydramine, is an ethanolamine antihistamine which induces sleep through the blockade of histamine and muscarinic receptors. Therefore, adverse effects and duration of sedation are similar to diphenhydramine. There are currently no studies demonstrating enhanced efficacy or safety of doxylamine compared to diphenhydramine.
      (a) Doxylamine is dosed as **25 mg/night.**
      (b) Doxylamine is the active ingredient in Unisom Nighttime Sleep Aid Tablets. However, it should be noted that Unisom SleepGels contain diphenhydramine.
   (3) Melatonin, a nocturnal neurohormone secreted by the pineal gland, has a **sleep-phase-shifting effect on circadian rhythm.** Recent trials have observed effectiveness of melatonin for sleep onset in patients with misaligned circadian rhythms attributable to shift work or jet lag.
      (a) Melatonin production decreases with age, possibly attributing to sleep disorders noted in elderly patients.
      (b) Melatonin production can be decreased by tobacco, alcohol, and certain medications (nonsteroidal anti-inflammatory drugs, calcium channel blockers, steroids, benzodiazepines, and fluoxetine).
      (c) When exogenous melatonin is **given in the early evening, the circadian phase will be advanced.** Although this may be beneficial for individuals who experience difficulty in initiating sleep, melatonin given in this manner may worsen the problem of individuals who complain of difficulty in reinitiating sleep after awakening too early.
      (d) If melatonin is **given in the morning, the circadian phase is delayed,** offering the possibility that the patient may become sleepier earlier and awaken earlier.

At present, it is unclear if continued administration of exogenous melatonin will suppress endogenous production.

(e) Melatonin may be dosed as **0.3–5 mg during the day or at night,** depending on the desired effect. A physiologic dose of melatonin is 0.1 mg, an intermediate dose is 0.3 mg, and a pharmacologic dose is 3 mg. **Doses > 1 mg** may improve sleep efficiency but **have not demonstrated the ability to provide quality sleep restoration** as well as the intermediate dose.

(f) Attributable to its short half-life (30–50 min), melatonin should have **minimal, if any, residual effects the following morning.**

(4) **Valerian root,** derived from *Valeriana officinalis,* is classified as generally recognized as safe (GRAS) for food use in the United States. In doses of **600 mg/day,** valerian root is purported to induce sedation through its blockade of γ-aminobutyric acid (GABA) breakdown. Adverse reactions of valerian root include vivid dreaming. Further research is necessary to determine the safety and efficacy of valerian root as a sleep aid.

(5) **Kava,** derived from *Piper methysticum,* is one of the most common dietary supplements used in the self-management of anxiety. It is theorized that if insomnia is caused by a state of hyperarousal, then management of anxiety and nervousness will help induce the desired sleep.

(a) A typical dose of kava is **120 mg/day.**

(b) Reported adverse effects of kava are significant, including diarrhea, extrapyramidal side effects, and hepatotoxicity. A recent FDA advisory has **recommended against the use of kava because of the reports of hepatotoxicity,** including hepatitis, cirrhosis, and liver failure.

(6) **L-Tryptophan** was **banned in 1989** owing to its **association with eosinophilia-myalgia syndrome;** however, it remains available as a 500-mg capsule. The safety and efficacy of L-tryptophan as a sleep aid has not been studied and should not be recommended at this time.

III. SMOKING CESSATION

A. **Introduction.** More than 400,000 deaths annually are attributable to diseases directly linked to cigarette smoking, including atherosclerotic vascular disease, lung cancer, and chronic obstructive pulmonary disease. It is the most preventable contributor to morbidity and mortality in the United States and yet nearly one third of the adult population (approximately 48 million adults) continues to smoke. The resulting economic burden is startling, estimated at $50 billion annually to treat smoking-related disorders and $47 billion for the loss of wages and productivity.

B. **Physiologic effects** of nicotine involve the CNS (e.g., enhanced relaxation, improved attention) and the cardiovascular system (e.g., elevated blood pressure, tachycardia). The manifestations of smoking become more pronounced as one ages and may include any or all of the following: deepening of the voice (an untoward effect in women); a constant, hacking cough; yellowed fingernails and surrounding skin from substances found in cigarette smoke; and premature aging of the skin, most noticeable on the face.

C. **Benefits of smoking cessation** are evident for both the patient and society.

1. Patient
   a. Decreased carbon monoxide levels
   b. Restoration of olfactory and gustatory senses within days
   c. Increased self-respect, sense of accomplishment
   d. Improved lung function (up to 30%) within 2–3 months
   e. Reduction in the risk of coronary heart disease (50%) after 1 year. After 2 years, the risk is equivalent to individuals who never smoked.
   f. Parallel risk of stroke to that of a nonsmoker within 5–15 years
   g. Progressive decline in the risk of lung cancer as number of years of abstinence increases. However, the risk will never be equivalent to one who never smoked.

2. Society
   a. Decreased healthcare costs for treatment of diseases directly linked to smoking
   b. Decreased work absenteeism owing to smoking related disease

    c. Cleaner environment from decreased secondhand smoke and cigarette remains (e.g., ashes or butts of cigarettes) in public places

D. Complications of smoking cessation. Smoking is an addiction and, therefore, not easy to give up. Nicotine withdrawal symptoms include tobacco cravings, depressed mood, insomnia, irritability, inability to concentrate, anxiety, decreased heart rate, and increased hunger. In a 1991 study in which individuals tried to stop smoking without aid, all symptoms of nicotine withdrawal resolved within 30 days, except increased hunger, which persisted past the 30-day cessation period.

E. Tailored interventions for smoking cessation should be offered to every patient who smokes. The U.S. Public Health Service endorses an approach known as the 5As, developed in 1996 by the Agency for Health Care Policy and Research:

1. **Ask** patients if they smoke.

2. **Advise** patients who smoke to quit.

3. **Assess** the patient's willingness to quit.

4. **Assist** the patient in efforts to quit through counseling and/or pharmacologic therapy. (The combination of counseling and pharmacologic therapy has proven to be the most successful method.)

5. **Arrange** follow-up within a short time frame.

6. To assess the patient's willingness to quit, the transtheoretical model of behavior change may be a useful tool. According to this model, patients are in one of five motivational stages to change their current behavior—that is, to stop smoking:
   a. **Pre-contemplation.** Patient is not ready to change current behavior.
   b. **Contemplation.** Patient is considering a change in current behavior in the future but not at the present time.
   c. **Preparation.** Patient is actively considering a change in current behavior and is actively engaged in seeking more information.
   d. **Action.** Patient is actively attempting to change behavior or has changed behavior within the last 6 months
   e. **Maintenance.** Patient has sustained changed behavior for at least 6 months.

7. For patients in the precontemplation and contemplation stages, the healthcare professional should still advise the patient to quit smoking and repeat the assessment at future visits. For patients in the contemplation stage, the healthcare professional should assist the patient by offering a referral for smoking-cessation counseling and/or pharmacologic therapy. Behavior modification works best as a multidisciplinary approach, involving the healthcare provider, pharmacist, nurse, and dentist.

F. Nicotine-Replacement Therapy

1. **Overview.** Nicotine-replacement therapy (NRT) is a smoking-cessation aid used to ameliorate nicotine withdrawal symptoms by providing a **nontobacco, controlled-release amount of nicotine.**
   a. Research has demonstrated that the use of NRT in individuals who smoke > 10 cigarettes a day **can double the chances of successful smoking cessation;** but it is most successful when combined with other nonpharmacologic measures, such as counseling.
   b. Currently, three available dosage forms of NRT are approved by the FDA (gum, lozenges, and patches); however, **none is effective if the patient is not mentally ready to quit.** Furthermore, NRT is **not effective for the cessation of smokeless tobacco** (e.g., chewing tobacco, cigars, and pipes).

2. **Safety.** Though it is recommended by the U.S. Public Health Service that all people trying to abstain from smoking should receive pharmacotherapy support, not everyone is an ideal candidate.
   a. For patients with **acute cardiovascular disease** (e.g., stroke, acute myocardial infarction, unstable angina) and **pregnant or breastfeeding women, absolute abstainment from nicotine should be recommended.** However, if the patient makes an informed decision,

under the supervision of a provider, a rapidly reversible preparation is advisable (e.g., gum or lozenge).

b. In recent studies, NRT **appears to be safe in patients with stable cardiovascular disease.** Blood pressure should be monitored closely.

c. The sale of NRT is **restricted to those over age 18.** Therefore adolescents desiring smoking cessation, should consult a medical provider.

d. Patients with **asthma or depression** are instructed to consult their physician before the use of NRT. The levels of certain medications used for management of these disease states (e.g., theophylline, imipramine) may be altered by smoking cessation. The nicotine found in NRT does not alter these levels.

e. It is recommended that patients **do not smoke while using NRT** because the purpose of NRT is to alleviate symptoms while weaning from cigarettes. Although some studies have indicated that the combination may be safe, until further research is conducted, concomitant use of NRT and cigarettes should not be seen as permissible.

f. Patients are advised on the labeling of NRT products not to combine two forms of NRT. However, a few small studies have shown combinations of NRT to be superior to either agent alone. Therefore, some specialists in the field do recommend combination therapy. However, until further research is conducted in the form of well-developed, large trials, combination therapy with NRT should be discouraged unless prescribed by the supervising medical provider.

3. **Available forms of NRT**
   a. **Nicotine polacrilex gum** received FDA approval for prescription sales in 1984 and nonprescription status in 1995.
      (1) **Dosing.** Sold under the trade name Nicorette, the gum is available in a **2-mg dose** for people who smoke < 25 cigarettes daily and a **4-mg dose** for those who smoke > 25 cigarettes daily. The typical usage is **10 pieces daily,** with a maximum recommended usage of 60 mg/day for up to 3 months. The **strength of gum purchased does not change;** instead, the number of pieces used decreases over the course of treatment (Table 31-1).
      (2) **Chew-and-park method.** The gum should be chewed slowly, releasing a peppery, tingling sensation, at which point the gum should be "parked" between the cheek and the gum to enhance buccal absorption of the nicotine.
      (3) **Adverse effects** most commonly reported are sore jaw and mouth, mouth ulcers, and dyspepsia.
      (4) **Counseling tips**
         (a) Slowly chew the gum until a peppery, tingling sensation is felt, then park the polacrilex gum between the cheek and the gum. Once the peppery, tingling sensation disappears, begin to slowly chew the gum again until the sensation returns. The gum should be parked in a different area than before. Once the gum looses the ability to produce the peppery, tingling sensation (approximately 30 min), discard the gum.
         (b) **Do not eat or drink for 15 min before using nicotine gum** because it requires a basic pH for proper release and absorption of the nicotine.
         (c) **Do not use other forms of NRT or smoke** while using the gum product, unless otherwise directed by a supervising provider.
         (d) The gum may be chewed at the beginning of the first day or at least 30 min after the last cigarette was smoked.
   b. **Nicotine lozenges,** currently sold only under the trade name Commit, delivers nicotine into the buccal mucosa when the individual sucks on the tablet, similar to a cough drop.

Table 31-1. Recommended Scheduling of Nicotine Gum and Lozenges[a]

Weeks	Dose
1–6	1 piece gum or 1 lozenge every 1–2 hr (at least 9/day)
7–9	1 piece gum or 1 lozenge every 2–4 hr
10–12	1 piece gum or 1 lozenge every 4–8 hr

[a]The recommended scheduling of nicotine polacrilex gum (Nicorette) and lozenges (Commit) is identical. If nicotine is needed past the 12-week schedule, a medical provider should be consulted.

(1) Dosing. Commit has a unique **dosing strategy, based on the timing of the first ciga-rette.** If the first cigarette is craved within 30 min of waking, the **4-mg** lozenge may be recommended. If the first cigarette craving is after 30 min of waking, the **2-mg** lozenge may be recommended. The **strength chosen will not change** throughout the course of cessation; instead fewer lozenges will be consumed each day during the **12-week proposed schedule** (Table 31-1).

(2) Adverse effects. If the lozenge is consumed too quickly or swallowed (rather than dissolved) dyspepsia may be experienced. Other reported adverse effects include insomnia, nausea, hiccups, coughing, headache, and flatulence.

(3) Counseling tips

    (a) Avoid chewing or biting the lozenge. Rather suck on the lozenge slowly, moving it from side to side, until it is completely dissolved (20–30 min). If accidentally swallowed, wait at least 1 hr before using another lozenge.

    (b) Do not use other forms of NRT and do not smoke cigarettes while using this product, unless otherwise directed by a supervising provider.

    (c) The first lozenge may be taken at the beginning of the first day or at least 30 min after the last cigarette was smoked.

    (d) Do not take more than 20 lozenges per day of either the 2-mg or 4-mg dose.

c. Nicotine patches were introduced in 1992 and acquired nonprescription status n 1996. Comparative studies of the available formulations of NRT have revealed that most individ-uals prefer the patch over the gum or a prescription nicotine inhaler. The patch must be **placed on a clean, dry, and hair-free area** (e.g., stomach, thigh, back), but not over joints (e.g., ankles, knees, elbows). The patch should never be placed over wounds or open areas and caution must be used in the patient with severe psoriasis and eczema. The most common adverse effect of the patches is **skin irritation,** but this may be reduced by rotating the patch site. Two trade name nonprescription nicotine patches are available: NicoDerm CQ and Nicotrol.

(1) NicoDerm CQ may be worn for **16–24 hr/day.** Patients with early-morning cigarette cravings may require 24-hr use. However, if insomnia or vivid dreaming occurs, the patch may be removed after 16 hr.

    (a) Dosing: NicoDerm CQ is available in three strengths: **21-, 14-, and 7-mg patches.** The patch should be **tapered over 2–4 months,** depending on the starting dose.

        (i) NicoDerm CQ 21-mg patch may be recommended to an individual who smokes > 10 cigarettes/day and then tapered as follows:

            {**1**} Step 1: 21 mg/day for 6 weeks

            {**2**} Step 2: 14 mg/day for 2 weeks

            {**3**} Step 3: 7 mg/day for 2 weeks

        (ii) Those who smoke < 10 cigarettes/day may begin with the NicoDerm CQ 14-mg patch and taper as follows:

            {**1**} Step 1: 14 mg/day for 6 weeks

            {**2**} Step 2: 7 mg/day for 2 weeks

(2) Nicotrol patches were formerly available only as a non-tapering single 15-mg dose to be used over a 6 week period. The new Nicotrol patches are available in a stepping pattern similar to Nicoderm CQ and are recommended to be worn for 16 hours and removed at bedtime.

Weeks 1–6: Step 1 (15 mg)

Weeks 7–8: Step 2 (10 mg)

Weeks 9–10: Step 3 (5 mg)

STUDY QUESTIONS

Directions: Each of the questions, statements, or incomplete statements can be correctly answered or completed by **one** of the suggested answers or phrases. Choose the **best** answer.

1. All of the following statements about dietary supplements are true *except* which one?

(A) Manufacturers are not required to demonstrate product safety and efficacy before marketing supplements.
(B) Adherence to good manufacturing practices is mandatory for manufacturers of dietary supplements.
(C) The U.S. Food and Drug Administration (FDA) files action against supplements determined unsafe.
(D) The Federal Trade Commission (FTC) takes action against manufacturers who present misleading product advertising.

2. All of the following statements about chitosan are true *except* which one?

(A) It is a common ingredient found in fat-trapper supplements.
(B) It is derived from the Indian cluster bean.
(C) Its safety is questionable for individuals with shellfish allergies.
(D) It is purported to inhibit dietary fat absorption.

3. Jane is 36 years old and wants to lose weight. Her current body mass index (BMI) is 32 kg/m^2, and her waist circumference is 40 inches. She has lost a minimal amount of weight in the past using fad diets and nonprescription weight loss products but has been unable to maintain the weight loss. Which of the following is true regarding Jane?

(A) Based on her BMI, Jane is considered obese.
(B) Her waist circumference of 40 inches increases her risk for cardiovascular disease.
(C) A safe rate of weight loss for Jane would be 1–2 lb/week.
(D) Exercise will provide only a modest amount of weight loss but will help her maintain the weight loss.
(E) All of the above

4. Since the sudden death of his father 2 weeks ago, Bob has been unable to sleep at night. He has difficulty going to sleep and awakens early in the morning, unable to return to sleep. Which of the following would be the correct classification of Bob's current insomnia?

(A) transient, primary insomnia
(B) short-term, primary insomnia
(C) transient, secondary insomnia
(D) short-term, secondary insomnia

5. William works the swing shift at the local manufacturing plant. Based on a recommendation from a friend at work, William would like to try melatonin to help him get to sleep faster. Which of the following is true regarding William's use of melatonin?

(A) An appropriate starting dose of melatonin is 5 mg/night.
(B) William may experience continued drowsiness the following morning owing to melatonin's long half-life.
(C) Recent trials have noted the effectiveness of melatonin in individuals participating in shift work.
(D) All of the above

6. Which of the following complementary alternative medicines (CAM) has been banned because of its association with eosinophilia-myalgia syndrome?

(A) melatonin
(B) kava
(C) L-tryptophan
(D) valerian root

7. Sylvia is 33 years old and wishes to purchase a sleep aid for her recent bout of insomnia (duration 2 days). She has linked it to an overwhelming amount of stress she has been under lately at work, trying to meet deadlines, and her recent lack of sleep is not helping. She has no current medical conditions and takes a multivitamin daily. All of the following are true regarding Sylvia's taking diphenhydramine and doxylamine *except* which one?

(A) Sylvia may benefit from diphenhydramine 50 mg used nightly.
(B) Sylvia should limit the use of diphenhydramine for insomnia to 10 consecutive nights.
(C) Sylvia may benefit from doxylamine 50 mg used nightly as needed.
(D) Sylvia may experience anticholinergic side effects with the use of doxylamine.

8. Jill, a 22-year-old college student, has been encouraged by her healthcare provider to stop smoking. She tells her doctor that she wants to quit but she does not want to gain weight right now or to sacrifice her grades as a result of an inability to concentrate during the day. According to the 5As and the transtheoretical model of change, what is the next step Jill's healthcare provider should take?

(A) Jill is in the precontemplation stage of change. Her provider should reassess her willingness to quit at the next visit.

(B) Jill is in the contemplation stage of change. Her provider should reassess her willingness to quit at the next visit.

(C) Jill is in the preparation stage of change. Her provider should reassess her willingness to quit at the next visit.

(D) Jill is in the preparation stage of change. Her provider should offer her counseling and/or pharmacologic therapy for smoking cessation.

9. Zack is 55 years old and wishes to start taking nicotine lozenges to quit smoking. Which of the following is important in the recommendation and selection of nicotine lozenges?

(A) number of cigarettes smoked daily

(B) timing of his first urge for a cigarette

(C) concomitant disease states and therapies

(D) both the number of cigarettes smoked daily and concomitant disease states and therapies

(E) both the timing of his first urge for a cigarette and concomitant disease states and therapies

10. All of the following are important counseling tips for the use of nicotine replacement therapies *except* which one?

(A) Do not eat or drink within 15 min of chewing nicotine gum.

(B) The initial start of nicotine replacement therapy may be 30 min after the last cigarette.

(C) Skin irritation associated with the use of a patch may be minimized by rotating the patch site.

(D) All nicotine patches should be removed and replaced every morning.

ANSWERS AND EXPLANATIONS

1. The answer is B *[see I.C].*
Manufacturers of dietary supplements are not required to demonstrate product safety and efficacy before marketing, nor are they required to adhere to good manufacturing practices.

2. The answer is B *[see I.C.5].*
Derived from the exoskeleton of shellfish, chitosan is purported to block dietary fat absorption and thus is a common ingredient found in fat-trapper supplements. Because it is derived from the exoskeleton of shellfish, the safety of chitosan in individuals with shellfish allergies remains in question.

3. The answer is E *[see I.A.1–2; I.B.1.b–c; I.B.2].*
A BMI > 30 kg/m² but < 40 kg/m² is considered obese, but not morbidly obese. Women with a waist circumference > 35 inches are at increased risk of developing cardiovascular disease, as well as type 2 diabetes, sleep apnea, and osteoarthritis. If Jane's BMI had been > 35 kg/m², her waist circumference measurement would not be valid for determining an increased cardiovascular risk. Diet and exercise are the best approach to weight loss. A reasonable weight loss is 1–2 lb./week. Although exercise is beneficial, it adds a only modest amount to the weight loss; it has greater effect in the maintenance of the weight loss.

4. The answer is D *[see II.B.3–4].*
Transient insomnia is insomnia lasting < 1 week, and short-term insomnia is insomnia lasting from 1 to 4 weeks. Primary insomnia is a pathological condition in which the patient experiences continued insomnia in the absence of a related medical or psychiatric condition. Secondary insomnia can be attributed to a variety of situations, especially situational stress, such as the death of a loved one.

5. The answer is C *[see II.B.5.b.(3)].*
Melatonin effectiveness for sleep onset has been observed in recent trials in individuals participating in shift work. However, melatonin is not FDA approved for this purpose. An initial starting dose of melatonin is 0.1–0.3 mg in the evening for patients desiring improved sleep onset. Doses > 1 mg daily have not been able to demonstrate the quality sleep restoration seen in 0.3-mg doses. Melatonin has minimal, if any, residual effects the following morning, owing to its short half-life of 30–50 min.

6. The answer is C *[see II.B.5.b.(6)].*
L-Tryptophan was banned in 1989 because of its association with eosinophilia-myalgia syndrome. However, it remains available for sale as a 500-mg capsule.

7. The answer is C *[see II.B.5.b.(1)–(2)].*
Diphenhydramine may be dosed as 25–50 mg nightly for a sleep aid used for up to 7–10 consecutive nights. The recommended dosage for doxylamine is 25 mg nightly. Both diphenhydramine and doxylamine are ethanolamine antihistamines. Therefore, anticholinergic effects may be experienced with the use of either agent.

8. The answer is B *[see III.E].*
Jill is in the contemplation stage, as she is considering a change in the future, but she does not feel that this is the right time to begin a smoking cessation program. Therefore, Jill's provider should reassess her willingness to quit at her next visit, when, it is hoped that Jill will be ready to quit.

9. The answer is E *[see III.F.3.b].*
The only currently available nicotine lozenge is Commit, which is unique in its dosing strategy. Dosing is based on the timing of the first urge for a cigarette, either within or after 30 min of waking up. Concomitant disease states should be considered as well. If the patient has hypertension, he will need to be monitored more closely while using nicotine replacement therapy. If he uses certain prescription medications for asthma or depression, his medication may need to be adjusted when he stops smoking.

10. The answer is D *[see III.F.3.a–c].*
Nicotrol nicotine patches are to be used only during the daytime for 16 hr and removed before bed. NicoDerm CQ patches may be worn for 24 hr if early-morning cravings for cigarettes are strong. If the patient develops insomnia or vivid dreams from NicoDerm CQ, he or she may benefit from removing the patch before bed, thus allowing only 16 hr of exposure to the nicotine.

OTC Agents for Fever, Pain, Cough, Cold, and Allergic Rhinitis

Gerald E. Schumacher

Jennifer D. Smith

I. ANALGESIC, ANTI-INFLAMMATORY, AND ANTIPYRETIC AGENTS. Over-the-counter (OTC) analgesics and antipyretics relieve mild to moderate pain and reduce inflammation and fever. These agents are effective for somatic pain (e.g., musculoskeletal pain in the joints; pain from headache, myalgia, and dysmenorrhea; discomfort resulting from generalized inflammation), but they are not effective in reducing discomfort from the visceral organs (e.g., stomach, lungs, heart). Salicylates and nonsteroidal anti-inflammatory drugs (NSAIDs) reduce pain, inflammation, and fever, but acetaminophen generally is effective for only pain and fever.

A. **Pathogenesis of pain.** Intense stimulus (e.g., tissue injury) releases substances that sensitize pain receptors to mechanical, thermal, and chemical stimulation. This triggers pain receptors to send pain impulses over afferent nerve fibers to the central nervous system (CNS).

1. **Awareness** of pain occurs in the thalamus.

2. Pain **recognition** and **localization** occur in the cortex.

3. **Mechanism of analgesic, anti-inflammatory, and antipyretic action.** These agents inhibit (centrally, peripherally, or both) the biosynthesis of various **prostaglandins,** substances involved in the development of pain and inflammation as well as in the regulation of body temperature.

B. **Salicylates**

1. **Therapeutic uses.**
   a. Salicylates are used to relieve mild to moderate pain and reduce inflammation and fever.
   b. Aspirin (acetylsalicylic acid), specifically, is also used to reduce the incidence of some forms of cardiovascular disease. Current evidence supports a modest reduction in the risk of strokes in women but notes less effect in men. On the other hand, evidence supports a significant reduction in the risk of myocardial infarction in men and women > 65 years but shows little effect on younger women.
   c. Men and women who have had a previous myocardial infarction, stable and unstable angina pectoris, or coronary artery bypass surgery, are candidates for aspirin use.
   d. No consensus has emerged on the prophylactic use of aspirin in healthy adults. The risks associated with aspirin use (see I.B.e.d) may outweigh the benefits of its widespread use.

2. **Mechanism of action**
   a. **Analgesic and anti-inflammatory actions.** The action of aspirin results from both the acetyl and the salicylate portions of the drug. Actions of other salicylates (e.g., sodium salicylate, salicylsalicylic acid, choline salicylate) result only from the salicylate portion of the agents.
      (1) These drugs **inhibit cyclooxygenase,** the enzyme that is responsible for the formation of precursors of prostaglandins (PGs) and thromboxanes from arachidonic acid (Figure 32-1).

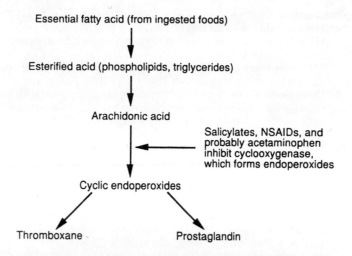

Figure 32-1. Inhibition of prostaglandin formation by aspirin, nonsteroidal anti-inflammatory drugs (NSAIDs), and acetaminophen.

   (2) Analgesia is produced mainly by **blocking the peripheral generation of pain impulses** mediated by prostaglandins and other chemicals. Analgesia probably secondarily involves a reduction in the awareness of pain in the CNS.
   b. Antipyretic action. The principal antipyretic action occurs in the CNS. Salicylates act on the hypothalamic heat-regulating center to produce peripheral vasodilation, which results from the inhibition of prostaglandin synthesis.
   c. Antiplatelet and antithrombotic actions
      (1) Antiplatelet. Aspirin (but not other salicylates, acetaminophen, or NSAIDs) **irreversibly inhibits cyclooxygenase in platelets,** which prevents the formation of the aggregating agent thromboxane A_2.
      (2) Antithrombotic. At low doses, aspirin inhibits thromboxane A_2 formation but has a relatively small effect on prostacyclin. This results in blocking the platelet aggregating agent thromboxane A_2 while preserving the action of the aggregation inhibitor prostacyclin (prostaglandin I_2; PGI_2).

3. Administration and dosage
   a. For **analgesia** or **antipyresis in adults,** 325–650 mg every 4 hr or 650–1000 mg every 6 hr should be administered as needed. The maximum daily dose is 4000 mg for no longer than 10 days for pain or 3 days for fever without consulting a physician.
   b. Child dosage depends on age. The dosages are 160 mg every 4 hr for children 2–4 years of age and 400–480 mg every 4 hr for children 9–12 years of age. Salicylates should be given for no longer than 5 days for pain, 3 days for fever, and 2 days for sore throat without consulting a physician.
   c. The **antirheumatic dosage for adults** is 3600–4500 mg daily in divided doses.
   d. For patients with **ischemic heart disease,** a 325-mg dose is given daily. Every other day is recommended for individuals with stable or unstable angina and evolving myocardial infarction. For patients without clinically apparent ischemic heart disease, the hemorrhagic complications associated with routine aspirin use may outweigh its benefit, unless individuals have established risk factors for atherosclerotic disease.
   e. For patients at risk of stroke, an 81-mg dose is given daily or every other day. As described earlier (see I.B.3.d), the risks may outweigh the benefits.
   f. Anti-inflammatory dosages. Although antipyretic and analgesic effects should appear within the first few doses, the anti-inflammatory effect may take 2 weeks or more to appear, even at high doses. The usual anti-inflammatory dosage of aspirin is 4000–6000 mg/day. The usual anti-inflammatory dosage of ibuprofen is 1200–3200 mg/day.

4. Precautions
   a. Hypersensitivity to aspirin occurs in up to 0.5% of the population.
      (1) Allergic reactions resulting in bronchoconstriction occur most frequently in people with **nasal polyps.**
      (2) Cross-reactivity with other NSAIDs occurs in > 90% of people. Cross-reactivity with acetaminophen occurs in 5% of people.
   b. Contraindications. Aspirin is contraindicated in patients with bleeding disorders or peptic ulcers. Also, aspirin should not be given to children or teenagers who have a viral illness, because Reye syndrome (i.e., fatty liver degeneration accompanied by encephalopathy) may occur.
   c. Pregnancy. Salicylates in chronic high doses are recommended with extreme caution during the last trimester of pregnancy because of:
      (1) Potential bleeding problems in the mother, fetus, or neonate
      (2) Prolonging or complicating delivery
   d. Gastrointestinal (GI) disturbances resulting from the inhibition of the gastric prostaglandins occur in 10%–20% of people at analgesic and antipyretic dosages. Anti-inflammatory regimens affect up to 40% of people. These effects decrease by using enteric-coated dosage forms and by taking salicylates with food or large doses of antacids. Buffered aspirin products contain insufficient buffers to counteract the adverse GI effects of aspirin.
   e. CNS disturbances such as tinnitus, dizziness, or headache may occur at anti-inflammatory doses in some patients.
   f. Salicylism (salicylate toxicity) may occur at anti-inflammatory doses. In addition to the CNS disturbances (see I.B.4.e), respiratory alkalosis, nausea, hyperthermia, confusion, and convulsions may occur.

5. Significant interactions
   a. Salicylates potentiate the effect of **anticoagulants** and **thrombolytic agents.**
   b. Salicylates potentiate (at anti-inflammatory doses) the effect of **hypoglycemics.**
   c. Salicylates potentiate the adverse gastrointestinal reaction resulting from chronic **alcohol** or **NSAID** use.
   d. Aspirin may competitively inhibit the metabolism of **zidovudine,** resulting in potentiation of zidovudine or aspirin toxicity.
   e. Caffeine taken in conjunction with salicylates appears to enhance the analgesic effect.

C. Acetaminophen

1. Therapeutic uses. Acetaminophen is used to relieve mild to moderate pain and to reduce fever. Guidelines from the American College of Rheumatology now recommend it as first-line therapy for osteoarthritis of the knee and hip. Because it has minimal anti-inflammatory activity, it cannot be used to treat the swelling or stiffness resulting from rheumatoid arthritis.

2. Mechanism of action. The analgesic and antipyretic actions of acetaminophen are the same as those for aspirin (see I.B.2.a–b).

3. Administration and dosage. Available dosage forms are 325 mg and 500 mg. A prolonged-dosage-form caplet of 650 mg is also available.
   a. For **analgesia** or **antipyresis in adults,** the dosage is 500–1000 mg three times daily as needed. The maximum daily dose is 4000 mg for no longer than 10 days for pain or 3 days for fever without consulting a physician. For osteoarthritis, 1000 mg four times daily is recommended.
   b. For **children age 6 years or older,** 325 mg is administered every 4–6 hr as needed. The maximum daily dose is 1600 mg for no longer than 5 days for pain, 3 days for fever, or 2 days for sore throat without consulting a physician.
   c. Routine use. Acetaminophen is routinely used in patients who are
      (1) Sensitive to the GI disturbances caused by salicylates and NSAIDs
      (2) Prone to bleeding disorders
      (3) Hypersensitive to salicylates

4. Precautions.
   a. Patients with active alcoholism, hepatic disease, or viral hepatitis are at risk from chronic administration of acetaminophen. Toxicity is rare, but chronic daily ingestion of 5 g or more for longer than 1 month is likely to result in liver damage. Acute doses of 10 g or more are hepatotoxic.

     b. Many OTC products contain acetaminophen in addition to other ingredients. It is important to counsel patients that the daily dosage limits cited in I.C.3.a–b apply to the total acetaminophen consumed from all products daily.

  5. Significant interactions. Acetaminophen may competitively inhibit the metabolism of **zidovudine,** resulting in potentiation of zidovudine or acetaminophen toxicity.

D. NSAIDs. Currently, **ibuprofen, naproxen,** and **ketoprofen** are the only NSAIDs available without a prescription.

  1. Therapeutic uses. NSAIDs are used to relieve mild to moderate pain and to reduce inflammation and fever. OTC drug use largely focuses on the analgesic and antipyretic indications of these agents. Maximum OTC drug dosage is generally recommended for osteoarthritis.

  2. Mechanism of action
    a. Analgesic and anti-inflammatory actions. NSAIDs inhibit prostaglandin synthesis both peripherally and centrally. Like salicylates, these drugs inhibit cyclooxygenase (Figure 32-1). NSAIDs produce analgesia mainly by blocking the peripheral generation of pain impulses that are mediated by prostaglandins and other chemicals. Secondarily, analgesia probably involves a reduction in the awareness of pain in the CNS.
    b. Antipyretic action. The principal antipyretic action is central. NSAIDs act on the hypothalamic heat-regulating center to produce peripheral vasodilation, which results from the inhibition of prostaglandin synthesis.

  3. Administration and dosage. The available OTC dosage forms of ibuprofen are a 200-mg tablet and a 100-mg per 5-mL oral suspension. Naproxen sodium OTC is available as a 220-mg (200 mg of naproxen) tablet. Ketoprofen OTC is sold in a 12.5-mg tablet.
    a. For **analgesia** or **antipyresis in adults,** the dosage of **ibuprofen** is 200–400 mg every 4–6 hr as needed. The maximum daily dose is 1200 mg for no longer than 10 days for pain or 3 days for fever without consulting a physician. For **naproxen sodium,** the recommended dose is 220 mg every 8–12 hr as needed. The maximum daily dose is 660 mg. **Ketoprofen** is recommended as 12.5 mg every 4–6 hr as needed, with a maximum daily dose of 75 mg. The limitations on the duration of treatment without consulting a physician recommended for ibuprofen also apply to naproxen and ketoprofen.
    b. For **rheumatoid arthritis dosage in adults, ibuprofen** is recommended to a maximum daily dosage of 3200 mg (administered on a 4- to 6-hr basis), **naproxen sodium** to a daily maximum of 1100 mg (divided doses every 8–12 hr), and **ketoprofen** to a maximum of 300 mg per day (administered every 4–6 hr).
    c. Naproxen sodium and **ketoprofen** are not recommended for children < 12 years of age. **Ibuprofen** is available as a suspension for children 2–11 years of age.

  4. Precautions
    a. NSAIDs are contraindicated in patients with **bleeding disorders** or **peptic ulcers.**
    b. NSAIDs are recommended with extreme caution during the last trimester of **pregnancy** because of:
      (1) Potential adverse effects on fetal blood flow
      (2) The possibility of prolonging pregnancy
    c. GI disturbances resulting from the inhibition of the gastric prostaglandins occur in 5%–10% of people at analgesic and antipyretic doses. Anti-inflammatory regimens (i.e., higher doses) affect up to 20% of people. These effects decrease when NSAIDs are taken with food or large doses of antacids. Ibuprofen is often preferred to aspirin by patients because ibuprofen causes fewer GI disturbances and bleeding events.
    d. Renal toxicity during chronic administration is a significant concern and may occur in the form of nephrotic syndrome, hyperkalemia, or interstitial nephritis.

  5. Significant interactions
    a. NSAIDs potentiate the effect of **anticoagulants** and **thrombolytic agents.**
    b. NSAIDs potentiate (at anti-inflammatory doses) the effect of **hypoglycemics.**
    c. NSAIDs potentiate the adverse GI reactions resulting from chronic **alcohol** or **salicylate** use.
    d. Caffeine taken in conjunction with ibuprofen appears to enhance the analgesic effect.
    e. Hypersensitivity to **aspirin** can occur with NSAID use.
    f. OTC labeling for these agents cautions against use of combining NSAIDs.

II. THE COMMON COLD

A. General

1. The common cold is generally a mild and self-limiting viral infection of the upper respiratory tract, though its economic burden of lost productivity and expenditures in symptom relief has a significant impact in the United States.

2. Rather than typical epidemiologic measures, the prevalence of the common cold is expressed as the number of incidences per individual, per year. Adults typically experience 2–3 colds per year; preschool children typically experience 5–7 colds per year. Children < 5 years old who attend daycare or have frequent interactions with a number of other children may experience as many as 12 colds per year.

3. Approximately $2 billion is spent each year in the United States on OTC cough and cold medications by patients seeking symptom relief.

4. The common cold accounts for approximately 26 million days of school (people aged 5–17 years) and 23 million days of work missed annually.

B. Etiology

1. The coronaviruses, respiratory syncytial virus (RSV), and rhinoviruses are the most contributing pathogens of the common cold, and the rhinovirus is the most frequently associated pathogen. Other pathogens involved include influenza, parainfluenza, and adenoviruses.

2. Three accepted general modes of transmission of the common cold exist: small-particle aerosols, large-particle aerosols, and direct contact. Direct contact between the virus and the nasal mucosa is the most prevalent mechanism of transmission of the rhinovirus.

3. Colds occur year-round, but peak incidences of the common cold are September, October, and early spring (March and April).

C. Pathogenesis. Pathogenic events of the common cold caused by the rhinovirus begin when a small dose of virus is deposited into the nose or the eye either by direct contact or by aerosol transmission (Figure 32.2).

1. Mucociliary action transports the virus to the adenoid where the virus is able to attach to the intracellular adhesion molecule (ICAM) receptors on lymphoepithelial cells. There, the virus begins to replicate, triggering the release of inflammatory mediators, including histamines, kinins, certain prostaglandins, and several interleukins (e.g., interleukin 1 [IL-1], IL-6, and IL-8).

2. Within 8–12 hr of viral entry into the nose or eye, the inflammatory mediators and parasympathetic nervous system reflex mechanisms lead to nasal congestion, rhinorrhea, sore throat, headache, and stimulation of cough and sneezing reflexes.

3. Cold symptoms decline and the risk of transmission of the virus is minimized after 3 days of infection.

D. Symptoms

1. Once viral contact has been made, individuals may begin to notice a scratchy throat 1–2 days after contact.

2. A sore throat is followed by a thin, watery discharge, known as rhinorrhea, and sneezing. Within 1–2 days, the thin, watery discharge may become thick and purulent.

3. A dry, nonproductive cough may develop between days 3 and 5, often evolving into a productive cough.

4. The general peak of cold symptoms is 2–4 days, and the median duration of the common cold is 7–13 days.

5. The pharmacist may recommend self-treatment for the following conditions: rhinorrhea, congestion, cough, headache, and sore throat.

Figure 32-2. Pathogenesis of the common cold.

E. Nonpharmacologic treatment

   1. Adequate fluid intake

   2. Adequate rest

   3. Increased humidification

   4. Nasal irrigation

F. Pharmacologic treatment

   1. Decongestants, also known as sympathomimetics, are the primary treatment for nasal congestion.

      a. Both oral and topical decongestants produce vasoconstriction by stimulating α-adrenergic receptors, thereby reducing the volume of blood circulated to the nasal mucosa and decreasing mucosal edema.

      b. Only **under the advice of a medical provider,** and **with extreme caution** should decongestants be **recommended to patients with disease states that are sensitive to adrenergic stimulation,** including coronary heart disease, hypertension, thyroid disease, diabetes, narrow-angle glaucoma, and difficulty in urination owing to an enlarged prostate gland.

      c. Patients currently taking monoamine oxidase inhibitors (MAOIs) **or who are within 2 weeks of discontinuation should avoid the use of oral and topical decongestants** owing to an increased effect on blood pressure (Table 32-1).

      d. Intranasal decongestants cause localized vasoconstriction by binding directly to adrenergic receptors. If the medication is used appropriately, systemic side effects should be

Table 32-1. Available Topical and Oral Decongestants

Agent	Products	Dosing	Avoid Use In . . .	Comments/Counseling Points
			Topical decongestants	
Oxymetazoline	Afrin; Neo-Synephrine 12 hr	2–3 sprays q10–12h	Questionable use in hypertension or receiving MAOI	Use for only 3–5 days owing to potential for rebound congestion (rhinitis medicamentosa)
Phenylephrine	Neo-Synephrine	2–3 gtt q4h	*May exacerbate:* hyperthyroidism, intraocular pressure, coronary heart disease, prostatic hypertrophy	Oxymetazoline is long acting *Adverse effects:* cardiovascular and CNS stimulation; burning; stinging; sneezing
				Xylometazoline discontinued, but generics available
				Naphazoline (previously sold as Otrivin) has been removed from market, but generics may still be available
Levmetamfetamine	Vicks Vapor Inhaler	*6–12 years:* 1 inhalation, no more than every 2 hr *12+ years:* 2 inhalations, no more than every 2 hr		Does not cause rhinitis medicamentosa within a 7-day period; thus approved for up to 7-day use Lacks vasopressor effect; thus not contraindicated in patients with hypertension, thyroid disease, diabetes, narrow-angle glaucoma, or difficulty in urination owing to enlarged prostate
			Oral decongestants	
Pseudoephedrine	Sudafed; Drixoral	*2–6 years:* 15 mg q4–6h *6–12 years:* 30 mg q4–6h *12+ years:* 60 mg q4–6h	Hypertension *May exacerbate:* hyperthyroidism, intraocular pressure, coronary heart disease, prostatic hypertrophy	Pseudoephedrine is absorbed well orally; however, phenylephrine has low oral bioavailability *Adverse effects:* cardiovascular (↑ BP, arrhythmias, tachycardia) and CNS stimulation (restlessness, insomnia, anxiety, hallucinations)
Phenylephrine	Sudafed PE	2–6y: 2.5 mg q4h 6–12y: 5 mg q4h 12+y: 10 mg q4h		Concomitant use with TCA may affect BP (↑ or↓), depending on specific decongestant

BP, blood pressure; *CNS,* central nervous system; *MAOI,* monoamine oxidase inhibitor; *TCA,* tricyclic antidepressant.

Table 32-2. Patient Counseling Information for Nasal Decongestants

Drops	Spray (Atomizer)	Inhalers	Metered-Dose Pump (Spray)
• Blow nose • Squeeze rubber bulb on dropper and withdraw medication from bottle • Recline on bed and hang head over side (preferred) *or* tilt head back while standing or sitting • Place drops into each nostril and gently tilt head from side to side to distribute drug • Keep head tilted back for several minutes after instilling drops • Rinse dropper with hot water	• Blow nose • Remove cap from spray container • For best results, do not shake squeeze bottle • Administer one spray with head in upright position • Sniff deeply while squeezing bottle • Wait 3–5 min, then blow nose • Administer another spray if necessary • Rinse spray tip with hot water, taking care not to allow water to enter bottle • Replace cap	• Blow nose • Warm inhaler in hand to increase volatility of medication • Remove protective cap • Inhale medicated vapor in one nostril while closing off other nostril; repeat in other nostril • Wipe inhaler clean after each use • Replace cap immediately • *Note:* Inhaler loses its potency after 2–3 months even though aroma may linger	• Blow nose. • Remove protective cap • Prime metered pump by depressing several times (for first use), pointing away from face • Hold bottle with thumb at base and nozzle between first and second fingers • Insert pump gently into nose with head upright • Depress pump completely, and sniff deeply • Wait 3–5 min, then blow nose • Administer another spray if necessary • Rinse spray tip with hot water, taking care not to allow water to enter bottle • Replace cap

minimal. However, given the difficulty of administration, systemic side effects are often seen with topical decongestants. Table 32-2 provides advice for patient counseling on device selected.

(1) Intranasal decongestants available in sprays and drops include phenylephrine and the imidazolines (oxymetazoline, naphazoline, and xylometazoline). Xylometazoline and naphazoline, previously sold under the trade names of Otrivin and Privine, respectively, have been removed from the market, but some generic formulations may be available.

(2) Intranasal decongestants approved by the U.S. Food and Drug Administration (FDA) are as follows:

   (a) Ephedrine (topical): 0.5%, every 4–6 hr; not less than (NLT) age 6 years

   (b) Naphazoline (topical): 0.025%–0.05%, every 4–6 hr; NLT age 12 years

   (c) Phenylephrine (topical; Neo-Synephrine, Nostril)

      (i) 0.25%–1%, every 4–6 hr; NLT age 6 years

      (ii) 0.125%, every 4–6 hr; NLT age 2 years

   (d) Xylometazoline (topical)

      (i) 0.05%, every 8–10 hr; NLT age 2 years

      (ii) 0.1%, every 8–10 hr; NLT age 12 years

   (e) Oxymetazoline (topical; Afrin, Neo-Synephrine 12 Hour, Nostrilla)

      (i) 0.05%, every 10–12 hr; NLT age 6 years

      (ii) 0.025%, every 10–12 hr; NLT age 2 years

(3) **Side effects.** Topical nasal decongestants may cause a temporary burning or stinging sensation when used and may also increase nasal discharge.

(4) **Counseling tips**

   (a) Patients using topical nasal decongestants should be cautioned to **limit use of the product to 3–5 days** to avoid rhinitis medicamentosa, a worsening of symptoms directly related to extended use and then discontinuation of the product. Treatment of this condition is to slowly withdraw the topical decongestant and begin oral decongestants. Topical normal saline may also be used to relieve irritated nasal passages.

    (b) To avoid spread of infection, patients should be counseled not to share topical nasal decongestants with others.

(5) Levmetamfetamine is an inhaler ingredient that has been deemed by the FDA as safe and effective as a nasal decongestant. It is currently found in Vick's Vapor inhalers.

    (a) Dosing

        (i) Ages 12 years and older: 2 inhalations in each nostril no more than every 2 hr

        (ii) Ages 6–12 years: 1 inhalation in each nostril no more than every 2 hr

    (b) Side effects. Levmetamfetamine lacks a vasopressor effect and, therefore, does not need to carry the warning for patients with cardiac conditions, hypertension, hyperthyroidism, diabetes, or difficulty in urination owing to an enlarged prostate gland.

    (c) Counseling tips

        (i) Unlike the imidazolines, levmetamfetamine has not demonstrated rebound congestion within a 7-day period; thus its use is approved for 7 days rather than carrying the 3- to 5-day limit. However, the manufacturers of the product voluntarily packaged the product with instructions to seek consultation with a provider if symptoms have not improved within 3 days.

        (ii) Once opened, nasal inhalers should be discarded after 2–3 months because the active ingredient dissipates, even when the product is tightly capped.

        (iii) Efficacy of this product may be diminished in the patient who has severely obstructed nasal passages because its use requires the ability of the medication to be delivered to the nasal mucosa.

  e. Oral decongestants available in the United States include pseudoephedrine and phenylephrine.

    (1) Phenylpropanolamine, a common ingredient found in weight-loss and cold products, was withdrawn from the market in recent years owing to an increased occurrence of stoke in certain populations (especially women).

    (2) Pseudoephedrine has quickly become known in all states and communities as the key ingredient in the illegal manufacturing of methamphetamine because of the simplicity of the diversion. The sale of pseudoephedrine has been restricted, placing it behind pharmacy counters in all states.

    (3) Phenylephrine is not as easily converted into methamphetamine and thus is more readily available to consumers who are seeking relief from congestion.

    (4) Pseudoephedrine acts directly on both α- and β-adrenergic receptors, producing vasoconstriction of respiratory mucosa, relaxation of the bronchioles, and increased heart rate and contractility. Pseudoephedrine also enters the CNS readily.

        (a) Dose

            (i) Patients < 2 years of age: 4 mg/kg/day in divided doses every 6 hr (only under medical advice)

            (ii) Patients 2–5 years of age: 15 mg every 4–6 hr; maximum dose 60 mg/24 hr

            (iii) Patients 6–12 years of age: 30 mg every 4–6 hr; maximum dose 120 mg/24 hr

            (iv) Patients > 12 years of age: 30–60 mg every 4–6 hr *or* for sustained release 120 mg every 12 hr; maximum dose 240 mg/24 hr

        (b) Side effects include central nervous stimulation (restlessness, insomnia, anxiety, or hallucinations), hypertension, and palpitations.

        (c) Drug interactions include MAOIs (see II.F.1.c)and tricyclic antidepressants owing to an increased pressor response.

        (d) Counseling tips

            (i) Notify a healthcare provider if symptoms worsen or do not improve within 7 days.

            (ii) Take the last dose no later than 4–6 hr before bedtime owing to the potential for insomnia.

(5) Oral **phenylephrine** is a more direct acting sympathomimetic agent than pseudoe-phedrine because it acts on α-adrenergic receptors and has weak action at β-adrener-gic receptors. This specificity of action allows for minimized cardiovascular side effects compared to pseudoephedrine, but such effects are still of concern when recommending its use in patients with coronary heart disease. Phenylephrine is also an ingredient found in products for the treatment of hemorrhoids and ophthalmic preparations for relief from redness of the eye.
  (a) Dose may be given every 4 hr, not to exceed six doses within 24 hr.
      (i) Patients 2–5 years of age: 2.5 mg every 4 hr
      (ii) Patients 6-12 years of age: 5 mg every 4 hr
      (iii) Patients > 12 years of age: 10 mg every 4 hr
  (b) **Side effects** may include increased heart rate and contractility, as with pseudoe-phedrine, and insomnia.
  (c) Drug interactions include MAOIs (see II.F.1.c and tricyclic antidepressants owing to an increased pressor response.
  (d) **Counseling tip.** Notify a healthcare provider if symptoms worsen or do not im-prove within 7 days.
  f. Nasal strips (Breathe Right) are **ideal in pregnancy, children,** and **in the elderly who take numerous medications.**
    (1) Bandage like in appearance, nasal strips function to physically open the nasal pas-sages.
    (2) Some strips are available with menthol.
    (3) The strip should be placed between the bridge and the tip of the nose.
    (4) As the strip attempts to resume a flattened shape, the nares are pulled into a more opened state.
  g. Decongestion alternatives (e.g., Coricidin HBP and its related line of products) are mar-keted for patients who are unable to take oral or topical nasal decongestants.
    (1) Chlorpheniramine, an antihistamine, is typically the ingredient found in these prod-ucts.
    (2) Antihistamines are advantageous since patients may only experience minimal side effects; however, antihistamines fail to target the primary problem, which is obstruc-tion of the nasal passages.

2. **Antihistamines**
  a. **Overview.**
    (1) **First-generation** antihistamines have been widely used in cough and cold prepara-tions for relief from rhinorrhea and sneezing, but have no effect on nasal congestion.
      (a) These agents are not FDA approved for use in children aged 2–5 years who are not under the supervision of a medical provider for such treatment. Many provid-ers advise against treating children for rhinorrhea and sneezing with the common cold owing to the increased risk of adverse effects.
      (b) The best advice to a caregiver seeking treatment of a runny nose for a child < 2 years of age is to simply let it run its course because the cold is a self-limiting viral infection.
    (2) **Second-generation** antihistamines have not demonstrated efficacy in the common cold, attributable to the lack of substantial anticholinergic activity of these products and should, therefore, not be recommended in the patient seeking relief from the common cold (Table 32-6).
  b. Common nonprescription first-generation antihistamines
    (1) Brompheniramine (Dimetapp)
      (a) Patients 6–12 years of age: 2 mg every 4–6 hr; maximum dose 12 mg/24 hr
      (b) Patients > 12 years of age: 4 mg every 4–6 hr; maximum dose i24 mg/24 hr
    (2) Chlorpheniramine (Chlor-Trimeton) is the least sedating of the first-generation antihis-tamines and is considered a drug of choice in pregnancy for rhinorrhea and sneezing.
      (a) Patients 2–5 years of age: 1 mg every 4–6 hr; maximum dose 6 mg/24 hr
      (b) Patients 6–12 years of age: 2 mg every 4–6 hr; maximum dose 12 mg/24 hr
      (c) Patients > 12 years of age: 4 mg every 4–6 hr; maximum dose 24 mg/24 hr
    (3) Clemastine (Tavist) is approved in only patients 12 years of age and older at a dose of 1.34 mg every 12 hr
    (4) Diphenhydramine (Benadryl)
      (a) Patients 2–5 years of age: 6.25 mg every 4–6 hr; maximum dose 37.5 mg/24 hr
      (b) Patients 6–12 years of age: 12.5–25 mg every 4–6 hr; maximum dose 150 mg/ 24 hr

(c) Patients > 12 years of age: 25–50 mg every 4–6 hr; maximum dose 300 mg/24 hr
(5) Triprolidine (Actifed)
  (a) Patients 6–12 years of age: 1.25 mg every 4–6 hr; maximum dose 5 mg/24 hr
  (b) Patients > 12 years of age: 2.5 mg every 4–6 hr; maximum dose 10 mg/24 hr
(6) Phenindamine (Nolahist)
  (a) Patients 6–12 years of age: 12.5 mg every 4–6 hr; maximum dose 75 mg/24 hr
  (b) Patients > 12 years of age: 25 mg every 4–6 hr; maximum dose 150 mg/24 hr
(7) Dexbrompheniramine (Drixoral)
  (a) Patients 6–12 years of age: 1 mg every 4–6 hr; maximum dose 6 mg/24 hr
  (b) Patients > 12 years of age: 2 mg every 4–6 hours; maximum dose 12 mg/24 hr
c. Side effects
  (1) Owing to anticholinergic properties, first-generation antihistamines may cause dry mouth (cotton mouth), blurred vision, difficulty in urination, constipation, irritability, and dizziness.
  (2) Patients with narrow-angle glaucoma and benign prostatic hypertrophy should avoid first-generation antihistamines because the anticholinergic activities may exacerbate their condition.
  (3) Patients taking first-generation antihistamines typically experience sedation, so caution should be taken driving or operating heavy machinery until one can identify how he or she will react to the ingredients.
  (4) Though first-generation antihistamines cause sedation in the adult patient, children may experience paradoxical CNS stimulation.

3. Expectorants, also known as mucolytic agents, work to loosen sputum and thin bronchial secretions by irritating the gastric mucosa and stimulating secretions of the respiratory tract. This increases the volume of the respiratory fluid and thins mucus. Therefore, it is logical to use expectorants only to treat a productive cough. The only available expectorant is guaifenesin, approved for patients aged 2 years and older.
  a. Dosing
    (1) Adults
      (a) Syrup: 200–400 mg every 4 hr; maximum dose 2.4 g/day
      (b) Extended-release tablet: 600–1200 mg every 12 hr; maximum dose **2.**4 g/day
    (2) Pediatric
      (a) Patients 2–5 years of age: 50–100 mg every 4 hr; maximum dose 300 mg/day
      (b) Patients 6–12 years of age: 100–200 mg every 4 hr; maximum dose 1.2 g/day
  b. Side effects. Guaifenesin is generally well tolerated, but side effects may include nausea and vomiting, dizziness, headache, rash, or diarrhea.
  c. Counseling tips
    (1) For enhanced efficacy in the loosening of mucus or phlegm in the lungs, patients should drink an ample amount of water when taking guaifenesin.
    (2) If symptoms worsen (development of fever, rash, or unremitting headache) or no improvement is noted in 7 days, consult a medical provider.

4. Antitussives are recommended for a nonproductive cough.
  a. Dextromethorphan, though a relative of morphine, is a nonnarcotic, having no analgesic or addictive properties, except in overdose. It is considered equipotent to codeine as a cough suppressant.
    (1) Dextromethorphan works centrally in the medulla to increase the cough threshold.
    (2) Dosing
      (a) Patients 2-5 years of age: 2.5–5 mg every 4 hr or 7.5 mg every 6–8 hr (one quarter of adult dose); maximum dose 30 mg/day
      (b) Patients 6–12 years of age: 5–10 mg every 4 hr or 15 mg every 6–8 hr,; extended-release form 30 mg twice daily (half of adult dose); maximum 60 mg/day
      (c) Patients > 12 years of age: 10–20 mg every 4 hr or 30 mg every 6–8 hr, extended-release form is 60 mg twice daily; maximum dose 120 mg/day
    (3) Adverse effects are not generally seen at typical doses, but constipation, GI upset, abdominal discomfort, and dizziness may occur.
    (4) Dextromethorphan should not be recommended for patients taking an MAOI (Nardil or Parnate) or who are within 2 weeks of discontinuation of these agents because the combination may cause serotonergic syndrome.

      (5) Reports of abuse of dextromethorphan in powder form (capsules) for a euphoric effect have recently increased in the adolescent population in the United States. Though adverse effects of dextromethorphan are generally benign in recommended doses, brain damage, seizures, loss of consciousness, irregular heart beat, and death have been reported with abuse of the drug.

   b. Codeine is a schedule C-V drug in a cough syrup, thus its sale may be restricted in some states.

      (1) Codeine, like dextromethorphan, works centrally in the medulla to increase the cough threshold.

      (2) Dosing of codeine is not recommended for children < the age of 6 years.

        (a) Patients 6–12 years of age: 5–10 mg every 4–6 hr; maximum dose 60 mg/day

        (b) Patients > 12 years of age: 10–20 mg every 4–6 hr; maximum dose 120 mg/day

      (3) Adverse effects include drowsiness, nausea and vomiting, excitement, abdominal discomfort, or worsening/aggravation of constipation. An overdose of codeine may cause death from respiratory depression and cardiovascular collapse. Caution should be used in recommending this product for patients with pulmonary disease or shortness of breath.

   c. Diphenhydramine is an antitussive and an antihistamine, though doses for an antitussive effect are much lower than those required for antihistaminic actions.

      (1) Newer, safer agents are available as antitussives, but diphenhydramine may be considered as a nighttime agent to induce sleep in the patient with a nonproductive cough.

      (2) As with dextromethorphan and codeine, diphenhydramine exhibits an antitussive effect by acting centrally in the medulla to suppress the cough threshold.

      (3) Diphenhydramine is not recommended for use in children < 6 years of age as an antitussive. Dose required for an antitussive action is 25 mg every 4 hr in individuals > 6 years of age.

      (4) Adverse effects include somnolence; sedation; and anticholinergic effects, such as dry mouth, blurred vision, difficulty in urination, and constipation.

   d. Camphor and menthol are the only FDA-approved topical antitussives.

      (1) Topical ointments containing 4.7–5.3% camphor or 2.6–2.8% menthol are FDA approved for alleviation of cough. Likewise, steam inhalants containing 6.2% camphor or 3.2% menthol are approved for use in steam vaporizers.

      (2) Menthol or camphor ointment may be applied as a thick layer rubbed into the throat and chest. A warm, dry cloth may be used to cover the area. Application may be repeated up to three times daily or as directed by supervising physician.

      (3) A menthol and camphor patch may be applied to the throat or chest of patients > 2 years of age. If the patient has sensitive skin, the patch may be applied to clothing covering the throat or chest, but the patch may not adhere to some types of polyester clothing. Clothing should be left loose so that vapors reach the nose and mouth. The patch should be removed and a new patch applied, if needed, up to three times daily.

      (4) Menthol or camphor steam inhalants may be added directly to the water (1 tablespoon per 1 quart of water) in a hot steam vaporizer, bowl, or basin. Vapors should be breathed in. This process may be repeated up to three times daily or as directed by supervising provider.

      (5) In 2002, the FDA ruled that all topical or inhalant products containing camphor or menthol must warn patients that their use near a flame, in hot water, or in a microwave oven may cause the products to splatter and cause serious burns to the user.

      (6) Menthol (5–10 mg) is also effective as an antitussive available in oral lozenges or compressed tablets. Menthol stimulates cold sensory receptors, producing a sensation of coolness and a local anesthetic effect on the respiratory passageways, thus engendering a soothing, antitussive effect.

5. Intranasal normal saline, available in drops and sprays, may be used to moisten nasal membranes and assist in the removal of encrusted secretions.

   a. Typical use of most intranasal normal saline products is 2–3 sprays in each nostril as needed.

    b. Some products may be used as a spray when held upright, or as drops when held upside down.

    c. Intranasal normal saline may be recommended for use in all patients, including infants and pregnant women, unless directed otherwise by a physician.

6. Local anesthetics in the form of lozenges and sprays may be useful in the alleviation of a sore throat. Mouthwashes have been recommended for use in the past; however, owing to localized action in the oral cavity, the pharyngeal wall may not be affected by these products.

    a. Because a sore throat is the initial symptom of many other illnesses, care should be taken to recommend products for sore throat alleviation only to patients who have concurrent symptoms of the common cold. If the throat is red and inflamed, unusually painful, or has persisted for several days, the patient should be referred to a primary-care provider for further evaluation.

    b. Throat sprays containing phenol (Chloraseptic) or dyclonine (Cepacol) are approved for use every 3–4 hr.

    c. Throat lozenges, approved for patients older than 2 years, may be used every 2 hr. Counsel caregivers that lozenges are potential choking hazards in young children.

7. Analgesics are occasionally indicated in the treatment of common cold symptoms when sore throat, myalgia, and/or headache exist. Aspirin, acetaminophen, ibuprofen, or naproxen sodium may be recommended, with consideration given to patient allergies, concurrent medications and disease states, and age.

8. Combination products (Tables 32-3 and 32-4)

    a. Numerous products are available that containing various combinations of antihistamines, decongestants, analgesics, expectorants, and antitussives. Certain product name designations help identify the ingredients.

        (1) *Nighttime* and *P.M.* usually signify that the product contains diphenhydramine, chlorpheniramine, or doxylamine.

        (2) *Sinus* usually signifies a decongestant (e.g., pseudoephedrine, phenylephrine) and/or an analgesic (e.g., acetaminophen).

        (3) *Cough* usually signifies that the product contains dextromethorphan, but some also contain guaifenesin in combination with dextromethorphan.

        (4) *Nondrowsy, A.M.,* and *daytime* usually indicate that the product contains a decongestant (e.g., pseudoephedrine, phenylephrine) and typically does not contain an antihistamine.

        (5) *Allergy* signifies that the product contains an antihistamine.

        (6) *Cold* and *flu* indicate that the product may contain any combination of ingredients, including a decongestant, antihistamine, cough suppressant, and/or antipyretic.

    b. Combination products may be useful for simplicity of dosing and adherence if patients are experiencing a variety of symptoms that can be alleviated by one product. For example, if a patient has a dry, hacking, nonproductive cough, headache, and nasal congestion, he or she may benefit from a combination product of dextromethorphan, acetaminophen, and pseudoephedrine. However, it would be a shotgun approach to recommend a product containing an antihistamine and expectorant in combination with other ingredients for this patient.

    c. Disadvantages to combination products occur when previously treated symptoms resolve, but the patient continues to treat other symptoms with the same product. This adds unnecessary medication(s) to the regimen, increasing the risk of adverse events. Combination products can also be difficult to recommend when selecting the appropriate product for patients with coexisting medical conditions.

9. Complementary therapy

    a. Zinc gluconate's effects on the duration or severity of the common cold have been studied. Results have been mixed, lending to what remains a controversial subject.

        (1) Current literature describes several possible mechanisms by which zinc may exert its effect, but such means remain unclear.

        (2) Despite its controversial use, a number of zinc products have been formulated, including tablets, capsules, chewing gums, lozenges, nasal gels, nasal sprays, and nasal swabs.

Table 32-3. Common OTC Products for Relief of Cough and Cold Symptoms

Product	Pain/Fever	Antitussive	Expectorant	Decongestant	Antihistamine	Sleep Agent
Alka-Seltzer Plus Cold and Cough		Dextromethorphan		Phenylephrine	Chlorpheniramine	
Alka-Seltzer Plus Cold and Cough Medicine Liqui-Gels	Acetaminophen	Dextromethorphan		Pseudoephedrine	Chlorpheniramine	
Alka-Seltzer Plus Night-Time Cold Liqui-Gels	Acetaminophen	Dextromethorphan		Pseudoephedrine		Doxylamine
Children's Tylenol Cold Plus Cough Multi Symptom	Acetaminophen	Dextromethorphan		Pseudoephedrine	Chlorpheniramine	
Comtrex Cough & Cold	Acetaminophen	Dextromethorphan		Phenylephrine		
Contac Cold/Flu Day Caplets	Acetaminophen	Dextromethorphan		Pseudoephedrine		
Contac Severe Cold and Flu Caplets	Acetaminophen	Dextromethorphan		Pseudoephedrine	Chlorpheniramine	
PediaCare Cough-Cold		Dextromethorphan		Pseudoephedrine	Chlorpheniramine	
PediaCare Night Rest Cough-Cold Liquid		Dextromethorphan		Pseudoephedrine	Chlorpheniramine	
Robitussin A-C		Codeine	Guaifenesin			
Robitussin Cold and Cough Liqui-Gels		Dextromethorphan	Guaifenesin	Pseudoephedrine		
Robitussin Cold, Cough and Flu Liqui-Gels	Acetaminophen	Dextromethorphan	Guaifenesin	Pseudoephedrine		
Robitussin-DM		Dextromethorphan	Guaifenesin			
Robitussin Night-Time Relief	Acetaminophen	Dextromethorphan		Pseudoephedrine		Pyrilamine
Robitussin-PE		Dextromethorphan	Guaifenesin	Phenylephrine		
Robitussin Pediatric Cough and Cold Long-Acting		Dextromethorphan			Chlorpheniramine	
Robitussin Severe Congestion Liqui-Gels			Guaifenesin	Pseudoephedrine		

(Continued on next page)

Table 32-3. Continued.

Product	Pain/Fever	Antitussive	Expectorant	Decongestant	Antihistamine	Sleep Agent
Mucinex			Guaifenesin			
Mucinex DM		Dextromethorphan	Guaifenesin			
Sudafed Children's Non-Drowsy Cold and Cough		Dextromethorphan		Pseudoephedrine		
Sudafed Cold and Cough Liquid Caps	Acetaminophen	Dextromethorphan	Guaifenesin	Pseudoephedrine		
TheraFlu Severe Cold	Acetaminophen			Phenylephrine		
TheraFlu Nighttime Severe Cold	Acetaminophen			Phenylephrine	Pheniramine	
Triaminic AM Non-Drowsy Cough and Decongestant		Dextromethorphan		Pseudoephedrine		
Triaminic Night Time	Acetaminophen	Dextromethorphan		Pseudoephedrine	Chlorpheniramine	
Triaminic Sore Throat Formula	Acetaminophen	Dextromethorphan		Pseudoephedrine		
Tylenol Cold and Flu No Drowsiness Powder	Acetaminophen	Dextromethorphan		Pseudoephedrine		
Tylenol Cold Medication, Nighttime	Acetaminophen	Dextromethorphan		Pseudoephedrine	Chlorpheniramine	
Tylenol Cold Medication, Daytime	Acetaminophen	Dextromethorphan		Pseudoephedrine		
Tylenol Severe Cold	Acetaminophen	Dextromethorphan	Guaifenesin	Phenylephrine		
Tylenol Flu Daytime	Acetaminophen	Dextromethorphan		Pseudoephedrine		
Tylenol Multi-Symptom Cough	Acetaminophen	Dextromethorphan		Pseudoephedrine		
Vicks Children's NyQuil Cold/Cough Relief		Dextromethorphan		Pseudoephedrine	Chlorpheniramine	
Vicks 44 Cough and Cold Relief Non-Drowsy LiquiCaps		Dextromethorphan		Pseudoephedrine		
Vicks 44D Cough and Head Congestion		Dextromethorphan		Pseudoephedrine		
Vicks DayQuil Multi-Symptom Cold/Flu LiquiCaps	Acetaminophen	Dextromethorphan		Pseudoephedrine		
Vicks 44E Cough and Chest Congestion		Dextromethorphan	Guaifenesin			
Vicks 44M Cough, Cold and Flu Relief	Acetaminophen	Dextromethorphan		Pseudoephedrine	Chlorpheniramine	

Product	Analgesic	Antitussive / Topical	Expectorant	Decongestant	Antihistamine
Vicks NyQuil Hot Therapy	Acetaminophen	Dextromethorphan		Pseudoephedrine	Doxylamine
Vicks NyQuil Multi-Symptom Cold/Flu	Acetaminophen	Dextromethorphan		Pseudoephedrine	Doxylamine
Vicks Pediatric 44D Cough and Head Decongestion		Dextromethorphan		Pseudoephedrine	
Vicks Children's Cough Syrup		Dextromethorphan	Guaifenesin		
Vicks Casero Rub		Camphor; menthol; eucalyptus			
Vicks Casero Chest Congestion Relief			Guaifenesin		
Vicks Sinex Nasal Spray				Phenylephrine	
Vicks Pediatric 44M Multi-Symptom Cough and Cold		Dextromethorphan		Pseudoephedrine	Chlorpheniramine

Table 32-4. Common Pediatric Cough and Cold Products by Category

Agent	Active Ingredient(s)	FDA-Approved Age
Antitussive		
Robitussin Pediatric Cough Long-Acting	Dextromethorphan 7.5 mg	2+
Delsym	Dextromethorphan 7.5 mg	2+
ElixSure Cough	Dextromethorphan 7.5 mg	2+
PediaCare Children's Medicated Freezer Pops Long-Acting Cough	Dextromethorphan 7.5 mg	2+
PediaCare Infant Drops Long-Acting Cough	Dextromethorphan 3. 75 mg	2+
Triaminic Thin Strips Long Acting Cough	Dextromethorphan 5.5 mg (equivalent to 7.5 mg)	6–12
Robitussin Honey Cough	Dextromethorphan 10 mg	6+
Triaminic Vapor Patch Cough	Camphor 4.7%, menthol 2.6%	2+
Vicks VapoRub	Camphor 4.8%, menthol 2.6%, eucalyptus 1.2%	2+
Vicks Casero Rub	Camphor 4.7%, menthol 2.6%, eucalyptus 1.2%	2+
Expectorant		
Vicks Casero Chest Congestion Relief	Guaifenesin 100 mg	2+
Antitussive & Expectorant		
Robitussin Infant Cough DM	Guaifenesin 100 mg, dextromethorphan 5 mg	2–6
Pediatric Vicks 44E	Guaifenesin 100 mg; dextromethorphan 10 mg	2–12
Decongestant		
PediaCare Gentle Vapors—Vapor Plug		
PediaCare Infant Drops—Decongestant	Pseudoephedrine 7.5 mg	2–6
ElixSure Congestion	Pseudoephedrine 15 mg	2+
Antitussive and decongestant		
PediaCare Infant Drops Decongestant & Cough	Dextromethorphan 2.5mg, pseudoephedrine 7.5mg	2–6
Robitussin Pediatric Cough & Cold Long-Acting	Dextromethorphan 7.5 mg, pseudoephedrine 15 mg	2+
Triaminic Cough	Dextromethorphan 7.5 mg	2–12
Triaminic Cough and Nasal Congestion	Dextromethorphan 7.5 mg, pseudoephedrine 15 mg	2–12
Expectorant and decongestant		
Triaminic Chest and Nasal Congestion	Guaifenesin 50 mg, pseudoephedrine 15 mg	
Antitussive, expectorant, and decongestant		
Robitussin Infant Cough & Cold CF	Guaifenesin 100 mg, dextromethorphan 5 mg, pseudoephedrine 15 mg	2–6
Antitussive and antihistamine		
Triaminic Cough & Runny Nose Thin Strips	Diphenhydramine 12.5 mg	6+

(*Continued on next page*)

Table 32-4. Continued.

Agent	Active Ingredient(s)	FDA-Approved Age
Antitussive, decongestant, and antihistamine		
Robitussin Pediatric Cough and Cold Nighttime	Chlorpheniramine 1 mg, dextromethorphan 7.5 mg, pseudoephedrine 15 mg	6+
Children's Vicks NyQuil	Chlorpheniramine 1 mg, dextromethorphan 15 mg, pseudoephedrine 30 mg	6+
Pediatric Vicks 44m	Chlorpheniramine 2 mg, dextromethorphan 15 mg, pseudoephedrine 30 mg	6+
Triaminic Cough and Cold	Chlorpheniramine 1 mg, dextromethorphan 5 mg, pseudoephedrine 15 mg	6+
Triaminic Nighttime Cough and Cold	Chlorpheniramine 1 mg, dextromethorphan 7.5 mg. pseudoephedrine 15 mg	
Triaminic Softchews Cold & Cough	Chlorpheniramine 1 mg. dextromethorphan 5 mg. pseudoephedrine 15 mg	6+
Antitussive, decongestant, and antipyretic		
Triaminic Softchews Cough & Sore Throat	Acetaminophen 160 mg. dextromethorphan 5 mg. pseudoephedrine 15 mg	2–12
Antitussive, decongestant, antihistamine, and antipyretic		
Triaminic Flu, Cough, & Fever	Acetaminophen 160 mg. chlorpheniramine 1 mg; dextromethorphan 7.5 mg. pseudoephedrine 15 mg	6–12
Decongestant and antihistamine		
Triaminic Cold and Allergy	Chlorpheniramine 1 mg, pseudoephedrine 15 mg	6+
PediaCare Cold & Allergy	Chlorpheniramine 1 mg, pseudoephedrine 15 mg	6+

(3) In studies showing the efficacy of zinc, formulations were begun within 24–48 hr of the onset of symptoms. Lozenges are recommended every 2 hr for the duration of the cold, and the nasal spray is recommended four times daily.

(4) Side effects reported with products containing zinc include nausea, GI upset, and unpleasant taste.

b. **Vitamin C.** Only a small number of studies have demonstrated the ability of vitamin C (dose > 1 g per day) to reduce the frequency or severity of the common cold. The clinical significance of the results of these studies remains questionable.

c. Echinacea has been used as a popular remedy for the common cold since the late 1800s. Unfortunately, current literature does not give definitive supportive evidence for the efficacy of Echinacea in the prevention and/or treatment of the common cold.

(1) Obstacles in studying echinacea lie in the fact that three different species of *Echinacea* exist, each with a different phytochemical composition. The composition may further be altered, depending on the part of the plant used and the time of year the plant is harvested.

(2) Current literature suggests that for echinacea to retain an immunostimulant effect, it should not be taken for longer than 2–3 weeks at a time.

G. Exclusions to self-treatment of the common cold

1. Fever > 101.5°F

2. Chest pain

3. Shortness of breath

4. Worsening of symptoms or development of additional symptoms

5. Concurrent underlying chronic cardiopulmonary diseases

6. AIDS or chronic immunosuppressant therapy

7. Frail patients of advanced age

Note: Since the original submission of this chapter, the American College of Chest Physicians (ACCP) has provided updated recommendations for the treatment of cough associated with the common cold. Focusing on evidence-based recommendations, the new guidelines stress the use of first generation antihistamines combined with a decongestant for the treatment of acute cough or upper airway cough syndrome in adults, rather than OTC expectorants or suppressants. The guidelines further advise against the recommendation of OTC cough and cold medications for children age 14 and younger.

III. ALLERGIC RHINITIS

A. Introduction. Rhinitis is an inflammation of nasal membranes, characterized by the four cardinal symptoms: nasal congestion, rhinorrhea, sneezing, and nasal itching.

1. Between 20 and 40 million people in the United States are affected by allergic rhinitis: 10–30% of the adult population and 40% of children. Allergic rhinitis typically develops before age 20, but its frequency increases with age until adulthood.

2. Treatment expenditures for allergic rhinitis and loss of productivity owing to absence from work or school are reported to be slightly over $5 billion.

3. Risk factors for allergic rhinitis include the following:
   a. Family history of atopy
   b. Higher socioeconomic class
   c. Exposure to indoor allergens (animals and dust mites)
   d. Positive allergy skin prick test

4. Allergic rhinitis may be classified as seasonal, perennial, episodic, or occupational. Seasonal and perennial, or a combination of the two, are the most frequent classifications.
   a. Seasonal allergic rhinitis. Symptoms may occur with repetitive and predictable seasonal symptoms.
   b. Perennial allergic rhinitis. Symptoms persist throughout the year without regard to changes in seasons.
   c. Combination seasonal and perennial allergic rhinitis. Symptoms persist throughout the year with seasonal exacerbations.

B. Etiology. There are five main triggers for allergic rhinitis: pollens, molds, dust mites, animal allergens, and insect allergens. These allergens trigger an immunoglobulin E (IgE) mediated immunological reaction.

1. Seasonal allergic rhinitis is typically caused by pollens and molds.

2. Perennial allergic rhinitis is typically caused by dust mites, molds, and animal allergens.

C. Pathogenesis. Patients become sensitized to allergens; on subsequent exposure, the allergens trigger a genetically predetermined immune response that results in the symptoms of allergic rhinitis. Allergic rhinitis may then be characterized by early- or late-phase responses.

1. Early-phase response
   a. Reexposure to the allergen triggers mast cells and eosinophils to generate inflammatory mediators (e.g., PGD_2 and leukotrienes) and release preformed mediators (e.g., histamine, tryptase, chymase, and kininogenase).

    b. Generation and release of the inflammatory mediators results in increased vascular permeability, mucosal edema, and watery rhinorrhea. Dilated blood vessels cause sinusoidal filling and the subsequent nasal congestion.

    c. Sensory nerves are stimulated, engendering a sensation of nasal itch, and thus sneezing.

  2. Late-phase response

    (a) Mast-cell-derived mediators lead to a migration and activation of eosinophils, neutrophils, and basophils, T lymphocytes, and macrophages within the nasal mucosa.

    b. During the 4–8 hr after allergen exposure, these cells become activated and release inflammatory mediators, providing reoccurrence of initial symptoms, with the predominant symptom of congestion.

D. Signs and symptoms. The four classic symptoms of allergic rhinitis include rhinorrhea, nasal congestion, sneezing, and nasal pruritus. Nasal pruritus is typically not a symptom of the common cold. Because children often cannot verbalize the symptoms of allergic rhinitis, it is important to recognize the signs.

  1. Repercussions of nasal pruritus include the following:

    a. Gothic arch, a steady upward movement of the upper lip and teeth which may result in an overbite, as a result of the "allergic salute," characterized by the constant upward rubbing of the nose with the palm of the hand.

    b. Allergic crease: a visible transverse line appearing between the tip and the bridge of the nose, caused by constant rubbing.

  2. Ophthalmic conditions present in the individual with allergic rhinitis include allergic shiners, a darkening of the lower eyelid attributable to chronic nasal obstruction, and Morgan lines (also known as the Dennie sign), which are seen as pleats under the eyes, running parallel to the lower eyelid margins.

  3. Individuals with allergic rhinitis may also experience fatigue, irritability, and malaise. Owing to these symptoms, allergic rhinitis may be a contributing factor to poor schoolwork in children afflicted by this condition.

E. Treatment. The primary goal in the treatment of allergic rhinitis is to control the symptoms without altering the patient's ability to function. Treatment options include environmental control, nonprescription pharmacologic treatment, and prescription treatment. This section focuses on environmental control and nonprescription treatment (Tables 32-5 and 32-6).

Table 32-5. Environmental Control Measures for Indoor and Outdoor Allergens

Allergen	Environmental Control Measure
Indoor	
Dust Mites	Encase bedding *or* wash at least weekly in hot (130°F) water
	Remove carpets (especially in bedrooms)
	Remove upholstered furniture
	Remove stuffed animals from home that cannot be laundered
Animal Dander	Avoid pets with fur if established allergen
	Some patients are allergic to long-haired dogs but are not affected by short-haired breeds
Cockroaches	Use of pesticides or professional extermination
Mold	Check houseplants often for mold growth; move outdoors if source of problem
	Use of HEPA filter
	Lower household humidity
	Vent food preparation areas and bathrooms
	Repair damp basements and crawl spaces
	Apply fungicide to obvious molded areas
Outdoor	
Pollen	Avoid outdoor activities when pollen counts are high
	Close house and car windows
	HEPA filters

HEPA, high-efficiency particulate air.

Table 32-6. OTC Treatment of Allergic Rhinitis

Agent	Product(s)	Dosing	Avoid Use In . . .	Comments/Counseling Points
		Nonsedating (second-generation) antihistamine		
Loratadine	Claritin Alavert Tavist ND Triaminic AllerChews	*2–6 years:* 5 mg q24h *6+ years:* 10 mg q24h		No anticholinergic activity Penetrates poorly into CNS; free of sedating effects at usual doses Liver/kidney disease may need lower dosage
		Sedating (first-generation) antihistamines		
Chlorpheniramine	Chlor-Trimeton	*2–6 years:* 1mg q4–6h *6–12 years:* 2 mg q4–6h *12+ years:* 4 mg q4–6h	Narrow-angle glaucoma MAOI use Prostatic hypertrophy Use caution in emphysema and chronic bronchitis	Largest side effect is drowsiness, followed by typical anticholinergic side effects Phenindamine may cause nervousness and insomnia Children and elderly may experience paradoxical stimulation Older adults are likely to have CNS depressive side effects, including confusion and hypotension *Photosensitizing:* Advise patients to wear sunscreen and protective clothing Chlorpheniramine is least sedating and is antihistamine of choice during pregnancy
Diphenhydramine	Benadryl	*2–6 years:* 12.5–25 mg q4–6h *12+ years:* 25–50 mg q4–6h		
Brompheniramine	Dimetapp	*6–12 years:* 2 mg q4–6h *12+ years:* 4 mg q4–6h		

Clemastine	Tavist	12+ years: 1.34 mg q12h 6–12 years: 1.25 mg q4–6h		
Triprolidine	Actifed	12+ years: 2.5 mg q4–6h 6–12 years: 12.5 mg q4–6h		
Phenindamine	Nolahist			
Dexbrompheniramine	Drixoral	12+ years: 25mg q4–6h 6–12 years: 1 mg q4–6h 12+ years: 2 mg q4–6h		
Ocular antihistamines (available only in combination with decongestants)				
Pheniramine	Naphcon A Opcon-A Visine-A	1–2 gtt TID–QID	Narrow-angle glaucoma: pupil dilation can cause angle-closure glaucoma	*Side effects:* burning, stinging, itching, foreign body sensation, dry eye, lid edema, and pupil dilation
Antazoline	Vasocon A	1–2 gtt TID–QID		
Mast cell stabilizer				
Cromolyn sodium	Nasalcrom	6+ years: 1 spray in each nostril 3–6 times daily		Most efficacious if started before seasonal symptoms May take 3–7 days for initial response and 2–4 weeks for maximal response *Side effects:* sneezing, nasal stinging, burning Drug of choice in pregnancy for sneezing and rhinorrhea

CNS, central nervous system; *MAOI*, monoamine oxidase inhibitor.

1. The best treatment remains avoidance of the allergen(s), once determined, though this is sometimes impractical. Environmental controls directed toward particular allergens can be the first initiative toward resolution of symptoms.

2. Antihistamines, both first and second generation, are the mainstay of treatment for allergic rhinitis.
   a. First-generation antihistamines are limited in continuous treatment of allergic rhinitis owing to their frequent dosing and related sedation. These agents remain the least expensive treatment option at this time; however, this aspect must be weighed against the ability to remain alert for work and school activities.
      (1) Owing to their lipophilicity, first-generation antihistamines easily cross the blood–brain barrier, causing significant sedation. Though patients may not notice sedation, studies have clearly demonstrated a reduction in intellectual and motor function in patients taking first-generation antihistamines.
      (2) Children and the elderly are most susceptible to the adverse effects of antihistamines; thus they are at increased risk of experiencing nightmares, anxiety, restlessness, unusual excitement, or irritability.
   b. Second-generation antihistamines are advantageous because of their preferential peripheral H_1-receptor binding. This allows for minimal CNS effects, minimal sedative effects, and minimal anticholinergic activity.

3. Oral decongestants are effective in relieving symptoms of nasal congestion but have no effect on other symptoms of allergic rhinitis, such as rhinorrhea, pruritus, or sneezing.
   a. Because treatment of allergic rhinitis is for extended periods of time, oral decongestants should be used for nasal congestion rather than topical decongestants owing to the potential for rhinitis medicamentosa.
   b. The combination of a decongestant and an antihistamine has proven to be an optimal treatment regimen for allergic rhinitis.
   c. Consideration must be taken into account when recommending products containing pseudoephedrine to adolescents and adults participating in sports programs, because of the "doping" effect of these agents.

4. Ocular antihistamines may be used for the treatment of ophthalmic conditions associated with allergic rhinitis, though their use has been classified by the FDA as less than effective owing to a lack of data demonstrating clinical effectiveness.
   a. There are two available nonprescription ocular antihistamines: pheniramine maleate and antazoline phosphate. Both of these agents are available only in combination with naphazoline (a decongestant).
   b. Avoid use in glaucoma, as pupil dilation may cause angle-closure glaucoma.
   c. Side effects may include burning, stinging, itching, foreign body sensation, dry eye, lid edema, and pupil dilation.

5. Cromolyn sodium (e.g., Nasalcrom) is best used as a preventive measure for the symptoms of allergic rhinitis but may also be used as treatment for all symptoms except nasal congestion. However, maximum benefit, when used as treatment, will not be seen for 1–2 weeks. When used for prevention, cromolyn sodium should be initiated approximately 1 week before allergen contact.
   a. Cromolyn sodium has a short duration of action and, therefore, must be dosed three to four times daily. This frequency in dosing may result in diminished adherence.
   b. Cromolyn sodium is approved for use in patients 2 years of age and older and should be dosed as one spray in each nostril three to four times daily. It should not be used more than six times daily. A provider should be consulted if symptoms worsen or no improvement is seen within 2 weeks.
   c. Adverse effects may include a brief stinging or sneezing directly after administration.
   d. Cromolyn sodium is considered a preferred initial drug of choice during pregnancy for rhinorrhea and sneezing.

F. **Exclusions to self-treatment of allergic rhinitis**

1. Symptoms of otitis media or sinusitis

2. Symptoms that suggest lower-respiratory tract problems

3. History of nonallergic rhinitis

STUDY QUESTIONS

Directions: Each of the questions, statements, or incomplete statements can be correctly answered or completed by **one** of the suggested answers or phrases. Choose the **best** answer.

1. Which statement concerning the use of over-the-counter (OTC) analgesic agents is true?

(A) Aspirin is indicated for mild to moderate analgesia, inflammatory diseases, antipyresis, and prophylaxis for patients with ischemic heart disease.
(B) Ibuprofen is indicated for mild to moderate analgesia, reduction of fever, and prophylaxis for patients with ischemic heart disease but not for inflammatory disorders.
(C) Acetaminophen is indicated for mild to moderate analgesia but not for reduction of fever and arthritis.
(D) Naproxen sodium is indicated for mild to moderate analgesia, antipyresis, and prophylaxis for patients with ischemic heart disease.

2. Which statement concerning drug interactions with over-the-counter (OTC) analgesic agents is true?

(A) Aspirin potentiates the effects of antihypertensives, cardiac glycosides, and anticoagulants.
(B) Ibuprofen potentiates the effect of zidovudine, hypoglycemics, and aminoglycosides.
(C) Acetaminophen potentiates the effect of zidovudine.
(D) For naproxen sodium, the OTC dosage recommendations are similar to the prescription dosage.

3. All of the following statements concerning contraindications with *chronic* use of over-the-counter (OTC) analgesic agents are correct *except* which one?

(A) Aspirin, ibuprofen, naproxen sodium, and ketoprofen are contraindicated in patients with bleeding disorders, peptic ulcer, and the third trimester of pregnancy.
(B) Aspirin, acetaminophen, and ibuprofen are implicated in Reye syndrome.
(C) Acetaminophen is contraindicated in patients with active alcoholism, hepatic disease, or viral hepatitis.

4. Which statement concerning dosage recommendations for over-the-counter (OTC) analgesic agents is true?

(A) Aspirin for analgesia or antipyresis in adults is 325–650 mg every 4 hr or 650–1000 mg every 6 hr, with a maximum daily dose of 4000 mg for no longer than 10 days for pain or 3 days for fever without consulting a physician; the antirheumatic dosage for adults is 3600–4500 mg daily in divided doses; and patients with ischemic heart disease should take 325 mg daily or every other day.
(B) Ibuprofen for analgesia or antipyresis in adults is 300–600 mg every 6–8 hr, with a maximum daily dose of 1800 mg for no longer than 10 days for pain or 3 days for fever without consulting a physician; the anti-inflammatory dosage for adults is 1800–3600 mg daily in divided doses.
(C) Acetaminophen for analgesia or antipyresis in adults is 325 mg every 8–12 hr, with a maximum daily dose of 2000 mg for no longer than 10 days for pain and 3 days for fever without consulting a physician; patients with ischemic heart disease take 325 mg daily or every other day.

5. Which of the following is an inhaler ingredient deemed safe and effective as a nasal decongestant?

(A) oxymetazoline
(B) phenylephrine
(C) levmetamfetamine
(D) ephedrine

6. Alice is 27 years old and in the first trimester of her pregnancy. She needs a recommendation for sneezing, rhinorrhea, and nasal itching, which started 2 days ago. She feels miserable with her symptoms, which worsen when she cleans the house. Her current medications include calcium carbonate and docusate sodium. Which of the following would be the *best* recommendation for Alice's symptoms?

(A) chlorpheniramine
(B) pseudoephedrine
(C) Breathe Right Nasal Strips
(D) intranasal cromolyn

7. John is 64 years old, whose chief complaint is of a dry, hacking cough. He states the cough started yesterday, but he has not had any fever, chills, sore throat, or congestion. His only medical condition is hypertension, which is controlled with hydrochlorothiazide (HCTZ). What would be the *best* recommendation for John's cough?

(A) dextromethorphan
(B) codeine
(C) diphenhydramine
(D) guaifenesin

8. The appropriate dose of pseudoephedrine for a 3-year-old child is

(A) 2.5 mg q4–6h.
(B) 5 mg q4–6h.
(C) 15 mg q4–6h.
(D) 30 mg q4–6h.

For questions 9–10: JB, a 42-year-old white male, complains of a scratchy throat, nasal congestion, and a cough that started 2 days ago. When he coughs, he brings up yellow-white phlegm. He has hypertension and dyslipidemia.

9. Which of the following would be the *best* recommendation for JB's cough?

(A) codeine
(B) dextromethorphan
(C) diphenhydramine
(D) guaifenesin

10. Which of the following would be the *most* appropriate over-the-counter (OTC) product for JBs nasal congestion?

(A) pseudoephedrine
(B) phenylephrine
(C) oxymetazoline
(D) levmetamfetamine

11. SO, a 22-year-old female, asks for a recommendation for sneezing, watery and itchy eyes, and a runny nose. She has no significant medical history. She is in the midst of final exams and must remain alert. What would be the *best* recommendation for SO?

(A) Alavert
(B) Benadryl
(C) Tavist
(D) Actifed

ANSWERS AND EXPLANATIONS

1. The answer is A *[see I.B]*.
Aspirin is the only analgesic agent with an approved labeling for analgesia, antipyresis, inflammation, and prophylaxis for ischemic heart disease.

2. The answer is C *[see I.C]*.
Acetaminophen may competitively inhibit the metabolism of zidovudine, resulting in potentiation of zidovudine or acetaminophen toxicity. As for the other choices, OTC dosage levels are generally one half the prescription dosage; aspirin is not commonly recognized to interact with antihypertensives or cardiac glycosides; nor is acetaminophen expected to interact with aminoglycosides.

3. The answer is B *[see I.B.4.b]*.
Aspirin is the only analgesic agent associated with the development of Reye syndrome.

4. The answer is A *[see I.B.3; I.C.3; I.D.3]*.
The aspirin dosage OTC recommendations are correct; the levels for acetaminophen are too low, and for ibuprofen, too high. In addition, acetaminophen does not carry an ischemic heart disease prophylaxis recommendation.

5. The answer is C *[see II.F.1.a.(2)]*.
Levmetamfetamine is an inhaler ingredient that has been deemed by the FDA as safe and effective as a nasal decongestant. It is currently found in Vicks Vapor Inhaler. Oxymetazoline, ephedrine, and phenylephrine are topical nasal decongestants found in pumps and drops, but not in inhalers.

6. The answer is A *[see II.F.2.b.(2); III.E.5.d]*.
Rhinorrhea, sneezing, and nasal itching are symptoms of allergic rhinitis, differentiated from the common cold by the nasal itching. Pseudoephedrine and Breathe Right Nasal Strips are indicated for nasal congestion, which she does not have. Both chlorpheniramine and intranasal cromolyn sodium are recommended treatments for the relief of sneezing and rhinorrhea in pregnancy. However, this patient needs relief from symptoms now. Cromolyn sodium may be used for treatment, but will take 1–2 weeks for noticeable symptom improvement. Chlorpheniramine will produce symptom improvement within hours.

7. The answer is A *[see II.F.3–4]*.
The complaint is a dry, hacking cough, warranting the use of an antitussive rather than an expectorant (e.g., guaifenesin). Dextromethorphan, diphenhydramine, and codeine are all antitussives used for relief of a dry, hacking cough. However, diphenhydramine should not be recommended as an antitussive unless the patient is experiencing difficulty in sleep initiation owing to the cough. Codeine, though a good option, may be limited because of its restricted sale in some states, adverse effects, and the potential for allergic reactions. Dextromethorphan has minimal adverse effects when used at recommended doses and is equipotent to codeine when used as a cough suppressant.

8. The answer is C *[see II.F.1.b.(1).(a)]*.
Pseudoephedrine should be dosed as 15 mg every 4–6 hr up to a maximum of 60 mg in 24 hr for patients 2–5 years of age. Patients aged 6–12 years may be safely recommended 30 mg every 4–6 hr, with a maximum recommended dose of 120 mg in 24 hr. Pseudoephedrine is not recommended for children < 2 years of age, unless under medical advice.

9. The answer is D *[see II.F.3]*.
The patient is experiencing a productive cough, as noted by the yellow-white phlegm. An expectorant is the best agent for relief of a productive cough. The only available expectorant is guaifenesin, which works to loosen sputum and to thin bronchial secretions by irritating the gastric mucosa and stimulates secretions of the respiratory tract.

10. The answer is D *[see II.F.1.a–b]*.
Pseudoephedrine is an oral decongestant, whereas phenylephrine can be found as an active ingredient in oral and topical products for nasal congestion. Oxymetazoline and levmetamfetamine are topical decongestants. Pseudoephedrine, phenylephrine, and oxymetazoline should be used cautiously in the patient with hypertension or diabetes, despite adequate control, owing to stimulation of adrenergic receptors. Levmetamfetamine lacks a vasopressor effect and, therefore, does not need to carry the warning for patients with cardiac conditions, hypertension, or diabetes.

11. The answer is A *[see II.F.2.b–c; III.E.2]*
The active ingredient in Alavert is loratadine, a second-generation antihistamine. Benadryl, Tavist, and Actifed all contain first-generation antihistamines as the active ingredient. Though the least expensive treatment option, the use of first-generation antihistamines is limited owing to significant sedation. Studies have clearly demonstrated a reduction in intellectual and motor function in patients taking first-generation antihistamines. Second-generation antihistamines are advantageous because their preference for peripheral H_1-receptor binding. This allows for minimal CNS effects, sedative effects, and anticholinergic activity.

OTC Agents for Constipation, Diarrhea, Hemorrhoids, and Heartburn

Laura K. Williford Owens

I. CONSTIPATION

A. General information

1. **Definition.** Constipation is defined as a decrease in the frequency of fecal elimination and is characterized by the passage of hard, dry, and sometimes painful stools. Normal stool frequency ranges from three times daily to three times per week. Patients may experience abdominal bloating, headaches, low back pain, and/or a sense of rectal fullness from incomplete evacuation of feces.

2. **Epidemiology**
   a. **Age.** Constipation is common in all age groups, however; there is a higher prevalence in people > 65 years of age.
   b. **Gender.** Women suffer from constipation more often than men.

3. **Causes.** Constipation can be caused by many factors, including the following:
   a. **Diet**
      (1) Insufficient dietary fiber
      (2) Inadequate fluid intake
   b. **Lack of exercise**
   c. **Poor bowel habits,** such as failure to respond to the defecatory urge or hurried bowels (i.e., incomplete evacuation)
   d. **Medications,** such as narcotic analgesics, diuretics, or anticholinergics (e.g., antidepressants, antihypertensives, antihistamines, phenothiazines, antispasmodics). In addition, nonprescription medications such as iron supplements, calcium- or aluminum-containing antacids, nonprescription NSAIDs, and histamine-2 receptor antagonists (H_2RAs) (i.e., ranitidine) may contribute to constipation.
   e. **Pregnancy** is a common contributor to constipation. The increased size of the uterus, hormonal changes, intake of calcium- and iron-containing prenatal vitamins, and a reduction in physical activity are all considered contributing factors.
   f. **Organic problems,** such as intestinal obstruction, tumor, inflammatory bowel disease, diverticulitis, hypothyroidism, hyperglycemia, irritable bowel syndrome, cerebrovascular disease, or Parkinson disease

4. **Practitioners should question the patient about the following:**
   a. Normal stool frequency
   b. Duration of the constipation
   c. Frequency of constipation episodes
   d. Exercise routine
   e. Amount of dietary fiber consumed and fluid intake
   f. Presence of other symptoms
   g. Current medications
   h. Medications used to relieve constipation and their effectiveness

B. Treatment

1. **Nonpharmacological**
   a. Increase intake of fluids (at least eight 8-oz. servings of noncaffeinated fluids daily) and fiber (e.g., whole-grain breads and cereals, beans, prunes, raisins, peas, carrots, corn).
   b. Increase exercise to increase and maintain bowel tone.

c. Bowel training to increase regularity (i.e. allowing regular and adequate time for defecation).

2. Pharmacological. Therapeutic agents are classified according to their mechanism of action. Refer patients taking prescription medications that might cause constipation to their provider. Laxatives should not be taken if symptoms of appendicitis are present (i.e. nausea, vomiting, or abdominal pain).

a. Bulk-forming laxatives. These medications are natural or synthetic polysaccharide derivatives that adsorb water to soften the stool and increase bulk, which stimulates peristalsis. Bulk-forming laxatives work in both the small and the large intestines. The onset of action of these agents is slow (12–24 hr and up to 72 hr), which is why they are best used to prevent constipation rather than to treat severe acute constipation.

(1) **Administration guidelines.** All bulk-forming agents must be given with at least 8 oz. of water to minimize the possible esophagus, stomach, small intestine, and colon obstruction experienced by some patients. Some bulk-forming medications may contain sugar, so patients with diabetes should use sugar-free products.

(2) **Adverse effects.** Abdominal cramping and flatulence are the most common adverse effects experienced by patients.

(3) **Warnings**
  (a) Bulk-forming agents should not be used if patients have an obstructing bowel lesion, intestinal strictures, or Crohn disease because they can make this situation worse and possibly result in bowel perforation.
  (b) Do not recommend sugar-free bulk-forming agents to patients with phenylketonuria.
  (c) Patients should be advised not to use bulk-forming laxatives for more than 1 week to treat constipation; however, they can be used on a long-term basis for prevention.

(4) **Natural bulk-forming laxatives**
  (a) **Psyllium** (e.g., Metamucil, Konsyl-D, Fiberall, Perdiem Fiber Granules). Adults: 3.5 g (1 rounded teaspoon) in 8 oz. of water one to three times per day; children: half the adult dosage one to three times per day
  (b) **Malt soup extract** (e.g., Maltsupex). Adults: 8–16 g (1–2 scoops) two to four times per day; children: 16 g one to two times per day

(5) **Synthetic bulk-forming laxatives**
  (a) **Methylcellulose** (e.g., Citrucel). Adults: 1–2 g (1 tablespoon) one to three times per day; children: 0.5 g one to three times per day
  (b) **Polycarbophil** (e.g., Konsyl Fiber, Fiber Con, Mitrolan, Perdiem). Adults: 1 g (2 tablets) one to four times per day; children: 0.5 g one to three times per day. Calcium polycarbophil may impair the absorption of tetracyclines if the drugs are taken concurrently.

b. Saline and **osmotic laxatives** work by creating an osmotic gradient to pull water into the small and large intestines. This increased volume results in distention of the intestinal lumen, causing increased peristalsis and bowel motility. These laxatives also increase the activity of cholecystokinin-pancreozymin, which is an enzyme that increases the secretion of fluids into the gastrointestinal (GI) tract. The **onset of action** depends on the ingredient and dosage form. Rectal formulations (e.g., enemas, suppositories) have an onset of action of 5–30 min, whereas oral preparations work within 3–6 hr.

(1) **Administration guidelines.** Patients should be advised to consume 8 oz. of water with each dose to prevent possible dehydration.

(2) **Adverse effects.** Diarrhea and abdominal cramping are common adverse effects. Less common adverse effects include excessive diuresis, nausea, vomiting, and dehydration.

(3) **Warnings**
  (a) Patients with hypertension or congestive heart failure should not receive saline laxatives on a prolonged basis owing to fluid retention from sodium absorption.
  (b) Patients with severe kidney disease should not use products containing magnesium unless advised by a physician.

(4) **Saline laxatives** include sodium and magnesium salts. As much as 20% of magnesium may be absorbed from these products, which may lead to hypermagnesemia in patients with preexisting renal impairment. Products include the following:

(a) **Magnesium citrate** (e.g., Magnesia Citrate). Adults: one full bottle; children 6–12 years of age: one third to one half bottle. Advise patients to refrigerate to increase palatability and help prevent crystallization.
(b) **Magnesium hydroxide** (e.g., Phillips' Milk of Magnesia). Adults: 30–60 mL; children 6–12 years of age: 15–30 mL; children 2–5 years of age: 5–15 mL
(c) **Magnesium sulfate** (e.g., Epsom salt). Adults: 10–30 g in 8 oz. of water; children 6–12 years of age: 5–10 g
(d) **Sodium phosphate** (e.g., Fleet Phospho-Soda). Adults: 20–45 mL; children 6–12 years of age: 5–20 mL

(5) **Osmotic laxatives**
(a) **Glycerin** is available in rectal products in suppository or enema form (e.g., Fleet Babylax).
(i) The only safe and effective use of glycerin is rectal. Rectal burning may occur with glycerin products. In addition to the osmotic effect, sodium stearate in these products can produce a local irritant effect.
(ii) Adults: 3 g in suppository form or 5–15 mL as an enema; children ≥ 6 years of age: 1–1.5 g in suppository form or 2–5 mL as an enema
(b) **Lactulose** (e.g., Chronulac, Enulose) is available only by prescription and is used to decrease blood ammonia levels in hepatic encephalopathy.
(i) It may cause flatulence and cramping and should be taken with fruit juice, water, or milk to increase the palatability. Onset of action is 24–48 hr.
(ii) Adults: 15–30 mL one to two times daily; children: 7.5 mL once daily, usually given after breakfast
(c) **Sorbitol,** a nonabsorbable sugar, is similar in efficacy to lactulose, which can be administered orally (70% solution) or rectally (25% solution).
(i) The **adverse effects** are the same as for lactulose and include flatulence, cramping, and abdominal pain over the first few days.
(ii) Adults: 30–150 mL orally (70% solution) or 120 mL rectally (25% solution); children 2–11 years of age: 15 mL orally (70% solution) or 30–60 mL of a rectal solution (25%)
(d) **Polyethylene glycol 3350 (Miralax)** is available only by prescription and can be used for bowel evacuation if other products have not worked.
(i) It has been shown to be more effective than lactulose in short-term trials with less abdominal cramping. Onset of action is 48–96 hr.
(ii) Adults: 17 g (1 cap) dissolved in 8 oz. of clear fluid (water, juice, cola, or tea) once daily for up to 2 weeks; children: 0.8 g/kg/day

c. **Stimulant laxatives.** These medications work in the small and large intestines to stimulate bowel motility (i.e., propulsive peristaltic activity) and increase the secretion of fluids into the bowel. The oral preparations usually have an onset of action within 6–12 hr; rectal preparations usually have an onset of action within 15–60 min. Stimulant laxatives are effective as initial drug therapy to treat constipation but should not be used for more than 1 week.
(1) **Administration guidelines.** Patients with undiagnosed rectal bleeding or signs of intestinal obstruction should not use stimulant laxatives.
(2) **Adverse effects.** All stimulant laxatives can cause abdominal cramping. Electrolyte and fluid deficiencies, enteric loss of protein, malabsorption, and hypokalemia are additional possible adverse effects. The suppository form may cause rectal burning.
(3) **Warnings**
(a) Chronic use of stimulant laxatives can lead to **cathartic colon,** which results in a poorly functioning colon and resembles the symptoms of ulcerative colitis. However, most cases of cathartic colon were published before 1960, when more toxic ingredients (e.g., podophyllin) were used in laxative products.
(b) Another issue surrounds the possible carcinogenicity of stimulant laxatives. Phenolphthalein was removed from the market as suggested by the U.S. Food and Drug Administration (FDA) when data of carcinogenic tumors and genetic damage in rats were reported. Subsequently, senna and the structurally similar products aloe and cascara sagrada are now considered category 3 drugs; more data are needed to assess their safety.
(4) **Anthraquinone laxatives** include senna (sennosides)
(a) **Melanosis coli,** which is a dark pigmentation of the colonic mucosa, can result with long-term use of anthraquinone laxatives. This usually disappears 6–12

months after discontinuing the medication. It was previously thought that melanosis did not result in adverse consequences; however, patients with melanosis have a threefold higher risk of cancer.

(b) Discoloration (pink/red, yellow, or brown) of the urine may occur.

(c) Additional anthraquinone laxatives (cascara, casanthranol, and aloe) were removed from the U.S. market because of carcinogenicity concerns.

(d) Anthraquinone products include the **sennosides** (e.g., Senokot, Ex-Lax, Fletcher's Castoria), which are considered to be potent and cause abdominal cramping.

(i) Sennosides can also be combined with docusate (stool softener) for relief of constipation (Peri-Colace, Senokot-S).

(ii) Adults: 12–50 mg twice daily; children: 6–25 mg twice daily

(5) Bisacodyl (e.g., Dulcolax, Doxidan, Correctol) is a **diphenylmethane derivative.**

(a) The tablet formulations of bisacodyl are enteric coated, so they should not be crushed or chewed. Also, bisacodyl-containing products should not be taken within 1 hr of ingesting antacids or milk.

(b) Adults (oral): is 5–15 mg daily; children ≥ 6 years of age (oral): 5 mg daily; adults (rectal): 10 mg (1 suppository); children > 2 years of age (rectal): 5 mg (1/2 suppository).

(6) Castor oil (e.g., Purge) has an onset of action within 2–6 hr.

(a) Castor oil works primarily at the small intestine, which can result in strong cathartic effects (e.g., excessive fluid and electrolyte loss). These cathartic effects can lead to dehydration.

(b) Castor oil should not be used in pregnant patients because it may induce premature labor.

(c) Adults: 15–60 mL; children 2–12 years of age: 5–15 mL

d. Emollient laxatives act as surfactants by allowing absorption of water into the stool, which makes the softened stool easier to pass. Emollient laxatives have a **slow onset of action** (24–72 hr), which is why they are not considered the drug of choice for severe acute constipation, and they are more useful for preventing constipation.

(1) Administration guidelines. These medications are particularly useful in patients who must avoid straining to pass hard stools, such as those who recently had a myocardial infarction or rectal surgery. However, clinical trials evaluating emollient stool-softening laxatives show that these products, when compared to placebo, do not affect the weight or water content of the stool or the frequency of stool passing.

(2) Adverse effects. Diarrhea and mild abdominal cramping are potential adverse effects.

(3) Warnings. Use should be avoided if nausea and vomiting, symptoms of appendicitis, or undetermined abdominal pain exist. Docusate products may facilitate the systemic absorption of mineral oil, so these agents should not be used concurrently.

(4) Products. Emollient laxatives are salts of the surfactant **docusate.** These products contain insignificant amounts of calcium, sodium, or potassium, and there are no specific guidelines for the selection of any one product. The products include

(a) Docusate sodium (Colace, Exlax stool softener)

(b) Docusate calcium (Surfak)

(c) Docusate potassium (Kasof)

(5) Dosage information

(a) Adults: 50–300 mg per day; children ≥ 2 years of age: 50–150 mg per day

(b) Each dose must be taken with at least 8 oz. of water. Liquid preparations should be taken in fruit juice or infant formula to increase palatability.

e. Lubricant laxative (mineral oil). Mineral oil works at the colon to increase water retention in the stool to soften the stool. It has an **onset of action** of 6–8 hr with oral administration and 5–15 min after rectal administration.

(1) Administration guidelines

(a) Mineral oil should be taken on an empty stomach. Because of possible aspiration of mineral oil into the lungs, patients should not take mineral oil at bedtime or recline after administration.

(b) Adults: 15–45 mL per day; children: 5–15 mL per day

(2) Adverse effects. Mineral oil products may cause anal seepage, which results in itching (i.e. pruritus ani) and perianal discomfort.

(3) Warnings

(a) Mineral oil can **decrease absorption of fat-soluble vitamins** (i.e., vitamins A, D, E, and K), so it should not be used on a chronic basis.

(b) Elderly, young, debilitated, and dysphagic patients are at the greatest risk of **lipid pneumonitis** from mineral oil aspiration.

(c) Emollients (e.g., docusate) may increase the systemic absorption of mineral oil, which can lead to **hepatotoxicity.**

(d) Mineral oil should not be given to patients with rectal bleeding or appendicitis.

(e) Mineral oil should not be given to children < 6 years of age.

C. Special patient issues

1. **Pediatric patients.** The bowel patterns of pediatric patients vary. During the first weeks of life, infants pass approximately four stools per day. As children get older, approximately one to three stools are passed per day. Constipation should be expected if there is a drastic change from a child's baseline bowel function.

   a. Nonpharmacological methods, such as increasing the amount of fluid or sugar in a child's formula in younger children or increasing the bulk content of the child's diet (fruit, fiber cereals, vegetables), should be tried before medications are used.

   b. If nonpharmacological methods do not work, rectal stimulation may be useful. Pharmacological agents that can be used for acute relief include glycerin suppositories and magnesium laxatives. Stimulant laxatives should be administered as a last resort, but enemas should not be used in children < 2 years of age and with extreme caution in children 2–5 years of age (see I.C.4). Bulk-forming agents and stool softeners can be used if the constipation does not need immediate relief.

2. **Pregnant patients.** Constipation in pregnancy is common and is often the result of compression of the colon by the enlarged uterus. Pregnant patients should avoid any preparation that may be absorbed systemically (e.g., stimulant laxatives), any preparation that can interfere with vitamin absorption (e.g., mineral oil), or any preparation that can induce premature labor (e.g., castor oil). Pregnant patients should use bulk-forming agents or stool softeners.

3. **Geriatric patients** tend to be at risk for constipation because of insufficient dietary (fiber) and fluid ingestion, failure to establish a regular bowel time habit, and abuse of stimulant laxatives resulting in a loss of smooth muscle tone in the bowel, which promotes constipation (see I.C.5). These causes should be investigated in addition to primary disease states (e.g., hypothyroidism) and medications (e.g., opiates, anticholinergics) that may lead to constipation in elderly patients. A **major concern** with geriatric patients is the possible loss of fluid that can be induced by aggressive laxative treatment (e.g., enemas, high-dose saline laxatives). Geriatric patients should not use stimulant laxatives on a chronic basis, and patients with renal impairment should not use magnesium products. Glycerin suppositories or orally administered lactulose may be useful for initial treatment of constipation and bulk-forming agents used to prevent constipation.

4. **Use of enemas.** Enemas are useful for evacuation of the bowel before surgery, childbirth, and for the treatment of acute constipation that has not responded to other medications (e.g., bisacodyl suppositories).

   a. An enema is the dosage route, and the enema fluid determines the mechanism of evacuation (e.g., stimulant, osmotic). When administered correctly, an enema evacuates only the distal colon, similar to a normal bowel movement. This is accomplished by having the patient lie on his or her side with the knees tucked toward the chest. While in this position, 1 pint (500 mL) of enema solution should be slowly squeezed into the rectum. This should be retained up to 1 hr or until definite lower abdominal cramping is felt. At this point, the bowel movement is ready for expulsion.

   b. Although all enemas cause abdominal cramping, some may have more serious **adverse effects** than others. Soap suds enemas can cause much rectal irritation and have been reported to cause anaphylaxis and rectal gangrene.

   c. The popular sodium phosphate enemas (e.g., Fleet) are very effective but have resulted in hyperphosphatasemia, hypocalcemia (tetany), hypokalemia, metabolic acidosis, and cardiac death, usually owing to conduction abnormalities in very small children. This has mainly occurred in children < 2 years of age or from 2 to 5 years of age with predisposing factors.

   (1) The factors include chronic renal disease, anorectal malformations, and/or Hirschsprung disease, which allow phosphate blood concentrations to become abnormally high and potassium and calcium to become low, predisposing these patients to cardiac arrhythmias and potentially death.

(2) Therefore, the use of enemas is highly discouraged in children < 5 years of age.

5. **Laxative abuse** is a term to describe the routine, chronic use of laxatives on a daily basis (e.g., elderly patients) to the administration of high doses several times daily by patients with anorexia nervosa or bulimia for weight control. Excessive use of laxatives can lead to excessive diarrhea and vomiting, resulting in fluid and electrolyte abnormalities. In addition to the risks to patients from hypokalemia (e.g., metabolic alkalosis, cardiac conduction problems), patients can also develop osteomalacia, liver disease, and cathartic colon. Cathartic colon results from superficial ulcerations in the colon as well as damage to the muscularis mucosa and submucosa. This results in a loss of tone of the smooth and striated muscle and causes poor bowel function.

II. DIARRHEA

A. General Information

1. **Definition.** Diarrhea is defined as an increase in the frequency and looseness of stools compared to one's normal bowel pattern. The overall weight and volume of the stool is increased (> 200 g or mL/day), and the water content is increased to 60%–90%. In general, diarrhea results when some factor impairs the ability of the intestine to absorb water from the stool, which causes excess water in the stool.

2. **Classification.** Diarrhea can be classified based on mechanisms or origin.
   a. **Classification by mechanism**
      (1) **Osmotic diarrhea** occurs when a nonabsorbable solute pulls excess water into the intestinal tract. Osmotic diarrhea ceases when the patient converts to a fasting state.
         (a) Ingestion of large meals or certain osmotic substances (e.g., sorbitol, glycerin) can lead to diarrhea.
         (b) Disaccharidase deficiency which is a lack of enzymes needed to break down disaccharides in the gut for absorption (e.g., lactase deficiency), results in an increase in osmotic sugars (i.e., lactose, sucrose) in the intestinal tract.
         (c) Medications that can induce osmotic diarrhea include lactulose and magnesium-containing antacids and laxatives.
      (2) **Secretory diarrhea** occurs when the intestinal wall is damaged, resulting in an increased secretion rather than absorption of electrolytes into the intestinal tract. Common sources include
         (a) **Bacterial endotoxins** (e.g., *Escherichia coli, Vibrio cholerae, Shigella, Staphylococcus aureus*)
         (b) **Bacterial infections** (e.g., *Shigella, Salmonella*)
         (c) **Viral infections** (e.g., rotavirus, Norwalk virus)
         (d) **Protozoal infections** (e.g., *Giardia lamblia, Entamoeba histolytica*)
         (e) **Miscellaneous causes.** Inflammatory bowel disease and medications (e.g., prostaglandins, antibiotics, colchicine, chemotherapeutic agents)
      (3) **Motility disorders.** Diarrhea induced by motility disorders results from decreased contact time of the fecal mass with the intestinal wall, so less water is absorbed from the feces.
         (a) **Motility disorders** include irritable bowel syndrome, scleroderma, diabetic neuropathy, gastric/intestinal resection, and vagotomy.
         (b) **Medications** that can induce motility disorders include parasympathomimetic agents that enhance the effects of acetylcholine (e.g., metoclopramide, bethanechol), digitalis, quinidine, and antibiotics.
            (i) Antibiotics cause diarrhea by causing intestinal irritation, increased bowel motility, and altered bowel microbial flora.
            (ii) Most antibiotic-induced diarrhea can be minimized by taking the agent with food.
   b. **Classification by origin**
      (1) **Acute diarrhea** (usually self-limiting for 2–3 days but may last up to 2 weeks)
         (a) **Infection. Most common** sources include viral and bacterial, but protozoal diarrhea also occurs. Organisms include the following:

  (i) Viruses that commonly cause diarrhea are rotaviruses and the Norwalk virus.

    {a} Rotaviruses usually affect children < 2 years of age. The virus has an onset of 1–2 days and lasts 5–8 days. Patients usually have vomiting and a mild fever, and may experience severe dehydration. There is usually no blood or pus in the stool.

    {b} The **Norwalk virus** affects older children and adults. It has an onset of 1–2 days and lasts 24–48 hr (the "24-hr bug"). As with rotaviruses, there is mild fever but no blood or pus in the stool.

  (ii) Bacteria. Most bacterial diarrhea results from consumption of contaminated water or food, with an onset of diarrhea in 8 hr to several days. Diarrhea caused by the consumption of contaminated food or water that occurs in a foreign country (e.g., Mexico, third-world countries) is referred to as "traveler's diarrhea."

    {a} Toxigenic bacteria. Diarrhea caused by toxigenic *E. coli, Staphylococcus aureus, V. cholerae,* and *Shigella* results from the secretory effects of enterotoxins released by these organisms in the small intestine. Patients usually experience large-volume stools that are watery or greasy.

    {b} Invasive bacteria. Diarrhea caused by invasive *E. coli, Shigella, Salmonella, Campylobacter,* and *Clostridium difficile* results from mucosal invasion of the colon. This results in a dysentery-like diarrhea, which is characterized by an extreme urgency to defecate, abdominal cramping, tenesmus, fever, chills, and small-volume stools that contain blood or pus.

  (iii) Protozoa. *G. lamblia, Entamoeba histolytica,* and *Cryptosporidium* cause explosive, foul-smelling, large-volume, watery stools. This is thought to be caused by invasion of the small intestine, which causes damage to the microvilli and, therefore, decreases absorption of fluids. This type of diarrhea can result in large fluid losses, and patients are at risk for dehydration. Although protozoan-induced diarrhea is self-limiting, it may persist for several months, so therapy should be considered to eradicate the organism.

 (b) Diet-induced diarrhea. Diarrhea induced by foods results from food allergies, high-fiber diets, fatty or spicy foods, large amounts of caffeine, or milk intolerance. The best treatment is prevention, by avoiding troublesome foods.

 (c) Drug-induced diarrhea (see II.A.2.a)

(2) Chronic diarrhea (lasts longer than 2 weeks). If a patient suffers from diarrhea for long periods of time, or from recurrent episodes of diarrhea, the following causes must be considered: protozoal organisms, food-induced diarrhea (e.g., lactose intolerance), irritable bowel syndrome, malabsorption syndromes (e.g., celiac sprue, diverticulosis, short bowel syndrome), inflammatory bowel disease, pancreatic disease, and hyperthyroidism.

B. Patient evaluation

1. Pharmacists who are consulted by patients should ask the patient for the following information before recommending a therapy:
   a. Age of the patient
   b. Onset and duration of the diarrhea
   c. Description of stool (i.e., frequency, volume, blood, pus, watery)
   d. Other symptoms (e.g., abdominal cramping, fever, nausea, vomiting, weight loss)
   e. Medications recently started or medications used to relieve the diarrhea
   f. Recent travel (where and how long ago)
   g. Medical history (history of GI disorders)

2. **Referrals to a physician** should be made by the pharmacist who encounters a patient with diarrhea that meets the following criteria:
   a. **Younger than 3 years** of age or **older than 60 years** of age (with multiple medical problems), pregnant or breast-feeding patients, and patients with HIV.
   b. **Blood or mucus in the stools**
   c. **High fever** (> 101°F or 38°C)
   d. **Dehydration or weight loss** > 5% of total body weight; signs of dehydration—dry mouth, sunken eyes, crying without tears, dry skin that is not elastic like normal skin
   e. **Duration of diarrhea** > 2 days
   f. **Vomiting**

Table 33-1. Guidelines for Oral-Replacement Therapy Established by the World Health Organization (WHO)

Ingredients	Dose
Sodium chloride (table salt)	90 mEq (1/2 teaspoon)
Potassium chloride (potassium salt)	20 mEq (1/4 teaspoon)
Sodium bicarbonate (baking soda)	30 mEq (1/2 teaspoon)
Glucose (sugar)	20 g (2 teaspoons)
Water	Enough to make 1 L of solution

C. **Treatment**

1. **Nonpharmacological**

   a. **Food/breast-feeding.** In the past, there was much controversy regarding the decision to feed or not to feed children during acute episodes of diarrhea. Originally, parents were told that children should not receive food, milk products, or breast–feed for 6–48 hr after the onset of diarrhea. Parents were also told that if children did receive food, they should receive the BRAT diet, which consists of bananas, rice, applesauce, and toast. This diet does not work and is deficient in calories, protein, and fat. All patients should receive their normal diet or breast–feeding during bouts of diarrhea because these do not make the diarrhea worse and may actually improve the condition. Fatty foods, foods rich in simple sugars (can cause osmotic diarrhea), and spicy foods (may cause GI upset) should be avoided. Caffeine-containing beverages, which may worsen the diarrhea, should also be avoided.

   b. **Fluids.** The most important part of treating acute diarrhea is the replacement of lost fluids and electrolytes. If patients experience mild to moderate fluid loss, fluid replacement can be achieved with oral-rehydration solutions (ORS). If fluid loss is severe (> 10% loss of body weight) and/or severe vomiting persists, then patients may need intravenous rehydration before oral maintenance fluids can be administered. ORSs can be easily made at home (Table 33-1) or purchased ready-to-use (e.g., Pedialyte, Rehydra-lyte). All of these solutions are considered equally safe and effective but have no effect on the duration of the diarrhea. The secretory and absorptive mechanisms of the bowel function separately, and this allows these ORS to be absorbed during acute episodes of diarrhea, preventing severe dehydration and complications. Not every patient needs ORS. For a child without evidence of dehydration (see II.B.2.d), administer 10 mL/kg or 1/2–1 cup of ORS for each loose stool. If a child is vomiting, administer smaller amounts (1–2 teaspoonsful) every 2–5 min as tolerated.

      (1) **Fluid and electrolyte replacement.** Fluid and electrolyte therapy is aimed at replacing what the body has lost. During this situation, the patient's fluid input and output as well as weight should be monitored. The World Health Organization (WHO) has established guidelines for oral-replacement therapy (Table 33-1). Recommended doses are given in Table 33-2.

      (2) **Fluids to be avoided** include hypertonic fruit juices and drinks (e.g., apple juice, powdered drink mixes, gelatin water), carbonated beverages, and caffeine-containing beverages, which can make diarrhea worse and do not contain needed electrolytes (i.e., Na^+, K^+). Gatorade diluted in water (1:1) is adequate and provides the necessary combination of glucose, sodium, and potassium.

Table 33-2. Guidelines for Fluid- and Electrolyte-Replacement Therapy

Age Group	Dose	
	Mild (2–3 stools/day)	Moderate (4–5 stools/day)
> 5 years of age	2 L/first 4 hr, then replace ongoing losses	2–4 L/first 4 hr, then replace ongoing losses
< 5 years of age	50 mL/kg/first 4 hr, then 10 mL/kg or 1/2–1 cup per stool	100 mL/kg/4 hr, then 10 mL/kg or 1/2–1 cup per stool

2. **Pharmacologic. Antidiarrheals** may serve to prevent an attack of diarrhea or to relieve existing symptoms. Based on the FDA review of antidiarrheal products, three agents have been identified as category 1 (i.e., safe and effective) ingredients: **kaolin, bismuth subsalicylate,** and **loperamide.** In April 2003, the FDA reclassified attapulgite and polycarbophil products from category 1 to category 3 because of insufficient effectiveness data. Antidiarrheal agents are classified in different categories on the basis of their chemical class or pharmacologic mechanism of action.

   a. **Antiperistaltic drugs**

      (1) **Mechanism of action.** Antiperistaltic drugs act by stimulating μ opioid receptors on the circular and longitudinal musculature of the small and large intestines to normalize peristaltic intestinal movements. They slow intestinal motility and affect water and electrolyte movement through the bowel. Loperamide is considered two to three times more potent than diphenoxylate and 50 times more potent than morphine in its ability to slow GI motility. Loperamide does not appreciably penetrate the central nervous system (CNS) and thus has a low risk for CNS side effects. Loperamide is effective in acute, nonspecific diarrhea, traveler's diarrhea, and chronic diarrhea associated with inflammatory bowel disease. The frequency of bowel movements is decreased, and the consistency of stools is increased. However, replacement of fluids (through ORS) and dietary management are still the main focus of therapy for diarrhea.

      (2) **Contraindication.** Antiperistaltic medications have always been restricted in patients with acute bacterial diarrhea associated with fecal leukocytes, high fever, or blood or mucus in the stool because of the potential for these drugs to decrease clearance of the organism and enhance systemic invasion of the organism. Most information shows that this is not significant and probably will cause no harm. However, these medications should not be used in patients with colitis (potential for the development of toxic megacolon) or in children < 2 years of age.

      (3) **Prescription agents** in this class include the opiate-related agent diphenoxylate/atropine (e.g., Lomotil).

      (4) **Nonprescription agents. Loperamide** (e.g., Imodium A-D, Maalox Anti-Diarrheal, Pepto Diarrhea Control) provides effective control of diarrhea as quickly as 1 hr after administration. Antiperistaltic drugs should not be used for more than 48 hr in acute diarrhea.

         (a) **Administration guidelines.** Adults: 4 mg followed by 2 mg after each loose stool, not to exceed 16 mg/day; children: 1–2 mg up to three times per day, depending on weight and age.

         (b) **Adverse effects.** At recommended doses, loperamide is generally well tolerated. Side effects are infrequent and consist primarily of abdominal pain, distention, or discomfort; drowsiness; dizziness; and dry mouth.

   b. **Adsorbents.** These medications are not selective and adsorb toxins, bacteria, gases, and fluids. In addition, adsorbents may adsorb drugs in the GI tract. They are not absorbed systemically, so they produce **few adverse effects.** These products are given for symptomatic relief and are usually administered in large doses immediately following a loose stool. They are generally not effective for severe acute diarrhea.

      (1) **Kaolin**

         (a) **Administration guidelines**

            (i) Adults and children 12 years of age and older (oral): 26.2 g after each loose stool.

            (ii) Continue to take every 6 hr until stool is firm but not for more than 2 days.

            (iii) Do not exceed 262 g in 24 hr.

         (b) **Adverse effects.** Because activated kaolin is inert and is not absorbed systemically, adverse effects are minor with few patients experiencing constipation, bloating, and fullness.

         (c) **Warnings.** It is recommended that this product not be given within 3 hr of other medications because it may decrease the absorption of other orally administered medications.

   c. **Miscellaneous agents**

      (1) **Bismuth subsalicylate** (e.g., Pepto-Bismol, Kaopectate). Bismuth salts work as adsorbents but also are believed to decrease secretion of water into the bowel. It is effective and can reduce the number of stools by 50%. Bismuth preparations have moderate effectiveness against the prevention and treatment of traveler's diarrhea and nonspe-

cific diarrhea, but doses required for relief are large and must be administered frequently, so these preparations may be inconvenient.
- **(a) Administration guidelines**
    - **(i)** Adults: 2 tablets or 30–60 mL (524 mg) every hour as needed to a maximum of 8 doses in a 24-hr period; children > 2 years of age: one third to one half of adult dose.
    - **(ii)** Bismuth subsalicylate can prevent traveler's diarrhea when 2 tablets are taken four times per day.
    - **(iii)** Shake the suspension well before use.
- **(b) Adverse effects** may include harmless grayish charcoal coloring of stools or tongue. Ringing in the ears (i.e. tinnitus) can occur with high doses, especially if the patient is simultaneously taking other salicylate products.
- **(c) Warnings/Contrandications**
    - **(i)** Patients with black or bloody stools should not use this product.
    - **(ii)** Bismuth subsalicylate should not be given to children or teenagers during or after recovery from chickenpox or flu because of the possible association of salicylates with Reye syndrome.
    - **(iii)** Patients with documented allergies to salicylates should not take this product.
    - **(iv)** Patients on anticoagulants should be monitored closely if taking these products.
    - **(v)** Pregnant or breast-feeding patients should not take these products.
- **(2) Lactobacillus** (e.g., Bacid, Lactinex) products are intended to replace the normal bacterial flora that is lost during the administration of oral antibiotics. However, there is little information to show that these products are useful for antibiotic-induced diarrhea; with the increase in bowel organisms, patients can experience flatulence. Most clinicians do not recommend their use.
- **(3) Lactase** (e.g., LactAid, Lactrase, Dairy Ease) is indicated for individuals who have insufficient amounts of lactase in the small intestine. Lactose (a disaccharide present in dairy products) must be broken down to glucose and galactose to be fully digested. If it is not, lactose draws water into the GI tract, and diarrhea results. Lactase is the enzyme responsible for digesting lactose. The dose is 1–2 capsules taken with milk or dairy products or added to milk before drinking. Titration of doses to higher levels may be required in some patients.
- **(4) Anti-infectives.** Depending on the suspected origin of the infectious diarrhea, prescription antibiotics and antiprotozoal medications can be used to eradicate the organisms and decrease the duration of symptoms (Table 33-3). If antibiotics are used to prevent traveler's diarrhea, therapy should be started 1 day before arrival in high-incidence regions and continued until 2 days after departure. If diarrhea has occurred, antibiotic treatment should last for 3–5 days.
- **(5) Anticholinergics** (e.g., atropine, hyoscyamine) decrease bowel motility, which results in an increase of fluid absorption from the intestinal tract and a decrease in abdominal cramping. These products are found in combination with adsorbents or opiates.

Table 33-3. Drugs and Doses Used to Treat Infectious Diarrhea

Antibacterials	Antiprotozoal	Dose[a]
Azithromycin	N/A	500 mg, then 250 mg daily
Ciprofloxacin	N/A	500 mg twice daily
Doxycycline	N/A	100 mg twice daily
Metronidazole[b]	—	250–750 mg three times daily
Norfloxacin	N/A	400 mg twice daily
Ofloxacin	N/A	300 mg twice daily
Quinacrine	—	100 mg three times daily
Trimethoprim/sulfamethoxazole DS[c]	N/A	1 tablet twice daily
Vancomycin[b]	N/A	125 mg four times daily

[a]Antibiotics are used for 3–5 days for bacterial- and protozoal-induced diarrhea.
[b]Metronidazole and vancomycin are used for 10–14 days for clostridial diarrhea.
[c]Trimethoprim/sulfamethoxazole is not considered first line because of resistance problems.

However, the amount of anticholinergic found in most products is not considered to be enough to alter the course of severe acute diarrhea. **Adverse effects** include dry mouth, blurred vision, and tachycardia. These products should not be used in patients with narrow-angle glaucoma.

III. HEMORRHOIDS

A. General Information

1. **Definition.** Hemorrhoids (also known as piles) are defined as abnormally large, bulging, symptomatic clusters of dilated blood vessels, supporting tissues, and overlying mucosus membranes. Hemorrhoids can present in the lower rectum (internal hemorrhoids) or anus (external hemorrhoids). Simply, hemorrhoids represent downward displacement of anal cushions that contain arteriovenous anastomoses.

2. **Epidemiology.** Hemorrhoids are common, with approximately 10%–25% of the U.S. population afflicted. The risk of developing hemorrhoids increases with advancing age and peaks in individuals 45–65 years of age. The incidence of hemorrhoids in pregnant women is higher than that of nonpregnant women of similar age. Although they are considered a minor medical problem, they may cause considerable discomfort and anxiety.

B. Types of hemorrhoids are determined by their anatomical position and vascular origin.

1. An **internal** hemorrhoid is an exaggerated vascular cushion with an engorged internal hemorrhoidal plexus located above the dentate line and covered with a mucous membrane.

2. An **external** hemorrhoid is a dilated vein of the inferior hemorrhoidal plexus located below the dentate line and covered with squamous epithelium.

3. A **mixed** hemorrhoid appears as a baggy swelling and exhibits simultaneous characteristics of internal and external hemorrhoids.

C. Origin. Although heredity may predispose a person to hemorrhoids, the exact cause is probably related to acquired factors.

1. Situations that result in **increased venous pressure** in the hemorrhoidal plexus (e.g., chronic straining during defecation; small, hard stools; prolonged sitting on the toilet; occupations that routinely require heavy lifting; pelvic tumors; pregnancy) can transform an asymptomatic hemorrhoid into a problem. Pregnancy is the most frequent cause of hemorrhoids in women of childbearing age.

2. The hemorrhoidal veins are pushed downward during defecation or straining; with increased venous pressure, they **dilate** and **become engorged.** Over time, the **fibers** that anchor the hemorrhoidal veins to their underlying muscular coats **stretch,** which results in **prolapse.**

D. Signs/symptoms

1. The **most common** sign/symptom of hemorrhoids is **painless bleeding** occurring during a bowel movement. The blood is usually bright red and may be visible on the stool, on the toilet tissue, or coloring the water in the toilet.

2. **Prolapse** is the **second most common** sign/symptom of hemorrhoids. A temporary protrusion may occur during defecation, and it may need to be replaced manually. A permanently prolapsed hemorrhoid may give rise to chronic, moist soiling of the underwear. These patients may complain of a dull, aching feeling.

3. **Pain** is unusual unless **thrombosis** involving external tissue is present, and then the pain can be excruciating.

4. **Discomfort, soreness, pruritus, swelling, burning,** and **seepage** may also occur with hemorrhoids.

E. A proper diagnosis is important, because there are a number of conditions that may produce symptoms that mimic those of hemorrhoids. **Other conditions** that may **mimic** hemorrhoids include the following, which usually require a physician's intervention:

1. An **anal abscess,** usually a *Staphylococcus* infection

2. **Cryptitis,** which is inflammation of the crypts (small indentations at the mucocutaneous junction)

3. An **anal fissure,** which is a small tear in the lining of the anus

4. An **anal fistula,** which is an abnormal communication between the mucosa of the rectum and the skin adjacent to the anus

5. **Inflammatory bowel diseases**

6. A **polyp,** which is a tumor of the large intestine

7. **Colorectal cancer**

F. **Internal** hemorrhoids are graded and classified into one of four groups.

1. A **first-degree** hemorrhoid (grade 1) does not descend or prolapse during straining on defecation. Painless bleeding is present.

2. A **second-degree** hemorrhoid (grade 2) descends with defecation but returns spontaneously with relaxation. Mild discomfort and bleeding are present.

3. A **third-degree** hemorrhoid (grade 3) requires manual replacement into the rectum after prolapse (which occurs during defecation or exertion related to work). Pain, bleeding, and discharge of mucus are present.

4. A **fourth-degree** hemorrhoid (grade 4) is permanently prolapsed and cannot be manipulated manually. Thrombosis often occurs.

G. **Treatment.** The symptoms of hemorrhoids are produced by a cycle of events: the protrusion of the vascular submucosal cushion through a tight anal canal, which becomes further congested and hypertrophic, which causes the cushion to protrude farther. All treatments of hemorrhoids aim to break this cycle, and they fall into a number of broad groups.

1. For **first-** and **second-degree internal** hemorrhoids that bleed minimally, a conservative approach can usually be taken.
   a. To **reduce straining** and **downward pressure** on the hemorrhoids, patients should avoid straining when defecating and avoid sitting on the toilet longer than necessary (suggest removing all reading materials from the bathroom).
   b. **Correction of constipation is of paramount importance.** This can be accomplished by eating a high-fiber diet and increasing water intake and physical activity. Bulk-forming laxatives, such as psyllium, and stool softeners, such as docusate, may be helpful.
   c. **Sitz baths** for 15 min, three to four times a day, can soothe the anal mucosa. Tepid water should be used, and prolonged bathing should be avoided. Epsom salts (magnesium sulfate) added to the bath or the application of an ice pack can help reduce the swelling of an edematous or clotted hemorrhoid.
   d. **OTC hemorrhoidal ointments, creams, foams,** and **suppositories** may also help relieve symptoms (see III.H).

2. **Higher-grade internal hemorrhoids** usually require physician expertise and specialized procedures for treatment.
   a. Symptomatic grades 2 or 3 hemorrhoids are often best treated with **hemorrhoid banding** (rubber band ligation). This procedure is performed through an anoscope; a rubber band ligature is placed on the rectal mucosa above the hemorrhoid, well above the dentate line to avoid excessive discomfort. The ligated area sloughs off in a few days.
   b. **Infrared photocoagulation** can be used for grade 2 hemorrhoids; it is less effective than banding with large hemorrhoids. Infrared light is focused at the base of the hemorrhoid, thereby destroying the varicosity secondary to the formation of a white coagulum.
   c. **Sclerotherapy** (injection of a sclerosing agent into the hemorrhoid) or cryotherapy ("freezing" the hemorrhoid) are older therapies that have been used.
   d. **Surgical hemorrhoidectomy** should be undertaken only for grades 3 or 4 hemorrhoids. Whether the procedure is done traditionally or with a laser, most patients have significant discomfort and a period of postoperative disability.

Table 33-4. Guide to Hemorrhoidal Therapy Based on Approved Indication for OTC Anorectal Drug Products

Therapy	Burning	Discomfort	Irritation	Itching	Pain	Soreness	Swelling
Analgesic, anesthetic, antipruritic	Yes	Yes		Yes	Yes	Yes	
Astringent	Yes	Yes	Yes	Yes			
Keratolytic		Yes		Yes			
Local anesthetic	Yes	Yes		Yes	Yes	Yes	
Protectant	Yes	Yes	Yes	Yes			
Vasoconstrictor		Yes	Yes	Yes			Yes
Hydrocortisone		Yes		Yes			Yes

3. An **external, thrombosed hemorrhoid** can be completely excised in an office setting, clinic, or operating room.

H. Nonprescription medication for hemorrhoidal and other anorectal diseases (Table 33-4). The FDA has identified several ingredients as safe and effective to alleviate burning, discomfort, inflammation, irritation, itching, pain, and swelling. These products are simply palliative; they are not meant to cure hemorrhoids or other anorectal disease. If these products do not improve symptoms within 7 days, a physician should be consulted. A physician should also be consulted if bleeding, prolapse, seepage of feces or mucus, thrombosis, or severe pain occurs. Patients < 12 years of age should not rely on self-treatment but should seek medical attention immediately.

1. **Ointments versus suppositories.** Generally, the ointment or cream dosage form is believed to be superior to a suppository, which may bypass the affected area. Patients should wash the anorectal area with mild soap and warm water and pat (not wipe) the area dry before applying a product. Alternatively, patients can use an OTC anal-cleansing pad (e.g., Tucks). Some ointments come with rectal pipes (pile pipes) that allow the patient to insert and apply the medication directly in the rectum. The openings in the rectal pipe allow the ointment to cover large areas of the rectal mucosa unreachable with the finger. The rectal pipe should be lubricated by spreading ointment around the tip of the pipe before insertion. Some clinicians advise against the use of the rectal pipe because the anal canal could be traumatized if the pipe is not inserted properly.

2. **Local anesthetics** work by blocking nerve-impulse transmission. **Agents** deemed safe and effective include benzocaine 5%–20% (e.g., Lanacane), pramoxine 1% (e.g., ProctoFoam), benzyl alcohol 1%–4% (e.g., Tucks Clear Gel), dibucaine 0.25%–1% (e.g., Nupercainal), dyclonine 0.5%–1% (e.g., Dyclone), lidocaine 2%–5% (e.g., Xylocaine), and tetracaine 0.5%–1% (e.g., Pontocaine).
   a. **Administration guidelines.** Local anesthetics should be used for symptoms of pain, itching, burning, discomfort, and irritation in the perianal region or lower anal canal (not in the rectum). The rectum contains no sensory pain receptors. The products should not be applied to abraded skin as this will increase absorption systemically.
   b. **Adverse effects.** These agents may produce a hypersensitivity reaction with burning and itching similar to that of anorectal disease. Systemic absorption is minimal unless the perianal skin is abraded. As a result of its unique chemical structure, pramoxine exhibits little cross-sensitivity compared to the other local anesthetics.
   c. **Warnings**
      (1) Allergic reactions may occur in some patients.
      (2) Advise patients not to use preparations longer than 7 days.

3. **Vasoconstrictors** decrease mucosal perfusion by causing arteriole constriction in the anorectal area after topical application. However, because bleeding in this area may be a sign of more serious disease, vasoconstrictors are not approved for control of minor bleeding. For temporary relief of itching, discomfort, and irritation, these agents have a local anesthetic effect of unknown mechanism.

    a. Agents deemed safe and effective include ephedrine sulfate 0.1%–1.25% in aqueous solution, epinephrine HCl 0.005%–0.01% in aqueous solution, and phenylephrine HCl 0.25% in aqueous solution. These agents are present in various ointments (e.g., Pazo) and suppositories (e.g., Preparation H).

    b. Adverse effects. Topical vasoconstrictors, at recommended doses, may cause nervousness, tremor, sleeplessness, nausea, and loss of appetite. Cardiac arrhythmias, irregular heart rate, and elevation of blood pressure are potentially serious adverse effects, but less likely at recommended doses.

    c. Warnings/contraindications apply to people with cardiovascular disease, high blood pressure, hyperthyroidism, diabetes, and prostate enlargement because of the possibility of systemic absorption.

4. Protectants provide a **physical barrier,** forming a protective coating over skin or mucous membranes, for temporary relief of itching, irritation, discomfort, and burning. They prevent irritation of anorectal tissue and prevent water loss from the stratum corneum. Protectants are often the bases or vehicles for other agents used for anorectal disease. Products include aluminum hydroxide gel, cocoa butter, kaolin, lanolin, hard fat, mineral oil, white petrolatum, petrolatum, glycerin (external use only), topical starch, cod liver oil, shark liver oil, and zinc oxide. When protectants are incorporated into the formulation of an OTC product, they should make up at least 50% of the dosage unit. If two to four protectants are used, their total concentration should represent at least 50% of the whole product. Lanolin, a derivative of wool alcohol, may be allergenic to susceptible individuals.

    a. Absorbents take up fluids that are on or secreted by skin or mucous membranes.

    b. Adsorbents attach to substances secreted by skin or mucous membranes.

    c. Demulcents combine with water to form a colloidal solution, which protects the skin in a way similar to mucus.

    d. Emollients, which are derived from animal or vegetable fats or petroleum products, soften or protect internal or external body surfaces.

5. Astringents lessen mucus and other secretions and protect underlying tissue through a local and limited protein coagulant effect. Action is limited to surface cells, but astringents provide temporary relief of itching, discomfort, irritation, and burning. Products considered to be safe and effective include calamine 5%–25%, witch hazel 10%–50% (external use only), and zinc oxide 5%–25%.

6. Keratolytics cause desquamation and débridement of the surface cells of the epidermis and provide temporary relief of discomfort and itching. Theoretically, keratolytics expose underlying tissue to other therapeutic agents. Products considered to be safe and effective include aluminum chlorhydroxyallantoinate (alcloxa) 0.2%–2.0% and resorcinol 1%–3%. Resorcinol should not be used on an open wound owing to the potential for a serious hypersensitivity reaction. Keratolytics are reserved for external use only.

7. Analgesics, anesthetics, and **antipruritics** provide temporary relief of burning, discomfort, itching, pain, and soreness. The FDA has redesignated several ingredients into this category that were formerly classified as **counterirritants.** Ingredients considered to be safe and effective for external use in the anorectal area include menthol (0.1%–1%), juniper tar (1%–5%), and camphor (0.1%–3%). These agents should not be used to treat internal hemorrhoids.

8. Wound-healing agents. Live yeast cell derivative (LYCD; skin-respiratory factor), which is a water-soluble extract of brewer's yeast, was present in Preparation H in the past. LYCD was removed from the list of **safe and effective** active ingredients by the FDA, which determined that studies have not proven this agent effective. Preparation H products have been reformulated without LYCD. Preparation H Ointment now contains protectants (petrolatum, mineral oil, shark liver oil, lanolin, and glycerin) and the vasoconstrictor phenylephrine.

9. Hydrocortisone (0.25%–1%) causes vasoconstriction, stabilization of lysosomal membranes, and antimitotic activity. These agents have the potential to reduce itching, inflammation, and discomfort in the anorectal area. Until recently, hydrocortisone-containing hemorrhoidal products were available by prescription only. As with any steroid cogener, hydrocortisone may mask the symptoms of bacterial or fungal infections. Hydrocortisone concentrations > 1% are available by prescription only.

IV. GASTROESOPHAGEAL REFLUX DISEASE (HEARTBURN)

A. General information

1. **Definition.** Gastroesophageal reflux disease (GERD) is defined as the retrograde movement of gastric contents into the esophagus (i.e. gastroesophageal reflux). Gastroesophageal reflux is generally a benign physiological process that occurs in normal individuals multiple times throughout the day. However, patients with GERD may experience esophageal tissue damage (reflux esophagitis) and/or symptoms of heartburn when the acidic gastric contents stay in prolonged contact with the esophagus.

2. **Epidemiology.** Between 30% and 50% of the population has experienced occasional episodes of heartburn. The following are predisposing factors for this condition:
   a. **Age.** Patients of any age can experience heartburn; however, this condition is most common in people > 50 years of age.
   b. **Gender,** males are more likely to experience GERD.
   c. **Pregnancy.** Between 30% and 50% of pregnant patients experience heartburn during the course of pregnancy; 25% experiencing daily symptoms. It has been suggested that hormonal changes as well as the increase in intra-abdominal pressure contribute to the high incidence of heartburn during pregnancy.
   d. **Obesity** may correlate to heartburn owing to the increase in intra-abdominal pressure or lower esophageal sphincter (LES) pressure. This predisposing factor can be voluntarily modified (i.e., weight loss) to reduce the patients risk of heartburn.

3. **Symptoms.** Heartburn (pyrosis) typically is described as a burning sensation or pain located in the lower chest. The pain may radiate higher in the chest, into the back, and into the throat or neck. Because the pain may radiate up into the chest, heartburn may be confused with pain associated with myocardial infarction (sweating associated with severe, crushing chest pain suggests a myocardial infarction and medical attention must be sought immediately). Symptoms usually occur soon after meals and when lying down at bedtime; patients may be awakened during the night with the pain. Pain on swallowing (odynophagia) may suggest severe mucosal damage in the esophagus.

4. **Complications.** Patients with severe, uncontrolled GERD may suffer bleeding from esophageal ulcers and pulmonary complications resulting from the aspiration of refluxed material into the upper airways and lungs. Patients who describe difficulty swallowing (i.e., dysphagia) may have an esophageal stricture, cancer, or a motility disorder.

5. **Causes.** There is an imbalance of aggressive forces (promote the development of GERD) and protective forces (prevent the development of GERD). Aggressive forces include acid and pepsin. The most important protective force is probably the LES. Many patients with GERD have a weak LES. As a result, the high pressure in the stomach creates enough force to overcome the weak squeeze of the LES and allows reflux to occur. Other protective forces include esophageal clearance, gastric-emptying rate, saliva, and esophageal mucosal defense.
   a. Drugs that reduce LES tone include calcium channel antagonists (e.g., nifedipine, verapamil, diltiazem), nitrates, anticholinergic agents (e.g., tricyclic antidepressants, antihistamines), and oral contraceptives and estrogen.
   b. Foods that reduce LES tone include chocolate, fatty foods, onions, peppermint, and garlic.
   c. Smoking (nicotine) reduces LES tone.

6. Pharmacists who are consulted by patients should ask for the following information before recommending a therapy:
   a. Duration and frequency of symptoms
   b. Severity of the pain and symptoms
   c. Timing of the symptoms (especially in relation to meals and at bedtime)
   d. Presence of other symptoms (nausea, vomiting, bloody stools, weight loss)
   e. Use of alcohol or tobacco
   f. Amount of high-fat foods, caffeine-containing products, chocolate, and tomato-based foods consumed
   g. Medications used currently, including nonprescription medications
   h. Medications used to relieve heartburn and their effectiveness

7. Patients with the following symptoms or conditions should be referred to a physician for evaluation rather than treated with nonprescription agents:
a. Severe abdominal or back pain
b. Unexplained weight loss
c. Chest pain that is indistinguishable from ischemic pain
d. Difficulty or pain on swallowing
e. Presence or history of vomiting blood
f. Black tarry bowel movements (if not taking iron or bismuth subsalicylate)
g. Children < 12 years of age
h. Possibility of being pregnant
i. Symptoms not responding to antacids or nonprescription H$_2$RAs within 2 weeks or recurring soon after stopping

B. Treatment

1. Nonpharmacological interventions for GERD attempt to reduce or eliminate dietary and lifestyle factors that promote reflux. Specific recommendations include the following:
a. Elevate the head of the bed 6–10 inches with blocks. This position improves esophageal clearance and reduces the duration of reflux. Try to avoid just propping a patient's head up with pillows because this may worsen symptoms by increasing abdominal pressure.
b. Eat evening meals at least 3–5 hr before going to bed to allow adequate time for gastric emptying.
c. Avoid foods that reduce LES tone.
d. Avoid foods that irritate the esophagus such as tomato-based products, coffee, citrus juices, and carbonated beverages (with or without caffeine).
e. Reduce the size of meals.
f. Avoid lying down for at least 2 hr after meals.
g. Stop use of tobacco products.
h. Limit alcohol intake.
i. Limit caffeine-containing beverages.
j. Lose weight if appropriate.
k. Avoid wearing tight-fitting clothing.

2. Pharmacological. The management of GERD may be viewed as a stepped-care approach, with antacids, nonprescription H$_2$RAs, and nondrug measures forming the basis for the first step (Figure 33-1). These measures may help alleviate symptoms in patients with mild to moderate GERD but cannot be expected to heal damaged esophageal mucosa or prevent complications. Steps 2 and higher use prescription-strength H$_2$RAs and other prescription medications as well as interventions such as surgery.
a. Antacids. Antacids are basic compounds that neutralize gastric acid, which increases the pH of refluxed gastric contents. As a result, the refluxed contents are not as damaging to the esophageal mucosa and alkalinization of gastric contents increase LES tone.
(1) Antacids generally relieve heartburn within 5–15 min of administration. Antacid suspensions generally dissolve more easily in gastric acid and thereby work quicker. In additio, sodium bicarbonate and magnesium hydroxide dissolve quickly at gastric pH and provide rapid relief; however, calcium carbonate and aluminum hydroxide dissolve slowly in stomach acid with a longer time frame for symptom relief (10–30 min).
(2) The duration of relief ranges from 1 to 3 hr if taken 1 hr after meals (duration of neutralization lasts only 20–40 min if taken without food). Because of their short duration, patients may need to take 4–5 doses throughout the day for adequate symptom relief. Antacids will not provide sustained neutralization of acid throughout the night.
(3) Adults: 40–80 mEq acid-neutralizing capacity (ANC) taken as needed for symptoms. If necessary, these doses may be titrated to a scheduled regimen, such as 40–80 mEq after meals and at bedtime.
(4) Sodium bicarbonate (e.g., Alka-Seltzer, Bromo-Seltzer) should be used for only short-term relief of symptoms. Because each gram of sodium bicarbonate contains 12 mEq of sodium, it is contraindicated in patients with edema, congestive heart failure, renal failure, cirrhosis, and patients on low-salt diets. It is the only systemic antacid available and can thus alter systemic pH.

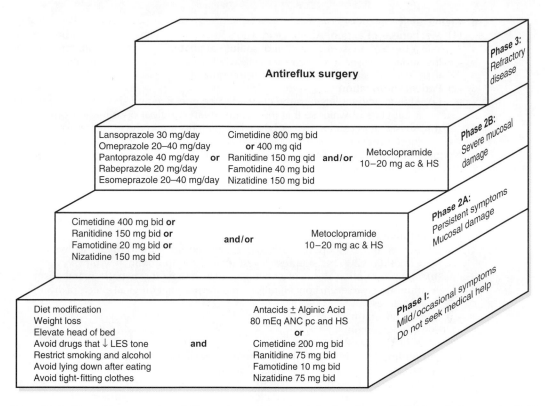

Figure 33-1. Step-wise progression of therapy for gastroesophageal reflux disease (GERD.) *ac,* before meals; *ANC,* acid-neutralizing capacity; *bid,* twice daily; *HS,* bedtime; *pc,* after meals; *qid,* four times daily.

(5) **Calcium carbonate** (e.g., Tums) is the most potent antacid ingredient but may cause constipation or, less likely, diarrhea. It is a good source of elemental calcium.

(6) **Aluminum hydroxide** (e.g., Amphojel, ALternaGEL) often causes constipation and should be avoided in patients with hemorrhoids or constipation, which is common in the elderly. Aluminum hydroxide has the lowest neutralizing capacity of all the antacids. Aluminum accumulation can be a problem in patients with chronic renal insufficiency.

(7) **Magnesium hydroxide** (e.g., Milk of Magnesia) rarely is used alone for heartburn because it frequently causes diarrhea. If used in renal failure patients, hypermagnesemia can occur rapidly.

(8) **Magnesium–aluminum** combination antacids (e.g., Maalox, Mylanta) provide the highest ANC per volume of antacid and are used most frequently. The predominant adverse effect of these combinations is diarrhea.

(9) **Patient information**

   (a) Patients with renal failure should avoid the use of all antacids. Potassium and magnesium content of antacids should be considered for patients with cardiac disease.

   (b) Patients should not take > 500–600 mEq ANC of antacid per day.

   (c) Palatability with antacid liquids may be increased with refrigeration (do not freeze).

   (d) Tablets must be chewed thoroughly to achieve optimal effect.

   (e) Antacids can interfere with the absorption of many drugs. In general, antacids should be spaced at least 2 hr apart from the administration of interacting drugs. This is often quite difficult to accomplish. Important clinical interactions with antacids may occur with the following drugs:

   (i) Tetracycline antibiotics

   (ii) Quinolone antibiotics (e.g., ciprofloxacin, levofloxacin)

   (iii) Iron supplements

   (iv) Digoxin

b. Alginic acid
(1) **Mechanism of action.** Alginic acid works by reacting with sodium bicarbonate and saliva to form a viscous solution of **sodium alginate.** This viscous solution floats on the surface of gastric contents so that, when reflux occurs, sodium alginate rather than acid is refluxed, and irritation is minimized.
(2) **Patient information**
  (a) Alginic-acid tablets must be chewed to be effective and should be followed by a full glass of water so that the viscous foam can float on it in the stomach.
  (b) Alginic-acid products work best when patients are in the upright position. Thus these products should not be taken at bedtime or just before lying down.
c. Nonprescription H$_2$RAs. These medications inhibit gastric acid secretion by competitively blocking H$_2$-receptors on the parietal cell. By decreasing gastric acid secretion, the refluxed material is less damaging to the esophagus. The onset of symptom relief with H$_2$RAs is 1–2 hr, which is considerably longer than antacids; however, the duration of action can last up to 10 hr. All H$_2$RAs are contraindicated in children < 12 years of age. Nonprescription H$_2$RAs can be used for relief or prevention of heartburn.
(1) **Cimetidine (Tagamet-HB)**
  (a) Adults (nonprescription): 200 mg as needed for symptoms, up to twice daily. Cimetidine 200 mg suppresses gastric acid for approximately 6 hr.
  (b) Nonprescription doses of cimetidine may **impair** the **hepatic metabolism** and thus increase serum concentrations and the pharmacological effects of the following drugs:
      (i) Warfarin
      (ii) Phenytoin
      (iii) Theophylline
(2) **Famotidine (Pepcid-AC, Pepcid Complete, Maximum Strength Pepcid-AC).** Unlike cimetidine, famotidine rarely impairs hepatic metabolism of other drugs
  (a) Adults (nonprescription): 10–20 mg as needed for symptoms, up to twice daily; maximum dose 40 mg/day. Patients who anticipate heartburn or indigestion may take 10–20 mg (1 tablet) 1 hr before eating; maximum of 2 tablets within a 24-hr period. Famotidine 10 mg suppresses acid secretion for 8–10 hr.
  (b) Famotidine, calcium carbonate, magnesium hydroxide (Pepcid Complete). A chewable combination of an H$_2$RA and an antacid.
(3) **Ranitidine (Zantac 75, Zantac 150 Maximum Strength).**
  (a) Adults (nonprescription): 75–150 mg as needed for symptoms, up to twice daily; maximum 150 mg/day
  (b) Ranitidine inhibits hepatic metabolism 5–10 times less than cimetidine; therefore, the potential for drug interactions is very small.
(4) **Nizatidine (Axid-AR).** Adults: 75 mg as needed for symptoms, up to twice daily. Nizatidine rarely impairs hepatic metabolism of other drugs.
(5) **Adverse effects.** These agents are extremely well tolerated. The **most common** adverse effects reported with nonprescription doses are headache, diarrhea, dizziness, and nausea.
d. Prescription H$_2$RAs. Patients with moderate to severe symptoms and/or esophageal mucosal lesions require higher doses of H$_2$RAs than are available over the counter. Unlike patients with peptic ulcer disease, patients with GERD respond best to multiple daily doses of H$_2$RAs rather than to single bedtime doses.
e. Prokinetic agents. Patients with moderate to severe GERD may benefit from the addition of these medications, which stimulate esophageal motility and increase LES tone. Prokinetic agents are available only by prescription.
(1) **Metoclopramide (Reglan, generic). Adverse effects,** such as sedation, depression, and extrapyramidal effects, limit the usefulness of this agent for many patients.
(2) **Cisapride (Propulsid).** The numerous drug interactions with this product have caused the manufacturer to voluntarily remove it from the market. Propulsid may still be obtained through an investigational limited-access program.
f. Proton pump inhibitors. These prescription-only agents (except omeprazole) provide complete acid suppression by inhibiting the hydrogen-potassium ATPase pump on the surface of the parietal cell. The duration of acid suppression with these agents is about 3 days. Proton pump inhibitors are the most potent and effective agents available for relieving severe GERD symptoms and healing esophageal lesions. In June 2003, the FDA switched omeprazole to OTC status for the prevention of symptoms of frequent (occurring

2 or more days per week) heartburn. These OTC drugs should be used for no more than 14 days every 4 months, unless directed by a physician.

(1) Omeprazole (Prilosec)
  (a) This drug may inhibit hepatic metabolism and thus increase serum concentration/pharmacologic effects of the following drugs: phenytoin, warfarin, and diazepam.
  (b) Adverse effects. Although rare, these may include headache, diarrhea, constipation, or dizziness.
(2) Lansoprazole (Prevacid) has no clinically significant drug interactions.
(3) Pantoprazole (Protonix) is the only proton pump inhibitor with an oral and intravenous formulation.
(4) Rabeprazole (Aciphex)
(5) Esomeprazole (Nexium)

C. **Special patient populations**

1. **Pediatric patients.** Gastroesophageal reflux occurs commonly in infants and children. Signs and symptoms in pediatric patients include vomiting, chest pain, irritability, feeding refusal, belching, and apnea. Serious complications (e.g., failure to thrive, esophageal strictures) can occur in infants and children.
    a. Antacids, with or without alginic acid, have been widely used in infants and children, but their safety has not been clearly established.
    b. H_2RAs have been used safely in children under the supervision of healthcare providers. However, the nonprescription H_2RAs are not approved for use in children < 12 years of age unless directed by a physician.

2. **Pregnant patients.** Heartburn occurs commonly during pregnancy because of increased abdominal pressure owing to the expanding uterus, as well as reduced LES pressure resulting from high concentrations of estrogen and progesterone. Nearly half of pregnant women experience GERD, especially during the third trimester.
    a. Antacids are generally considered safe in pregnancy as long as chronic high doses are avoided. It is best to avoid sodium bicarbonate because of the risks of systemic alkalosis and the sodium load leading to edema and weight gain.
    b. Data regarding the **safety** of **alginic acid** during pregnancy are not available.
    c. Controlled data regarding the safety of **H_2RAs** in pregnancy are limited. Pregnant women seeking a nonprescription H_2RA for GERD should be directed to use antacids, unless a physician has instructed her otherwise.

3. **Elderly patients.** Antacids and nonprescription H_2RAs may be safely used in elderly patients without any dosage adjustments.
    a. Dosage reduction of prescription H_2RAs may be necessary in elderly patients with reduced renal function.
    b. Elderly patients are more likely to be taking drugs that interact with antacids, H_2RAs, omeprazole, and/or cisapride.
    c. Elderly patients are also more likely to have symptoms or conditions that require referral to a physician before beginning nonprescription therapy.

STUDY QUESTIONS

Directions for questions 1–20: Each of the questions, statements, or incomplete statements in this section can be correctly answered or completed by **one** of the suggested answers or phrases. Choose the **best** answer.

1. Which laxative should *not* be used to treat acute constipation because of its slow onset of action?

(A) glycerin
(B) bisacodyl suppository
(C) psyllium
(D) milk of magnesia

2. Which is *not* a risk factor for hyperphosphatemia and death from sodium phosphate enemas when used in children?

(A) renal insufficiency
(B) Hirschsprung disease
(C) anorectal malformations
(D) children 6–12 years of age

3. All of the following statements about emollient stool softener laxatives are true *except* which one?

(A) They are not good for acute constipation.
(B) They are good for patients who should not strain by passing a hard stool (e.g., post-surgical patients).
(C) They never have been found to be better than placebo for long-term use.
(D) They are more effective than placebo for long-term use.

4. Which of the following statements adequately describes bulk-forming laxatives?

(A) can cause diarrhea if not taken with water
(B) are derived from polysaccharides and resemble fiber (bran) in mechanism of action
(C) onset of action in 4–8 hr
(D) produce much more complete evacuation of constipation than stimulant products

5. Which of the following statements about non-drug therapies for acute diarrhea is *not* correct?

(A) Breast-feeding should be continued as normal.
(B) Even if the patient is not vomiting, food should be withheld for 6–12 hr.
(C) Fluids can be given to patients who experience vomiting, but small amounts of fluid should be used.
(D) Replacement fluids mainly consist of water, sugar, potassium, sodium, and bicarbonate.

6. Which of the following products should *not* be used to replenish lost fluids from acute diarrhea?

(A) pedialyte solution
(B) Kool-Aid
(C) Gatorade (half-strength diluted with water)
(D) The World Health Organization (WHO) solution

7. Which of the following statements about adsorbent drugs used for diarrhea is true?

(A) useful for treatment of severe diarrhea
(B) very unsafe because not absorbed systemically
(C) in general, small doses needed to relieve diarrhea
(D) kaolin now generally recognized as a safe and effective OTC antidiarrheal agent

8. Which of the following statements concerning traveler's diarrhea is true?

(A) It can usually be avoided by not eating raw vegetables, seafood, or eggs when traveling to third world countries.
(B) It can be prevented by taking one dose of antibiotic 1 day before a trip.
(C) *Helicobacter pylori* is the primary pathogen responsible.
(D) Phillips' Milk of Magnesia is used to prevent and treat the condition.

9. All of the following agents are considered close to ideal laxatives *except*

(A) emollient laxatives.
(B) bulk-forming laxatives.
(C) fiber.
(D) stimulant laxatives.

10. A patient suffering from acute infectious diarrhea caused by *Shigella* can be managed in all of the following ways *except* which one?

(A) No treatment necessary because signs and symptoms usually resolve in 48 hr.
(B) Use glucose solutions (e.g., soda, apple juice) to settle the stomach and decrease the number of stools.
(C) Avoid food for at least 6 hr, then slowly increase fluid intake.
(D) Use antibiotics (e.g., Bactrim, doxycycline) for 7 days.

11. Which local anesthetic should be used to treat symptoms of pain, itching, burning, and discomfort in patients with an established lidocaine allergy?

(A) tetracaine
(B) dibucaine
(C) pramoxine
(D) benzocaine

12. All of the following items are part of a standard conservative approach to the treatment of first- or second-degree hemorrhoids except

(A) topical anesthetic (hemorrhoidal ointment).
(B) stool softener.
(C) sitz baths.
(D) rubber band ligation.

13. What is the most common sign/symptom of hemorrhoids?

(A) bleeding
(B) pain
(C) seepage
(D) pruritus

14. Which of the following agents is designated as a safe and effective analgesic, anesthetic, and antipruritic by the Food and Drug Administration?

(A) witch hazel
(B) juniper tar
(C) hydrocortisone
(D) phenylephrine

15. All of the following vasoconstrictors are deemed safe and effective for the temporary relief of itching and swelling except

(A) ephedrine 0.1%–1.25%.
(B) epinephrine 0.005%–0.01%.
(C) phenylpropanolamine 1%–10%.
(D) phenylephrine 0.25%.

16. All of the following symptoms associated with gastroesophageal reflux disease (GERD) may be treated with nonprescription agents except

(A) burning sensation located in the lower chest.
(B) pain that is worse after meals.
(C) pain or difficulty when swallowing.
(D) pain that is worse on lying down at bedtime.

17. Which of the following is an appropriate non-pharmacological recommendation for patients with gastroesophageal reflux disease (GERD)?

(A) Eat larger but fewer meals.
(B) Avoid meals high in protein.
(C) Eat evening meals at least 3 hr before bed.
(D) Prop a patient's head up with two pillows at night.

18. All of the following statements regarding antacid use in gastroesophageal reflux disease (GERD) are correct except which one?

(A) The onset of symptom relief with antacids is 1–2 hr.
(B) Antacids will relieve symptoms for 1–3 hr.
(C) Sodium bicarbonate should not be used in patients with edema, congestive heart failure, or those on low-salt diets
(D) The most frequent side effect of aluminum-magnesium combination antacids is diarrhea.

19. All of the following statements regarding use of nonprescription H_2RAs in gastroesophageal reflux disease (GERD) are correct except which one?

(A) The most common adverse effects of nonprescription H_2RAs are headache, diarrhea, dizziness, and nausea,
(B) Cimetidine may increase serum concentrations of warfarin, theophylline, and phenytoin,
(C) The onset of symptom relief with these agents is 1–2 hr.
(D) Nonprescription H_2RAs will heal severely damaged esophageal mucosa.

20. All of the following statements regarding use of nonprescription products for gastroesophageal reflux disease (GERD) in special populations are correct except which one?

(A) Nonprescription H_2RAs are not approved for use in children < 12 years of age.
(B) Antacids may be safely used in pregnant patients as long as chronic high doses are avoided.
(C) Sodium bicarbonate is the preferred antacid in pregnant patients.
(D) Doses of nonprescription H_2RAs do not need to be reduced in elderly patients.

Directions for questions 21–23: The questions and incomplete statements in this section can be correctly answered or completed by **one or more** of the suggested answers. Choose the answer, **A–E.**

> A   if **I only** is correct
> B   if **III only** is correct
> C   if **I and II** are correct
> D   if **II and III** are correct
> E   if **I, II, and III** are correct

21. Which of the following drugs most commonly causes constipation?

  I. ampicillin

 II. narcotic analgesics

III. drugs possessing anticholinergic properties

22. Which of the following statements about stimulant laxatives is correct?

  I. They produce a stool more quickly than any other type of laxative.

 II. They are associated with more adverse effects than any other type of laxative.

III. They work by irritating the lining of the colon wall to increase peristalsis and produce a stool.

23. When should a patient experiencing diarrhea be referred to a physician by a pharmacist?

  I. If the patient has pus or blood in the stool.

 II. If the patient also suffers from vomiting.

III. If the patient has a fever.

ANSWERS AND EXPLANATIONS

1. The answer is C *[see I.B.2.a].*
Glycerin and the bisacodyl suppository all produce stools in 30 min to a few hours, whereas psyllium, a bulk-forming laxative, produces stool in 24–72 hr in the same manner as a normal bolus of food or fiber.

2. The answer is D *[see I.C.4].*
The popular sodium phosphate enemas (e.g., Fleet) are very effective but have resulted in hyperphosphatemia, hypocalcemia (tetany), hypokalemia, metabolic acidosis, and cardiac death usually owing to conduction abnormalities in very small children. This has mainly occurred in children < 2 years of age or between 2 and 5 years of age with predisposing factors, such as chronic renal disease, anorectal malformations, and/or Hirschsprung disease. The use of enemas is highly discouraged in children < 5 years of age.

3. The answer is D *[see I.B.2.d].*
These agents have a long onset of action (24–48 hr); thus they should never be used for acute constipation but should be used mainly for patients who should not strain to pass hard stools (e.g., pregnant patients, postsurgical patients, post–myocardial infarction). However, they have never been found to be more effective than placebo in long-term use.

4. The answer is B *[see I.B.2.a; I.B.2.c].*
Stimulant products result in a quicker, more complete, and often more violent evacuation of the bowel than do the bulk-forming agents. Bulk-forming agents are developed from complex sugars, similar to fiber, that provide bulk to increase gastrointestinal motility and water absorption into the bowel. However, patients must drink plenty of water to facilitate the absorption of water into the bowel, or they may become more constipated.

5. The answer is B *[see II.C.1].*
The most important part of treating acute diarrhea is the replacement of lost fluids. If patients experience mild to moderate fluid loss, replacement can be done with oral-rehydration solutions. If fluid loss is severe (> 10% loss of body weight) and/or severe vomiting, then patients may need intravenous rehydration before oral-maintenance fluids can be administered. There has been much controversy regarding the decision to feed or not feed children during acute episodes of diarrhea. Recent information shows that children should remain on their normal diet or breast-feeding during episodes of diarrhea; these do not make the diarrhea worse and may actually improve the condition.

6. The answer is B *[see II.C.1.b].*
Replacement fluids for diarrhea should contain the appropriate amount of electrolytes (K^+, Na^+, Cl^-, citrate) and glucose per specified amount of water, as found in commercially available oral-rehydration solutions such as Pedialyte and Rehydralyte. The World Health Organization (WHO) solution, which can easily be made at home, and half-strength Gatorade provide the necessary electrolytes and glucose to replenish lost fluids. Kool-Aid does not contain potassium. Carbonated beverages are low in potassium, and some are too high in glucose.

7. The answer is D *[see II.C.2.b].*
Adsorbents are not effective for severe diarrhea because they simply cannot adsorb enough water and do not reverse the cause of the diarrhea. Large doses may decrease symptoms. Of all the adsorbents, kaolin is the most effective and is now recognized by the FDA as safe and effective. All adsorbents are safe because they are not adsorbed systemically.

8. The answer is A *[see II.A.2.b; II.C.2].*
Traveler's diarrhea is primarily caused by bacteria (mainly enterotoxin *Escherichia coli*). Prophylaxis and treatment regimens include oral antibiotics (fluoroquinolones, sulfonamides, doxycycline) and bismuth subsalicylate (Pepto-Bismol). *Helicobacter pylori* is the organism shown to contribute to refractory peptic ulcer disease.

9. The answer is D *[see I.B.2].*
The ideal laxative is natural (i.e., similar to food) and produces stool on a regular basis. The product produces stool quickly (i.e., in several hours) without adverse effects. such as abdominal cramping or the formation of a hard stool, which may be difficult to pass. Products such as fiber or bulk-forming agents produce a stool similar to a bolus of food, without adverse effects. Emollient laxatives (i.e., stool softeners) produce soft stools without difficult defecation. Stimulants produce a stool quickly, but patients often experience severe abdominal cramping and hard stools.

10. The answer is B *[see II.C; Table 33-3].*
Giving highly osmotic solutions of glucose (e.g., soda, fruit juice) can result in more water absorbed into the intestinal tract and thus further diarrhea. Many cases of diarrhea resolve within 48 hr without treatment. People with diarrhea can avoid food for at least 6 hr, then increase their fluid intake slowly. Severe cases of infectious diarrhea can be treated with antibiotics or antiprotozoals, depending on the organism that caused the episode.

11. The answer is C *[see III.H.2.b].*
Because of its chemically distinct structure, pramoxine exhibits less cross-sensitivity compared to the other anesthetics and should be used in patients with a lidocaine allergy.

12. The answer is D *[see III.G.1].*
A conservative approach to treatment includes sitz baths, the use of stool softeners to prevent straining when passing a stool, and the use of an anesthetic hemorrhoidal preparation. If improvement is not seen, more aggressive therapy may be pursued (e.g., rubber band ligation).

13. The answer is A *[see III.D.1].*
The most common sign/symptom of hemorrhoids is painless bleeding occurring during a bowel movement.

14. The answer is B *[see III.H.7].*
Juniper tar, menthol, and camphor are the only three agents deemed safe and effective as analgesics, anesthetics, and antipruritics by the FDA. These agents were formerly classified as counterirritants.

15. The answer is C *[see III.H.3.a].*
Vasoconstrictors deemed safe and effective by the FDA are ephedrine HCl, epinephrine, and phenylephrine.

16. The answer is C *[see IV.A.2–3; IV.A.6].*
Pain on swallowing often suggests severe esophageal mucosal damage, which would require prescription medications for healing. Difficulty on swallowing may indicate an esophageal stricture, cancer, or motor disorder. All of these conditions require diagnosis and treatment by a healthcare provider.

17. The answer is C *[see IV.B.1.a–k].*
Patients should be instructed to eat evening meals at least 3 hr before going to bed. This allows sufficient time for gastric emptying, so that the volume of refluxed material will be smaller and less irritating to the esophagus.

18. The answer is A *[see IV.B.2.a].*
One of the major advantages of antacid use in heartburn is its quick onset of action. Most patients with mild GERD will experience relief from antacids within 5–15 min of administration.

19. The answer is D *[see IV.B.2.c–d].*
Nonprescription doses of H_2RAs are too low to heal esophageal damage. Esophageal mucosal damage is difficult to heal and requires high doses of H_2Ras, which are available only by prescription. Alternatively, proton pump inhibitors, which completely suppress acid secretion, may be used to heal esophageal mucosal damage.

20. The answer is C *[see IV.C.2].*
Sodium bicarbonate should be avoided in pregnant patients because the high sodium load may cause systemic alkalosis, edema, and/or weight gain.

21. The answer is D (II, III) *[see I.A.3.d]*.
Opiate analgesics (e.g., narcotics) and drugs with anticholinergic properties decrease bowel motility, which results in increased water absorption from the intestinal tract. This can cause a harder, drier stool, which results in constipation. Ampicillin is often poorly absorbed from the intestinal tract and can alter the flora of the intestinal bowel. This destruction of bowel organisms causes increased secretions into the bowel, which results in diarrhea.

22. The answer is D (II, III) *[see I.B.2.c]*.
Stimulant laxatives do have a quick onset of action but not any quicker than the saline laxatives, which usually work in 4–6 hr. The mechanism of action for stimulant laxatives is that they irritate the lining of the colon wall, which increases peristalsis and produces a stool. These laxatives are associated with more adverse effects than other laxatives.

23. The answer is E (I, II, III) *[see II.B.2]*.
Patients with pus or blood in the stool, vomiting, or fever may be suffering from severe bacterial diarrhea and may lose large amounts of fluid, which could result in severe dehydration.

34
OTC Menstrual, Vaginal, and Contraceptive Agents

Laura K. Williford Owens

I. MENSTRUATION AND MENSTRUAL PRODUCTS

A. **Introduction. Menstruation** is a physiological discharge of blood, endometrial cellular debris, and mucus through the vagina of a nonpregnant woman and is a result of the monthly cycling of female reproductive hormones. The menstrual cycle eliminates a mature, unfertilized egg and prepares the endometrium for the possible implantation of a fertilized egg the following month.

1. **Onset.** The average age at which the initial menstrual cycle occurs in U.S. women is 12 years. Normal menarche (initial menstrual cycle) can occur between the ages of 9 and 16 years. Factors such as race, genetics, nutritional status, and body mass determine the onset.

2. **Duration.** The **average** duration of the menstrual cycle is 28 days (the time between the onset of one menstrual flow and the beginning of the next) and the normal range is 21–35 days. Day 1 is the first day of menstrual flow, which can last for 3–7 days (average duration of flow is 5 days).

3. **Physiology.** The menstrual cycle results from a complex interplay of hormones produced by the hypothalamus, pituitary gland, and the ovaries (hypothalamic–pituitary–ovarian axis).

B. **Menstrual abnormalities**

1. **Dysmenorrhea** is painful menstruation. It is the most common gynecologic problem in the United States.
    a. **Types**
        (1) **Primary dysmenorrhea** is pain associated with menstruation in the absence of identifiable pelvic disease. It is prompted by increased levels of prostaglandins in the menstrual fluids.
        (2) **Secondary dysmenorrhea** is associated with an underlying pelvic disorder. Possible causes include endometriosis, pelvic inflammatory disease (PID), and ovarian cysts.
    b. **Symptoms** of dysmenorrhea are primarily lower abdominal cramping and can often include nausea, vomiting, diarrhea, headache, and dizziness. Abdominal cramping usually begins at onset of menstrual flow or a few hours before onset.
    c. Practitioners should **question the patient** about the following:
        (1) Current medications
        (2) Age
        (3) Duration of dysmenorrhea
        (4) A description of the dysmenorrhea symptoms
        (5) History of pelvic disease (endometriosis, PID, ovarian cysts, infertility)
        (6) Allergy to aspirin or nonsteroidal anti-inflammatory drug (NSAID)
        (7) Bleeding disorder
        (8) Exercise routine
    d. **Treatment**
        (1) **Recommendation of therapy** should be based on the patient's assessment of the degree of pain. Pain associated with dysmenorrhea generally tapers within 2 days. Prolonged pain may be associated with an underlying problem, and patients should be referred to a physician.
        (2) **Nonpharmacological** recommendations include rest, heat, wearing loose-fitting clothing, and exercise.
        (3) **Agents** for the relief of dysmenorrhea include
            (a) **Analgesics** are used as primary treatment of dysmenorrhea and for relief of cramping associated with premenstrual syndrome (PMS; see I.B.4]. Analgesic

treatment provides relief for mild to moderate symptoms but will probably not help patients with severe symptoms.

    (i) Nonsteroidal anti-inflammatory drugs inhibit the synthesis and action of prostaglandins. Because prostaglandins are responsible for the cramping of dysmenorrhea it makes logical sense to recommend NSAIDs to a patient.

    For women who do not receive relief from over-the-counter (OTC) analgesics, prescription NSAIDs may prove more useful.

    {a} Administration guidelines. Begin therapy at the onset of pain; there is no proven value in beginning therapy in anticipation of dysmenorrhea.

- Ibuprofen (e.g., Advil, Midol IB, Nuprin): 200 mg every 4–6 hr; maximum 1200 mg/day
- Ketoprofen: 12.5 mg every 4–6 hr; maximum 25 mg in a 4- to 6-hr period or 75 mg in 24 hr
- Naproxen (Aleve): 200 mg every 8–12 hr; maximum 600 mg/day

    {b} Adverse effects. From a few days of use, adverse effects are limited. Common adverse effects associated with NSAIDs include upset stomach, vomiting, heartburn, abdominal pain, diarrhea, constipation, and dizziness. NSAIDs should be taken with food to decrease adverse gastrointestinal (GI) effects or bleeding.

    {c} Warnings. Patients should be advised to use the lowest effective dose for the shortest duration needed to lessen the potential risk for cardiovascular events. Patients with an allergy to NSAIDs or active GI disease should not take any NSAID.

    (ii) Treatment with **aspirin** or **acetaminophen** can prove of benefit for the symptoms associated with primary dysmenorrhea, however; aspirin is not as potent as the other NSAIDs and acetaminophen is not thought to prevent prostaglandin production to a great extent, although it can be helpful for treating the headache and backache that may occur with menstrual cramping.

(b) Diuretics are **recommended** by the U.S. Food and Drug Administration (FDA) for use in eliminating water during premenstrual and menstrual periods. When administered approximately 5 days before menses, diuretics help relieve bloating, excess water, cramps, and tension. Included in this category are ammonium chloride, caffeine, and pamabrom.

    (i) Ammonium chloride (Aqua-Ban) is an acid-forming salt often used in combination with caffeine.

    {a} Up to 3 g of ammonium chloride (NH_4Cl) per day can be administered in three divided doses for no longer than 6 days.

    {b} Larger doses are often associated with GI symptoms.

    {c} Aqua-Ban Plus contains both ammonium chloride and caffeine.

    (ii) Caffeine, a xanthine derivative, promotes diuresis by inhibiting tubular reabsorption of sodium and chloride.

    {a} The **recommended dosage** is 100–200 mg every 3–4 hr.

    {b} Side effects associated with caffeine use are GI disturbances and central nervous system (CNS) stimulation.

    {c} Patients should be counseled to limit the consumption of caffeine-containing foods or beverages while taking this product.

    (iii) Pamabrom (Midol PMS, Pamprin) is a theophylline derivative often used in combination with analgesics and antihistamines. The recommended dosage is 50 mg four times daily, not to exceed 200 mg/day.

2. Amenorrhea is the absence of menstruation. The development of primary or secondary amenorrhea requires physician evaluation.

3. Intermenstrual pain and **bleeding** generally occur at midcycle and may last from several hours to days. Pain is often associated with ovulation (mittelschmerz). Therapy consists of nonprescription analgesics. Patients with pain lasting longer than 2 days should be referred to a physician.

4. PMS

    a. Symptoms (e.g., marked mood swings, fatigue, appetite changes, bloating, breast tenderness, irritability, feelings of depression) begin 1–7 days before the onset of menses.

    b. Nonpharmacological therapy includes regular exercise, dietary modifications, and reduction of stress factors. Dietary modifications include avoiding alcohol and caffeine, which can increase irritability, and consuming a balanced diet of fruits, vegetables, and complex carbohydrates while avoiding salty foods and simple sugars (can exacerbate fluid retention). Patients experiencing symptoms abnormal to their cycle should be referred to a physician.

    c. Pharmacological treatment. The efficacy and safety of pharmacological treatment of PMS are aimed at the proposed causes (e.g., a drop in progesterone concentrations, high levels of prolactin, elevated estrogen concentrations, deficiencies of vitamins A or B_6, or an underlying disorder) and are not well studied. Although clinical trials do not support the efficacy of vitamins A or B_6, both have been used for the treatment of PMS.

        (1) Prescription drug products that have been studied in the management of PMS include benzodiazepines, monoamine oxidase inhibitors (MAOIs), tricyclic antidepressants (TCAs), and selective serotonin reuptake inhibitors (SSRIs). Fluoxetine (under the brand name Sarafem) has recently been approved for the treatment of premenstrual dysphoric disorder.

        (2) Combination products are marketed for women with PMS symptoms. These products contain acetaminophen, pamabrom, and pyrilamine (Midol and Pamprin). Nonprescription diuretics such as pamabrom are commonly used to reduce fluid accumulation associated with PMS. Pain is an uncommon symptom of PMS, and the sedative effect of an antihistamine is unlikely to provide relief of the emotional symptoms associated with PMS. Combination products should be recommended only with caution.

        (3) Daily **calcium supplementation** (equivalent to the recommended daily calcium intake for women of reproductive age) has been shown to reduce the emotional and physical symptoms of PMS.

  5. Menorrhagia is excessive menstrual blood loss. Low hematocrit, low hemoglobin, and low serum iron levels may occur. Treatment for menorrhagia is usually an estrogen–progestin combination (i.e., oral contraceptive).

C. Toxic shock syndrome (TSS) is a rare but sometimes fatal illness often associated with menstruation.

  1. TSS can be categorized either as menstrual or nonmenstrual, with approximately two thirds of cases associated with menstruation. TSS is known to occur in both men and women.

  2. The condition usually affects women < 30 years of age who use tampons. Women between the ages of 15 and 19 years are at the highest risk.

  3. TSS is characterized by an abrupt onset (8–12 hr) of flu-like symptoms (e.g., high fever, myalgia, vomiting, diarrhea). Neurologic symptoms such as headache, agitation, lethargy, seizures, and confusion can also occur.

  4. TSS results from an exotoxin produced by *Staphylococcus aureus.*

  5. The **primary risk factor** for TSS is the **use of tampons.** Additional risk factors include barrier contraceptives (e.g., diaphragms, cervical sponges).

  6. When TSS is suspected, patients should be hospitalized immediately. To lower the risk of TSS, women should use lower-absorbency tampons and alternate the use of tampons with feminine hygiene pads; however, to lower the risk to nearly zero, women should use sanitary pads instead of tampons.

D. Menstrual products like feminine hygiene pads and tampons are used to absorb menstrual and other vaginal discharges.

  1. Feminine hygiene pads are available in a wide variety of sizes and absorbencies. Super or maxi pads may be used for the heaviest menstrual flow (usually occurring on day 2 of the cycle). Mini or light pads and junior or teen pads are designed for women with smaller anatomy and/or lighter flow. Frequent changing of sanitary pads minimizes the occurrence of unpleasant odors and helps minimize irritation and chafing.

  2. Tampons are intravaginal inserts designed to absorb vaginal discharge. Many women prefer tampons because they are worn internally, which lessens chafing, odor, bulkiness, and irritation. Super tampons are designed for heavier flow. Junior or regular tampons are designed for moderate to light menstrual flow. Frequent changing of tampons will minimize the risks associated with TSS.

II. VAGINAL PRODUCTS

A. Vulvovaginal candidiasis

1. **General considerations**
   a. **Occurrence.** Approximately 75% of all women will experience vulvovaginal candidiasis (yeast infection) at least once, and 50% will have a second episode. Only 5% of women experience recurrent infections (four or more infections within a 1-year period).
   b. **Cause.** *Candida albicans* is responsible for up to 92% of infections. Infections owing to *C. glabrata* are increasing.
   c. **Predisposing factors.** Antibiotics, oral contraceptives containing high-dose estrogen, pregnancy, diabetes, and immunosuppression increase the risk for infection.
   d. **Symptoms.** Can include a thick, white, "cottage cheese–like," nonmalodorous vaginal discharge; dysuria; vaginal burning; and pruritus.

2. **Patient assessment**
   a. Patients should be questioned about presence of symptoms, medication use, medical conditions, and history of vaginal yeast infections.
   b. The following patients should be referred to a primary-care provider for diagnosis and treatment:
      (1) First episode of symptoms
      (2) Pregnant
      (3) Younger than 12 years of age
      (4) Systemic symptoms such as fever
      (5) History of recurrent vaginal yeast infections
      (6) Discharge with a fishy odor (indicates bacterial vaginosis, most often caused by anaerobic bacteria) or a thin, malodorous purulent discharge (indicates of *Trichomonas* infection)

3. **Pharmacological treatment**
   a. **Nonprescription agents** are recommended only for patients who have had a prior yeast infection and who can potentially recognize the infection and self-medicate.
   b. The choice of nonprescription therapy is based on patient preference.
   c. Available formulations include intravaginal creams, suppositories, and ointments.
   d. External vaginal creams can be used in combination with intravaginal products to treat vulvar symptoms of pruritus.
   e. Intravaginal products are used at bedtime, whereas the external creams can be used any time of day.
   f. Available nonprescription therapies include the antifungal agents Gyne-Lotrimin (clotrimazole), Monistat 3 and Monistat 7 (miconazole), Femstat 3 (butoconazole), and Monistat 1 and Vagistat 1 (tioconazole).
      (1) Gyne-Lotrimin and Monistat 7 are used for 7 consecutive days; Monistat 3 and Femstat 3 are used for 3 consecutive days; Monistat 1 and Vagistat 1 are used for 1 day.
      (2) Efficacy rates approach 80%–90%.

4. **Patient counseling**
   a. **Nonpharmacological**
      (1) Dry vaginal area well after bathing with a towel or a hairdryer on a low setting.
      (2) Avoid tight or damp clothing.
      (3) Wear cotton underwear.
      (4) Use unscented soap to avoid irritation.
      (5) Avoid douching.
      (6) Decrease consumption of sucrose and simple sugars.

b. **Pharmacological**
  (1) Complete the course of therapy even if symptoms improve.
  (2) Wash vaginal area with mild soap before application.
  (3) Avoid sexual intercourse during therapy.
  (4) Avoid condoms and diaphragm use for 72 hr after therapy is completed.
  (5) Continue use during menstrual period.
  (6) Avoid tampons during use.
  (7) Sanitary pads can be used for leakage of intravaginal products.
  (8) Side effects can include burning or irritation.

B. **Feminine hygiene products.** There are a variety of feminine hygiene products available for cleansing and controlling odor associated with normal vaginal discharge. These products are not used to treat vaginal infections.

  1. Vaginal douches (Summer's Eve) irrigate the vagina and can be used for cleansing, for soothing, as an astringent, or to produce a mucolytic effect.

  2. Vaginal suppositories (Betadine-medicated suppositories) are used for soothing, to relieve minor irritations, and to reduce the number of pathogenic microorganisms.

III. OTC CONTRACEPTIVES

A. **Introduction.** The **efficacy** and **pregnancy rates** for various means of contraception depend greatly on the **degree of compliance.** Table 34-1 lists ranges of pregnancy rates reported for a variety of contraceptives.

Table 34-1. Pregnancy Rates for Various Means of Contraception (%)[a]

Method of Contraception	Typical[b]	Lowest[c]
Oral contraceptives		
Combination (estrogen–progestin)	0.1–0.34	0.1
Progestin only	0.5–1.5	0.5
Mechanical/chemical		
Cervical cap[d]		
Multiparous	40	26
Nulliparous	20	9
Male condom without spermicide	12–14	3
Male condom with spermicide	4–6	1.8
Diaphragm[d]	20	6
Female condom	21	5
Intrauterine device	≤ 1–2	≤ 1–1.5
Levonorgestrel implants	≤ 1	≤ 1
Medroxyprogesterone injection	≤ 1	≤ 1
Spermicide alone	20–22	6
Other		
Rhythm (all types)	25	1–9
Vasectomy/tubal ligation	≤ 1	≤ 1
Withdrawal	40–50	30
No contraception	85	85

[a]During first year of continuous use.
[b]A typical couple who initiated a method that either was not always used correctly or was not used with every act of sexual intercourse, and who experienced an accidental pregnancy.
[c]The method of birth control was always used correctly with every act of sexual intercourse but the couple still experienced an accidental pregnancy.
[d]Used with spermicide.
Adapted with permission from Nonprescription Drug Therapy Guiding Patient Self-Care, 4th ed. St. Louis, MO, Wolters Kluwer Health, 2005.

B. Methods of contraception that may make use of nonprescription products or devices include the following:

1. **Fertility awareness methods** make use of information concerning the menstrual cycle to determine the days when intercourse is most likely to result in a pregnancy. **Periodic abstinence** is also referred to as the **rhythm method, natural family planning,** or **ovulation detection method.** The various natural family planning methods allow the patient to monitor the natural physiological signs that can, in many women, predict the fertile period (periovulatory phase of the menstrual cycle), enabling the couple to avoid coital exposure at that time. These methods are based on reproductive anatomy and physiology and are applied according to the signs and symptoms naturally occurring in the menstrual cycle.

   a. Calculations of the period of fertility take into account the **sperm viability** in the female reproductive tract, which is estimated to average **2–3 days** (up to 5 days), and the **fertile period of the ovum,** which is estimated to be **24 hr.** Recent studies indicate that conception is most likely to occur when couples have intercourse during a 6-day period ending on the day of ovulation. **Conception is highly unlikely if sexual intercourse occurs 6 or more days before ovulation or the day after ovulation.**

   b. **Disadvantages** to the rhythm method (but necessary to ensure efficacy) include both the **long periods of abstinence** and the **charting of menses.** Methods of natural family planning and periodic abstinence include the temperature method, calendar method, Billings method, and symptothermal method.

   c. **Temperature method. Basal body temperature** (BBT) determination makes use of a **basal thermometer,** which can be purchased without a prescription. The thermometer covers the range of temperature from 96°F to 100°F in 0.1° gradations.

      (1) The significance of basal temperature determination lies in the fact that within 24 hr preceding ovulation, there is a **moderate drop in the basal temperature** followed by a **noticeable rise in the body temperature,** usually about 24 hr after ovulation. This rise is usually maintained for the remainder of the cycle and is thought to be the result of the thermogenic properties of **progesterone,** the hormone indicating the transition from the ovulatory phase to the luteal phase. Therefore, ovulation is marked by the transition of the falling temperature to the rising temperature.

      (2) For many women, **abstinence** should be practiced from approximately **5 days after the onset of menses until 3 days after the transition in temperature.**

      (3) Because the basal temperature reflects the amount of heat radiation when the body is at its metabolic low, the temperature should be taken first thing in the morning (i.e., before any activity). The thermometer may be placed under the tongue, in the rectum, or in the vagina (the temperature should always be taken from the same place) and should be left undisturbed for at least 5 min (mercury thermometer). Electronic digital thermometers are also available that have shorter recording times (45–90 sec). Infection, tension, a restless night, or any type of excessive movement can cause variations in temperature readings that do not reflect the BBT.

   d. The **calendar method** estimates the possible day of ovulation. **Abstinence** should be practiced during the period around ovulation when there may be a fertilizable egg present. Whereas the calendar rhythm method was used for several decades, it has not been promoted as a method of natural family planning for many years. Although women who have regular menstrual cycles are able to use the calendar rhythm method successfully, women with irregular cycles, women who are breast-feeding, or women with postponed ovulation cannot depend on the calendar rhythm method.

      (1) For a span of **approximately 1 year,** the patient records her menstruation dates on a calendar.

      (2) Calendar charting allows the patient to calculate the onset and duration of her fertile period—the time during which a viable egg is available for fertilization by sperm. Calculation of the fertile period rests on three assumptions:

         (a) **Ovulation** occurs on day **14 (± 2 days) before the onset of the next menses.**
         (b) **Sperm remain viable for 2–3 days.**
         (c) **The ovum survives for 24 hr.**

      (3) The calendar is then reviewed to determine the length of her shortest and longest cycle.

         (a) The patient then subtracts 18 days from the number of days of her shortest cycle. This number should correspond to the first possible fertile day in any given cycle—14 + 2 = 16 days; 16 + 2 = 18 days (viability of sperm); see III.B.1.b.

        (b) Next, the patient subtracts 11 days from the number of days of the longest cycle. This number should correspond to the last possible fertile day in any given cycle—14 − 2 = 12 days; 12 − 1 = 11 days (viability of ova); see III.B.1.b.

    (4) **Abstinence** should be practiced from the first possible fertile day through the last possible fertile day.

    (5) **Example.** Assume the shortest number of days between two consecutive menses is 25 and the longest number of days between two consecutive menses is 32. Then, 25 days (the shortest cycle) − 18 days = 7 (or day 7), and 32 days (the longest cycle) − 11 days = 21 (or day 21). Therefore, abstinence should be practiced from day 7 through and including day 21 of each cycle.

  e. The **cervical mucus (Billings or cervical secretions)** method of rhythm is based on the principle that the normal, thick, creamy white vaginal mucus becomes clear and tenacious around the time of ovulation (much like a raw egg white).

    (1) The woman should watch for this change in mucus consistency and practice abstinence around the time of ovulation.

    (2) The woman should consider herself fertile for 3–4 days after the peak change.

  f. The **symptothermal** method, rather than relying on a single physiological index, uses several indices to determine the fertile period.

    (1) The **most common** calendar calculations and **changes in the cervical mucus** are used to estimate the **onset of the fertile period.**

    (2) Changes in the mucus or basal temperature are used to estimate the end of the fertile period.

    (3) Because several indices need to be monitored, this method is more difficult to learn than the single-index method, but it is more effective than the cervical mucus method (i.e., Billings method) alone.

2. **Spermicidal agents** are composed of an **active spermicidal chemical,** which immobilizes or kills sperm, and an **inert base** (e.g., foam, cream, jelly, gel, tablet, or suppository), which localizes the spermicidal chemical in proximity to the cervical os. These agents work by disrupting the sperm membrane and by decreasing the ability of sperm to metabolize fructose. Two forms of inert bases (gels and foams) act as a physical barrier against sperm.

  a. **The active ingredient** includes **nonoxynol-9.** which is considered safe and effective by the FDA.

    (1) **Administration guidelines.** Applicators may be prefilled before use.

    (2) **Side effects**—for example, sensation of warmth, rare allergic reactions (**contact dermatitis** with rash, stinging, itching, and swelling)—are minimal. If a suspected reaction occurs, one should be instructed to use another product because the issue might be the concentration of the spermicide or an additive specific to a given brand. There are no significant differences in birth-defect rates between users and nonusers.

  b. **Effects against sexually transmitted diseases (STDs).** Nonoxynol-9 is lethal to selected microbes in the laboratory setting and may help inhibit a variety of sexually transmissible organisms, including those responsible for gonorrhea, chlamydial infection, candidiasis, genital herpes, syphilis, trichomoniasis, and HIV/AIDS. There have been inconsistent results in human studies, however. One concern relates to the fact that frequent use of spermicides can cause vulvovaginal epithelial disruption, which may increase susceptibility to HIV. In addition, **spermicides** may alter the vaginal flora and, therefore, **should not be relied on alone for STD prevention.**

  c. **Dosage forms. Contraceptive spermicides,** which are available in several forms, offer the greatest variety within one specific method of contraception (Table 34-2).

    (1) **Creams, jellies, and gels** are used with a diaphragm. The concentration of spermicide is less than the necessary 8% to be employed as a single contraceptive method.

    (2) **Foams** disperse better into the vagina and over the cervical opening but provide less lubrication than creams, jellies, and gels. They usually contain a higher concentration of spermicide (i.e., **the optimal concentration of 8% or higher**). Because of volume differences among brands, the dosage amounts vary. If vaginal or penile irritation develops, another brand should be tried.

      (a) The can should be shaken vigorously 20 times before use.

      (b) The foam should be inserted intravaginally about two thirds the length of the applicator, and the contents should be discharged.

      (c) Foam should be reapplied during prolonged intercourse (i.e., lasting > 1 hr) and before every subsequent act of intercourse.

Table 34-2. Spermicides[a]

Type (Product)	Comments
Film (VCF)	Inserted by the female directly over the cervix; insert not less than 15 min and not more than 3 hr before intercourse; contraceptive protection begins 5–15 min after insertion and remains effective no more than 3 hr
Foam (Ortho Options Delfen foam, VCF Vaginal Contraceptive foam)	Contraceptive protection is immediate; remains effective no more than 1 hr, additional dose is needed before any subsequent intercourse
Jellies, creams, gels (KY Plus Lubricating, Ortho Options Gynol II jelly, Ortho Options Conceptrol gel, Advantage-S)	Contraceptive protection is immediate; used alone remains effective no more than 1 hr; when used with diaphragm or cap, keep diaphragm or cap in place for at least 6 hr after last intercourse
Suppositories and tablets (Encare Insert)	Contraceptive protection begins 10–15 min after insertion; remains effective no more than 1 hr

[a]The spermicidal agent in all listed products is nonoxynol-9.
Reprinted with permission from Hatcher RA. Contraceptive Technology 1994–1996, 16th ed. New York, Irvington, 1994:180.

    (d) To ensure efficacy, the patient should wait at least 8 hr before douching to avoid diluting the spermicide effect or "forcing" sperm into the cervix.
  (3) Suppositories and foaming tablets. These agents are both small and convenient. Although solid at room temperature, suppositories melt at body temperature, whereas foaming tablets effervesce.
    (a) The tablets should be wetted before insertion, which may create a sensation of warmth.
    (b) The tablet or suppository should be inserted high into the vagina, 10–15 min before intercourse.
    (c) Intercourse must occur within 1 hr or the dose must be repeated.
    (d) Another tablet or suppository should be inserted before each repeated act of intercourse.
    (e) To ensure efficacy, the patient should wait 6–8 hr after the last act of intercourse before douching.
  (4) Film comes as small paper-thin sheets (e.g., VCF). It is inserted on the tip of the finger into the vagina and placed at the cervical opening 5–15 min before intercourse.
  (5) Sponge. This fairly popular product was removed from the market in the mid-1990s because of cost issues related to its manufacture. The new owner of the Today sponge (Allendale Pharmaceuticals) is currently remarketing this product. It is a doughnut-shaped polyurethane device containing the spermicide nonoxynol-9; it is inserted into the vagina before sexual intercourse. Efficacy is approximately comparable to that of a cervical cap. It is believed to act as a contraceptive in three ways: (1) mechanically blocking the cervical entrance, (2) absorbing semen, and (3) providing a spermicide. It can remain in place for 24 hr. Concerns are a higher risk for TSS and a higher pregnancy rate for women who have never given birth (nulliparous women).

  3. Condoms are used to prevent transmission of sperm into the vagina.
    a. Types. They are made of latex rubber, processed collagenous lamb caecum sheaths (lambskin), or polyurethane.
    (1) Latex condoms may help prevent the transmission of many STDs. They are usually packaged with the following label "when used properly, the latex condom may prevent the transmission of many STDs such as syphilis, gonorrhea, chlamydia infections, genital herpes, and AIDS."
      (a) Latex affords greater elasticity than lambskin, and latex condoms are more likely to remain in place on the penis.
      (b) A variety of types are available (e.g., lubricated, ribbed, colored), including some with spermicide (concentration much less than that of a vaginal spermicide prod-

uct). It is doubtful that spermicide-lubricated condoms offer any better protection than plain latex condoms, and they have a shorter shelf life. There is a standard size, but smaller and larger versions are available.

(i) Latex condoms are available with a plain end or with a reservoir tip (sometimes designated as "enz"). The reservoir tip provides room for the ejaculate; however, a space may be left when using the plain-end condom, which accommodates the fluid just as effectively.

(ii) The **prelubricated condom** helps prevent dyspareunia in a couple with insufficient natural lubrication. Prelubrication decreases the risk of tearing the condom. However, the extra lubrication may be excessive, lessening sexual fulfillment for a couple who have adequate natural lubrication or when contraceptive foam is also used.

(iii) Latex rubber may cause an allergic reaction. An estimated 1%–2% of the population is sensitized to natural rubber latex, and higher percentages are likely for those frequently exposed to latex (e.g., healthcare workers). The most common symptoms are genital inflammation with redness, itching, and burning. Sometimes, antioxidants or accelerators used during the manufacturing process may be the cause of the allergy.

(2) **Lambskin** condoms are **not** considered as effective as latex condoms (and cannot be labeled as such) in preventing the transmission of STDs, including AIDS. The lambskin condoms are structured to consist of membranes that reveal layers of fibers crisscrossing in various patterns. This gives the lambskin strength, but also allows for an occasional pore. Therefore, lambskin may allow HIV and hepatitis B virus, which are smaller than sperm, to pass through.

(a) Lambskin has less elasticity than latex, and lambskin condoms may slip off the penis.

(b) Lambskin affords **greater sensitivity** than latex.

(c) Lambskin condoms are more expensive than latex condoms.

(3) A **polyurethane condom** (e.g., Avanti, Trojan Supra) is available for men and is marketed for individuals who are allergic to latex. Some evidence exists that slippage and breakage rates may be higher than for latex condoms. In contrast to the latex condom, petroleum-based products will not degrade the polyurethane.

b. **Advantages and disadvantages.** The relative accessibility, ease of transport, and low cost make condoms an attractive method of contraception. However, the coital act must be interrupted to apply the condom, and often one or both partners complain of a partial or complete decrease in sensation.

c. Use

(1) The female external genitalia should not be touched with the exposed penis, and the vagina should not be penetrated, until the condom is unrolled onto the erect penis.

(2) The condom should be unrolled onto the penis as far as it will go. With the plain-end condom, a space between the tip of the penis and the tip of the condom should be left to catch the ejaculate.

(3) With either reservoir-tip or plain-end condoms, the tip of the condom must be held between the thumb and index finger to avoid trapping air while unrolling the condom onto the penis. (The space will decrease the likelihood of both rupture secondary to pressure and regurgitation of the ejaculate onto the external genitalia.)

(4) Proper lubrication to minimize the possibility of tearing can be ensured by using either a lubricated condom or by applying KY jelly or spermicidal cream or jelly to either the condom or the woman's genitalia. (*Note:* Petroleum jelly [Vaseline] should never be used because it causes deterioration of the rubber [latex] and is a poor lubricant.) Spermicidal foam, cream, or jelly is an excellent adjunctive contraceptive.

(5) **Before the penis becomes flaccid,** it must be withdrawn from the vagina and the condom eased off. The **condom** should be handled with special care so as not to lose it into the vagina or spill any of the ejaculatory fluid onto the external genitalia.

(6) A condom should never be reused.

(7) Condoms should not be stored near excessive heat.

(8) If the condom should break or leak, spermicide foam should be immediately inserted vaginally.

(9) Do not buy or use condoms that have passed their expiration date.

(10) Be sure to store condoms in a cool, dry place, out of direct sunlight. The glove compartment of a car is not a good place to store condoms. Do not store condoms in pockets, purses, or wallets for more than a few hours.

4. The **female condom** (Reality) is a **disposable polyurethane sheath** that fits into the vagina and **provides protection from pregnancy and STDs.**

   a. The sheath resembles a plastic vaginal pouch and consists of an **inner ring,** which is inserted into the vagina near the cervix much like a diaphragm, whereas the **outer ring** remains outside the vagina, covering the labia. The condom is prelubricated, and additional lubricant is provided for use if needed. The polyurethane sheath is **stronger** and probably **less likely to tear or break** than the latex sheath of male condoms. It should be removed immediately after intercourse (before the woman stands up). It may be inserted up to 8 hr before intercourse.

   b. If it is used properly, it provides the woman with a method of preventing the transmission of STDs. However, with the noted pregnancy failure rate (Table 34-1), it is certainly not that reliable for disease transmission. It has not been very popular; some women complain that it interferes with sensation and that it makes unpleasant noises during use.

5. The **diaphragm** is a contraceptive device that is self-inserted into the vagina to block access of sperm to the cervix. It requires a prescription and must be used in conjunction with a nonprescription spermicide to seal off crevices between the vaginal wall and the device.

   a. The diaphragm is held in place by the spring tension of a wire rim encased by rubber. When positioned properly, the diaphragm forms a flexible dome to cover the cervix, the sides pressing against the vaginal muscle wall and the pubic bone.

   b. There are **four types** of diaphragms: the **coil spring, the flat spring,** the **arcing spring,** and a **wide-seal rim.** The tone of vaginal muscles as well as the position of the uterus and adjacent organs usually determine the type of diaphragm necessary.

   c. Sizes of the diaphragm range from 50 to 95 mm in diameter, in 5-mm gradations.

   d. Use

      (1) The diaphragm plus spermicide can be inserted as long as 6 hr before coitus. The device should be left in place for 6–8 hr after intercourse, but no longer than 24 hr. Additional spermicide is required for repeated intercourse.

      (2) Before inserting the diaphragm, 1 teaspoonful (a 2- to 3-inch ribbon) of spermicidal cream or jelly should be spread over the inside of the rubber dome.

      (3) Also, spermicide should be spread around the rim to permit a good seal between the diaphragm and the vaginal wall. (For added protection, it can be applied outside the dome.)

   e. Proper care

      (1) The diaphragm should be washed with soap and water, rinsed thoroughly, and dried with a towel.

      (2) It should be dusted with cornstarch and kept in its original container (away from heat).

6. The **cervical cap** is a prescription rubber device smaller than a diaphragm that fits over the cervix like a thimble. It is more difficult to fit than the diaphragm.

   a. It remains effective for more than one episode of intercourse, without adding more spermicide.

   b. The cap should be filled one third full of spermicide cream or jelly; the spermicide is then applied to the rim.

   c. The cervical cap may be left in place for a maximum of 48 hr and should be left in place for at least 8 hr after intercourse.

STUDY QUESTIONS

Directions for questions 1–8: Each of the questions, statements, or incomplete statements in this section can be correctly answered or completed by **one** of the suggested answers or phrases. Choose the **best** answer.

1. The most common cause of vaginal yeast infections is

(A) *Candida albicans.*
(B) *Candida glabrata.*
(C) *Trichomonas.*
(D) anaerobic bacteria.

2. The efficacy rate for nonprescription antifungal agents for vaginal yeast infections is

(A) 50%.
(B) 60%.
(C) 70%.
(D) 80%.

3. Which of the following statements about nonprescription antifungal agents for vaginal yeast infections is incorrect?

(A) Femstat 3 should be applied intravaginally for 3 consecutive nights.
(B) Antifungal agents should be continued during menstruation.
(C) Monistat 1 contains miconazole.
(D) The choice of formulation is based on patient preference.

4. The best product to treat vulvar pruritus in a woman with a vaginal yeast infection is

(A) external miconazole (Monistat).
(B) external miconazole and intravaginal miconazole (Monistat 7 combination pack).
(C) intravaginal tioconazole (Vagistat 1)
(D) intravaginal butoconazole (Femstat 3).

5. A patient complains of vaginal yeast infection symptoms. Under which of the following circumstances should she be referred to a physician?

(A) There is a history of recurrent vaginal yeast infections.
(B) She is pregnant.
(C) She is < 12 years of age.
(D) All of the above

6. All of the following statements regarding contraceptives are correct *except* which one?

(A) Using the basal temperature method, intercourse should be avoided for a full 6 days after the noted temperature transition.
(B) If a condom should break or leak, one could recommend immediate insertion of a vaginal spermicide foam.
(C) Vaginal spermicides may kill many of the causative agents of sexually transmitted diseases (STDs), but they should not be relied on alone for STD prevention.
(D) Latex condoms can be labeled for the prevention of HIV transmission.
(E) Nonoxynol-9 is a safe and effective vaginal spermicide.

7. All of the following statements concerning the vaginal spermicides are correct *except* which one?

(A) Used without a condom or diaphragm, it is recommended that the nonoxynol-9 concentration should be at least 8%.
(B) Foams probably disperse the spermicide throughout the vaginal canal better than cream or jelly forms.
(C) Douching should not occur for 6–8 hr after the last intercourse because it may dilute the spermicide effect or even force sperm into the cervix.
(D) Evidence to date shows no definite link between these agents and birth defects.
(E) None; all of the statements are correct

8. All of the following statements concerning contraception or contraceptive agents are correct *except* which one?

(A) Progesterone is apparently responsible for the increase in basal temperature after ovulation.
(B) Vaseline should not be used as a lubricant with latex condoms.
(C) Using a condom alone is more effective as a contraceptive than taking a combination oral contraceptive.
(D) According to the Billings method, vaginal mucus has an appearance similar to raw egg whites at around the time of ovulation.
(E) Sperm may be viable for up to 5 days in the female reproductive tract under the right conditions.

Directions for questions 9–10: Each statement in this section is most closely related to **one** of the following drug types. The drug types may be used more than once or not at all. Choose the **best** answer, A–E.

A	Diuretics
B	Salicylates
C	Nonsteroidal anti-inflammatory drugs (NSAIDs)
D	Narcotic analgesics

9. The primary nonprescription pharmacological treatment for pain associated with dysmenorrhea

10. Recommended by the Food and Drug Administration (FDA) for elimination of water before and during menstruation

ANSWERS AND EXPLANATIONS

1. The answer is A *[see II.A.1.b]*.
Candida albicans remains the most common cause. Infections caused by *C. glabrata* are increasing. *Trichomonas* and anaerobic bacteria cause other types of vaginal infections.

2. The answer is D *[see II.A.3.f.(2)]*.
Nonprescription antifungal agents' efficacy rates approach 80%–90%.

3. The answer is C *[see II.A.3.f]*.
Monistat 1 contains tioconazole, a long-acting ointment.

4. The answer is B *[see II.A.3.d]*.
External creams can be helpful for treating external itching. The vaginal yeast infection still must be treated with an intravaginal cream.

5. The answer is D *[see II.A.2.b]*.
All of these patients should be referred for diagnosis and treatment.

6. The answer is A *[see III.B.1.c.(2)]*.
Intercourse should be avoided for a full 3 days after the noted temperature transition. All of the other statements are correct.

7. The answer is E *[see III.B.2]*.
All the statements are correct.

8. The answer is C *[see Table 34-1]*.
The most effective contraceptive product available today is the combination oral contraceptive. All of the other statements are correct.

9. The answer is C *[see I.B.1.d.(3).(a)]*.

10. The answer is A *[see I.B.1.d.(3).(b)]*.
NSAIDs are approved by the FDA for the treatment of primary dysmenorrhea. For premenstrual and menstrual relief of water retention, bloating, and tension, the FDA has approved OTC diuretics.

35

Herbal Medicines and Nutritional Supplements

Teresa Klepser

I. INTRODUCTION. Many of the drugs available on the market are derived from plants. Some of those include aspirin, atropine, belladonna, capsaicin, cascara, colchicine, digoxin (Lanoxin), ephedrine, ergotamine, ipecac, opium, physostigmine, pilocarpine, podophyllum, psyllium, quinidine, reserpine, scopolamine, senna, Taxol, tubocurarine, vinblastine, and vincristine. Herb products are also derived from plants; however, these products are not considered drugs by the U.S. Food and Drug Administration (FDA).

A. Regulations

1. The **Federal Food, Drug, and Cosmetic Act of 1938** mandated pharmaceutical companies to test drugs for safety before marketing.

2. The **Kefauver-Harris Drug Amendments of 1962** mandated pharmaceutical companies to test drugs for efficacy before marketing.

3. The **Dietary Supplement Health and Education Act of 1994** mandated the following:
   a. Dietary supplements are not drugs or food. They are intended to supplement the diet.
   b. Herbs are considered dietary supplements.
   c. Dietary supplements do not have to be standardized.
   d. The secretary of Health and Human Services may remove a supplement from the market only when it has been shown to be hazardous to health.
   e. Dietary supplements may make claims only regarding the effects on structure or function of the body. No claims regarding a particular disease or condition may be made.
   f. The following statement is required on the product label: "This product has not been evaluated by the FDA. It is not intended to diagnose, treat, cure, or prevent."

4. **German Federal Health Agency**
   a. In 1978, the German Federal Health Agency established Commission E.
   b. Commission E evaluates the safety and efficacy of herbs through clinical trials and cases published in scientific literature.
   c. There are > 380 published monographs on herbs.

B. Herbs considered unsafe for human consumption

1. Carcinogenic herbs include borage, calamus, coltsfoot, comfrey, life root, and sassafras.

2. Hepatotoxic herbs include chaparral, germander, kava, and life root.

3. High doses of licorice for long periods may cause pseudoaldosteronism, a condition that may include headache, lethargy, sodium and water retention, hypokalemia, high blood pressure, heart failure, and cardiac arrest.

4. Ma huang may cause myocardial infarction, strokes or seizures.

5. Pokeroot may be fatal in children.

6. **Unsafe herbs according to the FDA.** In the 1990s, the FDA's Center for Food Safety and Applied Nutrition created the Special Nutritional Adverse Event Monitoring System Web site for dietary supplements. Unfortunately, by 1999 the site was no longer being updated and thus was eventually deleted. According to the last update from that Web site, the following dietary supplements were considered unsafe by the FDA:
   a. Arnica: muscle paralysis, death
   b. American and European mistletoe: seizures, coma
   c. Bittersweet and deadly nightshade: cardiac toxicity
   d. Bloodroot: hypotension, coma

   e. Broom: dehydration
   f. Comfrey: cancer
   g. Dutch and English tonka bean: hepatotoxicity
   h. Heliotrope: hepatotoxicity
   i. Horse chestnut: bleeding
   j. Jimson weed: anticholinergic, hallucinations
   k. Kava: hepatotoxicity
   l. Lily of the valley: cardiac toxicity
   m. Lobelia (nicotine): coma, death
   n. Mandrake/mayapple: severe gastrointestinal symptoms
   o. Morning glory: psychosis
   p. Periwinkle: renal and hepatotoxicity
   q. Snakeroot: reserpine derivative
   r. Spindle tree: seizures
   s. St. John's wort: drug interactions
   t. Sweet flag: hallucinations, liver cancer
   u. True jalap: purgative cathartic
   v. Wahoo: seizures
   w. Wormwood: seizures, paralysis
   x. Yohimbe: renal failure, hypertension

II. COMMONLY USED HERBS

A. Black cohosh (*Cimicifuga racemosa*)

1. **Commission E indications.** Premenstrual symptoms, painful or difficult menstruation, and neurovegetative symptoms (hot flashes) caused by menopause

2. **Mechanism of action**
   a. Black cohosh has estrogen-like effects that are exerted by an unknown mechanism, different from an estrogenic mechanism.
   b. It does not appear to bind to estrogen receptors. Nor does it appear to up-regulate estrogen-dependent genes.
   c. It does not affect the growth of estrogen-dependent tumors in experimental animals.

3. **Efficacy**
   a. Uncontrolled as well as double-blind, randomized, placebo-controlled clinical trials compared black cohosh to hormone therapy in perimenopausal and postmenopausal women with neurovegetative menopausal symptoms of different degrees of severity. The Kupperman menopausal index and psychiatric clinical and self-evaluation scales were significantly reduced after 3 months of treatment with black cohosh. Vaginal-cytological parameters also improved in regard to estrogen stimulation. Black cohosh was shown to be superior to placebo and comparable to estriol, conjugated estrogens, and estrogen–progesterone therapy (Mahady).
   b. Black cohosh may be effective in premenopausal breast cancer survivors with tamoxifen-induced hot flashes (Mahady).

4. **Contraindications/precautions**
   a. Pregnancy
   b. Unknown if suitable for patients for whom hormone-replacement therapy is contraindicated, such as estrogen-receptor-positive breast cancer
   c. Commission E recommends that length of use should not exceed 6 months.
   d. Use caution in liver disease, such as hepatitis and fulminant liver failure.

5. **Drug interactions**
   a. Cisplatin (Platinol) efficacy may be reduced.
   b. Theoretically, black cohosh may interact with hepatotoxic drugs, such as acetaminophen (Tylenol), carbamazepine (Tegretol), and isoniazid (Nydrazid) because it is an inhibitor of cytochrome P450 3A4 (CYP34A) isoenzyme.

6. **Side effects**
   a. Occasional intestinal problems may occur, such as nausea and vomiting; weight gain is possible.

    b. Liver toxicity may occur; liver function tests should be monitored periodically.

    c. Large doses of black cohosh may cause dizziness, nausea, severe headaches, stiffness, and trembling limbs.

  7. Dosage. Remifemin is a standardized product that contains 20 mg black cohosh and is taken twice daily. It is standardized to 1 mg of 27-deoxyactein per tablet.

B. Chaste tree berry (*Vitex agnus-castus*)

  1. Commission E indications. Disorders of the menstrual cycle, breast swelling, and premenstrual symptoms

  2. Mechanism of action

    a. Chaste tree berry binds to dopamine receptors and inhibits prolactin secretion.

    b. One of its ingredients, linoleic acid, binds to estrogen receptors.

    c. It increases the pituitary gland's production of luteinizing hormone and inhibits follicle-stimulating hormone (FSH).

  3. Efficacy. One randomized, double-blind, placebo-controlled, parallel group study included 170 women with premenstrual syndrome (Schellenberg). *Vitex* was given 20 mg daily for 3 cycles. Self-assessment and clinical global impression significantly improved.

  4. Contraindications/precautions

    a. Pregnancy

    b. Women receiving hormone-replacement therapy

  5. Drug interactions

    a. Theoretically, chaste tree berry may interact with medications that increase dopaminergic activity, such as bromocriptine (Parlodel) and levodopa.

    b. Theoretically, it may interact with medications that decrease dopaminergic activity, such as the antipsychotics.

    c. Theoretically, it may interact with hormone-replacement therapy and oral contraceptives.

  6. Side effects

    a. Mild gastrointestinal upset

    b. Skin rash

    c. Increased menstrual flow

  7. Dosage. Doses depend on the formulation. Typical dose range of chaste tree berry is 20–240 mg per day.

C. Cranberry (*Vaccinium macrocarpon*)

  1. Commission E indications. Recurrent urinary tract infections

  2. Mechanism of action

    a. Urinary acidification

    b. Benzoic and quinic acids break down and form hippuric acid (bacteriostatic).

    c. Inhibition of *Escherichia coli* adherence to epithelial cells of urinary tract

    d. Cranberry juice may suppress *Helicobacter pylori* infection.

  3. Efficacy

    a. A quasi-randomized, double-blind, placebo-controlled study included 153 women who received 300 mL of cranberry juice daily for 6 months (Avorn et al.). Bacteriuria with pyuria occurred less often in the cranberry group (15%) versus placebo (28%).

  4. Contraindications

    a. Benign prostatic hyperplasia

    b. Urinary obstruction

    c. Nephrolithiasis

    d. Cranberry juice contains high amounts of salicylic acid and may trigger an allergic reaction in patients with an aspirin allergy or asthma.

    e. Discontinue 2 weeks before surgery.

  5. Drug interactions

    a. Increased vitamin B_{12} absorption

    b. Potential to enhance elimination of renally excreted drugs by changing urine pH

    c. Cranberry juice may interact with warfarin, increasing the international normalized ratio (INR).

    d. May inhibit cytochrome P450 2C9. Drugs that are metabolized by CYP2C9 include amitriptyline (Elavil) and diazepam (Valium).

  6. Side effects

    a. Nausea, vomiting, diarrhea

    b. Nephrolithiasis

  7. Dosage. Recommended dose of cranberry is 300–400 mg twice daily using a standardized product to include 11%–12% quinic acid per dose. Patients may also take 8–16 oz. 100% cranberry juice daily. Drinking lots of fluids is recommended.

D. Dong quai (*Angelica senensis*)

  1. Traditional Chinese Medicine indications. Menstrual disorders, anemia, constipation, insomnia, rheumatism, neuralgia, and hypertension

  2. Mechanism of action

    a. Dong quai is only 1:400 as active as estrogen. However, it does not appear to produce any changes to the ovaries or vaginal tissue (Murray).

    b. It contains seven different coumarin derivatives: oxypeucedanin, osthole, psoralen, angelol, angelicone, bergapten, and 7-desmethylsuberosin. Many coumarins have been shown to have vasodilatory and antispasmodic effects. One of the coumarins (osthole) is a central nervous system (CNS) stimulant.

    c. It inhibits experimentally induced immunoglobulin E (IgE) titers, suggesting that components of the plant may have immunosuppressive activity.

    d. It inhibits prostaglandin E_2 (PGE_2) release and, therefore, possesses analgesic, antipyretic, and anti-inflammatory actions.

    e. It has a quinidine-type effect, so it may control tachycardia.

    f. It normalizes uterine contractions.

    g. It has antibiotic activity against gram-negative bacteria (*Bacillus dysenteriae, B. typhi, B. comma, B. paratyphi,* and *Escherichia coli*) and against gram-positive bacteria (hemolytic *Streptococcus* type A and B, *Corynebacterium diphtheriae*).

  3. Efficacy. A randomized, double-blind, placebo-controlled trial included 71 postmenopausal women (mean age, 52.4 years) who had FSH < 30 mIU/mL with hot flashes (Hirata et al.). Women received 3 capsules of dong quai three times daily (equivalent to 4.5 g of dong quai root daily) or placebo for 24 weeks. Dong quai did not produce estrogen-like responses in endometrial thickness or in vaginal maturation or relieve menopausal symptoms. The study is criticized for using dong quai alone, because in Traditional Chinese Medicine, dong quai is used in combination with four or more other herbs.

  4. Contraindications/precautions

    a. Pregnancy (uterine stimulant) and lactation

    b. Diarrhea

    c. Hemorrhagic disease; discontinue 2 weeks before surgery

    d. Hypermenorrhea

    e. Hypotension

    f. During colds or flus

    g. Allergy to parsley

  5. Drug interactions

    a. Dong quai interacts with anticoagulants, such as warfarin (Coumadin)

    b. Antihypertensives (hypotension)

    c. Theoretically, may interact with hormone-replacement therapy.

    d. Unknown if it interacts with other cardiovascular drugs such as procainamide (Pronestyl)

  6. Side effects

    a. Photodermatitis may occur in people collecting the plant.

    b. Burping, flatulence, and headache

    c. Safrole, found in the oil of dong quai, is carcinogenic and not recommended for ingestion.

  7. Dosage. A variety of doses are suggested. No standardized product is available. According to traditional Chinese medicine, dong quai alone may not be effective.

E. Echinacea (*Echinacea purpurea, E. angustifolia*)

1. **Commission E indications**
   a. Internal use: supportive therapy for infections of the upper respiratory tract (colds) and lower urinary tract
   b. External use: local application for the treatment of hard-to-heal superficial wounds and ulcers

2. **Mechanism of action.** Echinacea increases the body's resistance to bacteria by:
   a. Caffeic acid derivatives, which include cichoric acid, chlorogenic acid, and cynarin, increase phagocytosis and stimulate the production of immune-potentiating substances such as interferon, interleukins, and tumor necrosis factor.
   b. Polysaccharides, such as inulin, stimulate macrophages and inhibit hyaluronidase activity to decrease inflammation.
   c. Alkylamides, such as echinacein, have a local anesthetic effect and inhibit hyaluronidase activity to decrease inflammation.
   d. Echinacea has little or no direct bacteriocidal or bacteriostatic properties.

3. **Efficacy.** In a review of 26 controlled clinical trials evaluating echinacea's ability to strengthen the body's own defense mechanisms, it was found that 30 of 34 echinacea therapies were more effective compared to controls (Melchart et al.).

4. **Contraindications/precautions**
   a. Echinacea is contraindicated in infectious and autoimmune diseases such as tuberculosis, leukosis, collagenosis, multiple sclerosis, AIDS, HIV, and lupus.
   b. Caution should be used in patients who are allergic to members of the ragweed family.
   c. The effects of echinacea in pregnancy, lactation, and children are unknown. Comparison with a control group suggested no increased risk of major malformations in 206 pregnant women (Gallo et al.).
   d. Therapy should not exceed 8 weeks. Theoretically, prolonged use of echinacea may depress the immune system, possibly through overstimulation.

5. **Drug interactions**
   a. Unknown if echinacea interacts with immunosuppressants
   b. Echinacea inhibits cytochrome P450 1A2. Some drugs metabolized by CYP1A2 are caffeine (Cafcit) and theophylline.
   c. Echinacea induces and inhibits CYP3A4. Some drugs metabolized by CYP3A4 are midazolam (Versed), itraconazole (Sporanox) and fexofenadine (Allegra).

6. **Side effects**
   a. Nausea, vomiting, dizziness, tiredness, allergic reactions, and anaphylaxis.
   b. May interfere with male fertility.

7. **Dosage.** There are a variety of doses recommended. The most common dose is as the dried powder, 1 g or two 500-mg capsules orally three times daily. Recommended to use for 2 weeks only during a cold.

F. Feverfew (*Tanacetum parthenium*)

1. **Commission E indication.** Prophylaxis of migraine headaches

2. **Mechanism of action**
   a. Feverfew inhibits the release of 5-hydroxytryptamine (serotonin) from platelets, which may be the same mechanism as methysergide maleate (Sansert).
   b. It irreversibly inhibits prostaglandin synthesis through a different mechanism from that of the salicylates. It inhibits phospholipase A_2 by α-methylene butyrolactones (parthenolide and epoxyartemorin).
   c. There is an antithrombotic potential owing to a phospholipase inhibition that prevents the release of arachidonic acid.
   d. It inhibits polymorphonuclear leukocyte (PMN) degranulation, which reduces PMN-induced damage to the rheumatoid synovium.
   e. It inhibits phagocytosis of human neutrophils, which may reduce tissue damage from oxygen radicals.

    f. It inhibits mast cell release of histamine.

    g. It may have cytotoxic activity against human tumor cells.

    h. It may possess antimicrobial activity.

3. Efficacy. An evaluation of five trials for the efficacy of feverfew in the prevention of migraines compared to placebo was conducted (Cochrane Database of Systematic Reviews). A variety of doses and durations were used. Some trials showed the number and severity of migraine attacks and the degree of vomiting were reduced with feverfew. The duration of attacks was unaltered. Other trials showed no benefit.

4. Contraindications/precautions

    a. Feverfew should be avoided in pregnancy, lactation, and children < 2 years of age.

    b. Contraindicated in individuals with allergies to chrysanthemums.

    c. Contraindicated in patients with bleeding disorders. Discontinue 2 weeks before surgery.

5. Drug interactions

    a. Feverfew may interact with anticoagulants, increasing the risk of bleeding.

    b. Feverfew may inhibit the following cytochrome P450 isoenzymes: 1A2, 2C19, 2C9, and 3A4.

6. Side effects

    a. Gastric discomfort on oral consumption

    b. Contact dermatitis

    c. Minor ulcerations of oral mucosa, irritation of tongue, and swelling of lips may occur when fresh leaves are chewed.

    d. Palpitations.

    e. Post-feverfew syndrome: discontinuation of feverfew may produce muscle and joint stiffness and a cluster of nervous system reactions (rebound of migraines, anxiety, and insomnia).

7. Dosage. The usual dose of feverfew is 125 mg daily. A product containing at least 0.2% parthenolide is recommended.

G. Garlic (*Allium sativum*)

1. Commission E indications. Support dietary measures for the treatment of hyperlipoproteinemia and to prevent age-related changes in the blood vessels (arteriosclerosis)

2. Mechanism of action

    a. Garlic inhibits platelet function by interfering with thromboxane synthesis.

    b. It increases the levels of two antioxidant enzymes in the blood: catalase and glutathione peroxidase.

    c. Organic disulfides found in garlic oil inactivate the thiol enzymes such as coenzyme A (CoA) and hydroxymethyl glutaryl (HMG) CoA reductase.

3. Efficacy

    a. In a meta-analysis of eight studies evaluating the effect on blood pressure, the overall pooled difference in change of systolic blood pressure was 7.7 mm Hg lower with garlic than with placebo; diastolic blood pressure was 5.0 mm Hg lower with garlic (Silagy et al.).

    b. In a meta-analysis of five studies evaluating the effect on total serum cholesterol, patients were excluded if they were receiving lipid-lowering drugs (Warshafsky et al.). The overall pooled total cholesterol difference between garlic and placebo was -23 mg/dL (-29 to -17).

4. Contraindications/precautions

    a. Caution in diabetes. Garlic may increase the release of insulin or enhance the response to insulin.

    b. Caution in pregnancy (emmenagogue and abortifacient) and lactation

    c. Caution in peptic ulcer disease and gastroesophageal reflux

    d. Discontinue 2 weeks before surgery

5. Drug interactions

    a. Anticoagulants (increased bleeding)

    b. Protease inhibitors (decreased efficacy)

    c. Nonnucleoside reverse transcriptase inhibitors, such as nevirapine, efavirenz

    d. Increases amphotericin B (Fungizone) activity against *Cryptococcus neoformans*

    e. Antihypertensives (hypotension)

    f. Antidiabetic agents (hypoglycemia)

    g. May inhibit the following cytochrome P450 isoenzymes: 2C9, 2C19, 3A4.

    h. Caution should be used with contraceptive medications, cyclosporine, diltiazem, and verapamil.

6. Side effects. Gastrointestinal discomfort (heartburn, flatulence), sweating, light-headedness, allergic reactions, and menorrhagia

7. Dosage. Between 0.6 and 1.2 g dried powder (2–5 mg of allicin) daily or 2–4 g fresh garlic

8. Comments

    a. Alliinase (the enzyme that converts alliin to allicin) is inactivated by acids. Enteric-coated tablets or capsules allow more absorption because they pass through the stomach and release their contents in the alkaline medium of the small intestine.

    b. Odorless garlic preparations may not contain the active compounds.

H. Ginger (*Zingiber officinale*)

1. Commission E indications. Dyspepsia and prophylaxis of symptoms of travel sickness

2. Mechanism of action

    a. Ginger promotes saliva and gastric juice secretion, which increases peristalsis and the tone of the intestinal muscle.

    b. It acts on 5-hydroxytryptamine 3 (5-HT$_3$) receptors in the ileum, similar to ondansetron.

    c. It has positive inotropic activity.

    d. It inhibits thromboxane synthesis as a prostacyclin agonist.

3. Efficacy. A double-blind study included 36 blindfolded subjects with high susceptibility to motion sickness who were given ginger 940 mg, dimenhydrinate 100 mg, or placebo for the prevention of motion sickness induced by a tilted rotating chair. Ginger subjects remained in the chair an average of 5.5 min, dimenhydrinate 3.5 min, and placebo 1.5 min. The ginger group took longer to feel sick, but once sick, the sensations of nausea and vomiting progressed at the same rate in all groups (Mowrey et al.).

4. Contraindications/precautions

    a. Bleeding disorders. Discontinue 2 weeks before surgery

    b. It is contraindicated for gallstone pain.

    c. It is recommended by the American College of Obstetricians and Gynecologists (ACOG) for use in pregnancy < 17 weeks of gestation with the following cautions: ginger is a uterine relaxant in low doses and a uterine stimulant in high doses.

    d. Diabetes (hypoglycemia)

    e. Heart conditions

5. Drug interactions

    a. Antiplatelets and anticoagulants (increased bleeding)

    a. Diabetic agents (hypoglycemia)

    a. Calcium channel blockers (hypotension)

6. Side effects are dermatitis, heartburn, and diarrhea.

7. Dosage (for travel sickness). Daily dose is 2–4 g. Two 500-mg capsules taken 30 min before travel, then 1–2 more capsules every 4 hr as needed. The 1000 mg standardized extract is equivalent to:

    a. 1 teaspoon fresh grated rhizome

    b. 2 droppers liquid extract (2 mL)

    c. 2 teaspoons syrup (10 mL)

    d. 8 ounces ginger ale, made with real ginger

    e. 4 cups ginger tea (made by steeping 1/2 teaspoon grated ginger for 5–10 min in hot water)

I. **Ginkgo (*Ginkgo biloba*)**

1. **Commission E indications**

a. Treatment for cerebral circulatory disturbances resulting in reduced functional capacity and vigilance (vertigo, tinnitus, weakened memory, and mood swings accompanied by anxiety)

b. Treatment of peripheral arterial circulatory disturbance such as intermittent claudication

2. **Mechanism of action**

a. Ginkgo contains flavonoids (quercetin, kaempferol, and isorhamnetin) and terpenoids (ginkgolides A, B, and C and bilobalide).

b. Flavonoids provide the antioxidant activity, reduce capillary fragility, and increase the threshold of blood loss from capillaries.

c. Ginkgolides antagonize platelet-activating factor (PAF), which induces platelet aggregation, the degranulation of neutrophils, and the production of oxygen radicals.

d. Bilobalide protects nerve cells.

3. **Efficacy**

a. In a review of the clinical and pharmacological studies on ginkgo and cerebral insufficiency, eight were found to be of good quality (Kleijnen). Seven of the trials showed positive effects of ginkgo compared to placebo. Symptoms of cerebral insufficiency evaluated were difficulties of concentration and memory, absentmindedness, confusion, lack of energy, tiredness, decreased physical performance, depression, anxiety, dizziness, tinnitus, and headaches.

b. For intermittent claudication, there were 15 controlled trials, 2 of acceptable quality (Rittler et al.).

(1) One showed an increase in walking distance (Bauer et al.)—ginkgo, 112–222 m; placebo, 145–176 m.

(2) The other demonstrated amelioration of pain at rest (Saudreau et al.). The use of ginkgo showed a decrease on a 100-mm visual analog scale for pain from 61 to 30 mm (placebo 51 to 39 mm).

c. A randomized, double-blind, placebo-controlled study included 202 patients with either Alzheimer disease or multi-infarct dementia. These patients were given ginkgo 40 mg three times daily or placebo for 1 year. Ginkgo had a statistically significant improvement by at least two points or better on the Alzheimer Disease Assessment Scale—Cognitive (a 70-point subscale) compared to placebo (50% versus 29%). Ginkgo showed statistically significant improvement on the Geriatric Evaluation by Relative's Rating Instrument (37% versus 23%). There was no difference between ginkgo and placebo on the Clinical Global Impression of Change scale (LeBurs et al.).

4. **Contraindications/precautions.**

a. Epilepsy. Ginkgotoxin may cause neurotoxicity and seizures.

b. Bleeding disorders. Discontinue 2 weeks before surgery

c. Diabetes (hypoglycemia)

d. Infertility. Caution in difficulty conceiving.

4. **Drug interactions**

a. Ginkgo may potentiate the bleeding properties of antiplatelets—there is a case report of spontaneous hyphema (bleeding from the iris into the anterior chamber) from ginkgo and aspirin.

b. Aminoglycosides (increased ototoxicity)

c. Thiazide (increases blood pressure)

d. Trazodone (Desyrel) (coma)

e. Seizure threshold lowering drugs.

f. Anticonvulsants

g. Antidiabetic drugs (hypoglycemia)

h. Ginkgo may mildly affect the cytochrome P450 isoenzymes 1A2, 2C19, 2C9, 2D6, and 3A4.

5. **Side effects**

a. Gastric disturbances, headache, dizziness, and vertigo

b. Toxic ingestion may produce tonic–clonic seizures and loss of consciousness

6. **Dosage.** Recommended dose is 40 mg three times daily with meals for at least 4–6 weeks. Standardized preparations that contain 6% terpene lactones and 24% ginkgo flavone glycosides are recommended.

J. Asian ginseng (*Panax ginseng, P. quinquefolius*)

1. **Commission E indications.** Tonic to combat feelings of lassitude and debility, lack of energy, and ability to concentrate, and during convalescence

2. **Mechanism of action**
   a. At least 28 active ingredients, known as ginsenosides, have been identified.
   b. Ginseng effects vary with extract derivative, drying method, dose, duration of treatment, and animal species that was studied. Each ginsenoside produces different pharmacological effects on the central nervous system, cardiovascular system, and other body systems. Different ginsenosides are capable of producing biological effects in direct opposition with those produced by others. For example, the ginsenoside Rb_1 has been shown to have a suppressive effect on the central nervous system, whereas Rg_1 produces a stimulatory effect.

3. **Efficacy**
   a. A randomized, double-blind, placebo-controlled, crossover study included 50 male sports teachers who performed a treadmill exercise test. Volunteers received 2 ginseng capsules (Geriatric Pharmaton) daily for 6 weeks or placebo. Volunteers used energy more efficiently and had greater endurance while taking ginseng (Pieralisi et al.).
   b. A case-controlled study including 1987 pairs evaluated ginseng's effect on various human cancers. Individuals who took ginseng had a significant decreased risk for cancer compared with nonintakers. There may be a dose–response relationship; as the frequency and duration of ginseng use increased, the risk of cancer decreased. According to cancer site, ginseng significantly reduced the risk of cancer of the lip, oral cavity, and pharynx; esophagus; stomach; colon and rectum; liver; pancreas; lung; and ovaries. There was no risk reduction for cancers of the female breast, uterine cervix, urinary bladder, and thyroid gland (Yun et al.).

4. **Contraindications/precautions**
   a. Pregnancy and lactation
   b. Children
   c. Avoid in patients with hypertension, emotional/psychological imbalances, headaches, heart palpitations, insomnia, asthma, inflammation, or infections with high fever.
   d. Caution should be used in patients with a history of bleeding. Discontinue 2 weeks before surgery
   e. Diabetes (hypoglycemia)
   f. Schizophrenia
   g. Caution should be used in patients with a history of breast cancer. Ginseng may stimulate breast cancer cells.

5. **Drug interactions**
   a. Ginseng may interact with phenelzine (Nardil), producing hallucinations and psychosis.
   b. Ginseng may decrease the INR of warfarin (Coumadin).
   c. Ginseng may interact with stimulants, including caffeine (Cafcit).
   d. Ginseng may interact with hypoglycemics, causing hypoglycemia.
   e. It is unknown whether ginseng interacts with hormonal therapy, antihypertensives, or cardiac medications.
   f. It may inhibit cytochrome P450 2D6. Caution should be used with drugs that are metabolized via cytochrome P450 2D6, such as amitriptyline (Elavil) and fluoxetine (Prozac).
   g. It may interfere with immunosuppressants.

6. **Side effects**
   a. Nervousness and excitation for the first 4 days
   b. Inability to concentrate with long-term use
   c. Diffuse mammary nodularity and vaginal bleeding may be caused by ginseng's estrogen-like effect in women.
   d. Hypertension, euphoria, restlessness, nervousness, insomnia, skin eruptions, edema, and diarrhea have been reported with long-term ginseng use with an average dose of 3 g ginseng root daily.
   e. May increase the QT interval.

7. **Dosage.** 1–2 g crude herb daily or 100–300 mg ginseng extract three times daily. Standardized products that contain at least 4%–5% ginsenosides are recommended.

K. **Siberian ginseng (*Eleutherococcus senticosus*)**

1. **Commission E indications.** Tonic for fatigue, convalescence, decreased work capacity, or difficulty in concentration

2. **Mechanism of action.** Animal research suggests that Siberian ginseng may stimulate the hypothalamic–pituitary–adrenal cortex. It may bind to progestin, mineralocorticoid, and glucocorticoid receptors.

3. **Efficacy**
   a. A randomized, double-blind, placebo-controlled study evaluated 20 highly trained distance runners who received *E. senticosus* extract 60 drops daily for 6 weeks or placebo. Subjects underwent a maximal treadmill test and a 10K race. No significant difference was observed between treatment and placebo for heart rate, oxygen consumption, expired minute volume, ventilatory equivalent for oxygen, or respiratory exchange ratio (Dowling et al.).
   b. A randomized, placebo controlled prospective study evaluated 96 subjects with chronic, unexplained fatigue who received standardized *E. senticosus* 2000 mg daily for 2 months. No statistically significant difference was observed (Hartz et al.).

4. **Contraindications/precautions**
   a. Avoid in hypertension
   b. Not recommended in patients with febrile states, hypertonic crisis, or myocardial infarction
   c. Diabetes (hypoglycemia)
   d. Bleeding disorders. Discontinue 2 weeks before surgery
   e. Cardiovascular conditions: hypertension, tachycardia.
   f. Hormone-sensitive conditions.
   g. Psychiatric conditions: schizophrenia, mania

5. **Drug interactions**
   a. Serum levels of digoxin (Lanoxin) may increase when taken with Siberian ginseng.
   b. Barbiturates. Hexobarbital and Siberian ginseng increase sleep latency and duration.
   c. Siberian ginseng may increase the risk of hypoglycemia with diabetic agents
   d. Siberian ginseng may interact with anticoagulants.
   e. Theoretically, Siberian ginseng may interact with stimulants, such as caffeine.
   f. Theoretically, Siberian ginseng may interact with antihypertensives
   g. May inhibit the following cytochrome P450 isoenzymes: 1A2, 2C9, 2D6, and 3A4.

6. **Side effects**
   a. Mild, transient diarrhea, and insomnia
   b. Siberian ginseng may lower blood glucose.
   c. Tachycardia, hypertension, palpitations.

7. **Dosage.** Two capsules (each capsule containing 400–500 mg of powdered root) three times daily for a total of 2–3 g daily. Solid concentrated extract standardized on eleutherosides B and E 300–400 mg daily are recommended. Recommended not to use longer than 3 weeks.

L. **Milk thistle (*Silybum marianum*)**

1. **Commission E indications.** Chronic inflammatory liver conditions and cirrhosis

2. **Mechanism of action**
   a. Milk thistle produces antioxidants.
   b. It stimulates the activity of RNA polymerase A.
   c. It alters the outer liver membrane cell structure.

3. **Efficacy.** In an evaluation of 13 trials for the efficacy of milk thistle in the treatment of alcoholic and/or hepatitis B or C virus liver diseases, milk thistle had no significant effect on overall mortality, complications of liver disease, or liver histology (Cochrane Database of Systematic Reviews). Liver-related mortality was significantly reduced with milk thistle when all trials were evaluated but was not significantly reduced when only high-quality trials were evaluated.

4. **Contraindications/precautions**
   a. Avoid in pregnancy.
   b. Allergy to chrysanthemums
   c. Hormone-sensitive cancers

5. Drug interactions
a. Milk thistle may inhibit cytochrome P450 2C9 and 3A4.
b. Milk thistle does not interact with indinavir (Crixivan).

6. Side effects include diarrhea and other gastrointestinal reactions (nausea, dyspepsia, flatulence) and allergic reactions

7. Dosage. Recommended dose of milk thistle is 200–400 mg/day divided into three doses using a standardized product that includes 70%–80% silymarin.

M. Saw palmetto (*Serenoa repens*)

1. Commission E indications. Treatment of micturition difficulties associated with benign prostatic hyperplasia

2. Mechanism of action
a. Saw palmetto inhibits dihydrotestosterone to androgen receptors in prostate cells.
b. It may inhibit testosterone-5-α-reductase, the enzyme responsible for the conversion of testosterone to dihydrotestosterone.

3. Efficacy. A randomized, multicenter study evaluated 1069 men with moderate benign prostatic hyperplasia who received saw palmetto 160 mg twice daily or finasteride 5 mg daily for 6 months. There was no significant difference between saw palmetto and finasteride (Proscar) for the patients' self-rated quality-of-life score and the International Prostate Symptom score (Carraro et al.).

4. Contraindications/precautions
a. Avoid in pregnancy
b. Avoid in children
c. Discontinue 2 weeks before surgery

5. Drug interactions
a. Theoretically, saw palmetto may interact with anticoagulants.
b. Theoretically, saw palmetto may interact with contraceptive drugs or hormone-replacement therapy.

6. Side effects
a. Intraoperative hemorrhage
b. Headache
c. Stomach upset

7. Dosage. Recommended 1–2 g saw palmetto or 320 mg of lipophilic extract daily, usually given 160 mg twice daily and taken with food. Products standardized to contain 90% free and 7% esterified fatty acids are recommended.

N. St. John's wort (*Hypericum perforatum*)

1. Commission E indications. In supportive treatment for anxiety and depression

2. Mechanism of action
a. Active ingredients include hypericin, pseudohypericin, quercetin, quercitrin, isoquercitrin, hyperoside, rutin, amentoflavone, hyperin, hyperforin, adhyperforin, and xanthones.
b. Hypericin, flavonoids, and xanthones show in vitro irreversible monoamine oxidase inhibitor (MAOI) type A and B activity.
c. St. John's wort may inhibit serotonin reuptake.
d. St. John's wort may inhibit synaptic γ-aminobutyric acid (GABA) uptake and GABA-receptor binding.
e. It may reduce cytokine expression, such as interleukin 6. This may be helpful in depression because interleukins may induce depression.

3. Efficacy. An evaluation of 37 trials for the efficacy of St. John's wort in the treatment of depression showed the herb may be more effective than placebo for mild to moderate depression (Cochrane Database of Systematic Reviews). St. John's wort may be as effective as other antidepressants for mild to moderate depression. St. John's wort may not be effective for major depression.

4. Contraindications/precautions
   a. Caution in fair-skinned persons when exposed to bright sunlight
   b. Caution in pregnancy (emmenagogue and abortifacient)
   c. No negative influence on general performance or the ability to drive a car or operate heavy machinery has been reported.
   d. Psychiatric conditions such as bipolar, schizophrenia may be exacerbated.
   e. Hypothyroidism
   f. Anesthesia. St. John's wort may cause cardiovascular collapse.
   g. Infertility. St. John's wort may inhibit oocyte fertilization and alter sperm DNA.

5. Drug interactions
   a. Antidepressants such as paroxetine (Paxil), sertraline (Zoloft), and nefazodone have been reported to cause serotonin syndrome when taken with St. John's wort.
   b. Antiretroviral (protease inhibitors and nonnucleoside reverse transcriptase inhibitors) levels may decrease.
   c. St. John's wort may decrease the efficacy of barbiturates.
   d. St. John's wort may increase the efficacy of clopidogrel (Plavix).
   e. Cyclosporine (Sandimmune) levels may decrease.
   f. St. John's wort may interact with other drugs metabolized through the cytochrome P450 isoenzymes 1A2, 2C9, and 3A4.
   g. Digoxin (Lanoxin) levels may decrease.
   h. Irinotecan (Camptosar) and imatinib (Gleevec) levels may decrease.
   i. Methadone (Dolophine) levels may decrease.
   j. St. John's wort may decrease the efficacy of omeprazole (Prilosec).
   k. Oral contraceptives may have a decreased effect.
   l. St. John's wort may decrease the efficacy of HMG coenzyme reductase inhibitors.
   m. Tacrolimus (Prograf) levels may decrease.
   n. Theophylline levels may decrease.
   o. Theoretically, St. John's wort may interact with the triptans.
   p. Verapamil (Calan, Covera-HS, Isoptin, Verelan) levels may decrease.
   q. St. John's wort may decrease the INR of warfarin (Coumadin).

6. Food interactions
   a. Older studies suggested that St. John's wort was an MAOI (Suzuki et al.).
   b. Newer studies suggest St. John's wort is a weak MAOI (Muller et al.).
   c. No case reports published of MAO-type food interactions such as tyramine-containing foods: cheeses, beer, wine, herring, and yeast.

7. Side effects
   a. Photodermatitis
   b. Gastrointestinal irritations
   c. Allergic reactions
   d. Tiredness
   e. Restlessness
   f. Elevated thyroid-stimulating hormone
   g. Elevated blood pressure
   h. Mania

8. Dosage.
Recommended 2–4 g daily in two to three divided doses. Standardized products containing 0.4–2.7 mg hypericin/day or 0.3% hypericin are recommended.

O. Valerian (*Valeriana officinalis*)

1. Commission E indications.
Restlessness and nervous disturbance of sleep

2. Mechanism of action
   a. Several active compounds have been isolated from valerian and grouped into three categories: volatile oil, valepotriates, and alkaloids. It is believed that the sedative activity of valerian is secondary to the valepotriates.
   b. Valepotriates, valeranone 6, kessane derivatives 3a–f, valerenic acid 5a, and valerenal 5b have been reported to prolong barbiturate-induced sleeping time.

c. Valerenic acid 5a has been shown to possess pentobarbital-like central depressant activity rather than muscle relaxant or neuroleptic effects. It has also been shown to inhibit the enzyme that triggers the breakdown of GABA.

d. Valtrate and isovaltrate have exhibited antidepressant properties.

e. Didrovaltrate possesses a tranquilizing ability similar to the benzodiazepines.

3. Efficacy. A double-blind, randomized study included eight volunteers suffering from mild insomnia who received valerian aqueous extract 450 mg or 900 mg or placebo at bedtime. Valerian 450 mg significantly improved sleep quality, sleep latency, and sleep depth compared to placebo. The 900-mg dose offered no advantage over the 450-mg dose (Leathwood et al.).

4. Contraindications/precautions. Caution while driving or performing other tasks requiring alertness and coordination is recommended.

5. Drug interactions.
a. CNS depressants. Valerian may potentiate the sedative effect of barbiturates, benzodiazepines, opiates, alcohol, or other sedatives.
b. Valerian inhibits cytochrome P450 3A4.

5. Side effects
a. Headaches, hangover, excitability, insomnia, uneasiness, and cardiac disturbances
b. Hepatotoxicity
c. Toxicity includes ataxia, decreased sensibility, hypothermia, hallucinations, and increased muscle relaxation
d. Patients may experience a benzodiazepine-like withdrawal; so doses should be tapered down slowly.

6. Dosage. Dried root: 2–3 g per cup, one to three times daily. Standardized to contain 0.8%–1% valeremic acids/dose extract: 400–900 mg 30–60 min before bedtime.

III. OTHER DIETARY SUPPLEMENTS THAT ARE POTENTIALLY SAFE

A. Chondroitin

1. Nonapproved indications. Viscoelastic agent in ophthalmic procedures and the treatment of osteoarthritis

2. Mechanism of action
a. It concentrates in cartilage, where it can be used in the synthesis of new cartilaginous matrix.
b. It increases the RNA synthesis of chondrocytes, which may increase the synthesis of proteoglycans and collagens.
c. It may inhibit leukocyte elastase activity. Leukocyte elastase is found in high concentrations in the blood and synovial fluid of patients with rheumatic diseases.

3. Efficacy. One 6-month randomized, parallel study included 146 patients with knee osteoarthritis (Morreale et al.). Patients received either chondroitin sulfate 400 mg three times daily or diclofenac 50 mg three times daily for 3 months. Chondroitin was as effective for relieving symptoms associated with osteoarthritis, but the onset of action was much slower than diclofenac.

4. Contraindications/precautions
a. Previous hypersensitivity to chondroitin sulfate
b. Bleeding disorders
c. Use caution because chondroitin is usually produced from bovine cartilage (possible transmission of mad cow disease)

5. Drug interactions
a. May interact with heparin
b. Theoretically, may interact with warfarin (Coumadin)

6. Side effects. Nausea, epigastric pain, and headache

7. Dosage. Recommended: 400 mg three times daily

B. Coenzyme Q_{10} (ubiquinone or ubidecarenone)

1. **Nonapproved indications.** Heart failure (HF), hypertension, stable angina, ventricular arrhythmias, cancer, heart surgery, and periodontal disease

2. **Mechanism of action**
   a. It is a naturally occurring coenzyme that has a predominant role in oxidative phosphorylation and synthesis of adenosine triphosphate (ATP), which is needed for muscle contraction and relaxation.
   b. It may have antioxidant properties.
   c. It has been shown to reduce myocardial injury from ischemia and to reduce toxic myocardial damage from anthracyclines, such as doxorubicin (Adriamycin).

3. **Efficacy**
   a. **Heart failure.** One randomized, double-blind, placebo-controlled, multicenter study included 641 patients with New York Heart Association class III or IV chronic congestive heart failure who were receiving conventional treatment, such as digoxin (Lanoxin), diuretics, angiotensin-converting enzyme (ACE) inhibitors, and calcium-channel blockers (Morisco et al.). Patients received coenzyme Q_{10} 2 mg/kg/day for 1 year or placebo. The number of patients requiring hospitalization secondary to congestive HF was less in the coenzyme Q_{10} group ($n = 73$) versus placebo ($n = 118$); significance: $p < .001$. Episodes of pulmonary edema and cardiac asthma were reduced with coenzyme Q_{10} ($p < .001$).
   b. Studies suggest that there is a 20–50% reduction in serum levels of coenzyme Q_{10} in hypercholesterolemic patients after a statin has been initiated. The reduction in coenzyme Q_{10} concentration is believed to be dose related. However, it is still uncertain how much statins affect muscle coenzyme Q_{10} concentrations. Muscle coenzyme Q_{10} may affect statin-induced myopathy (Nawarskas).
   c. Several studies have evaluated the effect of coenzyme Q_{10} supplementation in patients taking statins. When coenzyme Q_{10} is given 30–300 mg per day, coenzyme Q_{10} serum concentrations significantly elevate. However, this elevation has not been evaluated to see whether it correlates to decreasing statin-related side effects (Nawarskas).

4. **Contraindications/precautions**
   a. Biliary obstruction
   b. Diabetes mellitus (hypoglycemia)
   c. Hepatic insufficiency
   d. Renal insufficiency
   e. Hyper and hypotension

5. **Drug interactions**
   a. Hypolipidemic agents lower plasma concentrations of coenzyme Q_{10}.
   b. Oral hypoglycemic agents potentially inhibit effects of exogenous administration.
   c. Doxorubicin toxicity may be increased.
   d. Antihypertensives (additive effect)
   e. Warfarin. Coenzyme Q_{10} is structurally related to vitamin K_2 so may have coagulant effects.

6. **Side effects**
   a. Rash and gastrointestinal disturbances, such as nausea, anorexia, epigastric pain, and diarrhea
   b. Elevations of serum aminotransferases have occurred with relatively high oral doses.

7. **Dosage.** Depends on indication: 100 mg daily, up to 3000 mg daily in 2–3 divided doses.

C. Glucosamine

1. **Nonapproved indication.** Osteoarthritis

2. **Mechanism of action**
   a. Glucosamine enhances cartilage proteoglycan synthesis.
   b. It inhibits the deterioration of cartilage secondary to osteoarthritis.
   c. It maintains an equilibrium between cartilage catabolic and anabolic processes.
   d. It may have an anti-inflammatory action unlike cyclooxygenase.

3. **Efficacy.** A double-blind trial included 40 patients with unilateral osteoarthritis of the knee. Patients were given glucosamine 500 mg three times daily or ibuprofen 400 mg three times daily for 8 weeks. Pain scores decreased faster during the first 2 weeks in the ibuprofen group than in the glucosamine group. No significant difference in swelling was observed between the two groups (Vaz).

4. **Contraindications/precautions**
   a. Hypersensitivity to glucosamine or shellfish
   b. Diabetes. Glucosamine may impair insulin secretion.

5. **Drug interactions**
   a. Fluoxetine (Prozac) may increase glucosamine serum concentrations.
   b. Glucosamine may interact with antidiabetic agents.
   c. Glucosamine may induce resistance to antimitotic chemotherapy (etoposide-VePesid), doxorubicin).
   d. Theoretically, glucosamine may interact with warfarin.

6. **Side effects**
   a. Gastrointestinal side effects such as epigastric pain and tenderness, heartburn, diarrhea, and nausea
   b. Central nervous system side effects such as drowsiness, headache, and insomnia
   c. Long-term side effects are unknown.

7. **Dosage.** Recommended: 500 mg three times daily

D. **Melatonin**

1. **Orphan drug status.** Treatment of circadian rhythm sleep disorders in blind people who have no light perception

2. **Nonapproved indications.** Jet lag, insomnia, depression, and cancer

3. **Mechanism of action**
   a. It is a hormone made from serotonin and secreted by the pineal gland. Melatonin controls the periods of sleepiness and wakefulness.
   b. It may possess antioxidant properties.

4. **Efficacy**
   a. **Jet lag.** A randomized, placebo-controlled trial evaluated the effect of melatonin in 52 aircraft personnel. Melatonin was given either 5 mg daily 3 days before departure until 5 days after arrival (early group) or 5 mg daily upon arrival and for 3 additional days (late group). The late group had significantly less jet lag, fewer overall sleep disturbances, and a faster recovery of energy compared to the placebo group and the early group (Petrie et al.).
   b. **Insomnia.** A meta-analysis on 17 randomized, double-blind, placebo-controlled trials that evaluated the sleep effect of melatonin in subjects showed that melatonin significantly decreased time to sleep onset, increased sleep efficiency, and increased total sleep duration compared to placebo (Brzezinski et al.). Unfortunately, melatonin preparations were varied and study designs differed.
   c. **Children.** Melatonin may be effective in decreasing the time to sleep onset in children with neurodevelopmental disabilities. Melatonin does not improve total sleep time or nighttime awakenings (Phillips et al.).

5. **Contraindications/precautions**
   a. Avoid in pregnancy
   b. Melatonin may aggravate depressive symptoms.
   c. Melatonin may increase the incidence of seizures.
   d. Diabetes (hyperglycemia)
   e. Hypertension (exacerbated)

6. **Drug interactions**
   a. Vitamin B_{12} influences melatonin secretion. Low levels of vitamin B_{12} will produce low levels of melatonin.
   b. MAOIs may increase melatonin serum concentrations.
   c. Selective serotonin reuptake inhibitors may increase melatonin serum concentrations.

   d. β-Blockers may decrease nocturnal secretion of melatonin.
   e. Other sedatives may exacerbate the sedative effects of melatonin.
   f. Melatonin may interact with immunosuppressants.
   g. Antidiabetic agents may be less effective.
   h. Anticoagulants (increased effect)
   i. Caffeine (theoretically, efficacy of melatonin may be decreased)
   j. Contraceptives (theoretically, efficacy of melatonin may be increased)
   k. Verapamil (increased melatonin excretion)

7. Side effects
   a. Side effects include drowsiness, daytime fatigue, headache, and transient depression.
   b. Long-term side effects are unknown.

8. Dosage. 0.3–5 mg at bedtime

STUDY QUESTIONS

Directions for questions: Each of the questions, statements, or incomplete statements can be correctly answered or completed by **one** of the suggested answers or phrases. Choose the **best** answer.

1. Which of the following herbs is known to cause cancer?

(A) chaparral
(B) comfrey
(C) Ma huang
(D) licorice
(E) St. John's wort

2. Which of the following is a correct statement?

(A) Dietary supplements must be proven safe and effective before marketing in the United States.
(B) The following statement is optional for labeling of herbal products: "This product has not been evaluated by the FDA. It is not intended to diagnose, treat, cure, or prevent."
(C) Herbs must be standardized to be considered dietary supplements.
(D) Dietary supplement manufacturers may claim that their products affect the structure and function of the human body.

3. Tom would like to try echinacea to prevent colds and flus during the winter months. Which of the following statements is true about echinacea?

(A) It is contraindicated in patients allergic to parsley.
(B) It should be taken continuously only for 3 months.
(C) It is contraindicated in patients with lupus and leukosis.
(D) Prolonged use of echinacea will upregulate the immune system.
(E) Side effects include headache, rash, and dizziness.

4. Mary has a family history of heart disease and wonders if garlic would be beneficial to her. Which of the following statements is correct about garlic?

(A) Enteric-coated tablets release their contents in the stomach.
(B) Side effects include heartburn, flatulence, and sweating.
(C) The safety of garlic in pregnancy is unknown.
(D) Garlic does not interact with warfarin.

5. An 80-year-old man takes warfarin for his mechanical heart valve. He would also like to take the following herbs: Asian ginseng, feverfew, Siberian ginseng, garlic, and dong quai. Which of the these herbs may decrease the effectiveness of warfarin?

(A) Asian ginseng
(B) feverfew
(C) Siberian ginseng
(D) garlic
(E) dong quai

6. A 30-year-old female is 10 weeks pregnant with her second child. During her first pregnancy, she became depressed and was started on Prozac 20 mg every day. She is already beginning to notice early symptoms of depression during her second pregnancy. She would like to try St. John's wort for her depression. Which of the following statements is correct regarding St. John's wort?

(A) The safety of St. John's wort in pregnancy is unknown.
(B) St. John's wort is not helpful in treating mild depression.
(C) St. John's wort may interact with serotonin reuptake inhibitors.
(D) St. John's wort may interact with dairy products like milk and eggs.

7. A 65-year-old is interested in taking ginkgo. Which of the following statements is correct regarding ginkgo?

(A) There are no contraindications with ginkgo.
(B) There is a drug–herb interaction between ginkgo and aspirin.
(C) Toxic effects include hypertension and cardiac arrest.
(D) There is a drug–herb interaction between ginkgo and phenelzine.
(E) Ginkgo is contraindicated in patients with gallstone pain.

8. A 20-year-old athletic man would like to take Asian and Siberian ginseng to increase his physical stamina. His girlfriend suggested that he ask a pharmacist about the safety of Asian and Siberian ginseng. Which of the following statements is correct?

(A) Asian ginseng may interact with phenelzine, warfarin, and digoxin.
(B) Asian ginseng is potentially harmful in patients with autoimmune diseases.
(C) Asian and Siberian ginseng are the same ginseng but grown in different countries.
(D) Asian and Siberian ginseng should be avoided in patients with hypertension.

ANSWERS AND EXPLANATIONS

1. The answer is B *[see I.B.1]*
Comfrey may be carcinogenic. Chaparral may be hepatotoxic. High doses of licorice for long periods may cause pseudoaldosteronism. Ma huang may cause myocardial infarction, strokes, or seizures. St. John's wort has many drug interactions.

2. The answer is D *[see I.A.3]*
The Dietary Supplement Health and Education Act of 1994 states that dietary supplements are not considered drugs or food. Since dietary supplements are not regulated as drugs, their safety and efficacy are not mandated by the FDA. Dietary supplements are intended to supplement the diet, do not have to be standardized, may make claims regarding only the effects on structure or function of the body. The following is the correct required labeling statement: "This product has not been evaluated by the FDA. It is not intended to diagnose, treat, cure, or prevent."

3. The answer is C *[see II.E.4]*
Echinacea is contraindicated in infectious and autoimmune diseases such as tuberculosis, leukosis, collagenosis, multiple sclerosis, AIDS, HIV, and lupus. Caution should be used in patients who are allergic to members of the ragweed family. Therapy should not exceed 8 weeks. Theoretically, prolonged use of echinacea may depress the immune system, possibly through over stimulation. Side effects include nausea, vomiting, allergic reactions, anaphylaxis, and interference with male fertility.

4. The answer is B *[see II.G.4]*
Garlic should be avoided in pregnancy because it is an emmenagogue and abortifacient. It may interact with anticoagulants, increasing the risk of bleeding. Side effects include gastrointestinal discomfort (heartburn, flatulence), sweating, lightheadedness, allergic reactions, and menorrhagia. Enteric-coated tablets or capsules allow more absorption because they pass through the stomach and release their contents in the alkaline medium of the small intestine.

5. The answer is A *[see II.J.5]*
Asian ginseng may decrease the INR of warfarin. Feverfew, garlic, Siberian ginseng, and dong quai may increase the INR of warfarin.

6. The answer is C *[see II.N.4]*
St. John's wort is indicated in by Commission E for depression and anxiety. St. John's wort should be avoided in pregnancy because it is an emmenagogue and abortifacient. St. John's wort interacts with many medications, including serotonin reuptake inhibitors. Food interactions may be similar to those of the MAOIs (tyramine-containing foods: cheese, beer, wine, herring, and yeast).

7. The answer is B *[see II.I.5]*
Contraindications and precautions for ginkgo include diabetes, epilepsy, bleeding disorders, and infertility. Ginkgo may potentiate the bleeding properties of antiplatelets. Side effects include gastric disturbances, headache, dizziness, and vertigo. Toxic ingestion may produce tonic-clonic seizures and loss of consciousness.

8. The answer is D *[see II.J.4; II.K.4]*
Asian ginseng's contraindications include patients with hypertension. Asian ginseng may interact with phenelzine, producing hallucinations and psychosis; may decrease the INR of warfarin; and may interfere with immunosuppressants. Siberian ginseng's contraindications/precautions include hypertension. It may interact with anticoagulants and antihypertensives and may inhibit cytochrome P450 isoenzymes. Asian and Siberian ginseng are not the same plant and are not of the same genus.

36

Clinical Pharmacokinetics and Therapeutic Drug Monitoring

Gerald E. Schumacher

I. INTRODUCTION

A. Objectives

1. **Therapeutic drug monitoring** (TDM) in a general sense is about using serum drug concentrations (SDCs), pharmacokinetics, and pharmacodynamics to individualize and optimize patient responses to drug therapy.

2. **TDM** aims to promote optimum drug treatment by maintaining SDC within a **therapeutic range,** above which drug-induced toxicity occurs too often and below which the drug is too often ineffective.

B. Definitions

1. Specifically, **TDM** is a practice applied to a small group of drugs in which there is a direct relation between SDCs and pharmacological response, as well as a narrow range of concentrations that are effective and safe and for which SDCs are used in conjunction with other measures of clinical observation to assess patient status.

2. **Clinical pharmacokinetics,** a term often used interchangeably with TDM, is more generally the application of pharmacokinetic principles for the rational design of an individualized dosage regimen.

3. For definitions of the terms used and the concepts applicable in basic and clinical pharmacokinetics, see Chapter 6 on pharmacokinetics.

C. Rationale and reasons

1. **The rationale** for TDM makes three assumptions.
   a. Measuring patient SDC provides an opportunity to adjust for variations in patient pharmacokinetics by individualizing drug dosage.
   b. The SDC is a better predictor of patient response than is dose.
   c. There is a good relation between SDCs and pharmacological response.

2. **Reasons for measuring SDC**
   a. Drug levels are used in conjunction with other clinical data to assist practitioners in determining how a patient is responding.
   b. Drug levels provide a basis for **individualizing** patient dosage regimens.
   c. Drug levels assist in determining if a change in **patient-specific** pharmacokinetics has occurred during a course of treatment, either as a result of a change in physiological state, a change in diet, or addition of other drugs.
   d. Assuring **drug compliance** is often cited as a reason for measuring SDC, but it is unreliable for this purpose. In truth, a noncompliant patient may outwit practitioners by manipulating preappointment behavior to induce an SDC that is nonreflective of the patient's drug-taking behavior.

II. APPLYING CLINICAL PHARMACOKINETICS IN TDM

A. What the practitioner controls and does not control in TDM

1. Figure 36-1 shows the relation between dose rate of drug administered, pharmacokinetic variables, SDC, and pharmacological response.

2. Note that the only variables that the practitioner controls are the amount of drug administered and how often it is given. These variables may be manipulated to compensate for the patient's pharmacokinetic and pharmacodynamic variables (i.e., bioavailability, clearance, steady-state SDC, pharmacological response), which the practitioner does not control, to achieve some designated SDC that yields a pharmacological response usually observed within the drug's commonly accepted therapeutic SDC range.

B. The concept of therapeutic range

1. For many drugs, a specific serum concentration range can be designated for each drug that maximizes effectiveness and minimizes toxicity. The range of SDC is called the **therapeutic range** for the drug.

2. The notion of a therapeutic range is more a **probabilistic concept** than an absolute entity. It is probable that the majority of patients will show effective and safe responses within the therapeutic range. However, a minority of patients will need SDC above or below the upper or lower limits, respectively, of the therapeutic range to achieve an effective response. Similarly, a minority of patients will not show toxicity at SDC modestly above the therapeutic range, whereas others will show toxicity below the therapeutic range.

3. Therefore, TDM is about **individualizing** patient dosage regimens to achieve SDC within patient-specific therapeutic ranges for a drug. More often than not, a patient-specific range will fall within the generally stated therapeutic range.

C. The concept of population pharmacokinetic values

1. **A population pharmacokinetic value or parameter** refers to the mean (average) value noted for a given cohort of people (e.g., adults 20–60 years of age, patients with a defined range of renal impairment). Usually, this population value is normalized on a weight basis (e.g., theophylline volume of distribution in adult normals of 0.5 L/kg). When a population parameter is stated without defining the target population, it usually refers to adults; further, when the value also is not normalized (e.g., volume of distribution of theophylline of 35 L), it usually refers to adults of average weight (approximately 60–80 kg).

2. Hardly anyone is average. Individual values of the population studied are summed to determine a mean value that is then reported as the **population value.** Individualizing patient dosage regimens takes this into account by adjusting observed patient-specific values and responses to expected population measures.

3. So the practitioner starts the determination of a patient-specific dosage regimen by assuming that the patient behaves like the average member of his or her population with respect to

Figure 36-1. Pharmacokinetic factors influencing serum drug concentration and pharmacological response. Bioavailability is f, clearance is Cl, steady-state serum drug concentration is C_{ss}, D is dose, and τ is frequency of administration of dose.

pharmacokinetics, serum level, and expected response, and uses population pharmacokinetic parameters to calculate the dosage regimen needed to meet the desired SDC objective.

4. If after administering the dosage regimen until steady state is reached, based on using population values, the patient is responding appropriately, then no adjustment in regimen is necessary.

5. If, however, the starting assumption of using average values turns out to be incorrect, because the patient's response is either subtherapeutic or toxic due to patient-specific pharmacokinetic and/or pharmacodynamic values that are atypical for the population, the practitioner's only option (except for changing the drug) is to manipulate the practitioner-controlled input variables, **dose and frequency,** to bring the pharmacological response within the desired range.

D. Timing of SDC measurements

1. SDCs are sometimes measured **early in a course of therapy,** before steady state is reached, to determine patient-specific pharmacokinetic parameters, rather than relying on population values.

2. More commonly, SDCs are measured **during a steady-state dosage interval** (τ_{ss}), because the objective is to determine if the SDC is within a desired therapeutic range, a range that has previously been determined almost invariably during τ_{ss}.

3. Because SDCs are most commonly measured at steady state and referenced to values obtained at steady state, it is necessary to wait after starting drug administration until at least three to four assumed half-life ($t_{1/2}$) values (88%–94% of reaching full steady state) so that SDC will be measured during a period when steady state may be assumed, for clinical purposes, to have been reached or approximated (e.g., approximately 90% of steady state or greater; so for an assumed $t_{1/2}$ of 6 hours, wait 18–24 hours after initiating drug treatment to measure SDC)

4. If there are no changes in patient response, there is usually **no need to take subsequent daily SDC measurements,** once an appropriate SDC has been achieved. Only if something occurs that may be expected to alter the patient's pharmacokinetic values (e.g., co-administration of another potentially modifying drug, change in physiological state), are frequent measurements necessary.

5. If a steady-state SDC (**C_{ss}**) is used appropriately to relate a patient's C_{ss} to a population or patient-specific therapeutic range, then it is important to note when during the steady-state dosage interval (τ_{ss}) the C_{ss} was measured in studies determining the therapeutic range. In other words, is the therapeutic range the practitioner is using as a basis for individualizing regimens based on C_{ss} measured **early** (apparent **$C_{max,ss}$**), near the **midpoint** (apparent **$C_{avg,ss}$**), or near the end (apparent **$C_{min,ss}$**) of τ_{ss}?

6. **Errors** in interpretation occur when C_{ss} for a patient is measured at a time during τ_{ss} that is markedly different than the time used for establishing the therapeutic range [e.g., measuring C_{ss} in a patient 1 hour after giving a dose on a q12h regimen when the C_{ss} for the referenced therapeutic range was actually taken at the end of τ_{ss} (**$C_{min,ss}$**)].

7. Errors in timing of C_{ss} are of greater concern for drugs with a short $t_{1/2}$ than for drugs with a long $t_{1/2}$. C_{ss} fluctuation during τ_{ss} is much greater in the former than the latter case.

III. TDM DRUGS AND COMMON CHARACTERISTICS

A. TDM drugs

1. Drugs for which TDM is commonly used are noted in Table 36-1, along with the population therapeutic range.

2. Drugs for which TDM is infrequently used in general situations, but perhaps commonly used by specialty practitioners or clinics, are noted in Table 36-2.

B. Common characteristics of TDM drugs. Drugs that qualify for TDM have, as a minimum, the following characteristics in common.

Table 36-1. Drugs Often Monitored Using Serum Drug Concentrations

Drug	Therapeutic Range for C_{ss}
Amikacin	$C_{max,ss}{}^{a} = 20\text{--}30\ \mu g/mL;\ C_{min,ss} <10\ mcg/mL$
Cyclosporine	Varies with transplanted organ, time after transplant, time of sampling during dosage interval, and method of analysis
Digoxin	$0.8\text{--}2^{b}\ ng/mL$
Gentamicin	$C_{max,ss}{}^{a} = 5\text{--}10\ \mu g/mL;\ C_{min,ss} <2\ mcg/mL$
Phenytoin	$10\text{--}20\ \mu cg/mL$
Theophylline	$5\text{--}20\ \mu cg/mL$
Tobramycin	$C_{max,ss}{}^{a} = 5\text{--}10\ \mu g/mL;\ C_{min,ss} <2\ mcg/mL$
Vancomycin	$C_{max,ss}{}^{a} = 30\text{--}50\ \mu g/mL;\ C_{min,ss} = 5\text{--}10\ mcg/mL$

[a]End of 30- to 60-min infusion.
[b]Levels for atrial fibrillation often exceed 2 ng/mL.

Table 36-2. Drugs Monitored Using Serum Drug Concentrations in Specialty Situations

Amitriptyline
Carbamazepine
Indinavin
Lidocaine
Lithium
Methotrexate
Nortriptyline
Salicylates
Valproic acid

1. SDC is the most practical intermediate end point to be used when there is no clearly observable therapeutic or toxic end point.

2. SDC is a reasonable proxy for drug concentration at the site of action.

3. The range of therapeutic and safe serum concentrations is narrow.

4. There is no predictable dose-response relation.

5. The pharmacological effect observed persists for a relatively long time. Acute, short, or intermittent effects are not well regulated by using serum drug levels.

6. A drug assay is available that is accurate, precise, specific, rapid, and relatively inexpensive.

IV. EQUATIONS FREQUENTLY USED IN TDM

A. **Linear pharmacokinetic drug clearance—normal renal function.** Linear clearance assumes that a **proportional** change in dose leads to the same **proportional** change in SDC. It also assumes that $t_{1/2}$ and drug clearance remain **constant** as the dose changes. See IV.D for an example of using some of the following equations.

1. **Estimating drug clearance (Cl):**

$$Cl = \frac{V}{1.4 t_{1/2}} \tag{1}$$

where V is the apparent volume of distribution of drug.

2. **Maximum concentration ($C_{max,ss}$)** during τ_{ss}, when absorption is assumed to be much faster than elimination:

$$C_{max,ss} = \frac{(S)(f)(dose/V)}{1 - 10^{-0.3(\tau/t_{1/2})}} \tag{2}$$

where S is the fraction of the dosage form that is the active moiety and f is the bioavailability.

3. **Minimum concentration ($C_{min,ss}$) during τ_{ss}, when absorption is assumed to be much faster than elimination:**

$$C_{min,ss} = (C_{max,ss})[10^{-0.3(\tau/t_{1/2})}] \tag{3}$$

4. **Average concentration resulting from intermittent administration ($C_{avg,ss}$) during τ_{ss}:**

$$C_{avg,ss} = \frac{(S)(f)(dose/\tau)}{Cl} \tag{4}$$

where dose/τ is the amount of drug administered during each selected unit of time (e.g., hours, minutes).

5. **Steady-state concentration resulting from continuous administration ($C_{inf,ss}$).** For the same dose rate (dose/τ), ($C_{avg,ss}$) for intermittent administration **is the same as** ($C_{inf,ss}$) for continuous administration:

$$C_{inf,ss} = \frac{(S)(f)(dose/t_{inf})}{Cl} \tag{5}$$

B. **Linear pharmacokinetic drug clearance—impaired renal function**

1. **Estimating creatinine clearance from serum creatinine** when serum creatinine is assumed to be stable, not changing daily, and weight is expressed by the patient's total weight, unless total weight is equal to or more than 20% of ideal (lean) body weight, in which case ideal weight should be used in the calculation:

$$Cl_{cr} \text{ (mL/min, males)} = \frac{(140 - age)(weight)}{(Cr_s)(72)} \tag{6}$$

where Cr_s denotes serum creatinine in mg/dl. The female value is 85% of the estimated male value in (6).

2. **Estimating prolonged drug $t_{1/2}$ or reduced drug Cl associated with reduced Cl_{cr}:**

$$\frac{(Cl)_{ri}}{(Cl)_n} = \frac{(t_{1/2})_n}{(t_{1/2})_{ri}} = 1 - F + F[(Cl_{cr})_{ri}/(Cl_{cr})_n] \tag{7}$$

where ri and n denote the renal impaired and normal conditions, respectively; F is the fraction of drug administered that is eliminated unchanged (unmetabolized); and Cl_{cr} represents creatinine clearance in mL/min. Important F values for some common TDM drugs are: aminoglycosides = 0.98, digoxin = 0.98, and vancomycin = 0.95.

3. **Using $C_{avg,ss}$ as a target** so that $C_{avg,ss}$ in the renal impaired patient is maintained the same as $C_{avg,ss}$ in normals: $\dfrac{(dose/\tau)_{ri}}{(dose/\tau)_n} = \dfrac{dose_{ri} \times \tau_n}{dose_n \times \tau_{ri}} = 1 - F + F[(Cl_{cr})_{ri}/(Cl_{cr})_n]$ (8)

4. **Using $C_{max,ss}$ as a target** so that $C_{max,ss}$ in the renal impaired is maintained the same as $C_{max,ss}$ in normals:

$$\text{dose per } \tau_{ri} = (dose_L)[1 - 10^{-0.3(\tau_{ri}/t_{1/2ri})}] \tag{9}$$

where $dose_L$ is a loading dose intended to achieve the same $C_{max,ss}$ in the renal impaired as in the normal patient.

C. **Nonlinear pharmacokinetic drug clearance—normal renal function. Nonlinear** clearance assumes that a proportional change in dose leads to a **disproportional** change in SDC. It also assumes that $t_{1/2}$ and Cl **change** as the dose changes and also as the amount of drug in the body from a given dose changes. Drugs exhibiting nonlinear clearance present a much greater challenge than linear clearance drugs because the assumptions in the latter case of proportional changes in dose yielding same proportional changes in C_{ss} and constant Cl and $t_{1/2}$ do not apply for nonlinear drugs. For nonlinear drugs, increases in dose lead to increases in $t_{1/2}$, decreases in Cl, and changes in C_{ss} that are excessive compared to the proportionate change in dose.

1. **Estimating drug clearance:**

$$Cl = \frac{V_{max}}{K_m + C_{avg,ss}} \tag{10}$$

where V_{max} is the maximum amount of drug that can be eliminated per unit of time (e.g., day) and K_m is the drug serum concentration at which the rate of elimination is 50% of V_{max}.

2. **Estimating $C_{avg,ss}$ resulting from a given dose/τ:**

$$C_{avg,ss} = \frac{(K_m)(S)(f)(dose/t)}{V_{max} - (S)(f)(dose/\tau)} \tag{11}$$

3. **Estimating dose/τ needed for a desired $C_{avg,ss}$:**

$$dose/\tau = \frac{(V_{max})(C_{avg,ss})}{(K_m + C_{avg,ss})(S)(f)} \tag{12}$$

D. **An example of applying some of the above equations to developing and modifying dosage regimens**

1. A common dosage regimen for intravenous (IV) gentamicin is 1.7 mg/kg q8h (as a 30-minute infusion). Regimens are usually adjusted to achieve $C_{max,ss}$ and $C_{min,ss}$ within 5–10 mcg/mL and less than 2 mcg/mL, respectively. Does the above regimen meet the target concentration objectives in normal patients? Assume the following population parameters in normals: Cl = 0.09 L/kg/hr, $t_{1/2}$ = 2.5 hr, V = 0.25 L/kg. For IV administration, f = 1, and S = 1 for the dosage form (label amount represents the actual amount of gentamicin).

2. **In normals,** using equations (2) and (3):

$$C_{max,ss} = \frac{(1)(1)(1.7 \text{ mg/kg})/(0.25 \text{ L/kg})}{1 - 10^{-0.3 \text{ (8 hr/2.5 hr)}}} = 7.6 \text{ mcg/mL}$$

$$C_{min,ss} = 7.6 \text{ mcg/mL} \times 10^{-0.3 \text{ (8 hr/2.5 hr)}} = 0.8 \text{ mcg/mL}$$

These values fall within the target concentration ranges for the average patient with normal renal function.

3. **In the renal impaired,** what should be done to modify the above regimen for a patient who is 60 years old, 70 kg, male, with a Cr_s of 2.5 mg/dl? In this patient, if the above regimen were used, the prolonged $t_{1/2}$ would yield $C_{max,ss}$ = 15.2 mcg/mL and $C_{min,ss}$ = 8.4 mcg/mL, values clearly above the target concentration ranges.

   a. Using equation (6) for estimating Cl_{cr} in this patient:

$$Cl_{cr} = \frac{(140 - 60 \text{ yr})(70 \text{ kg})}{(2.5 \text{ mg/dl})(72)} = 31 \text{ mL/min}$$

   b. Then using equation (7) for estimating $t_{1/2}$ in this patient, assuming F = 0.98 and $(Cl_{cr})_n$ = 120 mL/min:

$$\frac{(2.5 \text{ hr})}{(t_{1/2})_{ri}} = 1 - 0.98 + 0.98(31/120) = 0.27$$

$$(t_{1/2})_{ri} = 9.3 \text{ hr}$$

   c. Then using equation (9), first determine a loading dose (D_L) to achieve the same $C_{max,ss}$ of approximately 8 mcg/mL as estimated in IV.D.2 for a patient with normal renal function:

$$D_L = (C_{max,ss})(V)/(S)(f)$$

$$D_L = (8 \text{ mcg/mL})(0.25 \text{ L/kg})/(1)(1) = 2 \text{ mg/kg}$$

   Next, determine fraction of drug lost during τ, assuming a τ_{ri} of 24 hours, and using the $(t_{1/2})_{ri}$ of 9.3 hours estimated in IV.D.3.b:

$$\text{Fraction lost} = 1 - 10^{-0.3(\tau/t_{1/2})} = 1 - 10^{-0.3(24/9.3)} = 0.84$$

   Lastly, calculate D per τ_{ri}:

$$D \text{ per } \tau_{ri} = (D_L)[1 - 10^{-0.3(\tau/t_{1/2})}]$$

$$= (2 \text{ mg/kg})(0.84) = 1.7 \text{ mg/kg}$$

Thus, a D_L of 2 mg/kg followed by 1.7 mg/kg q24h is expected to maintain levels in this patient similar to that in normals.

V. EFFECT OF PHYSIOLOGICAL ALTERATIONS ON PHARMACOKINETIC VARIABLES

A. **General considerations.** It is apparent from Figure 36-1 and the equations in Section IV, that any changes in pharmacokinetic variables result in changes in C_{ss} and perhaps pharmacodynamic outcomes. This may necessitate changes in D/τ compared to normals. For renal impairment, **quantitative** estimates of resulting changes in Cl and $t_{1/2}$, compared to normal values, are available using the equations in Section IV. For hepatic, cardiac, pulmonary, and other impairments potentially inducing changes in normal pharmacokinetic variables, only **qualitative** estimates are possible.

B. **Renal impairment,** when marked, reduces drug clearance for drugs primarily dependent on the kidney for elimination. As noted in the equations in Section IV.B, physiological markers like serum creatinine and creatinine clearance are used to estimate the changes in Cl and $t_{1/2}$ resulting from reductions in Cr_s and Cl_{cr}.

C. **Hepatic impairment** exerts a complex influence on drug pharmacokinetics. Two processes may be altered, blood flow rate in delivering drug to the liver and the capacity of enzymes to metabolize the drug. In general terms, moderate to severe hepatic impairment is expected to slow overall Cl and prolong $t_{1/2}$ for drugs highly dependent on the liver for elimination.

D. **Cardiac impairment,** when substantial, decreases hepatic and renal clearances, reduces volume of distribution, and may slow absorption for some drugs. The effect of compromised perfusion is most critical for drugs that are both highly dependent on the liver for clearance and efficiently metabolized by the liver in normal patients.

E. **Aging** results in reductions in renal (consistently) and hepatic (inconsistently) clearances. The clearance of drugs primarily dependent on the kidney declines by nearly 50% and the half-life nearly doubles over a 40–50-year period from young adulthood. On the other hand, some drugs primarily dependent on the liver for clearance show no age-related changes, while others do. Changes with age in absorption, volume of distribution, and serum protein binding of drugs show no consistent pattern.

F. From a clinical viewpoint, serum **protein binding** of drugs becomes an important issue in TDM for drugs bound more than 80% to serum proteins. Because hepatic and renal clearances, volume of distribution, and pharmacological response are mediated by the free (unbound) form of the drug in serum, interpatient variations in protein binding not only result in variations in pharmacokinetics in normals, but also loss of serum proteins during renal and hepatic impairments may result in modified drug clearance and pharmacological response.

VI. THE TOTAL TESTING PROCESS APPLIED TO TDM

A. Defining the total testing process (TTP)

1. TDM involves both the laboratory for analysis and clinicians for interpretation of SDC. TTP refers to all aspects of the steps of laboratory testing beginning with a clinical question that is prompted by the patient–clinician encounter and concluding with the impact of the test result on patient care.

2. TTP emphasizes that TDM is a process involving a series of steps and interrelated activities and should not be viewed simply as a numerical value for an SDC.

3. TTP focuses on identifying all steps of the TDM testing process, highlighting where variations and errors can occur, interpreting SDC results in light of the steps involved, and improving the contribution of testing to achieving desired patient outcomes.

B. Components and steps in TTP. There are 4 components and 11 steps in TTP.

   1. The preanalytical component consists of four steps:

   (1) clinical question, (2) test selected, (3) test ordered, and (4) specimen collection.

   2. The analytical component then follows with three steps:

   (5) sample prepared, (6) analysis performed, and (7) result verified.

   3. The postanalytical component then concludes with four steps: (8) result reported, (9) clinical answer, (10) action taken, and (11) effect on patient care.

   4. The three components are affected by the fourth component, the **regulatory environment** within which TDM is performed.

C. Contributions of TDM to TTP

   1. TDM has the potential to improve many of the steps in TTP: providing education, drug information, interpretation of TDM results, assessing the appropriateness of the TDM order, scheduling specimen collection, developing drug dosage guidelines, and providing written and oral consultation concerning TDM results.

   2. The pharmacist's greatest involvement in TTP is in steps (2) assessing the appropriateness of TDM for a given situation, (4) timing of specimen collection, and (9) clinical interpretation of TDM results.

VII. USING TEST PERFORMANCE CHARACTERISTICS IN TDM

A. Rationale and reasons

   1. In TDM, the SDC functions like a diagnostic test to assist in classifying patient status.

   2. On the one hand, the patient's SDC may be used, in conjunction with a population SDC cutoff value measure for the drug, which acts as a separator, to classify the patient as a member of either drug-induced toxic (patient SDC > upper cutoff value) or therapeutic (within therapeutic range) subpopulations.

   3. Alternately, the patient's SDC may classify the patient as part of the therapeutic or subtherapeutic (SDC < lower cutoff value) subpopulations.

   4. Although classifying patients in subpopulations is the most common use of SDC in TDM, a more informed application of SDC is to use the result to modify the clinician's probability of patient status. This is the use of SDC as part of a Bayesian approach to diagnostic test interpretation.

B. Test performance characteristics. Test performance indices are not perfect classifiers of patient status and should never be used as the sole measure for determining how the patient is reacting to the drug. A number of test performance indices characterize the accuracy of a diagnostic test to accurately classify patients as toxic, therapeutic, or subtherapeutic. Four of these indices are most useful in interpreting SDC.

   1. Positive predictive value (PPV)
      a. Comparing drug-induced toxic versus nontoxic patients (using upper SDC cutoff level). PPV denotes the proportion of patients with a **positive test** (patient SDC > upper cutoff SDC) who are in a drug-induced **toxic** condition. So, the value of PPV represents the probability of a positive test being accurate in classifying the patient as toxic.
      b. Comparing therapeutic versus subtherapeutic patients (using lower SDC cutoff level). PPV denotes the proportion of patients with a **positive test** (patient SDC > lower cutoff SDC) who are **responding appropriately.** So, the value of PPV in this case represents the probability of a positive test being accurate in classifying the patient as therapeutic.

   2. Negative predictive value (NPV)
      a. Comparing drug-induced toxic versus nontoxic patients (using upper SDC cutoff level). NPV denotes the proportion of patients with a **negative test** (patient SDC < upper cutoff SDC) who are **not** manifesting drug-induced **toxicity.** So, the value of NPV represents the probability of a negative test being accurate in classifying the patient as nontoxic.

   b. Comparing therapeutic versus subtherapeutic patients (using lower SDC cutoff level). NPV denotes the proportion of patients with a **negative test** (patient SDC < lower cutoff SDC) who are **subtherapeutic.** So, the value of NPV in this case represents the probability of a negative test being accurate in classifying the patient as subtherapeutic.

3. **Positive likelihood ratio (PLR).** In defining conditions as + or - (as in + = toxic and − = negative, or + = therapeutic and − = subtherapeutic), **PLR** is the probability that a + **patient** has a + **test** divided by the probability that a − **patient** has a + **test** (e.g., the probability that a **toxic** patient has an SDC > cutoff divided by the probability that a **nontoxic** patient has an SDC > cutoff). The **higher** the **PLR,** the **more** discriminating the test.

4. **Negative likelihood ratio (NLR).** NLR is the probability that a + **patient** has a − **test** divided by the probability that a − **patient** has a − **test.** The **lower** the **NLR,** the **more** discriminating the test.

5. **Illustrating the use of PPV, NPV, PLR, and NLR.** For theophylline, using a test upper cutoff of 20 mcg/mL, PPV is 0.5, NPV is 0.95, PLR is 6, and NLR is 0.4.
   a. For PPV, this means that the proportion of patients with a positive test result (SDC > upper cutoff) who truly have theophylline-induced toxicity is 50%. For an individual patient with SDC > cutoff, the probability of toxicity is 0.5.
   b. For NPV, this means that the proportion of patients with a negative test result (SDC < upper cutoff) who truly are nontoxic is 95%. For an individual patient with SDC < cutoff, the probability of nontoxicity is 0.95.
   c. For PLR, toxic patients will have a positive test result six times more often than do nontoxic patients.
   d. For NLR, toxic patients will have a negative test result 40% as often as will nontoxic patients.
   e. These results suggest that a negative theophylline test result rules out toxicity (0.95) about twice as effectively as a positive test rules in toxicity (0.5). A positive test appears to be unreliable as an indicator of toxicity, but a negative test appears to be highly predictive of nontoxicity. Furthermore, the PLR suggests that a positive SDC test is six times more likely to come from a toxic than a nontoxic patient. On the other hand, the NLR implies that it is considerably less than one-half as likely (0.4) that a negative test comes from a toxic compared to a nontoxic patient.
   f. Knowledge of test performance characteristics of SDC measures provides the practitioner with an index of the usefulness of the SDC in categorizing patients.

C. **Using a Bayesian approach.** Using SDC in conjunction with likelihood ratio information enhances the application of the SDC in decision making. A Bayesian approach to probability revision allows the practitioner to make a pretest assessment of patient status, order a diagnostic test, and use the probability information contained in the test result to revise the assessment of status.

1. The relation between pretest, test, and posttest assessment is shown in the following equation:

$$\text{(pretest odds)(likelihood ratio)} = \text{(posttest odds)} \qquad \textbf{(13)}$$

   where pretest refers to the pretest odds of the condition being present prior to obtaining the patient's SDC and posttest refers to the posttest odds of the condition being present after learning the SDC.

2. **Odds** are defined as + results divided by − results (+/−). **Probability** is defined as + results divided by total results (+/total, where total is the sum of + and − results).

3. Odds are converted to probability as follows:

   Probability = odds/(1 + odds) $\qquad$ **(14)**

4. Probability is converted to odds as follows:

   Odds = probability/(1 − probability) $\qquad$ **(15)**

5. An example of applying a Bayesian approach to modifying the probability of patient status. Using the theophylline test performance characteristics noted in VII.B.5:

a. Assume that a practitioner assesses by visual inspection that the probability of theophylline-induced toxicity in a patient is 0.25 (the pretest probability). She orders a serum theophylline concentration (STC), and uses the measurement to revise her assessment of toxicity in the patient (the posttest probability).

b. Further assume that the test performance characteristics for the STC are: PLR = 6 and NLR = 0.4.

c. Using equations (13), (14), and (15), a pretest probability of 0.25 is the same as pretest odds of toxicity of 1/3 [0.25/(1 − 0.25)], using equation (15).

d. If the STC test for the patient comes back positive (STC > 20 mcg/mL), then PLR = 6 is used to revise the odds of toxicity. If the STC test is negative (STC ≤ 20 mcg/mL), then NLR = 0.4 is used.

e. Assume the patient's **STC =** 22 mcg/mL, then using equation (13) yields (1/3)(6) = 2. So, the posttest odds of toxicity are 2/1. Converting these odds to probability using equation (14): [2/(1 + 2)] = 0.67. The **posttest probability of toxicity is 0.67.** The pretest probability of 0.25 has nearly tripled using the STC as feedback.

f. Assume instead that the patient's STC = **14 mcg/mL;** then using equation (13) yields (1/3)(0.4) = 0.13. So, the posttest odds of toxicity are 0.13/1. Converting these odds to probability using equation (14): [0.13/(1 + 0.13)] = 0.12. **The posttest probability of toxicity is 0.12.**

g. While a positive STC test nearly tripled the probability of toxicity above, a negative test cuts the probability in half. This demonstrates the usefulness of using SDC in combination with practitioner assessment as a guide to quantifying the probability of patient status.

VIII. SUMMARY

A. TDM applies to a small number of drugs with a narrow range of effective and safe SDC wherein optimum drug treatment is promoted by maintaining SDC within a population or patient-specific therapeutic range, above which drug-induced toxicity occurs too often and below which the drug is too often ineffective.

B. A practitioner initiates drug treatment using a dose rate that assumes that the patient shows mean population values for the pharmacokinetic variables, even though it is expected that few patients will ever possess the mean value being used. If the resulting C_{ss} and/or pharmacological response is other than expected and the patient becomes at risk for subtherapeutic or drug-induced toxicity, it is likely due to the interpatient variability in pharmacokinetic values and pharmacodynamic response that characterizes the need for TDM; therefore, the dose rate is modified to produce a patient-specific C_{ss} that represents the best tradeoff of effectiveness and toxicity.

C. Timing of sampling of SDC is critical to reduce errors in interpretation of the measurement. SDC should be sampled at steady state, after postabsorption and postdistribution equilibrium is achieved, and a time during τ_{ss} that matches the time at which the therapeutic range was established.

D. The choice of $C_{max,ss}$, $C_{min,ss}$, $C_{avg,ss}$, or $C_{inf,ss}$ to estimate dosage regimens depends on the therapeutic range objective and, in the latter case, intravenous rather than intermittent administration.

E. For the renal-impaired patient, the dosage reduction factor is calculated to achieve, depending on the therapeutic range objective, a $C_{max,ss}$ or $C_{avg,ss}$ in the renal-impaired patient that is similar to that desired if the patient had normal renal function.

F. The TTP is the systematic sequence of events in which TDM is practiced from identification of the need for an SDC measurement, to proper timing of sample collection, laboratory analysis, interpretation of results, and dosage regimen modification, if indicated.

G. The SDC measure is more than a number used to relate the patient's value to a population therapeutic range. The SDC is a form of diagnostic test used (1) to assist in classifying patient status and (2) as feedback to revise practitioner estimates of patient status. Therefore, it is important to know the predictive values and likelihood ratios of SDC tests.

STUDY QUESTIONS

Directions: Each of the numbered items or incomplete statements in this section is followed by answers or by completions of the statement. Select the one lettered answer or completion that is **best** in each case.

1. Define therapeutic drug monitoring. What is meant by the term TDM?

(A) The use of drug serum concentration measurements, for drugs in which there is (1) a correlation between serum concentration and response, as well as (2) a narrow range of effective and safe concentrations, to assess patient status as an adjunct to clinical observation

(B) The use of drug serum concentration measurements to determine population values for a drug's half-life value

(C) The use of drug serum concentration measurements to assess the accuracy of the drug concentration assay

(D) Observing the effects of drugs in man

(E) Using drug serum concentration measurements to differentiate effective from ineffective drugs

2. The therapeutic range for theophylline is often stated as 10–20 mcg/mL. What does this mean?

(A) Fifty percent of people taking theophylline show a safe and effective response when the serum drug concentration is between 10–20 mcg/mL.

(B) Most people achieve the desired response to theophylline, with minimum adverse effects when the serum theophylline concentration is maintained between 10–20 mcg/mL. Fewer patients are managed effectively at <10 mcg/mL, but some may respond quite appropriately at lower levels. The frequency of adverse effects increases as the level increases above the upper limit of the therapeutic range, but a few patients are managed effectively, without adversity, above the range.

(C) Twenty-five percent of people show an effective response to theophylline at 10 mcg/mL, and 75% show an effective response at 20 mcg/mL.

(D) Twice daily administration of theophylline, but not three times daily, requires that serum drug concentrations stay within 10–20 mcg/mL.

(E) Theophylline serum drug concentrations outside of the 10–20 mcg/mL range are ineffective and/or unsafe.

3. Assume that for a digoxin, the therapeutic range is cited as $C_{avg,ss}$ = 0.8–2 ng/mL. If the patient is assumed to have an estimated digoxin $t_{1/2}$ of 48 hours, how long would you wait to take a serum digoxin concentration measurement, and when during τ would you schedule it?

(A) 28 days, then 3–4 hours after the dose is administered

(B) 14 days, then 6–8 hours after the dose is administered

(C) 7 days, then 10–14 hours after the dose is administered

(D) 3 days, then 1–2 hours after the dose is administered

(E) 1 day, then 18–22 hours after the dose is administered

4. Differentiate linear from nonlinear drug clearance. What is the effect on TDM?

(A) Linear drug clearance is first order, the Cl and $t_{1/2}$ are independent of drug dosage, and proportional changes in dose result in the same proportional changes in C_{ss}. Nonlinear drug clearance is zero order, Cl and $t_{1/2}$ change as dose changes (or as the amount of drug in the body changes), and proportional changes in dose yield disproportionate changes in C_{ss}.

(B) Linear drug clearance presents fewer serum concentration peaks and troughs during the dosage interval than does nonlinear drug clearance.

(C) Linear drug clearance is zero order, the Cl and $t_{1/2}$ are dependent on drug dosage, and proportional changes in dose do not result in the same proportional changes in C_{ss}. Nonlinear drug clearance is first order, and equations are not available to predict drug serum concentration from the dose rate.

(D) Drugs with linear clearance have shorter $t_{1/2}$ values than drugs with nonlinear clearance.

(E) Drugs with linear clearance are administered less often than drugs with nonlinear clearance.

5. What is the positive predictive value of a diagnostic test?

(A) The fraction of patients with a positive outcome who have a positive test result
(B) Being more than 50% correct in predicting success or failure upon using a drug regimen
(C) The fraction of patients who achieve a successful response in using a drug
(D) The fraction of patients with a positive test result who turn out to have a positive outcome
(E) The probability that knowledge of a drug serum concentration results in a successful response to treatment

6. A 70-year-old, 80-kg male, with serum creatinine of 3 mg/dL, is scheduled to start tobramycin therapy. What regimen is recommended to achieve $C_{max,ss}$ within 5–10 mcg/mL (use the midpoint of 7.5 mcg/mL for the calculation) and $C_{min,ss}$ <2 mcg/mL. Try a q24h regimen to start and, if unsuccessful in achieving the target concentration goals, alter τ and recalculate. Assume in normals the following values: $t_{1/2}$ = 2.5 hr, V = 0.25 L/kg, F = 0.98, S = 1, f = 1, Cl_{cr} = 120 mg/dL.

(A) A loading dose of 1.8–2.0 mg/kg followed by 1.0 mg/kg qd
(B) A loading dose of 1.8–2.0 mg/kg followed by 1.5 mg/kg qd
(C) 2.0 mg/kg qd
(D) 1.0 mg/kg qd
(E) 0.5 mg/kg qd

744   *Chapter 36*

ANSWERS AND EXPLANATIONS

1. The answer is A *[1.B].*

2. The answer is B *[II.B].*

3. The answer is C *[II.D.3].*
If the patient's estimated $t_{1/2}$ is 48 hours, 90% of steady state is expected to be achieved between 3–4 $t_{1/2}$ intervals or 6–8 days in this case. For clinical purposes, we choose 90% attainment of steady state as the minimum time to estimate drug accumulation. A level drawn at 7 days seems reasonable. Once a τ_{ss} has been selected, the time for scheduling a level should correspond with the reference time for the therapeutic range. In this case, $C_{avg,ss}$ was cited as the reference time, so a measurement scheduled for sometime near the midpoint of τ_{ss} (around 12 hours) is reasonable.

4. The answer is A *[IV.A, C].*
This presents challenges in TDM, because for linear drugs the clinician can expect a change in C_{ss} proportional to a change in dose, but for nonlinear drugs this is not true.

5. The answer is D *[VII.B.1].*
The positive predictive value of a diagnostic test is an index of how effective the test is in classifying patients correctly. For example, using a C_{ss} measure for a given drug, knowing that the positive predictive value is 0.8, given a group of patients with a C_{ss} above the test cutoff value, 80% of the patients will be accurately classified as having a positive outcome. If the test is being used to classify toxic versus nontoxic patients, 80% of the patients with C_{ss} above the test cutoff will experience drug-induced toxicity. If, instead, the test is being used to classify effective versus subeffective response in patients, 80% of the patients with C_{ss} above the test cutoff will experience effective response.

6. The answer is B *[IV.D.3].*
Using the equation for estimating Cl_{cr} in this patient from IV B 1:

$$Cl_{cr} = \frac{(140 - 70 \text{ yr})(80 \text{ kg})}{(3 \text{ mg/dL})(72)} = 26 \text{ mL/min}$$

then, using the equation for estimating $t_{1/2}$ in this patient from IV.B.2:

$$\frac{(2.5 \text{ hr})}{(t_{1/2})_{ri}} = 1 - 0.98 + 0.98 (26/120) = 0.23$$

$$(t_{1/2})_{ri} = 10.9 \text{ hr}$$

Then, using equation [IV.D.3.b], first determine a loading dose: (D_L) to achieve the desired $C_{max,ss}$ of 7.5 mcg/mL:

$$D_L = (C_{max,ss})(V)/(S)(f)$$

$$D_L = (7.5 \text{ mcg/mL})(0.25 \text{ L/kg})/(1)(1) = 1.9 \text{ mg/kg}$$

Then, determine fraction of drug lost during τ, assuming a τ_{ri} of 24 hr, and using the $(t_{1/2})_{ri}$ of 10.9 hr estimated above using the equation in IV.D.3.c:

$$\text{fraction lost} = 1 - 10^{-0.3(24/10.9)} = 0.78$$

Lastly, calculate D per τ_{ri}:

$$D \text{ per } \tau_{ri} = (D_L)(\text{fraction lost per } \tau_{ri})$$

$$= (1.9 \text{ mg/kg})(0.78) = 1.5 \text{ mg/kg}$$

Thus, a D_L of 1.9 mg/kg followed by 1.5 mg/kg q24h is expected to attain the desired $C_{max,ss}$ and $C_{min,ss}$ levels in this patient. Of course, many estimates were made along the way (Cl_{cr}, $t_{1/2}$, V), so if the patient's $C_{max,ss}$ and $C_{min,ss}$ vary from what has been expected from the calculations, it is likely due to the estimates being at variance with the actual value(s) in the patient.

37
Drug Use in Special Patient Populations: Pediatric, Pregnant, Geriatric

Marcia L. Buck

Julie J. Kelsey

I. PEDIATRIC PHARMACOTHERAPY

A. General considerations

1. Most pharmacists in community and hospital settings provide care for children. In the United States, children make up nearly one third of the total population. Although children typically require fewer medications than adults because of their relative good health, approximately 30% of all prescriptions filled in community pharmacies are for pediatric patients. As a result, **pharmacists need to have a basic knowledge of pediatric pharmacotherapy to appropriately assess and monitor drug therapy.**

2. Providing care for children is often a challenge. There is **limited information on the selection, dosing, and monitoring of drugs** in this population. It is estimated that only 25% of the drugs available on the market in the United States carry a Food and Drug Administration (FDA) approved indication for use in pediatric patients, although nearly 75% have been used to treat children. As a result, most pediatric dosing is considered off-label. Dosing information typically comes directly from case reports and small clinical trials published in the medical literature. In addition to being able to obtain pediatric-specific drug information, pharmacists must also be familiar with differences in pediatric pharmacokinetics and pharmacodynamics as well as the unique aspects of medication monitoring and compliance in this population.

B. Pharmacokinetic considerations

1. Unlike the relatively stable pharmacokinetic profile of most drugs in adults, children's **pharmacokinetic parameters change during maturation from neonates into adolescents** (Table 37-1). As a result, the pediatric population is a diverse and dynamic group. Each aspect of drug disposition is affected, including absorption, distribution, metabolism, and elimination. None of these processes is fully mature at birth, and they develop at different rates over the first years of life. The study of these changes is known as developmental pharmacology.

2. **Drug absorption.** For many routes of administration, the absorption of a drug is most greatly altered during infancy. Differences in drug absorption during this period may affect the choice of delivery method, dose, or monitoring.
   a. **Gastrointestinal absorption.** Oral drug absorption is most greatly altered during the first year of life. Several aspects of absorption are age dependent, including gastric pH, gastric emptying time, intestinal motility, bile salt production, and pancreatic enzyme function.
      (1) **Elevated gastric pH.** At birth, gastric pH is elevated (pH > 4). This results from a relative decrease in gastric acid production and an overall decrease in the volume of gastric secretions. As a result, acid-labile drugs such as penicillin G may have a greater bioavailability in neonates than in older infants. Conversely, drugs that are weak acids such as phenobarbital (Luminal) may not be as well absorbed. To compensate for this effect, neonates may require larger oral doses of these drugs than older infants to produce the desired therapeutic effect. Acid production rises steadily after birth, reaching adult levels within 2 months.

Table 37-1. Age Definitions

Age Group	Age
Newborn	
Preterm or premature	<36 weeks' gestation[a]
Term	>36 weeks' gestation[a]
Neonate	<1 month
Infant	1 month–1 year
Child	1–11 years
Adolescent	12–16 years

[a]Gestational age as measured from the time of the mother's last menstrual period.

(2) Prolonged gastric emptying and intestinal motility. The rate of passage of drugs through the gastrointestinal tract is also important in determining the rate and extent of their absorption. Coordination of contractions within the stomach begins to improve shortly after birth, while intestinal peristalsis increases more slowly, over the first 4 months of life. As a result of this prolonged transit time, absorption of drugs may be significantly slowed.

  (a) Preterm neonates typically have more delayed gastric emptying time than term neonates, so that changes in oral absorption may be most pronounced in these patients.

  (b) Breast-fed infants empty their stomachs approximately twice as fast as formula-fed infants. The increased caloric density of formula feedings delays gastric emptying.

(3) Bile salt and pancreatic enzyme production. The rate of bile salt synthesis in preterm and term infants is reduced to approximately 50% of adult values. Decreased fat absorption from enteral feedings, as well as decreased drug absorption, can occur. For example, when lipid-soluble vitamin D is administered to neonates, bioavailability is only 30% as compared with 70% in adults. The absorption of lipid-soluble drugs is further reduced as a result of lower levels of pancreatic enzymes.

(4) Other factors affecting oral drug absorption include reduced splanchnic blood flow in the 1st month of life and reduced activity of intestinal metabolic enzymes (altering the first-pass effect). In addition, neonates lack normal gut microflora. Although bacterial colonization normally occurs shortly after birth, it may be significantly delayed in preterm neonates who are being cared for in the sterile environment of an intensive care unit.

b. Percutaneous absorption

  (1) Absorption of drugs through the skin is enhanced in infants and young children owing to better hydration of the epidermis, greater perfusion of the subcutaneous layer, and the larger ratio of total body surface area to body mass compared to adults.

  (2) In preterm neonates, the stratum corneum is also thinner, further increasing the potential for the absorption of topical products.

  (3) This route of administration should be used with caution in infants and young children to avoid overdosage. There are numerous accounts of toxicity resulting from percutaneous absorption. For example, repeated applications of topical hydrocortisone cream for diaper rash or eczema can produce adrenal axis suppression after as little as 2 weeks of use in an infant.

c. Intramuscular absorption

  (1) The absorption of drugs administered by this route may be reduced in neonates as a result of reduced blood flow to skeletal muscles. In addition, weak or erratic muscle contractions in neonates may result in reduced drug distribution. These factors may be partially offset by the higher density of capillaries in skeletal muscle during infancy, which increases blood circulation.

  (2) Intramuscular administration of drugs is generally discouraged in the pediatric population because of the pain associated with the injection and the risk of nerve damage from inadvertent injection into nerve tissue.

(3) This route is generally reserved for the administration of vitamin K, vaccines, and occasionally antibiotics when intravenous access is not available. If it is used, the volume should not exceed 0.5 mL for infants and younger children and 1 mL for older children.

d. Rectal administration. Absorption by this route is fairly reliable, even for preterm neonates. Administration may be complicated in infants, however, by the increased number of pulsatile contractions in the rectum compared to adults, making expulsion of a suppository more likely.

e. Pulmonary administration. Inhalation of medications is increasingly being used in infants and older children to avoid systemic exposure. While developmental changes in the pulmonary vasculature and respiratory mechanics likely alter the pharmacokinetics of drugs given by inhalation, little is known about the effects of growth and maturation on this route of drug administration.

3. **Drug distribution.** Growth and maturation affect many of the factors that determine drug distribution. Body water content, fat stores, plasma protein concentrations, organ size and perfusion, hemodynamic stability, tissue perfusion, acid–base balance, and cell membrane permeability all undergo significant changes from infancy to adolescence.

  a. Body water and fat content. Total body water content decreases with increasing age. This is primarily the result of a larger extracellular body water content in neonates and young infants which decreases with age. Approximately 80% of a newborn's weight is body water. By 1 year of age, this value declines to 60%, similar to that of an adult. Highly water-soluble compounds, such as gentamicin (Garamycin), have a larger volume of distribution in neonates than in older children. As a result, larger milligram per kilogram doses are often needed to achieve desired therapeutic concentrations. Conversely, body fat increases with age, from 1–2% in a preterm neonate to 10–15% in a term neonate and 20–25% in a 1-year-old. Lipophilic drugs, such as diazepam (Valium), have a smaller volume of distribution in infants than in older children and adults.

  b. Protein binding. Acidic drugs bind to **albumin,** while basic substances bind primarily to α_1-acid glycoprotein (AGP). The quantity of total plasma proteins, including both of these substances, is reduced in neonates and young infants. In addition, the serum albumin of newborns may have a reduced binding affinity. These two factors result in an increase in the free fraction of many drugs (Table 37-2). The increase in the free fraction may result in enhanced pharmacological activity for a given dose. **The relative decrease in serum proteins may also produce increased competition by drugs and endogenous substances, such as bilirubin, for binding sites.** Drugs that are highly bound to albumin, such as the sulfonamides, may displace bilirubin from its binding sites and allow deposition in the brain, referred to as kernicterus. As a result, these drugs are considered contraindicated in the first 2 months of life.

  c. Metabolism. The most significant research in developmental pharmacology during the past decade has come in the area of drug metabolism. **Developmental changes have been identified for many phase I** (oxidation, reduction, hydroxylation, and hydrolysis) and **phase II** (conjugation) **reactions.** The maturation of metabolic function results in the need for age-related dosage alterations for many common therapies and may explain the increased risk for drug toxicity in infants and young children.

  (1) The activity of **phase I enzymes, such as the cytochrome P450 (CYP) enzymes, changes significantly during maturation.** The primary isoenzyme during the prenatal period, CYP3A7, peaks soon after birth and then declines rapidly. This enzyme exists in barely measurable quantities in adults. It may appear early in fetal life to detoxify

Table 37-2. Protein-Bound Drugs with a High Free Fraction in Neonates

Ampicillin (Principen)	Penicillin G (Pfizerpen)
Digoxin (Lanoxin)	Phenobarbital
Diazepam (Valium)	Phenytoin (Dilantin)
Lidocaine (Xylocaine)	Propranolol (Inderal)
Morphine (Duramorph)	Theophylline
Nafcillin (Nallpen)	

retinoic acid, a potential ratogen. Also at the time of birth, CYP2E1 and CYP2D6 levels begin to rise. Enzymes associated with the metabolism of many common drugs—CYP3A4, CYP2C9, and CYP2C19—appear within the first weeks of life, but their levels increase slowly. The last of the enzymes to develop, CYP1A2, is present by 1–3 months of life. The activity of these enzymes does not appear to increase in a direct linear manner with age, but varies over time. By 3–5 years of age, most patients have CYP isoenzyme activity levels similar to that of adults.

  (a) The altered pharmacokinetic profiles of drugs in children may, in large part, be explained by these developmental changes in the CYP enzyme system. One of the most well studied enzymes is **CYP1A2.** This enzyme is nearly nonexistent in fetal liver cells, and activity is minimal in neonates. As a result, the rate of metabolism of caffeine in the neonate is slow, resulting in an elimination half-life of 40–70 hr. Enzyme activity increases by 4–6 months of age. Within the first year of life it exceeds adult values, producing a caffeine half-life of approximately 5 hr. Infants receiving caffeine (Calfcit) for apnea of prematurity or chronic lung disease must have periodic adjustments in their dose to account for these changes in metabolism and maintain therapeutic serum concentrations.

  (b) **Alcohol dehydrogenase** activity is only 3%–4% of adult values at birth and does not achieve adult values until approximately 5 years of age. Because of this, newborns have a reduced ability to detoxify benzyl alcohol, a preservative found in many injectable products. Newborns exposed repeatedly to these products will accumulate benzyl alcohol, which may lead to a potentially fatal condition referred to as "gasping syndrome," with metabolic acidosis, respiratory failure, seizures, and cardiovascular collapse. Because of this risk, it is recommended that neonates receive preservative-free products or those containing alternative preservatives.

 (2) **Phase II reactions** (conjugation with glycine, glucuronide, or sulfate to form more water-soluble compounds) have not been studied as extensively in the pediatric population.

  (a) **Glucuronidation is generally decreased in neonates,** compared with older children and adults. The rate of metabolism increases with increasing age. This can be seen in the decreasing half-life of morphine (Duramorph) during the 1st year of life. The average half-life in a preterm neonate is 10–20 hr, compared to 4–13 hr in a neonate, 5–10 hr in infants between 1 and 3 months of age, and 1–8 hr in older infants and young children.

  (b) Unlike glucuronidation, **sulfation develops in utero and is well developed in the neonate.** The variation in the function of these two phase II reactions can be seen with the developmental changes in acetaminophen (Tylenol) metabolism. In early infancy, acetaminophen is converted primarily through formation of sulfate conjugates; but with increasing age, glucuronidation becomes the predominate form of metabolism.

 d. Elimination. Development of renal function is a complex and dynamic process. Nephrons begin forming as early as the 9th week of gestation and are complete by 36 weeks. Although the functional units of the kidneys are present, their capacity is significantly reduced at birth. Glomerular filtration rate in neonates is approximately half that of adults. Values are further reduced in preterm neonates. Glomerular filtration rate increases rapidly during the first 2 weeks of life and typically reaches adult values by 8–12 months of age. Tubular secretion rate is also reduced at birth to approximately 20% of adult capacity, but matures by 12 months of age.

 (1) **Immature renal function results in significant alterations in the elimination of many drugs.** Pharmacokinetic studies for several drugs, including the aminoglycosides and vancomycin (Vancocin), have shown a direct correlation between clearance and patient age. Prolongation of the half-life should be anticipated for all renally eliminated drugs administered to neonates and is most pronounced in preterm neonates.

 (2) **To account for the reduced ability of a neonate to eliminate these drugs, longer dosing intervals are often required.** Failure to account for the reduction in renal function may result in drug accumulation and toxicity.

C. Pharmacodynamic considerations. Unlike the rapidly accelerating knowledge of the pharmacokinetic changes associated with development, little is known of the pharmacodynamic changes associated with maturation. Preliminary investigations of warfarin (Coumadin) pharmacodynamics have demonstrated a relationship between anticoagulant response and patient age. Other examples include the increased incidence of certain adverse drug reactions in younger children, such as hepatoxicity with valproic acid (Depakene). Future research in age-related pharmacodynamic changes is needed to optimize the safe and effective use of drugs in infants and children.

D. Pediatric drug administration and monitoring. Drug administration, including the selection of agent and dose as well as the preparation of the dose and therapeutic drug monitoring are complicated in the pediatric population. Pharmacists caring for children must incorporate not only the changes in pharmacokinetics and pharmacodynamics described previously but also the need to carefully check dosage calculations and, if necessary, alter available dosage formulations to suit an infant or child's needs.

1. **Accurate dosage calculations are critical in the care of infants and children.** Pharmacists should use pediatric dosing information available in general drug references or pediatric-specific references such as *The Pediatric Dosage Handbook* (Lexi-Comp), or the *Harriet Lane Handbook* (Mosby). To account for differences in pharmacokinetic parameters, most pediatric doses are based on body weight. In the case of some drugs, such as chemotherapy, doses are based on body surface area (BSA). This value can be determined from the patient's height and weight, using either a nomogram or the following equation:

$$\text{BSA (m}^2\text{)} = \sqrt{\frac{\text{height (cm)} \times \text{weight (kg)}}{3600}}$$

There is no absolute rule for when adolescent patients should start to be dosed as adults. In general, adult dosing guidelines may be used in patients weighing more than 40–50 kg or when the calculated weight-based pediatric dose exceeds the standard adult dose.

2. **The need to calculate pediatric doses introduces a greater risk for dosage errors.** Dosing errors have been found to be more common in medication orders for children than in any other patient population. The need to calculate individual doses, along with potential decimal errors and transcription errors, increases the potential for mistakes. In addition, there is often a wide range of patient ages and weights within a single hospital or clinic. It is not uncommon to have patient doses vary by 10-fold, as an infant weighing 5 kg and an adolescent weighing 50 kg may be cared for by the same healthcare providers. All calculations should be double-checked, and orders outside of the normal pediatric dosage range verified with the prescriber.

3. **Dosage formulations may need to be altered to make them useful for infants and children.** Because young children cannot typically swallow tablets and capsules, these solid dosage formulations must often be converted to oral solutions or suspensions. Several compounding resources, including *Extemporaneous Formulations* (American Society of Health-System Pharmacists), are available to provide pharmacists with formulations that have been tested to ensure drug stability.

4. **Intravenous (IV) medications may be prepared as more concentrated solutions, because of the limits on fluid administration to infants and young children.** While a typical adult may receive up to 4–5 L of IV fluids per day, the total daily fluid requirements for a preterm neonate may be as little as 20–50 mL. Special equipment, such as syringe pumps and microbore tubing, is used to ensure accurate delivery of drugs in small fluid volumes. Currently available syringe pumps can deliver volumes as small as 0.1 mL over 1 hr. Microbore IV tubing is used to minimize the amount of dead space between the delivery device and the patient, further improving the accuracy of drug delivery. Pharmacists must also be capable of assessing literature on the compatibility with drugs and IV fluids because pediatric patients often have limited IV access, so that multiple solutions may need to be infused through the same IV site.

E. Therapeutic drug monitoring is often essential to optimizing drug therapy in infants and children. For most drugs, the therapeutic ranges developed for and used in adults are also appropriate for monitoring pediatric patients. A potential complication in interpreting serum drug concentrations is the **presence of endogenous substances,** which may cross-react with analytical drug assays. This has been demonstrated for digoxin (Lanoxin) in neonates and infants, for whom endogenous digoxin-like reactive substances (EDLRS) may produce falsely elevated serum digoxin concentrations. Standard assay techniques can be modified to exclude EDLRS as a complicating factor.

F. Pharmacists should also be aware of differences in adverse drug reactions between children and adults. Most of the adverse reaction information available in drug product labeling or cited in pharmacy references has been obtained from clinical trials in adults. As several studies have demonstrated, the adverse reaction profile in children may be significantly different from that observed in older subjects. For example, severe dermatologic reactions to lamotrigine (Lamictal), including Stevens-Johnson syndrome, were infrequent during premarketing phase III clinical trials. When the drug was introduced onto the market in the United States and began to be used in children off-label, a higher rate of dermatologic reactions was reported in children. Subsequent research revealed the incidence of severe dermatologic reactions to be 0.8% in children compared to 0.3% in adults. Differences such as these further highlight the need for clinical research in children.

G. In addition, **pharmacists should take an active role in promoting medication adherence (compliance) in children.** Several studies have shown compliance rates in pediatric patients to be 30%–70%. It is surprising that some of the poorest compliance rates have been associated with chronic diseases such as asthma, epilepsy, and diabetes and in children requiring immunosuppressive therapy after organ transplantation. As in adults, counseling about medication adherence should include efforts to identify and overcome barriers to therapy, education about the importance of medical management, and programs to incorporate medication regimens into normal daily tasks. When working with families of younger children, pharmacists should also explore problems with dosage formulation (taste or texture aversion), and dosing frequency, particularly with medications requiring administration at school or day care. In older children, pharmacists should be aware of their need for autonomy, and work with the patient's family to foster the goal of self-care. Pharmacists can serve a vital role in improving medication adherence in patients of all ages.

II. DRUG USE IN PREGNANT PATIENTS.
Most women would like to avoid pharmacologic therapy during pregnancy if at all possible. However, > 80% of women are exposed to substances, such as medication during their pregnancies. Preexisting conditions and other problems occurring during the pregnancy may require continuation or initiation of drug therapy. In rare circumstances, fetal therapy can be administered through the mother. It is important to understand maternal pharmacokinetic changes, placental drug transfer, eventual disposition of the drug, and limitations of the FDA classification system to safely treat pregnant women.

A. Fetal development. The effects of drug therapy in pregnancy depend largely on the stage of fetal development during which the exposure occurs. Pregnancies are normally dated from the first day of the last menstrual cycle; however, when discussing fetal development, fertilization occurs on day 1.

1. **Weeks 1–2.** During the first days after fertilization, the zygote forms in the fallopian tube. Over the next few days, division of the zygote eventually results in the formation of the blastocyst, which travels through the tube into the uterus. The blastocyst contains numerous types of relatively undifferentiated tissues that will ultimately become the fetus, the placenta, and the fetal membranes. Superficial implantation in the endometrium occurs within the first 5 days. During the 2nd week, differentiation begins and the placenta has started to form. During these weeks, there is an "all or none" phenomenon. With no placenta to transfer substances to the blastocyst, there is no susceptibility to teratogens. Exposure to environmental agents during this time will have either little or no effect on the embryo or will destroy most cells leading to pregnancy termination.

2. **Weeks 3–8.** It is during this time that the placenta becomes fully functional and organogenesis occurs. This is the most critical period of development, when the embryo is most susceptible to teratogens. All major organ systems develop structurally during these weeks. All are completely formed by the end of the 9th week, with the exception of the central nervous system. Major congenital anomalies, such as cardiac abnormalities, spina bifida, and limb defects occur during this time.

3. **Weeks 9–38 (the fetal period).** At the 9th week, the embryo is referred to as a fetus. Development during this time is primarily functional, with overall growth occurring throughout. The

fetus may be at risk during exposure to potentially fetotoxic drugs or viruses. Exposure to a drug is generally not associated with major congenital malformations; however, minor congenital anomalies and functional defects may occur during this time.

B. Placental transfer of drugs. The placenta is the functional unit between the fetal and the maternal blood supply. There is no mixing of the two systems, but exchange of nutrients, oxygen, and waste products occurs primarily via passive diffusion. This process is driven by the concentration gradient between the two systems. There are a few substances that are actively transported across the placenta (e.g., amino acids); drugs that are structurally similar to these compounds will also be transported by this mechanism.

1. **Placental metabolism.** The placenta produces a number of pregnancy-related hormones that are mainly secreted into the maternal circulation. Some of the other substances produced by the placenta are enzymes that metabolize drugs. A common example of this is prednisone metabolism, so that very little steroid reaches the fetus.

2. **Factors affecting placental drug transfer.** For a drug to cause a teratogenic or pharmacological effect in the embryo or fetus, it must cross from the maternal circulation to the fetal circulation or tissues. Generally, the principles that apply to drug transfer across any lipid membrane can be applied to placental transfer of a drug. Most substances administered for therapeutic purposes have, by design, the ability to cross the placenta to the fetus. The critical factor is whether the rate and extent of transfer are sufficient to cause significant drug concentrations in the fetus. There are many factors that affect the rate and extent of placental drug transfer.

    (a) **Molecular weight.** Low molecular weight drugs (< 500 Da) diffuse freely across the placenta. Drugs of a higher molecular weight (500–1000 Da) cross less easily. Drugs composed of very large molecules (e.g., heparin) do not cross the placental membranes.

    (b) **Drug pKa.** Weakly acidic and weakly basic drugs tend to rapidly diffuse across the placental membranes. Ionized compounds do not cross the placenta.

    (c) **Lipid solubility.** Moderately lipid-soluble drugs easily diffuse across the placental membranes. It is important to note that many drugs that have been formulated for oral administration and are designed for optimal lipid membrane transfer.

    (d) **Drug absorption.** During pregnancy, gastric tone and motility are decreased, which results in delayed gastrointestinal emptying time. This typically does not affect drug absorption. However, nausea and vomiting, which are most common in the first trimester but may continue throughout pregnancy, may affect absorption.

    (e) **Drug distribution.** The volume of distribution increases significantly during pregnancy and increases with advancing gestational age. The alteration in volume of distribution is the result of an increased plasma volume. Total body fluid (intravascular and extravascular volume) increases, as does adipose tissue. The placenta itself may also be a site for distribution. Hydrophilic drugs will have a higher volume of distribution leading to lower peak levels. Plasma concentrations of drugs that are widely distributed are usually lower than those with a small volume of distribution. Therefore, less drug is available to cross the placenta.

    (f) **Plasma protein binding.** Placental transfer of a highly plasma-protein-bound drug is less likely because only the free drug crosses the placenta. During pregnancy, a reduction in the levels of two major drug-binding proteins—albumin and AGP—is observed. A dilutional effect occurs with albumin and other protein concentrations, which can increase the free fraction of drugs.

    (g) **Physical characteristics of the placenta.** As a pregnancy progresses, the placental membranes become progressively thinner, resulting in a decrease in diffusion distance. The placenta also expands, causing a greater surface area for the transfer of substances.

    (h) **Maternal pharmacokinetic changes.** The dramatic increase in blood volume that occurs primarily during the first 30 weeks of pregnancy enhances blood flow through the kidneys and liver. Drugs that are excreted renally will experience a more rapid clearance, which could decrease the overall exposure time of the drug to the placenta. Metabolism of some drugs is increased; however, the elevated levels of estrogen and progesterone present during the pregnancy can competitively inhibit the metabolism of other drugs.

3. Teratogenic drugs

a. Teratogens are defined as agents that increase the risk of or cause a congenital anomaly to occur. These defects can be structural, functional, or behavioral in nature. Women may blame a specific exposure during their pregnancy as the cause of a fetal anomaly; however, the defect may have no known cause, as is the case in 3% of all births in the United States.

b. It may take years of exposures to actually link a specific drug to certain defects. Animal studies can only suggest potential problems in humans but are often the only source of information regarding safety of agents during early pregnancy. The dose that animals often receive exceeds the normal human dose, which diminishes the applicability of these data to humans.

c. The fetus is unable to metabolize or eliminate drugs as quickly as the mother. Some substances may be excreted into the amniotic fluid and then resorbed in the fetal intestines after the fluid is swallowed. Therefore, some drugs may have a longer exposure time in the fetus, whereas others are eliminated more rapidly.

c. Because fetal organ systems develop at different times, specific teratogenic effects depend mainly on the point of gestation when the drug was ingested.

d. The teratogenic rate of substances indicates how frequently anomalies occur and over what exposure period. For example, one of the most potent known teratogens, thalidomide, had a teratogenic rate of 20% with a single exposure, yet only one third of women who ingested the drug gave birth to affected infants. Other agents may increase the rate of specific defects over the general population, but the absolute incidence may be extremely low.

e. The FDA developed a classification system that groups drugs according to the degree of their potential risk during pregnancy.[1]

   (1) **Category A.** Adequate, well-controlled studies in pregnant women have not shown an increased risk of fetal abnormalities.

   (2) **Category B.** Animal studies have revealed no evidence of harm to the fetus; however, there are no adequate and well-controlled studies in pregnant women. Or animal studies have shown an adverse effect, but adequate and well-controlled studies in pregnant women have failed to demonstrate a risk to the fetus.

   (3) **Category C.** Animal studies have shown an adverse effect and there are no adequate and well-controlled studies in pregnant women. Or no animal studies have been conducted, and there are no adequate and well-controlled studies in pregnant women.

   (4) **Category D.** Studies, adequate well-controlled or observational, in pregnant women have demonstrated a risk to the fetus. However, the benefits of therapy may outweigh the potential risk.

   (5) **Category X.** Studies, adequate well-controlled or observational, in animals or pregnant women have demonstrated positive evidence of fetal abnormalities. The use of the product is contraindicated in women who are or may become pregnant.

d. **Problems with the current system.** The current system was created in 1979 and has not been revised since its inception. With many agents there is a paucity of human data, despite the fact the drug may carry a category B rating. Most newly marketed agents will be placed in category C, amid other agents with little data in humans or animals. This is the most difficult category to assess. Although there may be case reports of drug exposures, these tend to bias information toward fetal risk; most publish only outcomes with potential drug-related effects. Few drugs will ever be assigned a category A status because large, randomized, well-controlled trials are rarely conducted in pregnant women.

f. **Examples of teratogenic agents.**

   (1) **Vitamin A derivatives.** Drugs such as isotretinoin (Accutane) and etretinate (Tegison) are potent teratogens in humans. These agents should be discontinued several months before pregnancy.

   (2) **Warfarin** (Coumadin) is most teratogenic in the first trimester (weeks 6–9), but can also cause malformations during the second and third trimesters as well. Early exposure is associated with a pattern of defects known as fetal warfarin syndrome. These defects can include hypoplasia of the nose and extremities, congenital heart disease, and

---

[1] *Federal Register*, June 26, 1979, 44(124):37434–37467.

seizures. Central nervous system abnormalities are increased with later use. Heparins may be an appropriate substitute when anticoagulation is necessary; however, they are not as effective for preventing thrombosis in women with artificial heart valves.

(3) **Androgenic agents** can cause virilization of female fetuses, creating ambiguous genitalia. Finasteride (Propecia) can cause genital abnormalities in male offspring. Estrogen and progestins, fortunately, do not have this effect. Many women continue to take birth control pills during the first month or two after conception until the pregnancy is discovered.

(4) **Ethanol.** Alcohol consumed in large amounts for prolonged periods during pregnancy (> 4–5 drinks/day) is known to cause fetal alcohol syndrome (FAS). Features of FAS include growth restriction, craniofacial dysmorphology and central nervous system malfunctions, along with various other abnormalities. At least 30% of women who abuse alcohol will deliver an infant affected by FAS. Moderate alcohol consumption (2 drinks/day) can also lead to similar defects, although usually not the complete syndrome. Even though the most problematic time is during the first 2 months of pregnancy, moderate drinking during the second trimester is associated with an increased rate of spontaneous abortions.

(5) **Antineoplastics.** Many agents in this class are associated with fetal anomalies after first trimester chemotherapy administration. Growth restriction often occurs regardless of the timing of exposure. Owing to the mechanism of action of these agents, many are embryocidal.

(6) **Anticonvulsants.** Drugs such as phenytoin (Dilantin), valproic acid (Depakene), and carbamazepine (Tegretol) have all been associated with fetal anomalies. However, maternal benefit from these agents often outweighs the risk to the fetus. Anticonvulsants should not be stopped during pregnancy, but if appropriate, they should be discontinued several months before fertilization. Valproic acid and carbamazepine can increase the risk of neural tube defects; women taking these agents should receive folic acid supplementation starting before conception. Toxic epoxide radicals are thought to be the mechanism of teratogenicity with several of these agents. Genetic alterations in the epoxide hydrolase enzyme activity can reduce or increase the severity of abnormalities.

(7) **Infections.** Viral infections, such as rubella, cytomegalovirus, parvovirus, coxsackie, and varicella can be associated with growth restriction, congenital anomalies, premature delivery, and potential embryotoxicity or fetal demise. Nearly all maternal infections have been thought to cause growth restriction.

(8) **Cigarette smoking.** Cigarettes contain many toxic and carcinogenic compounds in addition to nicotine. Nicotine is a potent vasoconstricting agent capable of reducing uterine blood flow and increasing uterine vascular resistance. Smoking not only increases the risk of a growth restricted fetus but also increases the risk of spontaneous abortions, premature delivery, placental abruption, and premature rupture of the membranes. Small increases in defects of the heart, limbs and feet, skull, urinary system, abdomen, intestines, and muscles have also been associated with cigarettes. Smoking may also alter the effects of other substances, perhaps enhancing toxicity of both agents.

4. **Other problematic therapies.** Some agents given during pregnancy may result in pharmacological effects that are not necessarily toxic, yet need to be considered when medications are given during the later weeks of pregnancy.

a. **Central nervous system (CNS) depression** may occur with barbiturates, tranquilizers, antidepressants, and narcotics. Also, anesthetics and other agents commonly given during labor may cause significant CNS and respiratory depression in newborns (e.g., magnesium sulfate or opioid analgesics).

b. **Neonatal bleeding.** Maternal ingestion of agents such as nonsteroidal anti-inflammatory drugs (NSAIDs) and anticoagulants at therapeutic doses near term may cause bleeding problems in the newborn.

c. **Drug withdrawal.** Habitual maternal use of barbiturates, narcotics, benzodiazepines, alcohol, and other substances of abuse may lead to withdrawal symptoms in newborns.

d. **Constriction of the ductus arteriosus.** Maternal use of NSAIDs in the third trimester may cause the ductus arteriosus to close prematurely and could result in pulmonary hypertension in the newborn.

III. DRUG EXCRETION IN BREAST MILK. Today, > 60% of women choose to breast-feed their infants. Of these women, 90%–95% receive a medication during the first postpartum week, most commonly for pain control after delivery. It is important to understand the principles of drug excretion in breast milk and specific information on the various medications to minimize risks from drug effects in the nursing infant.

A. **Transfer of drugs from plasma to breast milk.** Drug transfer into breast milk is governed by many of the same principles that influence human placental drug transfer.

1. Most drugs cross into breast milk via passive diffusion along a concentration gradient formed by the un-ionized drug content on each side of the membrane.

2. Breast milk contents change throughout a feeding. Colostrum, the very first milk produced, is much higher in protein than mature milk and the fat content is minimal. Mature milk consists of fore-milk at the beginning of a feeding and hind-milk at the end. The protein and fat content increase throughout the nursing session. Therefore drugs that partition into more lipid solutions will have the highest concentration in hind milk.

3. A milk to plasma ratio can be determined for specific agents when both blood and milk concentrations are known. Most drugs have a ratio < 1; lower numbers indicate that less drug crosses into breast milk. Because the milk to plasma ratio may change within a feeding, the average breast milk concentration is usually used, if available.

4. It is possible to calculate the dose an infant receives if the breast milk concentration is known. A typical infant drinks 150 mL/kg per day. Multiplying the average concentration by the breast milk volume consumed will give the total daily exposure. It is important to remember that this drug must now be ingested by the infant, so the bioavailability of the drug is critical to calculate the actual daily dose. Doses < 10% of the maternal dose on a milligram per kilogram per day basis are preferable.

5. Some medications are not absorbed orally, but may pass into breast milk when administered intravenously to the mother. Although the drug may not enter the infant's blood, it may have effects on the gastrointestinal tract. For example, the bioavailability of gentamicin is negligible; however, it may cause diarrhea or sterilize the bowel.

B. **Drug factors.** The drug and its environment influence the rate and extent of drug passage into the breast milk.

1. **Molecular weight.** Drugs weighing < 200 Da cross into milk easily. Larger molecules can dissolve in the lipid membrane or pass through small pores. Large molecules, such as insulin, do not cross into breast milk.

2. **pH gradient.** Human milk is more acidic than plasma.
   a. Weak acids may diffuse across the membrane and remain un-ionized, allowing for passage back into the plasma. Lower amounts of these drugs will cross than those that are weak bases.
   b. Weak bases may diffuse into the breast milk and ionize, which causes drug trapping. This creates higher levels of drug in the breast milk; these drugs will have a milk to plasma ratio > 1. This effect though, is not usually clinical significant, especially when the maternal serum concentration is very low.

3. **Drug pKa.** Only the un-ionized form of a drug is able to pass through the lipid membrane.

4. **Plasma protein binding.** The free fraction of a drug is available to pass into the breast milk. In general, drugs with high plasma-protein-binding properties tend to remain in the plasma and pass into the milk in low concentrations. Milk proteins and lipids also may bind drugs when they are created in the mammary glands; this may represent another route of entry, rather than passive diffusion.

5. **Lipid solubility.** Lipid solubility is necessary for a drug to pass into the breast milk. Highly lipid-soluble drugs (e.g., diazepam, Valium) may pass into the breast milk in relatively high amounts and, therefore, may present a significant dose of drug to the nursing infant.

6. **Equilibration.** Some drugs may rapidly equilibrate between maternal plasma and breast milk. These agents will diffuse across the membrane as the drug concentration changes in the

maternal system. Other agents may never reach an equilibrium between milk and plasma. These drugs tend to slowly diffuse into breast milk and will respond gradually to changes in maternal concentrations.

C. Maternal factors. Maternal pharmacology plays a significant role in the rate and extent of drug passage into breast milk. The extent of plasma protein binding and changes in the mother's ability to metabolize or eliminate the drug influence the amount of drug that is available to pass into the breast milk. Equally important are the maternal dose of the drug, the dosing schedule or frequency, and the route of administration.

D. Drugs affecting hormonal influence of breast milk production. The primary hormone responsible for controlling breast milk production is prolactin. A decrease in milk production may result in diminished weight gain in the nursing infant, the need for supplementation, or premature cessation of breast-feeding.

    1. Drugs that decrease serum prolactin levels. Drugs such as bromocriptine have been used to suppress lactation in women who choose not to breast-feed. This practice has long been abandoned because myocardial infarctions, seizures, and stroke were attributed to its use. Other drugs include

        a. Ergot alkaloids

        b. L-dopa

    2. Drugs that increase serum prolactin levels. Metoclopramide (Reglan) has been useful therapeutically to enhance milk production. The following drugs are known to increase serum prolactin levels, but they are not used for this purpose. These drugs include

        a. Methyldopa (Aldomet)

        b. Haloperidol (Haldol)

        c. Phenothiazines

E. Factors to assess. In assessing the safety of an agent during breast-feeding, several considerations should be addressed:

    1. Inherent toxicity of the drug

    2. Drug safety data in infants

    3. Amount of drug ingested

    4. Duration of therapy

    5. Age of the infant or degree of prematurity

    6. Drug pharmacokinetics in the mother and child

F. Factors to minimize drug exposure to the infant. One of the goals when using medications in the breast-feeding mother is to maintain a natural, uninterrupted pattern of nursing. In many instances, it may be possible to withhold a drug when it is not essential or delay therapy until after weaning. Other factors include

    1. Medication selection. When a specific product is being selected, it is important to choose the agent that is distributed into the milk the least, if possible.

        a. Other desirable characteristics include a short half-life, inactive metabolites, and high protein binding.

        b. In addition, it is desirable to select agents with lower plasma concentrations, which may involve an alternative route of administration.

        c. Single doses may be preferable to a longer therapy course if the agent is contraindicated in breast-feeding. This can allow for the mother to pump and discard her milk for a defined period of time, often 12–24 hr, rather than discontinue breast-feeding altogether.

    2. Maternal dose relative to infant feeding. One of the goals of drug dosing in lactating women is minimal infant exposure to the drug. It is desirable to adjust the dosing and nursing schedules so that a drug dose is administered at the time of or immediately after the infant's feeding. Medications should be dosed before the infant's longest sleep.

G. Examples of drugs that readily enter breast milk. These agents should be used with caution in nursing mothers.

   1. **Narcotics, barbiturates, and benzodiazepines.** CNS active agents, such as diazepam, may have a hypnotic effect on the nursing infant. These effects are related to the maternal dose. Alcohol consumption may have a similar effect.

   2. **Antidepressants and antipsychotics.** These classes of drugs appear to pass into the breast milk; however, no serious adverse effects have been reported. The long-term behavioral effects of chronic exposure to these drugs on developing newborns are unknown.

   3. **Anticholinergic compounds.** These drugs may result in adverse CNS effects in the infant and may reduce milk volume in the mother. Dicyclomine (Bentyl) is contraindicated in nursing mothers because it may result in neonatal apnea.

IV. DRUG USE IN GERIATRIC PATIENTS. In 2000, more than 12% of the American population was > 65 years of age, representing more than 35 million Americans. It is estimated that three out of every four elderly people are taking prescription medications. Anticipated total drug usage, including nonprescription medications, reveals that 50% of all drugs used in the United States are used by the geriatric population.

   A. Adverse drug reactions. Geriatric patients are at increased risk for drug-induced adverse effects. Incidence of adverse drug reactions (ADRs) in patients over the age of 65 is two to three times greater compared to younger patients. The risk is five times higher in people approaching age 90. One in five of all elderly patients experiences an ADR. In some patients, these are overlooked because they mimic the characteristics of other diseases.

   1. Factors that are responsible for the higher prevalence of ADRs in the geriatric population include polypharmacy, poor relationship with healthcare providers, multiple disease states, increasing severity of illness, reduced drug elimination, and increased sensitivity to drug effects.
      a. Studies have shown that > 35% of geriatric patients living in the community use six or more medications; approximately one half of patients residing in long-term-care facilities use five or more medications. People 65 and older use approximately 40% of the drugs prescribed and 50% of the over-the-counter (OTC) medications taken.
      b. Patients taking multiple medications have a greater chance of experiencing ADRs owing to drug–drug interactions and the potential for overlap or synergy between adverse effect profiles.
      c. Patients with multiple disease states are at higher risk of having a drug–disease state interaction.
      d. In addition to the aforementioned risk factors for developing an ADR, it is difficult to predict how geriatric patients will respond to any given medication owing to altered pharmacokinetic and pharmacodynamic profiles.
      e. Another issue complicating geriatric drug therapy is adherence. Factors that have been shown to increase nonadherence include poor relationships with healthcare providers, lower socioeconomic status, living alone, polypharmacy, complicated drug regimens, and multiple comorbidities. As many as 60% of geriatric patients do not take their medications as prescribed and may self-medicate as often as once a week. If patients are hospitalized, their prescribed drug doses may represent a significant overdosage or underdosage, which could cause unintended effects.
      f. Elderly patients can have diseases that make adhering to drug therapy difficult. Conditions that affect vision, such as macular degeneration or cataract formation, can make reading prescription labels and medication instructions troublesome. Hearing loss can prevent patients from understanding and healthcare professionals from effectively communicating medication information and patient instructions. Arthritis can add to the difficulty of opening medication bottles. In these instances, providing patients with medication or "pill" boxes and written medication lists may limit potential barriers to patient adherence. Recognizing these factors, pharmacists can increase adherence in elderly patients.

   2. Pharmacists can provide recommendations to eliminate unnecessary drug therapy and monitor medication profiles to avoid potential drug–drug or drug–disease state interactions that may prove harmful. Efforts to optimize drug therapy, including simplifying and employing more cost-effective regimens, may ultimately afford better patient adherence.

Table 37-3. Age-Related Physiological Changes Affecting Drug Therapy

Factors	Change	Clinical Significance
	Pharmacokinetic	
Gastrointestinal motility	↓	May affect the rate but not the extent of drug absorption
Gastric pH	↑	No significant change in drug absorption
Renal function	↓	Reduced elimination of renally excreted drugs
Serum albumin	↓	Decreased protein binding leading to an increased free fraction of drug
Phase I hepatic metabolism	↓	Potential accumulation of drugs metabolized by oxidation, reduction, or hydrolysis reactions
Body fat to lean muscle mass ratio	↑	Increased volume of distribution of fat-soluble drugs
Total body water	↓	Decreased volume of distribution of water-soluble drugs
	Pharmacodynamic	
β-receptor sensitivity	↓	Potential diminished response to β-blockers
Baroreceptor sensitivity	↓	Greater risk of orthostatic hypotension
Response to benzodiazepines and opioid analgesics	↑	Increased risk of adverse effects with typical doses

B. **Pharmacokinetics.** Pharmacokinetic parameters may be altered in the elderly owing to age-related physiological changes. Specific age-related physiological changes affecting drug therapy are given in Table 37-3.

1. **Absorption.** Physiological changes that can alter absorption in the geriatric population include delayed gastric emptying, decreased splanchnic blood flow, elevated gastric pH, and impaired intestinal motility. Although the rate of drug absorption may be altered in some patients, the extent of absorption is rarely affected.

2. **Distribution.** Several age-related physiological changes may affect drug distribution.
   a. Elderly patients have a decrease in total body water, causing water-soluble drugs (e.g., acetaminophen, Tylenol) to have a smaller volume of distribution. Peak concentrations of these agents will be higher, and loading doses may need to be adjusted to incorporate this change.
   b. The volume of distribution of lipid-soluble drugs (e.g., diazepam, Valium; propranolol, Inderal) is increased because geriatric patients tend to have a greater ratio of adipose tissue to lean muscle mass. These medications may accumulate in fat stores, increasing their duration of action.
   c. Aging may also affect the pharmacokinetics of drugs that are highly protein bound. For example, drugs that are highly bound to albumin (e.g., warfarin, Coumadin; phenytoin, Dilantin) may have a greater free concentration because albumin can be decreased in the elderly who are chronically ill.
   d. Medications may have altered binding affinity in the elderly or albumin may experience a change in configuration, which can also lower binding capacity. Competition for acidic binding sites could occur with accumulated endogenous substances, altering the free fraction of drugs.
   e. Although AGP concentrations tend to increase with age, the increase in the concentrations of basic drugs (e.g., lidocaine, Xylocaine; propranolol, Inderal) that bind to AGP are usually clinically meaningful only in acutely ill patients.

3. **Renal excretion.** Perhaps the best documented age-related physiological change is the decline in renal function, specifically glomerular filtration rate and the tubular secretion rate.
   a. In patients without renal dysfunction, it is estimated that there is a 50% decline in renal function by age 80. Renal blood flow is reduced by approximately 10% each decade of life.
   b. Serum creatinine may not be a good predictor of renal function, as creatinine production also declines with age and lower activity levels (such as the bedridden or debilitated).

    c. Medications primarily eliminated by the kidneys may have increased concentrations of both the active drug and its metabolites, possibly leading to subsequent adverse effects. All renally eliminated drugs used in geriatric patients should be monitored for the need for dose reductions and potential toxicity.

 4. Hepatic metabolism. Age-related changes affecting the liver include a reduction in hepatic blood flow and a decline in hepatic metabolism.

    a. Phase II reactions (glucuronidation, acetylation, and sulfation) are relatively unchanged in the elderly.

    b. A reduction in phase I reactions (oxidation, reduction, and hydrolysis) can occur. Benzodiazepines and certain analgesics, which depend on phase I reactions for metabolism, represent situations in which changes in hepatic metabolism may be important. The elimination half-lives of these agents are prolonged and may result in drug accumulation and possible adverse effects.

    c. Liver volume and cell mass decrease in the elderly. It appears that this change in size enhances the reduced activity of oxidative and demethylation metabolism. Conjugation reactions do not appear to be affected by liver mass.

C. Pharmacodynamics

1. Geriatric patients can be more or less responsive to certain drugs, compared to younger patients. Reasons for this may include altered receptor sensitivity, receptor number, or receptor response. Studies have shown that elderly patients may show a diminished response to β-blockers.

2. In contrast, geriatric patients seem to have an exaggerated response to agents affecting the CNS, narcotic analgesics, benzodiazepines, and warfarin. Elderly patients should be monitored carefully when taking these medications. Initiation of any of these therapies should be at lower doses than recommended for younger patients. Avoidance of these drugs may not be possible, but if better alternatives exist they should be used first.

D. Drug therapy considerations

1. Drug therapy in geriatric patients is involved and can be very complex because of age-related changes in pharmacokinetics and pharmacodynamics.

2. A lack of clinical trials designed to evaluate the safety and efficacy of drug therapy in the elderly population increases the problem.

3. The higher incidence of adverse effects in geriatric patients may be in part the result of the complexity of drug therapy and the relative lack of clinical trials in this population. Table 37-4 lists several drugs and doses that should be avoided in the elderly owing to higher risks of adverse effects and/or lack of efficacy.

4. Owing to alterations in gait, balance, and mobility, falls and consequent adverse events are frequent occurrences in geriatric patients.

    a. The high prevalence of osteoporosis in the elderly results in an increased incidence of fractures. Complications associated with fractures, particularly hip fractures, are significant causes of morbidity and mortality.

    b. Medications causing orthostatic hypotension, drowsiness, dizziness, blurred vision, or confusion have the potential to cause or worsen postural instability and increase falls in the elderly.

    c. It is well established that many psychoactive agents, especially long-acting benzodiazepines, are associated with an increased risk of falls in the elderly. If a benzodiazepine must be prescribed, low-dose lorazepam (Ativan) or oxazepam (Serax) are better choices because of the lack of active metabolites and their metabolism involves phase II hepatic reactions only.

5. Geriatric patients tend to be sensitive to medications that possess anticholinergic effects. Dry mouth, urinary retention, blurry vision, constipation, tachycardia, memory impairment and confusion are typical anticholinergic adverse effects associated with several classes of drugs (Table 37-5). These agents can also induce delirium in some people.

    a. When possible, drugs with anticholinergic effects should be avoided in the elderly. In those instances when this is not an option, the least anticholinergic agent should be

Table 37-4. Target Drugs and Doses to Avoid in Geriatric Patients

Drug	Comments
Analgesics	
Pentazocine (Talwin)	Avoid; safer and more effective alternatives
Propoxyphene (Darvon)	Avoid; lack of efficacy (no more effective then acetaminophen and potential for accumulation and adverse narcotic effects
Meperidine (Demerol)	Avoid; safer and more effective alternatives
Antidepressants	
Amitriptyline (Elavil)	Avoid; anticholinergic adverse effects, increased risk of falls, and QT prolongation; use nortriptyline or desipramine as alternatives
Amitriptyline, perphenazine (Triavil)	Avoid; use separate antidepressant and antipsychotic agents in appropriate geriatric doses as necessary
Doxepin (Sinequan)	Avoid; safer and more effective alternatives
Antiemetics	
Trimethobenzamide (Tigan)	Avoid; more effective alternatives available
Antihistamines	
Sedating OTC agents, cold preparations	Avoid; potent anticholinergic effects
Hydroxyzine (Atarax)	Avoid; potent anticholinergic effects
Cyproheptadine (Periactin)	Avoid; potent anticholinergic effects
Chlorpheniramine (Chlor-Trimeton)	Avoid; potent anticholinergic effects
Antihypertensives	
Hydrochlorothiazide (HydroDIURIL)	Doses > 25 mg/day should be avoided
Methyldopa (Aldomet)	Avoid; safer alternatives
Propranolol (Inderal)	Lipophilic nonselective β-blocker with increased potential for adverse effects; avoid; use a cardioselective β-blocker instead
Reserpine	Avoid; risk of adverse effects (e.g., sedation, depression)
Antipsychotics	
Haloperidol (Haldol)	Avoid unless indicated for psychotic disorder; use in small doses (1 mg); risk of sudden death in higher doses
Thioridazine	Avoid unless indicated for psychotic disorder
Antispasmodics	
Belladonna	Avoid long-term use; anticholinergic adverse effects
Dicyclomine (Bentyl)	Avoid long-term use; anticholinergic adverse effects
Hyoscyamine (Pyridium)	Avoid long-term use; anticholinergic adverse effects
Decongestants	
Oxymetazoline (Afrin)	Daily use for > 3 days should be avoided
Phenylephrine (Neo-Synephrine)	Daily use for > 3 days should be avoided
Pseudoephedrine (Sudafed)	Avoid; anticholinergic effects and potential to raise blood pressure
Dementia treatments	

(*Continued on next page*)

Table 37-4. Continued.

Drug	Comments
Isoxsuprine	Avoid; lack of efficacy
H$_2$-antagonists	
Cimetidine (Tagamet)	Avoid; adverse CNS effects
Hypoglycemic agents	
Chlorpropamide (Diabinese)	Avoid; long half-life can cause prolonged hypoglycemic episodes and can induce SIADH
Muscle relaxants	
Carisoprodol (Soma)	Risk of adverse events greater than potential benefits; all use should be avoided
Cyclobenzaprine (Flexeril)	Risks of adverse events greater than potential benefits
Methocarbamol (Robaxin)	Risks of adverse events greater than potential benefits
Orphenadrine (Norflex)	Risks of adverse events greater than potential benefits
NSAIDs	
Indomethacin (Indocin)	Avoid; CNS adverse effects; use alternative NSAID
Phenylbutazone	Avoid; hematological adverse effects; use alternative NSAID
Non-cyclooxygenase selective NSAIDS	Avoid long-term use of naproxen, oxaprozin and piroxicam; increased risks of adverse effects
Platelet inhibitors	
Dipyridamole (Persantine)	Avoid; lack of efficacy and adverse effects (orthostatic hypotension) at high doses; aspirin is safer and more effective
Sedative hypnotics	
Long-acting benzodiazepines Chlordiazepoxide (Librium) Diazepam (Valium) Flurazepam (Dalmane)	Avoid; accumulation and increased risk of falls, sedation, and delirium
Short-acting benzodiazepines Alprazolam (Xanax) Oxazepam (Serax) Triazolam (Halcion)	Nightly use should be avoided; increased risk of falls, daytime sedation, and delirium
Meprobamate (Miltown)	All use should be avoided
Barbiturates	All use should be avoided; safer alternatives exist

CNS, central nervous system; *NSAIDs,* nonsteroidal anti-inflammatory drugs; *OCT,* over the counter; *SIADH,* syndrome of inappropriate antidiuretic hormone secretion.
Modified with permission from Fick DM, Cooper JW, Wade WE, et al. Updating the Beers criteria for potentially inappropriate medication use in older adults. Arch Int Med 2003;163:2716–2724.

Table 37-5. Drugs and Drug Classes Possessing Anticholinergic Effects

Antidiarrheal agents	Propantheline (Pro-Banthine)
Diphenoxylate/atropine (Lomotil)	Oxybutynin (XL formulation
Antiemetics/antivertigo agents	has fewer effects) (Ditropan)
Meclizine (Antivert)	Tolterodine (Detrol)
Scopolamine (Transderm	Class Ia antiarrhythmic agents
scopolamine)	Disopyramide (Norpace)
Trimethobenzamide (Tigan)	Quinidine
Promethazine (Phenergan)	Parkinson's agents
Prochlorperazine (Compazine)	Amantadine (Symmetrel)
Antihistamines, sedating types	Benztropine (Cogentin)
Antipsychotic agents	Procyclidine (Kemadrin)
Antispasmodics	Trihexyphenidyl
Belladonna alkaloids	Skeletal muscle relaxants
Clidinium bromide	Cyclobenzaprine (Flexeril)
Dicyclomine (Bentyl)	Orphenadrine (Norflex)
Hyoscyamine (Pyridium)	Tricyclic antidepressants

chosen and initiated at the lowest effective dose. For example, if a tricyclic antidepressant is needed, desipramine (Norpramin) and nortriptyline (Pamelor) possess less anticholinergic activity than amitriptyline (Elavil) and imipramine (Tofranil), and therefore would be better initial therapeutic options.

   b. Frequent monitoring for and patient and family education on signs and symptoms of possible anticholinergic adverse effects is always warranted when these drugs are prescribed in the elderly.

E. General principles. To aid clinicians in providing appropriate geriatric drug therapy, some general principles have been developed.

   a. Start with a low dose, and titrate the medication dose slowly.

   b. Owing to reduced renal and hepatic function, the half-lives of many drugs are prolonged in the elderly. Selection of agents should involve consideration of the specific pharmacokinetics of each drug in the geriatric population.

   c. Rapid dose escalations prevent attainment of the optimal therapeutic response because a steady-state concentration of the drug is not reached and increases the risks for developing an ADR.

   d. The fewest number of drugs should always be used to treat patients.

   e. Always evaluate possible drug toxicity. Geriatric patients can have atypical presentations of ADRs, which may manifest as CNS changes (e.g., altered mental status).

   f. Review concomitant medications and diseases to evaluate the possible interactions with new drugs.

   g. Reassess the need for each medication on a regular basis.

STUDY QUESTIONS

Directions for questions 1–14: Each of the questions, statements, or incomplete statements in this section can be correctly answered or completed by **one** of the suggested answers or phrases. Choose the **best** answer.

For questions 1–4: AH is a 1.2-kg female born prematurely at 30 weeks of gestational age. Her mother had an infection with a fever at the time of delivery. AH was admitted to the neonatal intensive care unit for presumed sepsis and placed on empiric antibiotic therapy with ampicillin (50 mg/kg IV every 12 hr) and gentamicin (2.5 mg/kg IV every 8 hr).

1. Which of the following variables will *most* likely be used to calculate doses for AH's antibiotics?

(A) height
(B) hepatic function
(C) weight
(D) age
(E) serum creatinine

2. After the administration of four doses of gentamicin, a serum concentration obtained 5 min before the next dose was 2.5 µg/mL. Which of the following answers best describes the pharmacokinetic differences observed in premature neonates (compared to older children and adults) that might explain this value?

(A) larger volume of distribution, longer half-life
(B) larger volume of distribution, shorter half-life
(C) smaller volume of distribution, longer half-life
(D) smaller volume of distribution, shorter half-life
(E) similar volume of distribution, shorter half-life

3. Ampicillin may exhibit pharmacokinetic differences in AH because of its protein binding characteristics. Which of the following answers best describes the effect of AH's age on ampicillin protein binding?

(A) increased protein binding, resulting in a greater free fraction
(B) increased protein binding, resulting in a reduced free fraction
(C) decreased protein binding, resulting in a greater free fraction
(D) decreased protein binding, resulting in a reduced free fraction
(E) decreased protein binding, resulting in no significant change in free fraction

4. As the pharmacist providing services for the neonatal intensive care unit, you evaluate medication orders and make recommendations to the medical team. Which of the following would be the *most* appropriate recommendation for AH's care?

(A) Change to oral antibiotics for better absorption.
(B) Double-check the calculations to avoid decimal errors.
(C) Dilute the gentamicin with a larger volume of IV fluids to make it easier to measure.
(D) Use a pediatric-specific therapeutic range for monitoring gentamicin.
(E) Change to sulfamethoxazole and trimethoprim (Bactrim) for single-agent antibacterial coverage.

5. You are counseling the grandmother of a 3-year-old boy who has a prescription for amoxicillin/clavulanate (Augmentin) to treat uncomplicated otitis media. Which of the following issues would be *least* likely to affect medication adherence (compliance)?

(A) lack of education about the medication
(B) cost
(C) dosing interval (frequency)
(D) taste
(E) autonomy

6. Which of the following medications is safe to use in the third trimester of pregnancy?

(A) acetaminophen
(B) nonsteroidal anti-inflammatory drugs
(C) warfarin
(D) OxyContin
(E) aspirin

7. Which of the following medications may have the potential to cause falls in a geriatric patient?

(A) amitriptyline (Elavil)
(B) trazodone (Desyrel)
(C) acetaminophen with codeine
(D) diazepam
(E) All of the above

8. Placental transfer of a drug is affected by all of the following characteristics *except*

(A) molecular weight.
(B) fetal gender.
(C) gestational age.
(D) lipid solubility of the drug.
(E) plasma protein binding.

9. When selecting a benzodiazepine product for a woman who has chronic panic disorder, all of the following drug properties are desirable for breast-feeding her 8-month-old infant who was born at term *except*

(A) hepatic metabolism to inactive metabolites.
(B) a short half-life.
(C) a rapid onset of action.
(D) high lipid solubility.

10. Drug safety in pregnancy of a specific agent can be assessed best by

(A) the FDA classification system, especially category C drugs.
(B) case reports.
(C) physician knowledge.
(D) databases, such as REPROTOX.

11. Which of the following drugs is expected to cause anticholinergic adverse effects in the elderly?

(A) propoxyphene (Darvon)
(B) ciprofloxacin (Cipro)
(C) amitriptyline (Elavil)
(D) propranolol (Inderal)
(E) cimetidine (Tagamet)

12. Which of the following antihypertensive agents should be avoided in elderly patients?

(A) amlodipine (Norvasc) 5 mg every day
(B) atenolol (Tenormin) 25 mg every day
(C) benazepril (Lotensin) 10 mg every day
(D) hydrochlorothiazide (HydroDIURIL) 25 mg every day
(E) methyldopa (Aldomet) 250 mg three times a day

13. Which of the following benzodiazepines is expected to cause the *least* amount of adverse effects in the elderly?

(A) chlordiazepoxide (Librium)
(B) diazepam (Valium)
(C) flurazepam (Dalmane)
(D) oxazepam (Serax)
(E) temazepam (Restoril)

14. Which of the following factors is associated with an increased risk of noncompliance in the elderly?

(A) polypharmacy
(B) hypertension
(C) living with a spouse in an isolated environment
(D) expensive medications
(E) good relationship with physician

Directions for questions 15–16: The questions and incomplete statements in this section can be correctly answered or completed by **one or more** of the suggested answers. Choose the answer, **A–E.**

A   if **I only** is correct
B   if **III only** is correct
C   if **I and II** are correct
D   if **II and III** are correct
E   if **I, II, and III** are correct

15. According to the principles of drug excretion into the breast milk, which combination of the following properties would result in the *highest* drug concentration in breast milk?

I. low molecular weight, moderately lipophilic
II. low plasma protein bound, weakly basic
III. highly plasma protein bound, weakly acidic

16. Following principles of teratogenicity, drug exposure during the following times could cause fetal abnormalities?

I. first 2 weeks of gestation
II. weeks 3–8 of gestation
III. the fetal period

ANSWERS AND EXPLANATIONS

1. The answer is C *[see I.D.1]*
Most pediatric doses are based on body weight. This single variable incorporates growth and maturation, while allowing a simple calculation for dose. Height is often difficult to measure accurately in children, and the calculation of body surface area is typically reserved for those drugs with narrow therapeutic indices, such as chemotherapy.

2. The answer is A *[see I.B.3.a; I.B.3.d]*
Aminoglycosides such as gentamicin exhibit a larger volume of distribution in neonates because of their larger body water content. Neonates also typically have a longer elimination half-life as the result of having reduced renal function during the first 6 months of life.

3. The answer is C *[see I.B.3.b; Table 37-2]*
Neonates have both a reduced quantity of plasma proteins, as well as a reduction in the affinity of albumin to bind to other substances. As a result, the free fraction of many drugs, including ampicillin, is increased.

4. The answer is B *[see I.D.1–2]*
All pediatric orders should be carefully checked for calculation errors. Errors are more common in the pediatric population as the result of weight-based dosing and the need for mathematical calculations. The use of the oral route would not be advisable in this patient, because of the potential reduced drug absorption. Likewise, the dilution of the dose with more IV fluid or the use of a sulfa drug would not be appropriate for this patient's age. Finally, the therapeutic range for gentamicin is the same in pediatric patients as in adults.

5. The answer is E *[see I.G]*
While the other options are all important aspects of counseling to enhance medication adherence in children, autonomy (the ability to provide self-care or give medications independently) would not be a consideration for a 3-year-old child. Autonomy becomes a much more critical issue in determining adherence in adolescence.

6. The answer is A *[see II.B.3.e.(1)–(2); II.4a–d].*
Acetaminophen is a safe and effective analgesic that can be used in therapeutic doses during pregnancy. NSAIDs may interfere with the onset or progress of labor when used in the third trimester. NSAIDs and warfarin, when used near delivery, may cause bleeding problems in the newborn infant. In addition, warfarin use in the third trimester may be associated with fetal CNS abnormalities. OxyContin use in the third trimester may induce neonatal withdrawal following delivery.

7. The answer is E *[see IV.D.4.b–c].*
Medications that can cause orthostatic hypotension, drowsiness, dizziness, blurred vision, or confusion have the potential to cause falls in geriatric patients. Thus all of the medications listed may put the patient at a fall risk.

8. The answer is B *[see II.B.2].*
Fetal gender does not affect placental transfer of a drug. The molecular weight and the lipid solubility of a drug greatly influence its ability to cross the placental membranes. Plasma protein binding affects the amount of free drug available to cross the placenta. Gestational age influences the volume of distribution of the drug as well as the thickness of the placental membranes.

9. The answer is D *[see III.C; III.F.1.a].*
When any drug is used by a nursing mother, it is desirable to have the least amount of active drug available in the maternal circulation to diffuse into the breast milk. A rapidly acting (for maternal onset of action), rapidly eliminated (i.e., short half-life) drug with inactive metabolites is optimal. If the drug is highly lipid soluble, it is more likely to pass into breast milk.

10. The answer is D *[see II.B.3.c–d]*
The FDA classification system does not assess risk well in category C drugs. Category A and to some extent category B drugs have been shown to be safest in pregnancy. Case reports of pregnancy exposures tend to bias data toward adverse outcomes. The best source of information is from available databases, such as REPROTOX or Teris, or with published books such as *Brigg's Drugs in Pregnancy and Lactation*.

11. The answer is C *[see IV.D.5.a; Table 37-5].*
Tricyclic antidepressants are an established cause of anticholinergic adverse effects in the elderly. When these agents are indicated, nortriptyline and desipramine are associated with a lower incidence of anticholinergic ADRs and are more desirable alternatives.

12. The answer is E *[see IV; Table 37-4].*
The use of methyldopa should be avoided in elderly patients owing to risk of CNS adverse effects and hypotension.

13. The answer is D *[see IV.D.4.c; Table 37-4].*
Chlordiazepoxide, diazepam, and flurazepam should be avoided in elderly patients owing to active metabolites and long-elimination half-lives. Oxazepam represents the safest alternative because of a relatively short half-life, absence of active metabolites, and it is devoid of phase I hepatic metabolism.

14. The answer is A *[see IV.A.1.e].*
Lower socioeconomic status, living alone, polypharmacy, complicated drug regimens, poor relationships with healthcare providers, and multiple disease states are all risk factors for noncompliance in the geriatric population.

15. The answer is C (I, II) *[see III.B.1–5].*
High-molecular-weight substances are less likely to pass into breast milk because of their size. Drugs that are highly plasma protein bound may reach the breast milk only in small amounts, because a large portion of the drug is bound to the maternal plasma proteins and, therefore, only a small amount is free to diffuse into breast milk. A low-molecular-weight, moderately lipophilic drug passes easily into breast milk. A drug that has a low degree of plasma protein binding has a significant amount of drug free to diffuse into breast milk. A weakly basic drug may ionize after reaching the breast milk and therefore remain trapped in the milk.

16. The answer is D (II, III) *[see II.A.1–3].*
During first 2 weeks after fertilization, the embryo is impervious to teratogens. Any exposure during this time will have either no effect or the embryo will be destroyed. During the remaining weeks of the pregnancy, teratogens may exert effects on the fetus. Teratogenic effects are not always structural in nature; they can be functional or behavioral. Therefore, exposures during the fetal period can also be problematic.

I. GENERAL PRINCIPLES

A. Laboratory test are performed for multiple purposes, including to discover a disease, confirm or differentiate a diagnosis, stage or classify a disease, and monitor effectiveness of therapy.

B. Laboratory tests are classified as screening or diagnostic. Screening tests are used in patients with no signs or symptoms of a disease (e.g., serum cholesterol for assessing cardiovascular disease risk). Diagnostic tests are done in patients with signs and symptoms of disease or with an abnormal screening test.

C. Monitoring drug therapy

1. **Laboratory test results** are used to investigate potential problems with a patient's anatomy or physiology. Pharmacists usually monitor laboratory tests to
   a. **Assess the therapeutic and adverse effects of a drug** (e.g., monitoring the serum uric acid level after allopurinol is administered, checking for increased liver function test values after administration of isoniazid)
   b. **Determine the proper drug dose** (e.g., assessment of the serum creatinine or creatinine clearance value before use of a renally excreted drug)
   c. **Assess the need for additional or alternate drug therapy** (e.g., assessment of white blood cell count after an antibiotic is administered)
   d. **Prevent test misinterpretation resulting from drug interference** (e.g., determination of a false-positive result for a urine glucose test after cephalosporin administration)

2. These tests can be **expensive,** and requests for them must be balanced against potential benefits for patients and how the laboratory test will affect your decision regarding therapy. Generally, lab tests should be ordered only if the results will affect the decisions about the management of the patient.

B. Definition of normal values

1. **Normal laboratory test results** fall within a predetermined range of values, and **abnormal values** fall outside that range. The normal range of a laboratory test is usually determined by applying statistical methods to results from a representative sample of the general population. Usually, the mean $\pm$ 2 standard deviations is taken as the normal range.
   a. **Normal limits may be defined somewhat arbitrarily;** thus values outside the normal range may not necessarily indicate disease or the need for treatment (e.g., asymptomatic hyperuricemia).
   b. Many factors (e.g., age, sex, time since last meal) must be taken into account when evaluating test results.
   c. **Normal values also vary among institutions** and may depend on the method used to perform the test.
   d. The goal is *not* to make all laboratory values normal; resist urges to do something in a clinically stable patient.
   e. Attempts have been made in recent years to standardize the presentation of laboratory data by using the International System of Units (SI units). Controversy surrounds this issue in the United States, and resistance to adopt this system continues. The SI unit of measure is a method of reporting clinical laboratory data in a standard metric format. The basic unit of mass for the SI is the mole. The mole is not influenced by the addition of excess weight of salt or ester formulations. Technically and pharmacologically, the mole is more meaningful than the gram because each physiological reaction occurs on a molecular level.

Efforts to implement the SI system began in the 1970s, resulting in the adoption of full SI-transition policies by a few major medical and pharmaceutical journals in the 1980s. Reluctance to use this system by many clinicians in the United States has forced changes in the policies by some journals to report both conventional and SI units or to report the conversion factor between the two systems. It is still controversial which method should be used to report clinical laboratory values. There are arguments for and against the universal conversion to the SI system. Readers should be aware that some journals report SI and/or conventional units in their text. Particular attention should be paid to the units associated with a reported laboratory value, and access to a conversion table may be necessary to avoid confusion in the interpretation of the data. When appropriate, both conventional and SI units will be reported in this chapter.

2. **Laboratory error** must always be considered when **test results do not correlate with expected results for a given patient.** If necessary, the test should be repeated. Common sources of laboratory error include spoiled specimens, incomplete specimens, specimens taken at the wrong time, faulty reagents, technical errors, incorrect procedures, and failure to take diet or medication into account.

3. During hospital admission or routine physical examination, a **battery of tests** is usually given to augment the history and physical examination. Basic tests may include an electrocardiogram (ECG), a chest x-ray, a sequential multiple analyzer **(SMA) profile, electrolyte tests, a complete blood count (CBC),** and **urinalysis.**

C. **Quantitative tests, qualitative tests, and analytical performance**

1. Tests with normal values reported in ranges (i.e., 3.5–5.0 mEq/L) are called **quantitative.**

2. Tests with positive (+) or negative (−) outcomes are called **qualitative.**

3. Those with varying degrees of positivity (e.g., 1 +, 2 +, 3 + glucose in the urine) are termed **semiquantitative.**

4. The quality of a quantitative assay is measured in terms of **accuracy** (accuracy is defined as the extent to which mean measurement is close to the true value). **Precision** refers to the reproducibility of the assay.

II. **HEMATOLOGICAL TESTS.** Blood contains three types of formed elements: red blood cells (RBCs), white blood cells (WBCs), and platelets (Figure 38-1). A CBC includes hemoglobin (Hb), hematocrit (Hct), total WBCs, total RBCs, mean cell volume (MCV), and platelet count.

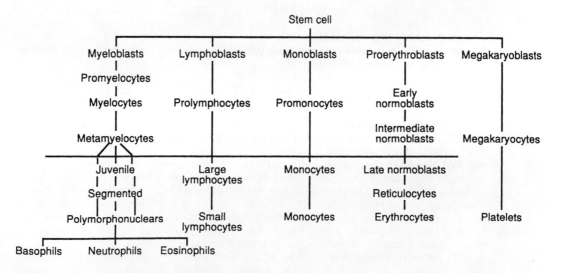

Figure 38-1. Derivation of blood elements from stem cells. Cells located below the *horizontal* line are found in normal peripheral blood, with the exception of the late normoblasts.

A. RBCs (erythrocytes)

1. The **RBC count,** which reports the number of RBCs found in a cubic millimeter (mm^3) of whole blood, provides an indirect estimate of the blood's Hb content. **Normal values** are
   a. 4.3–5.9 million/mm^3 of blood for men ($\times$ 10^{12}/L)
   b. 3.5–5.0 million/mm^3 of blood for women ($\times$ 10^{12}/L)

2. The **Hct or packed cell volume (PCV)** measures the percentage by volume of packed RBCs in a whole blood sample after centrifugation. The Hct value is usually three times the Hb value (see II.A.3) and is given as a percent or fraction of 1 (42%–52% or 0.42–0.52 for men; 37%–47% or 0.37–0.47 for women).
   a. **Low Hct** values indicate such conditions as anemia, overhydration, or blood loss.
   b. **High Hct** values indicate such conditions as polycythemia vera or dehydration.

3. The **Hb test** measures the grams of Hb contained in 100 mL (1 dL) or 1 L of whole blood and provides an estimate of the oxygen-carrying capacity of the RBCs. The Hb value depends on the **number of RBCs** and the **amount of Hb in each RBC.**
   a. **Normal values** are 14–18 g/dL for men and 12–16 g/dL for women.
   b. **Low Hb** values indicate anemia.

4. **RBC indices** (also known as **Wintrobe indices**) provide important information regarding RBC size, Hb concentration, and Hb weight. They are used primarily to categorize anemias, although they may be affected by average cell measurements. A peripheral blood smear can provide most of the information obtained through RBC indices. Observations of a smear may show variation in RBC shape (**poikilocytosis**), as might occur in sickle-cell anemia, or it may show a variation in RBC size (**anisocytosis**), as might occur in a mixed anemia (folic acid and iron deficiency).
   a. **MCV** is the ratio of the Hct to the RBC count. It essentially assesses average RBC size and reflects any anisocytosis.

   $$MCV = \frac{Hct\ (\%)\ \times\ 10}{RBC\ (millions)}$$

   (1) **Low MCV** indicates **microcytic** (undersize) **RBCs,** as occurs in iron deficiency.
   (2) **High MCV** indicates **macrocytic** (oversize) **RBCs,** as occurs in a vitamin B_{12} or folic acid deficiency.
   (3) **Normal range for MCV** is 90 $\pm$ 10.
   b. **Mean cell hemoglobin (MCHb)** assesses the amount of Hb in an average RBC.
   (1) MCHb is defined as:

   $$MCHb = \frac{Hb\ \times\ 10}{RBC\ (millions)}$$

   (2) **Normal range for MCH** is 30 $\pm$ 4.
   c. **Mean cell hemoglobin concentration (MCHbC)** represents the average concentration of Hb in an average RBC, defined as:

   $$MCHbC = \frac{Hb\ \times\ 100}{Hct}$$

   (1) **Normal range for MCHC** is 34 $\pm$ 3.
   (2) **Low MCHbC** indicates **hypochromia** (pale RBCs resulting from decreased Hb content), as occurs in iron deficiency.
   d. **Red blood cell distribution width (RDW)** is a relatively new index of RBCs. Normally, most RBCs are approximately equal in size, so that only one bell-shaped histogram peak is generated. Disease may change the size of some RBCs—for example, the gradual change in size of newly produced RBCs in folic acid or iron deficiency. The difference in size between the abnormal and the less abnormal RBCs produces either more than one histogram peak or a broadening of the normal peak. This value is used primarily with other tests to diagnose iron-deficiency anemia.
   (1) **An increased RDW** is found in factor-deficiency anemia (e.g., iron, folate, vitamin B_{12}).
   (2) **A normal RDW** is found in such conditions as anemia of chronic disease.
   (3) The **RDW index** is never decreased.

5. The **reticulocyte count** provides a measure of immature RBCs (reticulocytes), which contain remnants of nuclear material (reticulum). Normal RBCs circulate in the blood for about 1–2 days in this form. Hence, this test provides an index of bone marrow production of mature RBCs.

   a. Reticulocytes normally make up 0.1%–2.4% of the total RBC count.

   b. **Increased reticulocyte count** occurs with such conditions as hemolytic anemia, acute blood loss, and response to the treatment of a factor deficiency (e.g., an iron, vitamin B_{12}, or folate deficiency). **Polychromasia** (the tendency to stain with acidic or basic dyes) noted on a peripheral smear laboratory report usually indicates increased reticulocytes.

   c. **Decreased reticulocyte count** occurs with such conditions as drug-induced aplastic anemia.

6. The **erythrocyte sedimentation rate (ESR)** measures the rate of RBC settling of whole, uncoagulated blood over time, and it primarily reflects plasma composition. Most of the sedimentation effect results from alterations in plasma proteins.

   a. **Normal ESR rates** range from 0 to 20 mm/hr for males and from 0 to 30 mm/hr for females.

   b. **ESR values increase** with acute or chronic infection, tissue necrosis or infarction, well-established malignancy, and rheumatoid collagen diseases.

   c. **ESR values** are used to

      (1) Follow the clinical course of a disease

      (2) Demonstrate the presence of occult organic disease

      (3) Differentiate conditions with similar symptomatology—for example, angina pectoris (no change in ESR value) as opposed to a myocardial infarction (increase in ESR value)

B. WBCs (leukocytes)

1. The **WBC count** reports the number of WBCs in a cubic millimeter of whole blood.

   a. **Normal values** range from 4,000 to 11,000 WBC/mm^3.

   b. **Increased WBC count (leukocytosis)** usually signals infection; it may also result from leukemia or tissue necrosis. It is most often found with **bacterial infection.**

   c. **Decreased WBC count (leukopenia)** indicates bone marrow depression, which may result from metastatic carcinoma, lymphoma, or toxic reactions to substances such as antineoplastic agents.

2. The **WBC differential** evaluates the distribution and morphology of the five major types of WBCs: the **granulocytes** (**neutrophils, basophils, eosinophils**) and the **nongranulocytes** (**lymphocytes, monocytes**). A certain percentage of each type makes up the total WBC count (Table 38-1).

   a. **Neutrophils** may be mature or immature. Mature neutrophils are **polymorphonuclear leukocytes** (PMNs), also referred to as polys, segmented neutrophils, or segs; immature neutrophils are referred to as **bands** or stabs.

      (1) **Chemotaxis.** Neutrophils that **phagocytize and degrade many types of particles** serve as the body's first line of defense when tissue is damaged or foreign material gains entry. They congregate at sites in response to a specific stimulus, through a process known as chemotaxis.

      (2) **Neutrophilic leukocytosis.** This describes a response to an appropriate stimulus in which the total neutrophil count increases, often with an increase in the percentage

Table 38-1. Normal Percentage Values for White Blood Cell (WBC) Differential

Cell Type	Normal Range of Values (%)
Polymorphonuclear leukocytes	50–70
Bands	3–5
Lymphocytes	20–40
Monocytes	0–7
Eosinophils	0–5
Basophils	0–1

Table 38-2. Examples of Changes in Total White Blood Cell (WBC) Count and WBC Differential in Response to Bacterial Infection

Cell Type	WBC Count	
	Normal	**With Bacterial Infection**
Total WBCs	8,000 (100%)	15,500 (100%)
Neutrophils		
Polymorphonuclear leukocytes	60%	82%
Bands	3%	6%
Lymphocytes	30%	10%
Monocytes	4%	1%
Eosinophils	2%	1%
Basophils	1%	0%

of immature cells (**a shift to the left**). This may represent a systemic bacterial infection, such as pneumonia (Table 38-2).

    (a) Certain viruses (e.g., chickenpox, herpes zoster), some **rickettsial diseases** (e.g., Rocky Mountain spotted fever), some **fungi,** and **stress** (e.g., physical exercise, acute hemorrhage or hemolysis, acute emotional stress) may also cause this response.

    (b) Other causes include **inflammatory diseases** (e.g., acute rheumatic fever, rheumatoid arthritis, acute gout), **hypersensitivity reactions to drugs, tissue necrosis** (e.g., from myocardial infarction, burns, certain cancers), **metabolic disorders** (e.g., uremia, diabetic ketoacidosis), **myelogenous leukemia,** and **use of certain drugs** (e.g., epinephrine, lithium).

  (3) Neutropenia, a decreased number of neutrophils, may occur with an **overwhelming infection of any type** (bone marrow is unable to keep up with the demand). It may also occur with **certain viral infections** (e.g., mumps, measles), with **idiosyncratic drug reactions,** and as a result of chemotherapy. Neutropenia is defined as an absolute neutrophil count (ANC) of < 1000 cells/mm^3. Some define absolute neutropenia as an ANC of < 500 cells/mm^3. The ANC is calculated by multiplying the percent of neutrophils by the total WBC count:

WBC = 4000/mm^3
neutrophils = 60%
$$ANC = 4000 \times 0.6 = 2400 \text{ cells/mm}^3$$

 b. Basophils stain deeply with blue basic dye. Their function in the circulation is not clearly understood; in the tissues, they are referred to as **mast cells.**

  (1) Basophilia, an increased number of basophils, may occur with chronic myelogenous leukemia (CML) as well as other conditions.

  (2) A decrease in basophils is generally not apparent because of the small numbers of these cells in the blood.

 c. Eosinophils stain deep red with acid dye and are classically associated with immune reactions. **Eosinophilia,** an increased number of eosinophils, may occur with such conditions as **acute allergic reactions** (e.g., **asthma, hay fever, drug allergy**) and **parasitic infestations** (e.g., trichinosis, amebiasis).

 d. Lymphocytes play a dominant role in immunological activity and appear to produce antibodies. They are classified as B lymphocytes or T lymphocytes; T lymphocytes are further divided into helper-inducer cells (T_H4 cells) and suppressor cells (T_H8 cells).

  (1) Lymphocytosis, an increased number of lymphocytes, usually accompanies a normal or decreased total WBC count and is most commonly caused by **viral infection.**

  (2) Lymphopenia, a decreased number of lymphocytes, may result from **severe debilitating illness, immunodeficiency,** or from **AIDS,** which has a propensity to attack T_H4 cells.

  (3) Atypical lymphocytes (i.e., T lymphocytes in a state of immune activation) are classically associated with **infectious mononucleosis.**

e. **Monocytes** are phagocytic cells. **Monocytosis,** an increased number of monocytes, may occur with **tuberculosis (TB), subacute bacterial endocarditis,** and during the recovery phase of some **acute infections.**

C. **Platelets (thrombocytes).** These are the smallest formed elements in the blood, and they are involved in **blood clotting** and vital to the formation of a hemostatic plug after vascular injury.

1. **Normal values for a platelet count** are 150,000–300,000/mm^3 (1.5–3.0 $\times$ 10^{11}/L).

2. **Thrombocytopenia,** a decreased platelet count, can occur with a variety of conditions, such as idiopathic thrombocytopenic purpura or, occasionally, from such drugs as quinidine and sulfonamides.
   a. Thrombocytopenia is **moderate** when the platelet count is < 100,000/mm^3.
   b. Thrombocytopenia is **severe** when the platelet count is < 50,000/mm^3.

III. **COMMON SERUM ENZYME TESTS.** Small amounts of enzymes (catalysts) circulate in the blood at all times and are released into the blood in larger quantities when tissue damage occurs. Thus serum enzyme levels can be used to **aid in the diagnosis of certain diseases.**

A. **Creatine kinase (CK)**

1. Creatine kinase—formerly known as creatine phosphokinase (CPK)—is found primarily in heart muscle, skeletal muscle, and brain tissue.

2. CK levels are used primarily to **aid in the diagnosis of acute myocardial** (Figure 38-2) **or skeletal muscle damage.** However, vigorous exercise, a fall, or deep intramuscular injections can cause significant increases in CK levels.

3. The **isoenzymes** of CK—**CK-MM,** found in skeletal muscle; **CK-BB,** found in brain tissue; and **CK-MB,** found in heart muscle—can be used to differentiate the source of damage.
   a. Normally, serum CK levels are virtually all the **CK-MM isoenzyme.**
   b. Increase in **CK-MB** levels provides a sensitive indicator of myocardial necrosis.

Figure 38-2. The increase of serum creatine kinase (*CK*), lactate dehydrogenase (*LDH*), and aspartate aminotransferase (*AST*) levels after a myocardial infarction.

B. Lactate dehydrogenase (LDH)

1. LDH catalyzes the interconversion of lactate and pyruvate and represents a group of enzymes present in almost all metabolizing cells.

2. Five individual **isoenzymes** make up the total LDH serum level.
   a. **LDH$_1$** and **LDH$_2$** appear primarily in the heart.
   b. **LDH$_3$** appears primarily in the lungs.
   c. **LDH$_4$** and **LDH$_5$** appear primarily in the liver and skeletal muscles.

3. The distribution pattern of LDH isoenzymes may aid in diagnosing myocardial infarction, hepatic disease, and lung disease.

C. Alkaline phosphatase (ALP)

1. ALP is produced primarily in the **liver** and **bones.**

2. Serum ALP levels are **particularly sensitive to partial or mild biliary obstruction**—either extrahepatic (e.g., caused by a stone in the bile duct) or intrahepatic, both of which cause levels to increase.

3. **Increased osteoblastic activity,** as occurs in Paget disease, hyperparathyroidism, osteomalacia, and others, also increases serum ALP levels.

D. Aspartate aminotransferase (AST)

1. Aspartate aminotransferase—formerly known as **serum glutamic-oxaloacetic transaminase (SGOT)**—is found in a number of organs, primarily in heart and liver tissues and, to a lesser extent, in skeletal muscle, kidney tissue, and pancreatic tissue.

2. **Damage to the heart** (e.g., from **myocardial infarction**) results in increased AST levels about 8 hr after injury (Figure 38-2).
   a. Levels are **increased markedly** with **acute hepatitis;** they are **increased mildly** with **cirrhosis** and a **fatty liver.**
   b. Levels are also **increased** with **passive congestion of the liver,** such as occurs in congestive heart failure (CHF).

E. Alanine aminotransferase (ALT)

1. Alanine aminotransferase—formerly known as **serum glutamic-pyruvic transaminase (SGPT)**—is found in the liver, with lesser amounts in the heart, skeletal muscles, and kidney.

2. Although ALT values are **relatively specific for liver cell damage,** ALT is **less sensitive than AST,** and extensive or severe liver damage is necessary before abnormally increased levels are produced.

3. ALT also **increases less consistently and less markedly than AST after an acute myocardial infarction.**

F. Cardiac troponins (I, T, and C)

1. Troponins are a relatively new method to identify myocardial cell injury and thus assist in the diagnosis of acute myocardial infarction. These troponins may possess superior specificity in situations in which false-positive elevations of CK-MB are likely.

2. Troponin T is found in cardiac and skeletal muscle, troponin I is found only in cardiac muscle, and troponin C is present in two isoforms found in skeletal and cardiac muscle. Troponin T has shown prognostic value in unstable angina and in detecting minor myocardial cell injury with greater sensitivity than CK-MB.

3. The normal value for troponin T is < 0.1 ng/mL and I is < 1.5 ng/mL.

IV. LIVER FUNCTION TESTS

A. Liver enzymes

1. **Levels of certain enzymes** (e.g., LDH, ALP, AST, ALT) **increase with liver dysfunction** (see III).

2. These **enzyme tests indicate only that the liver has been damaged.** They do not assess the liver's ability to function. Other tests provide indications of liver dysfunction.

B. Serum bilirubin

1. Bilirubin, a breakdown product of Hb, is the **predominant pigment in bile.** Effective bilirubin conjugation and excretion depend on **hepatobiliary function** and on the **rate of RBC turnover.**

2. Serum bilirubin levels are reported as **total bilirubin** (conjugated and unconjugated) and as **direct bilirubin** (conjugated only).
   a. Bilirubin is released by Hb breakdown and is bound to albumin as water-insoluble **indirect bilirubin** (unconjugated bilirubin), which is not filtered by the glomerulus.
   b. **Unconjugated bilirubin** travels to the liver, where it is separated from albumin, conjugated with diglucuronide, and then actively secreted into the bile as **conjugated bilirubin** (direct bilirubin), which is filtered by the glomerulus (Figure 38-3).

3. **Normal values of total serum bilirubin** are 0.1–1.0 mg/dL (2–18 mmol/L); of **direct bilirubin,** 0.0–0.2 mg/dL (0–4 mmol/L).

4. **An increase in serum bilirubin** results in **jaundice** from bilirubin deposition in the tissues. There are three major causes of increased serum bilirubin.
   a. **Hemolysis** increases total bilirubin; direct bilirubin (conjugated) is usually normal or slightly increased. Urine color is normal, and no bilirubin is found in the urine.

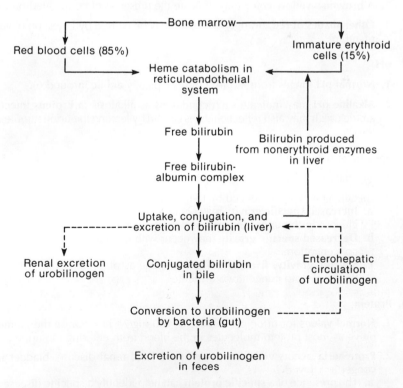

Figure 38-3. Bilirubin metabolism.

b. Biliary obstruction, which may be intrahepatic (as with a chlorpromazine reaction) or extrahepatic (as with a biliary stone), increases total bilirubin and direct bilirubin; intrahepatic cholestasis (e.g., from chlorpromazine) may increase direct bilirubin as well. Urine color is dark, and bilirubin is present in the urine.

c. Liver cell necrosis, as occurs in viral hepatitis, may cause an increase in both direct bilirubin (because inflammation causes some bile sinusoid blockage) and indirect bilirubin (because the liver's ability to conjugate is altered). Urine color is dark, and bilirubin is present in the urine.

C. Serum proteins

1. **Primary serum proteins** measured are **albumin** and the **globulins** (i.e., α, β, γ).
    a. **Albumin** (4.0–6.0 g/dL) maintains serum oncotic pressure and serves as a transport agent. Because it is primarily manufactured by the liver, liver disease can decrease albumin levels.
    b. **Globulins** (23–35 g/L) function as transport agents and play a role in certain immunological mechanisms. A decrease in albumin levels usually results in a compensatory increase in globulin production.

2. **Normal values** for total serum protein levels are 6.0–8.0 g/dL (60–80 g/L).

V. URINALYSIS.

Standard urinalysis provides basic information regarding renal function, urinary tract disease, and the presence of certain systemic diseases. Components of a standard urinalysis include appearance, pH, specific gravity, protein level, glucose level, ketone level, and microscopic examination.

A. Appearance. Normal urine is **clear** and ranges in color from **pale yellow to deep gold. Changes in color** can result from drugs, diet, or disease.

1. A **red color** may indicate, among other things, the presence of blood or phenolphthalein (a laxative).

2. A **brownish yellow color** may indicate the presence of conjugated bilirubin.

3. **Other shades of red, orange, or brown** may be caused by ingestion of various drugs (e.g., rifampin).

B. pH

1. **Normal pH** ranges from 4.5 to 9 but is typically **acidic** (around 6).

2. **Alkaline pH** may indicate such conditions as alkalosis, a **Proteus** infection, or acetazolamide use. It may also reflect changes caused by leaving the urine sample at room temperature.

C. Specific gravity

1. **Normal range** for specific gravity is 1.003–1.035; it is usually between 1.010 and 1.025.

2. Specific gravity is influenced by the number and nature of solute particles in the urine.
    a. **Increased specific gravity** may occur with such conditions as diabetes mellitus (excess glucose in the urine) or nephrosis (excess protein in the urine).
    b. **Decreased specific gravity** may occur with diabetes insipidus, which decreases urine concentration.
    c. **Specific gravity, fixed at 1.010** (the same as plasma), occurs when the kidneys lose their power to concentrate or dilute.

D. Protein

1. **Normal values** for urine protein are 50–80 mg/24 hr because the glomerular membrane prevents most protein molecules in the blood from entering the urine.

2. **Proteinuria** occurs with many conditions (e.g., renal disease, bladder infection, venous congestion, fever).
    a. The presence of a **specific protein** can help identify a specific disease state (e.g., Bence Jones protein may indicate multiple myeloma).

    b. Most often, the protein in urine is **albumin.** Albuminuria may indicate abnormal glomerular permeability.

E. Glucose

    1. The normal **renal threshold** for glucose is a blood glucose level of about 180 mg/dL; **glucose does not normally appear in urine** as detected by popular testing methods.

    2. Glycosuria usually indicates diabetes mellitus (DM). There are certain less common causes (e.g., a lowered renal threshold for glucose).

F. Ketones

    1. Ketones **do not normally appear in urine.** They are excreted when the body has used available glucose stores and begins to metabolize fat stores.

    2. The **three ketone bodies** are **β-hydroxybutyric acid** (80%), **acetoacetic acid** (about 20%), and acetone (a small percentage). Some commercial tests (e.g., Ames products) measure only acetoacetic acid, but usually all three are excreted in parallel proportions.

    3. Ketonuria usually indicates uncontrolled DM, but it may also occur with starvation and with zero- or low-carbohydrate diets.

G. Evaluation. Microscopic examination of centrifuged urine sediment normally reveals 0–1 RBC, 0–4 WBCs, and only an occasional cast per high-power field (HPF).

    1. Hematuria (i.e., the presence of RBCs) may indicate such conditions as trauma, a tumor, or a systemic bleeding disorder. In women, a significant number of **squamous cells** suggests vaginal contamination (menstruation).

    2. Casts (i.e., protein conglomerations outlining the shape of the renal tubules in which they were formed) may or may not be significant. Excessive numbers of certain types of casts indicate renal disease.

    3. Crystals, which are pH dependent, may occur normally in acid or alkaline urine. **Uric acid crystals** may form in acid urine; **phosphate crystals** may form in alkaline urine.

    4. Bacteria do not normally appear in urine. The finding of 50 or more bacteria per HPF may indicate a urinary tract infection (UTI); smaller values may indicate urethral contamination.

VI. COMMON RENAL FUNCTION TESTS

A. Introduction

    1. Renal function may be assessed by measuring **blood urea nitrogen (BUN)** and **serum creatinine.** Renal function decreases with age, which must be taken into account when interpreting test values.

        a. These tests primarily evaluate glomerular function by assessing the **glomerular filtration rate (GFR).**

        b. In many **renal diseases,** urea and creatinine accumulate in the blood because they are not excreted properly.

        c. These tests also aid in determining **drug dosage** for drugs excreted through the kidneys.

    2. Azotemia describes excessive retention of nitrogenous waste products (BUN and creatinine) in the blood. The clinical syndrome resulting from decreased renal function and azotemia is called **uremia.**

        a. Renal azotemia results from renal disease, such as glomerulonephritis and chronic pyelonephritis.

        b. Prerenal azotemia results from such conditions as severe dehydration, hemorrhagic shock, and excessive protein intake.

        c. Postrenal azotemia results from such conditions as ureteral or urethral stones or tumors and prostatic obstructions.

    3. Clearance—a theoretical concept defined as the volume of plasma from which a measured amount of substance can be completely eliminated, or cleared, into the urine per unit time—can be used to estimate glomerular function.

B. BUN

1. **Urea,** an end product of protein metabolism, is produced in the liver. From there, it travels through the blood and is excreted by the kidneys. Urea is **filtered at the glomerulus,** where the tubules reabsorb approximately 40%. Thus under normal conditions, **urea clearance** is about 60% of the true GFR.

2. **Normal values for BUN** range from 8 mg/dL to 18 mg/dL (3–6.5 mmol/L).
   a. **Decreased BUN levels** occur with **significant liver disease.**
   b. **Increased BUN levels** may indicate **renal disease.** However, factors other than glomerular function (e.g., protein intake, reduced renal blood flow, blood in the gastrointestinal tract) readily affect BUN levels, sometimes making interpretation of results difficult.

C. Serum creatinine

1. Creatinine (CR), the metabolic breakdown product of muscle creatine phosphate, has a relatively constant level of daily production. Blood levels vary little in a given individual.

2. Creatinine is **excreted** by glomerular filtration and tubular secretion. **Creatinine clearance** parallels the GFR within a range of ± 10% and is a **more sensitive indicator of renal damage than BUN levels** because renal impairment is almost the only cause of an increase in the serum creatinine level.

3. **Normal values for serum creatinine** range from 0.6 to 1.2 mg/dL (50 to 110 mmol/L).
   a. Values vary with the **amount of muscle mass**—a value of 1.2 mg/dL in a muscular athlete may represent normal renal function, whereas the same value in a small, sedentary person with little muscle mass may indicate significant renal impairment.
   b. Generally, the **serum creatinine value doubles with each 50% decrease in GFR.** For example, if a patient's normal serum creatinine is 1 mg/dL, 1 mg/dL represents 100% renal function, 2 mg/dL represents 50% function, and 4 mg/dL represents 25% function.

D. Creatinine clearance

1. Creatinine clearance, which represents the **rate at which creatinine is removed from the blood by the kidneys,** roughly approximates the GFR.
   a. The value is given in units of milliliters per minute, representing the volume of blood cleared of creatinine by the kidney per minute.
   b. **Normal values** for men range from 75 to 125 mL/min.

2. Calculation requires knowledge of **urinary creatinine excretion** (usually over 24 hr) and concurrent **serum creatinine levels. Creatinine clearance is calculated** as follows:

$$Cl_{CR} = \frac{C_U V}{C_{CR}}$$

where Cl_{CR} is the creatinine clearance in milliliters per minute, C_U is the concentration of creatinine in the urine, V is the volume of urine (in milliliters per minute of urine formed over the collection period), and C_{CR} is the serum creatinine concentration.

3. Suppose the serum creatinine concentration is 1 mg/dL, and 1440 mL of urine was collected in 24 hr (1440 min) for a urine volume of 1 mL/min. The urine contains 100 mg/dL of creatinine. Creatinine clearance is calculated as:

$$\frac{100 \text{ mg/mL} \times 1 \text{ mL/min}}{1 \text{ mg/dL}} = 100 \text{ mL/min}$$

4. Incomplete bladder emptying and other problems may interfere with obtaining an accurate timed urine specimen. Thus **estimations of creatinine clearance** may be necessary. These estimations require only a serum creatinine value. One estimation uses the method of **Cockroft and Gault,** which is based on body weight, age, and gender.
   a. This formula provides an **estimated value,** calculated for **males** as:

$$Cl_{CR} = \frac{[140 - \text{age (in years)}] \times \text{body weight (in kg)}}{72 \times C_{CR} \text{ (in mg/dL)}}$$

   b. For **females,** use 0.85 of the value calculated for males.

c. Example: A 20-year-old man weighing 72 kg has a C_{CR} of 1.0 mg/dL; thus

$$C_{CR} = \frac{(140 - 20 \text{ years}) \times 72 \text{ kg}}{72 \times 1 \text{ mg/mL}} = 120 \text{ mL/min}$$

5. Determination of GFR. The modified diet in renal disease (MDRD) equation is considered a more accurate measurement of GFR than other equations used to estimate renal function (e.g., Cockcroft-Gault) in patients with *reduced* GFR and is used in staging renal disease. Patients must have a serum creatinine concentration.

   a. The MDRD equation for **males** is as follows:

$$\text{GFR} = 186 \, (\text{Pcr})^{-1.154} \times \text{age}^{-0.203}$$

   where Pcr is serum creatinine. For **females,** multiply the result by 0.742; for **African Americans,** multiply by 1.210.

   b. The MDRD has been validated in Caucasians, patients with diabetic kidney disease, kidney transplant recipients, and African Americans and Asians with nondiabetic kidney disease.

   c. The MDRD equation has *not* been validated in patients < 18 years of age, pregnant women, patients > 70 years of age, other ethnic groups, patients with normal kidney function who are at an increased risk for chronic kidney disease, and patients with normal renal function.

   d. Many institutions are routinely reporting an MDRD-derived GFR estimation for patients as a routine component of a blood chemistry study. This value should be used to assist the clinician in staging a patient's degree of renal dysfunction and is not a substitute for creatinine clearance as estimated by the Cockroft and Gault equation, which should be used for drug dosing in renal impairment. The MDRD estimate has not been evaluated for the purpose of drug dosing.

VII. ELECTROLYTES

A. Sodium (Na)

   1. Sodium is the major cation of the **extracellular** fluid. Sodium along with chloride (Cl), potassium (K), and water is important in the regulation of osmotic pressure and water balance between intracellular and extracellular fluids. **Normal values** are 135–147 mEq/L or mmol/L.

   2. The sodium concentration is defined as the ratio of sodium to water, not the absolute amounts of either. Laboratory tests for sodium are used mainly to detect disturbances in water balance and body osmolality. The kidneys are the major organs of sodium and water balance.

   3. An increase in sodium concentration (**hypernatremia**) may indicate impaired sodium excretion or dehydration. A decrease in sodium concentration (hyponatremia) may reflect overhydration, abnormal sodium loss, or decreased sodium intake.

   4. Patients with kidney, heart, or pulmonary disease may have difficulty with sodium and water balance. In adults, changes in sodium concentrations most often reflect changes in water balance, not salt imbalances. Therefore, sodium concentration is often used as an indicator of fluid status, rather than salt imbalance.

   5. Control of sodium by the body is accomplished mainly through the hormones aldosterone and antidiuretic hormone (ADH).

   a. ADH is released from the pituitary gland in response to signals from the hypothalamus. ADH's presence in the distal tubules and collecting ducts of the kidney causes them to become more permeable to the reabsorption of water; therefore, concentrating urine.

   b. Aldosterone affects the distal tubular reabsorption of sodium as opposed to water. Aldosterone is released from the adrenal cortex in response to low sodium, high potassium, low blood volume, and angiotensin II. Aldosterone causes the spilling of potassium from the distal tubules into the urine in exchange for sodium reabsorption.

   6. Hyponatremia is usually related to total body depletion of sodium—as in mineralocorticoid deficiencies, sodium-wasting renal disease, replacement of fluid loss with nonsaline solutions, gastrointestinal (GI) losses, renal losses, or loss of sodium through the skin—or to dilution of serum sodium—as in cirrhosis, CHF, nephrosis, renal failure, excess water intake, or syndrome of inappropriate antidiuretic hormone (SIADH) secretion.

7. **Hypernatremia** usually results from a loss of free water or hypotonic fluid or through excessive sodium intake. Free water loss is most often associated with diabetes insipidus, but fluid loss can be via the GI tract, renal, skin, or respiratory systems. Excess sodium intake can occur through the administration of hypertonic intravenous (IV) solutions, mineralocorticoid excess, excessive sodium ingestion, or after administration of drugs high in sodium content [e.g., ticarcillin, sodium bicarbonate [HCO_3^-]).

B. Potassium (K)

1. Potassium is the most abundant **intracellular** cation (intracellular fluid potassium averages 141 mEq/L). Approximately 3500 mEq of potassium is contained in the body of a 70-kg adult. Only 10% of the body's potassium is extracellular. Normal values are 3.5–5.0 mEq/L or mmol/L.

2. The serum potassium concentration is not an adequate measure of the total body potassium because most of the body's potassium is intracellular. Fortunately, the clinical signs and symptoms of potassium deficiency—malaise, confusion, dizziness, electrocardiogram (ECG) changes, muscle weakness, and pain—correlate well with serum concentrations. The serum potassium concentration is buffered by the body and may be "normal" despite total body potassium loss. Potassium depletion causes a shift of intracellular potassium to the extracellular fluid to maintain potassium concentrations. There is approximately a 100 mEq total body potassium deficit when the serum potassium concentration decreases by 0.3 mEq/L. This may result in misinterpretation of serum potassium concentrations as they relate to total body potassium.

3. The role or function of potassium is in the maintenance of proper electrical conduction in cardiac and skeletal muscles (muscle and nerve excitability), it exerts an influence on the body's water balance (intracellular volume) and plays a role in acid–base equilibrium.

4. Potassium is regulated by:
   a. Kidneys (renal function)
   b. Aldosterone
   c. Arterial pH
   d. Insulin
   e. Potassium intake
   f. Sodium delivery to distal tubules

5. **Hypokalemia** can occur. The kidneys are responsible for approximately 90% of the daily potassium loss. Other losses occur mainly through the GI system. Even in states of no potassium intake, the kidneys still excrete up to 20 mEq of potassium daily. Therefore, prolonged periods of potassium deprivation can result in hypokalemia. Hypokalemia can also result from potassium loss through vomiting or diarrhea, nasogastric suction, laxative abuse, and by diuretic use (mannitol, thiazides, or loop diuretics). Excessive mineralocorticoid activity and glucosuria can also result in hypokalemia. Potassium can be shifted into cells with alkalemia and after administration of glucose and insulin.

6. **Hyperkalemia** most commonly results from decreased renal elimination, excessive intake, or from cellular breakdown (tissue damage, hemolysis, burns, infections). Metabolic acidosis may also result in a shift of potassium extracellularly as hydrogen ions move into cells and are exchanged for potassium and sodium ions. As a general guideline, for every 0.1 unit pH change from 7.4, the potassium concentration will change by about 0.6 mEq/L. If a patient has a pH of 7.1 and a measured potassium of 4.5 mEq/L, the actual potassium concentration would be

$$0.3 \text{ (units less than 7.4)} \times 0.6 = 1.8$$
$$\text{Potassium concentration} = 4.5 - 1.8 = 2.7 \text{ mEq/L}$$

Correction of the acidosis in this situation will result in a dramatic decrease in potassium unless supplementation is instituted.

C. Chloride (Cl)

1. Chloride is the major anion of the extracellular fluid and is important in the maintenance of acid–base balance. Alterations in the serum chloride concentration are rarely a primary indicator of major medical problems. Chloride itself is not of primary diagnostic significance. It is usually measured to confirm the serum sodium concentration. The relationship among sodium, chloride, and HCO_3^- is described by the following:

$$Cl^- + HCO_3^- + R = Na^+$$

where R is the anion gap. The **normal value** for Cl is 95–105 mEq/L or mmol/L.

2. **Hypochloremia** is a decreased chloride concentration, and it is often accompanied by metabolic alkalosis or acidosis caused by organic or other acids. Other causes include chronic renal failure, adrenal insufficiency, fasting, prolonged diarrhea, severe vomiting, and diuretic therapy.

3. **Hyperchloremia** is an increased chloride concentration that may indicate hyperchloremic metabolic acidosis. Hyperchloremia in the absence of metabolic acidosis is unusual because chloride retention is often accompanied by sodium and water retention. Other causes include acute renal failure, dehydration, and excess chloride administration.

D. Bicarbonate ([HCO$_3$)/carbon dioxide (CO$_2$) content

1. The carbon dioxide (CO_2) content represents the sum of the bicarbonate (HCO_3^-) concentration and the concentration of CO_2 dissolved in the serum. The HCO_3^-/CO_2 system is the most important buffering system to maintain pH within physiological limits. Most disturbances of acid–base balance can be considered in terms of this system. Normal values are 22–28 mEq/L or mmol/L.

2. The relationship among this system is defined as follows:

$$HCO_3^- + H^+ \times H_2CO_3 \times H_2O + CO_2$$

(bicarbonate ions bind hydrogen ions to form carbonic acid). Clinically, the serum HCO_3^- concentration is measured because acid–base balance can be inferred if the patient has normal pulmonary function.

3. **Hypobicarbonatemia** is usually caused by metabolic acidosis, renal failure, hyperventilation, severe diarrhea, drainage of intestinal fluid, and by drugs such as acetazolamide. Toxicity caused by salicylates, methanol, and ethylene glycol can also decrease the HCO_3^- level.

4. **Hyperbicarbonatemia** is usually caused by alkalosis, hypoventilation, pulmonary disease, persistent vomiting, excess HCO_3^- intake with poor renal function, and diuretics.

VIII. MINERALS

A. Calcium (Ca)

1. Calcium plays an important role in nerve impulse transmission, muscle contraction, pancreatic insulin release, hydrogen ion release from the stomach, as a cofactor for some enzyme reactions and blood coagulation, and most important bone and tooth structural integrity. Normal total calcium values are 8.8–10.3 mg/dL or 2.20–2.56 mmol/L.

2. The total calcium content of normal adults is 20–25 g/kg of fat-free tissue, and about 44% of this calcium is in the body skeleton. Approximately 1% of skeletal calcium is freely exchangeable with that of the extracellular fluid. The reservoir of calcium in bones maintains the concentration of calcium in the plasma constant. About 40% of the calcium in the extracellular fluid is bound to plasma proteins (especially albumin), 5%–15% is complexed with phosphate and citrate, and 45%–55% is in the unbound, ionized form. Most laboratories measure the total calcium concentration; however, it is the free, ionized calcium that is important physiologically. Ionized calcium levels may be obtained from the laboratory. Clinically, the most important determinant of ionized calcium is the amount of serum protein (albumin) available for binding. The normal serum calcium range is for

a serum albumin of 4 g/dL. A good approximation is that for every 1 g/dL decrease in albumin, 0.8 g/dL should be added to the calcium laboratory result. Doing this corrects the total plasma concentration to reflect the additional amount of free (active) calcium.

3. **Hypocalcemia** usually implies a deficiency in either the production or response to parathyroid hormone (PTH) or vitamin D. PTH abnormalities include hypoparathyroidism, pseudohypoparathyroidism, or hypomagnesemia. Vitamin D abnormalities can be caused by decreased nutritional intake, decreased absorption of vitamin D, a decrease in production, or an increase in metabolism. Administration of loop diuretics causing diuresis can also decrease serum calcium.

4. **Hypercalcemia** is an increased calcium concentration, and it is usually associated with malignancy or metastatic diseases. Other causes include hyperparathyroidism, Paget disease, milk-alkali syndrome, granulomatous disorders, thiazide diuretics, excessive calcium intake, or vitamin D intoxication.

B. Phosphate (PO_4)

1. Phosphate is a major intracellular anion and is the source of phosphate for adenosine triphosphate (ATP) and phospholipid synthesis. Serum calcium and PO_4 are influenced by many of the same factors. It is useful to consider calcium and PO_4 together when interpreting lab results. Normal PO_4 values are 2.5–5.0 mg/dL or 0.80–1.60 mmol/L.

2. **Hyperphosphatemia** and **hypophosphatemia** can occur. The extracellular fluid concentration of phosphate is influenced by PTH, intestinal absorption, renal function, nutrition, and bone metabolism. Hyperphosphatemia is usually caused by renal insufficiency, although increased vitamin D or phosphate intake, hypoparathyroidism, and hyperthyroidism are also causes. Hypophosphatemia can occur in malnutrition, especially when anabolism is induced, after administration of aluminum-containing antacids or calcium acetate, in chronic alcoholics, and in septic patients. Hyperparathyroidism and insufficient vitamin D intake can also induce hypophosphatemia.

C. Magnesium (Mg)

1. Magnesium is the second most abundant intracellular and extracellular cation. It is an activator of numerous enzyme systems that control carbohydrate, fat and electrolyte metabolism, protein synthesis, nerve conduction, muscular contractility, as well as membrane transport and integrity. Normal values are 1.6–2.4 mEq/L or 0.80–1.20 mmol/L.

2. **Hypomagnesemia** and **hypermagnesemia** can occur. **Hypomagnesemia** is found more often than hypermagnesemia. Depletion of magnesium usually results from excessive loss from the GI tract or the kidneys. Depletion can occur from either poor intestinal absorption or excessive GI fluid loss. Signs and symptoms include weakness, muscle fasciculations with tremor, tetany, and increased reflexes. Decreased intracardiac magnesium may manifest as an increased QT interval with an increased risk of arrhythmia. **Hypermagnesemia** is most commonly caused by increased magnesium intake in the setting of renal insufficiency. Other causes include excess magnesium intake, hepatitis, and Addison disease. Signs and symptoms of hypermagnesemia include bradycardia, flushing, sweating, nausea and vomiting, decreased calcium level, decreased deep-tendon reflexes, flaccid paralysis, increased pulse rate and QRS intervals, respiratory distress, and asystole.

STUDY QUESTIONS

Directions for questions 1–16: Each of the questions, statements, or incomplete statements in this section can be correctly answered or completed by **one** of the suggested answers or phrases. Choose the **best** answer.

1. Hematological testing of a patient with AIDS is most likely to show which of the following abnormalities?

(A) basophilia
(B) eosinophilia
(C) lymphopenia
(D) reticulocytosis
(E) agranulocytosis

2. Hematological studies are most likely to show a low reticulocyte count in a patient who has which of the following abnormalities?

(A) aplastic anemia secondary to cancer chemotherapy
(B) acute hemolytic anemia secondary to quinidine treatment
(C) severe bleeding secondary to an automobile accident
(D) iron-deficiency anemia 1 week after treatment with ferrous sulfate
(E) megaloblastic anemia owing to folate deficiency 1 week after treatment with folic acid

3. All of the following findings on a routine urinalysis would be considered normal *except* which one?

(A) pH: 6.5
(B) glucose: negative
(C) ketones: negative
(D) white blood cells (WBCs): 3 per high-power field (HPF), no casts
(E) red blood cells (RBCs): 5 per HPF

4. A 12-year-old boy is treated for otitis media with cefaclor (Ceclor). On the 7th day of therapy, he spikes a fever and develops an urticarial rash on his trunk. Which of the following laboratory tests could best confirm the physician's suspicion of a hypersensitivity (allergic) reaction?

(A) complete blood count (CBC) and differential
(B) serum hemoglobin (Hb) and reticulocyte count
(C) liver function test profile
(D) lactate dehydrogenase (LDH) isoenzyme profile
(E) red blood cell (RBC) count and serum bilirubin

5. An increased hematocrit (Hct) is a likely finding in all of the following individuals *except* which one?

(A) a man who has just returned from a 3-week skiing trip in the Colorado Rockies
(B) a woman who has polycythemia vera
(C) a hospitalized patient who mistakenly received 5 L of intravenous (IV) dextrose 5% in water (D_5W) over the last 24 hr
(D) a man who has been rescued from the Arizona desert after spending 4 days without water
(E) a woman who has chronic obstructive pulmonary disease

6. A 29-year-old white man is seen in the emergency room. His white blood cell (WBC) count is 14,200 with 80% polys. All of the following conditions could normally produce these laboratory findings *except* which one?

(A) a localized bacterial infection on the tip of the index finger
(B) acute bacterial pneumonia caused by *Streptococcus pneumoniae*
(C) a heart attack
(D) a gunshot wound to the abdomen with a loss of 2 pints of blood
(E) an attack of gout

7. A 52-year-old male construction worker who drinks "fairly heavily" when he gets off work is seen in the emergency room with, among other abnormal laboratory results, an increased creatine kinase (CK) level. All of the following circumstances could explain this increase *except* which one?

(A) he fell against the bumper of his car in a drunken stupor and bruised his right side
(B) he is showing evidence of some liver damage owing to the heavy alcohol intake
(C) he has experienced a heart attack
(D) he received an intramuscular (IM) injection a few hours before the blood sample was drawn
(E) he pulled a muscle that day when lifting a heavy concrete slab

8. A 45-year-old man with jaundice has spillage of bilirubin into his urine. All of the following statements could apply to this patient *except* which one?

(A) His total bilirubin is increased.
(B) His direct bilirubin is increased.
(C) He may have viral hepatitis.
(D) He may have hemolytic anemia.
(E) He may have cholestatic hepatitis.

For questions 9–11: A 70-year-old black man weighing 154 lb. complains of chronic fatigue. Several laboratory tests were performed with the following results:

blood urea nitrogen (BUN)	15 mg/dL
aspartate aminotransferase (AST)	within normal limits
white blood cell (WBC) count	7500/mm³
red blood cell (RBC) count	4.0 million/mm³
hematocrit (Hct)	29%
hemoglobin (Hb)	9.0 g/dL

9. This patient's mean cell hemoglobin concentration (MCHbC) is

(A) 27.5.
(B) 28.9.
(C) 31.0.
(D) 33.5.
(E) 35.4.

10. His mean cell volume (MCV) is

(A) 61.3.
(B) 72.5.
(C) 77.5.
(D) 90.2.
(E) 93.5.

11. From the data provided and from the calculations in questions 9 and 10, this patient is best described as

(A) normal except for a slightly increased blood urea nitrogen (BUN).
(B) having normochromic, microcytic anemia.
(C) having sickle-cell anemia.
(D) having hypochromic, normocytic anemia.
(E) having folic acid deficiency.

12. All of the following statements about sodium (Na) are true *except* which one?

(A) The normal range for sodium is 135–147 mEq/L.
(B) Sodium is the major cation of the extracellular fluid, and the laboratory test is used mainly to detect disturbances in water balance.
(C) Hyponatremia usually results from the total body depletion of sodium or through a dilutional effect.
(D) Control of the sodium concentration is mainly through regulation of arterial pH.

13. A 53-year-old woman with diabetes mellitus is seen in the emergency room. Her blood glucose is 673 mg/dL and ketones are present in her blood. A diagnosis of diabetic ketoacidosis (DKA) is made. Other important laboratory values are potassium of 4.8 mEq/L, 4+ glucose in urine, and an arterial pH of 7.1. All of the following statements apply to this patient *except* which one?

(A) Her potassium value is normal; therefore, no potassium supplementation is likely to be necessary.
(B) Her potassium value should be corrected owing to her acidosis; a corrected potassium would be 3.0 mEq/L.
(C) Potassium supplementation should be instituted because her total body potassium is depleted.
(D) Factors affecting potassium in this patient include glycosuria and arterial pH.

14. A 50-year-old man presents with bicarbonate of 18 mEq/L. All of the following could be a cause of his low bicarbonate level *except*

(A) metabolic acidosis.
(B) salicylate toxicity.
(C) diuretic therapy.
(D) diarrhea.

15. All of the following statements about calcium (Ca) and phosphorus (PO_4) are true *except* which one?

(A) An alcoholic with a serum albumin of 2 g/dL and a serum total calcium of 8.0 mg/dL has a corrected total calcium of 9.6 mg/dL.
(B) Calcium and PO_4 levels should be interpreted together because many of the same factors influence both minerals.
(C) Metastatic cancer often induces a decrease in serum calcium levels
(D) A patient with renal failure may present with hypocalcemia and hyperphosphatemia.

16. All of the following are important functions of magnesium (Mg) *except*

(A) nerve conduction.
(B) phospholipid synthesis.
(C) muscle contractility.
(D) carbohydrate, fat, and electrolyte metabolism.

Directions for questions 17–19: The questions and incomplete statements in this section can be correctly answered or completed by **one or more** of the suggested answers. Choose the answer, **A–E.**

A	if **I only** is correct
B	if **III only** is correct
C	if **I and II** are correct
D	if **II and III** are correct
E	if **I, II, and III** are correct

17. Factors likely to cause an increase in the blood urea nitrogen (BUN) level include

I. intramuscular (IM) injection of diazepam (Valium).
II. severe liver disease.
III. chronic kidney disease.

18. A patient who undergoes serum enzyme testing is found to have an increased aspartate aminotransferase (AST) level. Possible underlying causes of this abnormality include

I. methyldopa-induced hepatitis.
II. congestive heart failure (CHF).
III. pneumonia.

19. Serum enzyme tests that may aid in the diagnosis of myocardial infarction include

I. alkaline phosphatase.
II. creatine kinase (CK).
III. lactate dehydrogenase (LDH).

ANSWERS AND EXPLANATIONS

1. The answer is C *[see II.B.2.d.(2)].*
Valuable diagnostic information can be obtained through quantitative and qualitative testing of the cells of the blood. A finding of lymphopenia (i.e., decreased number of lymphocytes) suggests an attack on the immune system or some underlying immunodeficiency. AIDS attacks the T_H4 population of lymphocytes and thus may result in lymphopenia.

2. The answer is A *[see II.A.5].*
The reticulocyte count measures the amount of circulating immature RBCs, which provides information about bone marrow function. A low reticulocyte count is a likely finding in a patient with aplastic anemia—a disorder characterized by a deficiency of all cellular elements of the blood owing to a lack of hematopoietic stem cells in bone marrow. A variety of drugs (e.g., those used in anticancer therapy) and other agents produce marrow aplasia. A high reticulocyte count would likely be found in a patient with hemolytic anemia or acute blood loss or in a patient who has been treated for an iron, vitamin B_{12}, or folate deficiency.

3. The answer is E *[see V.B; V.E–G].*
Microscopic examination of the urine sediment normally shows < 1 RBC and from 0 to 4 WBCs per HPF. Other normal findings on urinalysis include an acid pH (i.e., around 6) and an absence of glucose and ketones.

4. The answer is A *[see II.B.2.c].*
An allergic drug reaction will usually produce an increase in the eosinophil count (eosinophilia). This could be determined by ordering a WBC differential.

5. The answer is C *[see II.A.2].*
Overhydration with an excess infusion of D_5W produces a low Hct. The other situations described in the question result in increases of the Hct.

6. The answer is A *[see II.B.2.a].*
The patient has leukocytosis with an increased neutrophil count (neutrophilia). A localized infection does not normally result in an increase in the total leukocyte count or neutrophil count. The other situations given in the question can produce a neutrophilic leukocytosis.

7. The answer is B *[see III.A].*
Because CK is not present in the liver, alcoholic liver damage would not result in an increase in the level of this enzyme. CK is present primarily in cardiac and skeletal muscle. The other situations described in the question could all result in the release of increased amounts of CK into the bloodstream.

8. The answer is D *[see IV.B].*
The patient with jaundice (deposition of bilirubin in the skin) usually has an increase in the total bilirubin serum level. Spillage of bilirubin into the urine requires an increased level of direct bilirubin, which is likely with viral hepatitis or cholestatic hepatitis. In hemolytic anemia, direct bilirubin is not usually increased, and therefore, there would be no spillage of bilirubin into the urine.

9. The answer is C *[see II.A.4.c]*

10. The answer is B *[see II.A.4.a]*

11. The answer is B *[see II.A.4; CI.B.2]*
The MCHbC is calculated as follows:

$$\text{MCHbC} = \frac{\text{Hb} \times 100}{\text{Hct}} = \frac{9 \times 100}{29} = 31.0$$

The mean cell volume (MCV) is calculated as follows:

$$\text{MCV} = \frac{\text{Hct (\%)} \times 10}{\text{RBC (millions)}} = \frac{29 \times 10}{4} = 72.5$$

The patient described in the question is anemic because his Hb is 9 (normal: 14–18). The anemia is normochromic because the patient's MCHbC of 31 is normal (normal range: 31–37), but the anemia is microcytic because the patient's MCV is 72.5 (normal: 80–100). The patient's BUN, 15 mg/dL, is within the normal range of 10–20 mg/dL.

12. The answer is D *[see VII.A.1; VII.A.5–7].*
Sodium, the major extracellular cation, is measured mainly to assist in the determination of fluid status and water balance. Regulation of sodium is mainly through the kidneys via aADH and aldosterone.

13. The answer is A *[see VII.B.2; VII.B.4; VII.B.6].*
A "normal" potassium level in the setting of metabolic acidosis, especially in a patient with DKA should be treated appropriately. If the serum potassium level is corrected for the patient's acidosis, the corrected level is 3.0 mEq/L. This corresponds to a depletion in total body potassium stores. Once the acidosis and hyperglycemia begin to correct with appropriate treatment, potassium levels will decrease precipitously unless supplementation is begun. It is important to recognize that a laboratory value in the "normal" range may not actually be normal, especially when potassium is involved.

14. The answer is C *[see VII.D.3–4].*
Low HCO_3^- is usually found in patients with acidosis or renal failure and after hyperventilation or severe diarrhea. In general, disturbances in acid–base balance cause alteration in the serum HCO_3^- or CO_2 content. Diuretic therapy can cause an alkalosis and an increase in HCO_3^-.

15. The answer is C *[see VIII.A.2–4; B.2].*
Malignancy or other metastatic diseases are most often associated with hypercalcemia, not hypocalcemia. Ionized calcium is the free active form, and this level is increased in the setting of a low albumin. Therefore, the total calcium level must be adjusted to account for an increased ionized calcium in this setting. Both minerals are influenced by many of the same factors and thus are often interpreted together. Renal function is one such factor whereby a decrease in renal function (i.e., renal failure) can result in a low level of calcium and a high level of PO_4.

16. The answer is B *[see VIII.C.1].*
Magnesium is the second most abundant intracellular and extracellular cation. It is an activator of numerous enzyme systems that control carbohydrate, fat, and electrolyte metabolism, protein synthesis, nerve conduction, muscular contractility, as well as membrane transport and integrity. PO_4, on the other hand, is important for ATP and phospholipid synthesis.

17. The answer is B (III) *[see VI.B.2].*
Chronic kidney disease can cause an increase in the BUN level; a heavy protein diet and bleeding into the GI tract are other factors that can produce this finding. Severe liver disease can prevent the formation of urea and, therefore, is likely to cause a decrease in the BUN level. Although an IM injection of diazepam (Valium) may cause an increase in the serum CK or AST level, it would have no effect on the BUN.

18. The answer is C (I, II) *[see III.D].*
A lung infection, such as pneumonia, normally would not cause an increase in the release of AST, an enzyme primarily found in the liver and heart. In acute hepatitis, a marked increase of AST is a likely finding. AST levels also can be increased with passive congestion of the liver, as occurs in CHF.

19. The answer is D (II, III) *[see III.A–C].*
Usually, the CK, aALT, AST, and LDH enzyme levels are increased after a myocardial infarction. Alkaline phosphatase is not present in cardiac tissue and, therefore, would not be useful in the diagnosis of a myocardial infarction.

39
Coronary Artery Disease

Alan H. Mutnick

Barbara Szymusiak-Mutnick

I. INTRODUCTION

A. **Definition. Coronary artery disease (CAD)** is a general term that refers to a number of diseases other than atherosclerosis, which causes a narrowing of the major epicardial coronary arteries. **Ischemic heart disease (IHD)** is a form of heart disease with primary manifestations that result from myocardial ischemia owing to atherosclerotic CAD. This term encompasses a spectrum of conditions, ranging from the asymptomatic preclinical phase to acute myocardial infarction and sudden cardiac death, and is used throughout the chapter.

B. **Incidence**

1. IHD continues to be the leading single cause of death in the United States (231.1–297.9 deaths per 100,000); cancer is the second leading cause of death (159.1–228.1 deaths per 100,000).

2. Each year more than 5 million patients present to emergency rooms with chest discomfort and related symptoms, and approximately 1.5 million are hospitalized for acute coronary syndromes. Each year in the United States, more than 1 million patients suffer an acute myocardial infarction (MI).

C. **Economics.** Based on models evaluating the costs associated with the treatment of Medicare patients with common IHD-related diagnosis, it has been estimated that the direct costs of hospitalization are > \$15 billion yearly, with an additional \$4.5 billion yearly in diagnostic procedures.

D. **Clinical guidelines.** Owing to the clinical, humanistic, and economic effect that IDH has in the United States, evidenced-based practice guidelines have evolved based on the differences in the diagnosis and management of IHD. The authors of this chapter have relied heavily on the use of those guidelines to ensure the most up-to-date recommendations based on the clinical literature. Guidelines that are pertinent to daily pharmacy practice include the following:

1. Gibbons RJ, Abrams J, Chatterjee K, Daley J, Deedwania PC, Douglas JS, Ferguson TB Jr, Fihn SD, Fraker TD Jr., Gardin JM, O'Rourke RA, Pasternak RC, Williams SV. ACC/AHA 2002 guideline update for management of patients with chronic stable angina: a report of the American College of Cardiology/American Heart Association Task Force on Practice Guidelines (Committee to Update the 1999 Guidelines for the Management of Patients with Chronic Stable Angina). 2002. J Am Coll Cardiol 2003; 41:159–168. Available at www.acc.org/clinical/guide lines/stable/stable.pdf.

2. Braunwald E, Antman EM, Beasley JW, Califf RM, Cheitlin MD, Hochman JS, Jones RH, Kereiakes D, Kupersmith J, Levin TN, Pepine CJ, Schaeffer JW, Smith EE III, Steward DE, Theroux P. ACC/AHA 2002 guideline update for management of patients with unstable angina and non-ST-segment elevation myocardial infarction: a report of the American College of Cardiology/American Heart Association Task Force on Practice Guidelines (Committee on the Management of Patients with Unstable Angina). 2002. J Am Coll Cardiol 2002; 40:366–374. Available at: http://www.acc.org/clinical/guidelines/unstable/ incorporated/index.htm.

3. Implications of Recent Clinical Trials for the National Cholesterol Education Program, Adult Treatment Panel III Guidelines for the Coordinating Committee of the National Cholesterol Education Program. Scott M. Grundy, James I. Cleeman, C. Noel Bairey Merz, H. Bryan Brewer, Jr, Luther T. Clark, Donald B. Hunninghake*, Richard C. Pasternak, Sidney C. Smith, Jr, Neil J. Stone, J Am Coll Cardiol 2004; 44:720–732.

4. National Cholesterol Education Program (NCEP). Third report of the National Cholesterol Education Program (NCEP): Detection, evaluation, and treatment of high blood cholesterol in adults (Adult Treatment Panel III). Final Report [NIH Publication 02–5215]. Bethesda, MD:

National Institutes of Health, 2002. Available at www.nhlbi.nih.gov/guidelines/cholesterol/atp3full.pdfC.

5. Antman EM, Anbe DT, Armstrong PW, Bates ER, Green LA, Hand M, Hochman JS, Kumholz HM, Kushner FG, Lamas GA, Mullany CJ, Ornato JP, Pearle DL, Sloan MA, Smith SC Jr. ACC/AHA guidelines for the management of patients with ST-elevation myocardial infarction: executive summary: a report of the ACC/AHA Task Force on Practice Guidelines (Committee to Revise the 1999 Guidelines on the Management of Patients With Acute Myocardial Infarction). J Am Coll Cardiol 2004; 44:671–719. Available at http://www.acc.org/qualityandscience/clinical/guidelines/stemi/exec_summ/index.htm.

6. W. Brian Gibler, Christopher P. Cannon, Andra L. Blomkalns, Douglas M. Char, Barbara J. Drew, Judd E. Hollander, Allan S. Jaffe, Robert L. Jesse, L. Kristin Newby, E. Magnus Ohman, Eric D. Peterson, and Charles V. Pollack. Practical implementation of the guidelines for unstable angina/non-ST-segment elevation myocardial infarction in the emergency department: a scientific statement from the American Heart Association Council on Clinical Cardiology (Subcommittee on Acute Cardiac Care), Council on Cardiovascular Nursing, and Quality of Care and Outcomes Research Interdisciplinary Working Group, in Collaboration With the Society of Chest Pain Centers. Circulation, May 2005; 111:2699–2710. Available at http://circ.ahajournals.org/cgi/citemap?id=circulationaha;111/20/2699.

E. Manifestations

1. **Angina pectoris,** an episodic, reversible oxygen insufficiency, is the most common form of IHD (see II).

2. The term **acute ischemic (coronary) syndromes** describes a group of clinical symptoms representing acute myocardial ischemia. The clinical symptoms include acute myocardial infarction, including ST-segment elevation or depression Q-wave or non–Q-wave infarction, and unstable angina (UA) (see III).

F. Etiology. The processes, singly or in combination, that produce IHD include decreased blood flow to the myocardium, increased oxygen demand, and decreased oxygenation of the blood. Generally, significant IHD is defined via angiography as a stenosis that is ≥ 70% of the diameter of at least one major coronary artery segment or 50% of the diameter of the left main coronary artery.

1. **Decreased blood flow** (Figure 39-1)
   a. **Atherosclerosis,** with or without coronary thrombosis, is the most common cause of IHD. In this condition, the coronary arteries are progressively narrowed by smooth muscle cell proliferation and the accumulation of lipid deposits (plaque) along the inner lining (intima) of the arteries.
   b. **Coronary artery spasm,** a sustained contraction of one or more coronary arteries, can occur spontaneously or be induced by irritation (e.g., by coronary catheter or intimal hemorrhage), exposure to the cold, and ergot-derivative drugs. One long-term study demonstrated that coronary spasm was most often associated with an atypical chest pain syndrome and cigarette smoking. These spasms can cause Prinzmetal angina and even MI. Variant angina (Prinzmetal angina) is a form of unstable angina that usually occurs spontaneously, is characterized by transient ST-segment elevation, and most commonly resolves without progression to MI.
   c. **Traumatic injury,** whether blunt or penetrating, can interfere with myocardial blood supply (e.g., the impact of a steering wheel on the chest causing a myocardial contusion in which the capillaries hemorrhage).
   d. **Embolic events,** even in otherwise normal coronary vessels, can abruptly restrict the oxygen supply to the myocardium.

2. **Increased oxygen demand usually in the presence of a fixed restricted oxygen supply** can occur with exertion (e.g., exercise, shoveling snow) and emotional stress as well as under circumstances external to the coronary arterial bed, which increases sympathetic stimulation and thus heart rate. Some factors affecting cardiac workload, and therefore myocardial oxygen supply and demand, are listed in Table 39-1.
   a. **Diastole.** Under normal circumstances, almost all of the oxygen is removed (during diastole) from the arterial blood as it passes through the heart. Thus little remains to be extracted if oxygen demand increases. To increase the coronary oxygen supply, blood

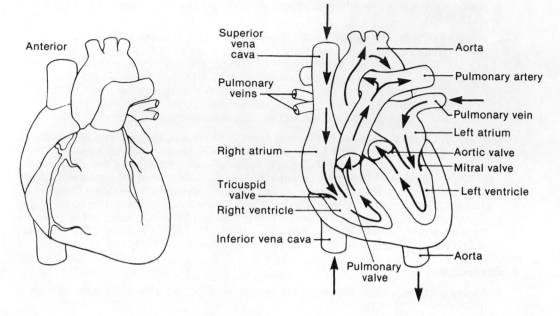

Anterior

Superior
vena
cava

Pulmonary
veins

Right atrium

Tricuspid
valve

Right ventricle

Inferior vena cava

Pulmonary
valve

Aorta

Pulmonary artery

Pulmonary vein

Left atrium

Aortic valve

Mitral valve

Left ventricle

Aorta

Figure 39-1. Oxygen and other nutrients are borne to the myocardium through the two major coronary arteries (the left and right) and their tributaries. The hemodynamic consequences of ischemic heart disease depend on which of the coronary vessels are involved and what part of the myocardium those vessels supply.

flow has to increase. The normal response mechanism is for the blood vessels, particularly the coronary arteries, to dilate, thereby increasing blood flow.

    b. Systole. The two phases of systole—contraction and ejection—strongly influence oxygen demand.

        (1) The **contractile (inotropic) state of the heart** influences the amount of oxygen it requires to perform.

        (2) Increases in systolic wall tension, influenced by left ventricular volume and systolic pressure, increase oxygen demand.

        (3) Lengthening of ejection time (i.e., the duration of systolic wall tension per cardiac cycle) also increases oxygen demand.

        (4) Changes in heart rate influence oxygen consumption by changing the ejection time.

  3. Reduced blood oxygenation. The oxygen-carrying capacity of the blood may be reduced, as occurs in various anemias or hypoxemia.

G. Risk factors for IHD and goals for modification, when applicable, are given in Table 39-2.

H. Therapeutic considerations. Because most IHD occurs secondary to atherosclerosis, which is a long-term, cumulative process, medical efforts focus on reducing risk factors through individual patient education and media campaigns. Once manifestations occur, treatment addresses their specific variables.

Table 39-1. Factors Affecting Cardiac Parameters That Control Myocardial Oxygen Demand

Factor	Heart Rate	Blood Pressure	Ejection Time	Ventricular Volume	Inotropic Effect
Exercise	Increase	Increase	Decrease	Increase or decrease	Increase
Cold	Increase	Increase	—	—	—
Smoking	Increase	Increase	Increase	—	Increase
Nitroglycerin	Increase	Decrease	Decrease	Decrease	Increase
β-blockers	Decrease	Decrease	Increase	Increase	Decrease

Table 39-2. Risk Factors for Ischemic Heart Disease and Guidelines for Their Modification, When Applicable

Hyperlipidemia
  Excess serum cholesterol > 200 mg/dL. Patients should be started on dietary therapy, and increased physical activity and weight management should be promoted.
  LDL cholesterol level > 130 mg/dL. An HMG-CoA reductase inhibitor should be used (class I[a] recommendation); lipid-lowering agents should be used if LDL cholesterol after diet remains > 100 mg/dL (class I recommendation).
  HDL cholesterol level < 40 mg/dL. As an isolated finding or in combination with other lipid abnormalities, a fibrate- or niacin-containing agent should be used (class I recommendation).
Hypertension. Control blood pressure to systolic/diastolic levels > 130/ 85 mm Hg (class I* recommendation)
Smoking. Stop smoking (class I recommendation)
Diabetes mellitus—Tight control of hyperglycemia (HbA1c <7.0%) in diabetics has been given a Class I* recommendation
Obesity—Achievement and maintenance has been given a Class I* recommendation
Family history of ischemic heart disease (IHD)
Sedentary life style—Daily exercise has been given a Class I* recommendation
Chronic stress or type A personality (i.e., aggressive, ambitious, chronically impatient, competitive)
Age and gender (i.e., prevalence is higher among men than among premenopausal women and increases for both genders with age)
Oral contraceptive use
Gout

*Class I recommendation: "Conditions for which there is evidence and/or general agreement that a given procedure or treatment is useful and effective."

II. ANGINA PECTORIS

A. **Definition.** The term **angina pectoris** is applied to varying forms of transient chest discomfort that are attributable to insufficient myocardial oxygen.

  1. Angina is a clinical syndrome characterized by discomfort in the chest, jaw, shoulder, back, and arms, which is usually aggravated by exertion or stress and relieved by nitroglycerin.

  2. Angina can occur in patients with valvular heart disease, uncontrolled hypertension, as well as in noncardiac organ systems such as the chest wall, esophagus, or lungs.

B. **Common causes.** Atherosclerotic lesions that produce a narrowing of the coronary arteries are the major cause of angina. However, tachycardia, anemia, hyperthyroidism, hypotension, and arterial hypoxemia can all cause an oxygen imbalance.

C. **Types**

  1. **Stable (classic) angina**
     a. In this most common form, has a more predictable pattern, which is brought on by exertion, emotional stress, or a heavy meal, which is usually relieved by rest, nitroglycerin, or both.
     b. Five components are usually considered: quality, location, and duration of pain; factors provoking pain; and factors that relieve pain.
     c. Pain has been referred to as "squeezing," "grip-like," "pressure-like," "suffocating," and "heavy," and is usually referred to as a discomfort rather than "pain."
     d. The anginal episode typically lasts for "minutes" and is usually substernal but has a tendency to radiate to the neck, jaw, epigastrium, or arms.
     e. Characteristically, the discomfort builds to a peak, radiating to the jaw, neck, shoulder, and arms, and then subsides without residual sensation. Angina is normally related to physical exertion, and the discomfort usually subsides quickly (i.e., in 3–5 min) with rest; if precipitated by emotional stress, the episode tends to last longer (i.e., about 10 min).
     f. Stable angina is characteristically the result of a fixed obstruction in a coronary artery.

2. Unstable angina. (See also III.)

a. In many patients who experience unstable angina, symptoms will be caused by significant coronary artery disease. Angina is considered unstable and requires further evaluation if patients experience

(1) Rest angina, which usually is prolonged > 20 min occurring within a week of presentation

(2) Severe new-onset angina refers to angina of at least Canadian Cardiovascular Society Classification (CCSC) to class III severity, with onset within 2 months of initial presentation

(3) Increasing angina refers to previously diagnosed angina that is distinctly more frequent, longer in duration, or lower in threshold

(4) Decreased response to rest or nitroglycerin

b. Unstable angina predicts a higher short-term risk, represents a progressive clinical entity, may signal incipient MI, is referred to as an acute coronary syndrome, and should be reported promptly to a physician.

3. Angina decubitus (nocturnal angina)

a. This angina occurs in the recumbent position and is not specifically related to either rest or exertion.

b. Gravitational forces shift fluids within the body with a resultant increase in ventricular volume, which increases oxygen needs and produces angina decubitus, and which may indicate cardiac decompensation.

c. Diuretics alone or in combination effectively reduce left ventricular volume and may aid the patient.

d. Nitrates such as nitroglycerin may relieve the paroxysmal nocturnal dyspnea associated with angina decubitus by reducing preload, owing to venous pooling, and improving left ventricular dysfunction.

4. Prinzmetal's angina (vasospastic or variant angina)

a. Coronary artery spasm that reduces blood flow precipitates this angina. The spasm may be superimposed on a coronary artery that already has a fixed obstruction owing to thrombi or plaque formation.

b. It usually occurs at rest (i.e., pain may disrupt sleep) rather than with exertion or emotional stress, and usually resolves without progression to an acute MI. However, if the attack is prolonged, MI, life-threatening ventricular arrhythmias, and sudden cardiac death can occur.

c. Characteristically, an electrocardiogram (ECG) taken during an attack reveals a transient ST-segment elevation, which returns toward normal after the acute attack.

d. Calcium-channel blockers, rather than β-blockers, are most effective for this form of angina. Nitroglycerin may not provide relief, depending on the cause of vasospasm.

D. Physical examination is usually not revealing, especially between attacks. However, the patient's history, risk factors, and full description of attacks—precipitation pattern, intensity, duration, relieving factors—usually prove diagnostic.

E. Diagnostic test results

1. The **ECG** is normal in 50% or more of patients with stable angina pectoris, and a normal resting ECG does not exclude severe IHD. However, an ECG with evidence of left ventricular hypertrophy or ST-T–wave changes consistent with myocardial ischemia favor the diagnosis of angina pectoris. The presence of Q waves from a previous MI makes the diagnosis of IHD very likely. An ECG obtained during chest pain is abnormal in 50% of patients with angina who have a normal resting ECG. The ST segment can be either elevated or depressed.

2. Stress testing (exercise ECG) is a well-established procedure, which aids the diagnosis in patients who have normal resting ECGs. The most commonly used definition for a positive test is a ≥ 1-mm ST-segment depression or elevation for ≥ 60–80 msec either during or after exercise. Exercise stress testing is preferable to other variations of the stress test (pharmacological) in patients who are able to exercise.

3. Pharmacological stress testing is useful in patients with suspected IHD who are unable to exercise.

a. Intravenous dipyridamole (coronary vasodilation), adenosine (coronary vasodilation) by inhibiting cellular uptake and degradation of adenosine increase coronary blood flow, and high-dose dobutamine (20–40 μg/kg/min) increase oxygen demand through increased heart rate, systolic blood pressure, and myocardial contractility causing an increase in myocardial blood flow are all able to induce detectable cardiac ischemia in conjunction with ECG testing.

   b. Side effects occur for each of the agents and include **dipyridamole** (angina, 18–42%; arrhythmias, 2%; headache, 5–23%; dizziness, 5–21%; nausea, 8–12%; and flushing, 3%), **adenosine** (chest pain, 57%; headache, 35%; flushing, 25%; shortness of breath, 15%; and first-degree atrioventricular [AV] heart block, 18%), **dobutamine** (premature ventricular beats, 15%; premature atrial beats, 8%; supraventricular tachycardia and nonsustained ventricular tachycardia, 3–4%; nausea, 8%; anxiety, 6%; headache, 4%; and tremor, 4%).

4. Stress perfusion imaging with thallium-201 or technetium-99m (^{99m}Tc) can diagnose multivessel disease, localized ischemia, and may be able to determine myocardial viability. The added expense of the test makes it reserved for patients who have ECG abnormalities at rest. Coronary arteriography and cardiac catheterization are very specific and sensitive but are also invasive, expensive, and risky (the mortality rate is 1%–2%); therefore, they must be used judiciously when trying to confirm suspected angina and to differentiate its origin.

5. Various drugs can have an effect on the ECG and should be considered before, during, and after an exercise test is carried out. Examples include

   a. Digoxin produces abnormal exercise-induced ST depression in 25%–40% of apparently healthy, normal subjects without ischemia.

   b. β-adrenergic blockers may delay the development of an abnormal ECG if patients receive them before or during a stress test. If possible, therapy should be slowly withheld from the patient at least four to five half-lives before the exercise testing. If it is not possible to withdraw therapy, the clinician needs to recognize that the test might be less reliable.

   c. Antihypertensives such as vasodilators can alter the stress test by altering the normal hemodynamic response of blood pressure. In addition, short-term use of nitrates can attenuate angina and ST-segment changes associated with myocardial ischemia.

F. Treatment goals

1. To prevent MI and death, thereby increasing a patient's quality of life

2. To reduce symptoms of angina and occurrence of ischemia, which should improve a patient's quality of life

3. To remove or reduce **risk factors**

4. The management of angina pectoris includes therapies aimed at reversing cardiac risk factors.

   a. Hyperlipidemia, if present, should be treated. Reducing cholesterol and low-density lipoprotein (LDL) is associated with a reduced risk of cardiovascular disease and incidence of ischemic cardiac events, as demonstrated by several recent studies using β-hydroxy-β-methylglutaryl–coenzyme A (HMG-CoA) reductase inhibitors. The NCEP has published updated guidelines for treatment of high blood cholesterol (Adult Treatment Panel III).

   (1) Total cholesterol is no longer the primary target of treatment; LDL cholesterol is now the primary target.

   (2) Current recommendations include the completion of a lipoprotein profile—total cholesterol, LDL cholesterol, high-density lipoprotein (HDL) cholesterol, and triglycerides—as the preferred initial test, rather than screening for total cholesterol and HDL alone.

   (3) Persons are categorized into one of four levels of risk, to identify group-specific treatment modalities: (1) *high-risk,* established IHD or IHD risk equivalents (diabetes, noncoronary forms of atherosclerotic disease); (2) *moderately high-risk,* multiple (more than two) risk factors and a calculated 10-year risk of 10%–20%; (3) *moderate risk,* multiple (more than two) risk factors and a calculated 10-year risk of 10%; and (4) *lower-risk,* zero to one risk factor.

   (4) All individuals with IHD or IHD risk equivalents have been called "high risk," and the treatment goals is to have LDL-cholesterol (LDL-C) levels < 100 mg/dL. Other recommendations are as follows:

   (a) If baseline LDL-C is < 100 mg/dL (goal of treatment), patients with IHD should be given instructions on diet and exercise and have levels monitored annually. Though the guidelines suggest an optional goal of obtaining an LDL-C of < 70 mg/dL.

(b) If baseline LDL-C is ≥ 100 mg/dL, an LDL-lowering drug should be started along with therapeutic lifestyle changes (TLCs). Lifestyle-related risk factors include things such as obesity, physical inactivity, elevated triglyceride, low-HDL-C, or metabolic syndrome.

(c) Adult Treatment Panel III did not mandate LDL-lowering drugs for patients with baseline LDL-C levels between 100 and 129 mg/dL but suggested intensifying lifestyle and the optional use of drug therapies to lower LDL to < 100 mg/dL. However, if the patient had elevated triglycerides or low high-density lipoprotein cholesterol (HDL-C), a drug should be started that targets these abnormalities—for example, nicotinic acid or fibric acid if the patient has elevated triglycerides (> 200 mg/dL) or low HDL levels (< 40 mg/dL). If triglycerides are ≥ 500 mg/dL, consider fibrate or niacin before LDL-lowering therapy.

(5) For moderately high risk patients, the recommended LDL-C goal is < 130 mg/dL, but a goal of < 100 mg/dL is an optional goal, based on recent clinical trial evidence. In addition, a recommendation to initiate TLCs when the patient has an LDL-C ≥ 130 mg/dL.

(6) For moderate risk patients, the recommended LDL-C goal is < 130 mg/dL. In addition, a recommendation to initiate TLC when the patient has an LDL-C ≥ 160 mg/dL.

(7) For lower risk patients, the recommended LDL-C goal is < 160 mg/dL, but again, a recommendation to initiate TLC for those patients with an LDL ≥ 190 mg/dL.

(8) The **metabolic syndrome** is closely linked to insulin resistance, when the normal actions of insulin are impaired. Excess body fat and physical inactivity promote the development of the syndrome; however, some individuals may be predisposed genetically. Patients with three or more of the following characteristics are referred to as having the metabolic syndrome and should be treated accordingly: abdominal obesity, triglycerides > 150 mg/dL, HDL levels of < 40 mg/dL for men and 50 mg/dL for women, blood pressure readings ≥ 130/85 mm Hg, and a fasting serum glucose level ≥ 110 mg/dL.

G. Individual drug classes

1. Bile acid sequestrant resins

a. Mechanism of action. These insoluble, nonabsorbable, anion-exchange resins bind bile acids within the intestines. Bile acids are synthesized from cholesterol.

b. Indications. These agents have been shown to be safe and effective in lowering LDL-C especially in patients with modestly elevated levels, in primary prevention, in young adult men, and postmenopausal women. They are effective in combination with other agents.

c. Currently available agents include the following:

(1) Cholestyramine (Questran): 2–8 g by mouth in two daily doses

(2) Colestipol (Colestid): 2–16 g by mouth in one or two daily doses

(3) Colesevelam (WelChol): 6–7 tablets (625 mg/tablet) by mouth in one daily dose

d. Precautions and monitoring effects

(1) These resins are taken just before meals and present palatability problems in patients.

(2) Gastrointestinal (GI) intolerance, especially constipation, flatulence, and dyspepsia are frequent.

(3) Absorption of many other drugs can be affected. Other drugs should be taken 1 hr before or 4–6 hr after resins.

2. Statins or HMG-CoA reductase inhibitors

a. Mechanism of action. These agents inhibit the enzyme HMG-CoA and reduce cholesterol production.

b. Indications. These agents are effective in lowering LDL levels, while increasing HDL levels and lowering triglyceride levels. They are primarily used to lower LDL cholesterol levels.

c. Currently available agents include the following:

(1) Atorvastatin (Lipitor): 10–80 mg by mouth daily

(2) Fluvastatin (Lescol): 20–80 mg by mouth at bedtime

(3) Lovastatin (Mevacor): 10–80 mg by mouth in the evening

(4) Pravastatin (Pravachol): 10–80 mg by mouth daily

(5) Rosuvastatin (Crestor): 5–40 mg by mouth daily

(6) Simvastatin (Zocor): 20–80 mg by mouth daily

d. Precautions and monitoring effects

(1) GI adverse effects are less frequently seen than with other classes of agents. Headache and dyspepsia frequently occur and should be evaluated, then followed up in 6–8 weeks, and then at each follow-up visit thereafter.

(2) These agents can elevate liver function tests—alanine aminotransferase (ALT) and aspartate aminotransferase (AST), which requires initial evaluation, then after approximately 12 weeks of therapy, then annually thereafter.

(3) Though the incidence of myopathy is believed to be low (0.08%) for lovastatin and simvastatin, elevations of creatine kinase (CK) > 10 times the upper limit of normal have been reported with pravastatin, with similar potential for the other members of the group. Most recently, cerivastatin (Baycol) was voluntarily removed from the market owing to the reported deaths of 31 patients from rhabdomyolysis while receiving the drug alone or in combination with gemfibrozil (Lopid). Consequently, routine monitoring is necessary in all patients, as follows:

(a) Evaluate muscle symptoms and check CK before starting therapy, evaluate in 6–12 weeks after starting therapy, and then at each follow-up visit.

(b) Patients presenting with muscle soreness, tenderness, or pain should have a CK measurement on presentation, to minimize the develop of myopathies.

(c) Concurrent therapy with other agents, including cyclosporine, macrolide antibiotics, azole antifungals, niacin, fibrates, or nefazodone, may increase the risk.

3. Fibric acid derivatives

a. Mechanism of action. These agents are presumed to inhibit cholesterol synthesis and lower LDL-C. They are effective at lowering triglycerides. In some patients, they modestly lower LDL-C and raise HDL-C.

b. Precautions and monitoring effects

(1) GI effects are the most commonly experienced adverse effect.

(2) These agents can elevate liver function tests; routine monitoring should be carried out.

(3) Use with statins can lead to elevated CK, and monitoring is necessary to identify myopathies or rhabdomyolysis.

c. Currently available agents include the following:

(1) Fenofibrate (Tricor): 200 mg by mouth daily

(2) Gemfibrozil (Lopid): 600 mg by mouth twice daily

4. Niacin

a. Mechanism of action. Numerous studies have demonstrated the role of niacin in the lowering of LDL-C and triglycerides through various mechanisms such as participation in tissue respiration oxidation–reduction reactions, which decreases hepatic LDL and very low-density lipoprotein (VLDL) production; inhibition of adipose tissue lipolysis, decreased hepatic triglyceride esterification, and increases in lipoprotein lipase activity. Table 39-3 presents several agents and their effects on lipoproteins.

b. Indications. Niacin is valuable in treating patients with elevated total cholesterol and low LDL-C levels. It is used in combination therapy.

c. Currently available agents include the following:

(1) Niacin controlled release (Niaspan): 1000–2000 mg by mouth at bedtime

(2) Niacin controlled release (Slo-Niacin): 250–750 mg by mouth 1–2 times daily

(3) Niacin immediate release: 1000–2000 mg by mouth 2–3 times daily.

d. Precautions

(1) Adverse GI effects are experienced with the use of niacin.

(2) Patients may experience flushing and itchy skin, which may be reduced with the administration of 325 mg aspirin about 30 min before the dose.

(3) Cases of severe liver toxicity have been reported. Liver function tests should be performed in patients receiving this drug.

5. Ezetimibe (Zetia)

a. Mechanism of action. First in a new class of lipid-lowering compounds approved by the U.S. Food and Drug Administration (FDA), which works by selectively inhibiting the intestinal absorption of cholesterol and related phytosterols, with a resultant decrease in intestinal cholesterol delivered to the liver, decreased hepatic cholesterol stores, and an increase in the clearance of cholesterol from the blood. Ezetimibe has demonstrated the

Table 39-3. Selected Agents and Their Effects on Lipoproteins

Class/Agent	Lipid/Lipoprotein Effects	Daily Dose	Adverse Drug Effects
HMG-CoA reductase inhibitors (statins)	LDL: 18–55% reduction HDL: 5–15% increase TG: 7–30% reduction	Lovastatin: 20–80 mg Pravastatin: 20–40 mg Simvastatin: 20–80 mg Fluvastatin: 20–80 mg Atorvastatin: 10–80 mg Rosuvastatin: 5–40 mg	Myopathy, increased liver enzymes
Bile acid sequestrants	LDL: 15–30% reduction HDL: 3–5% increase TG: No change or increase	Cholestyramine: 4–16 g Colestipol: 5–20 g Colesevelam: 2.6–3.8 g	GI distress, constipation, decreased absorption of other drugs
Nicotinic acid	LDL: 5–25% reduction HDL: 15–35% increase TG: 20–50% reduction	Immediate-release: 1.5–3 g Extended-release: 1–2 g Sustained-release: 1–2 g	Flushing, hyperglycemia, hyperuricemia (or gout), upper-GI distress, hepatotoxicity

Fibric acids	LDL: 5–20% reduction
	HDL: 10–20% increase
	TG: 20–50% reduction
		Gemfibrozil: 600 mg
		  twice daily
		Fenofibrate: 200 mg
		Clofibrate: 1000 mg
		  twice daily
			Dyspepsia, gallstones, myopathy, unexplained non-CHD deaths in WHO study

CHD, coronary heart disease; *GI,* gastrointestinal; *HDL,* high-density lipoprotein; *HMG-CoA,* β-hydroxy-β-methyl-glutaryl-coenzyme A; *LDL,* low-density lipoprotein; *TG,* triglycerides; *WHO,* World Health Organization.
Adapted from Grundy SM, Becher D, Clark LT et al. Third Report of the National Cholesterol Education Program (NCEP): Detection, Evaluation, and Treatment of High Blood Cholesterol in Adults (Adult Treatment Panel III) [NIH Publication No. 01-3670]. Washington DC, U.S. Department of Health and Human Services, May 2001. Available at: www.nhlbi.nih.gov/guidelines/cholesterol/atp3xsum.pdf.

ability to reduce total cholesterol, LDL-C, apolipoprotein B, and triglyceride levels while increasing HDL levels in patients with hypercholesterolemia.

   b. Indications. Ezetimibe as adjunctive therapy along with dietary measures, alone in patients with primary heterozygous familial and nonfamilial hypercholesterolemia, or in combination with the HMG-CoA reductase inhibitors (atorvastatin or simvastatin) in homozygous familial hypercholesterolemia.

   c. Dose. Normal dosing recommendations are a 10-mg dose given once daily.

   d. Precautions. As monotherapy, studies to date have not revealed significant side effects above those seen with placebo administration. However, when used in combination with HMG-CoA reductase inhibitors, reports have described an increased incidence (approximately 1.4%) in the elevation of liver transaminase levels (three times the upper limit of normal) as compared to the incidence of 0.4% with HMG-CoA agents used alone.

6. Combination products

   a. Ezetimibe/simvastatin (Vytorin) uses the individual class properties of the HMG-CoA reductase inhibitors (simvastatin) to reduce cholesterol production with the absorption-inhibiting properties of ezetimibe to target cholesterol with two differing mechanisms, which might aid in improving patient compliance.

   (1) Available product is supplied as 10/10, 10/20, 10/40, 10/80 combinations of ezetimibe and simvastatin, respectively, and the daily recommended dose is 1 tablet by mouth every morning.

   (2) Side effects reflect the additive side effect properties of ezetimibe and simvastatin and warrant consideration when occurring during therapy.

b. Lovastatin/niacin (Advicor) is a 24-hr, extended-release product that incorporates the actions of the HMG-CoA reductase inhibitor lovastatin with niacin into a single product, using differing mechanisms, which might aid in improving patient compliance.

    (1) Available product is supplied as 20/500, 20/1000 sustained-release tablet combinations of lovastatin and niacin, respectively. The recommended daily dose is 1–2 tablets by mouth at bedtime.

    (2) Side effects reflect the additive side effect properties for both lovastatin and niacin and warrant consideration during therapy.

c. Amlodipine/atorvastatin (Caduet) is a combination product that incorporates the actions of the dihydropyridine calcium channel blocker amlodipine with the lipid-lowering properties of the HMG-CoA reductase inhibitor atorvastatin. The calcium channel blocker offers no benefit for lipid lowering but represents a potentially beneficial product for a patient with coexisting disease states, such as IHD and hypertension, for which the use of a calcium channel blocker would be warranted.

    (1) Available product is supplied as 2.5/10, 2.5/20, 2.5/40, 5/10, 5/20, 5/40, 5/80, 10/10, 10/20, 10/40, and 10/80 tablet combinations of amlodipine and atorvastatin, respectively. The recommended daily dose is 1 tablet by mouth daily.

    (2) Side effects reflect the additive side effect properties for both amlodipine and atorvastatin and warrant consideration during therapy.

d. Aspirin, buffered/pravastatin (Pravigard PAC) is a combination product that incorporates the actions of the HMG-CoA reductase inhibitor pravastatin with the antiplatelet properties of aspirin.

    (1) Available product is supplied as 81/20, 81/40, 81/80, 325/20, 325/40, and 325/80 tablet combinations of buffered aspirin and pravastatin, respectively. The recommended daily dose is 1 tablet by mouth daily.

    (2) Side effects reflect the additive side effect properties for both aspirin and pravastatin and warrant consideration during therapy.

e. Omega-3-acid ethyl esters (Omacor) is the first FDA-approved omega 3-fatty acid, which is indicated for patients with elevated levels of triglycerides (> 500 mg/dL).

    (1) Available product is supplied as a 1-g capsule; the recommended daily dose is 4 capsules by mouth daily in one–two doses.

    (2) Side effects that have been reported include burping, infection, flu-like symptoms, upset stomach, change in one's sense of taste, back pain, and rash.

f. Hypertension. Treatment of hypertension according to the Joint National Conference VII guidelines has received a class I recommendation based on data from multiple randomized clinical trials with large numbers of patients (A, high) and should be controlled. Class I recommendations are based on evidence or general agreement that a given procedure or treatment is useful and effective (see Chapter 41).

g. Smoking should be stopped if at all possible and has received a class I recommendation based on data derived from a limited number of randomized trials with small numbers of patients (B, intermediate).

    (1) Transdermal use of nicotine-containing patches has become one strategy for aiding the cessation of smoking. Products such as Nicotrol, Habitrol, NicoDerm, and others are available in varying strengths to wean patients off the use of cigarettes over an 8- to 12-week period, using descending doses.

    (2) Nicotine gum (oral nicotine polacrilex chewing pieces) is available in 2-mg or 4-mg pieces. Nicorette is usually used for 3 months to aid in cessation of smoking.

    (3) Bupropion is a prescription antidepressant, which is also marketed under the brand name of Zyban as an aid to smoking cessation.

h. Obesity should be reduced through diet and an appropriate exercise program in patients with hypertension, hyperlipidemia, or diabetes mellitus and has received a class I recommendation based on expert consensus as the primary basis (C, low).

H. Therapeutic agents

1. Recent evidence-based guidelines have provided recommendations for the treatment of patients with stable angina. Recommendations use three classes of guidelines—class I (evidence or general agreement that a procedure or treatment is useful and effective), class II (conflicting evidence or a divergence of opinion about the usefulness/efficacy of a procedure or treatment), and class III (evidence and/or general agreement that the procedure/treatment is not useful/effective and in some cases may be harmful)—based on three levels of evidence—A (high; data obtained from multiple randomized clinical trials), B (intermediate; data obtained from a single randomized trial or nonrandomized studies), and C (low; consensus opinion of experts).

   a. Therapies with class IA recommendations are
   - **(1)** Aspirin in the absence of contraindications in patients with a prior MI
   - **(2)** β-Adrenergic blockers in the absence of contraindications in patients with a previous heart attack (myocardial infarction)
   - **(3)** Angiotensin-converting enzyme (ACE) inhibitors in all patients with IHD who also have diabetes and/or left ventricular systolic dysfunction.

   b. Therapies with class IB recommendations are
   - **(1)** β-Adrenergic blockers in the absence of contraindications in patients *without* a previous heart attack (MI)
   - **(2)** Sublingual nitroglycerin or nitroglycerin spray for the immediate relief of angina
   - **(3)** Calcium antagonists or long-acting nitrates as initial therapy for reduction of symptoms when β-adrenergic blockers are contraindicated

   c. Therapies with class IC recommendations are calcium antagonists and long-acting nitrates as a substitute for β-adrenergic blockers if initial treatment with β-adrenergic blockers leads to unacceptable side effects.

   d. Therapies with class IIa recommendations are
   - **(1)** Clopidogrel when aspirin is absolutely contraindicated
   - **(2)** Long-acting non–dihydropyridine calcium antagonists (diltiazem or verapamil) instead of β-adrenergic blockers as initial therapy
   - **(3)** ACE inhibitor in patients with IHD or other vascular disease

   e. Therapies with class IIb recommendations include low-intensity anticoagulation with warfarin in addition to aspirin.

   f. Therapies with class III levels of evidence are dipyridamole and chelation therapy.

2. Nitrates (e.g., nitroglycerin)
   a. Mechanism of action
   - **(1)** The primary value of nitrates is venous dilation, which reduces left ventricular volume (preload) and myocardial wall tension, decreasing oxygen requirements (demand).
   - **(2)** Nitrates may also reduce arteriolar resistance, helping reduce afterload, which decreases myocardial oxygen demand.
   - **(3)** By reducing pressure in cardiac tissues, nitrates also facilitate collateral circulation, which increases blood distribution to ischemic areas.
   - **(4)** Pharmacological effects have been shown to improve exercise tolerance, prolong the time to onset of angina, and the appearance of ST-segment depression during exercise testing.

   b. Indications
   - **(1)** Acute attacks of angina pectoris can be managed with sublingual, transmucosal (Nitrolingual spray or buccal tablets), or intravenous delivery.
   - **(2)** Indications include the prevention of anticipated attacks, using tablets (oral or buccal) or transdermal paste or patches. Sublingual nitrates (Nitrostat) can be used before eating, sexual activity, or a known stressful event.
   - **(3)** Nitrates are used in treatment of stable angina. They may not be effective as a single agent for treatment of Prinzmetal angina, although some studies have shown nitrates to prevent or reverse vasospasm at varying doses. Intravenous nitroglycerin is used in the immediate treatment of unstable angina and is used for long-term therapeutic relief.
   - **(4)** Nitrates used in combination with β-adrenergic blockers have been shown to be more effective than nitrates or β-adrenergic blockers used alone.

   c. Choice of preparation should be based on onset of action, duration of action, and patient compliance and preference because all nitrates have the same mechanism of action.

   d. Precautions and monitoring effects
   - **(1)** To maximize the therapeutic effect, patients should thoroughly understand the use of their specific dosage forms (e.g., sublingual tablets, transdermal patches or pastes, tablets, capsules).
   - **(2)** Blood pressure and heart rate should be monitored because all nitrates can increase heart rate while lowering blood pressure.
   - **(3)** Preload reduction can be assessed through reduction of pulmonary symptoms such as shortness of breath, paroxysmal nocturnal dyspnea, or dyspnea.

(4) Nitrate-induced headaches are the most common side effect.

    (a) Patients should be warned of the nature, suddenness, and potential strength of these headaches to minimize the anxiety that might otherwise occur.

    (b) Compliance can be enhanced if the patient understands that the effect is transient and that the headaches usually disappear with continued therapy.

    (c) Acetaminophen ingested 15–30 min before nitrate administration may prevent the headache.

  e. Effective therapy should result in fewer anginal attacks without inducing significant adverse effects (e.g., postural hypotension, hypoxia). If maximal doses are reached and the patient still experiences attacks, additional agents should be administered.

  f. Nitrate tolerance is a major problem with the long-term use of nitroglycerin and long-acting nitrates. Several agents such as ACE inhibitors (sulfhydryl-containing drugs), acetylcysteine, and diuretics have been shown to reverse nitrate tolerance by increasing the availability of sulfhydryl radicals. However, practical considerations suggest that less frequent administration (8–12 hr of nitrate-free intervals) is effective without introducing additional agents.

3. β-Adrenergic blockers

  a. Mechanism of action. β-Blockers reduce oxygen demand, both at rest and during exertion, by decreasing the heart rate and myocardial contractility, which also decreases arterial blood pressure.

  b. Indications

    (1) These agents reduce the frequency and severity of exertional angina that is not controlled by nitrates.

    (2) Nitrates have been combined with calcium antagonists, when slow-release dihydropyridines (e.g., felodipine-Plendil, amlodipine-Norvasc) are preferred over diltiazem (Cardizem) or verapamil (Calan). If patients need to receive a β-adrenergic blocker along with verapamil or diltiazem owing to the added effects, they have the potential to induce bradycardia, AV heart block, and fatigue.

  c. Precautions and monitoring effects

    (1) Doses should be increased until the anginal episodes have been reduced or until unacceptable side effects occur.

    (2) β-Blockers should be avoided in Prinzmetal angina (caused by coronary vasospasm) because they increase coronary resistance and may induce vasospasm.

    (3) Asthma is a relative contraindication because all β-blockers increase airway resistance and have the potential to induce bronchospasm in susceptible patients.

    (4) Patients with diabetes and others predisposed to hypoglycemia should be warned that β-blockers mask tachycardia, which is a key sign of developing hypoglycemia.

    (5) Patients should be monitored for excessive negative inotropic effects. Findings such as fatigue, shortness of breath, edema, and paroxysmal nocturnal dyspnea may signal developing cardiac decompensation, which also increases the metabolic demands of the heart.

    (6) Sudden cessation of β-blocker therapy may trigger a withdrawal syndrome that can exacerbate anginal attacks (especially in patients with IHD) or cause MI.

  d. Choice of preparations. All β-blockers are likely to be equally effective for stable (exertional) angina. For further review of β-adrenergic blockers, see Chapter 40. For a list of agents and doses, see Table 39-4.

4. Calcium-channel blockers

  a. Mechanism of action. Two actions are most pertinent in the treatment of angina.

    (1) These agents prevent and reverse coronary spasm by inhibiting calcium influx into vascular smooth muscle and myocardial muscle. This results in increased blood flow, which enhances myocardial oxygen supply.

    (2) Calcium-channel blockers decrease coronary vascular resistance and increase coronary blood flow, resulting in increased oxygen supply.

    (3) Calcium-channel blockers decrease systemic vascular resistance and arterial pressure; in addition, they decrease inotropic effects, resulting in decreased myocardial oxygen demand.

  b. Indications

    (1) Calcium-channel blockers are used in stable (exertional) angina that is not controlled by nitrates and β-blockers and in patients for whom β-blocker therapy is inadvisable. Combination therapy—with nitrates, β-blockers, or both—may be most effective.

Table 39-4. Selected Agents and Their Doses in the Treatment of Coronary Artery Disease

Class/Agent	Dose/Dosage Schedule	Comments
Nitrates		
Nitroglycerin sublingual tablets (Nitrostat)	0.3–0.6 mg up to 1.5 mg	Short-term effects: 1–7 min
Nitroglycerin spray (Nitrolingual)	0.4 mg as needed	Similar to sublingual tablets
Nitroglycerin transdermal (Nitro-Dur)	0.2–0.8 mg/hr every 12 hr	Remove patch for 8–12 hr to reduce tolerance
Nitroglycerin intravenous infusion (Various)	5–200 µg/min	Short acting requiring continuous infusion and monitoring
Isosorbide dinitrate oral tablets (Isordil)	5–80 mg, 2–3 times daily	Longer acting up to 8 hr
Isosorbide dinitrate slow-release tablets (Dilatrate-SR)	40 mg once or twice daily	Duration of activity up to 8 hr
β-adrenergic blockers		
Propranolol (Inderal)	20–80 mg twice daily	Possesses both β_1- and β_2-blocker effects
Metoprolol (Lopressor)	50–200 mg twice daily	Possesses β_1-blocker effects
Atenolol (Tenormin)	50–200 mg/day	Possesses β_1-blocker effects
Nadolol (Corgard)	40–80 mg/day	Possesses both β_1- and β_2-blocker effects
Timolol (Blocadren)	10 mg twice daily	Possesses both β_1- and β_2-blocker effects
Acebutolol (Sectral)	200–600 mg twice daily	Possesses β_1-blocker effects
Betaxolol (Kerlone)	10–20 mg/day	Possesses β_1-blocker effects
Bisoprolol (Zebeta)	10 mg/day	Possesses β_1-blocker effects
Esmolol (intravenous) (Brevibloc)	50–300 µg/kg/min	Possesses β_1-blocker effects
Labetalol (Trandate)	200–600 mg twice daily	Possesses both α_1-, β_1-, and β_2-blocker effects
Pindolol (Visken)	2.5–7.5 mg three times daily	Possesses both β_1- and β_2-blocker effects
Carvedilol (Coreg)	25 mg twice daily	Possesses both α_1- β_1-, and β_2-blocker effects
Penbutolol (Levatol)		Possesses both β_1- and β_2-blocker effects
Calcium-channel blockers		
Dihydropyridine derivatives		
Nifedipine (Procardia)	Immediate release; 30–90 mg daily	Short duration of action of 4–6 hr
Amlodipine (Norvasc)	5–10 mg once daily	Long duration of action
Felodipine (Plendil)	5–10 mg once daily	Long duration of action
Isradipine (Dynacirc)	2.5–10 mg twice daily	Intermediate duration of action
Nicardipine (Cardene)	20–40 mg three times daily	Short duration of action
Nisoldipine (Sular)	20–40 mg once daily	Short duration of action
Miscellaneous		
Diltiazem (Cardizem)	Immediate release: 30–80 mg four times daily	Short duration of action; important consideration necessary owing to hypotension, bradycardia, and edema
	Slow release: 120–320 mg once daily	Long duration of action; important consideration necessary owing to hypotension, bradycardia, and edema
Class/Agent		
Verapamil (Calan)	Immediate release: 80–160 mg three times daily	Short duration of action; important consideration necessary owing to hypotension, bradycardia, edema, myocardial depression, and heart failure
	Slow release: 120–480 mg once daily	Long duration of action; important consideration necessary owing to hypotension, bradycardia, edema, myocardial depression, and heart failure

(2) These agents, alone or with a nitrate, are particularly valuable in the treatment of Prinzmetal angina. They are considered the drug of choice in treatment of angina at rest.

c. Individual agents

(1) Diltiazem (Cardizem) and verapamil (Calan)

   (a) These drugs produce negative inotropic effects, and patients must be monitored closely for signs of developing cardiac decompensation (i.e., fatigue, shortness of breath, edema, paroxysmal nocturnal dyspnea). When coadministered with β-blockers or other agents that produce negative inotropic effects (e.g., disopyramide, quinidine, procainamide, flecainide), the negative effects are additive.

   (b) Patients should be monitored for signs of developing bradyarrhythmias and heart block because these agents have negative chronotropic effects.

   (c) Verapamil frequently causes constipation, which must be treated as needed to prevent straining at stool, which could cause an increased oxygen demand (Valsalva maneuver). Verapamil is not recommended in patients with sick sinus syndromes, AV nodal disease, or heart failure (HF).

(2) Nifedipine (Procardia)

   (a) This calcium-channel blocker is believed to possess the greatest degree of negative inotropic effects compared to the newer second-generation members of this group, amlodipine (Norvasc) and felodipine (Plendil); Nifedipine 10 mg (chewed or swallowed) has been used to treat Prinzmetal angina or refractory spasm in patients who are not hypotensive. Controversy still exists about the use of short-acting, rapid-release agents such as nifedipine in patients with IHD.

   (b) Because nifedipine increases the heart rate somewhat, it can produce tachycardia, which would increase oxygen demand. Coadministration of a β-blocker should prevent reflex tachycardia.

   (c) Its potent peripheral dilatory effects can decrease coronary perfusion and produce excessive hypotension, which can aggravate myocardial ischemia.

   (d) Dizziness, light-headedness, and lower extremity edema are the most common adverse effects, but these tend to disappear with time or dose adjustment.

(3) Amlodipine (Norvasc), felodipine (Plendil), isradipine (Dynacirc), nicardipine (Cardene), and nisoldipine (Sular) are second-generation dihydropyridine derivative, calcium-channel blockers. They have been used effectively as once- or twice-a-day agents owing to their long activity. Because of the potent negative inotropic effects of these agents, they are not recommended in patients with HF (amlodipine has been shown to have less negative potential in HF than other members of the class).

5. Antiplatelet agents

   a. Aspirin in doses of 75–325 mg daily should be routinely used in all patients with acute or chronic IHD with or without symptoms in the absence of any contraindications.

   b. Ticlopidine (Ticlid) is a thienopyridine derivative that inhibits platelet aggregation induced by adenosine diphosphate. However, unlike aspirin, it has not been shown to decrease adverse cardiovascular events in patients with stable angina and has been associated with thrombotic thrombocytopenic purpura on an infrequent basis.

   c. Clopidogrel (Plavix) is also a thienopyridine derivative related to ticlopidine, but it possesses antithrombotic effects that are greater than those of ticlopidine. Clopidogrel is a therapeutic option in those angina patients who can not take aspirin because of contraindications. Doses of 75 mg daily are recommended to prevent the development of acute coronary syndromes.

6. ACE inhibitors

   a. ACE inhibitors during the past 3–5 years have attracted continued attention as additional therapy in patients with IHD, as evidenced by the most recent guidelines, which provide a class IIa recommendation for their use in patients with IHD or other vascular diseases.

   b. The Heart Outcomes Prevention Evaluation (HOPE) trial demonstrated that the ACE inhibitor ramipril (Altace)—10 mg per day—reduced cardiovascular death, MI, and stroke in patients who were at high risk for or had vascular disease in the absence of heart failure.

   c. Current controversy on the use of ACE inhibitors centers around questions on therapeutic effects of each agent to determine if the beneficial effects seen in previous trials represent a class effect or if it is specific to those agents with proven benefit. Differences do exist among the currently available agents, and the need exists to determine the optimal dose necessary to induce the therapeutic effects appreciated from the HOPE trial, Survival and Ventricular Enlargement (SAVE) trial (captopril; Capoten), and Cooperative North Scandinavian Enalapril Survival Study (CONSENSUS I) trial (enalapril; Vasotec).

   d. Current guidelines do not suggest which agent to use, and it is anticipated that ongoing trials with additional agents will provide additional information regarding dosing regimens and potential differences that might exist among the class of drugs.

III. ACUTE CORONARY SYNDROME (ACS)

A. Definition. ACS is a relatively new term that has been introduced into the medical literature to describe any pattern of clinical symptoms that reflects the development of acute MI (Figure 39-2). This category includes the symptoms related to ST-segment elevated myocardial infarction (STEMI), non-ST-segment elevated myocardial infarction (NSTEMI), Q wave MI, non-Q wave MI, and unstable angina.

B. Incidence. It has been estimated that nearly 8 million patients seen in emergency departments each year in the United States are seen for chest pain, and that up to 5 million of these patients are admitted to the hospital. More than 2 million of the patients admitted to the hospital are admitted with an ACS (400,000 with STEMI, and 1.8 million with UA and NSTEMI).

C. Classification of patients presenting with presumed ACS is critical to the appropriate determination of prognosis as well as clinical interventions. In ACS owing to STEMI and NSTEMI, a portion of the cardiac muscle suffers a severe and prolonged restriction of oxygenated coronary blood. In the majority of patients, the cause is an occlusive or near-occlusive thrombus overlying or adjacent to a ruptured atherosclerotic plaque. This results in cellular ischemia, tissue injury, and tissue necrosis. About 1.5 million people suffer an AMI each year. UA is believed to indicated an impending AMI, and the goal of treatment is to prevent the development of the AMI.

   1. STEMI. A condition that requires immediate reperfusion therapy, if possible through either thrombolysis or percutaneous coronary intervention (PCI)

   a. The introduction of thrombolysis or PCI for the management of STEMI has demonstrated ability to remove the offending thrombus from the affected coronary artery.

   b. Damage to the myocardial tissue is not routinely reversible, as in the case of angina pectoris, owing to potential death of myocardial tissue if reperfusion does not take place early enough.

   2. UA and NSTEMI. Similar conditions for which there is no evidence showing the benefit to patients of reperfusion therapy. Specific guidelines have been developed for the diagnosis and management of these conditions. Up to 25% of patients who have both NSTEMI and elevated cardiac enzymes eventually develop Q-wave MI; the remaining patients develop non-Q-wave MI. Patients with UA carry a 10%–20% risk of progression to an MI if untreated; treatment has been shown to reduce the risk to 5%–7%.

D. Diagnosis. The ECG is at the center of the decision pathway for the evaluation and management of patients with ACS and is confirmed with serial cardiac markers in > 90% of patents presenting with significant ST-segment elevation. Patients who present without ST-segment elevation are considered to have either UA or NSTEMI; the final diagnosis is made later, after the presence or absence of serial cardiac markers is determined.

   1. Diagnostic test results. The development of an ACS is a life-threatening emergency; diagnosis is presumed—and treatment is instituted—based on the patient's complaints and the results of an immediate 12-lead ECG. Laboratory tests and further diagnostic tests can rule out or provide confirmation and help identify the locale and extent of myocardial damage.

   2. Serial 12-lead ECG. Abnormalities may be absent or inconclusive during the first few hours after presentation of the ACS and may not aid the diagnosis in about 15% of the cases. When present, characteristic findings show progressive changes.

   a. First, ST-segment elevation (injury current) appears in the leads, reflecting the injured area. Peaked upright or inverted T waves usually indicate acute myocardial injury, the early stages of a transmural Q-wave MI. Persistent ST depression may also indicate a non-Q-wave MI.

   b. Q waves developing (indicating necrosis) is generally diagnostic of an MI, but can be seen in other conditions.

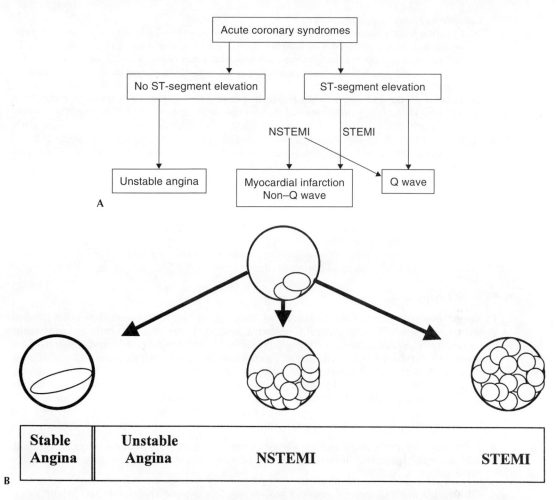

Figure 39-2. A. The spectrum of clinical conditions representing the acute coronary syndromes (ACSs). Patients with acute myocardial ischemia present with either an elevated or a nonelevated ST segment on electrocardiogram (ECG). Evidenced-based practice guidelines demonstrate that the majority of patients presenting with ST-segment elevated MI (STEMI) eventually develop a Q-wave myocardial infarction (MI); a smaller group of STEMI patients develop a non-Q-wave MI. The remaining ACS patients have either unstable angina or non-ST-segment elevated myocardial infarction (NSTEMI). Most NSTEMI patients experience a non-Q-wave MI; a smaller number eventually have a Q-wave MI. **B.** Evolutionary progression of ACSs. As atherosclerosis (most common cause of ischemic heart disease) advances, the reduction in myocardial perfusion results in the development of the ACS owing to either unstable angina, NSTEMI, or STEMI. The thrombi, which form in unstable angina, NSTEMI, STEMI, are rich in both fibrin and platelets. [Panel **A,** adapted from Braunwald E, Antman EM, Beasley JW et al. ACC/AHA 2002 guideline update for the management of patients with unstable angina and non-ST-segment elevation myocardial infarction-summary article: a report of the American College of Cardiology/American Heart Association Task Force on Practice Guidelines (Committee on the Management of Patients with Unstable Angina). Available at www.acc.org/clinical/guidelines/unstable/incorporated/index.htm. Panel **B,** adapted from Vanscoy G. Integrating new fibrinolytic findings into AMI reperfusion and combination therapy: 2002 and beyond." Paper presented at the meeting of the Delaware Valley Chapter of the Pennsylvania Society of Health-Systems Pharmacists, March 7, 2002.]

   c. Unequivocal diagnosis can be made only in the presence of all three abnormalities. However, the manifestations depend on the area of injury. For example, in non-Q-wave infarction, only ST-segment depression may appear.

   d. The most serious arrhythmic complication of an acute MI is ventricular fibrillation, which may occur without warning.

   e. Ventricular premature beats (VPBs) are the most commonly encountered arrhythmias and may require treatment.

3. Cardiac enzymes

a. Creatine kinase–heart muscle (CK-MB) is first elevated 3–12 hr after the onset of pain, peaks in 24 hr, and returns to baseline in 48–72 hr. Other conditions elevate the CK-MB enzyme but do not demonstrate the typical pattern of rise and fall as seen in an MI. Until recently, CK-MB had been the principal serum cardiac marker used in the evaluation of ACS.

b. Cardiac troponin I (cTnI) and **cardiac troponin T** (cTnT) are even more sensitive than MB-CK. They represent a powerful tool for risk stratification and have greater sensitivity and specificity than CK-MB. However, they do provide a low sensitivity in the early phases of an MI (< 6 hr after symptom onset) and require repeat measurements at 8–12 hr, if negative. Levels increase 3–12 hr after the onset of pain, peak at 24–48 hr, and return to baseline over 5–14 days.

c. Lactate dehydrogenase (LDH) is followed for its characteristic patterns of rise and fall. The ratio of $LDH_1:LDH_2$ is helpful in diagnosing an MI. LDH assays are being replaced by cTnT assays.

4. Cardiac imaging. As cardiac enzymes assays improve, the use of noninvasive cardiac imaging techniques are not indicated for initial diagnosis of an MI. Tests include ^{99m}Tc-pyrophosphate scintigraphy, myocardial perfusion imaging, radionucleotide ventriculography, two-dimensional echocardiography, and coronary angiography.

E. Signs and symptoms

1. Recent evidence-based clinical guidelines indicate a class I recommendation for patients with suspected ACS with chest discomfort at rest for longer than 20 min; hemodynamic instability or recent syncope or presyncope should be strongly considered for immediate referral to an emergency department or specialized chest pain unit. The foremost characteristic of ACS is persistent, severe chest pain or pressure, commonly described as crushing, squeezing, or heavy (likened to having an elephant sitting on the chest). The pain generally begins in the chest and, like angina, may radiate to the left arm, the abdomen, back, neck, jaw, or teeth. The onset of pain generally occurs at rest or with normal daily activities; it is not commonly associated with exertion.

2. Other common complaints include a sense of impending doom, sweating, nausea, vomiting, and difficulty breathing. In some patients, fainting and sudden death may be the initial presentation of ACS.

3. Observable findings include extreme anxiety, restless, agitated behavior, and ashen pallor.

4. Some patients, particularly those with diabetes or the elderly, may experience only mild or indigestion-like pain or a clinically silent MI, which may only manifest in worsening heart failure, loss of consciousness, acute confusion, dyspnea, a sudden drop in blood pressure, or a lethal arrhythmia.

F. Overall treatment goals in ACS

1. To relieve chest pain and anxiety

2. To reduce cardiac workload and stabilize cardiac rhythm

3. To prevent/reduce myocardial damage by limiting the area affected and preserving pump function

4. To prevent or arrest complications, such as lethal arrhythmias, AMI, HF, or sudden death

5. To reopen (or reperfuse) closed coronary vessels with thrombolytic drugs and/or PCI if indicated

G. Treatment of UA and NSTEMI

1. Anti-ischemic therapy

a. Current evidence-based clinical guidelines indicate class I recommendations for the following therapeutic interventions in patients with UA or NSTEMI:

(1) Bedrest with continuous ECG monitoring for ischemia and arrhythmia detection in patients with ongoing rest pain

(2) Nitroglycerin—sublingual, tablet, or spray followed by intravenous administration—for the immediate relief of ischemia and associated symptoms

(3) Supplemental oxygen for patients with cyanosis or respiratory distress and continued need for supplemental oxygen in the presence of hypoxemia

(4) Morphine sulfate intravenously when symptoms are not immediately relieved with nitroglycerin and a β-blocker, or when acute pulmonary congestion and/or severe agitation is present. Morphine has venodilation properties and will help patients with pulmonary congestion; it has the potential to reduce heart rate.

(5) A β-adrenergic blocker, with the first dose administered intravenously if there is ongoing chest pain, followed by oral administration in the absence of contraindications. Although there are no large studies on patients with UA, the proven benefits of β-blockers in patients with acute MI, HF, and angina have led to the recommendation of such drugs for UA patients as well.

(6) In patients with continuing or frequently recurring ischemia when β-adrenergic blockers are contraindicated, a non–dihydropyridine calcium antagonist (i.e., diltiazem or verapamil) is recommended as initial therapy in the absence of severe left ventricular dysfunction or other contraindications. In patients presenting with left ventricular dysfunction, current evidence shows that these agents might worsen the clinical status.

(7) An ACE inhibitor when hypertension persists despite treatment with nitroglycerin and a β-adrenergic blocker in patients with left ventricular dysfunction or HF and in ACS patients with diabetes. Angiotensin receptor blockers can be used in place of ACE inhibitors for patients intolerant to the ACE inhibitors.

b. Current evidence-based clinical practice guidelines indicate a class IIa recommendation for the following therapeutic interventions in patients with UA or NSTEMI:

(1) Oral long-acting calcium antagonists for recurrent ischemia in the absence of contraindications and when β-adrenergic blockers and nitrates are used at their maximal doses

(2) An ACE inhibitor for all post-ACS patients

(3) Intra-aortic balloon pump counterpulsation for severe ischemia that is continuing or recurs frequently despite intensive medical therapy or for hemodynamic instability in patients before or after coronary angiography

c. Current evidence-based clinical practice guidelines indicate a class IIb recommendation for the following therapeutic interventions in patients with UA or NSTEMI:

(1) Extended-release form of non–dihydropyridine calcium antagonists instead of a β-adrenergic blocker

(2) Immediate-release dihydropyridine (nifedipine-like) calcium antagonist in the presence of a β-adrenergic blocker

d. Current evidence-based clinical practice guidelines indicate a class III recommendation for the following therapeutic interventions in patients with UA or NSTEMI:

(1) Nitroglycerin or other nitrate within 24 hr of sildenafil (Viagra) use

(2) Immediate-release dihydropyridine calcium antagonist in the absence of a β-adrenergic blocker

2. Therapeutic agents. Table 39-4 lists selected agents and dosing regimens.

a. Nitrates (e.g., nitroglycerin). (See II.H.)

b. Morphine

(1) Mechanism of action. Morphine causes venous pooling and reduces preload, cardiac workload, and oxygen consumption. Morphine should be administered intravenously, starting with 2 mg and titrating at 5- to 15-min intervals until the pain is relieved or toxicity becomes evident.

(2) Indications. Morphine is the drug of choice for myocardial pain and anxiety.

(3) Precautions and monitoring effects

(a) Because morphine increases peripheral vasodilation and decreases peripheral resistance, it can produce orthostatic hypotension and fainting.

(b) Patients should be monitored for hypotension and signs of respiratory depression.

(c) Morphine has a vagomimetic effect that can produce bradyarrhythmias. If ECG monitoring reveals excess bradycardia, it should be reversed by administering atropine (0.5–1 mg).

(d) Nausea and vomiting may occur, especially with initial doses, and patients must be protected against aspiration of stomach contents.

(e) Severe constipation is a potential problem with ongoing morphine administration. The patient may need to use a Valsalva maneuver while straining at the stool, which can produce bradycardia or can overload the cardiac system and trigger cardiac arrest. Docusate (100 mg twice daily) is a useful prophylactic.

c. **Oxygen** is required at 2–4 L/min via nasal cannula in any patient who has chest pain and who may be ischemic. Mild hypoxemia is common in acute MI patients. Increasing the oxygen content of the blood, thus improving oxygenation of the myocardium, is a top priority as continuing hypoxia rapidly increases myocardial damage.

d. **Thrombolytic agents** have not demonstrated beneficial clinical outcomes in the absence of STEMI. Studies carried out to date have failed to show benefit with using thrombolytics in UA versus standard therapy to prevent MI. In addition, thrombolytic agents actually increased the risk of MI in such patients. Therefore, based on current evidence-based guidelines, thrombolytic agents are not recommended in the management of ACS without ST-segment elevation.

3. **Antiplatelet and anticoagulation therapy.** Table 39-5 lists selected agents and dosing regimens.

   a. Current evidence-based clinical guidelines indicate class I recommendations for the following therapeutic interventions in patients with UA or NSTEMI:

      (1) Antiplatelet therapy should be initiated promptly. Aspirin should be administered as soon as possible after presentation and continued indefinitely.

      (2) Clopidogrel should be administered to hospitalized patients who are unable to take aspirin because of hypersensitivity or major gastrointestinal intolerance.

      (3) In hospitalized patients for whom an early noninterventional approach is planned, clopidogrel should be added to aspirin as soon as possible on admission and administered for at least 1 month.

      (4) In patients for whom a PCI is planned, clopidogrel should be started and continued for at least 1 month and up to 9 months in patients who are not at high risk for bleeding.

      (5) In patients taking clopidogrel in whom elective coronary artery bypass grafting (CABG) is planned, the drug should be withheld for 5–7 days.

      (6) Anticoagulation with subcutaneous low molecular weight heparin (LMWH) or intravenous unfractionated heparin (UFH) should be added to antiplatelet therapy with aspirin and/or clopidogrel.

      (7) A platelet glycoprotein IIb/IIIa antagonist should be administered, in addition to aspirin and heparin, to patients for whom catheterization and PCI are planned. The agent may also be administered just before PCI.

   b. Current evidence-based clinical guidelines indicate a class IIa recommendation for the following therapeutic interventions in patients with UA or NSTEMI:

      (1) Eptifibatide or tirofiban should be administered, in addition to aspirin and LMWH or UFH, to patients with continuing ischemia, an elevated troponin, or other high-risk features for whom an invasive management strategy is not planned.

      (2) Enoxaparin is preferable to UFH as an anticoagulant in patients with UA or NSTEMI, unless CABG is planned within 24 hr.

      (3) A platelet glycoprotein IIb/IIIa antagonist should be administered to patients already receiving heparin, aspirin, and clopidogrel for whom catheterization and PCI are planned. The glycoprotein IIb/IIIa antagonist may also be administered just before PCI.

   c. Current evidence-based clinical practice guidelines indicate a class IIb recommendation for the following therapeutic intervention in patients with UA or NSTEMI: Eptifibatide or tirofiban, in addition to aspirin and LMWH or UFH, to patients without continuing ischemia who have no other high-risk features and for whom PCI is not planned.

   d. Current evidence-based clinical practice guidelines indicate a class III recommendation for the following therapeutic interventions in patients with UA or NSTEMI:

      (1) Intravenous (IV) thrombolytic therapy in patients without acute ST-segment elevation

      (2) Abciximab administration in patients for whom PCI is not planned

H. **STEMI.** Approximately 90% of patients with acute MI and ST-segment elevation have complete thrombotic occlusion of the infarct-related artery. Atherosclerotic plaques are made up of lipid and fibrous proteins. When the lesion ruptures, the release of adenosine diphosphate alteplase (ADP), serotonins, and thromboxane A_2 is triggered, leading to platelet aggregation and the

Table 39-5. Antithrombotic Agents Used in the Treatment of Ischemic Heart Disease

Class/Agent	Dosing Regimen	Level of Evidence (Guidelines)
Oral antiplatelets		
Aspirin	Initial dose of 162–325 mg followed by 75–160 mg/day	Class I
Clopidogrel (Plavix)	75 mg/day; loading dose of 4–8 tablets (300–600 mg) can be used when rapid onset of action required	Class I, if patient unable to tolerate aspirin
Ticlopidine (Ticlid)	250 mg twice daily; loading dose of 500 mg can be used when rapid onset of action required; monitoring of platelet and white cell counts during treatment required	Clopidogrel preferred over ticlopidine owing to its more rapid onset of action and better safety profile
Heparins		
Dalteparin, LMWH (Fragmin)	120 IU/kg SC every 12 hr (maximum 10,000 IU twice daily)	Class I
Enoxaparin, LMWH (Lovenox)	1 mg/kg subcutaneously every 12 hr; the first dose may be preceded by a 30-mg IV bolus dose	Class I
Heparin (UFH)	Bolus dose of 60–70 U/kg (maximum 5000 U) IV followed by infusion of 12–15 U/kg/hr (maximum 1000 U/hr) titrated to aPTT of 1.5–2.5 times control	Class I, current guidelines suggest that the evidence favors the use of enoxaparin over UHF as anticoagulant, unless CABG is planned within 24 hr
Intravenous antiplatelets		
Abciximab (Reopro)	0.25 mg/kg bolus followed by infusion of 0.125 mg/kg/min for 12–24 hr	Class I, for use in addition to aspirin and heparin in patients for whom catheterization and PCI are planned and in patients just before PCI Class III, in patients for whom PCI is not planned
Eptifibatide (Integrilin)	180 µg/kg bolus followed by infusion of 2.0 µg/kg/min for 72–96 hr	Class I, for use in addition to aspirin and heparin in patients for whom catheterization and PCI are planned, and in patients just before PCI Class IIa, in addition to aspirin and LMWH or UFH in patients with continuing ischemia, an elevated troponin, or with other high-risk features for whom an invasive management strategy is not planned Class IIb, in addition to aspirin and LMWH or UFH in patients without continuing ischemia who have no other high-risk features and for whom PCI is not planned
Tirofiban (Aggrastat)	0.4 µg/kg/min for 30 min followed by infusion of 0.1 µg/kg/min for 48–96 hr	Class I, in addition to aspirin and heparin in patients in whom catheterization and PCI are planned, and in patients just before PCI Class IIa, in addition to aspirin and LMWH or UFH in patients with continuing ischemia, an elevated troponin, or with other high-risk features for whom an invasive management strategy is not planned <Class IIb, in addition to aspirin and LMWH or UFH in patients without continuing ischemia who have no other high-risk features and for whom PCI is not planned

aPTT, activated partial thromboplastin time; *CABG,* coronary artery bypass graft; *IV,* intravenous; *LMWH,* low molecular weight heparin; *PCI,* percutaneous coronary intervention; *SC,* subcutaneous; *UFH,* intravenous unfractionated heparin.

formation of the primary clot. Thromboplastin released from the injured vessel initiates the clotting cascade. The resulting fibrin traps red blood cells (RBCs), platelets, and plasma protein to form an intraluminal thrombus. Clot dissolution is caused by the conversion of plasminogen to plasmin mediated by plasminogen activators. All patients with STEMI should be considered for antithrombotic therapy, which includes thrombolytics, heparin, LMWH, glycoprotein IIb/IIIa antagonists, warfarin, aspirin, and direct thrombin inhibitors.

1. **Mechanism of action.** Administration of thrombolytic agents causes the thrombus clot to be lysed when administered early after symptom onset ($< 6–12$ hr) and to restore blood flow. The conversion of plasminogen to plasmin promotes fibrinolysis and breakdown of the clot.

2. **Indications**
   a. Thrombolytic agents were used in patients with STEMI with chest pain $< 6–12$ hr. Successful early reperfusion has been shown to reduce infarct size, improve ventricular function, and improve mortality. However, benefits may be seen in patients using thrombolytic therapy as late as 12 hr after pain starts.
   b. Intravenous administration of a recombinant tissue-plasminogen activator (t-PA) such as alteplase (Activase), a recombinant plasminogen activator (r-PA) such as reteplase (Retavase), or tenecteplase (TNKase), may restore blood flow in an occluded artery if administered within 12 hr of an acute MI, although < 6 hr is optimal. The goal of treatment of STEMI patients is to initiate thrombolytic therapy within 30–60 min of arrival in an emergency room.
      (1) t-PA is relatively fibrin specific and is able to lyse clots without depleting fibrinogen, and TNKase has an even greater fibrin specificity. Streptokinase activates the fibrinolytic system and has a greater likelihood of causing systemic effects than t-PA. This effect may result in a greater degree of systemic bleeding compared with t-PA, r-PA, and TNK.
      (2) Though which agent—t-PA, r-PA, and TNK—is best is still controversial, most studies have shown that each agent, when used early, can reopen (reperfuse) occluded coronary arteries and reduce mortality from STEMI. However, considerations such as ease of use, onset of action, incidence of bleed, and cost are important factors in determining which agent to use for a given hospital and patient.

3. **Individual agents**
   a. **Alteplase (Activase)**
      (1) **Absolute contraindications** to t-PA include active internal bleeding; recent cerebrovascular accident (CVA); intracranial neoplasm; aneurysm; pregnancy; arteriovenous malformations; recent (within 2 months) intracranial surgery, spinal surgery, or trauma; and severe uncontrolled hypertension, bleeding diathesis, or hemorrhagic ophthalmic conditions.
      (2) A **front-loaded regimen**—an accelerated infusion that consists of a total dose of 100 mg or less that is given over 1.5 hr—may be more beneficial. The initial dose of 15 mg is given as an IV bolus, 1–2 min, while an infusion is begun to:
         (a) Infuse t-PA at the rate of 0.75 mg/kg over 30 min (not to exceed 50 mg)
         (b) Followed by t-PA infused at 0.5 mg/kg over 60 min (not to exceed 35 mg)
      (3) An alternate dosing regimen is based on the patient's weight.
         (a) **Dosage for patients > 65 kg.** A total of 100 mg of t-PA is generally administered to all patients who weigh > 65 kg over a 3-hr period. Though many regimens have been used, generally speaking, 6–10 mg of t-PA is given as an IV bolus over 1–2 min, followed by the remaining infusion rates over the next 3 hr: a 54–60-mg IV infusion over the 1st hr, a 20-mg IV infusion over the 2nd hr, and a 20-mg IV infusion over the 3rd hr.
         (b) **Dosage for patients < 65 kg.** A dose of 1.25 mg/kg is given over a 3-hr period, with 10% of the total dose given initially as a bolus dose over 1–2 min.
   b. **Reteplase (Retavase)**
      (1) **Absolute contraindications** to reteplase are similar to those for t-PA, though additional cautionary statements are given for patients with severely impaired renal function or liver function.
      (2) **Dosing** is initiated with the intravenous administration of 10 U over a 2-min period, and then repeated after 30 min, if there are no complications.

c. **Tenecteplase (TNKase)**
   (1) **Absolute contraindications** to tenecteplase are similar to those for t-PA and r-PA with the following addition: use with caution in patients recently receiving a glycoprotein IIb/IIIa agent, pregnant patients, elderly patients, patients with endocarditis, and patients with severe liver disease.
   (2) Tenecteplase is approved for use in acute treatment of MI at doses of 30–50 mg (based on the patient's weight) as a single IV bolus over 10-15 sec. Rapid rate of administration, fibrin specificity, fewer bleeding complications compared to t-PA, and superiority over t-PA in late-treated patients make tenecteplase a likely candidate to replace t-PA as the agent of choice in STEMI.

4. **Postthrombolysis adjunctive therapy.** Antiplatelet and anticoagulant therapy after successful reperfusion is necessary to prevent reocclusion, ischemia, and reinfarction.
   a. **Aspirin** administered (160–325 mg) during acute thrombolytic therapy has been shown to affect thrombolysis positively by preventing platelet aggregation and has reduced postinfarct mortality. Doses of aspirin, 75-162 mg daily have been recommended for long-term use at hospital discharge. Other agents include ticlopidine (Ticlid), and clopidogrel (Plavix).
   b. **Heparin** has been administered along with the thrombolytics to prevent reocclusion once a coronary artery has been opened. It also appears to decrease mortality in patients with an MI even if they have not received thrombolytic therapy.
      (1) In the United States, heparin has been given intravenously as a 4000-U bolus (60 U/kg), followed by a continuous infusion of 1000 U/hr (12 U/kg/hr); the goal of therapy is to maintain the activated partial thromboplastin time (aPTT) at 1.5–2 times control (50–70 sec).
      (2) Patients who have not received thrombolytic therapy but who are at risk for systemic or pulmonary embolism are candidates for continuous infusion of heparin. Other patients not receiving thrombolytic therapy may also benefit from low-dose subcutaneous heparin therapy until ambulatory.
      (3) LMWHs (e.g., enoxaparin, dalteparin) are currently being evaluated as alternatives to heparin.
   c. **Warfarin (Coumadin)** is approved for the treatment of acute MI to reduce mortality and prevent recurrent MI and other thromboembolic complications, such as stroke. The target international normalized ratio (INR) is 2.5–3.5.
   d. **Antiplatelet agents**—for example, abciximab (ReoPro) tirofiban (Aggrastat), eptifibatide (Integrilin)—act by inhibiting glycoprotein IIb/IIIa receptors. Fibrinogen acts with platelet glycoprotein IIb/IIIa receptors to mediate platelet aggregation. Combinations of these agents with thrombolytics have shown improved incidences and speed of reperfusion.
   e. **Heparin, enoxaparin (Lovenox), or dalteparin (Fragmin)** along with aspirin should be used in hospitalized patients with unstable angina for at least 48 hr, up to 5–8 days, or until the unstable angina has resolved.
   f. **β-Adrenergic blockers**
      (1) If administered early in the acute phase, β-adrenergic blockers have been shown to reduce ischemia, reduce the potential zone of infarction, decrease oxygen demands, preserve left ventricular function, and decrease cardiac workload.
      (2) β-adrenergic blocker therapy has also been shown to significantly reduce post-MI mortality owing to sudden death, risk of reinfarction, cardiac rupture, and ventricular arrhythmias.
   g. **ACE inhibitors**
      (1) Global left ventricular dysfunction has been determined to be an important marker of prognosis after MI. ACE inhibitors have clearly been shown to improve exercise capacity and reduce mortality in patients with moderate to severe congestive heart failure (CONSENSUS I trial, and Studies of Left Ventricular Dysfunction [SOLVD] trial).
      (2) ACE inhibitors are recommended in all patients indefinitely, starting as early as possible in stable patients who have high risks (e.g. anterior MI, previous MI, signs of HF). Angiotensin receptor blockers should be used in patients who cannot tolerate ACE inhibitors and who have signs of heart failure or an ejection fraction < 40%. ACE inhibitors are used after MI to prevent the development of progressive left ventricular dilation or "ventricular remodeling." These agents are beneficial in patients with MI presenting with left ventricular dysfunction.

(3) The HOPE trial was conducted to evaluate the effects of ramipril in preventing the primary end point, a composite of cardiovascular death, MI, and stroke. The results demonstrated that ramipril resulted in an reduction of 22% over placebo in the primary end points (cardiovascular mortality, MI, stroke). In addition, the benefits were observed in a broad range of patients without evidence of left ventricular dysfunction or heart failure who were at high risk for cardiovascular events.

h. Statins. Several large trials—Scandinavian Simvastatin Survival Study (4S), Long-Term Intervention with Pravastatin in Ischemic Disease (LIPID), and Cholesterol and Recurrent Events (CARE)—have shown that when HMG-CoA reductase inhibitors are used aggressively to lower cholesterol levels the result is a significant reduction in nonfatal MI or CHD (30%–40% reduction).

i. Lidocaine should not be administered prophylactically, but should be used in patients who develop ventricular arrhythmias.

j. Calcium-channel blocking agents are not used in acute phases of MI and may be harmful to patients with impaired left ventricular function. They may decrease the incidence of reinfarction in patients with non-Q-wave MIs.

k. Interventional therapy, coronary angiography, and percutaneous transluminal coronary angioplasty (PTCA) may be of use in patients who have contraindications to thrombolytic therapy, for those in cardiogenic shock, for those in whom thrombolytic therapy has failed, or for those with recurrent ischemia or hemodynamic instability.

(1) Adjunct therapy includes antiplatelet drugs, anticoagulants, use of intracoronary stents, and intra-aortic balloon pumping.

(2) Aspirin is given to reduce coronary reocclusion.

(3) Heparin in large doses continues to be administered 48–72 hr after the procedure.

(4) Intra-aortic balloon counter pulsation reduces recurrent ischemia and the incidence of reocclusion.

(5) Clopidogrel is administered with the aspirin in patients with intracoronary stent placement.

(6) Antiplatelet agents that bind to glycoprotein IIb/IIIa, such as abciximab, tirofiban, or eptifibatide, are used with heparin and aspirin.

I. Complications. MI potentiates many complications; the most common of these include the following:

1. Lethal arrhythmias. See Chapter 40 for a detailed discussion.

2. Heart failure. See Chapter 42 for a detailed discussion.
  a. Left ventricular failure causes pulmonary congestion. Diuretics, especially furosemide, help reduce the congestion.
  b. ACE inhibitors, β-adrenergic blockers, angiotensin receptor blockers, and direct-acting aldosterone antagonists play a key role in the treatment of heart failure.

3. Cardiogenic shock
  a. In this life-threatening complication, cardiac output is decreased and pulmonary artery and pulmonary capillary wedge pressures are increased. This typically occurs when the area of infarction exceeds 40% of muscle mass and compensatory mechanisms only strain the already compromised myocardium.
  b. Vasopressors—for example, norepinephrine (Levophed), epinephrine (Adrenalin), and dopamine (high doses)—enhance blood pressure through β-receptor stimulation and may be indicated.
  c. Inotropic drugs—for example, epinephrine, dopamine (middle doses), dobutamine, isoproterenol (Isuprel), and digoxin (Lanoxin)—are rapidly acting agents used to increase myocardial contractility and improve cardiac output.
  d. Vasodilators—for example, nitroprusside (Nipride)—reduce preload; they lower pulmonary capillary wedge pressure by dilating veins and reduce afterload by decreasing resistance to left ventricular ejection.
  e. Additional treatment may include invasive procedures such as intra-aortic balloon pumping.

STUDY QUESTIONS

Directions for questions 1–16: Each of the questions, statements, or incomplete statements in this section can be correctly answered or completed by **one** of the suggested answers or phrases. Choose the **best** answer.

1. Exertion-induced angina, which is relieved by rest, nitroglycerin, or both, is referred to as

   (A) Prinzmetal angina.
   (B) unstable angina.
   (C) stable angina.
   (D) variant angina.
   (E) preinfarction angina.

2. Myocardial oxygen demand is increased by all of the following factors *except*

   (A) exercise.
   (B) smoking.
   (C) cold temperatures.
   (D) isoproterenol.
   (E) metoprolol.

3. Which of the following agents used in Prinzmetal angina has spasmolytic actions, which increase coronary blood supply?

   (A) nitroglycerin
   (B) diltiazem
   (C) timolol
   (D) isosorbide mononitrate
   (E) propranolol

4. Patients with angina pectoris receiving propranolol plus diltiazem must be monitored for which adverse drug effect?

   (A) decreased cardiac output
   (B) decreased heart rate
   (C) increased heart rate
   (D) Both A and B
   (E) Both A and C

5. The development of ischemic pain occurs when the demand for oxygen exceeds the supply. Determinants of oxygen demand include all of the following choices *except* which one?

   (A) contractile state of the heart
   (B) myocardial ejection time
   (C) left ventricular volume
   (D) right atrial pressure
   (E) systolic pressure

6. Myopathy is an adverse effect of all the following agents *except*

   (A) lovastatin.
   (B) simvastatin.
   (C) pravastatin.
   (D) gemfibrozil.
   (E) colestipol.

7. Which of the following would not represent current therapeutic options in patients presenting with acute coronary syndrome (ACS) who are classified as having non-ST-segment elevated myocardial infarction (NSTEMI)?

   (A) sublingual nitroglycerin
   (B) β-adrenergic blockers
   (C) aspirin
   (D) morphine
   (E) tenecteplase

Directions for questions 8–9: The questions and incomplete statements in this section can be correctly answered or completed by **one or more** of the suggested answers. Choose the answer, **A–E.**

A	if **I only** is correct
B	if **III only** is correct
C	if **I and II** are correct
D	if **II and III** are correct
E	if **I, II, and III** are correct

For questions 8–9: A 55-year-old man arrives in the emergency room of the local hospital approximately 6 hr after developing chest pain with the signs and symptoms of an acute ST-segment elevated myocardial infarction (STEMI). This is the second such attack within the last 4 months, and the patient has not altered his lifestyle to eliminate important risk factors. Previous therapy included a thrombolytic agent (name unknown), a blood thinner, and daily aspirin.

8. Which of the following agents should be recommended during the acute myocardial infarction to help prevent sudden death?

   I. atenolol

   II. metoprolol

   III. ramipril

9. Which of the following is considered a component of acute coronary syndrome (ACS)?

   I. unstable angina

   II. non-ST-segment elevated myocardial infarction (NSTEMI)

   III. ST-segment elevated myocardial infarction (STEMI)

Directions for questions 10–14: Each of the following descriptions is most closely related to one of the following drugs. The descriptions may be used more than once or not at all. Choose the **best** answer, **A–E.**

(A) Inhibition of intestinal absorption of cholesterol

(B) Lowering of low-density lipoproteins (LDLs), triglycerides, and increased high-density lipoprotein (HDL) along with anti-inflammatory effects

(C) Glycoprotein IIb/IIIa antagonist that inhibits platelet aggregation

(D) Recommended for acute coronary syndrome (ACS) patients who cannot tolerate aspirin

(E) Recommended over unfractionated heparin (UFH) as an anticoagulant in patients with unstable angina (UA) or non-ST-segment elevated myocardial infarction (NSTEMI)

10. tirofiban

11. enoxaparin

12. simvastatin

13. clopidogrel

14. ezetimibe

ANSWERS AND EXPLANATIONS

1. The answer is C *[see II.C.1.a–f].*
Classic, or stable, angina refers to the syndrome in which physical activity or emotional excess causes chest discomfort, which may spread to the arms, legs, neck, and so forth. This type of angina is relieved promptly (within 1–10 mins) with rest, nitroglycerin, or both.

2. The answer is E *[see I.F.2; Table 39-1].*
Owing to the β-adrenergic blocking effects of metoprolol (e.g., decreased heart rate, decreased blood pressure, decreased inotropic effect), there is a net decrease in myocardial oxygen demand. This is the direct opposite of the effects seen with the β-agonist isoproterenol. Exercise, cigarette smoking, and exposure to cold temperatures have all been shown to increase myocardial oxygen demand.

3. The answer is B *[see II.H.4.c].*
Calcium-channel blocking agents such as diltiazem have been shown to be capable of reversing spasm and, therefore, increasing coronary blood flow in Prinzmetal angina. The calcium-channel blockers have proven benefit in the treatment of Prinzmetal angina, a syndrome believed due more to a spastic event than to a fixed coronary occlusion.

4. The answer is D *[see II.H.4.c.(1).(a); II.H.3.b.(2)].*
Because propranolol (a β-adrenergic blocker) and diltiazem (a calcium-channel blocker) both reduce heart rate (a negative chronotropic effect) and reduce cardiac contractility (negative inotropic effect), patients receiving both drugs must be monitored for signs of decompensation (reduced cardiac output) and bradyarrhythmias.

5. The answer is D *[see I.F.2].*
As with most muscles in the body, the contractile force of the heart dictates the amount of oxygen that the heart needs to perform efficiently. Consequently, as contractility decreases, the oxygen needs of the heart increase. As contractility continues to decrease, the volume of fluid in the left ventricle increases owing to poor muscle performance and increasing tension within the ventricle, resulting in additional oxygen requirements. As the amount of tension within the ventricle increases per cardiac cycle, there is again an added requirement for oxygen by the heart muscle.

6. The answer is E *[see II.G.2.d.(3)].*
Myopathy is an adverse effect of all the HMG-CoA reductase inhibitors (lovastatin, simvastatin, pravastatin, atorvastatin, and fluvastatin), and the combination of the fibric acid derivatives (gemfibrozil, fenofibrate, and clofibrate) has been shown to increase the creatine kinase levels and predispose patients to myopathies and rhabdomyolysis.

7. The answer is E *[see III.G.2.d].*
Tenecteplase is the newest of the thrombolytics available for clinical use. The most recent guidelines for the treatment of UA and NSTEMI have not demonstrated beneficial clinical outcomes of thrombolytic agents for these patients compared to standard therapy. In addition, thrombolytic agents actually increased the risk of MI in UA/NSTEMI patients. Therefore, based on current evidence-based guidelines, thrombolytic agents are not recommended in the management of ACS without ST-segment elevation.

8. The answer is C (I, II) *[see III.H.4.f].*
Recent studies have made it relatively clear that when atenolol, metoprolol, and propranolol are given during the acute phases of an MI, there is a significant reduction in sudden death and overall mortality in the patients treated. Each of these β-adrenergic blockers is given intravenously, followed by oral therapy, in an attempt to eliminate sudden death as a consequence of MI. Because of the negative inotropic and chronotropic effects, it is still imperative to monitor the patient closely for signs of cardiac decompensation and bradyarrhythmias.

9. The answer is E (I, II, III) *[see I.E.2].*
During recent years, there has been an attempt to link the various clinical symptoms of IHD into key categories, based on the presentation and symptoms at the time of evaluation. ACS refers to those situations that reflect an acute ischemic event and includes UA, NSTEMI, and STEMI. Clinical guidelines have incorporated treatment modalities based on these three presentations; UA and NSTEMI have similar recommended therapies and STEMI, has different treatment guidelines. Stable angina is not considered one of the ACS but represents the starting point for the progression of atherosclerosis, resulting in IHD.

10. The answer is C *[see III.H.4.d].*
Tirofiban is an antiplatelet that is referred to as a glycoprotein IIb/III, a receptor antagonist. This class of drugs works to prevent platelet aggregation by inhibiting the interaction between the primary binding site of platelets and has been shown to be effective in the prevention of thrombosis.

11. The answer is E *[see III.G.3.b.(2); Table 39-5].*
Enoxaparin is an example of a LMWH. As a group, the major advantage of these drugs over the more traditional heparin is that they exhibit a more predictable anticoagulant response. Owing to their lower molecular weight and decreased binding to plasma proteins, they have better bioavailability than heparin. In addition, their decrease in plasma protein binding and binding to the endothelium results in half-lives that are 2–4 times longer than that of heparin. Current clinical practice guidelines recommend enoxaparin over heparin in patients with UA or NSTEMI, unless CABG is planned within 24 hr.

12. The answer is B *[see II.G.2.b].*
Simvastatin is one of the five currently available HMG-CoA reductase inhibitors that have been shown to significantly reduce LDL levels and nonfatal MI or CHD (30%–40% reduction). Recent studies have demonstrated that inflammation is an important mechanism involved in ACS and that statins exert an important anti-inflammatory effect within coronary arteries (independent of their cholesterol-lowering effects).

13. The answer is D *[see II.H.5.c].*
Clopidogrel is a thienopyridine derivative related to ticlopidine that possesses antithrombotic effects that are greater than those of ticlopidine. Clopidogrel is a therapeutic option in those angina patients who cannot take aspirin. Doses of 75 mg daily are recommended to prevent the development of acute coronary syndromes.

14. The answer is A *[see II.G.5.a].*
Ezetimibe is the first in a new class of lipid-lowering compounds approved by the FDA, which reduces cholesterol levels via a different mechanism of action. By selectively blocking the intestinal absorption of cholesterol, it is able to stop one of the major pathways responsible for increasing available cholesterol within the body. Ezetimibe has demonstrated the ability to reduce total cholesterol, LDL, apolipoprotein B, and triglyceride levels while increasing HDL levels in patients with hypercholesterolemia. Simvastatin has recently been incorporated into a combination product with ezetimibe (Vytorin), which uses the individual class properties of the HMG-CoA reductase inhibitors (simvastatin) to reduce cholesterol production with the absorption-inhibiting properties of ezetimibe to target cholesterol with two different mechanisms, which might also aid in improving patient compliance with taking the medication.

40
Cardiac Arrhythmias
Alan H. Mutnick

I. INTRODUCTION. Sudden death from cardiac causes is believed to account for approximately 50% of all deaths from cardiovascular causes, with the majority of sudden deaths being caused by acute ventricular tachyarrhythmias. This would appear to create greater need for the knowledge necessary to appropriately use antiarrhythmics for this high-risk patient population. However, recently conducted studies have cast doubt on the true place of antiarrhythmics in the treatment and prevention of cardiac arrhythmias. Studies such as the Cardiac Arrhythmia Suppression Trial (CAST) have demonstrated that certain classes of antiarrhythmics increased mortality in patients treated with antiarrhythmics as compared to placebo. Since the release of the data from the CAST trial, subsequent studies have confirmed the finding that certain antiarrhythmics do possess "proarrhythmic" effects when used injudiciously. Consequently, the use of trial and error to determine antiarrhythmic therapy has given way to an era of outcome-based antiarrhythmic drug decision making. By understanding the causes of arrhythmias and being aware of drug–drug and drug–target interactions, we are more likely to understand the key considerations to maximize therapeutic strategies while minimizing drug-induced toxicities.

A. Definition. Cardiac arrhythmias are deviations from the normal heartbeat pattern. They include **abnormalities of impulse formation,** such as heart rate, rhythm, or site of impulse origin, and **conduction disturbances,** which disrupt the normal sequence of atrial and ventricular activation.

B. Electrophysiology

1. **Conduction system**
   a. **Two electrical sequences** that cause the heart chambers to fill with blood and contract are initiated by the conduction system of the heart.
      (1) **Impulse formation,** the first sequence, takes place when an electrical impulse is generated automatically.
      (2) **Impulse transmission,** the second sequence, occurs once the impulse has been generated, signaling the heart to contract.
   b. **Four main structures** composed of tissue that can generate or conduct electrical impulses make up the conduction system of the heart.
      (1) The **sinoatrial (SA) node,** in the wall of the right atrium, contains cells that spontaneously initiate an action potential. Serving as the main pacemaker of the heart, the SA node initiates 60–100 beats/min.
         (a) Impulses generated by the SA node trigger atrial contraction.
         (b) Impulses travel through internodal tracts—the anterior tract, middle tract (Wenckebach bundle), posterior tract (Thorel bundle), and anterior interatrial tract (Bachmann's bundle) (Figure 40-1).
      (2) At the **atrioventricular (AV) node,** situated in the lower interatrial septum, the impulses are delayed briefly to permit completion of atrial contraction before ventricular contraction begins.
      (3) At the **bundle of His**—muscle fibers arising from the AV junction—impulses travel along the left and right bundle branches, located on either side of the intraventricular septum.
      (4) The impulses reach the **Purkinje fibers,** a diffuse network extending from the bundle branches and ending in the ventricular endocardial surfaces. Ventricular contraction then occurs.
   c. **Latent pacemakers.** The AV junction, bundle of His, and Purkinje fibers are latent pacemakers; they contain cells capable of generating impulses. However, these regions have a slower firing rate than the SA node. Consequently, the SA node predominates except when it is depressed or injured, which is known as **overdrive suppression.**

2. **Myocardial action potential.** Before cardiac contraction can take place, cardiac cells must depolarize and repolarize.
   a. **Depolarization** and **repolarization** result from changes in the electrical potential across the cell membrane, caused by the exchange of sodium and potassium ions.

Figure 40-1. Electrical pathways of the heart. *AV,* atrioventricular; *SA,* sinoatrial.

b. **Action potential,** which reflects this electrical activity, has five phases (Figure 40-2).
   (1) **Phase 0 (rapid depolarization)** takes place as sodium ions enter the cell through fast channels; the cell membrane's electrical charge changes from negative to positive.
   (2) **Phase 1 (early rapid repolarization).** As fast sodium channels close and potassium ions leave the cell, the cell rapidly repolarizes (i.e., returns to resting potential).
   (3) **Phase 2 (plateau).** Calcium ions enter the cell through slow channels while potassium ions exit. As the cell membrane's electrical activity temporarily stabilizes, the action potential reaches a plateau (represented by the notch at the beginning of this phase in Figure 40-2).
   (4) **Phase 3 (final rapid repolarization).** Potassium ions are pumped out of the cell as the cell rapidly completes repolarization and resumes its initial negativity.

Figure 40-2. Myocardial action potential curve. This curve represents ventricular depolarization–repolarization. Phases: *0,* rapid depolarization; *1,* early rapid repolarization; *2,* plateau; *3,* final rapid repolarization; *4,* slow depolarization.

(5) Phase 4 (slow depolarization). The cell returns to its resting state with potassium ions inside the cell and sodium and calcium ions outside.
  c. During both depolarization and repolarization, a cell's ability to initiate an action potential varies.
    (1) The cell cannot respond to any stimulus during the **absolute refractory period** (beginning during phase 1 and ending at the start of phase 3).
    (2) A cell's ability to respond to stimuli increases as repolarization continues. During the **relative refractory period,** which occurs during phase 3, the cell can respond to a strong stimulus.
    (3) When the cell has been completely repolarized, it can again respond fully to stimuli.
  d. Cells in different cardiac regions depolarize at different speeds, depending on whether fast or slow channels predominate.
    (1) Sodium flows through fast channels; calcium flows through slow channels.
    (2) Where fast channels dominate (e.g., in cardiac muscle cells), depolarization occurs quickly. Where slow channels dominate (e.g., in the electrical cells of the SA node and AV junction), depolarization occurs slowly.

3. Electrocardiography. The electrical activity occurring during depolarization–repolarization can be transmitted through electrodes attached to the body and transformed by an **electrocardiograph (ECG) machine** into a series of waveforms (ECG waveform). Figure 40-3 shows a normal ECG waveform.
  a. The **P wave** reflects atrial depolarization.
  b. The **PR interval** represents the spread of the impulse from the atria through the Purkinje fibers.
  c. The **QRS complex** reflects ventricular depolarization.
  d. The **ST segment** represents phase 2 of the action potential—the absolute refractory period (part of ventricular repolarization).
  e. The **T wave** shows phase 3 of the action potential—ventricular repolarization.

C. Classification. Arrhythmias generally are classified by origin (i.e., supraventricular or ventricular).

1. Supraventricular arrhythmias stem from enhanced automaticity of the SA node (or another pacemaker region) or from reentry conduction.

2. Ventricular arrhythmias occur when an ectopic (abnormal) pacemaker triggers a ventricular contraction before the SA node fires (e.g., from a conduction disturbance or ventricular irritability).

3. Special note
  a. Torsades de pointes has received increased attention during the last few years as a major proarrhythmic event, which has been reported with antiarrhythmic drug therapy. It is defined as a polymorphic ventricular tachycardia with a twisting QRS complex morphology, which sometimes occurs with drugs that prolong ventricular repolarization (QT interval widening). Though initial reports of torsades de pointes centered around antiarrhythmic drugs (quinidine), today > 50 drugs, both antiarrhythmic agents and other classes of drugs such as antibiotics, have been shown to affect the duration of the QT interval and have been associated with this arrhythmia.
  b. A Web site devoted to providing education and research on drug-induced arrhythmias, especially those due to prolongation of the QT interval on the electrocardiogram (ECG), is available. The site, http://www.torsades.org/medical-pros/drug-lists/drug-lists.htm, is currently maintained by Dr. Raymond Woosley.

Figure 40-3. Normal ECG waveform.

    c. Woosley and colleagues have established the International Registry for Drug-Induced Arrhythmias, to which one can submit a suspected "drug-induced arrhythmia event." The registry also provides a list of drugs reported to prolong the QT interval or cause torsades de pointes (www.Torsades.org). Four drug lists were created based on the relative risk of inducing torsades de pointes (TdP) or a prolonged QT interval (Table 40-1).

D. Causes

  1. Precipitating causes. Arrhythmias result from various conditions, including
    a. Heart disease—for example, infection, coronary artery disease (CAD), valvular heart disease, rheumatic heart disease, ischemic heart disease
    b. Myocardial infarction (MI)
    c. Toxic doses of cardioactive drugs (e.g., digitalis preparations)
    d. Increased sympathetic tone
    e. Decreased parasympathetic tone
    f. Vagal stimulation (e.g., straining at stool)
    g. Increased oxygen demand (e.g., from stress, exercise, fever)
    h. Metabolic disturbances
    i. Cor pulmonale
    j. Systemic hypertension
    k. Hyperkalemia/hypokalemia
    l. Chronic obstructive pulmonary disease (COPD)—for example, chronic bronchitis, emphysema
    m. Thyroid disorders
    n. Drug therapy (both antiarrhythmic and non-antiarrhythmic drugs)

  2. Mechanisms of arrhythmias. Abnormal impulse formation, abnormal impulse conduction, or a combination of both may give rise to arrhythmias.
    a. Abnormal impulse formation may stem from:
      (1) Depressed automaticity, as in escape beats and bradycardia
      (2) Increased automaticity, as in premature beats, tachycardia, and extrasystole
      (3) Depolarization and triggered activity, leading to sustained ectopic firing
    b. Abnormal impulse conduction results from:
      (1) A conduction block or delay
      (2) Reentry occurs when an impulse is rerouted through certain regions in which it has already traveled. Thus the impulse depolarizes the same tissue more than once, producing an additional impulse (Figures 40-4 and 40-5). Reentry sites include the SA and AV nodes as well as various accessory pathways in the atria and ventricles (Figure 40-6). For reentry to occur, the following conditions must exist:
        (a) Markedly shortened refractoriness or a slow conduction area that allows an adequate delay so that depolarization recurs
        (b) Unidirectional conduction

E. Pathophysiology. Arrhythmias may decrease cardiac output, reduce blood pressure, and disrupt perfusion of vital organs. Specific pathophysiological consequences depend on the arrhythmia present.

F. Clinical evaluation

  1. Physical findings. Although some arrhythmias are silent, most produce signs and symptoms. Only an ECG can definitively identify an arrhythmia. However, physical findings may suggest which arrhythmia is present; they also yield information about the patient's clinical status and may help identify associated complications. **Signs and symptoms** that typically accompany arrhythmias include
    a. Chest pain
    b. Anxiety and confusion (from reduced brain perfusion)
    c. Dyspnea
    d. Skin pallor or cyanosis
    e. Abnormal pulse rate, rhythm, or amplitude
    f. Reduced blood pressure
    g. Palpitations
    h. Syncope

Table 40-1. Lists 1–4: Drugs That Prolong the QT Interval and/or Induce Torsades de Pointes

List 1. Drugs That Are Generally Accepted by Authorities to Have a Risk of Causing Torsades de Pointes

Drug (Generic)	Brand Name	Drug Class (Clinical Usage)	Comments[a]
Amiodarone	Cordarone	Antiarrhythmic: abnormal heart rhythm	F > M;TdP risk regarded as low
Arsenic trioxide	Trisenox	Anticancer: leukemia	
Bepridil	Vascor	Anti-anginal: heart pain	F > M
Chlorpromazine	Thorazine	Antipsychotic, antiemetic: schizophrenia, nausea	
Cisapride	Propulsid	GI stimulant: heartburn	Restricted availability; F > M
Clarithromycin	Biaxin	Antibiotic: bacterial infection	
Disopyramide	Norpace	Antiarrhythmic: abnormal heart rhythm	F > M
Dofetilide	Tikosyn	Antiarrhythmic: abnormal heart rhythm	
Domperidone	Motilium	Antinausea: nausea	
Droperidol	Inapsine	Sedative, antinausea: anesthesia adjunct, nausea	
Erythromycin	Erythrocin	Antibiotic, GI stimulant: bacterial infection, increase GI motility	F > M
Halofantrine	Halfan	Antimalarial: malaria infection	F > M
Haloperidol	Haldol	Antipsychotic: schizophrenia, agitation	
Ibutilide	Corvert	Antiarrhythmic: abnormal heart rhythm	F > M
Levomethadyl	Orlaam	Opiate agonist: pain control, narcotic dependence	
Mesoridazine	Serentil	Antipsychotic: schizophrenia	
Methadone	Dolophine	Opiate agonist: pain control, narcotic dependence	F > M
Methadone	Methadose	Opiate agonist: pain control, narcotic dependence	F > M
Pentamidine	NebuPent	Anti-infective: *Pneumocystis* pneumonia	F > M
Pimozide	Orap	Antipsychotic: Tourette tics	F > M
Procainamide	Pronestyl	Antiarrhythmic: abnormal heart rhythm	
Quinidine	Quinaglute	Antiarrhythmic: abnormal heart rhythm	F > M

List 2. Drugs That in Some Reports May Be Associated with Torsades de Pointes, but at This Time Lack Substantial Evidence for Causing Torsades de Pointes.

Drug (Generic)	Brand Name	Drug Class (Clinical Usage)
Amantadine	Symmetrel	Dopaminergic, antiviral, anti-infective: Parkinson disease
Azithromycin	Zithromax	Antibiotic: bacterial infection
Chloral hydrate	Noctec	Sedative: sedation: insomnia
Clozapine	Clozaril	Antipsychotic: schizophrenia
Dolasetron	Anzemet	Antinausea: nausea, vomiting
Felbamate	Felbatrol	Anticonvulsant: seizure
Flecainide	Tambocor	Antiarrhythmic: abnormal heart rhythm
Foscarnet	Foscavir	Antiviral: HIV infection
Fosphenytoin	Cerebyx	Anticonvulsant: seizure
Gatifloxacin	Tequin	Antibiotic: bacterial infection
Gemifloxacin	Factive	Antibiotic: bacterial infection
Granisetron	Kytril	Antinausea: nausea and vomiting

(*Continued on next page*)

Table 40-1. Continued.

Drug (Generic)	Brand Name	Drug Class (Clinical Usage)
Indapamide	Lozol	Diuretic: stimulate urine and salt loss
Isradipine	DynaCirc	Antihypertensive: high blood pressure
Levofloxacin	Levaquin	Antibiotic: bacterial infection
Lithium	Eskalith,	Antimania: bipolar disorder
Moexipril/HCTZ	Uniretic	Antihypertensive: high blood pressure
Moxifloxacin	Avelox	Antibiotic: bacterial infection
Nicardipine	Cardene	Antihypertensive: high blood pressure
Octreotide	Sandostatin	Endocrine: acromegaly, carcinoid diarrhea
Ondansetron	Zofran	Antiemetic: nausea and vomiting
Quetiapine	Seroquel	Antipsychotic: schizophrenia
Risperidone	Risperdal	Antipsychotic: schizophrenia
Salmeterol	Serevent	Sympathomimetic: asthma, COPD
Tacrolimus	Prograf	Immunosuppressant
Tamoxifen	Nolvadex	Anticancer: breast cancer
Telithromycin	Ketek	Antibiotic: bacterial infection
Tizanidine	Zanaflex	Muscle relaxant
Venlafaxine	Effexor	Antidepressant: depression
Voriconazole	Vfend	Antifungal: antifungal
Ziprasidone	Geodon	Antipsychotic: schizophrenia

List 3. Drugs to Be Avoided for Use in Patients with Diagnosed or Suspected Congenital Long QT Syndrome (Including Drugs on Lists 1 and 2)

Drug (Generic)	Brand Names	Drug Class (Clinical Usage)	Comments	List
Albuterol	Proventil	Bronchodilator: asthma		3
Amantadine	Symmetrel	Dopaminergic, antiviral, anti-infective: Parkinson disease		2
Amiodarone	Cordarone	Antiarrhythmic: abnormal heart rhythm	F > M; TdP risk regarded as low	1
Arsenic trioxide	Trisenox	Anticancer: leukemia		1
Azithromycin	Zithromax	Antibiotic: bacterial infection		2
Bepridil	Vascor	Antianginal: heart pain	F > M	1
Chloral hydrate	Noctec	Sedative, sedation: insomnia		2
Chlorpromazine	Thorazine	Antipsychotic, antiemetic: schizophrenia, nausea	Restricted availability; F > M	1
Cisapride	Propulsid	GI stimulant: heartburn		1
Clarithromycin	Biaxin	Antibiotic: bacterial infection		1
Cocaine	Cocaine	Local anesthetic		3
Disopyramide	Norpace	Antiarrhythmic: abnormal heart rhythm	F > M	1
Dobutamine	Dobutrex	Catecholamine: heart failure and shock		3
Dofetilide	Tikosyn	Antiarrhythmic: abnormal heart rhythm		1
Dolasetron	Anzemet	Antinausea: nausea, vomiting		2
Domperidone	Motilium	Antinausea: nausea		1
Dopamine	Intropine	Antiarrhythmic: abnormal heart rhythm		3
Droperidol	Inapsine	Sedative, antinausea: anesthesia adjunct, nausea		1
Ephedrine	Rynatuss	Bronchodilator, decongestant: allergies, sinusitis, asthma		3
Epinephrine	Primatene	catecholamine, vasoconstrictor: anaphylaxis, allergic reactions		3

(Continued on next page)

Table 40-1. Continued.

Drug (Generic)	Brand Names	Drug Class (Clinical Usage)	Comments	List
Erythromycin	Erythrocin	Antibiotic, GI stimulant: bacterial infection, increase GI motility	F > M	1
Felbamate	Felbatrol	Anticonvulsant: seizure		2
Fenfluramine	Pondimin	Appetite suppressant: dieting, weight loss		3
Flecainide	Tambocor	Antiarrhythmic: abnormal heart rhythm		2
Foscarnet	Foscavir	Antiviral: HIV infection		2
Fosphenytoin	Cerebyx	Anticonvulsant: seizure		2
Gatifloxacin	Tequin	Antibiotic: bacterial infection		2
Granisetron	Kytril	Antinausea: nausea and vomiting		2
Halofantrine	Halfan	Antimalarial: malaria infection		1
Haloperidol	Haldol	Antipsychotic: schizophrenia, agitation	F > M	1
Ibutilide	Corvert	Antiarrhythmic: abnormal heart rhythm	F > M	1
Indapamide	Lozol	Diuretic: stimulate urine and salt loss		2
Isoproterenol	Isupres	Catecholamine: allergic reaction		3
Isradipine	DynaCirc	Antihypertensive: high blood pressure		2
Levalbuterol	Xopenex	Bronchodilator: asthma		3
Levofloxacin	Levaquin	Antibiotic: bacterial infection		2
Levomethadyl	Orlaam	Opiate agonist: pain control, narcotic dependence		1
Lithium	Eskalith	Antimania: bipolar disorder		2
Mesoridazine	Serentil	Antipsychotic: schizophrenia		1
Metaproterenol	Alupent	Bronchodilator: asthma		3
Methadone	Dolophine	Opiate agonist: pain control, narcotic dependence	F > M	1
Midodrine	ProAmatine	Vasoconstrictor: low blood pressure, fainting		3
Moexipril/HCTZ	Uniretic	Antihypertensive: high blood pressure		2
Moxifloxacin	Avelox	Antibiotic: bacterial infection		2
Nicardipine	Cardene	Antihypertensive: high blood pressure		2
Norepinephrine	Levophed	Vasoconstrictor, inotrope: shock, low blood pressure		3
Octreotide	Sandostatin	Endocrine: acromegaly, carcinoid diarrhea		2
Ondansetron	Zofran	Antiemetic: nausea and vomiting		2
Pentamidine	NebuPent	Anti-infective: *Pneumocystis* pneumonia	F > M	1
Phentermine	Fastin	Appetite suppressant: dieting, weight loss		3
Phenylephrine	Neo-Synephrine	Vasoconstrictor, decongestant: low blood pressure, allergies, sinusitis, asthma		3
Phenylpropanolamine	Acutrim	Decongestant: allergies, sinusitis, asthma		3
Pimozide	Orap	Antipsychotic: Tourette tics	F > M	1
Procainamide	Pronestyl	Antiarrhythmic: abnormal heart rhythm		1

(*Continued on next page*)

Table 40-1. Continued.

Drug (Generic)	Brand Names	Drug Class (Clinical Usage)	Comments	List
Procainamide	Procan	Antiarrhythmic: abnormal heart rhythm		1
Pseudoephedrine	PediaCare	Decongestant: allergies, sinusitis, asthma		3
Pseudoephedrine	Sudafed	Decongestant: allergies, sinusitis, asthma		3
Quetiapine	Seroquel	Antipsychotic: schizophrenia	F > M	2
Quinidine	Quinaglute	Antiarrhythmic: abnormal heart rhythm		1
Risperidone	Risperdal	Antipsychotic: schizophrenia		2
Ritodrine	Yutopar	Uterine relaxant: prevent premature labor		3
Salmeterol	Serevent	Sympathomimetic: asthma, COPD		2
Sibutramine	Meridia	Appetite suppressant: dieting, weight loss	F > M	3
Sotalol	Betapace	Antiarrhythmic: abnormal heart rhythm		1
Sparfloxacin	Zagam	Antibiotic: bacterial infection		1
Tacrolimus	Prograf	Immunosuppressant		2
Tamoxifen	Nolvadex	Anticancer: breast cancer		2
Telithromycin	Ketek	Antibiotic: bacterial infection		2
Terbutaline	Brethine	Bronchodilator: asthma		3
Thioridazine	Mellaril	Antipsychotic: schizophrenia		1
Tizanidine	Zanaflex	Muscle relaxant		2
Venlafaxine	Effexor	Antidepressant: depression		2
Voriconazole	Vfend	Antifungal: antifungal		2
Ziprasidone	Geodon	Antipsychotic: schizophrenia		2

List 4. Drugs That in Some Reports Have Been Weakly Associated with Torsades de Pointes, but That When Used in Usual Dosages Are Unlikely to Be a Risk for Torsades de Pointes

Drug (Generic)	Brand Names	Drug Class (Clinical Usage)
Amitriptyline	Elavil	Tricyclic antidepressant: depression
Amoxapine	Asendin	Tricyclic antidepressant: depression
Ampicillin	Principen	Antibiotic: infection
Ciprofloxacin	Cipro	Antibiotic: bacterial infection
Citalopram	Celexa	Antidepressant : depression
Clomipramine	Anafranil	Tricyclic antidepressant: depression
Desipramine	Pertofrane	Tricyclic antidepressant: depression
Doxepin	Sinequan	Tricyclic antidepressant: depression
Fluconazole	Diflucan	Antifungal: fungal infection
Fluoxetine	Prozac	Antidepressant: depression
Galantamine	Reminyl	Cholinesterase inhibitor: dementia, Alzheimer
Imipramine	Norfranil	Tricyclic antidepressant: depression
Itraconazole	Sporanox	Antifungal: fungal infection
Ketoconazole	Nizoral	Antifungal: fungal infection
Mexiletine	Mexitil	Antiarrhythmic: abnormal heart rhythm
Nortriptyline	Pamelor	Tricyclic antidepressant: depression
Paroxetine	Paxil	Antidepressant: depression
Protriptyline	Vivactil	Tricyclic antidepressant: depression
Sertraline	Zoloft	Antidepressant: depression
Trimethoprim-Sulfamethoxazole	Bactrim	Antibiotic: bacterial infection
Trimipramine	Surmontil	Tricyclic antidepressant: depression

COPD, chronic obstructive pulmonary disease; *GI,* gastrointestinal.
[a]*TdP,* U.S. Food and Drug Administration–approved labeling includes mention of cases or a risk of torsades de pointes.
F > M, Substantial evidence indicates a greater risk (usually more than twofold) of TdP in females than in males.
Reproduced with permission from R. Woosley, vice president for health sciences, University of Arizona Health Sciences Center, Tucson, AZ. Drug lists available at http://www.torsades.org/medical-pros/drug-lists/drug-lists.htm.

Figure 40-4. Reentry arrhythmias. **A.** Two waves of excitation going in opposite directions. **B.** A unidirectional wave of excitation. **C.** Reexcitation of tissue in a slow conduction area.

     i. Weakness
     j. Convulsions
     k. Hypotension
     l. Decreased urinary output

2. Diagnostic test results
    a. An **ECG** can identify a specific arrhythmia; usually, a 12-lead ECG is used.
    b. Electrophysiological (EP) testing. This intracardiac procedure determines the location of ectopic foci and bypass tracts and may help assess therapeutic response to antiarrhythmic drug therapy. It also can determine the need for a pacemaker or surgical intervention.
       (1) Intracardiac catheters and pacing wires are placed transvenously or transarterially.
       (2) The heart is divided into imaginary sections, and each section is stimulated until an arrhythmia is induced. The section in which the arrhythmia occurs is identified as the origin of the ectopic foci.
    c. His bundle study, a type of EP testing, can locate the origin of a heart block or reentry pattern.

Figure 40-5. Ventricular reentry: a branched Purkinje fiber joining ventricular muscle. The *dark area* represents the site of a unidirectional block. In this depolarization region, the impulse heading toward the atrioventricular node continues upward, whereas the impulse traveling toward the muscle is blocked. Because retrograde conduction in *branch B* is slow, cells in *branch A* have time to recover and respond to the reentrant impulse.

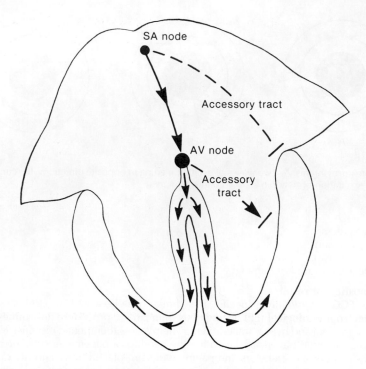

Figure 40-6. Reentry sites. *AV,* atrioventricular; *SA,* sinoatrial.

    d. Laboratory findings. Some arrhythmias result from electrolyte abnormalities—most commonly, hyperkalemia and hypocalcemia.
        (1) A serum potassium level > 5 mEq/L reflects hyperkalemia; a serum calcium level < 4.5 mEq/L signifies hypocalcemia.
        (2) An ECG tracing may suggest an electrolyte abnormality. For example, prolonged QRS complexes, tented T waves, and lengthened PR intervals may signal hyperkalemia; prolonged QT intervals and flattened, or inverted, T waves suggest hypocalcemia.

G. Treatment objectives

    1. Terminate or **suppress the arrhythmia** if it causes hemodynamic compromise or disturbing symptoms.

    2. Maintain adequate cardiac output and tissue perfusion.

    3. Correct or maintain fluid balance (some arrhythmias cause hypervolemia).

II. THERAPY. Antiarrhythmic agents directly or indirectly alter the duration of the myocardial action potential. Most antiarrhythmics fall into one of four classes, depending on their specific effects on the heart's electrical activity (Table 40-2).

A. Class I antiarrhythmics

    1. Indications
        a. Class IA drugs
            (1) Quinidine is used to treat and prevent acute and chronic ventricular and supraventricular arrhythmias, especially paroxysmal supraventricular tachycardias (PSVTs), premature ventricular contractions (PVCs), premature atrial contractions (PACs), and ventricular tachycardia.
            (2) Procainamide is used for the same arrhythmias for which quinidine is given. It is used more frequently than quinidine because it can be administered intravenously

Table 40-2. Williams's Classification of Antiarrhythmic Drugs Currently Available in the United States

Class	Action	Drugs
IA (fast-channel blockers)	Moderate depression of conduction, prolongation of repolarization, which results in an increase in the QRS interval and an increase in the QT interval	Disopyramide (Norpace), procainamide (Pronestyl), quinidine
IB	Modest depression of conduction, shortening of repolarization, which results in a decrease in the QT interval	Lidocaine (Xylocaine), mexiletine (Mexitil), phenytoin (Dilantin),
IC	Strong depression of conduction, with mild or no effect on repolarization, which results in a very large increase in the QRS interval	Flecainide (Tambocor), moricizine (Ethmozine), propafenone (Rythmol)
II (β-blockers)	β-adrenergic blockers slow sinus as well as AV nodal conduction, which results in a decrease in heart rate and a prolongation in the PR interval (atrial depolarization)	Propranolol (Inderal), esmolol (Brevibloc), acebutolol (Sectral)[a]
III	Prolongation of repolarization, which results in prolongation of the QT interval	Amiodarone (Cordarone), sotalol[b] (Betapace), ibutilide (Corvert), dofetilide (Tikosyn)
IV (slow-channel blockers)	Calcium-channel blockade in calcium-dependent channels, which results in reduced heart rate and an increase in the PR interval	Verapamil (Calan), diltiazem (Cardizem)
Other		Adenosine (Adenocard), atropine, digoxin (Lanoxin), magnesium

[a]Singh BN, Vaughan Williams EM. Classification of antiarrhythmic drugs. In: Sandoe E, Flensted-Jensen E, Olesen KH, eds. Symposium on Cardiac Arrythmias. Sodertalige: AB Astra, 1970.
[b]Sotalol is a β-adrenergic blocker that prolongs the action potential of phase 3 and is classified as type III.

and in sustained-release oral preparations. Quinidine poses added concern when used intravenously because of increased cardiovascular effects (i.e., hypotension, syncope, myocardial depression).

    (3) Disopyramide may be used as an alternative to quinidine or procainamide for treating ventricular arrhythmias (e.g., PVCs, moderate ventricular tachycardia).

  b. Class IB drugs

    (1) Lidocaine is used therapeutically for ventricular arrhythmias (especially PVCs and ventricular tachycardia) that result from acute MI and open-heart surgery. Controversy still exists as to the benefits of lidocaine when used prophylactically in patients with acute MI to prevent ventricular fibrillation. A recent analysis showed an increase in the number of deaths in patients receiving lidocaine during an acute MI as compared to placebo. Many feel that its current use prophylactically post-MI is no longer justified.

    (2) Phenytoin is most commonly used to treat digitalis-induced ventricular and supraventricular arrhythmias. It is also given to suppress ventricular arrhythmias associated with acute MI, open-heart surgery, or ventricular arrhythmias that are refractory to lidocaine or procainamide, but its efficacy is less significant for these indications than it is for digitalis-induced arrhythmias.

    (3) Mexiletine is closely related to lidocaine, structurally with modifications, which reduce first-pass liver metabolism, making oral therapy possible. It is most commonly used to treat patients in whom a class I agent has failed and is moderately effective in suppressing ventricular ectopy, although comparable to quinidine.

  c. Class IC drugs

    (1) Flecainide suppresses PVCs and ventricular tachycardia; it may be used to treat some arrhythmias that are refractory to other agents. Flecainide is reserved for patients with refractory life-threatening ventricular arrhythmias who do not have CAD. It has also been shown to be effective in the treatment of supraventricular arrhythmias.

(2) **Propafenone** also suppresses PVCs and ventricular tachycardia and has been used successfully for treating sustained ventricular tachycardia when the arrhythmia is life-threatening. It has also been shown to be effective in the treatment of supraventricular arrhythmias.

(3) **Moricizine** is a difficult antiarrhythmic to classify based on the fact that it has properties of all three class I antiarrhythmic groups. Because it prolongs the QRS interval like other class IC agents, it has been classified as a class IC agent throughout this discussion. Moricizine is effective for suppressing PVCs and may offer some benefits over other agents because of a lower incidence of proarrhythmic effects.

2. **Mechanism of action.** As a class, all of the agents work by blocking the rapid inward sodium current and thereby slow down the rate of rise of the cardiac tissue's action potential. However, though this is a similar effect for all class I agents, differences in EP effects had led to a subclassification of the class I agents into three subsets (IA, IB, and IC), based on these EP effects.

   a. **Class IA drugs** moderately reduce the depolarization rate and prolong repolarization (refractory period).

   b. **Class IB drugs** shorten repolarization (refractory period); they also weakly affect the repolarization rate.

   c. **Class IC drugs** strongly depress depolarization but have a negligible effect on the duration of repolarization or refractoriness.

3. **Administration and dosage**

   a. **Quinidine** is administered orally, usually in 3–4 daily doses of 200–400 mg as a rapid-release sulfate salt (83% quinidine). However, sustained-release products in the form of a gluconate (62% quinidine) salt or a polygalacturonate (60% quinidine) salt in doses of 324–648 mg, which corresponds to 300–600 mg of the sulfate salt, may be given every 8 hr (polygalacturonate) or 12 hr (gluconate). (In special circumstances, it has been given intravenously or intramuscularly with caution.) To achieve an effective plasma concentration rapidly, a loading dose of 600–1000 mg may be administered in doses of 200 mg every 2 hr to a maximum of 1000 mg, or a 5–8 mg/kg intravenous infusion can be given at a rate of 0.3 mg/kg/min.

   b. **Procainamide (Pronestyl)** is available for oral, intravenous, or intramuscular use.

      (1) For **acute therapy,** intravenous administration is preferred.

         (a) Intermittent intravenous administration calls for the administration of an intravenous dose of 3–6 mg/kg infusion (up to 100 mg) over 2–4 min, repeated every 5–10 min until the arrhythmia is abolished, side effects occur, or 1 g has been given. The usual effective dose is 500–1000 mg.

         (b) Rapid intravenous administration calls for infusion of 1–1.5 g at a rate of 20–50 mg/min.

         (c) Once the arrhythmia is terminated, 1.5–5 mg/min is given as a continuous infusion.

      (2) For **long-term therapy,** oral administration is used. The usual daily dosage is 50 mg/kg in divided doses given every 6 hr as a sustained-release product or 3–6 g daily.

         (a) Capsules and tablets (Pronestyl) available as 250, 375, and 500 mg given in 4–6 divided doses

         (b) Sustained-release tablets (Pronestyl-SR) available as 250, 500, 750, and 1000 mg given in 6-hr doses

         (c) Sustained-release tablets (Procanbid) available as 500 and 1000 mg given in 12-hr doses

   c. **Disopyramide (Norpace)** is available in oral form.

      (1) Usually, 300–400 mg is given as a loading dose to attain an effective plasma level rapidly.

      (2) For maintenance therapy, doses of 400–800 mg/day are given in 4 doses every 6 hr (non–sustained-release capsule) or in 2 doses every 12 hr (sustained-release capsule).

   d. **Lidocaine (Xylocaine)** may be administered intravenously or intramuscularly.

      (1) An intravenous loading dose rapidly achieves a therapeutic plasma level.

         (a) Initially, 1–1.5 mg/kg (100 mg) is administered.

         (b) A second injection of half the initial dose may be required 5 min later, up to a maximum of 300 mg.

(2) Continuous intravenous infusion of 2–4 mg/min produces an effective plasma level in 7–10 hr.

(3) In an emergency, an intramuscular injection rapidly achieves an effective plasma level. The usual dosage is 300–400 mg injected into the deltoid muscle.

e. Phenytoin (Dilantin) is given orally or in intermittent intravenous doses.

(1) For oral administration, a loading dose of 1 g is divided over the first 24 hr; for the next 2 days, 300–500 mg/day is administered. The maintenance dosage is 300–400 mg/day.

(2) For intermittent intravenous administration, 100 mg is given every 5 min at a rate not exceeding 25–50 mg/min, until the arrhythmia disappears, adverse effects develop, or 1 g has been given. The usual effective dosage is 700 mg.

f. Mexiletine (Mexitil) is administered orally and should be initiated in the hospital setting.

(1) A loading dose of 400 mg followed by maintenance dosage in 8 hr.

(2) If this fails to control the arrhythmia, the dosage may be increased to 400 mg every 8 hr. (Alternatively, doses may be given every 12 hr.)

(3) Normal maintenance doses are 200–300 mg every 8 hr.

g. Flecainide (Tambocor) is administered orally and should be initiated in the hospital setting.

(1) Initial dosage is 50 mg every 12 hr, and the dosage may be increased in twice-daily increments of 50 mg every 4 days to a maximum of 300 mg/day.

(2) The usual maintenance dose is 100 mg every 12 hr.

h. Propafenone (Rythmol) is administered orally and should be initiated in the hospital setting.

(1) Initial dosage is 150 mg every 8 hr and can be increased every 3–4 days to the desired therapeutic effect or side effects.

(2) The usual maintenance dose is 150–200 mg every 8 hr, up to a maximum of 900 mg /day.

i. Moricizine (Ethmozine) is administered orally and should be initiated in the hospital setting.

(1) Initial dosage is 200 mg every 8 hr, increased every 3 days by 150 mg to the desired effect or side effects.

(2) The usual maintenance dose is 200–300 mg divided into 3 equal doses throughout the day.

4. Precautions and monitoring effects. Note: Proarrhythmia (the ability to cause an arrhythmia) is the most important risk associated with the use of antiarrhythmic drug therapy. Bradyarrhythmias and ventricular tachyarrhythmias, such as torsades de pointes, can occur. These often take place during the initiation of antiarrhythmic drug treatment and should be considered when decision makers choose between outpatient and inpatient initiation of antiarrhythmic therapy.

a. Quinidine

(1) This drug is contraindicated in patients with

(a) Complete AV block unless a ventricular pacemaker is in place

(b) Marked prolongation of the QT interval or prolonged QT syndrome because ventricular tachyarrhythmia (torsades de pointes) may arise, resulting in quinidine syncope (i.e., syncope or sudden death)

(2) An increase of 50% or more in the duration of the QRS complex necessitates dosage reduction.

(3) Quinidine has a narrow therapeutic index. Therapeutic serum levels are in the range of 2–6 μg/mL, depending on the specificity of the assay. Toxicity may cause acute cardiac effects, such as pronounced slowing of conduction in all heart regions; this, in turn, may lead to SA block or arrest, ventricular tachycardia, or asystole.

(4) The ECG should be monitored during quinidine therapy to detect signs of cardiotoxicity. To counteract quinidine-induced ventricular tachyarrhythmias, catecholamines, glucagon, or sodium lactate may be given.

(5) In patients receiving quinidine for atrial tachyarrhythmias, vagolytic effects may increase impulse conduction at the AV node, resulting in an accelerated ventricular response. To prevent this, agents that slow AV nodal conduction (e.g., verapamil, digoxin) may be administered.

(6) The dosage should be reduced in elderly patients (> 60 years old) and in patients with hepatic dysfunction or congestive heart failure (CHF).

(7) Embolism may occur on restoration of normal sinus rhythm after prolonged atrial fibrillation. To prevent or minimize this complication, anticoagulants may be administered before quinidine therapy begins.

(8) Quinidine may cause cinchonism at high serum concentrations, manifested by tinnitus, hearing loss, blurred vision, and gastrointestinal (GI) disturbances. In severe cases, nausea, vomiting, diarrhea, headache, confusion, delirium, photophobia, diplopia, and psychosis may occur.

(9) GI reactions are the most common adverse reactions to quinidine. About 30% of patients experience diarrhea; nausea and vomiting may also occur. Arising almost immediately after the first dose, these symptoms sometimes warrant discontinuing the drug. However, aluminum hydroxide or use of the polygalacturonate salt may reverse this.

(10) Hypersensitivity reactions include anaphylaxis, thrombocytopenia, respiratory distress, and vascular collapse.

b. Procainamide (Pronestyl)

(1) This drug is contraindicated in patients with hypersensitivity to procaine and related drugs, myasthenia gravis, second- or third-degree AV block with no pacemaker, a history of procainamide-induced systemic lupus erythematosus (SLE), prolonged QT syndrome, or torsades de pointes.

(2) An increase of 50% or more in the duration of the QRS complex necessitates dosage reduction.

(3) Procainamide has a narrow therapeutic index. Therapeutic serum levels are reported in the range of 4–10 μg/mL. *N*-acetyl procainamide (NAPA) levels of 15–25 μg/mL are considered therapeutic. The active metabolite, NAPA possesses differing pharmacological cardiovascular effects, and serum levels need to be evaluated independently of procainamide. Toxicity may cause acute cardiac effects (e.g., pronounced slowing of conduction in all heart regions), which, in turn, may lead to SA block or arrest, ventricular tachycardia, or asystole.

(4) High serum procainamide levels may induce ventricular arrhythmias (e.g., PVCs, ventricular tachycardia or fibrillation). The ECG should be monitored continuously to detect these problems. Catecholamines, glucagon, or sodium lactate may be administered to counteract these arrhythmias.

(5) Hypotension may occur with rapid intravenous administration.

(6) GI effects are less common than with quinidine therapy.

(7) Hypersensitivity reactions are the most severe adverse effects of procainamide. These reactions include drug fever, agranulocytosis, and an SLE-like syndrome.

    (a) An SLE-like syndrome is manifested by fatigue, arthralgia, myalgia, and low-grade fever.

    (b) Antinuclear antibody titer is positive in 50%–80% of patients receiving procainamide. However, only 20%–30% of these patients develop symptoms of the SLE-like syndrome.

    (c) Drug discontinuation usually is necessary when symptomatic SLE-like syndrome occurs.

(8) The dosage should be reduced and given over 6 hr to patients with renal or hepatic impairment, as the drug half-life is increased in these patients.

(9) Lower doses may be needed in patients with CHF to adjust for the lower volume of distribution.

(10) Embolism may occur on restoration of normal sinus rhythm after prolonged atrial fibrillation. An anticoagulant is frequently administered before procainamide therapy begins to prevent this complication.

c. Disopyramide (Norpace)

(1) This drug may cause marked hemodynamic compromise and ventricular dysfunction. It is contraindicated in patients with cardiogenic shock or second- or third-degree AV block with no pacemaker.

(2) Disopyramide should be avoided or used with extreme caution in patients with CHF. It should also be used cautiously in patients with urinary tract disorders, myasthenia gravis, and renal or hepatic dysfunction.

(3) In patients receiving this drug for atrial tachyarrhythmias, vagolytic effects may increase impulse conduction at the AV node, resulting in an accelerated ventricular response. To prevent this, agents that slow AV nodal conduction (e.g., verapamil, digoxin) may be given.

    (4) Anticholinergic effects of this drug include dry mouth, constipation, urinary hesitancy or retention, and blurred vision.

    (5) Therapeutic plasma levels range from 2 to 4 μg/mL.

d. Lidocaine (Lidocaine)

    (1) This drug may cause hemodynamic compromise in patients with severe cardiac dysfunction. Generally, however, it has few untoward cardiovascular effects.

    (2) Lidocaine should be used cautiously and in reduced dosage in patients with CHF or renal or hepatic impairment.

    (3) Central nervous system (CNS) reactions are the most pronounced adverse effects of lidocaine. These reactions may range from lightheadedness and restlessness to confusion, tremors, stupor, and convulsions.

    (4) Tinnitus, blurred vision, and anaphylaxis have been reported.

    (5) Plasma lidocaine levels of 1.5–6.5 μg/mL are therapeutic.

    (6) Lidocaine's metabolites—glycinexylidide and monoethylglycinexylidide—may have neurotoxic as well as antiarrhythmic effects.

e. Phenytoin (Dilantin)

    (1) This drug is contraindicated in patients with sinus bradycardia or heart block.

    (2) Phenytoin must be used cautiously in patients with heart failure (HF), renal or hepatic impairment, myocardial insufficiency, respiratory depression, or hypotension.

    (3) During acute therapy, this drug may cause CNS reactions (e.g., drowsiness, vertigo, nystagmus, ataxia, nausea). Cardiotoxicity also may occur, especially with fast intravenous infusion rates.

    (4) Chronic phenytoin may lead to vestibular and cerebellar effects, behavioral changes, GI distress, gingival hyperplasia, megaloblastic anemia, and osteomalacia.

    (5) Hypersensitivity reactions may be manifested by liver, skin, and hematological problems.

      (a) Toxic hepatitis may occur.

      (b) Skin reactions include exfoliative dermatitis, Stevens-Johnson syndrome, scarlatiniform or morbilliform rash, SLE, toxic epidermal necrolysis, eosinophilia, and erythema multiforme.

      (c) Hematological reactions include agranulocytosis, megaloblastic anemia, leukopenia, thrombocytopenia, and pancytopenia.

    (6) Therapeutic plasma phenytoin levels range from 10 to 18 μg/mL.

f. Mexiletine (Mexitil)

    (1) This drug is contraindicated in patients with cardiogenic shock or second- or third-degree AV block with no pacemaker.

    (2) Tremor is an early sign of mexiletine toxicity. Dizziness, ataxia, and nystagmus indicate an increasing plasma drug concentration.

    (3) Hypotension, bradycardia, and widened QRS complexes may develop during mexiletine therapy.

    (4) Adverse GI effects include nausea and vomiting.

    (5) Therapeutic serum levels range from 0.50 to 2.0 μg/mL.

g. Flecainide (Tambocor)

    (1) This drug is contraindicated in patients with cardiogenic shock or second- or third-degree AV block with no pacemaker.

    (2) The ECG should be monitored during flecainide therapy because this drug may exacerbate existing arrhythmias or precipitate new ones. Flecainide was shown in the CAST study to increase mortality in patients with asymptomatic ventricular arrhythmias and, therefore, should be reserved for patients with life-threatening ventricular arrhythmias that are refractory to other drugs.

    (3) This drug has a significant negative inotropic effect and may bring on or worsen CHF and cardiomyopathy.

    (4) Adverse CNS effects (e.g., dizziness, headache, tremor) and GI effects (e.g., nausea, abdominal pain) may occur.

    (5) Blurred vision and dyspnea have been reported.

    (6) Therapeutic serum levels recommended for flecainide are between 0.2 and 1.0 μg/mL.

h. Propafenone (Rythmol)

   (1) This drug, like other antiarrhythmic agents, may cause new or worsened arrhythmias. Such proarrhythmic properties range from an increased frequency of PVCs to the development of severe ventricular tachycardia, ventricular fibrillation, and torsades de pointes. This proarrhythmic effect has been under discussion for the class IC agents; thus, when used, these agents should be monitored closely. The findings from the CAST study must be weighed against the benefits of using these agents for treating significant ventricular arrhythmias.

   (2) Dizziness is a side effect that has been reported in as many as 10%–15% of patients taking the drug.

   (3) Other associated side effects include vomiting, a metallic bitter taste in the mouth, constipation, headache, and new or worsening CHF and asthma.

   (4) Therapeutic serum levels recommended for propafenone are between 0.06 and 1.0 μg/mL.

i. Moricizine (Ethmozine)

   (1) This drug has been reported to have proarrhythmic properties. However, it has been reported that the incidence of this effect may be less than with other antiarrhythmics. Patients predisposed to the development of such proarrhythmic effects include those with a history of coronary artery bypass surgery, pacemakers, CAD, CHF, and conduction abnormalities. As most patients receiving this agent have at least one of the previously mentioned risk factors, this agent must be used cautiously. The benefits of using this agent must be weighed against its associated risks.

   (2) Dizziness is the most commonly reported adverse effect associated with the drug and has been reported in up to 15% of all patients.

   (3) Other associated side effects include nausea, intraventricular conduction delays, headache, fatigue, palpitations, and shortness of breath.

   (4) Further studies are necessary, as no specific concentrations have generally been defined.

5. Significant interactions

   a. Quinidine

      (1) Quinidine may increase serum levels of **digoxin** and increase the effects of **digitalis** on the heart, with a resultant increase in toxicity.

      (2) Severe orthostatic hypotension may occur with concomitant administration of **vasodilators** (e.g., **nitroglycerin**).

      (3) **Phenytoin, rifampin (Rifadin),** and **barbiturates** may antagonize quinidine activity and reduce its therapeutic efficacy.

      (4) **Nifedipine (Procardia)** may reduce plasma quinidine levels.

      (5) **Antacids, sodium bicarbonate (Neut),** and **sodium acetazolamide (Diamox)** may increase plasma quinidine levels, possibly resulting in toxicity.

      (6) Quinidine may produce additive hypoprothrombinemic effects with **coumarin** anticoagulants.

   b. Amiodarone (Cordarone) and **cimetidine (Tagamet)** may increase plasma procainamide levels, possibly leading to drug toxicity.

   c. Phenytoin accelerates disopyramide metabolism, possibly reducing its therapeutic efficacy.

   d. Lidocaine

      (1) **Phenytoin** may increase the cardiodepressant effects of lidocaine.

      (2) **β-Blockers** (class II antiarrhythmics) may reduce lidocaine metabolism, possibly leading to drug toxicity.

   e. Phenytoin

      (1) The risk of phenytoin toxicity increases with concomitant administration of **diazepam (Valium), antihistamines, isoniazid (Nydrazid), chloramphenicol (Chloromycetin), cimetidine (Tagamet), salicylates, sulfisoxazole (Gantrisin), amiodarone (Cordarone),** and **valproate (Depacon).**

      (2) **Carbamazepine (Tegretol)** may enhance phenytoin metabolism and thus reduce plasma phenytoin levels and therapeutic efficacy. (Phenytoin has the same effect on carbamazepine.)

   f. Mexiletine (Mexitil). Phenobarbital, rifampin (Nydrazid), and **phenytoin (Dilantin)** reduce plasma mexiletine levels and may decrease therapeutic efficacy.

B. Class II antiarrhythmics

1. **Indications.** These drugs—**β-adrenergic blockers**—are used mainly to treat systemic hypertension. Among the drugs in this class, propranolol, esmolol, and acebutolol are approved for antiarrhythmic use.
   a. **Propranolol-(Inderal)** may be given to:
      (1) Control supraventricular arrhythmias (e.g., atrial fibrillation or flutter, PSVTs)
      (2) Treat tachyarrhythmias caused by catecholamine stimulation (e.g., in hyperthyroidism, during anesthesia)
      (3) Suppress severe ventricular arrhythmias in **prolonged QT syndrome**
      (4) Treat digitalis-induced ventricular arrhythmias
      (5) Terminate certain ventricular arrhythmias (e.g., PVCs in patients without structural heart disease)
   b. **Esmolol (Brevibloc)** is used to treat supraventricular tachycardias; it possesses a short (9-min) half-life and has been used to control the ventricular response to atrial fibrillation or flutter during or after surgery.

2. **Mechanism of action.** Class II antiarrhythmics reduce sympathetic stimulation of the heart, decreasing impulse conduction through the AV node and lengthening the refractory period. Additionally, this class of antiarrhythmics slow the sinus rhythm without significantly changing the QT or QRS intervals, resulting in a reduced heart rate and a decrease in myocardial oxygen demand.

3. **Administration and dosage**
   a. **Propranolol** may be given intravenously or orally when used as an antiarrhythmic.
      (1) Emergency therapy calls for slow intravenous administration of 1–3 mg diluted in 50 mL dextrose 5% in water or normal saline solution. This dose is infused slowly (no faster than 1 mg/min). A second dose of 1–3 mg may be given 2 min later.
      (2) For oral therapy, 10–80 mg/day is given in 3–4 doses. (However, 1000 mg or more may be required for resistant ventricular arrhythmias.)
   b. **Esmolol** is given intravenously. A loading dose of 500 μg/kg/min is infused over 1 min, followed by a 4-min maintenance infusion of 50 μg/kg/min. If a satisfactory response is not achieved within 5 min, the loading dose is repeated and followed by a maintenance infusion of 100 μg/kg/min.

4. **Precautions and monitoring effects**
   a. **Propranolol (Inderal)**
      (1) This drug is contraindicated in patients with sinus bradycardia, second- or third-degree AV block, cardiogenic shock, severe HF, or asthma.
      (2) The β-blocking effects of this drug may lead to marked hypotension, exacerbation of CHF and left ventricular failure, or cardiac arrest.
      (3) Blood pressure, heart rate, and the ECG should be monitored during intravenous infusion.
      (4) Embolism may occur upon restoration of normal sinus rhythm after sustained atrial fibrillation. An anticoagulant may be given before propranolol therapy begins to prevent this complication.
      (5) Propranolol may depress AV node conduction and ventricular pacemaker activity, resulting in AV block or asystole.
      (6) This drug may mask the signs and symptoms of hypoglycemia. It also may mask signs of shock.
      (7) Fatigue, lethargy, increased airway resistance, and skin rash have been reported.
      (8) Nausea, vomiting, and diarrhea may occur.
      (9) Sudden withdrawal of propranolol may lead to acute MI, arrhythmias, or angina in cardiac patients. Drug therapy is discontinued by tapering the dose over 4–7 days.
   b. **Esmolol (Brevibloc)**
      (1) This drug is contraindicated in patients with severe CHF or sinus bradycardia.
      (2) Hypotension occurs in approximately 30% of patients receiving esmolol. This effect can be reversed by reducing the dosage or stopping the infusion.
      (3) This drug is for short-term use only and should be replaced by a long-acting antiarrhythmic once the patient's heart stabilizes.
      (4) Dizziness, headache, fatigue, and agitation may occur.
      (5) Other adverse effects include nausea, vomiting, and bronchospasm.

5. **Significant interactions**
   a. **Propranolol**
      (1) Severe vasoconstriction may occur with concomitant **epinephrine** administration.
      (2) **Digitalis** preparations can cause excessive bradycardia.
      (3) **Calcium-channel blockers**—for example, **diltiazem (Cardizem)** and **verapamil (Calan)**—and other negative **inotropic** and **chronotropic drugs**—such as **disopyramide (Norpace)** and **quinidine**—add to the myocardial depressant effects of propranolol.
   b. **Esmolol. Morphine (MS Contin)** may raise plasma esmolol levels.

C. **Class III antiarrhythmics**

1. **Indications**
   a. **Amiodarone (Cordarone)** is given to control malignant ventricular arrhythmias and has most recently within the new advanced cardiac life support (ACLS) guidelines been recommended in the treatment of ventricular fibrillation and pulseless ventricular tachycardia, and may be used prophylactically against both atrial and ventricular tachycardia and fibrillation. Unlike most other antiarrhythmics, with the exception of the β-adrenergic blockers, amiodarone has been shown to reduce arrhythmic deaths in patients after an MI.
   b. **Sotalol (Betapace)** is used to treat supraventricular and ventricular tachyarrhythmias. Sotalol antagonizes both β_1- and β_2- adrenergic receptors, but also prolongs the phase 3 action potential. It is this property that distinguishes it from other β-adrenergic blockers and is the reason why it is classified as a type III antiarrhythmic drug rather than a type II agent (β-adrenergic blocker).
   c. **Ibutilide (Corvert)** is used in the conversion of atrial fibrillation and flutter of recent onset (duration < 30 days).
   d. **Dofetilide (Tikosyn)** is available in the United States under restricted access in the treatment of atrial fibrillation/flutter.

2. **Mechanism of action.** Class III antiarrhythmic drugs prolong the refractory period and action potential; they have no effect on myocardial contractility or conduction time.

3. **Administration and dosage**
   a. **Amiodarone (Cordarone)** Available for both oral and intravenous use and should only be initiated in the hospital setting. The Amiodarone in Out-of-Hospital Resuscitation of Refractory Sustained Ventricular Tachycardia (ARREST) study compared amiodarone with placebo in a blinded, randomized trial in patients with shock-refractory out-of-hospital ventricular fibrillation or pulseless ventricular tachycardia. This was the first large, randomized study to show a benefit of any antiarrhythmic drug over placebo in patients with out-of-hospital cardiac arrest. Amiodarone-treated patients had a significantly greater likelihood of surviving to hospital admission as compared to the placebo patients. Since publication of the ARREST trial, amiodarone has been incorporated into the most recent ACLS (2005) guidelines and recommended by the expert panel members as the first-choice antiarrhythmic for shock-refractory ventricular fibrillation/ventricular tachycardia.
      (1) It is available for oral use; 800–1600 mg every 12 hr is given for 7–14 days, then 200–400 mg daily thereafter.
      (2) Oral treatment is used to suppress ventricular and supraventricular arrhythmias but can take days or weeks to take effect. Oral doses of 100–600 mg/day (usually 300–400 mg/day) for maintenance therapy in ventricular tachycardia and 100–200 mg/day for maintenance therapy for supraventricular tachycardias are given.
      (3) Intravenous formulation is available for treatment and prophylaxis of recurrent ventricular fibrillation or hemodynamically unstable ventricular tachycardia in refractory patients.
      (4) The intravenous form is rapidly distributed throughout the body. Recommended doses include a rapid loading infusion of 150 mg over 10 min, followed by a slow infusion of 1 mg/min for 6 hr (360 mg), and then a maintenance infusion of 0.5 mg/min for the remainder of the 24-hr period. Patients usually receive 2–4 days of infusions before conversion to oral form. However, a maintenance infusion can be continued for 2–3 weeks.
   b. **Sotalol (Betapace)** is available commercially as an oral tablet, and therapy should be initiated within the hospital setting. Normal dosing of 80 mg twice daily initially and

increasing doses at 2- to 3-day intervals to a maximum dose of 640 mg/day, given in 2–3 doses throughout the day.

c. **Ibutilide (Corvert)** is available only for injection in a 0.1-mg/mL, 10-mL vial. Normal doses for the conversion of recent-onset atrial fibrillation to normal sinus rhythm is a dose of 1 mg (0.01 mg/kg for those < 60 kg) over 10 min, with a repeat dose in 10 min if the arrhythmia does not end.

d. **Dofetilide (Tikosyn)** is available only for oral administration in 0.125-, 0.25-, and 0.5-mg capsules under the trade name of Tikosyn and should only be initiated in a hospital setting with trained personnel and the equipment necessary to provide continuous cardiac monitoring during initiation of therapy.

   (1) A normal dose for the conversion of recent-onset atrial fibrillation to normal sinus rhythm is 0.5 mg twice daily for patients with creatinine clearance values > 60 mL/min; doses are reduced 50% (0.25 mg) for those with creatinine clearance values of 40–60 mL/min, and doses are reduced an additional 50% (0.125 mg) for those with creatinine clearance values of 20–40 mL/min.

   (2) Maintenance therapy is based on the ECG; with doses being reduced with QTc prolongation exceeding 15% of the baseline value. Any patient developing a QTc interval exceeding 500 msec should have therapy discontinued immediately.

   (3) Dofetilide should not be given to those with creatinine clearance values < 20 mL/min.

4. **Precautions and monitoring effects**
   a. **Amiodarone (Cordarone)**
      (1) Life-threatening pulmonary toxicity may occur during amiodarone therapy, especially in patients receiving > 400 mg/day. Baseline as well as routine pulmonary function tests reveal relevant pulmonary changes.
      (2) Most patients develop corneal microdeposits 1–4 months after amiodarone therapy begins. However, this reaction rarely causes visual disturbance, but the patient should be monitored with routine ophthalmological examinations.
      (3) Blood pressure and heart rate and rhythm should be monitored for hypotension and bradyarrhythmias.
      (4) Patients should be monitored routinely for the possible development of hepatic dysfunction, thyroid disorders (e.g., hyperthyroidism, hypothyroidism), and photosensitivity.
      (5) CNS reactions include fatigue, malaise, peripheral neuropathy, and extrapyramidal effects.
      (6) Nausea and vomiting have been reported.
      (7) This drug has an extremely long half-life (up to 60 days). Therapeutic response may be delayed for weeks after oral therapy begins; adverse reactions may persist up to 4 months after therapy ends.
   b. **Sotalol (Betapace)**
      (1) Side effects of this drug are directly related to β-blockade and prolongation of repolarization.
      (2) Transient hypotension, bradycardia, myocardial depression, and bronchospasm have all been associated with this drug.
      (3) This drug carries all the contraindications associated with other β-blockers along with those owing to its electrophysiologic properties.
   c. **Ibutilide (Corvert)**
      (1) Infusion should be discontinued as soon as the atrial arrhythmia is terminated or if sustained or nonsustained ventricular arrhythmia or marked QT prolongation is documented.
      (2) Continuous ECG monitoring is required for at least 4 hr after discontinuing the infusion or until the QT interval returns to baseline.
   d. **Dofetilide (Tikosyn)**
      (1) Patients need to be monitored closely for the subsequent development of ventricular arrhythmias with increasing doses of dofetilide or with declining renal status. In clinical trials, ventricular tachycardias, including torsades de pointes, are the most frequently occurring arrhythmias due to dofetilide.
      (2) Hypokalemia and those situations that might cause hypotension will predispose a patient to prolongation of the QT interval, which could put a dofetilide patient at risk for toxic arrhythmias.

5. Significant interactions
   a. Amiodarone
      (1) Amiodarone may increase the plasma levels of **quinidine, procainamide, diltiazem, digitalis,** and **flecainide.**
      (2) It may increase the pharmacological effect of β-blockers, **calcium-channel blockers,** and **warfarin.**
      (3) Special note: Amiodarone has been reported to have numerous drug–drug interactions among all categories of drugs. To avoid the development of a significant drug–drug interaction a thorough patient medication profile should be carried out for each patient having amiodarone therapy initiated, as well as each time a patient currently receiving amiodarone is given an additional drug.
   b. Sotalol
      (1) Sotalol must be used cautiously in those patients receiving agents with cardiac-depressant properties.
      (2) Agents such as sotalol, which prolong the QT interval, may induce malignant arrhythmias when used in combination with other type IA antiarrhythmics, especially in the presence of low potassium levels.
   c. Ibutilide should be avoided with other agents that prolong repolarization or within 4 hr of administration.
   d. Dofetilide should be avoided in patients who have hypokalemia or preexisting QT prolongation.

D. Class IV antiarrhythmics

1. Indications
   a. Calcium-channel blockers (e.g., verapamil, Calan; diltiazem, Cardizem) are used mainly to treat and prevent supraventricular arrhythmias.
      (1) They are first-line agents for the suppression of PSVTs stemming from AV nodal re-entry.
      (2) They can rapidly control the ventricular response to atrial flutter and fibrillation.
   b. Other calcium-channel blockers available include nicardipine, nifedipine, bepridil, amlodipine, and felodipine, but these agents have primarily been used in the treatment of angina pectoris and hypertension. For information on these agents, see Chapters 39 and 41.

2. Mechanism of action. Class IV antiarrhythmics are calcium-channel blockers. They inhibit AV node conduction by depressing the SA and AV nodes, where calcium channels predominate.

3. Administration and dosage
   a. To control atrial arrhythmias, verapamil usually is administered intravenously. A dose of 2.5–10 mg is given over at least 2 min and may be repeated in 30 min, if necessary. A 5–10 mg/hr continuous intravenous infusion has also been used in treating arrhythmias.
   b. To prevent PSVTs, verapamil may be given orally in four daily doses of 80–120 mg each.
   c. To control atrial arrhythmias, diltiazem usually is administered intravenously. A dose of 20 mg (0.25 mg/kg) is given over 2 min. If an adequate response is not obtained, a second dose of 25 mg (0.35 mg/kg) is administered after 15 min. A 5–15 mg/hr intravenous continuous infusion has also been used in treating arrhythmias.

4. Precautions and monitoring effects
   a. Verapamil and diltiazem are contraindicated in patients with AV block; left ventricular dysfunction; severe hypotension,; concomitant, intravenous β-blockers; and atrial fibrillation with an accessory AV pathway.
   b. These drugs must be used cautiously in patients with CHF, sick sinus syndrome, MI, and hepatic or renal impairment.
   c. Because of the negative chronotropic effect, verapamil and diltiazem must be used cautiously in patients who have slow heart rates or who are receiving digitalis glycosides.
   d. The ECG (especially the RR interval) should be monitored during therapy.
   e. Patients > 60 years old should receive reduced dosages and slower injection rates.
   f. Constipation and nausea have been reported with verapamil.

5. Significant interactions
  a. Concomitant administration of β-**blockers** or **disopyramide** may precipitate heart failure.
  b. Quinidine may increase the risk of calcium-channel blocker–induced hypotension.
  c. Verapamil may increase serum **digoxin** concentrations, and diltiazem may do the same to a lesser extent.
  d. Rifampin may enhance the metabolism of calcium-channel blockers, with a resultant decrease in pharmacological effect.
  e. Verapamil and diltiazem may inhibit **theophylline** metabolism and may require reductions in theophylline dosage.
  f. Diltiazem and verapamil inhibit the metabolism of **cyclosporine (Gengraf)** and may require reductions in cyclosporine dosages.

E. Unclassified antiarrhythmics

1. Atropine
  a. Indications. Atropine is therapeutic for symptomatic sinus bradycardia and junctional rhythm.
  b. Mechanism of action. An anticholinergic, atropine blocks vagal effects on the SA node, promoting conduction through the AV node and increasing the heart rate.
  c. Administration and dosage. For antiarrhythmic use, atropine is administered in a dose of 0.4–1 mg by intravenous push; the dose is given every 5 min to a maximum of 2 mg.
  d. Precautions and monitoring effects
    (1) Thirst and dry mouth are the most common adverse effects of atropine.
    (2) CNS reactions (e.g., restlessness, headache, disorientation, dizziness) may occur with doses over 5 mg.
    (3) Tachycardia and ophthalmic disturbances (e.g., mydriasis, blurred vision, photophobia) may occur with doses of 1 mg or more.
    (4) Initial doses may induce a reflex bradycardia owing to incomplete suppression of vagal impulses.

2. Adenosine (Adenocard)
  a. Indications. Adenosine is indicated for the conversion of acute supraventricular tachycardia to normal sinus rhythm.
  b. Mechanism of action. Adenosine is a naturally occurring nucleoside, which is normally present in all cells of the body. It has been shown to:
    (1) Slow conduction through the AV node
    (2) Interrupt reentry pathways through the AV node
    (3) Restore normal sinus rhythm in patients with PSVTs
  c. Administration and dosage. For antiarrhythmic effects, adenosine is given as a rapid bolus intravenous injection in a 6-mg dose over 1–2 sec. If the first dose does not eliminate the arrhythmia within 1–2 min, the dose should be increased to 12 mg and again given as a rapid intravenous dose. An additional 12-mg dose may be repeated if necessary.
  d. Precautions and monitoring effects
    (1) The effects of adenosine are antagonized by methylxanthines, such as caffeine and theophylline. Theophylline has been successfully used for treating adenosine-induced side effects, such as hypotension, sweating, and palpitations. If side effects are encountered, aggressive therapy is not required because of the ultra-short half-life of the drug (10 sec or less).
    (2) The main side effect associated with adenosine use in up to 18% of patients is facial flushing, but this effect is normally very short-lived.
    (3) Other side effects associated with adenosine use include shortness of breath, chest pressure, nausea, headache, and a metallic taste.
  e. Additional use. Adenosine has been used as an adjunctive agent in patients undergoing various types of pharmacological stress testing (e.g., with thallium). In this situation, adenosine is given as a continuous infusion over a period of 4–6 min and is able to provide a form of exercise tolerance test in patients not able to exert themselves owing to age, fatigue, and various other physical handicaps.

STUDY QUESTIONS

Directions: Each of the questions, statements, or incomplete statements can be correctly answered or completed by **one** of the suggested answers or phrases. Choose the **best** answer.

1. Strong anticholinergic effects limit the antiarrhythmic use of

   (A) quinidine.
   (B) procainamide.
   (C) tocainide.
   (D) flecainide.
   (E) disopyramide.

2. A pronounced slowing of phase 0 of the myocardial action potential results in a prolongation of either atrial depolarization causing a prolonged P wave on the electrocardiogram (ECG) or ventricular depolarization causing a prolonged QRS complex characterized by which class of antiarrhythmics?

   (A) type I
   (B) type II
   (C) type III
   (D) type IV
   (E) type V

3. Which of the following type III antiarrhythmics has been reported as causing the torsades de pointes type of ventricular tachycardia?

   (A) lidocaine
   (B) amiodarone
   (C) quinidine
   (D) flecainide
   (E) diltiazem

4. A patient receiving a class I antiarrhythmic agent on a chronic basis complains of fatigue, low-grade fever, and joint pain suggestive of systemic lupus erythematosus (SLE). The patient is most likely receiving

   (A) lidocaine
   (B) procainamide
   (C) quinidine
   (D) flecainide
   (E) propranolol

5. Class IA antiarrhythmics do all of the following to the cardiac cell's action potential *except*

   (A) slow the rate of rise for phase 0 of depolarization.
   (B) delay the fast-channel conductance of sodium ions.
   (C) prolong phases 2 and 3 of repolarization.
   (D) inhibit the slow-channel conductance of calcium ions.
   (E) prolong the refractory period of the action potential.

6. Which of the following drugs is a class IV antiarrhythmic that is primarily indicated for the treatment of supraventricular tachyarrhythmias?

   (A) ibutilide
   (B) mexiletine
   (C) verapamil
   (D) quinidine
   (E) propranolol

7. Which of the following agents was involved in the ARREST trial and for which evidence-based practice justifies its addition as a first-line agent within the 2005 ACLS guidelines?

   (A) lidocaine
   (B) diltiazem
   (C) bretylium
   (D) amiodarone
   (E) dofetilide

8. Which of the following drugs is a class III antiarrhythmic agent that is effective in the acute management of atrial fibrillation or atrial flutter of recent onset?

   (A) propranolol
   (B) dofetilide
   (C) metoprolol
   (D) disopyramide
   (E) diltiazem

9. All of the following problems represent concerns when patients are started on amiodarone *except*

(A) extremely long elimination half-life.

(B) need for multiple daily doses.

(C) development of hyperthyroidism or hypothyroidism.

(D) development of pulmonary fibrosis.

(E) interactions with other antiarrhythmic drugs.

ANSWERS AND EXPLANATIONS

1. The answer is E *[see II.A.4.c.(4)].*
Disopyramide has anticholinergic actions about one tenth the potency of atropine. Effects include dry mouth, constipation, urinary retention, and blurred vision. Therefore, it cannot be used in patients with glaucoma or with conditions causing urinary retention. Moreover, disopyramide has a negative inotropic effect and must, therefore, be used with great caution, if at all, in patients with preexisting ventricular failure.

2. The answer is A *[see II.A.2].*
The class I antiarrhythmics (fast-channel blockers) slow impulse conduction by depressing the flow of sodium ions into cells during phase 0 of the action potential. Class II antiarrhythmics decrease impulse conduction through the AV node and lengthen the refractory period through their direct effects on the sympathetic nervous system. Class III antiarrhythmics prolong the refractory period and action potential and have no effect on conduction time throughout the AV and SA nodes. Class IV antiarrhythmics work directly on low-channel ion conduction, which is more likely to take place during phase 2 (plateau), when calcium ions enter the cell through slow channels. Current classification of antiarrhythmics does not include a group of class V agents.

3. The answer is B *[see I.C.3; Table 40-1].*
Torsades de pointes is a form of ventricular tachyarrhythmia characterized by electrocardiographic changes, which include a markedly prolonged QT interval. This potentially fatal reaction has now been reported for both antiarrhythmics and non-antiarrhythmics. Antiarrhythmics, which have been reported to cause torsades de points, include amiodarone, disopyramide, dofetilide, flecainide, ibutilide, procainamide, quinidine, and sotalol. In addition, drug classes such as antibiotics (e.g., erythromycin, levofloxacin, moxifloxacin, pentamidine, sparfloxacin), along with other agents (such as, dolasetron, felbamate, fluoxetine, fosphenytoin, indapamide, isradipine, paroxetine, sumatriptan, and tamoxifen) have been reported to be able to cause either a prolongation in the QT interval and/or induce torsades de pointes (Table 40-1). Of the agents listed, only amiodarone is a class III antiarrhythmic.

4. The answer is B *[see II.A.4.b.(7)].*
The patient's complaints are typical of a SLE-like hypersensitivity reaction to procainamide. Symptoms of an SLE-like syndrome include fatigue, arthralgia, myalgia, a low-grade fever, and a positive antinuclear antibody titer. The patient's symptoms should subside if procainamide therapy is stopped and an alternative antiarrhythmic agent is given instead.

5. The answer is D *[see II.A.2].*
Class IA antiarrhythmic agents delay phase 0 of depolarization. Fast-channel conduction of sodium and phases 2 and 3 of repolarization are also slowed. The net effect is to extend the refractory period of myocardial tissue. Class IA antiarrhythmic agents do not inhibit the slow-channel conductance of calcium ions—that is an action of class IV agents such as verapamil.

6. The answer is C *[see II.D.1.a].*
Of the agents listed, verapamil is a calcium-channel blocker and represents the class IV antiarrhythmics. Verapamil has been used for its direct-acting effects on impulse conduction throughout the heart. Thus verapamil is used to treat and prevent supraventricular arrhythmias. Ibutilide is a class III agent, quinidine is a class IA drug, mexiletine is a class IB agent, and propranolol, a β-adrenergic blocker, is class II. Mexiletine, quinidine, and propranolol are all also effective for supraventricular arrhythmias, and ibutilide is indicated for the treatment of atrial fibrillation/flutter of recent onset.

7. The answer is D *[see II.C.3.a].*
In the ARREST trial, 44% of amiodarone-treated patients versus 34% of placebo-treated patients survived to hospital admission ($p = 0.03$) after shock-refractory cardiac arrest. The benefit was consistently observed in all major subgroups, regardless of the presenting cardiac-arrest rhythm. As a result of the trial, evidence of its findings were cited within the ACLS 2000 Guidelines, describing the lack of similar data for other antiarrhythmics, and the agreement by the expert panel that they would consider amiodarone as a first-line agent for such patients. Lidocaine and bretylium are the only other agents listed, which have been used in this patient population for ventricular tachyarrhythmias. However, the data have been lacking as to their efficacy compared to placebo.

8. The answer is B *[see II.C.1.d].*
Dofetilide, ibutilide, amiodarone, and sotalol are class III antiarrhythmic agents. Class III agents, which prolong the refractory period and myocardial action potential, are used to treat ventricular arrhythmias. However, dofetilide and ibutilide are approved as type III agents indicated for the conversion from atrial fibrillation and flutter of recent onset to normal sinus rhythm. Propranolol, along with other β-blockers, is a class II antiarrhythmic; metoprolol is not routinely used in the treatment of arrhythmias; and disopyramide and diltiazem are class Ia and class IV antiarrhythmics, respectively.

9. The answer is B *[see II.C.3.a; II.C.4.a; II.C.5.a].*
Amiodarone, like ibutilide and sotalol, is a class III antiarrhythmic agent and acts by prolonging repolarization of cardiac cells. Amiodarone is given orally, often in once-a-day or twice-a-day maintenance dosage. Because of its very long elimination half-life, therapeutic response may be delayed for weeks. Therefore, an initial loading phase is often advisable. This requires hospitalization with close monitoring for desired effects, untoward reactions, and adjustments in dosage. Amiodarone may increase the plasma levels of quinidine, procainamide, diltiazem, and digitalis. During therapy with amiodarone, patients may develop hypothyroidism or hyperthyroidism, pulmonary disorders, hepatic dysfunction, and various other unwanted effects. Because of amiodarone's extremely long half-life, adverse reactions may persist for months after therapy ends.

41
Hypertension
Alan H. Mutnick

I. GENERAL CONSIDERATIONS

A. Definition. Hypertension is blood pressure elevated enough to perfuse tissues and organs. Elevated systemic blood pressure is usually defined as a systolic reading $\geq$ 140 mm Hg and a diastolic reading $\geq$ 90 mm Hg ($\geq$ 140/90). The "Seventh Report of the Joint National Committee on Detection, Evaluation, and Treatment of High Blood Pressure" (JNC-7) added a "prehypertension" category, which includes individuals with systolic blood pressure readings of 120–139 or diastolic blood pressure readings of 80–89 mm Hg; this category is now included in contemporary management strategies.

B. Classification of hypertension is shown in Table 41-1. The table reflects the recommendations of the JNC-7.

C. The **relationship between elevated blood pressure and cardiovascular disease** was addressed in the JNC-7, which formalizes the fact that the higher the blood pressure, the greater the chance of a myocardial infarction (MI), heart failure (HF), stroke, or kidney disease. Table 41-2 provides cardiovascular risk factors and/or lifestyle factors that affect the prognosis and treatment of hypertension and the various types of target-organ damage associated with hypertension.

D. Incidence. Hypertension is the most common cardiovascular disorder. Approximately 43 million Americans have blood pressure measurements > 140/90. This number translates to almost 25% of the adult population. The incidence increases with age—that is, 60%–71% of people > 60 years of age have hypertension, according to data obtained from the Third National Health and Nutrition Examination Survey (NHANES III).

1. Primary (or essential) hypertension, in which no specific cause can be identified, constitutes > 90% of all cases of systemic hypertension. The average age of onset is about 35 years.

2. Secondary hypertension, resulting from an identifiable cause, such as renal disease or adrenal hyperfunction, accounts for the remaining 2%–5% of cases of systemic hypertension. This type usually develops between the ages of 30 and 50.

E. Physiology

Blood pressure = (stroke volume $\times$ heart rate) $\times$ total peripheral vascular resistance (TPR)

Altering any of the factors on the right side of the blood pressure equation results in a change in blood pressure, as shown in Figure 41-1.

1. Sympathetic nervous system. Baroreceptors (pressure receptors) in the carotids and aortic arch respond to changes in blood pressure and influence arteriolar dilation and arteriolar constriction. When stimulated to constriction, the contractile force strengthens, increasing the heart rate and augmenting peripheral resistance, thus increasing cardiac output. If pressure remains elevated, the baroreceptors reset at the higher levels and so sustain the hypertension. Little evidence suggests that epinephrine and norepinephrine have a clear role in the cause of hypertension. However, many of the drugs used to treat hypertension lower blood pressure by blocking the sympathetic nervous system.

2. Renin–angiotensin–aldosterone system. Sympathetic stimulation, renal artery hypotension, and decreased sodium delivery to the distal tubules stimulate the release of renin by the kidney (juxtaglomerular apparatus of the kidney). Renin (an enzyme) reacts with circulating substrate, angiotensinogen to produce angiotensin I (a weak vasoconstrictor). Within the

Table 41-1. Classification of Hypertension for Adults ≥ 18 Years of Age

Classification	Systolic (mm Hg)[a]		Diastolic (mm Hg)[a]	Management			
				Lifestyle Modification	Initial Drug Therapy		
					Without Compelling Indication	With Compelling Indications	
Normal	< 120	and	< 80	Encourage			
Prehypertension	120–139	or	80–89	Yes	No antihypertensive drug indicated, unless presence of a compelling indication[b] requiring use of drug therapy	Drug(s) for compelling indications	
Stage 1 hypertension	140–159	or	90–99	Yes	Thiazide-type diuretics for most; may consider ACE inhibitor, ARB, β-blocker, CCB, or combination	Drug(s) for compelling indications; other antihypertensive drugs (diuretics, ACE inhibitor, ARB, β-blocker, CCB) as needed	
Stage 2 hypertension	≥ 160	or	≥ 100	Yes	Two-drug combination for most (usually thiazide-type diuretic and ACE inhibitor, ARB, β-blocker, or CCB)	Drug(s) for compelling indications; other antihypertensive drugs (diuretics, ACE inhibitor, ARB, β-blocker, CCB) as needed	

ACE, angiotensin-converting enzyme; *ARB*, angiotensin-receptor blocker; *CCB*, calcium-channel blocker.

[a]Treatment is determined by the patient's highest blood pressure category.

[b]Selected drug therapies have been identified from clinical trials to possess positive clinical outcomes for specific clinical situations and represent compelling indication for their use. Compelling indications (and drug therapies): heart failure (diuretics, β-blockers, ACE inhibitors, ARB, aldosterone antagonists), postmyocardial infarction (β-blockers, ACE inhibitors, and aldosterone antagonists), high coronary disease risk (diuretic, β-blocker, ACE inhibitors, CCB), diabetes (diuretic, β-blockers, ACE inhibitors, ARB, CCB), chronic kidney disease (ACE inhibitors, ARB), and recurrent stroke prevention (diuretic, ACE inhibitors).

Based on Joint National Committee on Detection, Evaluation, and Treatment of High Blood Pressure. The seventh report of the Joint National Committee on Detection, Evaluation, and Treatment of High Blood Pressure: The JNC-7 report [Special communication; Clinician's Corner]. JAMA 2003;289:2560–2572.

Table 41-2. Cardiovascular and/or Lifestyle Risk Factors for Consideration in the Management of Hypertension

Hypertension
Cigarette smoking
Obesity (BMI ≥ 30)
Physical inactivity
Dyslipidemia (as a component of the metabolic syndrome)
Diabetes mellitus (as a component of the metabolic syndrome)
Microalbuminuria or estimated glomerular filtration rate < 60 mL/min
Age (> 55 years for men; > 65 years for women)
Family history of premature cardiovascular disease (men < 55 years; women < 65 years)

BMI, body mass index (calculated as weight in kilograms divided by the square of height in meters).
Based on Joint National Committee on Detection, Evaluation, and Treatment of High Blood Pressure. The seventh report of the Joint National Committee on Detection, Evaluation, and Treatment of High Blood Pressure: The JNC-7 report [Special communication; Clinician's Corner]. JAMA 2003;289:2560–2572.

pulmonary endothelium is another enzyme, referred to as angiotensin-converting enzyme (ACE), which is able to hydrolyze the decapeptide angiotensin I to form the octapeptide angiotensin II (a potent natural vasoconstrictor). Angiotensin II has several important functions in the regulation of fluid volume:

a. It stimulates the release of aldosterone from the adrenal gland (zona glomerulosa), which results in increased sodium reabsorption, fluid volume, and blood pressure.
b. It constricts resistance vessels, which increases peripheral vascular resistance and arterial pressure.
c. It stimulates the release of vasopressin, or antidiuretic hormone (ADH), from the posterior pituitary, which acts within the kidneys to increase fluid retention.

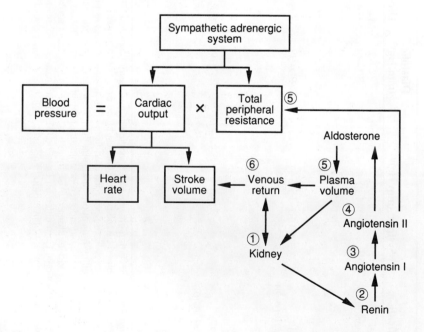

Figure 41-1. Blood pressure regulation: the determinants of blood pressure as they relate to cardiac output and total peripheral resistance. Angiotensin II, a potent vasopressor, not only increases total peripheral resistance but also, by stimulating aldosterone release, leads to an increase in plasma volume, venous return, stroke volume, and ultimately an increase in cardiac output.

d. It stimulates cardiac hypertrophy and vascular hypertrophy.

e. It facilitates norepinephrine release from sympathetic nerve endings and inhibits norepinephrine reuptake by nerve endings, which enhances sympathetic function.

3. Mosaic theory centers around the fact that multiple factors, rather than one factor alone, are responsible for sustaining hypertension. The interactions among the sympathetic nervous system, renin–angiotensin–aldosterone system, and potential defects in sodium transport within and outside the cell may all play a role in long-term hypertension. Additional factors contributing to the development include genetics, endothelial dysfunction, and neurovascular anomalies. Other vasoactive substances that are involved in the maintenance of normal blood pressure have also been identified; these include nitric oxide (vasodilating factor), endothelin (vasoconstrictor peptide), bradykinin (potent vasodilator inactivated by ACE), and atrial natriuretic peptide (naturally occurring diuretic).

4. Fluid volume regulation. Increased fluid volume increases venous system distention and venous return, affecting cardiac output and tissue perfusion. These changes **alter vascular resistance,** increasing the blood pressure.

F. Complications. Untreated systemic hypertension, regardless of cause, results in inflammation and necrosis of the arterioles, narrowing of the blood vessels, and restriction of the blood flow to major body organs (Table 41-3). When blood flow is severely compromised, target-organ damage ensues.

1. Cardiac effects

   a. Left ventricular hypertrophy (cardiac remodeling) compensates for the increased cardiac workload. Signs and symptoms of heart failure occur, and the increased oxygen requirements of the enlarged heart may produce angina pectoris.

Table 41-3. Target-Organ Damage Associated with Hypertension

Organ/System and Findings	Basis of Findings
Cardiovascular	
Blood pressure persistently $\geq$ 140 mm Hg systolic and/or $\geq$ 90 mm Hg diastolic	Constricted arterioles, causing abnormal resistance to blood flow
Angina pain	Insufficient blood flow to coronary vasculature
Left ventricular hypertrophy/dyspnea on exertion	Heart failure
Edema of extremities	Decrease in blood supply
Neurological	
Severe occipital headaches with nausea and vomiting, drowsiness, anxiety, and mental impairment	Vessel damage within brain characteristic of dizziness, severe mental impairment, hypertension, resulting in transient ischemic attacks or strokes
Renal	
Polyuria, nocturia, and diminished ability to concentrate urine; protein and red blood cells in urine; elevated serum creatinine	Arteriolar nephrosclerosis (hardening of arterioles within kidney)
Ocular	
Retinal hemorrhage and exudates	Damage to arterioles that supply retina
Peripheral vascular	Absence of pulses in extremities with or without intermittent claudication; development of aneurysm

Based on Joint National Committee on Detection, Evaluation, and Treatment of High Blood Pressure. The seventh report of the Joint National Committee on Detection, Evaluation, and Treatment of High Blood Pressure: The JNC-7 report [Special communication; Clinician's Corner]. JAMA 2003;289:2560–2572.

    b. Hypertension can be caused by accelerated atherosclerosis. Atheromatous lesions in the coronary arteries lead to decreased blood flow, resulting in angina pectoris. MI and sudden death may ensue.

2. Renal effects
    a. Decreased blood flow leads to an increase in renin–aldosterone secretion, which heightens the reabsorption of sodium and water and increases blood volume.
    b. Accelerated atherosclerosis decreases the oxygen supply, leading to renal parenchymal damage with decreased filtration capability and to azotemia. The atherosclerosis also decreases blood flow to the renal arterioles, leading to nephrosclerosis and, ultimately, renal failure (acute as well as chronic).

3. Cerebral effects. Decreased blood flow, decreased oxygen supply, and weakened blood vessel walls lead to transient ischemic attacks, cerebral thromboses, and the development of aneurysms with hemorrhage. There are alterations in mobility, weakness and paralysis, and memory deficits.

4. Retinal effects. Decreased blood flow with retinal vascular sclerosis and increased arteriolar pressure with the appearance of exudates and hemorrhage result in visual defects (e.g., blurred vision, spots, blindness).

II. SECONDARY HYPERTENSION

A. Clinical evaluation. Because most patients presenting with high blood pressure have primary rather than secondary hypertension, extensive screening is unwarranted. A thorough history and physical examination followed by an evaluation of common laboratory tests should rule out most causes of secondary hypertension. Patient age (primary hypertension is normally seen between 30 and 55 years of age), sudden onset of worsening of hypertension, and blood pressure elevations not responding to treatment are findings consistent with secondary hypertension. If a secondary cause is not found, the patient is considered to have essential (primary) hypertension.

1. A patient's **history** and **other physical findings** suggest an underlying cause of hypertension. These include the following:
    a. Weight gain, moon face, truncal obesity, osteoporosis, purple striae, hirsutism, hypokalemia, diabetes, and increased plasma cortisol may signal Cushing syndrome.
    b. Weight loss, episodic flushing, diaphoresis, increased urinary catecholamines, headaches, intermittent hypertension, tremors, and palpitations suggest pheochromocytoma.
    c. Steroid or estrogen intake, including oral contraceptives, nonsteroidal anti-inflammatory drugs (NSAIDs), nasal decongestants, tricyclic antidepressants, appetite suppressants, cyclosporine, erythropoietin, and monoamine oxidase (MAO) inhibitors, suggests drug-induced hypertension.
    d. Repeated urinary tract infections, elevated serum creatinine levels, nocturia, hematuria, and pain on urinating may signify renal involvement (e.g., chronic kidney disease).
    e. Abdominal bruits, recent onset, and accelerated hypertension indicate renal artery stenosis (e.g., renovascular disease).
    f. Muscle cramps, weakness, excess urination, and isolated hypokalemia may suggest primary aldosteronism.
    g. Sleep apnea, coarctation of the aorta, thyroid disease, and parathyroid disease have been included by the JNC-7 as additional secondary causes of hypertension.

2. Laboratory findings
    a. Blood urea nitrogen (BUN) and creatinine elevations suggest renal disease.
    b. Increased urinary excretion of catecholamine or its metabolites (e.g., vanillylmandelic acid, metanephrine) confirms pheochromocytoma.
    c. Serum potassium evaluation revealing hypokalemia suggests primary aldosteronism or Cushing syndrome.

3. Diagnostic tests
    a. Renal arteriography, ultrasound, or renal venography may show evidence of renal artery stenosis.
    b. Electrocardiography (ECG) may reveal left ventricular hypertrophy or ischemia.

B. Cause

1. **Primary aldosteronism.** Hypersecretion of aldosterone by the adrenal cortex increases distal tubular sodium retention, expanding the blood volume, which increases total peripheral resistance.

2. **Pheochromocytoma.** A tumor of the adrenal medulla stimulates hypersecretion of epinephrine and norepinephrine, which results in increased total peripheral resistance.

3. **Renal artery stenosis.** Decreased renal tissue perfusion activates the renin–angiotensin–aldosterone system (see I.E.2).

C. Treatment.
Secondary hypertension requires treatment of the underlying cause (e.g., surgical intervention accompanied by supplementary control of hypertensive effects; see III.B).

III. ESSENTIAL (PRIMARY) HYPERTENSION

A. Clinical evaluation
requires a thorough history and physical examination followed by a careful analysis of common laboratory test results.

1. **Objectives**
   a. To rule out uncommon secondary causes of hypertension
   b. To determine the presence and extent of target-organ damage
   c. To determine the presence of other cardiovascular risk factors in addition to high blood pressure
   d. To reduce morbidity and mortality through multiple strategies that reduce blood pressure through lifestyle modifications with or without pharmacological treatment with minimal side effects.

2. **Predisposing factors**
   a. **Family history** of essential hypertension, stroke, and premature cardiac disease
   b. **Patient history** of intermittent elevations in blood pressure
   c. **Racial predisposition.** Hypertension is more common among African Americans than whites.
   d. **Obesity.** Weight reduction has been shown to reduce blood pressure in a large proportion of hypertensive patients who are > 10% above ideal body weight.
   e. **Smoking,** resulting in vasoconstriction and activation of the sympathetic nervous system, is a major risk factor for cardiovascular disease.
   f. Stress
   g. High dietary intake of saturated fats or sodium
   h. Sedentary lifestyle
   i. Diabetes mellitus
   j. Hyperlipidemia
   k. Major risk factors according to the JNC-7 include smoking, diabetes mellitus, age (> 55 for men; > 65 for women), family history of cardiovascular disease, and dyslipidemia.
   l. Target-organ damage/clinical cardiovascular disease according to the JNC-7 includes heart disease (e.g., left ventricular hypertrophy, angina, prior MI, heart failure), stroke or transient ischemic attacks, nephropathy, peripheral artery disease, and retinopathy.

3. **Physical findings**
   a. Serial blood pressure readings ≥ 140/90 should be obtained on at least two occasions before specific therapy is begun, unless the initial blood pressure levels are markedly elevated (i.e., > 210 mm Hg systolic; > 120 mm Hg diastolic, or both) or are associated with target-organ damage. A single elevated reading is an insufficient basis for a diagnosis.
   b. Essential hypertension usually does not become clinically evident—other than through serial blood pressure elevations—until vascular changes affect the heart, brain, kidneys, or ocular fundi.
   c. Examination of the ocular fundi is valuable; their condition can indicate the duration and severity of the hypertension.
      (1) **Early stages.** Hard, shiny deposits; tiny hemorrhages; and elevated arterial blood pressure occur.

(2) **Late stages.** Cotton-wool patches, exudates, retinal edema, papilledema caused by ischemia and capillary insufficiency, hemorrhages, and microaneurysms become evident.

4. Untreated hypertension increases the likelihood of the development of numerous organ problems, which include left ventricular failure, MI, renal failure, cerebral hemorrhage or infarction, and severe changes in the retina of the eye.

B. **Treatment** (Tables 41-4 and 41-5; Figure 41-2)

1. **General principles.** Treatment primarily aims to lower blood pressure toward "normal" with minimal side effects and to prevent or reverse organ damage. Currently, there is no cure for primary hypertension. Treating systolic and diastolic blood pressures to targets that are < 140/90 mm Hg is associated with a decrease in cardiovascular complications. For patients

Table 41-4. Common Antihypertensive Drugs

I. Diuretics	**V. Sympatholytics**
A. Thiazide diuretics	**A.** β-Adrenergic blocking agents
Chlorothiazide (Diuril)	Acebutolol (Sectral)
Chlorthalidone (Hygroton)	Atenolol (Tenormin)
Hydrochlorothiazide (HydroDIURIL)	Betaxolol (Kerlone)
Indapamide (Lozol)	Bisoprolol (Zebeta)
Methyclothiazide (Enduron)	Carteolol (Cartrol)
Metolazone (Zaroxolyn)	Carvedilol (Coreg)
B. Loop diuretics	Labetalol (Normodyne, Trandate)
Bumetanide (Bumex)	Metoprolol (Lopressor, Toprol XL)
Ethacrynic acid (Edecrin)	Nadolol (Corgard)
Furosemide (Lasix)	Penbutolol (Levatol)
Torsemide (Demadex)	Pindolol (Visken)
C. Potassium-sparing diuretics	Propranolol (Inderal)
Amiloride (Midamor)	Timolol (Blocadren)
Spironolactone (Aldactone)	**B.** Centrally acting α-agonists
Triamterene (Dyrenium)	Clonidine (Catapres)
II. Vasodilators (direct acting)	Guanabenz (Wytensin)
Diazoxide (Hyperstat)	Guanfacine (Tenex)
Hydralazine (Apresoline)	Methyldopa (Aldomet)
Minoxidil (Loniten)	**C.** Postganglionic adrenergic neuron
Nitroprusside (Nitropress)	blockers
III. Angiotensin-converting enzyme (ACE)	Reserpine (various)
inhibitors	**D.** α-Adrenergic blocking agents
Benazepril (Lotensin)	Doxazosin (Cardura)
Captopril (Capoten)	Prazosin (Minipress)
Enalapril (Vasotec)	Terazosin (Hytrin)
Enalaprilat (IV) (Vasotec)	**E.** Calcium-channel blockers
Fosinopril (Monopril)	1. Benzodiazepine derivatives
Lisinopril (Prinivil, Zestril)	Diltiazem (Cardizem, Dilacor,
Moexipril (Univasc)	Tiazac)
Perindopril (Aceon)	2. Diphenylalkylamine derivatives
Quinapril (Accupril)	Verapamil (Isoptin, Calan)
Ramipril (Altace)	3. Dihydropyridines
Trandolapril (Mavik)	Amlodipine (Norvasc)
IV. Angiotensin II receptor antagonists	Felodipine (Plendil)
Candesartan cilexetil (Atacand)	Isradipine (DynaCirc)
Eprosartan (Teveten)	Nicardipine (Cardene)
Irbesartan (Avapro)	Nifedipine (Procardia XL, Adalat
Losartan (Cozaar)	CC)
Olmesartan (Benicar)	Nisoldipine (Sular)
Telmisartan (Micardis)	
Valsartan (Diovan)	

Table 41-5. Common Combination Products for Hypertension

I. Diuretics
Hydrochlorothiazide—spironolactone (Aldactazide)
Hydrochlorothiazide—triamterene (Dyazide, Maxzide)
Hydrochlorothiazide—amiloride (Moduretic)

II. Diuretics—β-adrenergic blockers
Bendroflumethiazide—nadolol (Corzide)
Chlorthalidone—atenolol (Tenoretic)
Hydrochlorothiazide—propranolol (Inderide)
Hydrochlorothiazide—metoprolol (Lopressor HCT)
Hydrochlorothiazide—timolol (Timolide)
Hydrochlorothiazide—bisoprolol (Ziac)

III. Diuretics—angiotensin-converting enzyme (ACE) inhibitors
Hydrochlorothiazide—captopril (Capozide)
Hydrochlorothiazide—benazepril (Lotensin HCT)
Hydrochlorothiazide—lisinopril (Prinzide, Zestoretic)
Hydrochlorothiazide—enalapril (Vaseretic)
Hydrochlorothiazide—fosinopril (Monopril HCT)
Hydrochlorothiazide—moexipril (Uniretic)
Hydrochlorothiazide—quinapril (Accuretic)

IV. Diuretics—angiotensin II receptor antagonists
Hydrochlorothiazide—losartan (Hyzaar)
Hydrochlorothiazide—irbesartan (Avalide)
Hydrochlorothiazide—valsartan (Diovan HCT)
Hydrochlorothiazide—telmisartan (Micardis HCT)
Hydrochlorothiazide—candesartan (Atacand HCT)
Hydrochlorothiazide—eprosartan (Teveten HCT)

V. Angiotensin-converting enzyme (ACE) inhibitors—Calcium-channel blockers
Enalapril—felodipine (Lexxel)
Trandolapril—verapamil (Tarka)
Benazepril—amlodipine (Lotrel)

VI. Other
Chlorthalidone—clonidine (Combipres)
Hydrochlorothiazide—hydralazine (Apresazide)
Polythiazide-prazosin (Minizide)

---

with hypertension who have diabetes or renal disease, the blood pressure goal recommended by the JNC-7 is 130/80 mm Hg.

a. Candidates for treatment

   (1) All patients with a diastolic pressure of > 90 mm Hg, a systolic pressure of > 140 mm Hg, or a combination of both should receive antihypertensive drug therapy.

   (2) For those patients with a diastolic pressure of 80–89 mm Hg or a systolic pressure of 120–139 mm Hg (prehypertension), no drug treatment is indicated unless the patient has a compelling indication. However, lifestyle modifications such as weight reduction, dietary sodium reduction, increased physical activity, and moderation of alcohol consumption should be initiated.

b. Nonspecific measures. Before initiating antihypertensive drug therapy, patients are encouraged to eliminate or minimize controllable risk factors (see III.A.2).

c. Pharmacological treatment. The recommendations of the JNC-7 suggest that recent clinical trials have demonstrated that most hypertensive patients will require two or more antihypertensive drugs.

   (1) Thiazide diuretics should be the initial choice of therapy because they have demonstrated a reduction in morbidity and mortality when used as initial monotherapy. They have been shown to lower morbidity and mortality rates, have shown adequate long-term safety data, and have demonstrated patient tolerability.

   (2) Thiazide diuretics should be considered initial agents for treatment unless there are compelling indications for other medications.

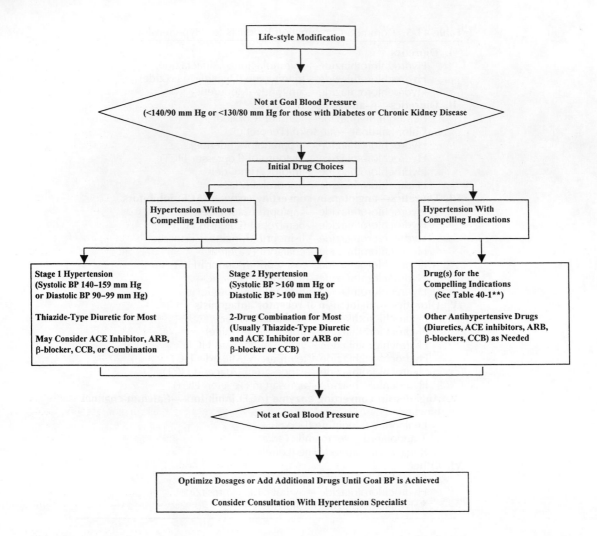

Figure 41-2. Algorithm for the treatment of hypertension. *ACE,* angiotensin-converting enzyme; *ARB,* angiotensin-receptor blocker; *CCB,* calcium-channel blocker. [Based on the recommendations from the Seventh Report of the Joint National Committee on Detection, Evaluation, and Treatment of High Blood Pressure (JNC-7).]

(3) Agents such as ACE inhibitors, angiotensin-receptor blockers, β-blockers, and calcium-channel blockers have all been recommended for patients who cannot receive a thiazide diuretic or in combination with a thiazide diuretic for adequate control of blood pressure. This may include the use of ACE inhibitors in hypertensive patients having systolic dysfunction after a myocardial infarction, a diabetic nephropathy patient who might benefit from an ACE inhibitor in combination with a diuretic, or a patient with HF.

d. Monitoring guidelines. Specific monitoring guidelines for the various drug categories are outlined in III.B.2–7.

(1) Blood pressure should be monitored routinely to determine the therapeutic response and to encourage patient compliance.

(2) Clinicians must be alert to indications of adverse drug effects. Many patients do not link side effects to drug therapy or are embarrassed to discuss them, especially effects related to sexual function or effects that appear late in therapy.

e. Patient compliance

(1) Because hypertension is usually a symptomless disease, how the patient "feels" does not reflect the blood pressure level. In fact, the patient may actually report "feeling normal" with an elevated blood pressure and "abnormal" during a hypotensive episode because of the light-headedness associated with a sudden drop in blood pressure. Because essential hypertension requires a lifelong drug regimen, it is extremely difficult but necessary to impress on patients the need for compliance with their therapeutic regimen.

(2) Recognizing the seriousness of the consequences of noncompliance is key. Patients should be told that prolonged, untreated hypertension, known as the "silent killer," can affect the heart, brain, kidneys, and ocular fundi.

2. Diuretics

a. Thiazide diuretics and their derivatives are currently recommended as initial therapy for hypertension. JNC-VII recommends initiating therapy with a low dose (12.5 mg of hydrochlorothiazide (HydroDIURIL or its equivalent), increasing the dose if necessary, and not exceeding a dose of 50 mg of hydrochlorothiazide or its equivalent.

(1) Actions. Antihypertensive effects are produced by directly dilating the arterioles and reducing the total fluid volume. Thiazide diuretics increase the following:

(a) Urinary excretion of sodium and water by inhibiting sodium and chloride reabsorption in the distal convoluted (renal) tubules

(b) Urinary excretion of potassium and, to a lesser extent, bicarbonate

(c) The effectiveness of other antihypertensive agents by preventing reexpansion of extracellular and plasma volumes

(2) Significant interactions. NSAIDs, such as the now common over-the-counter forms of ibuprofen (Advil, Motrin), interact to diminish the antihypertensive effects of the thiazide diuretics.

(3) Precautions and monitoring effects

(a) Potassium ion (K^+) depletion may require supplementation, increased dietary intake, or the use of a potassium-sparing diuretic such as spironolactone (Aldactone).

(b) Uric acid retention may occur; this is potentially significant in patients who are predisposed to gout and related disorders.

(c) Blood glucose levels may increase, which may be significant in patients with diabetes.

(d) Calcium levels may increase because of the potential for retaining calcium ions.

(e) Patients with known allergies to sulfa-type drugs should be questioned to determine the significance of the allergy.

(f) Other common effects include fatigue, headache, palpitations, rash, vertigo, and transitory impotence.

(g) Hyperlipidemia, including **hypertriglyceridemia,** hypercholesterolemia, increased low-density lipoprotein (LDL) cholesterol, and decreased high-density lipoprotein (HDL) cholesterol, must be evaluated routinely to prevent an added risk for coronary artery disease.

(h) Fluid losses must be evaluated and monitored to prevent dehydration, postural hypotension, and even hypovolemic shock.

(i) Alterations in fluids and electrolytes (e.g., hypokalemia, hypomagnesemia, hypercalcemia) may predispose patients to cardiac irritability, with a resultant increase in cardiac arrhythmias. ECG) is performed routinely to detect and prevent the development of life-threatening arrhythmias.

(4) Usual effective doses

(a) Chlorothiazide (Diuril): 250–500 mg daily or twice daily

(b) Chlorthalidone (Hygroton): 12.5–25 mg daily

(c) Hydrochlorothiazide (HydroDIURIL): 12.5–50 mg daily

(d) Indapamide (Lozol): 1.25–2.5 mg daily

(e) Methyclothiazide (Enduron): 2.5–5.0 mg daily

(f) Metolazone (Zaroxolyn): 2.5–5.0 mg daily

b. Loop (high-ceiling) diuretics

(1) Indications. These agents are indicated when patients are unable to tolerate thiazides, experience a loss of thiazide effectiveness, or have impaired renal function (clearance < 30 mL/min).

(2) Actions. Furosemide (Lasix), ethacrynic acid (Edecrin), bumetanide (Bumex), and torsemide (Demadex) act primarily in the ascending loop of Henle; hence they are called "loop" diuretics. By acting within the loop of Henle, they decrease sodium reabsorption. Their action is more intense but of shorter duration (1–4 hr) than that of the thiazides; they may also be more expensive.

(3) Significant interactions. As with the thiazides, the antihypertensive effect of loop diuretics may be diminished by **NSAIDs.**

(4) Precautions and monitoring effects. Loop diuretics have the same effects as thiazides (see III.B.2.a), in addition to the following:

   (a) Loop diuretics have a complex influence on renal hemodynamics; thus patients must be monitored closely for signs of hypovolemia.

   (b) Because these agents should be used cautiously in patients with episodic or chronic renal impairment, BUN and serum creatinine levels should be checked routinely.

   (c) Transient deafness has been reported. If the patient is taking a potentially ototoxic drug (e.g., an aminoglycoside antibiotic), another class of diuretic (e.g., a thiazide diuretic) should be substituted.

(5) Usual effective doses

   (a) Bumetanide (Bumex): 0.5–2.0 mg daily

   (b) Ethacrynic acid (Edecrin): 25–100 mg daily

   (c) Furosemide (Lasix): 20–80 mg daily

   (d) Torsemide (Demadex): 2.5–10 mg daily

c. Potassium-sparing diuretics

(1) Indications. The diuretics in this group—spironolactone (Aldactone), amiloride (Midamor), and triamterene (Dyrenium)—are indicated for patients in whom potassium loss is significant and supplementation is not feasible. These agents are often used in combination with a thiazide diuretic because they potentiate the effects of the thiazide while minimizing potassium loss. **Spironolactone** is particularly useful in patients with hyperaldosteronism, as it has direct antagonistic effects on aldosterone (aldosterone-receptor blocker). **Eplerenone** (Inspra), is another aldosterone-receptor blocker recently approved by the U.S. Food and Drug Administration (FDA) that, similar to spironolactone, blocks aldosterone binding at the mineralocorticoid receptor. Both of these agents have been used in hypertension, and have an increased level of use in the treatment of HF (see Chapter 42).

(2) Actions. Potassium-sparing diuretics achieve their diuretic effects differently and less potently than the thiazides and loop diuretics. Their most pertinent shared feature is that they promote potassium retention.

(3) Significant interactions. Coadministration with **ACE inhibitors** or **potassium supplements** significantly increases the risk of hyperkalemia.

(4) Precautions and monitoring effects

   (a) Potassium-sparing diuretics should be avoided in patients with acute renal failure and used with caution in patients with impaired renal function (monitor serum creatinine) because they can retain potassium.

   (b) Triamterene should not be used in patients with a history of kidney stones or hepatic disease.

   (c) Hyperkalemia is a major risk, requiring routine monitoring of serum electrolytes. BUN and serum creatinine levels should be checked routinely to signal incipient excess potassium retention and impaired renal function.

(5) Usual effective doses

   (a) Amiloride (Midamor): 5–10 mg daily

   (b) Spironolactone (Aldactone): 25–100 mg daily and 100–400 mg daily to treat hyperaldosteronism

   (c) Triamterene (Dyrenium): 50–100 mg daily

   (d) Eplerenone (Inspra): 50–100 mg daily

d. Combination products. Several products combine a thiazide and a potassium-sparing diuretic.

(1) Aldactazide: 25 mg spironolactone plus 25 mg hydrochlorothiazide (one to two tablets daily)

(2) Aldactazide-50: 50 mg spironolactone plus 50 mg hydrochlorothiazide (one tablet daily)

- **(3) Moduretic:** 5 mg amiloride plus 50 mg hydrochlorothiazide (one to two tablets daily)
- **(4) Dyazide:** 37.5 mg triamterene plus 25 mg hydrochlorothiazide (one to two capsules daily)
- **(5) Maxzide:** 75 mg triamterene plus 50 mg hydrochlorothiazide (one half to one tablet daily)
- **(6) Maxzide-25:** 37.5 triamterene plus 25 mg hydrochlorothiazide

3. **Sympatholytics**
   a. **β-Adrenergic blockers**
      - **(1) Indications.** β-Blockers are particularly effective in patients with rapid resting heart rates (i.e., atrial fibrillation, paroxysmal supraventricular tachycardia) or compelling indications such as heart failure, post-MI, high coronary disease risk, and diabetes.
      - **(2) Actions.** Proposed mechanisms of action include the following:
        - **(a)** Stimulation of renin secretion is blocked.
        - **(b)** Cardiac contractility is decreased, thus diminishing cardiac output.
        - **(c)** Sympathetic output is decreased centrally.
        - **(d)** Reduction in heart rate decreases cardiac output.
        - **(e)** β-Blocker action may combine all of the above mechanisms.
      - **(3) Epidemiology.** Young (< 45 years) whites with high cardiac output, high heart rate and normal vascular resistance respond best to β-blocker therapy.
      - **(4) Precautions and monitoring effects**
        - **(a)** Patients must be monitored for signs and symptoms of **cardiac decompensation** (i.e., reduction in cardiac output) owing to the fact that decreased myocardial contractility can trigger compensatory mechanisms, leading to HF (see Chapter 41).
        - **(b)** ECGs should be monitored routinely because all β-blockers can decrease electrical conduction within the heart and cause bradyarrhythmias.
        - **(c)** Relative cardioselectivity is dose dependent and is lost as dosages are increased. Therefore, **no β-blocker is totally safe in patients with bronchospastic disease**—for example asthma and chronic obstructive pulmonary disease (COPD).
        - **(d)** Abrupt stoppage in β-blocker therapy puts the patient at risk for a **withdrawal syndrome** that may produce
          - **(i)** Exacerbated anginal attacks, particularly in patients with coronary artery disease
          - **(ii)** Myocardial infarction
          - **(iii)** A life-threatening rebound of blood pressure to levels exceeding pretreatment readings
        - **(e)** β-Blocker therapy should be used with caution in patients with the following conditions:
          - **(i) Diabetes.** β-Blockers can mask hypoglycemic symptoms, such as tachycardia.
          - **(ii) Raynaud phenomenon or peripheral vascular disease.** Vasoconstriction can occur and, in predisposed patients, might result in a clinically significant problem.
          - **(iii) Neurological disorders.** Several β-blockers enter the central nervous system (CNS), potentiating related side effects (e.g., fatigue, lethargy, poor memory, weakness, or mental depression).
        - **(f)** Impotence and decreased libido may result in reduced patient compliance.
      - **(5) Significant interactions.** β-Adrenergic blockers interact with numerous agents, requiring cautious selection, administration, and monitoring.
      - **(6) β-Blocker terms**
        - **(a) Relative cardioselective activity.** Relative to propranolol, β-blockers have a greater tendency to occupy the β_1-receptor in the heart, rather than the β_2-receptors in the lungs.
        - **(b) Intrinsic sympathomimetic activity.** These agents have the ability to release catecholamines and to maintain a satisfactory heart rate. Intrinsic sympathomimetic activity may also prevent bronchoconstriction and other direct β-blocking actions.
      - **(7) Specific agents**
        - **(a) Propranolol (Inderal)** was the first β-adrenergic blocking agent shown to block both β_1- and β_2-receptors. The **usual daily dose range** is 40–160 mg. It is available

both as a rapid-acting product and a long-acting product (Inderal-LA); the usual daily dose range is 60–180 mg.

   (b) Metoprolol (Lopressor) was the first β-adrenergic blocking agent to show relative cardioselective blocking activity, with relatively less blockade of the β_2-receptors in the lung when compared to propranolol. The **usual daily dose** is 50–100 mg. A sustained-release form of the drug is now available, as the succinate salt (Toprol XL), which requires less frequent dosing, (daily versus once or twice daily for immediate-release metoprolol).

   (c) Nadolol (Corgard) was the first β-adrenergic blocking agent that allowed once-daily dosing. It blocks both β_1- and β_2-receptors similar to propranolol. The **usual daily dose** is 40–120 mg.

   (d) Atenolol (Tenormin) was the first β-adrenergic blocking agent to combine once-daily dosing (nadolol) with relative cardioselective blocking activity (metoprolol). The **usual daily dose** is 25–100 mg.

   (e) Timolol (Blocadren) was the first β-adrenergic blocking agent shown to be effective after an acute MI to prevent sudden death. It blocks both β_1- and β_2-receptors. The **usual daily dose** is 20–40 mg.

   (f) Pindolol (Visken) was the first β-adrenergic blocking agent shown to have high intrinsic sympathomimetic activity. The **usual daily dose** is 10–40 mg.

   (g) Labetalol (Trandate) was the first β-adrenergic blocking agent shown to possess both α- and β-adrenergic blocking activity. The **usual daily dose** is 200–800 mg. Labetalol is also effective for treating hypertensive crisis (Table 41-6).

   (h) Acebutolol (Sectral) was the first β-adrenergic blocking agent that combined efficacy with once-daily dosing (nadolol), possessing intrinsic sympathomimetic activity (pindolol) and having relative cardioselective blocking activity (metoprolol). The **usual daily dose** is 200–800 mg.

   (i) Esmolol (Brevibloc) was the first β-adrenergic blocking agent to have an ultrashort duration of action. This agent is not used routinely in treating hypertension owing to its duration of action and the need for intravenous administration. However, it has been used for hypertension and or tachycardia during and after surgical procedures. The **usual dose** is 150–300 μg/kg/min up to 300 μg/kg/min intravenously.

   (j) Betaxolol (Kerlone) is a β-adrenergic blocker that possesses relative cardioselective blocking activity similar to metoprolol but has a half-life that allows for once-daily dosing. The **usual daily dose** is 5–20 mg.

   (k) Penbutolol (Levatol) is a β-adrenergic blocking agent that has weak intrinsic sympathomimetic activity like pindolol and allows for once-daily dosing. The **usual daily dose** is 10–20 mg.

   (l) Bisoprolol (Zebeta) is a β-adrenergic blocking agent that is cardioselective and has no intrinsic sympathomimetic activity. It allows for once-daily dosing, and the **usual daily dose** is 2.5–10 mg.

   (m) Carvedilol (Coreg) is a β-adrenergic blocking agent that has β-blocking properties as well as α-blocking properties, with a resultant vasodilation. The drug is administered twice daily with a starting dose of 6.25 mg titrated at 7- to 14-day intervals to a dose of 25 mg twice daily. **Usual daily doses** are 12.5–50 mg daily.

  b. Peripheral α_1-adrenergic blockers—for example, prazosin (Minipress), terazosin (Hytrin), and doxazosin(Cardura)

   (1) Indications. This group of drugs is available for hypertensive patients who have not responded to initial antihypertensive therapy.

   (2) Actions. The α_1-blockers (indirect vasodilators) block the peripheral postsynaptic α_1-adrenergic receptor, causing vasodilation of both arteries and veins. Also, the incidence of reflex tachycardia is lower with these agents than with the vasodilator hydralazine. These hemodynamic changes reverse the abnormalities in hypertension and preserve organ perfusion. Recent studies have also shown that these agents have no adverse effect on serum lipids and other cardiac risk factors.

   (3) Precautions and monitoring effects

    (a) First-dose phenomenon. A syncopal episode may occur within 30–90 min of the first dose; similarly associated are postural hypotension, nausea, dizziness, headache, palpitations, and sweating. To minimize these effects, the first dose should be limited to a small dose (1 mg) and administered just before bedtime.

Table 41-6. Rapid-Acting Parenteral Antihypertensive Agents for Hypertensive Crisis

Drug	Dose/Route	Onset of Action	Duration of Action	Comments
Vasodilators				
Sodium nitroprusside (Nipride)	0.3–10 mg/kg/min as IV infusion	0.5–1 min	1–2 min	Immediate effect, very short duration; nausea, vomiting, muscle twitching, sweating, thiocyanate and cyanide intoxication
Nicardipine hydrochloride (Cardene)	5–15 mg/hr IV	< 5–15 min	1–4 hr	Intermediate onset and duration; tachycardia may occur, headache, flushing, local phlebitis
Fenoldopam mesylate (Corlopam)	0.1–0.3 μg/kg/min as IV infusion	< 5 min	30 min	Intermediate onset and duration; action on dopamine D_1- receptors (dilation of renal/mesenteric vessels might be preferred over nitroprusside for long-term or with renal dysfunction; tachycardia, headache, nausea, flushing
Nitroglycerin	5–200 μg/min (0.3–6.0 mg/hr) as IV infusion	2–5 min	3–5 min	Useful in coronary artery disease; headache, vomiting, methemoglobinemia, tolerance with prolonged use
Enalaprilat (Vasotec IV)	0.625–1.25 mg every 6 hr IV	15–30 min	4–6 hr	Useful in HF, but avoid in renal impairment; precipitous fall in blood pressure in high-renin states
Hydralazine	10–40 mg IV/IM	10–20 min	3–8 hr	Afterload reduction through arteriole dilation resulting in increased cardiac output; tachycardia, flushing headache, vomiting, aggravation of preexisting angina
Diazoxide (Hyperstat)	1–3 mg/kg over 30 sec as IV bolus, repeated every 5–15 min, or 10–30 mg/min infusion	2–4 min	3–12 hr	Useful in hypertensive encephalopathy, malignant hypertension, and eclampsia; flushing, nausea, tachycardia, and chest pain
Adrenergic inhibitors				
Labetalol hydrochloride (Trandate)	40–80 mg IV bolus every 10 min, or 0.5–2.0 mg/min IV infusion	5–10 min	3–6 hr	Contraindicated in HF, bronchospastic patients, or bradycardia; predictable hypotensive effect; vomiting, scalp tingling, burning in throat, heart block, orthostatic hypotension

(Continued on next page)

Table 41-6. Continued.

Drug	Dose/Route	Onset of Action	Duration of Action	Comments
Esmolol (Brevibloc)	250–500 µg/kg/ min for 2 min, then 50–100 µg/kg/min for 4 min; may repeat if needed	1–2 min	10–20 min	β-Adrenergic blocker with ultra-short duration of effect; primary use in perioperative situation owing to short duration and quick onset; hypotension, nausea
Phentolamine	5–15 mg IV	1–2 min	3–10 min	α-Adrenergic blocker causing peripheral dilation; tachycardia, flushing, headache

HF, heart failure; *IM*, intramuscular; *IV*, intravenous.

(b) Additional adverse effects include diarrhea, weight gain, peripheral edema, dry mouth, urinary urgency, constipation, and priapism. Doxazosin in doses of 2–8 mg/day was one of the treatment arms in the recent Antihypertensive and Lipid-Lowering Treatment to Prevent Heart Attack Trial (ALLHAT), and the treatment was discontinued prematurely owing to an apparent 25% increase in the incidence of combined cardiovascular disease outcomes than patients in the control group receiving the diuretic chlorthalidone. The added risk for HF, stroke, and coronary heart disease were the major outcomes affected in the doxazosin arm.

(4) The average daily doses are
    (a) Prazosin (Minipress): 2–20 mg
    (b) Terazosin (Hytrin): 1–20 mg
    (c) Doxazosin(Cardura): 1–16 mg

c. Centrally active α-agonists have been used in the past as alternatives to initial antihypertensives, but their use in mild to moderate hypertension has been reduced primarily owing to other available agents. They act primarily within the CNS on α_2-receptors to decrease sympathetic outflow to the cardiovascular system.

(1) Methyldopa (Aldomet)
    (a) Actions. Methyldopa decreases total peripheral resistance through the above mechanism while having little effect on cardiac output or heart rate (except in older patients).
    (b) Precautions and monitoring effects
        (i) Common untoward effects include orthostatic hypotension, fluid accumulation (in the absence of a diuretic), and rebound hypertension on abrupt withdrawal. Sedation is a common finding upon initiating therapy and when increasing doses; however, the sedative effect usually decreases with continued therapy.
        (ii) Fever and other flu-like symptoms occasionally occur and may represent hepatic dysfunction, which should be monitored by liver function tests.
        (iii) A positive Coombs test develops in 25% of patients with chronic use (> 6 months). Less than 1% of these patients develop a hemolytic anemia. (Red blood cells, hemoglobin, and blood count indices should be checked.) The anemia is reversible by discontinuing the drug.
        (iv) Other effects include dry mouth, subtly decreased mental activity, sleep disturbances, depression, impotence, and lactation in either gender.
    (c) The **usual daily dose** is 250 mg–1.0 g

(2) Clonidine (Catapres)
    (a) Indications. Clonidine is effective in patients with renal impairment, although they may require a reduced dose or a longer dosing interval.
    (b) Actions. Clonidine stimulates α_2-receptors centrally, decreasing vasomotor tone and heart rate.

(c) Precautions and monitoring effects
- **(i)** Intravenous administration causes an initial paradoxical increase in pressure (diastolic and systolic) that is followed by a prolonged drop. As with methyldopa, abrupt withdrawal can cause rebound hypertension.
- **(ii)** Sedation and dry mouth are common but usually disappear with continued therapy.
- **(iii)** Clonidine has a tendency to cause or worsen depression, and it heightens the depressant effects of alcohol and other sedating substances.

(d) The **usual daily dose** is 0.1–0.8 mg.

(e) Patient compliance is a major issue for most hypertensive patients. The recently released once-weekly patch (Catapres-TTS), which provides 0.1–0.3 mg per 24 hr, may improve compliance.

(3) Guanabenz (Wytensin) and **guanfacine (Tenex)**

(a) Indications. These agents are recommended as adjunctive therapy with other antihypertensives for additive effects when initial therapy has failed.

(b) Actions. Guanabenz and guanfacine are centrally active α_2-agonists that have actions similar to clonidine.

(c) Precautions and monitoring effects. These agents should be used cautiously with other sedating medications and in patients with severe coronary insufficiency, recent MI, cerebrovascular accident (CVA), and hepatic or renal disease. Side effects include sedation, dry mouth, dizziness, and reduced heart rate.

(d) The **usual daily doses** are 4–8 mg in two doses for guanabenz and 1–3 mg in one dose for guanfacine.

d. Postganglionic adrenergic neuron blockers. This class of antihypertensive drugs is best avoided unless it is necessary to treat severe refractory hypertension that is unresponsive to all other medications, because agents in this class are poorly tolerated by most patients.

(1) Reserpine

(a) General considerations. Because of the high incidence of adverse effects, other agents are usually chosen first. When used, reserpine is given in low doses and in conjunction with other antihypertensive agents. Reserpine in very low doses (0.05 mg) combined with a diuretic such as chlorothiazide (50–100 mg) may be an alternative to traditional doses of 0.05–0.25 mg/day.

(b) Actions. Reserpine acts centrally as well as peripherally by depleting catecholamine stores in the brain and in the peripheral adrenergic system.

(c) Precautions and monitoring effects
- **(i)** A history of depression is a contraindication for reserpine. Even low doses, such as 0.25 mg/day, can trigger a range of psychic responses, from nightmares to suicide attempts. Drug-induced depression may linger for months after the last dose.
- **(ii)** Peptic ulcer is also a contraindication for using reserpine. Even a single dose tends to increase gastric acid secretion.
- **(iii)** Common adverse effects include drowsiness, dizziness, weakness, lethargy, memory impairment, sleep disturbances, and weight gain. Nasal congestion is also common but may decrease with continued therapy.

(d) The **usual daily dose** of **reserpine** is 0.1–0.25 mg.

4. ACE inhibitors

a. General considerations. The ACE inhibitors—benazepril (Lotensin), captopril (Capoten), enalapril (Vasotec), fosinopril (Monopril), lisinopril (Zestril), moexipril (Univasc), perindopril (Aceon), quinapril (Accupril), ramipril (Altace), and trandolapril (Mavik)—are a rapidly growing group of drugs. The Heart Outcomes Prevention Evaluation (HOPE) project demonstrated substantial clinical benefits in patients receiving ramipril, which could not be explained through its blood pressure–lowering effects alone. Subsequently, studies, similar to HOPE have been completed, to date, which have demonstrated the benefit of ACE inhibitors in the treatment of hypertension and prevention of cardiac events, renal disease etc.

b. Indications. Previous guidelines used ACE inhibitors as first-line alternatives for treating hypertension in patients unable to tolerate thiazides or β-blockers. However, JNC-7 recommendations have identified specific patient populations that have compelling indications—such as diabetes, postmyocardial infarction, high coronary disease risk, chronic kidney disease, and recurrent stroke prevention—for which the ACE inhibitors are indicated in the treatment of hypertension or prehypertension. This has been primarily because of studies documenting their clinical efficacy as well as minimal effect on patients' abilities to maintain normal function.

   c. Actions
   - **(1)** These agents inhibit the conversion of angiotensin I (a weak vasoconstrictor) to angiotensin II (a potent vasoconstrictor), which decreases the availability of angiotensin II.
   - **(2)** ACE inhibitors indirectly inhibit fluid volume increases when interfering with angiotensin II by inhibiting angiotensin II–stimulated release of aldosterone, which promotes sodium and water retention. The net effect appears to be a decrease in fluid volume, along with peripheral vasodilation.

   d. Significant interactions
   - **(1)** The antihypertensive effect of ACE inhibitors may be diminished by **NSAIDs** (e.g., over-the-counter forms of ibuprofen).
   - **(2)** Potassium-sparing diuretics increase serum potassium levels when used with ACE inhibitors, and potassium levels need to be closely monitored in these patients.

   e. Precautions and monitoring effects
   - **(1)** Neutropenia is rare but serious; there is an increased incidence in patients with renal insufficiency or autoimmune disease.
   - **(2)** Proteinuria occurs, particularly in patients with a history of renal disease. Urinary proteins should be monitored regularly.
   - **(3)** Serum potassium levels should be monitored regularly for hyperkalemia. The mechanism of action tends to increase potassium levels somewhat. Patients with renal impairment are at increased risk.
   - **(4)** Renal insufficiency can occur in patients with predisposing factors, such as renal stenosis, and when ACE inhibitors are administered with thiazide diuretics. Renal function should be monitored (e.g., through monitoring levels of serum creatinine and BUN).
   - **(5)** A dry cough may occur but disappears within a few days after the ACE inhibitor is discontinued. All ACE inhibitors have the potential to cause this side effect, but switching to an alternative agent may improve the symptoms.
   - **(6)** Other untoward effects include rashes, an altered sense of taste (dysgeusia), vertigo, headache, fatigue, first-dose hypotension, and minor gastrointestinal disturbances.

   f. Specific agents
   - **(1) Captopril (Capoten).** The original ACE inhibitor is given initially as a 12.5–25 mg dose three times daily and is increased to a **usual daily dose** of 25–100 mg in two or three doses. Initial dose is usually lower if patient is on diuretics to avoid initial hypotensive response.
   - **(2) Enalapril (Vasotec)** is a prodrug, which is rapidly converted to its active metabolite, enalaprilat. Initial doses are 5.0 mg daily, with a **usual daily dose** of 5–40 mg in one to two doses. In addition, the enalaprilat form (Vasotec IV) of the drug has been used effectively for treating acute hypertensive crisis (Table 41-6).
   - **(3) Lisinopril (Zestril)** is a long-acting analog of enalapril, given initially as a 5–10 mg daily dose and adjusted to a **usual daily dose** of 10–40 mg in one dose.
   - **(4)** Benazepril (Lotensin), fosinopril (Monopril), moexipril (Univasc), perindopril (Aceon), quinapril (Accupril), ramipril (Altace), and trandolapril (Mavik) have as their major benefit a longer duration of action, which in many patients may result in once-daily dosing and improved compliance. **Average daily doses** for these agents are
      - **(a) Benazepril (Lotensin):** 10–40 mg in one to two doses
      - **(b) Fosinopril (Monopril):** 10–40 mg in one dose
      - **(c) Moexipril (Univasc):** 7.5–30 mg in one dose
      - **(d) Perindopril (Aceon):** 4–8 mg in one to two doses
      - **(e) Quinapril (Accupril):** 10–80 mg in one dose
      - **(f) Ramipril (Altace):** 2.5–20 mg in one dose
      - **(g) Trandolapril (Mavik):** 1–4 mg in one dose
   - **(5)** Further study of these agents continues, and their use in other cardiovascular as well as noncardiovascular diseases continues to expand.

5. Angiotensin II type I receptor antagonists
   - **a. Indications.** This class of drugs has been one of the fastest growing groups of drugs for the treatment of hypertension. Currently, seven agents are available: candesartan cilexetil

(Atacand), eprosartan (Teveten), irbesartan (Avaprol), losartan (Cozaar), olmesartan (Benicar), telmisartan (Micardis), and valsartan (Diovan).

b. Actions. This class of drugs works by blocking the binding of angiotensin II to the angiotensin II receptors. By blocking the receptor site, these agents inhibit the vasoconstrictor effects of angiotensin II as well as prevent the release of aldosterone owing to angiotensin II from the adrenal glands. These two properties of angiotensin II have been shown to be important causes for developing hypertension. Clinically, angiotensin receptor blockers appear to be equally effective for the treatment of hypertension as ACE inhibitors.

c. Precautions and monitoring effects

(1) Similar to ACE inhibitors, increases in serum potassium levels can occur, especially in patients receiving potassium-sparing diuretics. When used alone, hyperkalemia has not been reported to be severe enough to require stopping its use. However, as in patients receiving ACE inhibitors, potassium levels need to be monitored closely in those with compromised renal function.

(2) Renal function is an important consideration for patients receiving angiotensin-receptor blockers (ARBs). Similar to ACE inhibitors, declining renal function or acute renal failure will result in elevated serum potassium levels, owing to the kidneys inability to excrete potassium. BUN and serum creatinine levels should be monitored to prevent the development of hyperkalemia.

d. Dosage guidelines for the available agents are as follows:

(1) **Candesartan cilexetil (Atacand):** 8–32 mg in one to two doses
(2) **Eprosartan (Teveten):** 400–800 mg in one to two doses
(3) **Irbesartan (Avapro):** 150–300 mg in one dose
(4) **Losartan (Cozaar):** 25–100 mg in one to two doses
(5) **Olmesartan (Benicar):** 20–40 mg in one dose
(6) **Telmisartan (Micardis):** 20–80 mg in one dose
(7) **Valsartan (Diovan):** 80–320 mg in one-two doses

e. Current status

(1) Many authorities believe that in the treatment of hypertension, there do not appear to be significant differences between ACE inhibitors and angiotensin receptor blockers.
(2) Familiarity and cost might well provide the basis of the selection of one agent over another at this time.
(3) Angiotensin receptor blockers have found use in special hypertensive populations with compelling indications, such as diabetes, HF, and chronic kidney disease, especially in patients who cannot tolerate an ACE inhibitor.

6. Calcium-channel blockers

a. Indications. The calcium-channel blockers are considered alternative drugs for the initial treatment of hypertension in select patient populations that are unable to take β-adrenergic-receptor blockers, such as patients with a high coronary disease risk or diabetes mellitus who also have bronchospastic disease or Raynaud disease. Currently, eight agents—amlodipine (Norvasc), diltiazem (Cardizem), felodipine (Plendil), isradipine (DynaCirc CR), nicardipine (Cardene), nifedipine (Procardia), nisoldipine (Sular), and verapamil (Calan) are available.

b. Actions

(1) Calcium-channel blockers inhibit the influx of calcium through slow channels in vascular smooth muscle and cause relaxation. Low-renin hypertensive, black, and elderly patients respond well to these agents.
(2) Although the calcium-channel blockers share a similar mechanism of action, each agent produces different degrees of systemic and coronary arterial vasodilation, sinoatrial (SA) and atrioventricular (AV) nodal depression, and a decrease in myocardial contractility.

c. Significant interactions. β-Adrenergic blockers, when used with calcium-channel blockers, may have an additive effect on inducing HF and bradycardia. Electrical conduction to the AV node may be further depressed when patients are given agents such as verapamil or diltiazem along with β-blockers.

d. Precautions and monitoring effects

(1) Diltiazem and verapamil must be used with extreme caution or not at all in patients with conductive disturbances involving the SA or AV node, such as second- or third-degree AV block, sick sinus syndrome, and digitalis toxicity.

(2) Nifedipine use has been associated with flushing, headache, and peripheral edema; the patient may find these troublesome and thus may become noncompliant. Using the sustained-release product once daily has been shown to effectively reduce these effects.

(3) Verapamil use has been associated with a significant degree of constipation, which must be treated to prevent stool straining and noncompliance.

e. Specific agents

(1) Diltiazem (Cardizem). The release of several extended-release products (Cardizem CD, Cardizem-LA, Dilacor XR, Tiazac) has reduced the frequency of daily doses in the treatment of hypertension. A single daily dose of 120–540 mg is effective for treating mild to moderate hypertension. Diltiazem already has proven efficacy as an antiarrhythmic and an antianginal agent.

(2) Nifedipine (Procardia). The release of once-daily sustained-release preparations (Procardia XL, Adalat CC) has made this agent effective as a once-daily therapy for long-term treatment of hypertension. A previously reported long list of side effects has been reduced with the sustained-release product at a single daily dose of 30–90 mg. Immediate-release nifedipine has been reported to cause ischemic events, and the current recommendation is to avoid its use if at all possible.

(3) Verapamil (Calan). This drug is similar to diltiazem in its actions (though with more potent effects on electrical conduction depression). Sustained-release products (Calan SR, Isoptin SR, Covera-HS, Verelan) at doses of 120–480 mg daily have been shown to be efficacious for long-term management of mild to moderate hypertension, while side effects such as dizziness, constipation, and hypotension are reduced.

(4) Amlodipine (Norvasc), isradipine (DynaCirc), felodipine (Plendil), nicardipine (Cardene SR), and nisoldipine (Sular) are second-generation calcium-channel blockers. These agents have been developed to produce more selective effects on specific target tissues than the first-generation agents diltiazem, nifedipine, and verapamil. These agents are chemically similar to nifedipine and are referred to as dihydropyridine derivatives. The daily dose ranges are

(a) Amlodipine (Norvasc): 2.5–10.0 mg in one dose

(b) Isradipine (DynaCirc): 2.5–10 mg in one tp two doses

(c) Felodipine (Plendil): 2.5–20 mg in one dose

(d) Nicardipine (Cardene SR): 60–120 mg as an extended-release product twice daily

(e) Nisoldipine (Sular): 10–40 mg in one dose

7. Vasodilators. These drugs are used as second-line agents in patients refractory to initial therapy with diuretics, β-blockers, ACE inhibitors, ARBs, or calcium-channel blockers. Vasodilators directly relax peripheral vascular smooth muscle—arterial, venous, or both. The direct vasodilators should not be used alone owing to increases in plasma renin activity, cardiac output, and heart rate.

a. Hydralazine (Apresoline)

(1) Actions. Hydralazine directly relaxes arterioles, decreasing systemic vascular resistance. It is also used intravenously or intramuscularly in managing hypertensive crisis.

(2) Precautions and monitoring effects

(a) Because hydralazine triggers compensatory reactions that counteract its antihypertensive effects, it is most useful when combined with a β-blocker, central α-agonist, or diuretic as a latter-step agent.

(b) Reflex tachycardia is common and should be considered before initiating therapy.

(c) Hydralazine may induce angina, especially in patients with coronary artery disease and those not receiving a β-blocker.

(d) Drug-induced systemic lupus erythematosus (SLE) may occur.

    (i) Baseline and serial complete blood counts (CBCs) with antinuclear antibody titers should be followed routinely to detect SLE.

    (ii) Slow acetylators of this drug have an increased incidence of SLE. Their risk may be reduced by administering doses of < 200 mg/day.

    (iii) Fatigue, malaise, low-grade fever, and joint aches may signal SLE.

(e) Other adverse effects may include headache, peripheral neuropathy, nausea, vomiting, fluid retention, and postural hypotension.

(3) The **usual daily dose** is 25–100 mg.

b. **Minoxidil**
   (1) **Actions.** A more potent vasodilator than hydralazine, minoxidil relaxes arteriolar smooth muscle directly, decreasing peripheral resistance. It also decreases renal vascular resistance while preserving renal blood flow. Effective in most patients, minoxidil is commonly used to treat patients with severe hypertension that has been refractory to conventional drug regimens.
   (2) **Precautions and monitoring effects**
      (a) Peripheral dilation results in a reflex activation of the sympathetic nervous system and an increase in heart rate, cardiac output, and renin secretion.
      (b) Because this agent promotes sodium and water retention, particularly in the presence of renal impairment, patients should be monitored for fluid accumulation and signs of cardiac decompensation. Administering minoxidil along with a sympatholytic agent and a potent diuretic (e.g., furosemide) minimizes increased sympathetic stimulation and fluid retention.
      (c) Hypertrichosis (i.e., excessive hair growth) is a common side effect, particularly if the drug is continued for > 4 weeks.
   (3) The **usual daily dose** is 2.5–80 mg.
c. **Nitroprusside**
   (1) **Actions.** A direct-acting peripheral dilator, this agent has potent effects on both the arterial and venous systems. It is usually used only in short-term emergency treatment of acute hypertensive crisis, when a rapid effect is required. Onset of action is almost instantaneous and is maximal in 1–2 min. Nitroprusside is administered intravenously with continuous blood pressure monitoring.
   (2) **Precautions and monitoring effects.** To prevent acute hypotensive episodes, initial doses should be very low, followed by slow titration upward until the desired effect is achieved.
      (a) Once the solution is prepared, it should be protected from light. Color changes are a signal that replacement is needed.
      (b) Thiocyanate toxicity may develop with long-term treatment—particularly in patients with reduced renal activity—but can be treated with hemodialysis. Symptoms may include fatigue, anorexia, disorientation, nausea, psychotic behavior, or muscle spasms.
      (c) Cyanide toxicity can occur (rarely) with long-term, high-dose administration. It may present as altered consciousness, convulsions, tachypnea, or even coma.
   (3) The **usual dose** is 0.3–10 µg/kg/min as a continuous intravenous infusion.
d. **Diazoxide (Hyperstat)**
   (1) **Indications.** Diazoxide exerts a direct action on the arterioles but has little effect on venous capacity. It is used intravenously in the emergency treatment of acute hypertensive crisis.
   (2) **Administration**
      (a) Because the antihypertensive effect of diazoxide increases with the speed of infusion, recent recommendations suggest that the dose be administered over 30 sec and, if necessary, repeat doses given every 5–15 min.
   (3) **Precautions and monitoring effects**
      (a) Diazoxide is closely related to the thiazides chemically; therefore, patients with thiazide sensitivity cross-react to diazoxide. In patients with impaired cerebral or cardiac function, the risks may outweigh the benefits of diazoxide administration.
      (b) Diazoxide also produces transient hyperglycemia, requiring caution if administered to patients with diabetes.
      (c) Hypotensive reactions may be severe.
      (d) Unlike the thiazides, this agent promotes sodium and water retention, potentiating edema.

IV. HYPERTENSIVE EMERGENCIES

A. **Definition.** A hypertensive emergency is a severe elevation of blood pressure (i.e., > 200 mm Hg systolic or > 140 mm Hg diastolic) that demands reduction—either immediate (within minutes) or prompt (within hours) to prevent or limit target-organ damage.

1. Conditions requiring immediate reduction include hypertensive encephalopathy, acute left ventricular failure with pulmonary edema, eclampsia, dissecting aortic aneurysm, acute MI, stroke, and intracranial hemorrhage.

2. Conditions requiring prompt reduction include malignant or accelerated hypertension.

B. Treatment

1. The **reduction in blood pressure must be gradual** (e.g., a 15-mm Hg decrease in mean arterial pressure over the 1st hr) rather than precipitous to avoid compromising perfusion of critical organs, particularly cerebral perfusion.

2. **Specific agents** used in hypertensive crisis are shown in Table 41-6.

STUDY QUESTIONS

Directions for questions 1–6: Each of the questions, statements, or incomplete statements in this section can be correctly answered or completed by **one** of the suggested answers or phrases. Choose the **best** answer.

1. Which of the following agents represents a relatively new class of drugs used in treating hypertension?

(A) trandolapril (Mavik)
(B) carvedilol (Coreg)
(C) irbesartan (Avapro)
(D) moexipril (Univasc)
(E) nimodipine (Nimotop)

2. Reflex tachycardia, headache, and postural hypotension are adverse effects that limit the use of which of the following antihypertensive agents?

(A) prazosin (Minipress)
(B) captopril (Capoten)
(C) methyldopa (Aldomet)
(D) guanabenz (Wytensin)
(E) hydralazine (Apresoline)

3. A 65-year-old man presents with stage I hypertension. He has diabetes mellitus and chronic kidney disease and is intolerant to lisinopril. Which of the following agents would be an appropriate selection for initial treatment in this patient based on the guidelines from the "Seventh Report of the Joint National Committee on Detection, Evaluation, and Treatment of High Blood Pressure" (JNC-7)?

(A) chlorothiazide (Diuril)
(B) propranolol (Inderal)
(C) nitroprusside (Nipride)
(D) candesartan (Atacand)
(E) clonidine (Catapres)

4. A patient with stage I hypertension who has bronchospastic airway disease and who is noncompliant would be best treated with which of the following β-blocking agents?

(A) timolol (Blocadren)
(B) penbutolol (Levatol)
(C) esmolol (Brevibloc)
(D) acebutolol (Sectral)
(E) propranolol (Inderal)

5. Long-standing hypertension leads to tissue damage in all of the following organs *except* the

(A) heart.
(B) lungs.
(C) kidneys.
(D) brain.
(E) eyes.

6. According to the "Seventh Report of the Joint National Committee on Detection, Evaluation, and Treatment of High Blood Pressure" (JNC-7), which of the following agents is suitable as initial therapy for treating stage I hypertension (assuming no compelling indications for another type of drug)?

(A) chlorothiazide (Diuril)
(B) labetalol (Trandate)
(C) atenolol (Tenormin)
(D) propranolol (Inderal)
(E) bisoprolol (Zebeta)

Directions for questions 7–9: The questions and incomplete statements in this section can be correctly answered or completed by **one or more** of the suggested answers. Choose the answer, **A–E.**

A   if **I only** is correct
B   if **III only** is correct
C   if **I and II** are correct
D   if **II and III** are correct
E   if **I, II, and III** are correct

7. A patient treated with a spironolactone should be monitored regularly for altered plasma levels of

I. potassium.
II. serum creatinine.
III. blood urea nitrogen (BUN).

8. Before antihypertensive therapy begins, secondary causes of hypertension should be ruled out. Laboratory findings that suggest an underlying cause of hypertension include

I. a decreased serum potassium level.
II. an increased urinary catecholamine level.
III. an increased blood cortisol level.

9. In an otherwise healthy adult with stage I hypertension, appropriate initial antihypertensive therapy would be

 I. chlorthalidone (Diuril)
 II. metoprolol (Lopressor)
III. bisoprolol (Zebeta)

Directions for questions 10–14: Each list of adverse effects in this section is most closely associated with **one** of the following antihypertensive agents. The agents may be used more than once or not at all. Choose the **best** answer, **A–E.**

   (A)   clonidine (Catapres)
   (B)   olmesartan (Benicar)
   (C)   nitroprusside (Nipride)
   (D)   prazosin (Minipress)
   (E)   propranolol (Inderal)

10. thiocyanate intoxication, hypotension, and convulsions

11. bradycardia, bronchospasm, and cardiac decompensation

12. angioedema, cough, hyperkalemia,

13. rebound hypertension, dry mouth, drowsiness

14. first-dose syncope, postural hypotension, and palpitations

Directions for questions 15–19: Each description listed in this section is most closely associated with **one** of the following β-adrenergic blocking agents. The agents may be used more than once or not at all. Choose the **best** answer, **A–E.**

   (A)   esmolol (Brevibloc)
   (B)   labetalol (Trandate)
   (C)   bisoprolol (Zebeta)
   (D)   nadolol (Corgard)
   (E)   pindolol (Visken)

15. a β-blocker with intrinsic sympathomimetic activity

16. a β-blocker that also blocks α-adrenergic receptors

17. a β-blocker with an ultrashort duration of action

18. a β-blocker with a long duration of action and nonselective blocking activity

19. a β-blocker with relative cardioselective blocking activity

ANSWERS AND EXPLANATIONS

1. The answer is C *[see III.B.5.a].*
Irbesartan is one of the relatively new classes of drugs used in the treatment of hypertension referred to as an angiotensin II receptor antagonist, which blocks the production of angiotensin II and consequently its effects as a powerful vasoconstrictor and stimulant for aldosterone release. Trandolapril and moexipril are ACE inhibitors; carvedilol is a β-adrenergic blocking agent; and nimodipine is a calcium-channel blocker.

2. The answer is E *[see III.B.7.a].*
Hydralazine is a vasodilator that works by directly relaxing arterioles, thereby reducing peripheral vascular resistance. Its effectiveness as an antihypertensive agent is compromised, however, by the compensatory reactions it triggers (e.g., reflex tachycardia) and by its other adverse effects (e.g., headache, postural hypotension, nausea, palpitations). Fortunately, the unwanted effects of hydralazine are minimized when it is used in combination with a diuretic agent and a β-blocker. Thus hydralazine is most effective as a supplemental antihypertensive drug in combination with first-line therapy.

3. The answer is D *[see III.B.5.e.(3)].*
Candesartan, an angiotensin II receptor blocker, which acts by blocking the binding of angiotensin II to the angiotensin II receptors. By blocking the receptor site, this class of drugs inhibits the vasoconstrictor effects of angiotensin II and prevents the release of aldosterone owing to angiotensin II from the adrenal glands. JNC-7 guidelines call for the use of diuretics in the initial treatment of hypertension, unless the patient has compelling indications that have been shown to benefit from the use of specific classes of drugs. This patient has diabetes and chronic kidney disease and is unable to tolerate the ACE inhibitor lisinopril, therefore, an ARB would be an acceptable alternative for this patient rather than a β-blocker (propranolol) or diuretic (chlorothiazide). Nitroprusside and clonidine are not indicated for the initial treatment of hypertension.

4. The answer is D *[see III.B.3.a.(7).(a)–(m)].*
The β-adrenergic blocking agents continue to demonstrate effectiveness in the treatment of hypertension. A major feature of some of these agents is their relative selectivity for β₁-receptors (in the heart) rather than for β₂-receptors (in the lung), which provides advantages in the treatment of certain patients (e.g., those with bronchospastic airway or COPD). Of the β-blockers listed, acebutolol is less likely than the rest to block β₂-receptors because of its relative cardioselective-blocking activity. Acebutolol also has a long duration of action, which could be helpful in the noncompliant patient by requiring fewer doses per day. Penbutolol has weak intrinsic sympathomimetic activity like pindolol but lacks relative cardioselectivity, despite its long duration of action. Esmolol by nature of its continuous intravenous infusion would not lend itself to chronic ambulatory therapy. Timolol is a long-acting β-blocker and lacks the relative cardioselective properties that acebutolol possesses.

5. The answer is B *[see I.F; Table 41-3].*
Left untreated, hypertension can be lethal because of its progressively destructive effects on major organs, such as the heart, kidneys, and brain. The eyes also suffer damage; the lungs, however, do not. End-organ damage caused by hypertension includes left ventricular hypertrophy, heart failure, angina pectoris, myocardial infarction, renal insufficiency caused by atherosclerotic lesions, nephrosclerosis, cerebral aneurysm and hemorrhage, retinal hemorrhage, and papilledema.

6. The answer is A *[see III.B.2.a].*
Thiazide diuretics are considered the first-line treatment choice for hypertension and should be used alone or in combination with other antihypertensives, if necessary. β-Blockers such as labetalol, atenolol, bisoprolol, nifedipine, and propranolol are no longer considered initial agents for treating hypertension. β-blockers have shown positive clinical outcomes in patients with heart failure, post-myocardial infarction, high coronary disease risk, and diabetes (compelling indications) and would be acceptable options for patients presenting with prehypertension or hypertension with a compelling indication.

7. The answer is E (I, II, III) *[see III.B.2.c.(4)].*
Spironolactone is a direct-acting aldosterone-receptor blocker and decreases its effects on sodium and water retention. However, a benefit of spironolactone is its potassium-sparing effect, through the exchange of sodium for potassium in the kidney. Patients with reduced renal function and acute renal failure (evidenced by elevations in serum creatinine) lose their ability to excrete potassium, and this needs to be monitored when patients are started on spironolactone. BUN and creatinine are good indirect indicators of renal function.

8. The answer is E (I, II, III) *[see II.A.2].*
Low serum potassium levels in a hypertensive patient suggest primary aldosteronism. Elevated urinary catecholamines suggest a pheochromocytoma; other signs and symptoms of this tumor include weight loss, episodic flushing, and sweating. Elevated serum cortisol levels suggest Cushing syndrome; the patient is also likely to have a round (moon) face and truncal obesity. Secondary hypertension requires treatment of the underlying cause; supplementary antihypertensive drug therapy may also be needed.

9. The answer is A (I) *[see III.B.2.a].*
Thiazide diuretics such as chlorthalidone are now considered, based on the JNC-7, first-line therapy for hypertension, barring any compelling indications such as heart failure, diabetes, chronic kidney disease, or post-MI, when other antihypertensive agents would be indicated. β-Adrenergic blockers, such as metoprolol and bisoprolol, are no longer indicated as initial antihypertensive agents for treating hypertension.

10. The answer is C *[see III.B.7.c.(2)].*

11. The answer is E *[see III.B.3.a.(4)].*

12. The answer is B *[see III.B.5.c.(2)].*

13. The answer is A *[see III.B.3.c.(2).(c)].*

14. The answer is D *[see III.B.3.b.(3).(a)].*
The goal of treatment in hypertension is to lower blood pressure toward normal with minimal side effects. All antihypertensive drugs can cause adverse effects. The primary purpose of the JNC-7 guidelines is to acknowledge the long-term benefits of diuretics in the treatment of hypertension.

15. The answer is E *[see III.B.3.a.(7).(a)–(m)].*

16. The answer is B *[see III.B.3.a.(7).(a)–(m)].*

17. The answer is A *[see III.B.3.a.(7).(a)–(m)].*

18. The answer is D *[see III.B.3.a.(7).(a)–(m)].*

19. The answer is C *[see III.B.3.a.(7).(a)–(m)].*
The β-adrenergic blocking agents are valuable for managing hypertension and are used as initial antihypertensives. The β-blockers are sympathetic antagonists. They act by blocking various receptors of the sympathetic nervous system. They differ in their selectivity for these sympathetic receptors. For example, β_1-blockers have relative cardioselective activity—that is, they block β_1-receptors (in the heart) rather than β_2-receptors (in bronchial smooth muscle) and, therefore, are highly useful antihypertensive agents. Intrinsic sympathomimetic activity also appears to reduce the problem of bronchoconstriction; moreover, drugs with this property can also maintain a satisfactory heart rate.

42
Heart Failure
Alan H. Mutnick

I. INTRODUCTION

A. **Definition. Heart failure (HF)** is a complex clinical syndrome that can result from any cardiac disorder that impairs the ability of the ventricle to deliver adequate quantities of blood to the metabolizing tissues during normal activity or at rest. The condition in the past has been referred to as "congestive heart failure," owing to the **edematous state** commonly produced by the fluid backup resulting in shortness of breath, fatigue, limitation of exercise tolerance, and fluid retention. Fluid retention may lead to pulmonary and peripheral edema. More recently, because all patients do not necessarily present with fluid overload at the initial or follow-up evaluations, the term "heart failure" is used to more adequately reflect the clinical syndrome.

B. **Mortality rate.** Approximately 300,000 patients die as a result of the direct or indirect consequences of HF each year, and the number of deaths owing to HF (primary or secondary causes) has increased steadily, despite treatment advances. The risk of death is 5%–10% annually in patients with mild symptoms and is as high as 30%–40% in patients with advanced disease manifestations.

C. **Incidence of HF.** HF is a common medical condition that affects almost 5 million people in the United States, with > 500,000 new cases diagnosed each year. Between 1.5% and 2.0% of the population has HF, and the incidence increases to 6%–10% in patients older than age 65. HF makes up 20% of all hospitalizations in patients > 65 years of age. HF is the only major cardiovascular disorder that is increasing in incidence and prevalence. During the last 10 years, there has been a dramatic increase in the number of hospitalizations, primarily owing to HF (500,000 in 1991 to more then 1 million, currently). The reasons for the increased numbers of hospital admissions are listed in Table 42-1.

D. **Cost of HF.** The total costs (direct and indirect) for the treatment of HF in the United States during 2005 were approximately $27.9 billion. Currently in the United States, more than $2.9 billion is spent annually on drugs used in the treatment of HF.

E. **Causes**

1. Although the disease occurs most commonly among the elderly (80% of patients hospitalized with HF are > 65 years of age), it may appear at any age as a consequence of underlying cardiovascular disease.

2. There currently is no single diagnostic test for HF, and the clinical diagnosis is normally based on patient history and physical examination.

3. HF should not be considered an independent diagnosis because it is superimposed on an underlying cause.
   a. Coronary artery disease (CAD) is the cause of HF in about two thirds of patients with left ventricular systolic dysfunction.
   b. The remaining third of patients have a nonischemic cause of systolic dysfunction owing to other causes of myocardial stress, which included trauma, disease, or other abnormal states (e.g., pulmonary embolism, infection, anemia, pregnancy, drug use or abuse, fluid overload, arrhythmia, valvular heart disease, cardiomyopathies, congenital heart disease).

4. The New York Heart Association (NYHA) developed a classification system, still used today to quantify the functional limitations of HF patients. The NYHA classes are as follows:
   a. Class I: Degree of effort necessary to elicit HF symptoms equals those that would limit normal individuals.
   b. Class II: Degree of effort necessary to elicit HF symptoms occurs with ordinary exertion.

Table 42-1. Causes for Increased Hospitalization Rates of Heart Failure

Aging of the population in the United States
Rising incidence of chronic heart failure
Improved treatment results obtained for myocardial infarction, coronary
   artery bypass surgery, and stenting
Unavoidable progression of heart disease in an aging population
Incomplete treatment of heart failure in the hospital setting
Poor application of guidelines for treatment
Noncompliance with diet and drug therapy

Adapted with permission from Hobbs RE. Guidelines for the diagnosis and management of heart failure. Am J Ther 2004;11:467–472.

    c. Class III: Degree of effort necessary to elicit HF symptoms occurs with less-than-ordinary exertion.

    d. Class IV. Degree of effort necessary to elicit HF symptoms occurs while at rest.

  5. A criticism of the NYHA classification is its dependence on subjective assessments by the clinical practitioner, which changes frequently and might not accurately reflect different treatment options based on the degree of symptoms. Consequently, more recently, the "ACC/AHA Guidelines for the Evaluation and Management of Chronic Heart Failure" offered new classification scheme that depicts HF as an evolving clinical entity and details a progression based on risk factors and structural changes, which may be asymptomatic or symptomatic. Within this classification, specific treatments can be targeted at each stage to affect morbidity and mortality (Table 42-2). The introduction of the four stages of HF are not intended to replace the NYHA classification but rather to complement it.

F. Forms of HF. As mentioned, HF is a complex syndrome and has been described in various ways. The cardinal manifestations of HF are dyspnea and fatigue, which may limit exercise tolerance, result in fluid retention, and lead to pulmonary congestion and peripheral edema. However, the following sections provide several ways that have been used to describe the pathophysiology and the symptomatology involved in the condition. Though the terms *low-output* versus *high-output* and *left-sided* versus *right-sided* are not routinely used in the clinical setting, their use here is to help convey important educational aspects of HF and are presented only for the purpose of simplifying the discussion of the pathophysiology and symptomatology.

  1. Low-output versus high-output failure

    a. If metabolic demands are within normal limits but the heart is unable to meet them, the failure is designated **low output** (the most common type).

    b. If metabolic demands increase (e.g., hyperthyroidism, anemia) and the heart is unable to meet them, the failure is designated **high output.** Compared to low-output failure, correction of the underlying cause of high-output failure is paramount as the initial treatment modality.

  2. Left-sided versus right-sided failure

    a. General symptomatology. The signs and symptoms of HF usually result from the effects of blood backing up behind the failing ventricle (except in HF owing to increased body demands).

    b. Left-sided and right-sided HF do not routinely exist as separate entities; however, the use of separate terms best illustrates the systemic consequences.

    c. This progression occurs because the cardiovascular system is a closed system (Figure 42-1); thus, over time, right-sided failure causes left-sided failure and vice versa.

    d. Left-sided failure. If blood cannot be adequately pumped from the left ventricle to the peripheral circulation and it accumulates within the left ventricle, the patient is likely to exhibit signs of **left-sided HF.** As the fluid portion of the blood backs up into the pulmonary alveoli the result is the development of pulmonary edema that can present as, shortness of breath, dyspnea on exertion and a third heart sound.

    e. Right-sided failure. When blood is not pumped from the right ventricle, the fluid portion of the blood backs up throughout the body (e.g., in the veins, liver, legs, bowels), producing systemic edema. Such signs would include evidence of elevated pressures in the venous system (e.g., peripheral edema, jugular venous distension)

Table 42-2. Stages of Heart Failure (HF) Based on Evolution and Progression of Clinical Findings

Stage	Description	Examples
A	Patients at high risk of developing HF because of the presence of conditions that are strongly associated with the condition; such patients have no identified structural or functional abnormalities of the pericardium, myocardium, or cardiac valves and have never shown signs or symptoms of HF	Hypertension, atherosclerotic disease, diabetes mellitus, obesity, metabolic syndrome, history of cardiotoxic drug therapy or alcohol abuse, personal history of rheumatic fever, family history of cardiomyopathy
B	Patients who have developed structural heart disease that is strongly associated with the development of HF but who have never shown signs or symptoms of the condition	Left ventricular remodeling, including left ventricular hypertrophy or low ejection fraction; asymptomatic valvular disease; previous myocardial infarction
C	Patients who have current or prior symptoms of HF associated with underlying structural heart disease	Known structural heart disease, dyspnea or fatigue, reduced exercise tolerance
D	Patients with refractory HF who require specialized interventions	Patients with marked symptoms at rest despite maximal medical therapy (are frequently hospitalized for HF and cannot be safely discharged from the hospital, patients in the hospital awaiting heart transplantation, patients at home receiving continuous intravenous support for symptom relief or being supported with a mechanical circulatory assist device, patients in a hospice setting for the management of HF)

Adapted from Hunt SA, Abraham WT, Chin MH, et al. ACC/AHA 2005 guidelines for the diagnosis and management of chronic heart failure in the adult. A report of the American College of Cardiology/American Heart Association Task Force on Practice Guidelines (Writing Committee to Update the 2001 Guidelines for the Evaluation and Management of Heart Failure). J Am Coll Cardiol 2005;46:1–82.

3. **Progressive nature of HF**
   a. Injury to the myocardium or stress placed on it is generally required before the development of left ventricular dysfunction.
   b. The primary presentation for the associated signs and symptoms of HF is a change in the shape and structure of the left ventricle, where it dilates and/or hypertrophies into more of a spherical shape, referred to as cardiac remodeling. Such changes in the shape of the heart result in altered stresses on the cardiac walls owing to size as well as structural changes, which also lend themselves to altered blood flow through the various heart chambers.

G. **Treatment goals.** HF requires a two-pronged therapeutic approach, the overall goals of which are

1. **To remove or mitigate the underlying causes or risk factors**—for example, by eliminating ingestion of certain drugs or other substances that can produce or exacerbate HF or by correcting an anemic syndrome, which can increase cardiac demands (Table 42-3). In addition, modify risk factors that can cause cardiac injury by treating hypertension and diabetes; managing atherosclerotic disease; and controlling smoking, alcohol, and illicit drug use.

2. **To relieve the symptoms and improve pump function by:**
   a. Reducing metabolic demands through rest, relaxation, and pharmaceutical controls
   b. Reducing fluid volume excess through dietary and pharmaceutical controls
   c. Administering a combination of diuretics, angiotensin-converting enzyme inhibitors (ACEIs) β-adrenergic blockers, and angiotensin-receptor blockers (ARBs)
   d. Promoting patient compliance and self-regulation through education
   e. Selecting appropriate patients for cardiac transplantation

Figure 42-1. An overview of blood flow through the cardiovascular system.

Table 42-3. Substances That May Exacerbate Heart Failure

Promote Sodium Retention	Produce Osmotic Effect	Decrease Contractility
Androgens	Albumin	Antiarrhythmic agents (e.g., disopyramide,
Corticosteroids	Glucose	flecainide, quinidine)
Diazoxide	Mannitol	β-adrenergic blockers
Estrogens	Saline	Select calcium channel blockers (e.g.,
Licorice	Urea	diltiazem, nifedipine, verapamil)
Lithium carbonate		Direct cardiotoxins (e.g., doxorubicin,
NSAIDs		ethanol, cocaine, amphetamines)
		Tricyclic antidepressants

NSAIDs, nonsteroidal anti-inflammatory drugs.

3. During recent years, several sets of guidelines have been developed for the treatment of HF. Most recently, a panel of leading physicians and researchers in the field of HF provided recommendations. See within the following citation: Hunt SA, Abraham WT, Chin MH, et al. ACC/AHA 2005 guidelines for the diagnosis and management of chronic heart failure in the adult. A report of the American College of Cardiology/American Heart Association Task Force on Practice Guidelines (Writing Committee to Update the 2001 Guidelines for the Evaluation and Management of Heart Failure). J Am Coll Cardiol 2005;46:1–82; available at content.onlinejacc.org/cgi/reprint/46/6/e1.

4. These guidelines represent the most up-to-date standards for the prevention, diagnosis, and treatment of HF (Table 42-4).
   a. The guidelines focus on four stages in the development of HF; stages A and B include patients at risk for HF and stages C and D include patients who have developed HF.
   b. Paramount to the new guidelines is the role that ACEIs or ARBs and β-adrenergic blockers play, based on evidence-based practice.
   c. Treatment of patients with refractory end-stage HF (stage D) should include the primary therapeutic agents that are used for stages A, B, and C. However, lack of an acceptable response will require specialized nonpharmacologic modalities, such as mechanical circulatory support, transplantation, and end-of-life care for those exhibiting no benefit.

II. **PATHOPHYSIOLOGY.** HF and decreased cardiac output trigger a complex scheme of compensatory mechanisms designed to normalize cardiac output (cardiac output = stroke volume × heart rate). The principal manifestation of progression in cardiac dysfunction is a change in the geometry of the left ventricle, resulting in ventricular dilation and hypertrophy, with a resultant increase in a more spherical shape—referred to as *cardiac remodeling.* This results in increases in ventricular wall tension, depression in mechanical performance, and retention of normal cardiac fluid, which worsen the remodeling process.

A. **Compensation.** These mechanisms are shown in Figure 42-2.

1. **Sympathetic responses.** Inadequate cardiac output stimulates reflex (norepinephrine and epinephrine) activation of the sympathetic nervous system and an increase in circulating catecholamines. The heart rate increases, and blood flow is redistributed to ensure perfusion of the most vital organs (the brain and the heart).

2. **Hormonal stimulation.** The redistribution of blood flow results in reduced renal perfusion, which decreases the glomerular filtration rate (GFR). Reduction in GFR results in:
   a. Sodium and water retention
   b. Activation of the renin–angiotensin–aldosterone system, which further enhances sodium retention and thus volume expansion

3. **Concentric cardiac hypertrophy** describes a mechanism that thickens cardiac walls, providing larger contractile cells and diminishing the capacity of the cavity in an attempt to precipitate expulsion at lower volumes (ventricular remodeling; see II).

4. **Frank-Starling mechanism.** The premise of this response is that increased fiber dilation heightens the contractile force, which then increases the energy released.
   a. Within physiological limits, the heart pumps all the blood it receives without allowing excessive accumulation within the veins or cardiac chambers.
   b. As blood volume increases, the various cardiac chambers dilate (stretch) and enlarge in an attempt to accommodate the excess fluid.
   c. As these stretched muscles contract, the contractile force increases in proportion to their distention. Then the extended fibers snap back (as a rubber band would), expelling the extra fluid into the arteries.
   d. Additional evidence suggests that the release of cytokines (e.g., tumor necrosis factor) occurs in concert with elevated levels of circulating norepinephrine, angiotensin II, aldosterone, endothelin, and vasopressin, which may all play a role in adversely affecting the heart structure, resulting in depressed performance.

B. **Decompensation.** Over time, the compensatory mechanisms become exhausted and increasingly ineffective, entering a vicious spiral of decompensation in which the mechanisms surpass

Table 42-4. Approach to Heart Failure (HF)[a]

| | At Risk for Heart Failure | | Heart Failure | |
	Stage A	Stage B	Stage C	Stage D
Patients	Patients at high risk of developing HF because of presence of conditions that are strongly associated with development of condition; such patients have no identified structural or functional abnormalities of the pericardium, myocardium, or cardiac valves and have never shown signs or symptoms of HF	Patients who have developed structural heart disease that is strongly associated with development of HF but who have never shown signs or symptoms of the condition	Patients who have structural heart disease with current or prior symptoms of HF	Patients with refractory HF who require specialized interventions
Goals	Treat hypertension Encourage smoking cessation Treat lipid disorders Encourage regular exercise Discourage alcohol intake, illicit drug use Control metabolic syndrome	Same as stage A	Same as stage A Dietary salt restriction	Same as stages A and C Decision concerning appropriate level of care
Drugs	ACEIs to prevent HF in patients at high risk who have a history of atherosclerotic vascular disease, diabetes mellitus, or hypertension	ACEIs in patients with reduced ejection fractions and no symptoms of HF, even without previous MI	ACEIs and β-blockers, with one proven to reduce mortality (bisoprolol, carvedilol, and sustained-release metoprolol for all stable patients) with current or prior symptoms of HF and reduced LVEF	Referral to an HF program with expertise in the management of refractory HF

ARBs, as with ACEIs, though evidence not as strong

β-Blockers and ACEIs in all patients with recent or remote history of MI
ARBs should be administered to post-MI patients without HF who cannot tolerate ACEIs and have low LVEF, though evidence not as strong.
β-Blockers for all patients without MI who have reduced LVEF with no HF symptoms, though evidence not as strong.

ARBs in patients with current or prior symptoms of HF and reduced LVEF who cannot tolerate ACEIs
Diuretics and salt restriction in patients with current or prior symptoms of HF and reduced LVEF who have evidence of fluid retention, though evidence not as strong
Addition of an aldosterone antagonist in select patients with moderately severe to severe HF symptoms and reduced LVEF who can be carefully monitored for renal function and potassium concentrations, though evidence not as strong.
Current evidence favors combination of hydralazine and a nitrate in patients with reduced LVEF and persistent symptoms already receiving ACEIs and β-blockers

Drug therapy not considered, instead consideration is given for transplantation, when applicable
Continuous intravenous infusion of a positive inotropic agent for palliation of symptoms, though evidence not strong

ACEIs, angiotensin-converting enzyme inhibitors; *ARBs,* angiotensin-receptor blockers; *LVEF,* left ventricular ejection fraction; *MI,* myocardial infarction.
ªThe guidelines listed here are definitive, based on available evidence, and are not intended to reflect the entire set of guidelines with less-than-substantial evidence. A complete set of usage guidelines is available at content.onlinejacc.org/cgi/reprint/46/6/e1.
Adapted from Hunt SA, Abraham WT, Chin MH, et al. ACC/AHA 2005 gu delines for the diagnosis and management of chronic heart failure in the adult. A report of the American College of Cardiology/American Heart Association Task Force on Practice Guidelines (Writing Committee to Update the 2001 Guidelines for the Evaluation and Management of Heart Failure). J Am Coll Cardiol 2005;46:1–82.

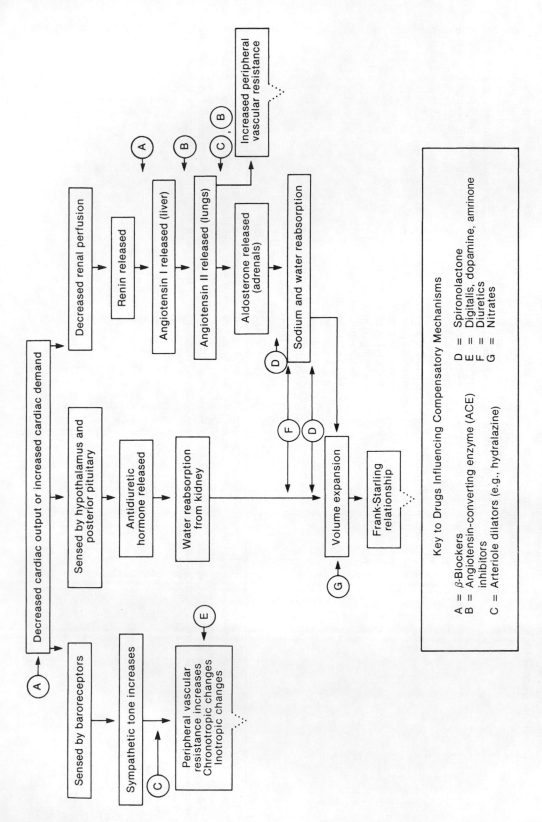

Figure 42-2. Compensatory mechanisms in heart failure.

their limits and become self-defeating—as they work harder, they only exhaust the system's capacity to respond.

1. As the strain continues, total peripheral resistance and afterload increase, thereby decreasing the percentage of blood ejected per unit of time. Afterload is determined by the amount of contractile force needed to overcome intraventricular pressure and eject the blood.

   a. **Afterload** is the tension in ventricular muscles during contraction. In the left ventricle, this tension is determined by the amount of force needed to overcome pressure in the aorta. Afterload (also known as intraventricular systolic pressure) is sometimes used to describe the amount of force needed in the right ventricle to overcome pressure in the pulmonary artery.

   b. **Preload** is the force exerted on the ventricular muscle at the end of diastole, which determines the degree of muscle fiber stretch. This concept is also known as ventricular end-diastolic pressure. Preload is a key factor in contractility because the more these muscles are stretched in diastole, the more powerfully they contract in systole.

2. As the fluid volume expands, so do the demands on an already exhausted pump, allowing increased volume to remain in the ventricle.

3. The resulting fluid backup (from the left ventricle into the lungs; from the right ventricle into peripheral circulation) produces the signs and symptoms of HF.

III. **CLINICAL EVALUATION.** Assessment of fluid status and left ventricular ejection fraction (usually < 40% in patients with HF (Table 42-4).

A. **Fluid accumulation behind the left ventricle**

   1. **Signs and symptoms**
      a. Dyspnea
         (1) As HF progresses, the amount of effort required to trigger **exertional dyspnea** lessens.
         (2) **Both paroxysmal nocturnal dyspnea** and **orthopnea** result from volume pooling in the recumbent position and can be relieved by propping up the patient with pillows or having the patient sit upright. (Orthopnea is often gauged by the number of pillows the patient needs to sleep comfortably.)
      b. Dry, wheezing cough
      c. Exertional fatigue and weakness
      d. Nocturia. Edematous fluids that accumulate during the day migrate from dependent areas when the patient is in a recumbent position and renal perfusion increases.

   2. **Physical findings**
      a. Rales (or crackles) indicate the movement of air through fluid-filled passages.
      b. Tachycardia is an early compensatory response detected through an increased pulse rate.
      c. S_3 ventricular gallop is a vibration produced by rapid filling of the left ventricle early in diastole.
      d. S_4 atrial gallop is a vibration produced by increased resistance to sudden, forceful ejection of atrial blood in late diastole; it does not vary with inspiration in left-sided failure and is more common in diastolic dysfunction.

   3. **Diagnostic test results**
      a. Cardiomegaly (heart enlargement), left ventricular hypertrophy, and pulmonary congestion may be evidenced by chest radiograph, electrocardiogram (ECG), and reduction in left ventricular function via echocardiography and radionuclide ventriculography.
      b. Arm-to-tongue circulation time is prolonged.
      c. Transudative pleural effusion may be suggested by radiograph and confirmed by analysis of aspirated pleural fluid.

B. **Fluid accumulation behind the right side of the heart**

   1. **Signs and symptoms**
      a. Complaints by the patient of tightness and swelling (e.g., ''My ring is too tight,'' ''My skin feels too tight'') suggest edema.
      b. Nausea, vomiting, anorexia, bloating, or abdominal pain on exertion may reflect hepatic and visceral engorgement, resulting from venous pressure elevation.

2. **Physical findings**
   a. Jugular vein distention reflects increased venous pressure and is a cardinal sign of HF.
   b. S_3 ventricular gallop (see III.A.2.c).
   c. S_4 atrial gallop intensifies on inspiration in right-sided failure.
   d. Hepatomegaly (a tender, enlarged liver) is revealed when pushing on the edge of the liver results in a fluid reflux into the jugular veins, causing bulging (positive hepatojugular reflux).
   e. Bilateral leg edema is an early sign of right-sided HF; pitting ankle edema signals more advanced HF. However, edema is common to many disorders, and a pattern of associated findings, such as concurrent neck vein distention, is required for differential diagnosis.

3. **Laboratory findings. Elevated levels of hepatic enzymes**—for example, alanine aminotransferase (ALT)—reflect hepatic congestion.

4. **Evaluation of natriuretic peptides.** Measurement of B-type natriuretic peptide (BNP) has been suggested in the evaluation of patients presenting in the acute care setting when a diagnosis of HF is uncertain. Elevated levels of BNP have been associated with a reduction in the left ventricular ejection fraction (LVEF) as well as in left ventricular hypertrophy, acute myocardial infarction, and ischemia, though they are not specific for HF and can occur in patients with obstructive lung disease, and pulmonary emboli.

IV. THERAPY

A. **Bedrest**

1. **Advantages**
   a. Bedrest decreases metabolic needs, which reduces cardiac workload.
   b. Reduced workload, in turn, reduces pulse rate and dyspnea.
   c. Bedrest also helps decrease excess fluid volume by promoting diuresis.

2. **Disadvantages.** Physical activity (except during acute decompensation) should be encouraged to avoid physical deconditioning and exercise intolerance. The risk of venous stasis increases with bedrest and can result in thromboembolism. Antiembolism stockings help minimize this risk, as do passive or active leg exercises, when the patient's condition permits.

3. **Progressive ambulation** should follow adequate bedrest.

B. **Dietary controls**

1. **Consuming small but frequent meals** (four to six daily) that are low in calories and residue provide nourishment without unduly increasing metabolic demands.

2. **Moderate sodium restriction** along with daily measurements of weight help maximize the lowest and safest doses of diuretics, a primary tool in reducing central volume in HF.
   a. Renal function should be evaluated to assess sodium conservation if severe sodium restriction is contemplated.
   b. Moderate sodium restriction (2–4 g of dietary sodium/day) can be achieved with relative ease by limiting the addition of salt during cooking and at the table.
   c. The patient should be advised about medications and common products that contain sodium and cautioned about their use (e.g., antacids, sodium bicarbonate or baking soda, commercial diet food products, water softeners). Table 42-3 lists other substances that promote sodium retention.

C. **Drug-related considerations.** Therapeutic interventions might improve cardiac performance in the following ways:

1. Drugs may increase the cardiac ejection fraction by directly stimulating cardiac contractility. The use of positive inotropic agents such as dopamine, dobutamine, and milrinone can produce immediate benefits; however, the long-term benefit has not been appreciated, and in some cases may actually increase morbidity and mortality.

2. Drugs may increase the ejection fraction by decreasing the impedance to ejection through relaxation of peripheral blood vessels. The use of vasodilators such as hydralazine and other

arterial dilators may produce short-term benefit but do not necessarily produce clinical benefits in the long term.

3. Drugs may improve the ejection fraction by affecting the cardiac remodeling process. Neuro-hormonal antagonists such as ACEIs, β-adrenergic receptor blockers, ARBs, and vasodilator-growth inhibitors such as nitrates may not produce immediate benefits, but long-term use might improve clinical status and decrease future cardiac events.

4. ACEIs, ARBs, diuretics, and β-adrenergic blockers usually form the basic core of treatment for HF.

D. ACEIs

1. Recent guidelines recommend the use of ACEIs in all patients with HF owing to left ventricular systolic dysfunction unless the patients have a contraindication to their use or have demonstrated intolerance to their use. Currently, ACEIs are considered the first-line agents in the treatment of HF and have been shown to have a beneficial effect on cardiac remodeling.

2. Relative contraindications include history of intolerance or adverse reactions, serum potassium > 5.5 mEq/L, serum creatinine levels > 3 mg/dL, symptomatic hypotension, severe renal artery stenosis, and pregnancy.

3. ACEIs have been shown to reduce symptoms, improve clinical status, enhance the overall quality of life, and reduce death as well as the risk of death or hospitalization in mild, moderate, and severe HF patients with or without coronary artery disease.

4. They inhibit the enzyme responsible for the conversion of angiotensin I (a weak vasoconstrictor) to angiotensin II (a potent vasoconstrictor). This action significantly decreases total peripheral resistance, which aids in reducing afterload.

5. Inhibiting the production of angiotensin II interferes with stimulation of aldosterone release, thus indirectly reducing retention of sodium and water, which decreases venous return and preload.

6. In patients with a history of fluid retention or who present with fluid retention, a diuretic can be added to an ACEI. ACEIs are also indicated for patients with left ventricular dysfunction without symptoms of HF.

7. ACEIs are indicated for the long-term management of chronic HF and are generally recommended in combination with a β-adrenergic blocker and diuretic.

8. All ACEIs that have been studied in the treatment of HF have shown benefit. The selection of agent and dose should be based on currently available large-scale studies in which target doses of ACEIs—captopril (Capoten), enalapril (Vasotec), lisinopril (Zestril), perindopril (Aceon), ramipril (Altace), and trandolapril (Mavik)—are different from those used to treat hypertension. Table 42-5 provides a comparative review of ACEIs currently used in the treatment of HF.

9. Common side effects to be monitored include hypotension (patients should be well hydrated before initiation of ACEIs), dizziness, reduced renal function (increased serum creatinine of 0.5 mg/dL or more requires reassessment), cough, and potassium retention (if potassium levels are high without supplementation, discontinue the ACEI for several days and then try to restart at lower dose).

10. Angioedema is a life-threatening side effect of ACEIs that has been reported to occur in < 1% of patients. It has been reported to occur at a more frequent rate in black patients, and the suspicion of the reaction would justify the avoidance of ACEIs in such patients.

E. ARBs

1. The newest in the class of drugs used to treat HF that has have been approved for use in the treatment of mild to moderate hypertension. However, this class of drugs is now considered a reasonable alternative to the use of ACEIs.

2. Currently available agents include candesartan cilexetil (Atacand), eprosartan (Teveten), irbesartan (Avapro), losartan (Cozaar), olmesartan (Benicar), telmisartan (Micardis), and valsartan (Diovan) and initial studies on several of the agents have shown potential benefits for treating HF.

Table 42-5. Comparative Doses of Select Agents Used in the Treatment of Heart Failure (HF)

Drug	Initial Daily Dose(s)	Maximal Total Daily Dose
Loop diuretics		
Bumetanide (Bumex)	0.5–1 mg once or twice	10 mg
Furosemide (Lasix)	20–40 mg once or twice	600 mg
Torsemide (Demadex)	10–20 mg once	200 mg
Thiazide diuretics		
Chlorthalidone (Hygroton)	12.5–25 mg once	200 mg
Chlorothiazide (Diuril)	250–500 mg once or twice	2000 mg
Hydrochlorothiazide (Hydrodiuril)	25 mg once or twice	200 mg
Metolazone (Zaroxolyn)	2.5 mg once	20 mg
Potassium-sparing diuretics		
Amiloride (Midamor)	5 mg once	20 mg
Spironolactone (Aldactone)	12.5–25 mg once	50 mg
Triamterene (Dyrenium)	50–75 mg twice	300 mg
ACEIs		
Captopril (Captoten)	6.25 mg three times	450 mg
Enalapril (Vasotec)	2.5 mg twice	40 mg
Fosinopril (Monopril)	5–10 mg once	80 mg
Lisinopril (Zestril)	2.5–5 mg once	40 mg
Perindopril (Aceon)	2 mg once	32 mg
Quinapril (Accupril)	5 mg twice	40 mg
Ramipril (Altace)	1.25–2.5 mg once	10 mg
Trandolapril (Mavik)	1 mg once	4 mg
Angiotensin II receptor blockers		
Candesartan (Atacand)	4–8 mg once	32 mg
Losartan (Cozaar)	25–50 mg once	100 mg
Valsartan (Avapro)	20–40 mg twice	320 mg
Aldosterone antagonists		
Spironolactone (Aldactone)	12.5 mg once	50 mg
Eplerenone (Inspra)	25 mg once	50 mg
β-Adrenergic receptor blockers		
Bisoprolol (Zebeta)	1.25 mg once	10 mg
Carvedilol (Coreg)	3.125 mg twice	50 mg; 100 mg for patients > 85 kg
Metoprolol succinate (Toprol XL) (extended release)	12.5–25 mg once	200 mg

3. Current guidelines suggest that ACEIs should be preferred over the ARBs. However, ARBs may be used in patients who initially responded to ACEIs and are intolerant to them.

F. β-Adrenergic blocking agents

1. Unlike ACEIs, which strictly work by blocking the effects of the renin–angiotensin system, β-adrenergic blockers interfere with the sympathetic nervous system—that is, norepinephrine-induced peripheral vasoconstriction, norepinephrine-induced sodium excretion by the kidney, norepinephrine-induced cardiac hypertrophy, norepinephrine induced arrhythmia generation, norepinephrine-induced hypokalemia, or norepinephrine-induced cell death (apoptosis) through increased stress owing to norepinephrine stimulation.

2. β-Adrenergic blockers, specifically, bisoprolol (Zebeta), sustained-release metoprolol (Toprol XL), and carvedilol (Coreg), have been shown to decrease the risk of death or hospitaliza-

tion as well as improve the clinical status of HF patients. However, doses for other select β-adrenergic blockers have been included in the current guidelines based on reported experience (Table 42-5).

3. Current guidelines recommend the use of β-adrenergic blockers in all patients with stable HF as a result of left ventricular dysfunction, unless they have a contraindication to their use or are unable to tolerate their effects owing to hypotension, bradycardia, bronchospasm, and the like.

4. β-adrenergic blockers are generally used in conjunction with diuretics, ACEIs, or ARBs. β-Adrenergic blockers should not be taken without diuretics in patients with a current or recent history of fluid retention to avoid its development and to maintain sodium balance.

5. Side effects of β-adrenergic blockers may occur during the early days of therapy but do not generally prevent their long-term use; and progression of the disease may be reduced, even if symptoms of the disease have not responded to β-adrenergic blocker therapy. Therapy should be initiated with low doses and titrated upward slowly as tolerated.

6. Patients should be monitored for signs of fluid retention by having patients weigh themselves daily and report any significant increases, which might warrant increases in diuretic doses or reductions in the dose of the β-adrenergic blocker. In addition, fatigue, hypotension, bradycardia, and heart block are reported sides effects, which should be monitored to ensure appropriate attention and management.

7. Studies support the use of β-adrenergic blockers in patients with stage C heart failure—and not in the acute management of patients, as in an intensive care unit (ICU). Patients should have no or minimal evidence of fluid retention and have no recent evidence for the use of an intravenous inotropic agent. In addition, β-adrenergic blockers should be considered in patients who develop HF post–myocardial infarction if they are able to tolerate the negative inotropic effects.

8. Initiation of β-adrenergic blockers should not be undertaken until the patient is stable without fluid overload or hypotension, and on concomitant medications, which include diuretics and/or ACEIs or ARBs.

9. Patient education is an important aspect for initiating β-adrenergic blockers therapy, and patients need to be informed that they might not see positive effects for several months after obtaining the target dosage of the agent.

G. Diuretics

1. Diuretics should be prescribed for all patients with symptoms of HF who have evidence of or who have experienced fluid retention because these drugs are the only ones that can correct fluid retention. Diuretics are generally best used in conjunction with an ACEI, ARB, and/or β-adrenergic blocker.

2. Diuretics have been shown to cause a reduction in jugular venous pressures, pulmonary congestion, peripheral edema, and body weight in short-term studies and have been shown to improve cardiac function and exercise tolerance in intermediate-term studies.

3. The goal of diuretic therapy is to reduce and eventually eliminate signs and symptoms of fluid retention as assessed by jugular venous distension (JVD), peripheral edema, or both. Slow titration upward in doses may be necessary to minimize hypotension and should be continued until fluid retention is eliminated.

4. Body weight is an effective method of monitoring fluid losses and is best done on a daily basis by the patient.

5. Patients who experience diuretic resistance or tolerance to their effects might need intravenous administration, a combination of two agents with differing mechanisms (furosemide and metolazone) or the addition of agents such as dopamine or dobutamine, which increase renal blood flow. Furthermore, evaluation of patient drug profiles may identify the addition of sodium-retaining agents such as nonsteroidal anti-inflammatory drugs (NSAIDs).

6. All diuretics increase urine volume and sodium excretion but differ in their pharmacological properties.

7. Select Diuretic Classes
  a. **Thiazide diuretics** include chlorothiazide (Diuril), hydrochlorothiazide (HydroDIURIL), chlorthalidone (Hygroton), and indapamide (Lozol). They are effective and commonly used in HF, specifically in patients with hypertension, but they deplete potassium stores in the process. These agents are relatively weak because they are able to increase the fractional excretion of sodium to only 5%–10% of the filtered load. However, they have been shown to lose their effectiveness in HF patients with moderately impaired renal function (creatinine clearance < 30 mL/min).
  b. **Loop diuretics** include furosemide (Lasix), ethacrynic acid (Edecrin), bumetanide (Bumex), and torsemide (Demadex) and have become the preferred diuretics. They have the ability to increase sodium excretion to 20%–25% of the filtered load and to maintain their efficacy until renal function is severely impaired (creatinine clearance < 5 mL/min) plus have the added advantage of reducing venous return independent of diuresis. In addition, furosemide's action is more intense, making it useful as a rapid-acting intravenous agent in reversing acute pulmonary edema, owing to its direct dilating effects on pulmonary vasculature (see Table 42-5 for dosing).
  c. **Potassium-sparing diuretics** include amiloride (Midamor), spironolactone (Aldactone) and triamterene (Dyrenium) and may help avoid the incidence of hypokalemia. However, they also possess a weaker diuretic effect than the other diuretics. As the number of HF patients receiving ACEIs or ARBs continues to increase, fewer patients may require supplemental potassium therapy.

8. Aldosterone antagonists. Spironolactone (Aldactone), is a potassium-sparing diuretic, but was the first aldosterone antagonist available for clinical use in the United States, when it had been shown to have direct blocking effects on the actions of aldosterone. Results from a large study, the Randomized Aldactone Evaluation Study (RALES), revealed that the addition of low doses (12.5–25 mg daily) of spironolactone to patients with class IV symptoms (NYHA) taking ACEIs reduced the risk of death and hospitalization.
  a. Current guidelines recommend that spironolactone be considered in patients with stage C heart failure—as add-on therapy to ACEIs or ARBs and a β-adrenergic blocker—who can be closely monitored for changes in renal function and potassium levels.
  b. Patients receiving spironolactone should have serum potassium levels evaluated and reduced to < 5.0 mmol/L along with a serum creatinine level < 2.5 mg/dL before initiation of therapy. Potassium levels should be routinely monitored to prevent the subsequent development of hyperkalemia.
  c. Eplerenone (Inspra) was the second aldosterone receptor antagonist introduced and is currently indicated in the treatment of hypertension and in post-MI patients with HF.

H. Vasodilators

1. These agents reduce pulmonary congestion and increase cardiac output by reducing preload and/or afterload. However, at the current time, there are no large-scale trials supporting the use of vasodilators (nitrates or hydralazine) alone in the treatment of HF.

2. Individual agents
  a. **Nitroprusside (Nipride)** is administered intravenously in doses of 0.3–10 μg/kg/min to provide potent dilation of both arteries and veins.
  b. **Hydralazine (Apresoline).** This arteriole dilator decreases afterload and increases cardiac output in patients with HF.
  c. **Prazosin (Minipress).** This α-adrenergic blocker acts as a balanced arteriovenous dilator.
  d. **Nitrates.** Venous dilation by nitrates increases venous pooling, which decreases preload.
    (1) Their arterial effects seem to result in decreased afterload with continued therapy.
    (2) Nitrates are available in many forms and doses. Because individual reactions to these agents vary widely, dosages have to be adjusted; but, in general, they are higher for HF than for angina. Table 42-6 provides examples of nitrate doses that have been used in HF.
  e. **Combination therapy.** Hydralazine has been used with isosorbide dinitrate (Isordil) to reduce afterload (or with nitroglycerin to reduce preload) for treating chronic HF.
    (1) The combination of these two agents—hydralazine and isosorbide dinitrate (BiDil) should not be used as initial therapy over ACEIs, ARBs, or β-adrenergic blockers, but could be considered in patients who have persistent symptoms despite the use of these agents.

Table 42-6. Examples of Nitrates That Have Been Used in Heart Failure

Form of Nitrate	Typical Dose	Dosing Interval
Intravenous nitroglycerin	5–200 µg/min	Continuous infusion
Nitroglycerin buccal tablets	1–3 mg	4–6 hr
Nitroglycerin capsules (sustained release)	6.5–19.5 mg	4–6 hr
Nitroglycerin ointment	1–3 inches	4–6 hr
Sublingual nitroglycerin	0.4 mg	1–2 hr
Oral isosorbide dinitrate	10–60 mg	4–6 hr
Sublingual isosorbide dinitrate	5–10 mg	4 hr

(2) A recently completed trial demonstrated that the addition of isosorbide dinitrate and hydralazine to standard medical therapy consisting of ACEIs and β-adrenergic blockers can be effective in black patients with NYHA functional class III or IV heart failure.

(3) Suggested dosing regimens include hydralazine 50–100 mg four times daily and isosorbide dinitrate 10–40 mg three times daily.

I. Digitalis glycosides

1. Digitalis, specifically digoxin, continues to play a role in the treatment of HF, but ongoing evaluations have altered its place in the long-term management of HF. It has been shown to be effective as a short-term therapy in improving symptoms, quality of life, and exercise tolerance in patients with mild to moderate HF. It is now recommended as add-on therapy in conjunction with diuretics, ACEIs or ARBs, and a β-adrenergic blocker to improve the symptoms and clinical status of patients with HF.

2. Digoxin (Lanoxin) had previously been recommended in patients with HF who had rapid atrial fibrillation to control the ventricular rate. However, β-adrenergic blockers have been shown to improve survival and may be more effective in controlling the rate alone. Current guidelines suggest use of alternative agents for ventricular rate control rather than digoxin.

3. Digoxin can be used early to reduce symptoms in HF patients who have been started on ACEIs or β-adrenergic blockers but have not yet responded to them.

4. Long-term trials of select patients with HF have demonstrated that treatment with digoxin had little effect on short-term mortality but reduced the risk of death and hospitalization.

5. Therapeutic effects
  a. Positive inotropic effects were previously felt to provide most of the benefits through increased cardiac output, decreased cardiac filling pressure, decreased venous and capillary pressure, increased renal blood flow, and decreased heart size.
  b. Recent evidence suggests that digitalis acts by furthering the activation of neurohormonal systems rather than as a positive inotropic agent. This results in deactivation of renin–angiotensin–aldosterone compensation, which promotes diuresis, reduces fluid volume, decreases renal sodium reabsorption, and diminishes edema.
  c. Negative chronotropic effects occur from the effect of digitalis on the sinoatrial (SA) node when given in doses that produce high total body stores (e.g., 15–18 µg/kg).

6. Choice of agent. All of the digitalis glycosides have similar properties; however, digoxin is the most commonly used preparation in the United States.
  a. Digoxin is available in tablet, injection, elixir, and capsule forms.
  b. Calculation of doses must factor in the differences in systemic availability among these forms. For example, digoxin solution in capsules is more bioavailable than digoxin tablets; therefore, 0.125-mg tablets are equivalent to 0.1-mg capsules. In the majority of patients, the dosage of digoxin should be the equivalent of 0.125–0.25 mg daily of the tablet formulation.

7. Dosage and administration. The range between therapeutic and toxic doses is extremely narrow. There is no magic threshold level for digoxin therapy, but serum concentrations of 0.8–1.0 ng/mL have been associated with therapeutic response and minimal toxicity.

a. **Rapid digitalization.** Though not routinely necessary in the treatment of HF, in this method, the effects (and steady-state levels) are achieved within 24 hr, but the actual administration rate is usually slow and delivered in divided doses.

b. **Slow digitalization.** For the average HF patient, oral administration of maintenance doses should achieve steady-state levels in 7–8 days (3–4 weeks in a patient with renal dysfunction).

8. **Precautions and monitoring effects**
   a. **Potassium** seems to antagonize digitalis preparations.
      (1) Decreased potassium levels favor digoxin binding to cardiac cells and increase its effect, thus increasing the likelihood of digitalis toxicity. This antagonism is particularly significant for the HF patient who is receiving a diuretic (many of which decrease potassium levels).
      (2) Conversely, increased potassium levels seem to decrease digoxin binding and decrease its effect. This is likely in patients taking potassium or an ACEI or ARB (which increase potassium reabsorption).
   b. **Calcium** ions act synergistically with digoxin, and increased levels increase the force of myocardial contraction. At excessive levels, arrhythmias and systolic standstill can develop.
   c. **Magnesium** levels are inversely related to digoxin activity. As magnesium levels decrease, the predisposition to toxicity increases and, within reason, vice versa.
   d. **Serum digoxin levels**
      (1) In cardiac glycoside therapy, the patient's clinical state is the most practical barometer of a successful regimen. However, should questions arise as to compliance, absorption, or a drug–drug interaction, serum digoxin levels may be helpful.
      (2) After oral ingestion of digoxin, serum levels rise rapidly, then drop sharply as the drug enters the myocardium and other tissues. Therefore, a meaningful evaluation requires a determination of the relationship between serum digoxin levels and myocardial tissue levels.
      (3) The most meaningful results are obtained if serum samples are taken after steady state has been reached and 6–8 hr after an oral dose (3–4 hr after an intravenous dose).
   e. **Renal function studies.** Because the kidney is the primary metabolic route for **digoxin,** renal function studies such as serum creatinine levels aid the evaluation of elimination kinetics for digoxin.

9. Digitalis toxicity is a fairly common occurrence because of the narrow therapeutic range and can be fatal in a significant percentage of patients experiencing a toxic reaction.
   a. **Risk of toxicity** increases with coadministration of quinidine, verapamil (Calan), itraconazole (Sporanox), erythromycin (Erythrocin), clarithromycin (Biaxin), propafenone (Rythmol), spironolactone (Aldactone), and amiodarone (Cordarone) and is influenced by the electrolyte (hypokalemia, hypomagnesemia) effects described previously.
   b. **Signs of toxicity** include
      (1) Anorexia, a common and early sign
      (2) Fatigue, headache, and malaise
      (3) Nausea and vomiting
      (4) Mental confusion and disorientation
      (5) Alterations in visual perception (e.g., blurring, yellowing, a halo effect)
      (6) Cardiac effects:
         (a) Premature ventricular contractions and ventricular tachycardia and fibrillation
         (b) SA and atrioventricular (AV) block
         (c) Atrial tachycardia with AV block
   c. **Treatment of toxicity**
      (1) Digitalis is discontinued immediately, as is any potassium-depleting diuretic.
      (2) If the patient is hypokalemic, potassium supplements are administered and serum levels are monitored to avoid hyperkalemia through overcompensation. However, potassium supplements are contraindicated in a patient with severe AV block.
      (3) Arrhythmias are treated with lidocaine (Xylocaine) (usually a 100-mg bolus, followed by infusion at 2–4 mg/min) or phenytoin (Dilantin) (as a slow intravenous infusion of 25–50 mg/min, to a maximum of 1.0 g).
      (4) Cholestyramine (Questran), which binds to digitalis glycosides, may help prevent absorption and reabsorption of digitalis in the bile.

(5) Patients with very high serum digoxin levels (such as those resulting from a suicidal overdose) may benefit from the use of purified digoxin-specific Fab fragment antibodies (Digibind). One vial (38 mg) will bind 0.6 mg of digitalis. The dosage is calculated based on the estimated total body store of digitalis.

J. Calcium-channel blockers

1. Owing to the lack of evidence supporting efficacy, calcium-channel blockers should not be used for the treatment of HF. Current guidelines list calcium channel blockers as a class III recommendation, which states: "Calcium-channel blocking drugs are not indicated as routine treatment for HF in patients with current or prior symptoms of HF and reduced LVEF."

2. Calcium channel blockers have been listed as one of three classes of drugs (with antiarrhythmics and NSAIDs) that can exacerbate HF and should be avoided in most patients.

K. Inotropic agents have been used in the emergency treatment of patients with HF. However, long-term oral therapy with these agents has not improved symptoms or clinical status, and has been reports to increase mortality, especially in patients with advanced HF.

1. Current guidelines provide a class III recommendation, which states: "Long-term use of an infusion of a positive inotropic drug may be harmful and is not recommended for patients with current or prior symptoms of HF and reduced LVEF, except as palliation for patients with end-stage disease who cannot be stabilized with standard medical treatment."

2. Dopamine (intravenous)
   a. **Low doses** of 2–5 μg/kg/min stimulate specific dopamine receptors within the kidney to increase renal blood flow and thus increase urine output.
   b. **Moderate doses** of 5–10 μg/kg/min increase cardiac output (positive inotropic effect) in HF patients.
   c. **High doses**
      (1) As doses are raised above 10 μg/kg/min, α peripheral activity increases, resulting in increased total peripheral resistance and pulmonary pressures.
      (2) When the infusion exceeds 8–9 μg/kg/min, the patient should be monitored for tachycardia. If the infusion is slowed or interrupted, the adverse effect should disappear, as dopamine has a very short half-life in plasma.

3. Dobutamine (intravenous)
   a. Patients who are unresponsive to, or adversely affected by, dopamine may benefit from dobutamine in doses of 5–20 μg/kg/min.
   b. Although dobutamine resembles dopamine chemically, its actions differ somewhat. For example, dobutamine does not directly affect renal receptors and, therefore, does not act as a renal vasodilator. It increases urinary output only through increased cardiac output.
   c. Serious arrhythmias are a potential occurrence, although less likely to occur than with dopamine. Slowing or interrupting the infusion usually reverses this effect, as it does for dopamine.
   d. Dobutamine and dopamine have been used together to treat cardiogenic shock, but similar use in HF has yet to be accepted.

4. Inamrinone (intravenous) is referred to as nonglycoside, nonsympathomimetic inotropic agents.
   a. A bipyridine derivative, inamrinone has both a positive inotropic effect and a vasodilating effect.
   b. By inhibiting phosphodiesterase located specifically in the cardiac cells, it increases the amount of cyclic adenosine monophosphate (cAMP).
   c. Inamrinone has been used in patients with HF that have been refractory to treatment with other inotropic agents.
   d. Effective regimens have used loading intravenous infusions of 0.75 mg/kg over 2–3 min followed by maintenance infusions of 5–10 μg/kg/min.
   e. **Precautions and monitoring effects**
      (1) Inamrinone is unstable in dextrose solutions and should be added to saline solutions instead. Because of fluid balance concerns, this can be a potential problem in patients with HF.

(2) Because of the peripheral dilating properties, patients should be monitored for hypotension.

(3) Thrombocytopenia has occurred and is dose dependent and asymptomatic.

(4) Ventricular rates may increase in patients with atrial flutter or fibrillation.

5. **Milrinone (Primacor), intravenous,** is similar to inamrinone. It possesses both inotropic and vasodilatory properties.

   a. This agent has been used as short-term management to treat patients with HF.

   b. Most milrinone patients in clinical trials have also been receiving digoxin and diuretics.

   c. Effective dosing regimens have used a loading dose of 50 μg/kg administered slowly over 10 minutes intravenously, followed by maintenance doses of 0.375 μg/kg/min by continuous infusion, based on the clinical status of the patient.

   d. Precautions and monitoring effects

   (1) Renal impairment significantly prolongs the elimination rate of milrinone, and infusions need to be reduced accordingly.

   (2) Monitoring is necessary for the potential arrhythmias occurring in HF, which may be increased by drugs such as milrinone and other inotropic agents.

   (3) Blood pressure and heart rate should be monitored when administering milrinone, owing to its vasodilatory effects and its potential to induce arrhythmias.

   (4) Additional side effects include mild to moderate headache, tremor, and thrombocytopenia.

6. **Nesiritide (Natrecor)** is a recombinant form of human BNP, which is a naturally occurring hormone secreted by the ventricles. It is the first of this drug class to become available for human use in the United States.

   a. Nesiritide is approved for the intravenous treatment of patients with acutely decompensated HF associated with shortness of breath at rest or with minimal activity.

   b. Nesiritide binds to natriuretic peptide receptors in blood vessels, resulting in increased production of cyclic guanosine monophosphate (cGMP) in target tissues, which mediates vasodilation. In HF, nesiritide reduces pulmonary capillary wedge pressure and systemic vascular resistance.

   c. Initial treatment involves a bolus dose of 2 μg/kg followed by a continuous intravenous infusion of 0.01 μg/kg/min to a maximum dose of 0.03 μg/kg/min.

   d. Monitoring for hypotension, elevated serum creatinine, headache, nausea, and dizziness is the key to successful use. Concomitant use of ACEIs may increase the risk of symptomatic hypotension (systolic blood pressure < 90 mm Hg and syncope).

   e. Nesiritide has been shown to improve symptoms in the setting of acute HF, but the effect on morbidity and mortality has not yet been proven. At this point in time, owing to lack of pivotal studies demonstrating its benefit, nesiritide's use as intermittent or continuous outpatient treatment is not recommended.

L. Patient education

1. Patient should be made aware of the importance of taking their medications exactly as prescribed and should be advised to watch for signs of toxicity.

2. Patients should be educated on the need for lifestyle modifications that will have a positive effect on reducing HF development and reducing HF symptoms, including daily weight monitoring, fluid management, sodium restriction, early intervention if symptoms appear, compliance with the treatment plan, modification of alcohol intake, exercise, and stress reduction.

3. The patient should understand the need for regular checkups and be able to recognize symptoms that require immediate physician notification—for example, an unusually irregular pulse rate, palpitations, shortness of breath, swollen ankles, visual disturbances, or weight gain exceeding 3–5 lb in 1 week.

4. The patient needs to be educated about drugs such as calcium channel blockers; NSAIDs, which may cause a problem in HF by retaining fluid; and sodium. In addition, the patient needs to be informed of the potential dangers of use of over-the-counter medications that might also predispose him or her to HF symptoms and loss of symptom control. A thorough review of all medications (both prescription and over-the-counter) should be carried out as frequently as possible to ensure compliance with the treatment regimen.

STUDY QUESTIONS

Directions for questions 1–8: Each of the questions, statements, or incomplete statements in this section can be correctly answered or completed by **one** of the suggested answers or phrases. Choose the **best** answer.

1. Which of the following combinations of drugs, when used together, particularly in black patients, reduce both preload and afterload angiotensin-converting enzyme and might provide an alternative to ACEIs in patients who are intolerant of them?

(A) nitroglycerin (Nitrostat) and isosorbide dinitrate (Isordil)
(B) hydralazine (Apresoline) and isosorbide dinitrate
(C) diltiazem (Cardizem) and verapamil (Calan)
(D) prazosin (Minipress) and angiotensin II
(E) hydralazine and methyldopa (Aldomet)

2. When spironolactone (Aldactone) is used in a patient with heart failure (HF), it works through what primary mechanism?

(A) positive inotropic effect
(B) positive chronotropic effect
(C) aldosterone antagonism
(D) negative inotropic effect
(E) angiotensin II blockade

For questions 3–4: A 60-year-old hypertensive woman is currently being treated with nitroglycerin, carvedilol, furosemide, nifedipine (Procardia), ramipril, aspirin, and digoxin. She is admitted with a diagnosis of stage C heart failure.

3. Which agent is most likely to be discontinued in this patient?

(A) nifedipine
(B) carvedilol
(C) aspirin
(D) digoxin
(E) furosemide

4. Which of the following best represents the goals of therapy for this patient?

(A) Treat underlying causes such as hypertension, cigarette smoking, lipid disorders.
(B) Discourage the use of alcohol intake, illicit drug use, and dietary salt intake.
(C) Control the metabolic syndrome.
(D) All of the above.
(E) None of the above.

5. Because of proven beneficial effects on cardiac remodeling, a particular group of agents is now indicated as first-line therapy in HF patients. Which of the following is a representative of this group of drugs?

(A) hydrochlorothiazide (HydroDIURIL)
(B) lisinopril (Zestril)
(C) losartan (Cozaar)
(D) carvedilol (Atacand)
(E) furosemide (Lasix)

6. Which of the following statements is *not* correct, as it relates to the current status of heart failure (HF) in the United States?

(A) HF is the one cardiovascular disorder that is increasing in incidence and prevalence.
(B) Medication costs for treating HF in the United States approaches $38 billion.
(C) Patients with advanced disease have a 30%–40% risk of death annually.
(D) Current figures reveal approximately 5 million people in the United States who suffer from HF.
(E) Approximately 500,000 people each year are diagnosed with HF in the United States.

7. If treating a patient with HF, which of the following dosages of dopamine would be used to elicit its positive inotropic effects?

(A) 2.0 μg/kg/min
(B) 5–10 μg/kg/min
(C) 10–20 μg/kg/min
(D) 40 μg/kg/min
(E) 40 mg/kg/min

8. The use of angiotensin-converting enzyme inhibitors (ACEIs) in heart failure (HF) centers around what pharmacologic effect?

(A) direct reduction in renin levels with a resultant decrease in angiotensin II and aldosterone levels
(B) indirect reduction in angiotensin II and aldosterone levels owing to inhibition of angiotensin-converting enzyme
(C) direct reduction in aldosterone secretion and angiotensin I production by inhibiting angiotensin-converting enzyme
(D) increase in afterload owing to an indirect decrease in angiotensin II as well as a decrease in preload owing to an indirect reduction in aldosterone secretion
(E) inhibition of the angiotensin II receptor, which results in reduced angiotensin II levels and reduced secretion of aldosterone

Directions for questions 9–12: The questions and incomplete statements in this section can be correctly answered or completed by **one or more** of the suggested answers. Choose the answer, **A–E.**

A   if **I only** is correct
B   if **III only** is correct
C   if **I and II** are correct
D   if **II and III** are correct
E   if **I, II, and III** are correct

9. Which of the following have been shown to be effective in the acute management of digitalis toxicity?

I. cholestyramine resin (Questran)
II. Fab fragment antibody (Digibind)
III. potassium administration

10. Situations that predispose a digitalis-treated patient to toxicity include

I. hypercalcemia.
II. hyperkalemia.
III. hypermagnesemia.

11. Correct statements about dobutamine include which of the following?

I. Doses of 5–20 μg/kg/min have been associated with a positive inotropic effect in treating the patient with heart failure (HF).
II. Patients receiving dobutamine should be monitored for increases in peripheral vascular resistance.
III. Dobutamine is considered a nonglycoside, nonsympathomimetic-positive inotropic agent.

12. Which statements accurately describe heart (HF) classification stage A?

I. Patients have a high risk for HF without structural heart disease or symptoms
II. Patients need to receive ACEIs or ARBs
III. Patients should be treated for any underlying causes that would be responsible for causing HF

ANSWERS AND EXPLANATIONS

1. The answer is B *[see IV.H.2.e].*
The venous dilating properties of isosorbide dinitrate (preload) in conjunction with the arteriolar dilating effects of hydralazine (afterload) make this combination effective in reducing both preload and afterload. Recent guidelines suggest that the combination of the vasodilators hydralazine and isosorbide dinitrate should not be considered as initial therapy over ACEIs but has been shown to be effective, particularly in black patients when added to standard therapy for HF.

2. The answer is C *[see IV.G.8].*
Spironolactone was the first aldosterone antagonist available for clinical use in the United States. In the completed RALES trial, spironolactone, given in 12.5- to 25-mg daily doses to HF patients with class IV symptoms who were taking ACEIs, reduced the risk of death and hospitalization. It is a weak diuretic but also works as a direct antagonist to the actions of aldosterone, which has demonstrated benefit in HF patients with moderately to severe symptoms.

3. The answer is A *[see IV.J.1–2].*
Because they have the potential to produce negative inotropic effects, calcium channel blockers such as nifedipine have been identified as one of three groups of drugs to avoid in most HF patients. Besides calcium channel blockers, antiarrhythmics, and NSAIDs should be avoided in most HF patients owing to their ability to induce HF symptoms.

4. The answer is D *[see Table 42-4].*
The updated classification system was introduced with the newly established guidelines to demonstrate the progressive nature of HF and to provide a continuum of goals and treatment options as it progresses. Stage C represents the first stage in which the patient presents with structural heart disease as well as current or prior symptoms of HF. Initial goals for earlier stages remain important goals for stage C, but the "restriction in dietary salt" is added to all of the previous goals.

5. The answer is B *[see IV.D.1]*
ACEIs have shown an ability to have a positive effect on cardiac remodeling, which is believed to be the underlying change that results in the increased stresses and pathologic events that eventually cause the symptoms associated with HF. Recent studies have shown the positive benefits for each of the ACEIs used in HF patients, and today they represent the initial therapy for HF patients.

6. The answer is B *[see I.B–D].*
The actual costs involved in the treatment of HF, including medical care, home health care, medication costs, and hospitalization costs, reported in 2005 were approximately $27.9 billion. Medication costs alone are a bit less but are still reported to be more than $2.9 billion annually.

7. The answer is B *[see IV.K.2.b].*
Dopamine has shown great versatility in its effects. At doses of 2–5 μg/kg/min, it increases renal blood flow through its dopaminergic effects. At doses of 5–10 μg/kg/min, it increases cardiac output through its β-adrenergic stimulating effect. At doses of 10–20 μg/kg/min, it increases peripheral vascular resistance through its β-adrenergic stimulating effects. There is no specific cutoff for any of these effects, so close titration is required to provide for individual response.

8. The answer is B *[see IV.D.4–5; Figure 42-2].*
By directly inhibiting the angiotensin-converting enzyme, production of angiotensin II is reduced, as is angiotensin II–mediated secretion of aldosterone from the adrenal gland. These effects are believed to have a beneficial effect on the prevention of cardiac remodeling, which has been shown to have a detrimental effect on cardiac function.

9. The answer is E (I, II, III) *[see IV.I.9.c.(5)].*
Cholestyramine resin has been used in the acute situation to decrease the absorption of digoxin within the gastrointestinal tract. This results in lower digoxin levels if the resin is administered before all the digoxin has been absorbed. Potassium administration has been shown to be effective in protecting the myocardium from the toxic effects of digoxin while toxic levels return to normal. Fab fragment antibody, though expensive, has been shown to be effective in the management of very high serum digoxin levels, by which 40 mg of drug is able to bind 0.6 mg of digitalis.

10. The answer is A (I) *[see IV.I.8.a–c].*
Calcium ions act synergistically with digitalis. Therefore, when hypercalcemia occurs, digitalis exerts an added pharmacological effect on the heart. This may present itself as toxic arrhythmias, cardiac standstill, and even death. Elevated potassium levels or elevated magnesium levels seem to aid in the prevention of digitalis-induced toxicity. There is building evidence that digitalis preparations need calcium ions to work, and consequently low calcium levels may negate the pharmacological potential of digoxin.

11. The answer is A (I) *[see IV.K.3.a].*
Dobutamine in doses of 5–20 μg/kg/min is an inotropic agent that is useful in the treatment of HF. Dobutamine does not have the versatility that dopamine offers, lacking comparable effects on renal blood flow and peripheral vascular resistance. Rather, dobutamine has a peripheral dilating effect that offers a benefit to patients who have reduced cardiac output due to elevated peripheral resistance.

12. The answer is E (I, II, III) *[see Table 42-4].*
The recent guidelines for the diagnosis and management of chronic heart failure recognize four stages in the progression of HF, and each stage is associated with clinical findings, goals of treatment, and medications that which should be considered. Stage A represents patients who are merely at risk for heart failure owing to underlying risk factors such as hypertension, hyperlipidemia, and smoking. ACEIs are recognized for their beneficial effects in cardiac remodeling and have been recommended as first-line therapy for select patients with stage A heart failure.

43
Thromboembolic Diseases

James B. Groce III

I. **Definition.** Venous thromboembolic disease (VTED) occurs when one or more of the elements of **Virchow's triad** are present, resulting in deep venous thrombosis (DVT) and/or pulmonary embolism (PE).

    A. Vascular injury

    B. Venous stasis

    C. Hypercoagulable state (i.e., decreased protein C, protein S, or antithrombin)

II. **Incidence.** It is estimated that the annual incidence of VTE events exceeds 600,000 and the number of VTE-associated deaths is 296,370 annually.

III. **Risk Factors for VTE**

    A. **Patient specific and those associated with medical illness and surgical procedures**

        1. Surgery

        2. Trauma (major or lower extremity)

        3. Immobility or paresis

        4. Malignancy

        5. Cancer therapy (hormonal, chemotherapy or radiotherapy)

        6. Previous VTE

        7. Increasing age (> 40 years of age)

        8. Pregnancy and the postpartum period

        9. Estrogen-containing oral contraceptives or hormone-replacement therapy

      10. Selective estrogen-receptor modulators

      11. Acute medical illness

      12. Heart or respiratory failure

      13. Inflammatory bowel disease

      14. Nephrotic syndrome

      15. Myeloproliferative disorders, i.e., diseases in which malignant (cancer) bone marrow cells multiply and spread to the blood.

      16. Paroxysmal nocturnal hemoglobinuria

      17. Obesity

      18. Smoking

      19. Varicose veins

      20. Central venous catheterization

      21. Inherited or acquired thrombophilia (e.g., deficiency of antithrombin, protein C, or protein S, activated protein C resistance, antiphospholipid antibody, lupus anticoagulant)

IV. Prevention and Treatment

A. **Nonpharmacologic prevention.** Mechanical methods of prophylaxis are recommended, primarily in patients who are at high risk of bleeding, and may include **external pneumatic compression, graduated compression stockings** or **venous foot pumps.** These devices **increase venous outflow and/or reduce stasis** within the leg veins.

B. **Pharmacologic prevention.** VTED can be prevented by counteracting increased blood coagulability with **unfractionated heparin (UFH)** (see V.A), **oral anticoagulant therapy with a vitamin K antagonist such as warfarin** (see V.B), **low molecular weight heparin (LMWH)** (see V.C), or a **synthetic pentasaccharide** (see V.D).

V. Pharmacologic Agents. New recommendations for treatment of VTED have been promulgated that suggest a hierarchical approach to selection of pharmacologic agents for managing VTED. These recommendations are listed in Table 43-1 and each of the recommended pharmacologic agents are discussed in the following sections.

Table 43-1. Guidelines for Initial Treatment of Venous Thromboembolic Disease

Clinical situation	Recommended treatment
Confirmed acute DVT of the leg High suspicion of DVT of the leg	SC LMWH, IV UFH, or SC UFH anticoagulants while awaiting the outcome of diagnostic tests

Selection	Treatment options
IV UFH	Continuous infusion Using weight-based dosing protocol, adjust dosage to prolong aPTT to a range that corresponds to a plasma heparin level of 0.3–0.7 units/mL antifactor Xa activity by amidolytic antifactor Xa assay If therapeutic levels of aPTT are not reached despite large daily doses of UFH, measure antifactor Xa levels for dosage guidance
SC UFH	An alternative to IV UFH Initial dose 35,000 units/24 hr, then maintain aPTT within therapeutic range
SC LMWH	Recommended initial treatment once or twice a day over UFH (as outpatient therapy if possible, as inpatient therapy if necessary) Routine monitoring with antifactor Xa levels not recommended

Further recommendations

Once UFH therapy commences, check aPTT or antifactor Xa heparin level at 6 hr for UFH and adjust to maintain aPTT corresponding to therapeutic antifactor Xa heparin level of 0.3–0.7 units/mL

Antifactor Xa heparin levels not recommended for LMWH therapy

Platelet count should be checked daily while on UFH or LMWM

Warfarin therapy should be commenced on day 1; adjust daily dosing based on PT/INR

Stop unfractionated heparin or LMWH after 5 days overlap with warfarin (minimally), when INR is stable and > 2.0

Anticoagulate (warfarin) for 6–12 months (depending on patient and disease state)

aPTT, activated partial thromboplastin time; *INR,* international normalized ratio; *IV,* intravenous; *LMWH,* low molecular weight heparin; *PT,* prothrombin time; *SC,* subcutaneous; *UFH,* unfractionated heparin.
Adapted with permission from Buller HR, Agnelli G, Hull R, et al. Antithrombotic therapy for venous thromboembolic disease. Paper presented at the Seventh ACCP Conference on Antithrombotic and Thrombolytic Therapy. Chest 2004;126(Suppl):401s–428s.

A. Unfractionated heparin

1. **Indications.** Patients with proven VTED may receive concomitant UFH for acute treatment and warfarin therapy acutely, followed by warfarin therapy for continued prevention of recurrence of VTED (Table 43.1), unless contraindications to warfarin (e.g., pregnancy) are present.

2. **Mechanism of action.** The major mechanism by which heparin blocks coagulation is by catalyzing the inhibition of thrombin. UFH acts as an anticoagulant by catalyzing the **inactivation of thrombin (factor IIa), activated factor X (factor Xa), and activated factor IX (factor IXa) by antithrombin.**

3. **Pharmacokinetics.** The mechanisms of heparin clearance are complex.
   a. Heparin binds to a number of plasma proteins other than antithrombin, which competes with antithrombin heparin binding.
   b. UFH is cleared by rapid-phase (cellular) elimination followed by a more gradual (renal) clearance, which can best be explained by a **combination of saturable and nonsaturable first-order kinetic models.**
   c. When administered in fixed doses, the anticoagulant response to UFH varies among patients and within the same patient (i.e., interpatient and intrapatient variability). This variability is caused by differences in patients' plasma concentrations of heparin-neutralizing proteins and rates of heparin clearance.

4. **Administration and dosage**
   a. UFH's therapeutic effect is hastened by administration of a **loading dose,** which may be **empirically selected** (e.g., 5000-units bolus given intravenously) or individualized by the patient's **dosing weight.**
      (1) The weight-based approach has resulted in the use of loading doses varying from 70 to 100 units/kg.
      (2) In some instances, the indication for which heparin therapy is being initiated is considered, with 70 units/kg being used for all thrombotic indications other than suspected or proved pulmonary embolism, for which up to 100 units/kg may be used.
   b. **Variable approaches** to continuous dosing have been employed.
      (1) **Empiric dosing of 1000 units/hr** may be used but may result in subtherapeutic or supratherapeutic outcomes (i.e., an activated partial thromboplastin time below or above the targeted range).
      (2) Another approach to continuous dosing includes commencing with a fixed dose (other than the empiric dose of 1000 units/hr). One such approach may see an initial loading dose followed by 32,000 units/24 hr by continuous infusion.
      (3) Yet another approach validated in the medical and pharmaceutical literature uses a **weight-based dosing nomogram** for commencing UFH therapy that varies between 15 and 25 units/kg/hr.
         (a) Lower doses are used initially for most thrombotic indications other than pulmonary embolism.
         (b) Pulmonary embolism requires more aggressive therapy (i.e., up to 25 units/kg/hr) based on the consideration that the clearance of heparin may be increased, thus necessitating an increased dose.
      (4) **Initial heparin weight-based dosing nomograms and subsequent adjustment protocols** have been developed to assist the initial weight-based dosing efforts. Such protocols should be developed for a specific aPTT reagent (Tables 43-2 and 43-3).

5. **Monitoring the effects of UFH.** The anticoagulant effects of UFH are usually monitored by the **aPTT.** The aPTT should be **obtained at baseline** before commencing therapy and then **monitored 6 hr** after commencing heparin therapy. Subsequent dosing adjustments are based on the results of this and additional aPTTs.
   a. The aPTT ratio used to determine therapeutic effect is measured by dividing the observed aPTT by the mean of the normal laboratory control aPTT.
   b. Traditionally, it was taught that for many aPTT reagents, a therapeutic effect was achieved with an **aPTT ratio of 1.5–2.5.**
   c. However, because aPTT reagents may vary in their sensitivity, it is **inappropriate to use the same aPTT ratio (i.e., 1.5–2.5) for all reagents.** The therapeutic range for each aPTT reagent should be calibrated to be equivalent to a heparin level of 0.2–0.4 units/mL by whole blood (protamine titration) or to an **antifactor Xa level (i.e., plasma heparin level) of 0.3–0.7 units/mL collected at the 6th hr for UFH.**

Table 43-2. Weight-Based Nomogram

aPTT	Dose
Initial dose	80 units/kg bolus, then 18 units/kg/hr
< 35 sec	80 units/kg bolus, then 4 units/kg/hr
35–45 sec	40 units/kg bolus, then 2 units/kg/hr
46–70 sec[a]	No change
71–90 sec	Decrease infusion rate by 2 units/kg/hr
90 sec	Hold infusion 1 hr, then decrease infusion rate by 3 units/kg/hr

[a]This therapeutic range corresponds to antifactor Xa activity of 0.3–0.7 units/mL. The therapeutic range at any institution should be established by correlation with antifactor Xa levels in the range of 0.3–0.7 units/mL.

Adapted with permission from Hirsch J, Raschke R. Heparin and low-molecular-weight heparin. Paper presented at the Seventh ACCP Conference on Antithrombotic and Thrombolytic Therapy. Chest 2004;126(Suppl):188s–203s.

B. Oral anticoagulants—warfarin

1. Indications

a. Warfarin is proven effective in the:

  (1) Primary and secondary prevention of VTED

  (2) Prevention of systemic arterial embolism in patients with tissue and mechanical prosthetic heart valves or atrial fibrillation

  (3) Prevention of acute myocardial infarction (MI) in patients with peripheral arterial disease

  (4) Prevention of stroke, recurrent infarction, and death in patients with acute MI

b. Warfarin may also be used in patients with valvular heart disease to prevent systemic arterial embolism, although its effectiveness has never been demonstrated by a randomized clinical trial.

2. Mechanism of action

a. Oral anticoagulants (e.g., warfarin) are vitamin K antagonists, producing their anticoagulant effect by **interfering with the cyclic interconversion of vitamin K and its 2,3-epoxide (vitamin K epoxide).**

b. Inhibition of this process leads to the depletion of vitamin K_{H2} and **results in the produc-**

Table 43-3. Heparin Dosage Adjustment Protocol[a]

Patient's aPTT (sec)[b]	Repeat Bolus Dose (units)	Stop Infusion (min)	Change Rate of Infusion (mL/hr)[c] [units/24 hr]	Timing of Next aPPT
< 50	5000	0	+3 [2880]	6 hr
50–59	0	0	+3 [2880]	6 hr
60–85[d]	0	0	0	Next morning
86–95	0	0	−2 [−1920]	Next morning
96–120	0	30	−2 [−1920]	6 hr
> 120	0	60	−4 [−3840]	6 hr

aPTT, activated partial thromboplastin time.
[a]Starting dose of 5000 units intravenous IV bolus followed by 32,000 units/24 hr as a continuous infusion. First aPTT performed 6 hr after the bolus injection; dosage adjustments are made according to protocol and the aPTT is repeated as indicated in the far-right column.
[b]The normal range for aPTT with Dade Actin FS reagent is 27–35 sec; the range may vary, depending on the sensitivity of the reagent.
[c]Concentration of heparin equal to 40 units/mL.
[d]A therapeutic range of 60–85 sec is equivalent to a heparin level of 0.2–0.4 units/mL by whole blood protamine titration or 0.3–0.7 units/mL as a plasma antifactor Xa level. The therapeutic range varies with the responsiveness of the aPTT reagent to heparin.
Adapted with permission from Hirsch J, Raschke R. Heparin and low-molecular-weight heparin. Paper presented at the Seventh ACCP Conference on Antithrombotic and Thrombolytic Therapy. Chest 2004;126(Suppl):188s–203s.

tion of hemostatically defective, vitamin K–dependent coagulant proteins or clotting factors (prothrombin or factors II, VII, IX, and X).

   c. These vitamin K–dependent coagulant proteins or clotting factors (factors VII, IX, X, and II, respectively) decline over 6–96 hr.

3. Pharmacokinetics

   a. Warfarin is a **racemic mixture** of roughly equal amounts of two optically active isomers: the **R and S forms.**

   b. Warfarin is rapidly absorbed from the gastrointestinal tract and reaches maximal blood concentrations in healthy volunteers in 90 min.

   c. Dose response to warfarin is influenced by:

   (1) Pharmacokinetic factors (i.e., differences in absorption and metabolic clearance)

   (2) Pharmacodynamic factors (i.e., differences in the hemostatic response to given concentrations of warfarin)

   (3) Technical factors—for example, inaccuracies in prothrombin time (PT) and international normalized ratio (INR) testing and reporting

   (4) Patient-specific factors—for example, diet (increased intake of green, leafy vegetables), poor patient compliance (missed doses, self-medication, alcohol consumption), poor communication between patient and physician (undisclosed use of drugs that may interact with warfarin) (Table 43-4)

4. Administration and dosage

   a. Warfarin, a coumarin compound, is the most widely used oral anticoagulant in North America. Although it is primarily **administered orally,** an injectable preparation is available in the United States.

   b. Commence oral anticoagulant therapy with the **anticipated daily maintenance dose of warfarin,** which can be variable.

Table 43-4. Factors that May Potentiate or Inhibit Warfarin Effects

Factor	Potentiate Anticoagulant Effect	Inhibit Anticoagulant Effect
Drugs	Phenylbutazone	Cholestyramine
	Metronidazole	Barbiturates
	Sulfinpyrazone	Rifampin
	Trimethoprim-sulfamethoxazole	Griseofulvin
	Disulfiram	Carbamazepine
	Amiodarone	
	Erythromycin	
	Anabolic steroids	
	Clofibrate	
	Cimetidine	
	Omeprazole	
	Thyroxine	
	Ketoconazole	
	Isoniazid	
	Fluconazole	
	Piroxicam	
	Tamoxifen	
	Quinidine	
	Vitamin E (large doses)	
	Phenytoin	
	Penicillin	
Other	Low vitamin K intake	High vitamin K intake
	Reduced vitamin K absorption	Alcohol (acute use)
	Liver disease	
	Hypermetabolic states (e.g., thyrotoxicosis)	
	Alcohol (chronic use)	

Adapted with permission from Ansell J, Hirsh J, Poller L, et al. The pharmacology and management of the vitamin K antagonists. Paper presented at the Seventh ACCP Conference on Antithrombotic and Thrombolytic Therapy. Chest 2004;126:204S–233S.

Table 43-5. Practical Oral Anticoagulation Dosing

Day	Rapid Anticoagulation	Anticoagulation[a]
1	5–10 mg	5 mg
2	5–10 mg	5 mg
3	2.5–7.5 mg (adjust based on INR)[b]	5 mg (adjust based on INR)[b]

[a]Rapid anticoagulation is not required or there is a risk of bleeding.
[b]Adjust dosage based on INR until the INR is stable and therapeutic.
Adapted with permission from Ansell J, Hirsh J, Poller L, et al. The pharmacology and management of the vitamin K antagonists. Paper presented at the Seventh ACCP Conference on Antithrombotic and Thrombolytic Therapy. Chest 2004;126: 204S–233S.

    c. The initial dose of warfarin therapy can be flexible. (Table 43-5)
        (1) Patient-specific parameters used to determine the initial dose of warfarin include the patient's weight (e.g., obesity, concurrent use of interacting drugs known to inhibit the anticoagulant effect of warfarin, and the desired rapid anticoagulant effect).
        (2) Based on these patient-specific parameters, some clinicians may use a larger initial dose of warfarin (e.g., 7.5–10 mg), which should not be misconstrued as a loading dose.
    d. The initial dose of warfarin should be **overlapped with UFH, LMWH or a pentasaccharide for 5–7 days** (Table 43-1).
    e. The **duration of warfarin therapy** depends on each patient's indication(s) for use (Table 43-6).
    f. Reversal of warfarin effects may be necessary owing to an elevated INR or complications associated with oral anticoagulant therapy (Table 43-7).
  5. Monitoring warfarin therapy. PT and INR monitoring are usually performed daily on commencing oral anticoagulant therapy (e.g., warfarin), until such time that the INR has been found to be therapeutic.
    a. Laboratory monitoring is performed by measuring the **PT** for calculation of the INR.
        (1) The PT is **responsive to depression of three** of the four vitamin K–dependent procoagulant **clotting factors (prothrombin** or **factors II, VII, and X).**
        (2) The common commercial PT reagents vary markedly in their responsiveness to coumarin-induced reduction in clotting factors; therefore, PT results reported using different reagents are not interchangeable among laboratories.
    b. The problem of variability in responsiveness of PT reagents has been overcome by the introduction of a standardized test known as the **INR.**
        (1) The INR is equal to:

$$INR = \left(\frac{patient\ PT}{mean\ laboratory\ control\ PT}\right)^{ISI}$$

Table 43-6. Duration of Warfarin Therapy[a]

Duration	Indications
3–6 months	First event with reversible[b] or time-limited risk factor
≥ 6 months	Idiopathic venous thromboembolism, first event
12 months to lifetime	First event[c] with cancer (until resolved), anticardiolipin antibody, antithrombin deficiency
	Recurrent event, idiopathic or with throbophilia

[a]See Table 43-4 for factors that may influence warfarin effects. All recommendations are subject to modification by individual characteristics, including patient preference, age, comorbidity, and likelihood of recurrence.
[b]Reversible or time-limited risk factors: surgery, trauma, immobilization, estrogen use.
[c]Proper duration of therapy is unclear in first event with homozygous factor V Leiden, homocystinemia, deficiency of protein C or S or multiple thrombophilias and in recurrent events with reversible risk factors.
Adapted with permission from Buller HR, Agnelli G, Hull R, et al. Antithrombotic therapy for venous thromboembolic disease. Paper presented at the Seventh ACCP Conference on Antithrombotic and Thrombolytic Therapy. Chest 2004;126(Suppl):401s–28s.

Table 43-7. Guidelines for Reversal of Warfarin Effects

Clinical Situation	Guidelines
INR > therapeutic range but < 5.0; no clinically significant bleeding, rapid reversal not indicated for reasons of surgical intervention	
INR significantly above therapeutic range	Lower the dose or omit the next dose; resume warfarin therapy at a lower dose when the INR approaches desired range
INR minimally above therapeutic range	Dose reduction may not be necessary
INR > 5.0 but < 9.0; no clinically significant bleeding	
No additional risk factors for bleeding	Omit the next dose or two of warfarin; monitor INR more frequently; resume warfarin therapy at a lower does when the INR is in therapeutic range
Increased risk of bleeding	Omit the next dose of warfarin; give vitamin K_1 (1.0–2.5 mg orally)
More rapid reversal needed before urgent surgery or dental extraction	Give vitamin K_1 (2–4 mg orally); closely monitor INR; repeat dose of vitamin K_1 if INR not substantially reduced by 24–48 hr
INR > 9.0; no clinically significant bleeding	Give vitamin K_1 (3–5 mg orally); closely monitor INR; repeat dose of vitamin K_1 if INR not substantially reduced by 24–48 hr
INR > 20.0; serious bleeding, major warfarin overdose requiring very rapid reversal of anticoagulant effect	Give vitamin K_1 (10 mg by slow intravenous infusion) with fresh frozen plasma transfusion or prothrombin complex concentrate, depending on urgency; vitamin K_1 injections may be needed every 12 hr
Life-threatening bleeding, serious warfarin overdose	Give prothrombin complex concentrate with vitamin K_1 (10 mg by slow intravenous infusion); repeat if necessary, depending on INR
Continuing warfarin therapy indicated after high doses of vitamin K_1	Give heparin until the effects of vitamin K_1 have been reversed and patient is responsive to warfarin

INR, international normalized ratio.
Adapted with permission from Ansell J, Hirsh J, Poller L, et al. The pharmacology and management of the vitamin K antagonists. Paper presented at the Seventh ACCP Conference on Antithrombotic and Thrombolytic Therapy. Chest 2004;126:204S–233S.

where ISI (international sensitivity index) is a measure of the responsiveness of a given thromboplastin to reduction of the vitamin K–dependent coagulation factors. The **lower the ISI,** the **more responsive the reagent** and the closer the derived INR will be to the observed PT ratio.

(2) Guidelines of the American College of Chest Physicians (ACCP) Conference on Antithrombotic and Thrombolytic Therapy recommend two levels of therapeutic intensity: a less-intense range corresponding to an INR of 2.0–3.0, and a more-intense range corresponding to an INR of 2.5–3.5. The range corresponds to the indication (Table 43-8).

(3) Once the desired therapeutic INR has been achieved for 2 consecutive days, (e.g., for concomitant heparin plus warfarin overlap therapy) follow-up INR monitoring can be performed according to the following protocol:
   (a) Week 1: monitor INR two or three times
   (b) Week 2: monitor INR two times
   (c) Weeks 3–6: monitor INR once a week
   (d) Weeks 7–14: monitor INR once every 2 weeks
   (e) Week 15 to end of therapy: monitor INR once every 4 weeks (if INR dose responsiveness remains stable; if dose adjustment is necessary, a more frequent monitoring schedule is employed until stable dose responsiveness is achieved)

Table 43-8. Recommended Therapeutic Goal and Range for Oral Anticoagulant Therapy

| | INR | |
Indication	Goal	Range
Prophylaxis of venous thrombosis (high-risk surgery)	2.5	2.0–3.0
Treatment of venous thrombosis	2.5	2.0–3.0
Treatment of pulmonary embolism	2.5	2.0–3.0
Prevention of systemic embolism	2.5	2.0–3.0
Tissue heart valves	2.5	2.0–3.0
Anterior myocardial infarction (to prevent systemic embolism)	2.5	2.0–3.0
Anterior myocardial infarction (to prevent recurrent infarction)	3.0	2.5–3.5
Valvular heart disease	2.5	2.0–3.0
Atrial fibrillation	2.5	2.0–3.0
Mechanical prosthetic valves (high risk)	3.0	2.5–3.5

Adapted with permission from Ansell J, Hirsh J, Poller L, et al. The pharmacology and management of the vitamin K antagonists. Paper presented at the Seventh ACCP Conference on Antithrombotic and Thrombolytic Therapy. Chest 2004;126:204S–233S.

    c. Upon commencing oral anticoagulant therapy, **prolongation of the PT/INR** does not occur until depletion of the vitamin K–dependent procoagulant clotting factors occurs. This delay is **variable over 2–4 days.** During this delay, if active venous thrombosis is present, either UFH or LMWH is concomitantly commenced to adequately anticoagulate the patient while awaiting the therapeutic effect of warfarin.

C. Low molecular weight heparin

  1. Indications
    a. LMWH indications vary by manufacturer.
    b. Each of the LMWHs have been evaluated in a large number of randomized clinical trials and have been proven to be safe and efficacious for **the prevention and treatment of venous thromboembolism.**
    c. To date, different LMWHs have been evaluated for their role in:
      (1) Prevention of venous thrombosis
      (2) Treatment of VTED
      (3) Management of unstable angina pectoris/non–Q wave MI

  2. Chemistry. LMWHs are fragments of standard commercial-grade heparin produced by either chemical or enzymatic depolymerization. LMWHs are approximately one third the size of heparin. Like **heparin,** which has a **mean molecular weight of 15,000 Da** (range 3000–30,000 Da), **LMWHs** are heterogeneous in size with a **mean molecular weight of 4000–5000 Da** (range 1000–10,000 Da).

  3. Mechanism of action
    a. LMWHs achieve their **major anticoagulant effect by binding to antithrombin** through a unique pentasaccharide sequence that enhances the ability of antithrombin **to inactivate factor IIa (thrombin) and factor Xa.**
      (1) Heparin and **LMWHs catalyze the inactivation of factor IIa (thrombin) by binding to antithrombin through the unique pentasaccharide sequence and to thrombin to form a ternary complex.** A minimum chain length of 18 saccharides (including the pentasaccharide sequence) is required for ternary complex formation.
        (a) Virtually all heparin molecules contain at least 18 saccharide units.
        (b) Only 20%–50% of the different LMWHs contain fragments with 18 or more saccharide units.
        (c) Therefore, **compared with heparin, which has an antifactor Xa to antifactor IIa binding affinity ratio of approximately 1:1,** the various commercial **LMWHs have an antifactor Xa to antifactor IIa binding affinity ratio varying from 2:1 up to 4:1,** depending on their molecular size distribution (Table 43-9).
      (2) In contrast, inactivation of factor Xa by antithrombin does not require binding of the heparin molecules to the clotting enzyme. Therefore, inactivation of factor Xa is

Table 43-9. Pharmacokinetic and Pharmacodynamic Parameters of Different Low Molecular Weight Heparins (LMWHs)

LMWH	Brand Name	Average Molecular Weight	Bioavailability	Half-Life	Xa:IIa Binding-Affinity Ratio
Dalteparin	Fragmin	6000 Da	87%	3–5 hr	2.7:1
Enoxaparin	Lovenox	4500 Da	92%	4.5 hr	3.8:1
Tinzaparin	Innohep	6500 Da	87%	3.9 hr	2.8:1

achieved by small molecular weight heparin fragments provided that they contain the high-affinity pentasaccharide.

   b. The **antithrombotic and hemorrhagic effects** of heparin have been compared with LMWHs in a variety of **experimental animal models.**

   (1) When compared on a gravimetric basis, **LMWHs are said to cause decreased** potential for **hemorrhagic episodes.**

   (2) These differences in the relative antithrombotic to hemorrhagic ratios among these polysaccharides could be explained by the observation that **LMWHs have less inhibitory effects on platelet function** and vascular permeability.

4. Pharmacokinetics. The plasma recoveries and pharmacokinetics of LMWHs differ from heparin because of differences in the binding properties of the two sulfated polysaccharides to plasma proteins and endothelial cells.

   a. LMWHs bind much less avidly to heparin-binding proteins than heparin, a property that contributes to the superior bioavailability of LMWHs at low doses and their more predictable anticoagulation effect.

   b. LMWHs do not bind to endothelial cells in culture, a property that could account for their longer plasma half-life and their dose-independent clearance. Principally, the renal route clears LMWHs; therefore, the biologic half-life of LMWHs is increased in patients with renal failure.

5. Administration and dosage

   a. Dosing of LMWHs is **disease-state** and **product specific;** different doses are administered based on the indication for use and the manufacturer of the specific LMWH. Table 43-10 shows manufacturer's suggested, U.S. Food and Drug Administration (FDA) approved dosing for specific indications.

D. Synthetic pentasaccharide

1. Indications

   a. Synthetic pentasaccharide [fondaparinux (Arixtra)] is indicated for:

   (1) Thromboprophylaxis against DVT/PE after

   (a) Hip fracture surgery

   (b) Hip fracture surgery; extended prophylaxis

   (c) Knee-replacement surgery

   (d) Hip-replacement surgery

   (e) Abdominal surgery

   (2) Treatment of

   (a) Acute DVT

   (b) Acute PE

2. Chemistry. Synthetic pentasaccharide is a selective **factor Xa inhibitor.** The molecular weight of the synthetic pentasaccharide product is 1728 Da.

3. Mechanism of action

   a. The antithrombotic activity of fondaparinux is the result of antithrombin-mediated selective inhibition of factor Xa. Neutralization of factor Xa interrupts the blood coagulation cascade and thus inhibits thrombin formation and thrombus development.

   b. Fondaparinux does not inactivate thrombin (activated factor II) and has no known effect on platelet function.

4. Pharmacokinetics

   a. After subcutaneous administration, the drug is completely bioavailable, and steady-state peak plasma levels are achieved in approximately 3 hr after administration of the dose.

Table 43-10. FDA-Approved Dosing of Low Molecular Weight Heparin (LMWH) Based on Disease State

Approved Labeling and Dosing[a]	Dalteparin	Enoxaparin	Tinzaparin
Hip-replacement surgery prophylaxis	5000 units q.d. for 5–10 days	30 mg every 12 hr, or 40 mg q.d. for 7–10 days	n/a
Extended hip-replacement prophylaxis	n/a	40 mg q.d. for 3 weeks	n/a
Knee-replacement surgery prophylaxis	n/a	30 mg every 12 hr for 7–10 days	n/a
General surgery prophylaxis	2500 units q.d. or 5000 units qd (high risk) for 5–10 days	40 mg q.d. for 7–10 days	n/a
Acute medically ill prophylaxis	5000 units q.d. for 12–14 days	40 mg q.d. for 6–14 days	n/a
Treatment of DVT with or without PE	n/a	As a bridge to warfarin until stable INR: 1 mg/kg every 12 h (outpatient treatment permitted) *or* 1.5 mg/kg every 24 h (inpatient only)	As a bridge to warfarin until stable INR: 175 units/kg every 24 hr
Unstable angina and NSTEMI	120 units/kg every 12 hr for 5–8 days plus aspirin indefinitely	1 mg/kg every 12 hr for 2–8 days plus aspirin indefinitely	n/a

DVT, deep-vein thrombosis; *INR,* international normalized ratio; *n/a,* not applicable; *NSTEMI,* non-ST-segment elevated myocardial infarction; *PE,* pulmonary embolism.
Adapted with permission from Rihn T, Vanscoy GJ. Low molecular weight heparin: Formulary drug class reviews. Pharm Ther 2001:26;486-492.

    b. The elimination half-life is 17–21 hr, enabling once-daily dosing.
    c. The drug does not seem to be metabolized and appears in the urine in active form and is renally eliminated.

  5. Administration and dosage
    a. Fondaparinux must not be administered intramuscularly.
    b. For prophylaxis against VTE, the drug should not be used in patients with body weight < 50 kg because the incidence of major bleeding was found to double in this patient population during clinical trials.
    c. For prophylaxis against VTE a usual **dose of 2.5 mg subcutaneously once daily for 5–9 days** is recommended for **all prophylaxis indications.** The initial dose should be started 6–8 hr after surgery when hemostasis is established.
    d. For treatment of established VTE, administer a once-daily subcutaneous dose as follows:
      (1) Patients with body weight between 50 and 100 kg: 7.5 mg
      (2) Patients with body weight < 50 kg: 5 mg
      (2) Patients with body weight > 100 kg: 10 mg

  6. Cautions
    a. Contraindications
      (1) Severe renal impairment
      (2) Patients weighing < 50 kg when used for prophylaxis
      (3) Patients with active major bleeding
      (4) Bacterial endocarditis
      (5) Thrombocytopenia associated with positive in vitro test for antiplatelet antibody in the presence of fondaparinux
      (6) Known hypersensitivity to fondaparinux

   b. Precautions
   (1) Conditions or procedures that may enhance the risk of severe bleeding (e.g., trauma, hemophilia, gastrointestinal ulceration, concurrent use of antiplatelet agents, history of cerebrovascular hemorrhage, severe uncontrolled hypertension)
   (2) Renal impairment
   (3) Heparin-induced thrombocytopenia
   (4) Neuraxial anesthesia and indwelling epidural catheter use
   (5) Elderly patients
   (6) Pregnancy category B and lactating (the drug is excreted into breast milk)
   (7) Protamine is **ineffective** as an antidote

STUDY QUESTIONS

Directions for questions 1–4: Each of the questions, statements, or incomplete statements in this section can be correctly answered or completed by **one** of the suggested answers or phrases. Choose the **best** answer.

1. A 67-year-old man who weighs 100 kg (212 lb) and is 60 in. tall presents to his physician after a transatlantic flight complaining of pain and swelling of his right lower extremity. The patient had total knee arthroplasty 2 weeks before his travel. His medical history reveals that he has an ejection fraction of 15%, he is in remission for non-Hodgkin lymphoma, and he has had a previous myocardial infarction. His mother, father, and sister are dead as a result of stroke, pulmonary embolism, and childbirth, respectively. Given this patient's history, he is most likely suffering from which of the following?

(A) ruptured Baker cyst
(B) deep venous thrombosis of the lower extremity
(C) torn medial meniscus
(D) septic arthritis

2. Prophylaxis against venous thromboembolic disease (VTED) may include

(A) nonpharmacological prophylaxis.
(B) pharmacological prophylaxis.
(C) nonpharmacological and pharmacological prophylaxis.
(D) neither nonpharmacological and pharmacological prophylaxis

3. Unfractionated heparin binds to antithrombin III and inactivates clotting factor(s)

(A) Xa
(B) IXa
(C) IIa
(D) All of the above
(E) None of the above

4. Initiation of unfractionated heparin therapy for the patient described in question 1 would best be achieved with

(A) 5000 U loading dose followed by 1000 U/hr
(B) 5000 U loading dose followed by 1800 U/hr
(C) 8000 U loading dose followed by 1800 U/hr
(D) 1000 U loading dose followed by 1000 U/hr

Directions for questions 5–11: The questions and incomplete statements in this section can be correctly answered or completed by **one or more** of the suggested answers. Choose the answer, **A–E.**

A if **I only** is correct
B if **III only** is correct
C if **I and II** are correct
D if **II and III** are correct
E if **I, II, and III** are correct

Directions for questions 5–10: Upon confirmation of diagnosis, the attending physician asks you, the pharmacist, to commence low molecular weight heparin therapy for the patient described in question 1 above. The following questions pertain to your pharmaceutical care for this patient.

5. When choosing an FDA-approved low molecular weight heparin to treat this patient, you would administer

I. enoxaparin 1 mg/kg/dose subcutaneously q 12 hr.
II. enoxaparin 1.5 mg/kg/dose subcutaneously q 24 hr.
III. tinzaparin 175 IU/kg/dose subcutaneously q 24 hr.

6. Which of the following tests are used to monitor heparin antithrombotic therapy?

I. international normalized ratio
II. activated partial thromboplastin time
III. heparin assay

7. A patient to be commenced on oral anticoagulant therapy for DVT would be treated with:

I. oral anticoagulant therapy with warfarin for a goal international normalized ratio (INR) of 2–3.
II. oral anticoagulant therapy with warfarin for a goal INR of 2.5–3.5.
III. oral anticoagulant therapy with aspirin for a goal INR of 2–3.

8. A patient on oral anticoagulant therapy is commenced on sulfamethoxazole-trimethoprim, double-strength twice daily. One may expect to see the international normalized ratio

I. increase.
II. decrease.
III. remain unchanged.

9. If a patient has an international normalized ratio (INR) > 20 and active bleeding that is clinically significant (i.e., hematuria), the pharmacist should

I. hold the drug therapy.
II. administer vitamin K.
III. administer fresh frozen plasma.

10. Compared to unfractionated heparin, low molecular weight heparins have

I. preferential binding affinity to factor Xa relative to IIa (thrombin).
II. shorter half-lives.
III. dose-dependent renal clearance.

11. An 87-year-old woman who weighs 49.0 kg (108 lb) and is 66 in tall has sustained a hip fracture requiring open reduction with internal fixation (ORIF) surgery. She has a documented serum creatine value recorded in the chart and in the laboratory results as 4.3 mg%. The orthopedic surgeon asks you, the pharmacist, about the appropriate fondaparinux dosing for this patient to prevent venous thromboembolism after the surgery. Which of the following are contraindications to the use of fondaparinux in this patient?

I. patient weighs < 50 kg
II. patient has severe renal impairment
III. patient is elderly

898 *Chapter 43*

ANSWERS AND EXPLANATIONS

1. The answer is B *[see I.A–C].*
The patient has the classic triad of risk factors predisposing him to DVT injury (recent knee arthroplasty), venous stasis (transatlantic travel), and hypercoagulable state (family history of venous thromboembolic disease). The patient has other risk factors as well, including age > 40, recent surgery, oncologic disease (though in remission), congestive heart failure, previous myocardial infarction with low ejection fraction, and obesity.

2. The answer is C *[see IV.A–B].*
Prophylaxis of VTED can involve a nonpharmacological approach, a pharmacological approach, or a combination of nonpharmacological and pharmacological approaches. The method of prophylaxis used is determined based on the patient's degree of risk. For example, a patient at high to extremely high risk for development of VTED requires nonpharmacological and pharmacological prophylaxis.

3. The answer is D *[see V.A.2].*
Unfractionated heparin acts as an anticoagulant by catalyzing the inactivation of factor IIa, factor Xa, and factor IXa by antithrombin III.

4. The answer is C *[see V.A.4.b.(4)].*
Several nomograms for dosing continuous infusion unfractionated heparin exist in the medical and pharmaceutical literature. The loading dose is typically 70–100 units/kg. In this case, the patient weighs 100 kg (212 lb) and the loading dose is 80 units/kg. Maintenance doses of 15–25 units/kg/hr are typically used. In this case, the maintenance dose is 18 units/kg/hr.

5. The answer is E *(I, II, III) [see Table 43-10].*
Primary literature reveals appropriate randomized prospective trials examining the role of LMWH compared to unfractionated heparin. From these trials, evidence of efficacy and safety for enoxaparin and tinzaparin at the treatment doses listed exists and has been approved by FDA for treatment of established VTE.

6. The answer is D *(II, III) [see V.A.5.a–c].*
Unfractionated heparin may be appropriately monitored by either the activated partial thromboplastin time (aPTT) or heparin assay. Because different laboratories use aPTT reagents with different sensitivities, the aPTT range and its corresponding ratio must be correlated to a heparin level of 0.2–0.4 units/mL by whole-blood (protamine titration) assay or 0.3–0.7 units/mL by plasma-amidolytic assay. The safety and efficacy of LMWH cannot be reliably evaluated by aPTT determinations. LMWH safety and efficacy can be evaluated by heparin assay. Because of the reliability of dose responsiveness seen with LMWH therapy, the need to perform heparin assays is controversial.

7. The answer is A *(I) [see V.B.5.a–b; Table 43-8].*
Oral anticoagulant therapy is monitored by measuring the PT. The PT is responsive to depression of three of the four vitamin K–dependent procoagulant clotting factors (prothrombin or factors II, VII, and X). These respective clotting factors take approximately 96 hr to be depleted, at which time the PT should be sufficient to arrive at an INR of 2.0–3.0 for patients with DVT (by appropriately converting the PT ratio to the power of the ISI). Patients with mechanical prosthetic heart valves have INRs targeted in the 2.5–3.5 range. Aspirin therapy is not monitored by INR determinations.

8. The answer is A *(I) [see Table 43-4].*
Oral anticoagulant therapy with warfarin may be complicated by myriad drug–drug interactions owing to the highly protein-bound state of warfarin. Such drug interactions may potentiate (prolong) PT:INR ratio, inhibit (shorten) the anticoagulant effect of warfarin, or have no effect on the actions of warfarin. Sulfamethoxazole-trimethoprim and other antibiotics have the potential to augment the anticoagulant effect of warfarin by eliminating bacterial flora and, thereby, producing vitamin K deficiency.

9. The answer is E *(I, II, III) [see Table 43-7].*
Pharmacists may be called on to offer advice regarding reversal of warfarin therapy or may be empowered using Pharmacy and Therapeutics Committee or Medical Board approved protocols to reverse warfarin's effect. In all instances, the pharmacist must critically and clinically evaluate the situation and communicate with the physician regarding management issues. A need for immediate surgery or invasive procedures will always hasten the urgency of warfarin reversal. In the setting of active bleeding, its clinical significance must be demonstrated by consultation with the patient's physician. If the INR is > 20 and the patient has active bleeding that is clinically significant, the pharmacist must hold drug therapy, consider the most appropriate dose and route of vitamin K delivery, and administer fresh frozen plasma to replete the vitamin K–dependent clotting factors.

10. The answer is A *(I) [see V.C.3.a.(1); V.C.4.b].*
UFH has an Xa:IIa binding-affinity ratio of approximately 1:1, and the various commercial LMWHs have Xa:IIa binding-affinity ratios of 2:1 up to 4:1, depending on their molecular size distribution. This increased binding affinity for factor Xa relative to factor IIa (thrombin) is said to account for the improved ability of LMWHs to catalyze inactivation of thrombin; the smaller fragments cannot bind to thrombin and, therefore, retain their ability to inactivate factor Xa. LMWHs have longer half-lives than unfractionated heparin. LMWHs are cleared primarily via the kidneys, and their biologic half-life is increased in patients with renal failure *independent* of dose.

11. The answer is C *(I, II) [see V.D.5.b; V.D.6.a.(1)–(2)].*
The synthetic pentasaccharide fondaparinux is contraindicated in patients who have severe renal impairment and who weigh < 50 kg. Calculation of the patient's estimated creatinine clearance by the Crockcoft-Gault method reveals an estimated clearance of approximately 8.5 mL/min, which would be defined as severe renal impairment. Her stated weight is 49 kg. Thus this patient's severe renal impairment and low weight constitute contraindications to the use of fondaparinux. Fondaparinux is recommended for use with *precaution* in the elderly patient population.

44
Infectious Diseases

Paul F. Souney

Anthony E. Zimmermann

Linda M. Spooner

Ronald J. DeBellis

I. Principles of Anti-Infective Therapy

A. Definition. Anti-infective agents treat infection by suppressing or destroying the causative microorganisms—bacteria, mycobacteria, fungi, protozoa, or viruses. Anti-infective agents derived from natural substances are called **antibiotics;** those produced from synthetic substances are called **antimicrobials.** These two terms are now used interchangeably.

B. Indications. Confirm the presence of infection by completing a careful history and physical examination, searching for signs and symptoms of infection as well as predisposing factors. Anti-infective agents should be used only when

1. A significant infection has been diagnosed or is strongly suspected

2. An established indication for prophylactic therapy exists

C. Gram stain, microbiological culturing, and **susceptibility tests** should be performed before anti-infective therapy is initiated. Test materials must be obtained by a method that avoids contamination of the specimen by the patient's own flora.

1. **Gram stain.** Performed on all specimens except blood cultures, the gram stain helps identify the cause of infection immediately. By determining if the causative agent is gram positive or gram negative, the test allows a better choice of drug therapy, particularly when an anti-infective regimen must begin without delay.
   a. **Gram-positive** microorganisms stain **blue** or **purple.**
   b. **Gram-negative** microorganisms stain **red** or **rose-pink.**
   c. **Fungi** may also be identified by gram stain.

2. **Microbiological cultures.** To identify the specific causative agent, specimens of body fluids or infected tissue are collected for analysis.

3. **Susceptibility tests.** Different strains of the same pathogenic species may have widely varying susceptibility to a particular anti-infective agent. Susceptibility tests determine microbial susceptibility to a given drug and thus can be used to predict whether the drug will combat the infection effectively.
   a. **Microdilution method.** The drug is diluted serially in various media containing the test microorganism.
      (1) The lowest drug concentration that prevents microbial growth after 18–24 hr of incubation is called the **minimum inhibitory concentration (MIC).**
      (2) The lowest drug concentration that reduces bacterial density by 99.9% is called the **minimum bactericidal concentration (MBC).**
      (3) **Breakpoint** concentrations of antibiotics are used to characterize antibiotic activity: The interpretive categories are **susceptible, moderately susceptible (intermediate),** and **resistant.** These concentrations are determined by considering pharmacokinetics, serum and tissue concentrations following normal doses, and the **population distribution** of MICs of a group of bacteria for a given drug.
   b. **Kirby-Bauer disk diffusion technique.** This test is less expensive but less reliable than the microdilution method; however, it provides qualitative susceptibility information.

    (1) Filter paper disks impregnated with specific drug quantities are placed on the surface of agar plates streaked with a microorganism culture. After 18 hr, the size of a clear inhibition zone is determined; drug activity against the test strain is then correlated to zone size.

    (2) The Kirby-Bauer technique does not reliably predict therapeutic effectiveness against certain microorganisms (e.g., *Staphylococcus aureus, Shigella*).

D. Choice of agent. An anti-infective agent should be chosen on the basis of its pharmacological properties and spectrum of activity as well as on various host (patient) factors (Figure 44-1).

  1. Pharmacological properties include the drug's ability to reach the infection site and to attain a desired level in the target tissue.

  2. Spectrum of activity. To treat an infectious disease effectively, an anti-infective drug must be active against the causative pathogen. Susceptibility testing or clinical experience in treating a given infection may suggest the effectiveness of a particular drug.

  3. Patient factors. Selection of an anti-infective drug regimen must take various patient factors into account to determine which type of drug should be administered, the correct drug dosage and administration route, and the potential for adverse drug effects.

    a. Immunological status. A patient with impaired immune mechanisms may require a drug that rapidly destroys pathogens (i.e., **bactericidal agent**) rather than one that merely suppresses a pathogen's growth or reproduction (i.e., **bacteriostatic agent**).

    b. Presence of a foreign body. The effectiveness of anti-infective therapy is reduced in patients who have prosthetic joints or valves, cardiac pacemakers, and various internal shunts.

    c. Age. A drug's pharmacokinetic properties may vary widely in patients of different ages. In very young and very old patients, drug metabolism and excretion commonly decrease. Elderly patients also have an increased risk of suffering ototoxicity when receiving certain antibiotics.

    d. Underlying disease

      (1) Preexisting **kidney** or **liver disease** increases the risk of nephrotoxicity or hepatotoxicity during the administration of some antibacterial drugs.

      (2) Patients with **central nervous system (CNS) disorders** may suffer neurotoxicity (motor seizures) during penicillin therapy.

      (3) Patients with **neuromuscular disorders** (e.g., myasthenia gravis) are at increased risk for developing neuromuscular blockade during aminoglycoside or polymyxin B therapy.

    e. History of drug allergy or adverse drug reactions. Patients who have had previous allergic or other untoward reactions to a particular antibiotic have a higher risk of experiencing the same reaction during subsequent administration of that drug. Except in life-threatening situations, patients who have had serious allergic reactions to penicillin, for example, should not receive the drug again.

    f. Pregnancy and lactation. Because drug therapy during pregnancy and lactation can cause unwanted effects, the mother's need for the antibiotic must be weighed against the drug's potential harm.

      (1) Pregnancy can increase the risk of adverse drug effects for both mother and fetus. Also, plasma drug concentrations tend to decrease in pregnant women, reducing a drug's therapeutic effectiveness.

      (2) Most drugs, including antibiotics, appear in the breast milk of nursing mothers and may cause adverse effects in infants. For example, sulfonamides may lead to toxic bilirubin accumulation in a newborn's brain.

    g. Genetic traits

      (1) Sulfonamides may cause hemolytic anemia in patients with glucose-6-phosphate dehydrogenase (G6PD) deficiency.

      (2) Patients who rapidly metabolize drugs (i.e., rapid acetylators) may develop hepatitis when receiving the antitubercular drug isoniazid.

E. Empiric therapy. In serious or life-threatening disease, anti-infective therapy must begin before the infecting organism has been identified. In this case, the choice of drug (or drugs) is based on clinical experience, suggesting that a particular agent is effective in a given setting.

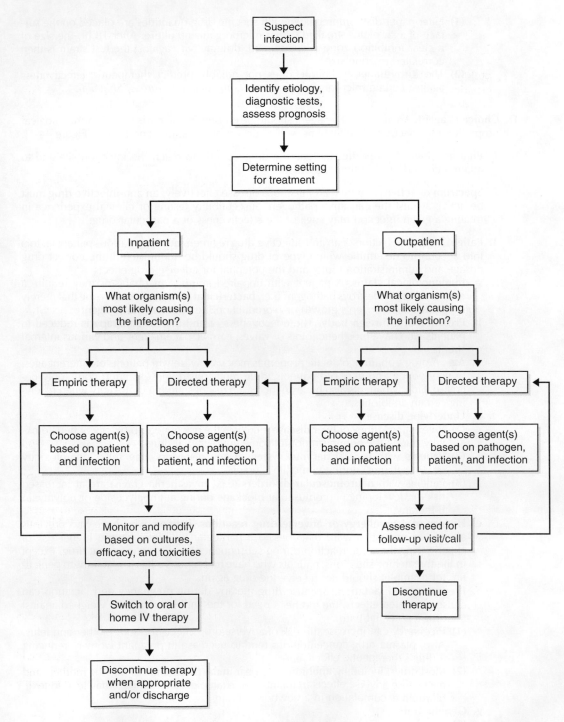

Figure 44-1. Approach to management of infection.

1. A **broad-spectrum antibiotic** usually is the most appropriate choice until the specific organism has been determined.

2. In all cases, **culture specimens must be obtained** before therapy begins.

F. **Multiple antibiotic therapy.** A combination of drugs should be given only when clinical experience has shown such therapy to be more effective than single-agent therapy in a particular setting. A multiple-agent regimen can increase the risk of toxic drug effects and, in a few cases, may result in drug antagonism and subsequent therapeutic ineffectiveness. Indications for multiple-agent therapy include

1. **Need for increased antibiotic effectiveness.** The **synergistic** (intensified) effect of two or more agents may allow a dosage reduction or a faster or enhanced drug effect.

2. **Treatment of an infection caused by multiple pathogens** (e.g., intra-abdominal infection)

3. **Prevention of proliferation of drug-resistant organisms** (e.g., during treatment of tuberculosis)

G. **Duration of anti-infective therapy.** To achieve the therapeutic goal, anti-infective therapy must continue for a sufficient duration.

1. **Acute uncomplicated infection.** Treatment generally should continue until the patient has been afebrile and asymptomatic for at least 72 hr.

2. **Chronic infection** (e.g., endocarditis, osteomyelitis). Treatment may require a longer duration (4–6 weeks) with follow-up culture analyses to assess therapeutic effectiveness.

H. **Monitoring therapeutic effectiveness.** To assess the patient's response to anti-infective therapy, appropriate specimens should be cultured and the following parameters monitored.

1. **Fever curve.** An important assessment tool, the fever curve may be a reliable indication of response to therapy. Defervescence usually indicates favorable response.

2. **White blood cell (WBC) count.** In the initial stage of infection, the neutrophil count from a peripheral blood smear may rise above normal (neutrophilia), and immature neutrophil forms ("bands") may appear ("left shift"). In patients who are elderly, debilitated, or suffering overwhelming infection, the WBC count may be normal or subnormal.

3. **Radiographic findings.** Small effusions, abscesses, or cavities that appear on radiographs indicate the focus of infection.

4. **Pain** and **inflammation** (as evidenced by swelling, erythema, and tenderness) may occur when the infection is superficial or within a joint or bone, also indicating a possible focus of infection.

5. **Erythrocyte sedimentation rate (ESR or "sed rate").** Large elevations in ESR are associated with acute or chronic infection, particularly endocarditis, chronic osteomyelitis, and intra-abdominal infections. A normal ESR does not exclude infection; more often, ESR is elevated as a result of noninfectious causes such as collagen vascular disease.

6. **Serum complement concentrations,** particularly the C3 component, are often reduced in serious infections because of consumption during the host defense process.

I. **Lack of therapeutic effectiveness.** When an antibiotic drug regimen fails, other drugs should not be added indiscriminately or the regimen otherwise changed. Instead, the situation should be reassessed and diagnostic efforts intensified. Causes of therapeutic ineffectiveness include the following:

1. **Misdiagnosis.** The isolated organism may have been misidentified by the laboratory or may not be the causative agent for infection (e.g., the patient may have an unsuspected infection).

2. **Improper drug regimen.** The drug dosage, administration route, dosing frequency, or duration of therapy may be inadequate or inappropriate.

3. **Inappropriate choice of antibiotic agent.** As discussed in I.D, patient factors and the pharmacological properties and spectrum of activity of a given drug must be considered when planning anti-infective drug therapy.

4. **Microbial resistance.** By acquiring resistance to a specific antibiotic, microorganisms can survive in the drug's presence. Many gonococcal strains, for instance, now resist penicillin. Drug resistance is particularly common in geographical areas in which a specific drug has been used excessively (and perhaps improperly).

5. **Unrealistic expectations.** Antibiotics are ineffective in certain circumstances.
    a. Patients with conditions that require **surgical drainage** frequently cannot be cured by anti-infective drugs until the drain has been removed. For example, the presence of necrotic tissue or pus in patients with pneumonia, empyema, or renal calculi is a common cause of antibiotic failure.
    b. **Fever** should not be treated with anti-infective drugs unless infection has been identified as the cause. Although fever frequently signifies infection, it sometimes stems from noninfectious conditions (e.g., drug reactions, phlebitis, neoplasms, metabolic disorders, arthritis). These conditions do not respond to antibiotics. One exception to this position is neutropenic cancer patients; such patients with no signs or symptoms of infection other than fever are widely treated with antimicrobial agents.

6. **Infection by two or more types of microorganisms.** If not detected initially, an additional cause of infection may lead to therapeutic failure.

J. Antimicrobial prophylaxis for surgery

1. **Definition.** Antibiotic prophylaxis is a short course of antibiotic administered before there is clinical evidence of infection.

2. **General considerations**
    a. **Timing.** The antibiotic should be administered to ensure that appropriate antibiotic levels are available at the site of contamination before the incision. Initiation of prophylaxis is often at induction of anesthesia, within 1 hr or just before the surgical incision. This ensures peak serum and tissue antibiotic levels.
    b. **Duration.** Prophylaxis should be maintained for the duration of surgery. Long surgical procedures (e.g., > 3 hr) may require additional doses. There is little evidence to support continuation of prophylaxis beyond 24 hr.
    c. **Antibiotic spectrum** should be appropriate for the usual pathogens.
       (1) In general, **first-generation cephalosporins** (e.g., cefazolin) are the drugs of choice for most procedures and patients. These agents have an appropriate spectrum, a low frequency of side effects, a favorable half-life, and a low cost.
       (2) **Vancomycin** is a suitable alternative in penicillin-sensitive patients and in situations in which methicillin-resistant *S. aureus* is a concern.
    d. **Route of administration.** Intravenous (IV) or intramuscular (IM) routes are preferred to guarantee good serum and tissue levels at the time of incision.

II. Antibacterial Agents

A. **Definition and classification**. Used to treat infections caused by **bacteria,** antibacterial agents fall into several major categories: **aminoglycosides, carbapenems, cephalosporins, erythromycins, penicillins** (including various subgroups), **sulfonamides, tetracyclines, fluoroquinolones, metronidazole** (see V.C.2.b)**, urinary tract antiseptics,** and **miscellaneous anti-infectives** (Table 44-1).

B. **Aminoglycosides.** These drugs, containing amino sugars, are used primarily in infections caused by gram-negative enterobacteria and in suspected sepsis. They have little activity against anaerobic and facultative organisms. The toxic potential of these drugs limits their use. Major aminoglycosides include **amikacin (Amikin), gentamicin (Garamycin), kanamycin, neomycin, netilmicin, streptomycin,** and **tobramycin (Nebcin).**

1. **Mechanism of action.** Aminoglycosides are **bactericidal;** they inhibit bacterial protein synthesis by binding to and impeding the function of the 30S ribosomal subunit. (Some aminoglycosides also bind to the 50S ribosomal subunit.) Their mechanism of action is not fully known.

2. **Spectrum of activity**
    a. **Streptomycin** is active against both gram-positive and gram-negative bacteria. However, widespread resistance to this drug has restricted its use to the organisms that cause

Table 44-1. Some Important Parameters of Anti-Infective Drugs

Agent	Elimination Route	Half-Life	Administration Route	Common Dosage Range (Adults)
Aminoglycosides				
Amikacin	Renal	2–3 hr	IV, IM	15 mg/kg/day, (once daily dose)
Gentamicin	Renal	2 hr	IV, IM	3 mg/kg/day (standard dose); 6–7 mg/kg/day (once daily dose)
Kanamycin	Renal	2–4 hr	Oral, IV	15 mg/kg every 8–12 hr
Neomycin	Renal	2–3 hr	Oral, topical	50–100 mg/kg/day (oral); 10–15 mg/kg/day (topical)
Netilmicin	Renal	2–7 hr	IV, IM	3–6 mg/kg/day
Streptomycin	Renal	2–3 hr	IM	15 mg/kg/day[a]
Tobramycin	Renal	2–5 hr	IV, IM	3 mg/kg/day (standard dose); 6–7 mg/kg/day, (once daily dose)
Carbapenems				
Imipenem	Renal	1 hr	IV	250 mg–1 g every 6 hr
Ertapenem	Renal	4 hr	IV, IM	1 g/day
Meropenem	Renal	1.5 hr	IV, IM	0.5–2 g every 8 hr
Cephalosporins				
First-generation				
Cefadroxil	Renal	1.5 hr	Oral	1–2 g/day
Cefazolin	Renal	1.4–2.2 hr	IV	250 mg–1 g every 8 hr
Cephalexin	Renal	0.9–1.3 hr	Oral	250–500 mg every 6 hr
Cephapirin	Renal (H)	0.6–0.8 hr	IV, IM	500 mg–2 g every 4–6 hr
Cephradine	Renal	1.3 hr	Oral, IV	250–500 mg every 6 hr
Second-generation				
Cefaclor	Renal (H)	0.8 hr	Oral	250–500 mg every 8 hr
Cefmetazole	Renal	72 min	IV	2 g every 6–12 hr
Cefotetan	Renal	2.8–4.6 hr	IV, IM	1–2 g every 12 hr
Cefoxitin	Renal	0.8 hr	IV	1–2 g every 6–8 hr
Cefprozil	Renal	78 min	Oral	250–500 mg every 12–24 hr
Cefuroxime	Renal	1.5–2.2 hr	IV, IM	750 mg–1.5 g every 8 hr
Loracarbef	Renal	1 hr	Oral	200 mg every 12 hr or 400 mg/day
Third-generation				
Cefixime	Renal	3–4 hr	Oral	400 mg/day
Cefdinir	Renal	1.7–1.8 hr	Oral	300 mg every 12 hr
Cefoperazone	Hepatic	1.6–2.4 hr	IV	2–4 g every 12 hr
Cefotaxime	Renal (H)	1.5 hr	IV	1–2 g every 6–8 hr
Cefpodoxime	Renal	2.5 hr	Oral	100–400 mg every 12 hr
Ceftazidime	Renal	1.8 hr	IV, IM	1–2 g every 8–12 hr
Ceftibuten	Renal	2.5 hr	Oral	400 mg/day
Ceftizoxime	Renal	1.7 hr	IV	1–2 g every 8–12 hr
Ceftriaxone	Renal	8 hr	IV, IM	1–2 g/day
Fourth-generation				
Cefepime	Renal	2–2.3 hr	IV, IM	1–2 g every 8–12 hr
Erythromycins and other macrolides				
Azithromycin	Hepatic	68 hr	Oral	250 mg/day
Clarithromycin	Renal	3–7 hr	Oral	250–500 mg every 12 hr
Dirithromycin	Hepatic	8 hr	Oral	500 mg/day
Erythromycin base estolate, ethylsuccinate, and stearate	Hepatic	1.2–2.6 hr	Oral	250–500 mg every 6 hr

(*Continued on next page*)

Table 44-1. Continued.

Agent	Elimination Route	Half-Life	Administration Route	Common Dosage Range (Adults)
Erythromycins and other macrolides (continued)				
Erythromycin gluceptate and lactobionate			IV	0.5–2 g every 6 hr
Natural penicillins				
Penicillin G	Renal (H)	0.5 hr	Oral, IV, IM	200,000–500,000 U every 6–8 hr
Penicillin V	Renal	1 hr	Oral	500 mg–2 g/day
Penicillin G procaine	Renal	24–60 hr	IM	300,000–600,000 U/day
Penicillin G benzathine	Renal	24–60 hr	IM	300,000–600,000 U/day
Penicillinase-resistant penicillins				
Cloxacillin	Renal (H)	0.5 hr	Oral	250–500 mg every 6 hr
Dicloxacillin	Renal (H)	0.5–0.9 hr	Oral	500 mg–1 g/day
Methicillin	Renal (H)	0.5–1 hr	IV, IM	1–2 g every 4–6 hr
Nafcillin	Hepatic (R)	0.5 hr	Oral, IV, IM	0.25–2 g every 6 hr
Oxacillin	Renal (H)	0.5 hr	Oral, IV, IM	500 mg–2 g every 4–6 hr 500–875 mg every 12 hr
Aminopenicillins				
Amoxicillin	Renal (H)	0.9–2.3 hr	Oral	250–500 mg every 8 hr
Amoxicillin/ clavulanic acid	Renal	1 hr	Oral	250–500 mg every 8 hr
Ampicillin	Renal (H)	0.8–1.5 hr	Oral, IV, IM	250 mg–2 g every 4–6 hr
Ampicillin/ sulbactam	Renal	1–1.8 hr	IV, IM	1.5–3 g every 6 hr
Extended-spectrum penicillins				
Mezlocillin	Renal (H)	0.6–1.2 hr	IV, IM	1–3 g every 4–6 hr
Piperacillin	Renal (H)	0.8–1.4 hr	IV, IM	1–1.5 mg/kg every 6–12 hr
Piperacillin/ tazobactam	Renal	0.7–1.2 hr	IV	3.375 g every 6 hr
Ticarcillin	Renal	0.9–1.5 hr	IV, IM	1–3 g every 4–6 hr
Ticarcillin/ clavulanic acid	Renal	1–1.5 hr	IV	3.1 g every 4–6 hr
Sulfonamides				
Sulfacytine	Renal	4–4.5 hr	Oral	250 mg every 6 hr
Sulfadiazine	Renal (H)	6 hr	Oral, IV	2–4 g/day
Sulfamethoxazole	Hepatic (R)	9–11 hr	Oral	1–3 g/day
Sulfisoxazole	Renal (H)	3–7 hr	Oral, IV	2–8 g/day
Sulfamethizole	Renal	—	Oral	0.5–1 g every 6–8 hr
Tetracyclines				
Demeclocycline	Renal	10–17 hr	Oral	300 mg–1 g/day
Doxycycline	Hepatic	14–25 hr	Oral, IV	100–200 mg every 12 hr
Minocycline	Hepatic	12–15 hr	Oral, IV	100–200 mg every 12 hr
Oxytetracycline	Renal	6–12 hr	Oral, IM	250–500 mg every 6 hr 250–500 mg q.i.d. or 300 mg/day in 1 or 2 divided doses
Tetracycline[b]	Renal	6–12 hr	Oral, IV, IM	1–2 g/day
Fluoroquinolones				
Alatrofloxacin[c]	Hepatic/ fecal	11 hr	IV	200–300 mg IV followed by 200 mg oral therapy
Ciprofloxacin	Renal (H)	5–6 hr	IV	200–600 mg every 12 hr

(*Continued on next page*)

Table 44-1. Continued.

Agent	Elimination Route	Half-Life	Administration Route	Common Dosage Range (Adults)
Fluoroquinolones (continued)				
Enoxacin	Renal (H)	3–6 hr	Oral	200 mg/day–400 mg every 12 hr
Gatifloxacin	Renal	7 hr	Oral, IV	400 mg once daily
Gemifloxacin	Fecal (R)	4-12 hr	Oral	320 mg once daily
Lomefloxacin	Renal	6.35–7.77 hr	Oral	400 mg/day
Levofloxacin	Renal	8 hr	IV, Oral	250–500 mg every 24 hr
Moxifloxacin	Hepatic	12 hr	Oral	400 mg once daily
Ofloxacin	Renal	5–7.5 hr	Oral	100 mg/day–400 mg
Sparfloxacin	Renal	20 hr	Oral	200 mg every 24 hr
Trovafloxacin[c]	Hepatic/fecal	11 hr	Oral	100–300 mg every 24 hr
Urinary tract antiseptics				
Cinoxacin	Renal	1–1.5 hr	Oral	250 mg every 6 hr or 500 mg every 12 hr
Fosfomycin	Renal/fecal	5.7 hr	Oral	One packet (3 g) in 90–120 mL water × 1 dose
Methenamine hippurate and mandelate	Renal	1–3 hr	Oral	0.5–2 g q.i.d.
Nalidixic acid	Renal	8 hr	Oral	4 g/day
Nitrofurantoin	Renal	0.3–1 hr	Oral	5–7 mg/kg/day
Norfloxacin	Hepatic	3–4 hr	Oral	400 b.i.d.
Miscellaneous anti-infectives				
Atovaquone	Fecal	50–84 hr	Oral	750 mg b.i.d. × 21 days
Aztreonam	Renal	1.7 hr	Oral, IV	50–100 mg/kg/day
Clindamycin	Hepatic	2–4 hr	Oral, IM, IV	300–900 mg every 6–8 hr
Clofazimine	Hepatic	70 days	Oral	50–100 mg/day
Dapsone	Hepatic (R)	28 hr	Oral	50–100 mg/day
Daptomycin	Renal	8 hr	IV	4 mg/kg/day
Lincomycin	Hepatic (R)	4.4–6.4 hr	IV, IM	600 mg–1 g every 8–12 hr
Linezolid	Renal	4–6 hr	Oral, IV	600 mg every 12 hr
Mupirocin	Renal	19–35 min	Topical	Apply every 8–12 hr
Quinupristin/dalfopristin	Hepatic	1 hr/0.4–0.5 hr	IV	7.5 mg/kg every 8 hr
Spectinomycin	Renal	1.2–2.8 hr	IM	2–4 g (single dose)
Telithromycin	Hepatic (R)	10 hr	Oral	800 mg/day
Tigecycline	Biliary (R)	42 hr	IV	100 mg load, 50 mg every 12 hr
Trimethoprim	Renal (H)	8–15 hr	Oral	100–200 mg/day
Vancomycin	Renal	6–8 hr	Oral, IV	500 mg every 6 hr
Antifungal agents				
Amphotericin B	Unknown	24 hr	IV	1–1.5 mg/kg/day
Anidulafungin	Fecal (R)	40–50 hr	IV	Candidemia: 200 mg day 1, then 100 mg/day Esophageal candidiasis: 100 mg day 1, then 50 mg/day
Caspofungin	Hepatic	9–11 hr	IV	70 mg on day 1, then 50 mg q.d.
Fluconazole	Renal	22–37 hr	IV, Oral	100–800 mg/day
Flucytosine	Renal	6 hr	Oral	50–150 mg/kg/day
Griseofulvin	Hepatic (R)	9–24 hr	Oral	300–375 mg/day
Itraconazole	Hepatic	24–42 hr	Oral	200–600 mg/day

(*Continued on next page*)

Table 44-1. Continued.

Agent	Elimination Route	Half-Life	Administration Route	Common Dosage Range (Adults)
Antifungal agents (continued)				
Ketoconazole	Hepatic/fecal	3.3 hr	Oral	200–400 mg/day bid
Micafungin	Hepatic	11–17 hr	IV	Esophageal candidiasis: 150 mg/day; HSCT prophylasis: 50 mg/day
Miconazole	Hepatic	20–24 hr	Oral	200–400 mg/day
Nystatin	Fecal	—	Oral	500,000–1,000,000 U t.i.d.
Terbinafine	Hepatic (R)	11–16 hr	Oral	250 mg/day
Voriconazole	Hepatic	6 hr	IV, Oral	IV: 6 mg/kg every 12 hr × 2 doses, then 4 mg/kg every 12 h; oral: 200 mg every 12 h for > 40 kg, 100 mg every 12 h for < 40 kg
Antiprotozoal agents				
Atovaquone	Hepatic	67 hr	Oral	750 mg b.i.d.
Chloroquine	Renal/fecal	72–120 hr	IM, Oral	Depends on disease
Diloxanide	Renal	—	IM	500 mg tid
Eflornithine	Renal	3 hr	IV	100 mg/kg/dose every 6 hr
Fansidar	Renal	100–231 hr	Oral	1 tablet every week
Halofantrine	Hepatic	3–4 days	Oral	500 mg every 6 hr × 3 doses; repeat in 7 days
Hydroxychloroquine	Renal	72–120 hr	Oral	310 mg every week
Iodoquinol	Fecal	—	Oral	650 mg t.i.d. for 20 days
Mefloquine	Hepatic	15–33 days	Oral	1250 mg single dose
Metronidazole	Hepatic (R)	6–14 hr	Oral, IV	250–500 mg every 6–8 hr
Nitazoxanide	Hepatic	1–1.6 hr	Oral	100–200 mg b.i.d. based on age
Paromomycin	Fecal	—	Oral	25–35 mg/kg/day
Pentamidine	Renal	6–9 hr	IM, IV, inhalation	IV, IM: 3–4 mg/kg every day; inhalation: 300 mg every 4 weeks
Primaquine	Hepatic	3.7–9.6 hr	Oral	15 mg (base)/day
Pyrimethamine	Renal	111 hr	Oral	25 mg every week
Quinacrine		5 days	Oral	100 mg/day
Quinine	Renal	12 hr	Oral	325 mg b.i.d.
Tinidazole	Hepatic (R)	13.2 hr	Oral	2 g q.d. × 1–3 days
Antitubercular agents				
Aminosalicylic acid	Renal	1 hr	Oral	150 mg/kg daily (maximum 12 g/day)
Capreomycin	Renal	4–6 hr	IM	15 mg/kg/day to 1 g/day maximum
Cycloserine	Renal	10 hr	Oral	15–20 mg/kg (maximum 1 g/day)
Ethambutol	Hepatic	3.3 hr	Oral	15–25 mg/kg/day
Ethionamide	Hepatic	3 hr	Oral	500 mg–1 g/day
Isoniazid	Hepatic	1–4 hr	Oral, IV	5–10 mg/kg daily (maximum dose = 300 mg)
Pyrazinamide	Hepatic	9–10 hr	Oral	15–30 mg/kg daily (maximum 2 g/day)
Rifampin	Hepatic	2–3 hr	Oral, IV	10 mg/kg (up to 600 mg) q.d.

(*Continued on next page*)

Table 44-1. Continued.

Agent	Elimination Route	Half-Life	Administration Route	Common Dosage Range (Adults)
Antitubercular agents (continued)				
Rifabutin	Hepatic	45 hr	Oral	300 mg q.d.
Rifepentine	Hepatic	13.9 hr (active metabolite \13.4 hr)	Oral	600 mg every 3 days
Antiviral agents				
Abacavir	Hepatic	1.5 hr	Oral	300 mg b.i.d. or 600 mg every day
Adefovir	Renal	7.5 hr	Oral	10 mg every day
Acyclovir	Renal	2.2 hr	Oral, IV, topical	IV: 5–10 mg/kg every 8 hr ; oral: 200–800 mg every 4 hr
Amprenavir	Hepatic	7–10 hr	Oral	1200 mg b.i.d.
Atazanavir	Hepatic	7 hr	Oral	400 mg every day
Amantadine	Renal	17 hr	Oral	100 mg b.i.d. or 200 mg every day
Cidofovir	Renal	6.5 hr	IV	5 mg/kg week × 2 (induction); 5 mg/kg every 2 weeks (maintenance)
Darunavir	Hepatic	15 hr	Oral	600 mg plus 100 mg ritonavin b.i.d.
Delavirdine	Hepatic (R)	2–11 hr	Oral	400 mg t.i.d.
Didanosine	Renal	1.5 hr	Oral	> 60 kg: 400 mg every day (EC caps); < 60 kg: 250 mg every day (EC caps)
Emtricitabine	Renal	10 hr	Oral	200 mg every day
Enfuvirtide	n/a	3.8 hr	SC	90 mg b.i.d.
Entecavir	Renal	128–149 hr	Oral	0.5 mg every day
Efavirenz	Hepatic	40–55 hr	Oral	600 mg every day
Famciclovir	Renal	2–2.3 hr	Oral	250–500 mg every 8–12 hr
Foscarnet	Renal	3–6 hr	IV	90 mg/kg every 12 hr (CMV induction); 90 mg/kg every day (CMV maintenance)
Ganciclovir	Renal	2.9 hr	IV	5 mg/kg every 12 hr (induction)
		4.8 hr	Oral	1000 mg t.i.d. (after induction)
Indinavir	Hepatic	1.4–2.2 hr	Oral	800 mg every 8 hr
Lamivudine	Renal	3–7 hr	Oral	150 mg b.i.d. or 300 mg daily
Lopinavir/ ritonavir	Hepatic	4.4–6.1 hr	Oral	200 mg/50 mg per tab (4 tablets every day)
Nelfinavir	Hepatic	3.5–5 hr	Oral	750 mg t.i.d. or 1250 mg b.i.d.
Nevirapine	Renal (H)	25–30 hr	Oral	200 mg every day × 14 days, then 200 mg b.i.d.
Oseltamivir	Renal	6–10 hr	Oral	75 mg b.i.d.
Rimantadine	Renal	25 hr	Oral	100 mg b.i.d.
Ritonavir	Hepatic	3–5 hr	Oral	100-400 mg daily, divided in 1 or 2 doses (as booster agent with other PIs)
Ribavirin	Renal	298 hr	Oral	800–1000 mg daily, divided into 2 doses

(Continued on next page)

Table 44-1. Continued.

Agent	Elimination Route	Half-Life	Administration Route	Common Dosage Range (Adults)
Antiviral agents (continued)				
Saquinavir	Hepatic	13 hr	Oral	1200 mg t.i.d. (Fortovase); 1000 mg (Invirase) plus 100 mg ritonavir b.i.d.
Stavudine	Renal	1.5 hr	Oral	> 60 kg: 40 mg every 12 hr; < 60 kg: 30 mg every 12 hr
Tenofovir	Renal	10–14 hr	Oral	300 mg daily
Tipranavir	Hepatic	6 hr	Oral	500 mg plus 200 mg ritonavir b.i.d.
Valacyclovir	Renal	2.5–3.6 hr	Oral	1 g every day or b.i.d. or t.i.d.
Valganciclovir	Renal	4 hr	Oral	900 mg b.i.d. (induction), 900 mg every day (maintenance)
Zalcitabine	Renal	1–3 hr	Oral	0.75 mg t.i.d.
Zanamivir	Renal	2.5–5.1 hr	Inhalation (Diskhaler)	2 inhalations (10 mg) b.i.d. × 5 days
Zidovudine	Renal (H)	1.5–3.1 hr	Oral	300 mg b.i.d.
			IV	2 mg/kg over 1 hr, then 1 mg/kg/hr until cord clamping (intrapartum perinatal prophylaxis for pregnant women)
Anthelmintics				
Albendazole	Hepatic	8–12 hr	Oral	400–800 mg daily
Diethylcarba-mazine	Renal	8 hr	Oral	25 mg/day for 3 days, then 50 mg/day for 5 days, then 100 mg/day for 3 days, then 150 mg/day for 12 days
Ivermectin	Hepatic	16–35 hr	Oral	150-200 mcg/kg × 1 dose
Mebendazole	Hepatic	8 hr	Oral	100 mg b.i.d.
Praziquantel	Hepatic	0.8–3 hr	Oral	60–75 mg/kg in 3 divided doses on the same day
Pyrantel	Hepatic	—	Oral	11 mg/kg (maximum = 1 g) as a single dose
Thiabendazole	Hepatic	—	Oral	< 70 kg: 22 mg/kg b.i.d.; > 70 kg: 1.5 g b.i.d.

CMV, cytomegalovirus; *EC cap*, enteric-coated capsule; *H*, additional significant hepatic elimination; HSCT, hematopoietic stem cell transplant; *IM*, intramuscular; *IV*, intravenous; *PIs*, protease inhibitors *R*, additional significant renal elimination; *SC*, subcutaneous.

[a] Dosage applies to infections other than tuberculosis; for tuberculosis, dosage is 1 g/day.
[b] Intravenous agent withdrawn from U.S. market.
[c] Trovafloxacin has a black box warning associated with its use.

plague and tularemia, gram-positive streptococci (given in combination with penicillin), and *Mycobacterium tuberculosis* (given in combination with other antitubercular agents, as described in VI.C.2).

b. **Amikacin, kanamycin, gentamicin, tobramycin, neomycin,** and **netilmicin** are active against many gram-negative bacteria (e.g., *Proteus, Serratia,* and *Pseudomonas* organisms).

   (1) **Gentamicin** is active against some *Staphylococcus* strains; it is more active than tobramycin against *Serratia* organisms.

(2) **Amikacin** is the broadest spectrum aminoglycoside with activity against most aerobic gram-negative bacilli as well as many anaerobic gram-negative bacterial strains that resist gentamicin and tobramycin. It is also active against *M. tuberculosis* and *Mycobacterium avium-intracellulare* (MAI).

(3) **Tobramycin** may be more active against *Pseudomonas aeruginosa* than gentamicin.

(4) **Netilmicin** may be active against gentamicin-resistant organisms; it appears to be less ototoxic than other aminoglycosides.

(5) **Neomycin,** in addition to its activity against such gram-negative organisms as *Escherichia coli* and *Klebsiella pneumoniae,* is active against several gram-positive organisms (e.g., *S. aureus*). *P. aeruginosa* and most streptococci are now neomycin resistant.

3. Therapeutic uses

a. Streptomycin is used to treat plague, tularemia, acute brucellosis (given in combination with tetracycline), bacterial endocarditis caused by *Streptococcus viridans* (given in combination with penicillin), and tuberculosis (given in combination with other antitubercular agents, as described in VI.C.2).

b. Gentamicin, tobramycin, amikacin, and **netilmicin** are therapeutic for serious gram-negative bacillary infections (e.g., those caused by *Enterobacter, Serratia, Klebsiella,* and *P. aeruginosa*), pneumonia (given in combination with a cephalosporin or penicillin), meningitis, complicated urinary tract infections, osteomyelitis, bacteremia, and peritonitis.

c. Neomycin is used for preoperative bowel sterilization; hepatic coma (as adjunctive therapy); and, in topical form, for skin and mucous membrane infections (e.g., burns).

4. Precautions and monitoring effects. Aminoglycosides can cause serious adverse effects. To prevent or minimize such problems, blood drug concentrations and blood urea nitrogen (BUN) and serum creatinine levels should be monitored during therapy.

a. Ototoxicity. Aminoglycosides can cause vestibular or auditory damage. The relative ototoxicity is as follows:

streptomycin = kanamycin > amikacin = gentamicin = tobramycin > netilmicin

(1) Gentamicin and streptomycin cause primarily **vestibular** damage (manifested by tinnitus, vertigo, and ataxia). Such damage may be bilateral and irreversible.

(2) Amikacin, kanamycin, and neomycin cause mainly **auditory** damage (hearing loss).

(3) Tobramycin can result in both vestibular and auditory damage.

b. Nephrotoxicity. Because aminoglycosides accumulate in the proximal tubule, mild renal dysfunction develops in up to 25% of patients receiving these drugs for several days or more. Usually, this adverse effect is reversible. Use of once-daily administration (ODA) has been reported in the literature to be as effective and less nephrotoxic than traditional dosing.

(1) Neomycin is the most nephrotoxic aminoglycoside; streptomycin is the least nephrotoxic. Gentamicin and tobramycin are nephrotoxic to approximately the same degree.

(2) **Risk factors** for increased nephrotoxic effects include the following:

(a) Preexisting renal disease

(b) Previous or prolonged aminoglycoside therapy

(c) Concurrent administration of another nephrotoxic drug

(d) Impaired renal flow unrelated to renal disease (e.g., from hypotension, severe hepatic disease)

(3) Trough levels > 2 μg/mL for gentamicin and tobramycin and > 10 μg/mL for amikacin are associated with nephrotoxicity.

c. Neuromuscular blockade. This problem may arise in patients receiving high-dose aminoglycoside therapy.

(1) **Risk factors** for neuromuscular blockade include the following:

(a) Concurrent administration of a neuromuscular blocking agent or an anesthetic

(b) Preexisting hypocalcemia or myasthenia gravis

(c) Intraperitoneal or rapid IV drug administration

(2) Apnea and respiratory depression may be reversed with administration of calcium or an anticholinesterase.

d. Hypersensitivity and **local reactions** are rare adverse effects of aminoglycosides.

e. Therapeutic levels

(1) Gentamicin and tobramycin peak at 6–10 μg/mL for traditional dosing; when using the ODA method, the peak is 16–20 μg/mL or 8–10 times the MIC of targeted bacteria. Their trough level is 0.5–1.5 μg/mL for traditional or once-daily regimens.

(2) Amikacin peaks at 25–30 μg/mL. The trough level is 5–8 μg/mL.

5. **Significant interactions**
   a. **IV loop diuretics** can result in increased ototoxicity.
   b. **Other aminoglycosides, cephalothin, cisplatin, amphotericin B,** and **methoxyflurane** can cause increased nephrotoxicity when given concurrently with streptomycin.

C. **Carbapenems.** These agents are β-lactams that contain a fused β-lactam ring and a 5-membered ring system that differs from penicillins in being unsaturated and containing a carbon atom instead of a sulfur atom. The class has a broader spectrum of activity than do most β-lactams. Formerly known as thienamycin, **imipenem (Primaxin)** was the first carbapenem compound introduced in the United States, followed by **meropenem (Merrem)** and, most recently, **ertapenem (Invanz).** Because it is inhibited by renal dipeptidases, imipenem must be combined with **cilastatin** sodium, a dipeptidase inhibitor (cilastatin is not required with meropenem or ertapenem because these are not sensitive to renal dipeptidase).

1. **Mechanism of action.** Carbapenems are **bactericidal,** inhibiting bacterial cell wall synthesis.

2. **Spectrum of activity.** These drugs have the broadest spectrum of all β-lactam antibiotics. The group is active against most gram-positive cocci (including many enterococci), gram-negative rods (including many *P. aeruginosa* strains), and anaerobes. This class has good activity against many bacterial strains that resist other antibiotics. Ertapenem has a narrower spectrum of activity than the other carbapenems. It has little or no activity against *P. aeruginosa* and *Acinetobacter.* These β-lactam antibiotics resist destruction by most β-lactamases.

3. **Therapeutic uses.** Carbapenems are most valued in the treatment of severe infections caused by drug-resistant organisms susceptible to these agents. These agents are effective against urinary tract and lower respiratory infections, intra-abdominal and gynecological infections, and skin, soft-tissue, bone, and joint infections.

4. **Precautions and monitoring effects**
   a. Carbapenems may cause nausea, vomiting, diarrhea, and pseudomembranous colitis.
   b. Seizures, dizziness, and hypotension may develop; seizures appear less frequently with meropenem or ertapenem (1.5% of patients receiving imipenem versus 0.5% of those receiving meropenem or ertapenem).
   c. Patients who are allergic to penicillin or cephalosporins may suffer cross-sensitivity reactions during carbapenem therapy.

D. **Cephalosporins.** These agents are known as **β-lactam antibiotics** because their chemical structure consists of a β-lactam ring adjoined to a thiazolidine ring. Cephalosporins generally are classified in four major groups based mainly on their spectrum of activity (Table 44-2).

1. **Mechanism of action.** Cephalosporins are **bactericidal;** they inhibit bacterial cell wall synthesis, reducing cell wall stability and thus causing membrane lysis.

2. **Spectrum of activity**
   a. **First-generation** cephalosporins are active against most gram-positive cocci (except enterococci) as well as enteric aerobic gram-negative bacilli (e.g., *E. coli, K. pneumoniae, Proteus mirabilis*).
   b. **Second-generation** cephalosporins are active against the organisms covered by first-generation cephalosporins and have extended gram-negative coverage, including β-lactamase-producing strains of *Haemophilus influenzae.*
   c. **Third-generation** cephalosporins have wider activity against most gram-negative bacteria, for example, *Enterobacter, Citrobacter, Serratia, Providencia, Neisseria,* and *Haemophilus* organisms, including β-lactamase–producing strains.
   d. **Fourth-generation** cephalosporins include **cefepime (Maxipime),** which is the first member of this group to be marketed. However, its designation as a fourth-generation cephalosporin is debatable. Cefepime is highly resistant to β-lactamases and has a low propensity for selection of β-lactam-resistant mutant strains. It shows evidence of greater

Table 44-2. Classification of Cephalosporins

First Generation	Second Generation	Third Generation	Fourth Generation
Cefadroxil (Duricef, Ultracef)[a]	Cefaclor (Ceclor)[a]	Cefdinir (Omnicef)[a]	Cefepime (Maxipime)
Cefazolin (Ancef, Kefzol)	Cefmetazole (Zefazone)	Cefixime (Suprax)[a]	
Cephalexin (Keflex)[a]	Cefotetan (Cefotan)[b]	Cefoperazone (Cefobid)	
Cephapirin (Cefadyl)	Cefoxitin (Mefoxin)	Cefotaxime (Claforan)	
Cephradine (Anspor, Velosef)[a]	Cefuroxime(Zinacef)	Cefpodoxime proxetil (Vantin)[a]	
	Cefuroxime axetil (Ceftin)[a]	Ceftazidime (Fortex, Tazicef, Tazidime)	
	Cefprozil (Cefzil)[a]	Ceftibuten (Cedax)[a]	
	Loracarbef (Lorabid)[a]	Ceftizoxime (Cefizox)	
		Ceftriaxone (Rocephin)	
		Cefditoren (Spectracef)[a]	

[a]Oral agent.
[b]Discontinued in the U.S. market 2005.

activity versus gram-positive cocci, *Enterobacteriaceae,* and *Pseudomonas* than third-generation cephalosporins.

   e. Each generation of cephalosporin has shifted toward increased gram-negative activity but has lost activity toward gram-positive organisms. Fourth-generation agents have improved activity toward gram-positive organisms over third-generation agents.

3. Therapeutic uses

   a. First-generation cephalosporins commonly are administered to treat serious *Klebsiella* infections and gram-positive and some gram-negative infections in patients with mild penicillin allergy. These agents also are used widely in perioperative prophylaxis. For most other indications, they are not the preferred drugs.

   b. Second-generation cephalosporins are valuable in the treatment of urinary tract infections resulting from *E. coli* organisms, acute otitis media, sinusitis, and gonococcal disease caused by organisms that resist other agents.

   (1) Cefaclor (Ceclor) is useful in otitis media and sinusitis in patients who are allergic to ampicillin and amoxicillin. **Cefprozil (Cefzil)** and **loracarbef (Lorabid)** are second-generation cephalosporins that can be administered twice daily but offer no important spectrum differences.

   (2) Cefoxitin (Mefoxin) is therapeutic for mixed aerobic–anaerobic infections, such as intra-abdominal infection. The **cefotetan (Cefotan)** spectrum is similar but this agent can be given twice daily.

   (3) Cefuroxime (Zinacef) is commonly administered for outpatient community-acquired pneumonia.

   c. Third-generation cephalosporins penetrate the cerebrospinal fluid (CSF) and thus are valuable in the treatment of meningitis caused by such organisms as meningococci, pneumococci, *H. influenzae,* and enteric gram-negative bacilli.

   (1) These agents also are used to treat sepsis of unknown origin in immunosuppressed patients and to treat fever in neutropenic immunosuppressed patients (given in combination with an aminoglycoside).

   (2) Third-generation cephalosporins are useful in infections caused by many organisms resistant to older cephalosporins.

   (3) These agents are frequently administered as empiric therapy for life-threatening infection in which resistant organisms are the most likely cause.

   (4) Initial therapy of mixed bacterial infections (e.g., sepsis) commonly involves third-generation cephalosporins.

   d. The **fourth-generation** agent, cefepime, is approved for treatment of urinary tract infections, uncomplicated skin and skin structure infections, pneumonia, and empiric use in febrile neutropenic patients. Cefepime has a spectrum of activity similar to third-generation agents but is more resistant to some β-lactamases.

4. **Precautions and monitoring effects**
   a. Because all cephalosporins (except cefoperazone) are eliminated renally, doses must be adjusted for patients with renal impairment.
   b. Cross-sensitivity with penicillin has been reported in up to 10% of patients receiving cephalosporins. More recent information indicates that true cross-reactivity is rare.
   c. Cephalosporins can cause hypersensitivity reactions similar to those resulting from penicillin (see II.E.1.e.(1)). Manifestations include fever, maculopapular rash, anaphylaxis, and hemolytic anemia.
   d. Other adverse effects include nausea, vomiting, diarrhea, superinfection, nephrotoxicity, and *Clostridium difficile*–induced colitis; with cefoperazone, cefmetazole, and cefotetan (and formerly moxalactam and cefamandole), bleeding diatheses may occur. Bleeding can be reversed by vitamin K administration.
   e. Cephalosporins may cause false-positive glycosuria results on tests using the copper-reduction method.

5. **Significant interactions**
   a. **Probenecid** may impair the excretion of cephalosporins (except ceftazidime), causing increased cephalosporin levels and possible toxicity.
   b. **Alcohol consumption** may result in a disulfiram-type reaction in patients receiving cefmetazole, cefotetan, and cefoperazone.
   c. **Aminoglycosides or loop diuretics** may cause additive toxicity when administered with cephalothin.
   d. Plasma concentrations of cefaclor extended-release tablets, cefdinir, and cefpodoxime may be reduced by coadministration with **antacids.**
   e. **H$_2$-antagonists** may reduce plasma levels of cefpodoxime and cefuroxime.
   f. **Iron supplements** and **iron-fortified foods** reduce absorption of cefdinir by 80% and 30%, respectively.

E. **Erythromycins.** The chemical structure of these macrolide antibiotics is characterized by a lactone ring to which sugars are attached. Erythromycin base and the estolate, ethylsuccinate, and stearate salts are given orally; erythromycin lactobionate and gluceptate are given parenterally.

1. **Mechanism of action.** Erythromycins may be **bactericidal** or **bacteriostatic;** they bind to the 50S ribosomal subunit, inhibiting bacterial protein synthesis.

2. **Spectrum of activity.** Erythromycins are active against many gram-positive organisms, including streptococci (e.g., *Streptococcus pneumoniae*), and *Corynebacterium* and *Neisseria* species as well as some strains of *Mycoplasma, Legionella, Treponema,* and *Bordetella.* Some *S. aureus* strains that resist penicillin G are susceptible to erythromycins.

3. **Therapeutic uses**
   a. Erythromycins are the preferred drugs for the treatment of *Mycoplasma pneumoniae* and *Campylobacter* infections, Legionnaires disease, chlamydial infections, diphtheria, and pertussis.
   b. In patients with penicillin allergy, erythromycins are important alternatives in the treatment of pneumococcal pneumonia, *S. aureus* infections, syphilis, and gonorrhea.
   c. Erythromycins may be given prophylactically before dental procedures to prevent bacterial endocarditis.

4. **Precautions and monitoring parameters**
   a. Gastrointestinal (GI) distress (e.g., nausea, vomiting, diarrhea, epigastric discomfort) may occur with all erythromycin forms and are the most common adverse effects.
   b. Allergic reactions (rare) may present as skin eruptions, fever, and eosinophilia.
   c. Cholestatic hepatitis may arise in patients treated for 1 week or longer with erythromycin estolate; symptoms usually disappear within a few days after drug therapy ends. There have been infrequent reports of hepatotoxicity with other salts of erythromycin.
   d. IM injections of more than 100 mg produce severe pain persisting for hours.
   e. Transient hearing impairment may develop with high-dose erythromycin therapy.

5. **Significant interactions**
   a. Erythromycin inhibits the hepatic metabolism of **theophylline,** resulting in toxic accumulation.

b. Erythromycin interferes with the metabolism of **digoxin, corticosteroids, carbamaze-pine, cyclosporin,** and **lovastatin,** possibly potentiating the effect and toxicity of these drugs.

c. **Clarithromycin (Biaxin)** may potentiate **oral anticoagulants** (monitor prothrombin time), increase **cyclosporine** levels with increased toxicity, and increase **digoxin** and **theophylline** levels.

d. Co-administration of clarithromycin and **cisapride** may increase risk of serious cardiac arrhythmias; coadministration is contraindicated.

e. Sudden deaths have been reported when clarithromycin was added to ongoing **pimozide** therapy; co-administration is contraindicated.

6. Alternatives to erythromycin

a. Clarithromycin, azithromycin (Zithromax), and **dirithromycin (Dynabac)** are semisynthetic macrolide antibiotics. These expensive but well-tolerated alternatives to erythromycin are administered once daily.

  (1) Clarithromycin

   (a) Spectrum of activity. Clarithromycin is more active than erythromycin against staphylococci and streptococci. In addition to activity against other organisms covered by erythromycin, it is also active in vitro against MAI, *Toxoplasma gondii,* and *Cryptosporidium* spp.

   (b) Therapeutic uses. This agent is indicated for the prevention of *Mycobacterium avium* complex (MAC) infection and is useful in otitis media, sinusitis, mycoplasmal pneumonia, and pharyngitis. Clarithromycin is also used with proton pump inhibitors (PPIs) for *Helicobacter pylori* eradication.

  (2) Azithromycin

   (a) Spectrum of activity. Azithromycin is less active than erythromycin against gram-positive cocci but more active against *H. influenzae* and other gram-negative organisms. Azithromycin concentrates within cells, and tissue levels are higher than serum levels.

   (b) Therapeutic uses. This agent is useful in nongonococcal urethritis caused by chlamydia, lower respiratory tract infections, (MAC) infection and prophylaxis, pharyngitis, pelvic inflammatory disease, and legionnaires' disease. Azithromycin is also indicated for pediatric use.

  (3) Dirithromycin is indicated for the treatment of acute exacerbations of chronic bronchitis, pharyngitis and tonsillitis caused by *Streptococcus pyogenes,* and uncomplicated skin and skin structure infections caused by *S. aureus.*

F. Penicillins

1. Natural penicillins. As with cephalosporins and all other penicillins, natural penicillins are β-lactam antibiotics. Among the most important antibiotics, natural penicillins are the preferred drugs in the treatment of many infectious diseases.

  a. Available agents

   (1) Penicillin G sodium and potassium salts can be administered orally, intravenously, or intramuscularly.

   (2) Penicillin V (Pen-Vee K), a soluble drug form, is administered orally.

   (3) Penicillin G procaine and **penicillin G benzathine** are repository drug forms. Administered intramuscularly, these insoluble salts allow slow drug absorption from the injection site and thus have a longer duration of action (12–24 hr).

  b. Mechanism of action. Penicillins are **bactericidal;** they inhibit bacterial cell wall synthesis in a manner similar to that of the cephalosporins.

  c. Spectrum of activity

   (1) Natural penicillins are highly active against gram-positive cocci and against some gram-negative cocci.

   (2) Penicillin G is 5–10 times more active than penicillin V against gram-negative organisms and some anaerobic organisms.

   (3) Because natural penicillins are readily hydrolyzed by penicillinases (β-lactamases), they are ineffective against *S. aureus* and other organisms that resist penicillin.

  d. Therapeutic uses

   (1) Penicillin G is the preferred agent for all infections caused by penicillin-susceptible *S. pneumoniae* organisms, including

(a) Pneumonia
(b) Arthritis
(c) Meningitis
(d) Peritonitis
(e) Pericarditis
(f) Osteomyelitis
(g) Mastoiditis

(2) Penicillins G and V are highly effective against other streptococcal infections, such as pharyngitis, otitis media, sinusitis, and bacteremia.
(3) Penicillin G is the preferred agent in gonococcal infections, syphilis, anthrax, actinomycosis, gas gangrene, and *Listeria* infections.
(4) Administered when an oral penicillin is needed, penicillin V is most useful in skin, soft-tissue, and mild respiratory infections.
(5) Penicillin G procaine is effective against syphilis and uncomplicated gonorrhea.
(6) Used to treat syphilis infections outside the CNS, penicillin G benzathine also is effective against group Aβ-hemolytic streptococcal infections.
(7) Penicillins G and V may be used prophylactically to prevent streptococcal infection, rheumatic fever, and neonatal gonorrhea ophthalmia. Patients with valvular heart disease may receive these drugs preoperatively.
(8) There is emerging resistance to penicillin G by *S. pneumoniae* in some areas of the United States. The alternative therapy is vancomycin.

e. Precautions and monitoring effects
(1) Hypersensitivity reactions. These occur in up to 10% of patients receiving penicillin. Manifestations range from mild rash to anaphylaxis.
  (a) The rash may be urticarial, vesicular, bullous, scarlatiniform, or maculopapular. Rarely, thrombopenic purpura develops.
  (b) Anaphylaxis is a life-threatening reaction that most commonly occurs with parenteral administration. Signs and symptoms include severe hypotension, bronchoconstriction, nausea, vomiting, abdominal pain, and extreme weakness.
  (c) Other manifestations of hypersensitivity reactions include fever, eosinophilia, angioedema, and serum sickness.
  (d) Before penicillin therapy begins, the patient's history should be evaluated for reactions to penicillin. A positive history places the patient at heightened risk for a subsequent reaction. In most cases, such patients should receive a substitute antibiotic. (However, hypersensitivity reactions may occur even in patients with a negative history.)
(2) Other adverse effects of natural penicillins include GI distress (e.g., nausea, diarrhea), bone marrow suppression (e.g., impaired platelet aggregation, agranulocytosis), and superinfection. With high-dose therapy, seizures may occur, particularly in patients with renal impairment.

f. Significant interactions
(1) Probenecid increases blood levels of natural penicillins and may be given concurrently for this purpose.
(2) Antibiotic antagonism occurs when **erythromycins, tetracyclines,** or **chloramphenicol** is given within 1 hr of the administration of penicillin. The clinical significance of such antagonism is not clear.
(3) With penicillin G procaine and benzathine, precaution must be used in patients with a history of hypersensitivity reactions to penicillins because prolonged reactions may occur. Intravascular injection should be avoided. Procaine hypersensitivity is a contraindication to the use of procaine penicillin G.
(4) Parenteral products contain either potassium (1.7 mEq/million units) or sodium (2 mEq/million units).

2. Penicillinase-resistant penicillins. These penicillins are not hydrolyzed by staphylococcal penicillinases (β-lactamases). These agents include **methicillin, nafcillin,** and the **isoxazolyl penicillins—cloxacillin, dicloxacillin (Dynapen),** and **oxacillin.**
a. Mechanism of action (see II.E.1.b)
b. Spectrum of activity. Because these penicillins resist penicillinases, they are active against staphylococci that produce these enzymes.

c. **Therapeutic uses**
   (1) Penicillinase-resistant penicillins are used solely in staphylococcal infections resulting from organisms that resist natural penicillins.
   (2) These agents are less potent than natural penicillins against organisms susceptible to natural penicillins and thus make poor substitutes in the treatment of infections caused by these organisms.
   (3) Nafcillin is excreted by the liver and thus may be useful in treating staphylococcal infections in patients with renal impairment.
   (4) Oxacillin, cloxacillin, and **dicloxacillin** are most valuable in long-term therapy of serious staphylococcal infections (e.g., endocarditis, osteomyelitis) and in the treatment of minor staphylococcal infections of the skin and soft tissues.
d. **Precautions and monitoring effects**
   (1) As with all penicillins, the penicillinase-resistant group can cause hypersensitivity reactions (see II.E.1.e.(1)).
   (2) Methicillin may cause nephrotoxicity and interstitial nephritis.
   (3) Oxacillin may be hepatotoxic.
   (4) Complete cross-resistance exists among the penicillinase-resistant penicillins.
e. **Significant interactions. Probenecid** increases blood levels of these penicillins and may be given concurrently for that purpose.

3. **Aminopenicillins.** This penicillin group includes the semisynthetic agents **ampicillin** and **amoxicillin (Amoxil).** Because of their wider antibacterial spectrum, these drugs are also known as **broad-spectrum penicillins.**
   a. **Mechanism of action** (see II.E.1.b)
   b. **Spectrum of activity.** Aminopenicillins have a spectrum that is similar to but broader than that of the natural and penicillinase-resistant penicillins. Easily destroyed by staphylococcal penicillinases, aminopenicillins are ineffective against most staphylococcal organisms. Against most bacteria sensitive to penicillin G, aminopenicillins are slightly less effective than this agent.
   c. **Therapeutic uses.** Aminopenicillins are used to treat gonococcal infections, upper respiratory infections, uncomplicated urinary tract infections, and otitis media caused by susceptible organisms.
      (1) For infections resulting from penicillin-resistant organisms, **ampicillin** may be given in combination with sulbactam (**Unasyn**).
      (2) Amoxicillin is less effective than ampicillin against shigellosis.
      (3) Amoxicillin is more effective against *S. aureus, Klebsiella,* and *Bacteroides fragilis* infections when administered in combination with clavulanic acid—amoxicillin/potassium clavulanate (**Augmentin**) because clavulanic acid inactivates penicillinases.
   d. **Precautions and monitoring effects**
      (1) Hypersensitivity reactions may occur (see II.E.1.e.(1)).
      (2) Diarrhea is most common with ampicillin.
      (3) In addition to the urticarial hypersensitivity rash seen with all penicillins, ampicillin and amoxicillin frequently cause a generalized erythematous, maculopapular rash. (This occurs in 5%–10% of patients receiving ampicillin.)
   e. **Significant interactions** (see II.E.2.e)

4. **Extended-spectrum penicillins.** These agents have the widest antibacterial spectrum of all penicillins. Also called **antipseudomonal penicillins,** this group includes the **carboxypenicillin** (e.g., **ticarcillin**) and the **ureidopenicillins** (e.g., **mezlocillin, piperacillin**).
   a. **Mechanism of action** (see II.E.1.b)
   b. **Spectrum of activity.** These drugs have a spectrum similar to that of the aminopenicillins but also are effective against *Klebsiella* and *Enterobacter* spp., some *B. fragilis* organisms, and indole-positive *Proteus* and *Pseudomonas* organisms.
      (1) Ticarcillin is active against *P. aeruginosa.* Combined with clavulanic acid (**Timentin**), ticarcillin has enhanced activity against organisms that resist ticarcillin alone.
      (2) Piperacillin is more active than ticarcillin against *Pseudomonas* organisms.
      (3) Piperacillin and tazobactam (Zosyn). Tazobactam is a β-lactamase inhibitor that expands the spectrum of activity to include some organisms not sensitive to piperacillin alone (if resistance is the result of β-lactamase production), including strains of staphylococci, *Haemophilus, Bacteroides,* and *Enterobacteriaceae.* Generally, tazobactam does not enhance activity against *Pseudomonas.*

   c. **Therapeutic uses.** Extended-spectrum penicillins are used mainly to treat serious infections caused by gram-negative organisms (e.g., sepsis; pneumonia; infections of the abdomen, bone, and soft tissues). Piperacillin/tazobactam is effective in the treatment of nosocomial pneumonia.
   d. **Precautions and monitoring effects**
      (1) Hypersensitivity reactions may occur (see II.E.1.e.(1)).
      (2) Ticarcillin may cause hypokalemia.
      (3) The high sodium content of ticarcillin may pose a danger to patients with heart failure (HF).
      (4) All inhibit platelet aggregation, which may result in bleeding.
   e. **Significant interactions** (see II.E.2.e)

G. **Sulfonamides.** Derivatives of sulfanilamide, these agents were the first drugs to prevent and cure human bacterial infection successfully. Although their current usefulness is limited by the introduction of more effective antibiotics and the emergence of resistant bacterial strains, sulfonamides remain the drugs of choice for certain infections. The major sulfonamides are **sulfadiazine, sulfamethoxazole, sulfisoxazole,** and **sulfamethizole.**

1. **Mechanism of action.** Sulfonamides are **bacteriostatic;** they suppress bacterial growth by triggering a mechanism that blocks folic acid synthesis, thereby forcing bacteria to synthesize their own folic acid.

2. **Spectrum of activity.** Sulfonamides are broad-spectrum agents with activity against many gram-positive organisms (e.g., *S. pyogenes, S. pneumoniae*) and certain gram-negative organisms (e.g., *H. influenzae, E. coli, P. mirabilis*). They also are effective against certain strains of *Chlamydia trachomatis, Nocardia, Actinomyces,* and *Bacillus anthracis.*

3. **Therapeutic uses**
   a. Sulfonamides most often are used to treat urinary tract infections caused by *E. coli,* including acute and chronic cystitis, and chronic upper urinary tract infections.
   b. These agents have value in the treatment of nocardiosis, trachoma and inclusion conjunctivitis, and dermatitis herpetiformis.
   c. **Sulfadiazine** may be administered in combination with pyrimethamine to treat toxoplasmosis.
   d. **Sulfamethoxazole** may be given in combination with trimethoprim (**Bactrim**) to treat such infections as *Pneumocystis carinii* pneumonia, *Shigella* enteritis, *Serratia* sepsis, urinary tract infections, respiratory infections, and gonococcal urethritis (see II.J.7.c). It is the drug of choice in the treatment of *Stenotrophomonas maltophilia.*
   e. **Sulfisoxazole** is sometimes used in combination with erythromycin ethylsuccinate to treat acute otitis media caused by *H. influenzae* organisms. For the initial treatment of uncomplicated urinary tract infections, sulfisoxazole may be given in combination with phenazopyridine for relief of symptoms of pain, burning, or urgency.
   f. Prophylactic sulfonamide therapy has been used successfully to prevent streptococcal infections and rheumatic fever recurrences.

4. **Precautions and monitoring effects**
   a. Sulfonamides may cause blood dyscrasias (e.g., hemolytic anemia—particularly in patients with G6PD deficiency, aplastic anemia, thrombocytopenia, agranulocytosis, and eosinophilia).
   b. Hypersensitivity reactions to sulfonamides probably result from sensitization and most commonly involve the skin and mucous membranes. Manifestations include various types of skin rash, exfoliative dermatitis, and photosensitivity. Drug fever and serum sickness also may develop.
   c. Crystalluria and hematuria may occur, possibly leading to urinary tract obstruction. (Adequate fluid intake and urine alkalinization can prevent or minimize this risk.) Sulfonamides should be used cautiously in patients with renal impairment.
   d. Life-threatening hepatitis caused by drug toxicity or sensitization is a rare adverse effect. Signs and symptoms include headache, nausea, vomiting, and jaundice.
   e. AIDS patients have increased frequency of cutaneous hypersensitivity reactions to sulfamethoxazole.

5. **Significant interactions.** Sulfonamides may potentiate the effects of **phenytoin, oral anticoagulants,** and **sulfonylureas.**

H. Tetracyclines. These broad-spectrum agents are effective against certain bacterial strains that resist other antibiotics. Nonetheless, they are the preferred drugs in only a few situations. The major tetracyclines include **demeclocycline (Declomycin), doxycycline (Vibramycin), minocycline (Minocin),** and **chlortetracycline.**

1. **Mechanism of action.** Tetracyclines are **bacteriostatic;** they inhibit bacterial protein synthesis by binding to the 30S ribosomal subunit.

2. **Spectrum of activity.** Tetracyclines are active against gram-negative and gram-positive organisms, spirochetes, *Mycoplasma* and *Chlamydia* organisms, rickettsial species, and certain protozoa.
   a. *Pseudomonas* and *Proteus* organisms are now resistant to tetracyclines. Many coliform bacteria, pneumococci, staphylococci, streptococci, and *Shigella* strains are increasingly resistant.
   b. Cross-resistance within the tetracycline group is extensive.

3. **Therapeutic uses**
   a. Tetracyclines are the agents of choice in rickettsial (Rocky Mountain spotted fever), chlamydial, and mycoplasmal infections; amebiasis; and bacillary infections (e.g., cholera, brucellosis, tularemia, some *Salmonella* and *Shigella* infections).
   b. Tetracyclines are useful alternatives to penicillin in the treatment of anthrax, syphilis, gonorrhea, Lyme disease, nocardiosis, and *H. influenzae* respiratory infections.
   c. Oral or topical tetracycline may be administered as a treatment for acne.
   d. **Doxycycline** is highly effective in the prophylaxis of "traveler's diarrhea" (commonly caused by *E. coli*). Because the drug is excreted mainly in the feces, it is the safest tetracycline for the treatment of extrarenal infections in patients with renal impairment.
   e. **Demeclocycline** is used commonly as an adjunctive agent to treat the **syndrome of inappropriate antidiuretic hormone (SIADH)** secretion.

4. **Precautions and monitoring effects**
   a. GI distress (e.g., diarrhea, abdominal discomfort, nausea, anorexia) is a common adverse effect of tetracyclines. This problem can be minimized by administering the drug with food or temporarily decreasing the dosage.
   b. Skin rash, urticaria, and generalized exfoliative dermatitis signify a hypersensitivity reaction. Rarely, angioedema and anaphylaxis occur.
   c. Cross-sensitivity within the tetracycline group is common.
   d. Phototoxic reactions (severe skin lesions) can develop with exposure to sunlight. This reaction is most common with demeclocycline and doxycycline.
   e. Tetracyclines may cause hepatotoxicity, particularly in pregnant women. Manifestations include jaundice, acidosis, and fatty liver infiltration.
   f. Renally impaired patients may experience a significant increase in BUN secondary to catabolic effects of tetracyclines.
   g. Tetracyclines may induce permanent tooth discoloration, tooth enamel defects, and retarded bone growth in infants and children.
   h. Use of outdated and degraded tetracyclines can lead to renal tubular dysfunction, possibly resulting in renal failure.
   i. Minocycline can cause vestibular toxicity (e.g., ataxia, dizziness, nausea, vomiting).
   j. IV tetracyclines are irritating and may cause phlebitis.

5. **Significant interactions**
   a. **Dairy products** and other foods, **iron preparations,** and **antacids** and **laxatives** containing aluminum, calcium, or magnesium can cause reduced tetracycline absorption. Absorption of doxycycline is not inhibited by these factors.
   b. **Methoxyflurane** may exacerbate the tetracyclines' nephrotoxic effects.
   c. **Barbiturates** and **phenytoin** decrease the antibiotic effectiveness of tetracyclines.
   d. Demeclocycline antagonizes the action of **antidiuretic hormone (ADH)** and may be given as a diuretic in patients with SIADH.

I. Fluoroquinolones are agents related to nalidixic acid—see II.I.1.c; II.2.c.(1);II.4.c.(1)—and include **ciprofloxacin (Cipro), enoxacin (Penetrex), lomefloxacin (Maxaquin), norfloxacin (Noroxin), ofloxacin (Floxin), sparfloxacin (Zagam), gatifloxacin (Tequin), moxifloxacin (Avelox), levofloxacin (Levaquin),** and **trovafloxacin (Trovan).** They are bactericidal for growing bacteria.

1. **Mechanism of action.** Fluoroquinolones inhibit DNA gyrase.

2. **Spectrum of activity.** Fluoroquinolones are highly active against enteric gram-negative bacilli, *Salmonella, Shigella, Campylobacter, Haemophilus,* and *Neisseria.*
   a. **Ciprofloxacin** has activity against *P. aeruginosa,* but the fluoroquinolones as a group have variable activity against non–*P. aeruginosa.* Ciprofloxacin is active against some anaerobes; it has moderate activity against *M. tuberculosis.*
   b. Gram-positive organisms are less susceptible than gram-negative organisms but usually are sensitive, except for *Enterococcus faecalis* and methicillin-resistant staphylococci.
   c. **Ofloxacin** has the greatest activity against *Chlamydia.*
   d. **Trovafloxacin** has a broad spectrum including gram-positive and gram-negative anaerobes, *Chlamydia* spp., and *M. pneumoniae.*

3. **Therapeutic uses** (Table 44-3)
   a. Norfloxacin is indicated for the oral treatment of urinary tract infections, uncomplicated gonococcal infections, and prostatitis.
   b. Ciprofloxacin, ofloxacin, levofloxacin, gatifloxacin, and trovafloxacin are available orally and intravenously. Ciprofloxacin is approved for use in urinary tract infections; lower respiratory infections; sinusitis; bone, joint, and skin structure infections; empiric use in febrile neutropenic patients; typhoid fever; urethral and cervical gonococcal infections; and infectious diarrhea. Ofloxacin is approved for use in lower respiratory infections, uncomplicated gonococcal and chlamydial cervicitis and urethritis, skin and skin structure infections, prostatitis, and urinary tract infections.
   c. Lomefloxacin, levofloxacin, gatifloxacin, trovafloxacin, and enoxacin are approved for the treatment of urinary tract infections. Lomefloxacin, sparfloxacin, gatifloxacin, moxifloxacin, levofloxacin, and trovafloxacin are also used in lower respiratory infections.
   d. Moxifloxacin is approved for the treatment of complicated intra-abdominal infections but should not be used for urinary tract infections.

4. **Precautions and monitoring effects**
   a. Occasional adverse effects include nausea, dyspepsia, headache, dizziness, insomnia, cardiac QT prolongation, arthropathy, tendonitis, CNS effects, photosensitivity, and hypoglycemia.
   b. Infrequent adverse effects include rash, urticaria, leukopenia, and elevated liver enzymes. Crystalluria occurs with high doses at alkaline pH.
   c. Gatifloxacin is contraindicated in diabetic patients.

Table 44-3. Quinolone Agents Classified by Generation

	Agent	Spectrum of Coverage	Site of Infection
First-generation	Cinoxacin (Cinoxacin, Cinobac) Enoxacin (Penetrex) Nalidixic acid (NegGram) Norfloxacin (Noroxin)	Gram negatives	Urinary tract
Second-generation	Lomefloxacin (Maxaquin) Ciprofloxacin (Cipro) Ofloxacin (Floxin)	Gram negatives Gram positives	Urinary tract Systemic, urinary tract
Third-generation	Gatifloxacin (Tequin) Levofloxacin (Levaquin) Sparfloxacin (Zagam) Moxifloxacin (Avelox)	Gram negatives Atypicals	Systemic, urinary tract Systemic only
Fourth-generation	Trovafloxacin (Trovan)	Gram negatives Gram positives Atypicals Anaerobes	Systemic, urinary tract

d. Cartilage erosion has been observed in young animals; thus fluoroquinolones should not be used in children or in women who are pregnant or nursing.

e. **Trovafloxacin has a black box warning**. It is reserved for those who meet **all** the treatment restriction criteria outlined in the package insert. It has been associated with serious liver injury leading to liver transplantation and/or death. Liver injury has been reported with both short-term and long-term drug exposure. Trovafloxacin use longer than 2 weeks significantly increases risk. **This agent should be reserved for serious life or limb-threatening infections.**

5. Significant interactions

a. Ciprofloxacin has been shown to increase **theophylline** levels. Variable effects on theophylline levels have been reported from other members of the group. In patients requiring fluoroquinolones, theophylline levels should be monitored.

b. **Antacids** and **sucralfate** and divalent or trivalent cations such as iron significantly decrease the absorption of fluoroquinolones.

c. Fluoroquinolones may increase prothrombin times in patients receiving **warfarin.**

d. Concurrent use with **nonsteroidal anti-inflammatory drugs** (NSAIDs) may increase the risk of CNS stimulation (seizures).

e. Fluoroquinolones may produce prolonged QT interval when administered with **cisapride** and **antiarrhythmic agents.** Some fluoroquinolones (i.e., gatifloxacin, moxifloxacin) should be avoided in patients with known prolongation of the QTC interval, with uncorrected hypocalcemia, or who are receiving class IA or class III antiarrhythmic drugs.

f. Some fluoroquinolones have been reported to enhance the effects of oral anticoagulants.

g. Hyperglycemia and hypoglycemia have been reported in patients receiving quinolones and an antidiabetic agent. Blood glucose monitoring is recommended in such patients.

h. Didanosine should be administered at least 4 hr after gatifloxacin.

J. **Urinary tract antiseptics.** Concentrating in the renal tubules and bladder, these agents exert local antibacterial effects; most do not achieve blood levels high enough to treat systemic infections. However, some new quinolone derivatives, such as ciprofloxacin and ofloxacin, are valuable in the treatment of certain infections outside the urinary tract (see II.H.3.b).

1. Mechanism of action

a. **Methenamine** is hydrolyzed to ammonia and formaldehyde in acidic urine; formaldehyde is antibacterial against gram-positive and gram-negative organisms. Mandelic and hippuric acids, with which methenamine is combined, provide supplementary antibacterial action.

b. **Nitrofurantoin** is **bacteriostatic;** in high concentrations, it may be **bactericidal.** Presumably, it disrupts bacterial enzyme systems.

c. **Quinolones. Nalidixic acid** and its analogs and derivatives—**oxolinic acid, norfloxacin, cinoxacin, ciprofloxacin,** and others—interfere with DNA gyrase and inhibit DNA synthesis during bacterial replication.

d. **Fosfomycin tromethamine** is bactericidal in the urine at therapeutic doses. The bactericidal action is because of its inactivation of the enzyme enolpyruvyl transferase, thereby blocking the condensation of uridine diphosphate-*N*-acetylglucosamine with p-enolpyruvate, one of the first steps in bacterial cell wall synthesis.

2. Spectrum of activity

a. **Methenamine** is active against both gram-positive and gram-negative organisms (e.g., *Enterobacter, Klebsiella, Proteus, P. aeruginosa, S. aureus*).

b. **Nitrofurantoin** is active against many gram-positive and gram-negative organisms, including some strains of *E. coli, S. aureus, Proteus, Enterobacter,* and *Klebsiella.*

c. **Quinolones** (see II.H)

(1) **Nalidixic acid** and **oxolinic acid** are active against most gram-negative organisms that cause urinary tract infections, including *P. mirabilis, E. coli, Klebsiella,* and *Enterobacter* organisms. These drugs are not effective against *Pseudomonas* organisms.

(2) **Norfloxacin** is active against *E. coli, Enterobacter, Klebsiella, Proteus, P. aeruginosa, S. aureus, Citrobacter,* and some *Streptococcus* organisms.

(3) **Cinoxacin** is active against *E. coli, Klebsiella, P. mirabilis, Proteus vulgaris, Proteus morganii, Serratia,* and *Citrobacter* organisms.

3. Therapeutic uses

   a. Methenamine and **nitrofurantoin** are used to prevent and treat urinary tract infections.

   b. Quinolones are administered to treat urinary tract infections; some also are used in such diseases as osteomyelitis and respiratory tract infections.

   c. Fosfomycin is indicated for treatment of uncomplicated urinary tract infection (acute cystitis) in women caused by susceptible strains of *E. coli* or *E. faecalis.*

4. Precautions and monitoring effects

   a. Methenamine may cause nausea, vomiting, and diarrhea; in high doses, it may lead to urinary tract irritation (e.g., dysuria, frequency, hematuria, albuminuria). Skin rash also may develop.

   b. Nitrofurantoin may cause various adverse effects.

   (1) GI distress (e.g., nausea, vomiting, diarrhea) is relatively common.

   (2) Hypersensitivity reactions to nitrofurantoin may involve the skin, lungs, blood, or liver; manifestations include fever, chills, hepatitis, jaundice, leukopenia, hemolytic anemia, granulocytopenia, and pneumonitis.

   (3) Adverse CNS effects include headache, vertigo, and dizziness. Polyneuropathy may develop with high doses or in patients with renal impairment.

   c. Quinolones

   (1) Nalidixic acid and **oxolinic acid** may cause nausea, vomiting, abdominal pain, urticaria, pruritus, skin rash, fever, eosinophilia, and CNS effects, such as headache, dizziness, confusion, vertigo, drowsiness, and weakness.

   (2) Cinoxacin may induce nausea, vomiting, diarrhea, headache, insomnia, skin rash, pruritus, and urticaria.

5. Significant interactions

   a. The effects of methenamine are inhibited by **alkalinizing agents** and are antagonized by **acetazolamide.**

   b. Nitrofurantoin absorption is decreased by **magnesium-containing antacids.** Nitrofurantoin blood levels are increased and urine levels decreased by **sulfinpyrazone** and **probenecid,** leading to increased toxicity and reduced therapeutic effectiveness.

   c. Quinolones

   (1) Cinoxacin urine levels are decreased by **probenecid,** reducing therapeutic effectiveness.

   (2) Norfloxacin is rendered less effective by **antacids.**

K. Miscellaneous antibacterial agents

1. Aztreonam (Azactam). This agent was the first commercially available monobactam (monocyclic β-lactam compound). It resembles the aminoglycosides in its efficacy against many gram-negative organisms but does not cause nephrotoxicity or ototoxicity. Other advantages of this drug include its ability to preserve the body's normal gram-positive and anaerobic flora, activity against many gentamicin-resistant organisms, and lack of cross-allergenicity with penicillin.

   a. Mechanism of action. Aztreonam is **bactericidal;** it inhibits bacterial cell wall synthesis.

   b. Spectrum of activity. This drug is active against many gram-negative organisms, including *Enterobacter* and *P. aeruginosa.*

   c. Therapeutic uses. Aztreonam is therapeutic for urinary tract infections, septicemia, skin infections, lower respiratory tract infections, and intra-abdominal infections resulting from gram-negative organisms. Increased incidence of *P. aeruginosa* resistant to aztreonam have been reported.

   d. Precautions and monitoring effects

   (1) Aztreonam sometimes causes nausea, vomiting, and diarrhea.

   (2) Liver enzymes may increase transiently during aztreonam therapy.

   (3) This drug may induce skin rash.

2. Chloramphenicol. A nitrobenzene derivative, this drug has broad activity against rickettsia as well as many gram-positive and gram-negative organisms. It also is effective against many ampicillin-resistant strains of *H. influenzae.*

   a. Mechanism of action. Chloramphenicol is primarily **bacteriostatic,** although it may be bactericidal against a few bacterial strains.

b. **Spectrum of activity.** This agent is active against rickettsia and a wide range of bacteria, including *H. influenzae, Salmonella typhi, Neisseria meningitidis, Bordetella pertussis, Clostridium, B. fragilis, S. pyogenes,* and *S. pneumoniae.*

c. **Therapeutic uses.** Because of its toxic side effects, chloramphenicol is used only to suppress infections that cannot be treated effectively with other antibiotics. Such infections typically include

   (1) Typhoid fever
   (2) Meningococcal infections in cephalosporin-allergic patients
   (3) Serious *H. influenzae* infections, particularly in cephalosporin-allergic patients
   (4) Anaerobic infections (e.g., those originating in the pelvis or intestines)
   (5) Anaerobic or mixed infections of the CNS
   (6) Rickettsial infections in pregnant patients, tetracycline-allergic patients, and renally impaired patients

d. **Precautions and monitoring effects**

   (1) Chloramphenicol can cause bone marrow suppression (dose-related) with resulting pancytopenia; rarely, the drug leads to aplastic anemia (not related to dose).
   (2) Hypersensitivity reactions may include skin rash and, in extremely rare cases, angioedema or anaphylaxis.
   (3) Chloramphenicol therapy may lead to gray baby syndrome in neonates (especially premature infants). This dangerous reaction, which stems partly from inadequate liver detoxification of the drug, is manifested by vomiting, gray cyanosis, rapid and irregular respirations, vasomotor collapse, and in some cases death.

e. **Significant interactions**

   (1) Chloramphenicol inhibits the metabolism of **phenytoin, tolbutamide, chlorpropamide,** and **dicumarol,** leading to prolonged action and intensified effect of these drugs.
   (2) **Phenobarbital** shortens chloramphenicol's half-life, thereby reducing its therapeutic effectiveness.
   (3) **Penicillins** can cause antibiotic antagonism.
   (4) **Acetaminophen** elevates chloramphenicol levels and may cause toxicity.

3. **Clindamycin (Cleocin).** This agent has essentially replaced lincomycin, the drug from which it is derived. It is used to treat skin, respiratory tract, and soft-tissue infections caused by staphylococci, pneumococci, and streptococci.

   a. **Mechanism of action.** Clindamycin is **bacteriostatic;** it binds to the 50S ribosomal subunit, thereby suppressing bacterial protein synthesis.
   b. **Spectrum of activity.** This agent is active against most gram-positive and many anaerobic organisms, including *B. fragilis.*
   c. **Therapeutic uses.** Because of its marked toxicity, clindamycin is used only against infections for which it has proven to be the most effective drug. Typically, such infections include abdominal and female genitourinary tract infections caused by *B. fragilis.*
   d. **Precautions and monitoring effects**

      (1) Clindamycin may cause rash, nausea, vomiting, diarrhea, and pseudomembranous colitis as evidenced by fever, abdominal pain, and bloody stools.
      (2) Blood dyscrasias (e.g., eosinophilia, thrombocytopenia, leukopenia) may occur.
   e. **Significant interactions.** Clindamycin may potentiate the effects of **neuromuscular blocking agents.**

4. **Dapsone.** A member of the sulfone class, this drug is the primary agent in the treatment of all forms of leprosy.

   a. **Mechanism of action.** Dapsone is **bacteriostatic** for *Mycobacterium leprae;* its mechanism of action probably resembles that of the sulfonamides.
   b. **Spectrum of activity.** This drug is active against *M. leprae;* however, drug resistance develops in up to 40% of patients. Dapsone also has some activity against *P. carinii* organisms and the malarial parasite *Plasmodium.*
   c. **Therapeutic uses**

      (1) Dapsone is the drug of choice for treating leprosy.
      (2) This agent may be used to treat dermatitis herpetiformis, a skin disorder.
      (3) Maloprim, a dapsone–pyrimethamine product, is valuable in the prophylaxis and treatment of malaria.
      (4) Dapsone, with or without trimethoprim, is used for prophylaxis of *P. carinii* pneumonia in patients with AIDS.

d. Precautions and monitoring effects
  (1) Hemolytic anemia can occur with daily doses > 200 mg. Other adverse hematological effects include methemoglobinemia and leukopenia.
  (2) Nausea, vomiting, and anorexia may develop.
  (3) Adverse CNS effects include headache, dizziness, nervousness, lethargy, paresthesias, and psychosis.
  (4) Dapsone occasionally results in a potentially lethal mononucleosis-like syndrome.
  (5) Paradoxically, this drug sometimes exacerbates leprosy.
  (6) Other adverse effects include skin rash, peripheral neuropathy, blurred vision, tinnitus, hepatitis, and cholestatic jaundice.
e. Significant interactions. Probenecid elevates blood levels of dapsone, possibly resulting in toxicity.

5. **Linezolid (Zyvox)** is a synthetic oxazolidinone that has clinical use in the treatment of infections caused by aerobic gram-positive bacteria.
  a. Mechanism of action. Linezolid is bacteriostatic against *Enterococci* and *Staphylococci,* and bactericidal against *Streptococci.* Linezolid binds to the 23S ribosomal RNA of the 50S subunit and thus inhibits protein synthesis.
  b. Spectrum of activity. The drug is active against vancomycin-resistant *Enterococcus faecium* and *S. aureus* (methicillin-susceptible and -resistant strains) as well as other aerobic gram-positive bacteria.
  c. Therapeutic uses. Linezolid is indicated for treatment of infections caused by vancomycin-resistant *E. faecium,* nosocomial pneumonia caused by methicillin-susceptible and -resistant strains of *S. aureus,* community-acquired pneumonia caused by penicillin-susceptible strains of *S. pneumoniae,* and skin and skin structure infections owing to these organisms.
  d. Precautions and monitoring effects
    (1) Safety data are limited. Adverse effects generally are minor (e.g., gastrointestinal complaints, headache, rash).
    (2) Thrombocytopenia or a significant reduction in platelet count has been reported (2.4%) and is related to duration of therapy. Monitor platelets in patients with risk of bleeding, preexisting thrombocytopenia, platelet disorders (including those caused by concurrent medications) and in patients receiving linezolid lasting longer than 2 weeks.
    (3) Myelosuppression owing to direct bone marrow suppression has been reported rarely.
  e. Significant interactions. Patients receiving concomitant therapy with adrenergic or serotonergic agents or consuming more than 100 mg of tyramine a day may experience an enhancement of the drug's effect or serotonin syndrome.

6. **Spectinomycin.** An aminocyclitol agent related to the aminoglycosides, this antibiotic is useful against penicillin-resistant strains of gonorrhea.
  a. Mechanism of action. Spectinomycin is **bacteriostatic;** it selectively inhibits protein synthesis by binding to the 30S ribosomal subunit.
  b. Spectrum of activity. This agent is active against various gram-negative organisms.
  c. Therapeutic uses. Spectinomycin is used only to treat gonococcal infections in patients with penicillin allergy or when such infection stems from penicillinase-producing gonococci (PPNG).
  d. Precautions and monitoring effects. Because spectinomycin is given only as a single-dose IM injection, it causes few adverse effects. Nausea, vomiting, urticaria, chills, dizziness, and insomnia occur rarely.

7. **Trimethoprim.** A substituted pyrimidine, trimethoprim is most commonly combined with sulfamethoxazole (a sulfonamide discussed in II.F) in a preparation called co-trimoxazole. However, it may be used alone for certain urinary tract infections.
  a. Mechanism of action. Trimethoprim inhibits dihydrofolate reductase, thus blocking bacterial synthesis of folic acid.
  b. Spectrum of activity
    (1) Trimethoprim is active against most gram-negative and gram-positive organisms. However, drug resistance may develop when this drug is used alone.
    (2) Trimethoprim–sulfamethoxazole is active against a variety of organisms, including *S. pneumoniae, N. meningitidis,* and *Corynebacterium diphtheriae;* some strains

of *S. aureus, Staphylococcus epidermidis, P. mirabilis, Enterobacter, Salmonella, Shigella, Serratia,* and *Klebsiella* spp.; and *E. coli.*

    (3) The trimethoprim–sulfamethoxazole combination is synergistic; many organisms resistant to one component are susceptible to the combination.

  c. Therapeutic uses

    (1) Trimethoprim may be used alone or in combination with sulfamethoxazole to treat uncomplicated urinary tract infections caused by *E. coli, P. mirabilis,* and *Klebsiella* and *Enterobacter* organisms.

    (2) Trimethoprim–sulfamethoxazole is therapeutic for acute gonococcal urethritis, acute exacerbation of chronic bronchitis, shigellosis, and *Salmonella* infections.

    (3) Trimethoprim–sulfamethoxazole may be given as prophylactic or suppressive therapy in *P. carinii* pneumonia. It is the drug of choice for the treatment of *Stenotrophomonas maltophilia* infections.

  d. Precautions and monitoring effects

    (1) Most adverse effects involve the skin (possibly from sensitization). These include rash, pruritus, and exfoliative dermatitis.

    (2) Rarely, trimethoprim–sulfamethoxazole causes blood dyscrasias (e.g., acute hemolytic anemia, leukopenia, thrombocytopenia, methemoglobinemia, agranulocytosis, aplastic anemia).

    (3) Adverse GI effects including nausea, vomiting, and epigastric distress glossitis may occur.

    (4) Neonates may develop kernicterus.

    (5) Patients with AIDS sometimes suffer fever, rash, malaise, and pancytopenia during trimethoprim therapy.

8. Vancomycin. This glycopeptide destroys most gram-positive organisms.

  a. Mechanism of action. Vancomycin is **bactericidal;** it inhibits bacterial cell wall synthesis.

  b. Spectrum of activity. This drug is active against most gram-positive organisms, including methicillin-resistant strains of *S. aureus and Enterococci.*

  c. Therapeutic uses. Vancomycin usually is reserved for serious infections, especially those caused by methicillin-resistant staphylococci. It is particularly useful in patients who are allergic to penicillin or cephalosporins. Typical uses include endocarditis, osteomyelitis, and staphylococcal pneumonia.

    (1) Oral vancomycin is valuable in the treatment of antibiotic-induced pseudomembranous colitis caused by *C. difficile* or *S. aureus* enterocolitis. Because vancomycin is not absorbed after oral administration, it is not useful for systemic infections. Because of resistance, the Centers for Disease Control and Prevention (CDC) recommend vancomycin as the second choice to metronidazole for *C. difficile* infections.

    (2) Because 1 g provides adequate blood levels for 7–10 days, IV vancomycin is particularly useful in the treatment of anephric patients with gram-positive bacterial infections.

  d. Precautions and monitoring effects

    (1) Ototoxicity may arise; nephrotoxicity is rare but can occur with high doses.

    (2) Vancomycin may cause hypersensitivity reactions, manifested by such symptoms as anaphylaxis and skin rash.

    (3) Therapeutic levels peak at 20–40 μg/mL. The trough is $<$ 15 μg/mL.

    (4) Red man's syndrome may occur. This is facial flushing and hypotension owing to too rapid infusion of the drug. Infusion should be over a minimum of 60 min for a 1-g dose.

    (5) IV solutions are very irritating to the vein.

  e. Vancomycin-resistant enterococci. A few strains of vancomycin-resistant enterococci are susceptible to teicoplanin (investigational by Hoechst Marion Roussel), linezolid (Zyvox), or quinupristin/dalfopristin (Synercid). These agents may be useful for multiple-drug–resistant *E. faecium.*

9. Clofazimine is phenazine dye with antimycobacterial and anti-inflammatory activity.

  a. Mechanism of action. Clofazimine appears to bind preferentially to mycobacterial DNA, inhibiting replication and growth. It is **bactericidal** against *M. leprae,* and it appears to be **bacteriostatic** against MAI.

  b. Spectrum of activity. Clofazimine is active against various mycobacteria, including *M. leprae, M. tuberculosis,* and MAI.

c. Therapeutic uses. Clofazimine is used to treat leprosy and a variety of atypical *Mycobacterium* infections.

d. Precautions and monitoring effects

(1) Pigmentation (pink to brownish) occurs in 75%–100% of patients within a few weeks. This skin discoloration has led to severe depression (and suicide).

(2) Urine, sweat, and other body fluids may be discolored.

(3) Other effects include ichthyosis and dryness of skin (8%–28%), rash and pruritus (1%–5%), and GI intolerance (e.g., abdominal/epigastric pain, diarrhea, nausea, vomiting) in 40%–50% of patients. Clofazimine should be taken with food.

10. **Quinupristin/dalfopristin (Synercid)** is an intravenous streptogramin antibiotic composed of two chemically distinct compounds.

a. **Mechanism of action.** Quinupristin binds to the 50S subunit, and dalfopristin binds tightly to the 70S ribosomal particle.

b. **Spectrum of activity.** Synercid has activity against *Staphylococci* spp., including resistant strains. This combination has better activity against *E. faecium* than *Enterococcus faecalis* and is also active against some gram-negative organisms and anaerobes; activity has not been shown against *Enterobacteriaceae*.

c. **Therapeutic uses.** It is used for treatment of vancomycin-resistant *E. faecium* (VREF) bacteremia and skin and skin structure infections caused by *S. aureus* and *S. pyogenes*.

d. **Precautions and monitoring effects**

(1) Reported side effects are generally mild and infusion related: pain, erythema, or itching at the infusion site; increases in pulse and diastolic pressure; headache; nausea or vomiting; and diarrhea. It may increase liver function tests slightly.

(2) Drug interactions are a result of cytochrome P450 3A4 inhibition. Potential drug interactions include **cyclosporin, nifedipine,** and **midazolam.**

(3) Concomitant use of medications that may prolong QTc interval should be avoided.

(4) Mild to life-threatening pseudomembranous colitis has been reported.

11. **Daptomycin (Cubicin)** is a unique lipopeptide antibiotic with clinical activity in the treatment of resistant gram-positive infections.

a. **Mechanism of action**. Daptomycin is bactericidal; unlike other antibiotics, it binds to the bacterial cell membrane, causing depolarization of the membrane potential leading to inhibition of RNA, DNA, and protein synthesis.

b. **Spectrum of activity**. This drug is active against vancomycin-susceptible *E. faecium* and *S. aureus* (including methicillin-resistant strains) as well as other aerobic gram-positive bacteria.

c. **Therapeutic uses**. Daptomycin is indicated for the treatment of complicated skin and skin structure infections and S. aureus bacteremia. It is *not* indicated for the treatment of pneumonia.

d. **Precautions and monitoring effects**

(1) Reported side effects are generally mild and self-limiting and include constipation, abnormal liver function tests, and renal failure.

(2) Cases of myalgia and/or muscle weakness, exacerbations of myasthenia gravis, and increases in creatine phosphokinase (CPK) have been reported.

12. **Telithromycin (Ketek)** is the first of a new class of antimicrobials called the ketolides. It is an oral semisynthetic derivative of erythromycin.

a. **Mechanism of action**. Telithromycin may be bactericidal or bacteriostatic; it inhibits bacterial protein synthesis.

b. **Spectrum of activity.** This drug is active against many aerobic and anaerobic gram-positive organisms, including multidrug- resistant *S. pneumoniae*, some gram-negative organisms as well as atypical pathogens.

c. **Therapeutic uses.** Telithromycin is indicated for the treatment of community-acquired pneumonia, acute sinusitis, and acute exacerbations of chronic bronchitis.

d. **Precautions and monitoring effects**

(1) GI effects (including diarrhea, nausea, and vomiting) were the most common side effects followed by dizziness and visual disturbances (such as diplopia and blurred and abnormal vision); serious liver toxicity has been reported.

(2) Cross-sensitivity with the other macrolides occurs.

(3) Concomitant use of drugs or conditions that may prolong the QTc interval should be avoided.

e. **Significant interactions**
  (1) Co-administration of telithromycin with either cisapride or pimozide is contraindicated.
  (2) Concomitant administration of drugs metabolized by cytochrome P450 3A4 in patients with telithromycin should be closely monitored.
  (3) Patients on bepridil, mesoridazine, terfenadine, thioridazine, or ziprasidone should not be prescribed telithromycin owing to the high potential for toxicity.
  (4) **This agent has a high potential to interact with many drugs. Check product information for the most current interaction information.**

13. **Tigecycline (Tygacil).** An intravenous glycylcycline antibiotic developed as a semisynthetic analogue of tetracycline with a broad spectrum of activity.
  a. **Mechanism of action.** Tigecycline is bacteriostatic; it inhibits bacterial protein synthesis by reversibly binding to the 30S ribosome subunit.
  b. **Spectrum of activity.** The drug is active against vancomycin-susceptible *E. faecalis,* methicillin-resistant *S. epidermidis,* and *S. aureus* (methicillin-susceptible and -resistant strains) as well as some gram-negative aerobes and anaerobes.
  c. **Therapeutic uses.** Tigecycline is indicated for the treatment of complicated intra-abdominal infections caused by *E. coli,* vancomycin-susceptible *E. faecalis, S. aureus* (methicillin-susceptible strains only) and *B. fragilis.* Also indicated for the treatment of complicated skin and skin structure infections caused by *E. faecalis* (vancomycin-susceptible strains), *S. pyogenes* and *S. aureus* (methicillin-susceptible and -resistant strains).
  d. **Precautions and monitoring effects.**
    (1) Safety data are limited. Side effects are generally mild with GI disturbances—for example, nausea (22%–35%) and vomiting (13%–19%)—the most commonly reported. The mechanism of these reactions is uncertain.
    (2) May cause permanent discoloration of the teeth similar to the tetracyclines.
    (3) Caution in patients with a history of hypersensitivity reactions to tetracyclines.
    (4) Phototoxic reactions, pancreatitis, and increases in BUN may occur.
  e. **Significant interactions.** Closely monitor the prothrombin time or international sensitivity index (INR) in patients on warfarin during concomitant administration of tigecycline.

III. Systemic Antifungal Agents

A. **Definition.** These agents treat systemic and local fungal (mycotic) infections—diseases that resist treatment with antibacterial drugs.

B. **Amphotericin B (Fungizone).** This polyene antifungal antibiotic is therapeutic for various fungal infections that frequently proved fatal before the drug became available. It is used increasingly in the empiric treatment of severely immunocompromised patients in certain clinical situations.

1. **Mechanism of action.** Amphotericin B is both **fungistatic** in clinically obtained concentrations and may be fungicidal in the presence of susceptible organisms. It binds to sterols in the fungal cell membrane, thereby increasing membrane permeability and permitting leakage of intracellular contents. Other mechanisms may be involved as well.

2. **Spectrum of activity.** Amphotericin B is a broad-spectrum antifungal agent with activity against *Aspergillus, Blastomyces, Candida* spp. (*albicans, krusei tropicalis,* and *glabrata*), *Cryptococcus, Coccidioides, Histoplasma, Paracoccidioides, Phycomycetes* (*mucor*), and *Sporothrix.* It is also useful against some protozoa such as *Leishmania, Naegleria,* and *Acanthamoeba.*

3. **Therapeutic uses.** Amphotericin B is the most effective antifungal agent in the treatment of systemic fungal infections, especially in immunocompromised patients.
  a. It is the treatment of choice for pulmonary *Aspergillus* infections; *Blastomyces* infections, which are life-threatening with AIDS or CNS involvement; deep-organ infections with *Candida; Coccidioides* infections with severe pulmonary involvement or with disseminated nonmeningeal immunocompetent or immunocompromised patients; all *Cryptococcus* infections; disseminated *Histoplasma* infections involving CNS or immu-

nosuppressed patients; *Malassezia furfur* fungemia; pulmonary and extrapulmonary *Phycomycetes* (mucormycosis); *Penicillium marneffei;* and extracutaneous *Sporothrix.*
   b. This agent may be used to treat coccidioidal arthritis.
   c. Topical preparations are given to eradicate cutaneous and mucocutaneous candidiasis.
   d. It may be used as empiric therapy in febrile, neutropenic patients.
   e. It is used as secondary prophylaxis of fungal infections in HIV-positive patients, guarding against recurrence of infection.
   f. It may be used prophylactically in neutropenic cancer patients and bone marrow transplant or solid-organ transplant patients to reduce the incidence of *Aspergillus* and *Candida* infections.

4. Precautions and monitoring effects. Because amphotericin B can cause many serious adverse effects, it should be administered in a hospital setting—at least during the initial therapeutic stage. The adverse effects are divided into infusion reactions and others.
   a. Infusion reactions occur while the drug is being administered and include fever, shaking chills, hypotension, anorexia, nausea, vomiting, headache, dyspnea, and tachypnea. Premedication with acetaminophen and diphenhydramine has been helpful in prophylaxing against infusion reactions. In addition, hydrocortisone 10–50 mg may be added to the infusion as prophylaxis against infusion-related reactions. Meperidine 25–50 mg IV is effective treatment of active shaking chills/rigors. Meperidine is also effective in prophylaxis of rigors.
   b. Nephrotoxicity frequently occurs. Dosage adjustment or drug discontinuation or changing to a liposomal amphotericin B product may be necessary as renal impairment progresses.
   c. Electrolyte abnormalities, including hypokalemia, hypomagnesemia, and hypocalcemia, are common. Monitor and replace electrolytes as needed.
   d. Normocytic, normochromic anemia will develop over long-term use (10 weeks). Monitor hematocrit periodically.
   e. Bronchospasm, wheezing, and anaphylaxis or anaphylactoid reactions have occurred. A test dose of 1 mg of amphotericin B is often administered before infusion of large quantities of the drug.
   f. Phlebitis or thrombophlebitis is reported with conventional amphotericin B. Heparin (500–1000 U) can be added to the infusion to aid in prevention.
   g. CNS effects include headache, peripheral neuropathy, malaise, depression, seizure, myasthenia, and hallucinations.
   h. Elevated liver transaminases, aspartate aminotransferase (AST), alanine aminotransferase (ALT), alkaline phosphatase, bilirubin, γ-glutamyltransferase (GGT), and lactate dehydrogenase (LDH) may occur.
   i. Amphotericin B parenteral use should be mixed only in dextrose 5% in water (D$_5$W) and should be protected from light.

5. Significant interactions. Other nephrotoxic drugs (aminoglycosides, capreomycin, colistin, cisplatin, cyclosporine, methoxyflurane, pentamidine, polymyxin B, and vancomycin) may cause additive nephrotoxicity.

6. Amphotericin B lipid complex (Abelcet), amphotericin B cholesterol sulfate complex (Amphotec), and liposomal amphotericin B (AmBisome) offer alternative formulations of amphotericin B for the treatment of severe fungal infections in patients who are intolerant of or whose disease is refractory to conventional treatment.

C. Caspofungin (Cancidas). This echinocandin systemic antifungal agent is used in patients with refractory aspergillosis and candida esophagitis. Micafungin and anidulafungin (Eraxis) are recently approved additions to this class.

1. Mechanism of action. Caspofungin works by causing fungal cell wall lysis. By being a noncompetitive inhibitor of β (1,3) synthase, which is an essential component of fungal cell wall synthesis, it causes osmotic instability within the fungus and fungal cell wall lysis.

2. Spectrum of activity. Good in vitro activity has been demonstrated with caspofungin against *Aspergillus* spp., *Candida* spp. and *Histoplasma* spp. Caspofungin has also been shown to be effective against *Candida* spp. resistant to azoles and amphotericin B.

3. Therapeutic uses. Caspofungin may be used as an alternative to amphotericin B when treating patients with *Aspergillus.* It also plays a role in treating patients with resistant *Aspergillus* infections.

a. Caspofungin is effective in treating patients with aspergillosis, particularly when using a prolonged course of therapy (approximately 1 month) with resistant strains of *Aspergillus*. Caspofungin may be used alone or in combination with itraconazole for this indication.

b. More published data are necessary; however, good preliminary data exist for the use of caspofungin in treating *Candida* esophagitis. The duration of therapy is less with this disease (approximately 14 days).

4. Precautions and monitoring effects. Although this drug has adverse events associated with its use, the overall toxicity profile is significantly better than that of amphotericin B. The side effects may appear similar for the two drugs; however, these occur much more frequently with amphotericin B.

a. Infusion vein complications (not defined by manufacturer) and thrombophlebitis have been seen on infusion of caspofungin.

b. Hematological decreases in hemoglobin and hematocrit may occur; however, the incidence does not differ from that of having a fungal disease.

c. Headache may occur.

d. Slight decreases in serum potassium may occur, but nowhere near the magnitude of that caused by amphotericin B.

e. Anorexia, nausea, vomiting, and diarrhea have occurred.

f. Rare increases in serum creatinine; however, there have been no reported cases of nephrotoxicity.

g. Possible slight increases in serum aminotransferases

h. Allergic reactions occur in < 5% of patients and anaphylaxis in < 2% of patients.

i. Pregnancy category C embryotoxic reactions have occurred in animals.

5. Significant interactions

a. When cyclosporine is combined with caspofungin, clinically significant rises in ALT were observed. Serum transaminases should be monitored, and this combination should be avoided in patients with preexisting liver disease.

b. When used in combination, carbamazepine, nelfinavir, nevirapine, phenytoin, and rifampin increases the clearance of caspofungin. Higher doses of caspofungin (70 mg every day) should be considered when this combination is administered.

c. Tacrolimus clearance will be increased when the combination is used; monitor tacrolimus serum levels closely.

D. Flucytosine (Ancobon). This fluorinated pyrimidine usually is given in combination with amphotericin B.

1. Mechanism of action. Flucytosine penetrates fungal cells and is converted to fluorouracil, a metabolic antagonist. Incorporated into the RNA of the fungal cell, flucytosine causes defective protein synthesis. It is either **fungistatic** or **fungicidal,** depending on the concentration of the drug.

2. Spectrum of activity. This drug is primarily active against *Cryptococcus* and *Candida*. It is most commonly used in conjunction with amphotericin B. Fungal resistance against flucytosine alone has been well documented. Flucytosine may also possess some activity against chromomycosis and some strains of *Aspergillus* (in vitro testing only).

3. Therapeutic uses. Flucytosine is adjunctively used with amphotericin B for severe systemic infections (e.g., septicemia, endocarditis, pulmonary and urinary tract infections, meningitis). Use of flucytosine alone is not recommended.

4. Precautions and monitoring effects

a. Frequent adverse effects include GI intolerance with nausea, vomiting, and diarrhea.

b. Occasional adverse reactions are more severe and include marrow suppression with leukopenia or thrombocytopenia (dose related, especially with renal failure or concurrent amphotericin B use). Confusion, rash, hepatitis, enterocolitis, headache, and photosensitivity reactions can also occur.

c. Rare reactions include hallucinations, blood dyscrasias with agranulocytosis and pancytopenia, fatal hepatitis, anaphylaxis, and anemia.

d. Flucytosine may cause a markedly false elevation of serum creatinine if an Ektachem analyzer is used.

5. Significant interactions. Beneficial drug interactions occur with flucytosine. Flucytosine has demonstrated synergy with **amphotericin B** and **fluconazole** against *Cryptococcus* and *Candida* spp.

E. Griseofulvin (Fulvicin). Produced from *Penicillium griseofulvin Dierckx,* this drug is deposited in the skin, bound to keratin.

1. Mechanism of action. This agent is **fungistatic;** it inhibits fungal cell activity by interfering with mitotic spindle structure. Its mechanism of action is similar to colchicine.

2. Spectrum of activity. Griseofulvin is active against various strains of *Microsporum, Epidermophyton,* and *Trichophyton.*

3. Therapeutic uses. Griseofulvin is effective in tinea infections of the skin, hair, and nails (including athlete's foot, jock itch, and ringworm) caused by *Microsporum, Epidermophyton,* and *Trichophyton.*
  a. Generally, this agent is given only for infections that do not respond to topical antifungal agents.
  b. Griseofulvin is available only in oral form.
  c. It possesses vasodilatory activity and may be used in Raynaud disease.
  d. It may be used to treat gout.

4. Precautions and monitoring effects
  a. Griseofulvin rarely results in serious adverse effects. However, the following problems have been reported.
     (1) *Common:* headache, fatigue, confusion, impaired performance, syncope, and lethargy, which generally resolve with continued use
     (2) *Occasional:* leukopenia, neutropenia, and granulocytopenia
     (3) *Rare:* serum sickness, angioedema, urticaria, erythema, and hepatotoxicity
  b. The dosage depends on the particle size of the product: 250 mg of ultramicrosize (Fulvicin P/G) is equivalent in therapeutic effects to 500 mg of microsize (Fulvicin U/F).

5. Significant interactions
  a. Griseofulvin may increase the metabolism of **warfarin,** leading to decreased prothrombin time.
  b. **Barbiturates** may reduce griseofulvin absorption.
  c. **Alcohol consumption** may cause tachycardia and flushing.
  d. **Oral contraceptives** may cause amenorrhea or increased breakthrough bleeding.

F. Imidazoles. The substituted imidazole derivatives **ketoconazole (Nizoral), miconazole (Monistat), fluconazole (Diflucan), itraconazole (Sporanox),** and **voriconazole (Vfend)** are valuable in the treatment of a wide range of systemic fungal infections.

1. Mechanism of action. Imidazoles inhibit sterol synthesis in fungal cell membranes and increase cell wall permeability; this, in turn, makes the cell more vulnerable to osmotic pressure. These agents are **fungistatic.**

2. Spectrum of activity. These agents are active against many fungi, including yeasts, dermatophytes, actinomycetes, and some *Phycomycetes.*

3. Therapeutic uses
  a. Ketoconazole, an oral agent, successfully treats many fungal infections that previously yielded only to parenteral agents.
     (1) It is therapeutic for systemic and vaginal candidiasis, mucocandidiasis, candiduria, oral thrush, histoplasmosis, coccidioidomycosis, chromomycosis, dermatophytosis (tinea), and paracoccidioidomycosis.
     (2) Because ketoconazole is slow acting and requires a long duration of therapy (up to 6 months for some chronic infections), it is less effective than other antifungal agents for the treatment of severe and acute systemic infections.
  b. Miconazole, primarily administered as a topical agent, The parenteral form has been discontinued in the United States. It was a relatively toxic formulation which has been replaced by other members of this class (e.g., fluconazole).

(1) Topical miconazole is highly effective in vulvovaginal candidiasis, ringworm, and other skin infections.

c. **Fluconazole.** Available in oral and parenteral forms, fluconazole can be used against systemic and CNS infections involving *Cryptococcus* and *Candida*. *Candida* oropharyngeal infection and esophagitis may also be treated with fluconazole. *Aspergillus, Coccidioides,* and *Histoplasma* have demonstrated in vitro sensitivity.

d. **Itraconazole** is available as an oral agent with activity against systemic and invasive pulmonary aspergillosis without the hematological toxicity of amphotericin B. Other deep mycotic infections susceptible to itraconazole include blastomycosis, coccidioidomycosis, cryptococcosis, and histoplasmosis.

e. **Voriconazole.** Voriconazole is available as both an intravenous and an oral agent for the treatment of fungal infections involving invasive aspergillosis, *Scedosporium apiospermum,* and *Fusarium* spp., including those species that are refractory to other therapy.

4. **Precautions and monitoring effects**
   a. **Ketoconazole** may cause nausea, vomiting, diarrhea, abdominal pain, and constipation. Rarely, it leads to headache, dizziness, gynecomastia, and fatal hepatotoxicity.
   b. **Fluconazole** commonly causes GI disturbances (e.g., nausea, vomiting, epigastric pain, diarrhea). Reversible elevations in serum aminotransferase, exfoliative skin reactions, and headaches have been reported.
   c. **Itraconazole** may cause nausea, vomiting, hypertriglyceridemia, hypokalemia, rash, and elevations in liver enzymes.
   d. **Voriconazole.** Visual disturbances, fever, rash, vomiting, nausea, diarrhea, headache, sepsis, peripheral edema, abdominal pain, and respiratory disorders rarely occurred. Liver function test abnormalities have occurred.

5. **Significant interactions**
   a. Both **ketoconazole** and **miconazole** may enhance the anticoagulant effect of **warfarin.**
   b. **Ketoconazole** may antagonize the antibiotic effects of **amphotericin B.**
   c. **Fluconazole** has been shown to elevate serum levels of **phenytoin, cyclosporine, warfarin,** and **sulfonylureas.** Concurrent hepatic enzyme inducers, such as **rifampin,** have resulted in increased elimination of both fluconazole and itraconazole.
   d. Coadministration of **itraconazole** or **ketoconazole** with **astemizole** or **terfenadine** may result in increased astemizole or terfenadine levels, possibly leading to life-threatening dysrhythmias and death.
   e. Both **ketoconazole** and **itraconazole** need the presence of stomach acid for adequate absorption. Use with antacids, H_2-blockers, or proton pump inhibitors is contraindicated.
   f. Concomitant use of imidazole antifungal agents with **cisapride** may result in increased concentrations of cisapride, which has been associated with adverse cardiac events such as torsades de pointes leading to sudden death.
   g. **Voriconazole.** Cytochrome P450 2C19 is the major enzyme involved in metabolism. Voriconazole inhibits cytochrome P450 2C19, 2C9, and 3A4. Any medication that is metabolized via these routes may be affected, and monitoring of blood levels (if appropriate) or clinical signs and symptoms is necessary when taking concomitant medications.

G. **Nystatin (Mycostatin).** A polyene antibiotic, nystatin has a chemical structure similar to that of amphotericin B.

1. **Mechanism of action.** Nystatin is **fungicidal** and **fungistatic;** binding to sterols in the fungal cell membrane, it increases membrane permeability and permits leakage of intracellular contents.

2. **Spectrum of activity.** Nystatin is active primarily against *Candida* spp.

3. **Therapeutic uses**
   a. This drug is used primarily as a topical agent in vaginal and oral *Candida* infections.
   b. Oral nystatin is therapeutic for *Candida* infections of the GI tract, especially oral and esophageal infections; because the drug is not readily absorbed, it maintains good local activity.

4. **Precautions and monitoring effects.** Oral nystatin occasionally causes GI distress (e.g., nausea, vomiting, diarrhea). Rarely, hypersensitivity reactions occur.

H. Terbinafine (Lamisil) is a synthetic allylamine with structure and activity related to naftifine.

 1. **Mechanism of action.** Terbinafine inhibits squalene monooxygenase, leading to an interruption of fungal sterol biosynthesis. Terbinafine may be **fungicidal** or **fungistatic,** depending on drug concentration and species.

 2. **Spectrum of activity.** Terbinafine has activity against dermatophytic fungi (*Trichophyton, Microsporum,* and *Epidermophyton*), filamentous fungi (*Aspergillus*), and dimorphic fungi (*Blastomyces*). It may also possess some activity against yeasts.

 3. **Therapeutic uses**
    a. Oral terbinafine is useful against infections of the toenail and fingernail (onychomycosis, tinea unguium). Time to cure is reduced over imidazole antifungals for these indications. It is useful in patients who may not tolerate the adverse effect profile of imidazole antifungals.
    b. It is also used in tinea capitis and tinea corporis infections.

 4. **Precautions and monitoring effects.** Adverse effects include taste or ocular disturbances, symptomatic hepatobiliary dysfunction, decrease in lymphocyte count and neutropenia, and serious skin reactions.

IV. Topical Antifungal Agents

 A. Definition. These agents are for topical use for fungal infections.

 B. Amphotericin B (Fungizone) is available as a 3% cream or lotion or an oral suspension that is not absorbed through the GI tract.

 1. **Mechanism of action.** See III.B.1.

 2. **Spectrum of activity.** See III.B.2.

 3. **Therapeutic uses.** Amphotericin B is used for oropharyngeal candidiasis, cutaneous and mucocutaneous candidal infections, or as a local irrigant for the bladder and intrapleural or intraperitoneal areas.

 4. **Precautions and monitoring effects.** Compared with systemic administration, the topical formulations have relatively low toxicity.
    a. Dry skin and local irritation with erythema, pruritus, or burning, along with mild skin discoloration, has occurred with the lotion and cream.
    b. Rash and GI effects (e.g., nausea, vomiting, steatorrhea, diarrhea) tend to occur with the suspension. In addition, there have been case reports of urticaria, angioedema, Stevens-Johnson syndrome, and toxic epidermal necrolysis.

 C. Butenafine (Mentax) is a synthetic benzylamine related to the allylamine antifungal agents (naftifine, terbinafine).

 1. **Mechanism of action.** Butenafine alters fungal membrane permeability and growth inhibition, interferes with sterol biosynthesis by allowing squalene to accumulate within the cell, and may be fungicidal in certain concentrations against susceptible organisms such as the dermatophytes.

 2. **Spectrum of activity.** Butenafine is active against *Trichophyton rubrum, Trichophyton mentagrophytes, Microsporum canis, Sporothrix schenckii,* and yeasts including *Candida parapsilosis* and *C. albicans.*

 3. **Therapeutic uses.** The 1% cream is used in dermatophytoses, including tinea corporis, tinea cruris, and tinea pedis.

 4. **Precautions and monitoring effects.** If clinical improvement of fungal infection does not improve after the treatment period, the diagnosis should be reevaluated.

 D. Butoconazole (Mycelex) is an azole antifungal cream available for vaginal use.

 1. **Mechanism of action.** Butoconazole has fungistatic activity against susceptible organisms. The drug interferes with membrane permeability, secondary metabolic effects, and growth

inhibition. Butoconazole contains antibacterial effects against some gram-positive organisms.

2. **Spectrum of activity.** Butoconazole is active against dermatophytes (*Trichophyton concentricum, T. mentagrophytes, T. rubrum, Trichophyton tonsurans, Epidermophyton floccosum, M. canis, Microsporum gypseum*), yeasts (*C. albicans, C. glabrata*), and some gram-positive organisms (*S. aureus, E. faecalis,* and *S. pyogenes*).

3. **Therapeutic uses.** A 2% cream is used for vulvovaginal candidiasis and complicated, recurrent vulvovaginal candidiasis.

4. **Precautions and monitoring effects**
   a. Vulvovaginal burning and itching are the most common; however, their incidence is low. Headache; itching of fingers; urinary frequency and burning; and vulvovaginal discharge, irritation, soreness, stinging, odor, and swelling rarely occur.
   b. Butoconazole may damage birth-control devices such as condoms and diaphragms, leading to inadequate protection. Consider alternative methods of birth control.
   c. Tampon use should be avoided with the use of butoconazole.

E. **Ciclopirox (Loprox)** is a synthetic antifungal agent that is chemically unrelated to any other antifungal agent. The ethanolamine contained in ciclopirox appears to enhance epidermal penetration.

1. **Mechanism of action.** Ciclopirox causes intracellular depletion of amino acids and ions necessary for normal cellular function.

2. **Spectrum of activity.** Ciclopirox is active against dermatophytes, yeasts, some gram-positive and gram-negative bacteria, *Mycoplasma,* and *Trichomonas vaginalis.* Specifically, ciclopirox has activity against *T. mentagrophytes, T. rubrum, E. floccosum, M. canis, M. furfur,* and *C. albicans.*

3. **Therapeutic uses.** Ciclopirox is used topically for the treatment of tinea pedis, tinea cruris, tinea corporis, tinea versicolor (from *Malassezia*), and cutaneous candidiasis (moniliasis) from *C. albicans.*

4. **Precautions and monitoring effects.** Local irritation manifested by erythema, pruritus, burning, blistering, swelling, and oozing has occurred. If this occurs, ciclopirox should be discontinued.

F. **Clioquinol** (formerly iodochlorhydroxyquin) is a topical antifungal in a 3% ointment that can be used alone or in combination with hydrocortisone.

1. **Mechanism of action.** Unknown

2. **Spectrum of activity.** It is active against dermatophytic fungi.

3. **Therapeutic uses.** It is used topically against the following:
   a. Tinea pedis and tinea cruris (ringworm infections)
   b. Previously used to treat diaper rash; however, it is no longer recommended, and use in children < 2 years of age is contraindicated

4. **Precautions and monitoring effects**
   a. Local irritation, rash, and sensitivity reactions are common.
   b. Systemic absorption after topical application may occur.
   c. High doses of clioquinol over long periods of time have been associated with oculotoxic/neurotoxic effects, including optic neuritis, optic atrophy, and subacute myelo-optic neuropathy.

G. **Clotrimazole (Lotrimin)** is an azole antifungal agent that is an imidazole derivative. It is related to other azole antifungal agents such as **butoconazole, econazole, ketoconazole, miconazole, oxiconazole, sulconazole,** and **tioconazole.**

1. **Mechanism of action.** Clotrimazole alters fungal cell membrane permeability by binding with phospholipids in the membrane.

2. **Spectrum of activity.** It is active against yeasts, dermatophytes (*T. rubrum, T. mentagrophytes, E. floccosum, M. canis*), and some gram-positive bacteria. At higher concentrations,

clotrimazole inhibits *M. furfur, Aspergillus fumigatus, C. albicans,* and some strains of *S. aureus, S. pyogenes, Proteus vulgaris,* and *Salmonella.* At very high concentrations, clotrimazole has an effect on *Sporothrix, Cryptococcus, Cephalosporium, Fusarium,* and *T. vaginalis.*

3. Therapeutic uses
   a. The lozenges, which are administered 5 times per day, are useful in treating oropharyngeal candidiasis. Lozenges are also used for primary prophylaxis of mucocutaneous candidiasis in HIV-infected infants or children with severe immunosuppression.
   b. The cream, lotion, or solution is used to treat dermatophytoses, superficial mycoses, and cutaneous candidiasis.
   c. Intravaginal dosage forms are useful in treating vulvovaginal candidiasis.

4. Precautions and monitoring effects
   a. Cutaneous reactions with topical administration may include blistering, erythema, edema, pruritus, burning, stinging, peeling, skin fissures, and general irritation.
   b. The vaginal tablets are associated with mild burning, skin rash, itching, vulval irritation, lower abdominal cramps, bloating, slight cramping, vaginal soreness during intercourse, and an increase in urinary frequency.
   c. Cross-sensitization occurs with imidazole; however, it is unpredictable.
   d. Abnormal liver function tests (elevated AST) have occurred in patients taking the lozenges.

H. Econazole (Spectazole) is an azole antifungal agent that is an imidazole derivative.

1. Mechanism of action. Econazole alters cell membranes and increases permeability (like many other azole agents).

2. Spectrum of activity. Econazole is active against dermatophytes, yeasts, some gram-positive bacteria, and *T. vaginalis.*

3. Therapeutic uses
   a. The 1% topical cream, lotion, or solution is useful in treating dermatophytoses and cutaneous candidiasis (tinea corporis and tinea cruris).
   b. Econazole is also used to treat pityriasis (tinea) versicolor (*M. furfur*).

4. Precautions and monitoring effects. In general, there is a low incidence of toxicity. Topically, a patient may experience burning, stinging sensations, pruritus, and erythema (after 2–4 days).

I. Gentian violet is a dye that possesses the ability to kill fungi, yeasts, and some gram-positive bacteria.

1. Mechanism of action. None known

2. Spectrum of activity. Gentian violet is active against *Candida, Epidermophyton, Cryptococcus, Trichophyton,* and some *Staphylococcus* spp.

3. Therapeutic uses. It is used to treat cutaneous *C. albicans* infections (monilia or thrush).

4. Precautions and monitoring effects
   a. Gentian violet may cause irritation or sensitivity reactions or possibly ulceration of the mucous membranes. If the solution is swallowed, esophagitis, laryngitis, or tracheitis may occur.
   b. Skin tattooing may occur if gentian violet is applied to granulation tissue.
   c. Gentian violet should not be used in areas of extensive ulceration.
   d. This drug is a dye and will stain clothing.

J. Ketoconazole (Nizoral) is an imidazole-derived antifungal drug that is available topically as a cream and a shampoo.

1. Mechanism of action. See III.E.1.

2. Spectrum of activity. See III.E.2.

3. Therapeutic uses
   a. The 2% topical cream is used in treating tinea corporis, tinea cruris, and tinea pedis caused by the dermatophytes (*E. floccosum, T. mentagrophytes,* and *T. rubrum*).

b. It is used for cutaneous candidiasis.

c. The 2% topical cream or 2% shampoo may be used in treating tinea versicolor (*M. furfur*). Selenium-based shampoos may also be useful in this area.

d. The 2% topical cream is useful against seborrheic dermatitis. The 2% shampoo is useful in reducing scaling caused by dandruff.

e. When combined with a steroid, ketoconazole is useful in treating the following: atopic dermatitis, diaper rash, eczema, folliculitis, impetigo, intertrigo, lichenoid dermatitis, and psoriasis.

f. An ophthalmic suspension can be extemporaneously prepared to treat fungal keratitis.

4. Precautions and monitoring effects

a. Reactions from the 2% topical cream include local irritation, pruritus, and stinging. Contact dermatitis is possible and occurs with other imidazole derivatives.

b. The 2% shampoo may lead to increased hair loss, irritation, abnormal hair texture, scalp pustules, dry skin, pruritus, and oiliness or dryness of hair and scalp. It may in addition straighten otherwise curly hair.

K. Miconazole (Monistat) is an imidazole-derived antifungal drug that is available topically as a 2% aerosol, 2% aerosol powder, 2% cream, a kit, 2% powder and 2% tincture, 2% vaginal cream, and 100 mg and 200 mg vaginal suppositories.

1. Mechanism of action. See III.E.1.

2. Spectrum of activity. See III.E.2.

3. Therapeutic uses. Miconazole is advantageous over other agents such as nystatin and tolnaftate in that its activity covers dermatophytes as well as *Candida*.

a. Topical use is effective against tinea pedis, tinea cruris, and tinea corporis caused by dermatophytes (*T. mentagrophytes, T. rubrum,* and *E. floccosum*).

b. It is also effective against tinea versicolor from *M. furfur.*

c. Like other imidazole derivatives, it is useful in treating cutaneous fungal infections.

d. The vaginal cream and vaginal suppositories are effective in treating vulvovaginal candidiasis.

4. Precautions and monitoring parameters

a. Topical creams have caused local irritation and burning.

b. Vaginal preparations have led to vulvovaginal burning, itching, irritation, pelvic cramps, vaginal burning, headache, hives, and skin rash.

c. If vulvovaginal candidiasis persists for longer than 3 days, seek further medical attention.

d. Tampons should be avoided in patients using vaginal suppositories or cream; sanitary pads should be substituted.

e. Vaginal suppositories are manufactured from a vegetable oil base that may interact with latex products. Avoid using diaphragms or condoms concurrently with suppositories. Seek an alternative form of birth control.

L. Naftifine (Naftin) is a synthetic allylamine similar to terbinafine. It is available as a 1% topical cream and a 1% topical gel.

1. Mechanism of action. Naftifine is **fungistatic** and interferes with sterol biosynthesis by accumulating squalene in the fungal cell. Naftifine also possesses some local anti-inflammatory activity.

2. Spectrum of activity

a. Naftifine is active against *T. mentagrophytes, T. rubrum, T. tonsurans, Trichophyton verrucosum, Trichophyton violaceum, E. floccosum, Microsporum audouinii, M. canis,* and *M. gypseum.*

b. *C. albicans, Candida krusei, Candida parapsilosis,* and *Candida tropicalis* are affected by naftifine; however, the concentrations of naftifine vary for *Candida* killing, depending on the species.

c. In vitro activity has been demonstrated against *Aspergillus flavus* and *Aspergillus fumigatus.* Others include *Sporothrix schenckii, Cryptococcus neoformans, Petriellidium boydii, Blastomyces dermatitidis,* and *Histoplasma capsulatum.*

3. Therapeutic uses. Naftifine is active against dermatophytoses and cutaneous candidiasis.
   a. It is also used to treat tinea cruris, tinea pedis, tinea corporis, and tinea manus (*T. mentagrophytes, T. rubrum, T. verrucosum, T. violaceum, E. floccosum,* or *M. canis*).
   b. It is also useful in treating tinea unguium (onychomycosis).

4. Precautions and monitoring effects. Transient burning and stinging

M. Nystatin (Mycostatin). A polyene antibiotic, nystatin has a chemical structure similar to that of amphotericin B. It is available as an oral suspension, tablet, lozenge, topical cream, ointment, topical powder, and vaginal tablet.

1. Mechanism of action. Nystatin is **fungicidal** and **fungistatic;** binding to sterols in the fungal cell membrane, it increases membrane permeability and permits leakage of intracellular contents.

2. Spectrum of activity. Nystatin is active primarily against *Candida* spp.

3. Therapeutic uses. This drug is used primarily as a topical agent in vaginal and oral *Candida* infections.

4. Precautions and monitoring effects. Irritation has occurred in extremely rare instances.

N. Oxiconazole (Oxistat) is an imidazole-derived antifungal drug that is available as a 1% topical cream or 1% topical lotion.

1. Mechanism of action. See III.E.1.

2. Spectrum of activity. See III.E.2.

3. Therapeutic uses
   a. The 1% cream or lotion is useful in treating tinea cruris, tinea corporis, tinea manus, and tinea pedis from dermatophytes.
   b. Oxiconazole is also effective against tinea versicolor caused by *M. furfur.*

4. Precautions and monitoring effects. Adverse effects are rare and are confined to local irritation.

O. Sulconazole (Exelderm) is an imidazole-derived antifungal drug that is available as a 1% topical cream and a 1% topical solution.

1. Mechanism of action (see III.E.1). The antibacterial effects exerted by sulconazole are thought to be the result of a direct physicochemical effect on the destruction of unsaturated fatty acids present in bacterial cell membranes.

2. Spectrum of activity
   a. Sulconazole has activity against dermatophytes, including *E. floccosum, M. audouinii, M. canis, M. gypseum, T. mentagrophytes, T. rubrum, T. tonsurans,* and *T. violaceum.* It also has activity against *M. furfur.*
   b. Sulconazole also has activity against selected gram-positive aerobes (*S. aureus, S. epidermidis, Staphylococcus saprophyticus, E. faecalis, Micrococcus luteus,* and *Bacillus subtilis*) and anaerobes (*Clostridium* and *Propionibacterium acnes, Clostridium perfringens, Clostridium tetani,* and *Clostridium botulinum*).

3. Therapeutic uses
   a. The 1% topical cream or 1% topical solution is useful in treating tinea corporis and tinea cruris.
   b. The 1% topical cream has been studied for use against tinea pedis; the solution has not been evaluated for this indication.
   c. The 1% cream is useful against tinea versicolor (*M. furfur*).
   d. There is not an approved indication for cutaneous candidiasis; however, sulconazole 1% is as effective as miconazole 2% or clotrimazole 1% in treating cutaneous candidiasis.
   e. Sulconazole is useful in treating infections caused by bacteria such as impetigo (*S. pyogenes*) and ecthyma (*S. aureus*).

4. Precautions and monitoring effects. Adverse reactions include local effects such as burning and irritation, skin edema, dryness, scaling, fissuring, cracking, generalized red papules, and severe eczema.

P. Terbinafine (Lamisil AT) is a synthetic allylamine available as a 1% cream with structure and activity related to naftifine.

1. **Mechanism of action.** Terbinafine inhibits squalene monooxygenase, leading to an interruption of fungal sterol biosynthesis. Terbinafine may be **fungicidal** or **fungistatic,** depending on drug concentration and species.

2. **Spectrum of activity.** Terbinafine has activity against dermatophytic fungi (*Trichophyton, Microsporum,* and *Epidermophyton*), filamentous fungi (*Aspergillus*), and dimorphic fungi (*Blastomyces*). It may also possess some activity against yeasts.

3. **Therapeutic uses.** It is useful for tinea pedis, tinea corporis, and tinea cruris.

4. **Precautions and monitoring effects.** It can cause local irritation.

Q. Terconazole (Terazol-7) is an imidazole-derived antifungal drug that is available as a 0.4% and 0.8% vaginal cream and an 80-mg vaginal suppository.

1. **Mechanism of action.** It is **fungicidal** against *C. albicans.* Like other imidazole agents, terconazole alters cellular membranes, resulting in increased membrane permeability.

2. **Spectrum of activity.** It is active against dermatophytes; yeasts; and, at high concentrations, gram-positive and gram-negative bacteria.

3. **Therapeutic uses** are for complicated and uncomplicated vulvovaginal candidiasis.

4. **Precautions and monitoring effects.** Adverse reactions include burning, pruritus, irritation, headache, body pain, and pain of female genitalia.

R. Tioconazole (Vagistat-1) is an imidazole-derived antifungal drug that is available as a 6.5% vaginal ointment.

1. **Mechanism of action.** Tioconazole is **fungicidal** against *C. albicans.* Like other imidazole agents, tioconazole alters cellular membranes, resulting in increased membrane permeability.

2. **Spectrum of activity**
   a. Activity against fungi includes most strains of *Candida* and the dermatophytes. There is also activity against *Aspergillus* and *C. neoformans.*
   b. Tioconazole is active against the following aerobic gram-positive bacteria: *Gardnerella vaginalis, Corynebacterium minutissimum, E. faecalis, S. aureus, S. epidermidis,* and some *Streptococci* spp. Gram-negative bacteria: it is active against *H. pylori, Haemophilus ducreyi, Moraxella catarrhalis, Neisseria gonorrhoeae,* and *N. meningitidis.*
   c. Other organisms that tioconazole has activity against are *T. vaginalis, Lymphogranuloma venereum,* and *Chlamydia trachomatis.*

3. **Therapeutic uses.** Tioconazole is used for simple and complicated vulvovaginal candidiasis. Other uses have been explored; however, topical creams for use in those scenarios are not available in the United States.

4. **Precautions and monitoring effects.** Local irritation has been manifested as vulvovaginal burning, vaginitis, and pruritus.

S. Tolnaftate (Tinactin) is available topically as a 1% aerosol, 1% powder, 1% cream, and 1% solution.

1. **Mechanism of action.** It may distort hyphae and stunt mycelial growth in susceptible fungi.

2. **Spectrum of activity.** Tolnaftate may be either **fungistatic** or **fungicidal** to the following organisms: *M. gypseum, M. canis, M. audouinii, Microsporum japonicum, T. rubrum, T. mentagrophytes, Trichophyton schoenleinii, T. tonsurans, E. floccosum, Aspergillus niger, C. albicans, C. neoformans,* and *A. fumigatus.*

3. **Therapeutic uses.** Tolnaftate is used for dermatophytoses and tinea versicolor.

4. **Precautions and monitoring effects.** There may be slight local irritation.

V. Antiprotozoal Agents

A. **Classification.** These drugs fall into two main categories: **antimalarial agents,** used to treat malaria infection, and **amebicides** and **trichomonacides,** used to treat amebic and trichomonal infections.

B. **Antimalarial agents.** Still a leading cause of illness and death in tropical and subtropical countries, malaria results from infection by any of four species of the protozoal genus *Plasmodium.* Antimalarial agents are selectively active during different phases of the protozoan life cycle. Major antimalarial drugs include **chloroquine (Aralen), halofantrine (Halfan), hydroxychloroquine (Plaquenil), primaquine, pyrimethamine (Daraprim), quinine,** and **mefloquine (Lariam).** In addition, two combination brands are available: sulfadoxine plus pyrimethamine (Fansidar) and atovaquone plus proguanil (Malarone).

1. **Mechanism of action**
   a. **Chloroquine** and **hydroxychloroquine** bind to and alter the properties of microbial and mammalian DNA.
   b. The mechanism of action of **primaquine, quinine, Fansidar,** and **mefloquine** is unknown.
   c. **Pyrimethamine** impedes folic acid reduction by inhibiting the enzyme dihydrofolate reductase.

2. **Spectrum of activity**
   a. **Chloroquine** and **hydroxychloroquine** are suppressive blood **schizonticidal** agents and are active against the asexual erythrocyte forms of *Plasmodium vivax* and *Plasmodium falciparum* and gametocytes of *P. vivax, Plasmodium malariae,* and *Plasmodium ovale.*
   b. **Primaquine,** a curative agent, is active against liver forms of *P. vivax* and *P. ovale* and the primary exoerythrocyte forms of *P. falciparum.*
   c. **Pyrimethamine** is active against chloroquine-resistant strains of *P. falciparum* and some strains of *P. vivax.*
   d. **Quinine,** a generalized protoplasmic poison, is toxic to a wide range of organisms. In malaria, this drug has both suppressive and curative action against chloroquine-resistant strains.
   e. **Fansidar** (sulfadoxine plus pyrimethamine) is a blood **schizonticidal** agent that is active against the erythrocytic forms of susceptible plasmodia. It is also active against *T. gondii.*
   e. **Malarone** (atovaquone plus proguanil) is active against the erythrocytic and exoerythrocytic forms of *Plasmodium* spp.
   f. **Mefloquine** is a blood **schizonticidal** agent that is active against *P. falciparum* (both chloroquine-susceptible and -resistant strains) and *P. vivax.*
   g. **Halofantrine** is a blood schizonticidal agent active against *P. falciparum* and *P. vivax.*

3. **Therapeutic uses**
   a. **Chloroquine** is the preferred agent used to suppress malaria symptoms and to terminate acute malaria attacks resulting from *P. falciparum* and *P. malariae* infections.
      (1) It is more potent and less toxic than quinine.
      (2) Except where drug-resistant *P. falciparum* strains are prevalent, chloroquine is the most useful antimalarial agent.
   b. **Hydroxychloroquine** is used as an alternative to chloroquine in patients who cannot tolerate chloroquine or when chloroquine is unavailable.
   c. **Primaquine** is used to cure relapses of *P. vivax* and *P. ovale* malaria and to prevent malaria in exposed persons returning from regions where malaria is endemic.
   d. **Pyrimethamine** is effective in the prevention and treatment of chloroquine-resistant strains of *P. falciparum.* It is now used almost exclusively in combination with a sulfonamide or sulfone.
   e. **Quinine**
      (1) Quinine sulfate, an oral form, is therapeutic for acute malaria caused by chloroquine-resistant strains.
      (2) Quinine dihydrochloride, a parenteral form, is used in severe cases of chloroquine-resistant malaria. (It is available only from the CDC.)
      (3) Quinine is almost always given in combination with another antimalarial agent.
   f. **Fansidar**
      (1) Fansidar is used for the suppression or prophylaxis of chloroquine-resistant *P. falciparum* malaria.

(2) It has been used for the prophylaxis of *P. carinii* infections in AIDS patients unable to tolerate cotrimoxazole (trimethoprim–sulfamethoxazole).

g. **Mefloquine** is indicated for the treatment of acute malaria and the prevention of *P. falciparum* and *P. vivax* infections.

h. **Halofantrine** is indicated for treatment of malaria in adults who can tolerate oral medication and who have mild to moderate malaria ($\geq$ 100,000 parasites/mm^3) caused by *P. falciparum* or *P. vivax*.

i. **Malarone**

(1) Prophylaxis of *P. falciparum* malaria, including areas where chloroquine resistance has been reported.

(2) Treatment of acute, uncomplicated *P. falciparum* malaria. This combination has been shown to be effective in regions where the drugs chloroquine, halofantrine, mefloquine, and amodiaquine may have unacceptable failure rates, presumably because of drug resistance.

4. **Precautions and monitoring effects**

a. **Chloroquine and hydroxychloroquine**

(1) Because these drugs concentrate in the liver, they should be used cautiously in patients with hepatic disease.

(2) Chloroquine must be administered with extreme caution in patients with neurological, hematological, or severe GI disorders.

(3) Visual disturbances, headache, skin rash, and GI distress have been reported.

b. **Primaquine**

(1) This agent is contraindicated in patients with rheumatoid arthritis and lupus erythematosus and in those receiving other potentially hemolytic drugs or bone marrow suppressants.

(2) Primaquine may cause agranulocytosis, granulocytopenia, and mild anemia. In patients with G6PD deficiency, it may cause hemolytic anemia.

(3) Abdominal cramps, nausea, vomiting, and epigastric distress sometimes occur.

c. **Pyrimethamine**

(1) In high doses, this drug may cause agranulocytosis, megaloblastic anemia, aplastic anemia, and thrombocytopenia.

(2) Erythema multiforme (Stevens-Johnson syndrome), nausea, vomiting, and anorexia may develop during pyrimethamine therapy.

d. **Quinine**

(1) Quinine is contraindicated in patients with G6PD deficiency, tinnitus, and optic neuritis.

(2) Quinine overdose or hypersensitivity reactions may be fatal. Manifestations of quinine poisoning include visual and hearing disturbances; GI symptoms (e.g., nausea, vomiting); hot, flushed skin; headache; fever; syncope; confusion; shallow, then depressed, respirations; and cardiovascular collapse.

(3) Quinine must be used cautiously in patients with atrial fibrillation.

(4) Renal damage and anuria have been reported.

e. **Fansidar**

(1) Severe, sometimes fatal, hypersensitivity reactions have occurred. In most cases, death resulted from severe cutaneous reactions, including erythema multiforme, Stevens-Johnson syndrome, and toxic epidermal necrolysis.

(2) Adverse hematological and hepatic effects as seen with sulfonamides have been reported.

f. **Mefloquine**

(1) Concomitant use of mefloquine with quinine, quinidine, or β-adrenergic blockade may produce electrocardiographic abnormalities or cardiac arrest.

(2) Concomitant use of mefloquine and quinine or chloroquine may increase the risk of convulsions.

g. **Halofantrine**

(1) Do not administer with drugs known to prolong the QTc interval; interaction with mefloquine further prolongs the QTc interval.

(2) A sevenfold increase in peak plasma level and threefold increase in the area under the curve (AUC) occurred when given with high-fat food. Similar increases occur when doses are administered 2 hr after a meal. Administer halofantrine on an empty stomach.

> **h. Malarone**
>> **(1)** Concomitant administration with tetracycline has been associated with 40% reduction in plasma concentrations of atovaquone. Similarly, concurrent rifampin is known to reduce atovaquone levels by 50%.
>> **(2)** Take malarone with food or milk.

C. Amebicides and trichomonacides. These agents are crucial in the treatment of amebiasis, giardiasis, and trichomoniases—the most common protozoal infections in the United States. The major amebicides include **diloxanide, iodoquinol (Yodoxin), metronidazole (Flagyl), nitazoxanide (Alinia), paromomycin (Humatin), quinacrine,** and **tinidazole (Tindamax).**

1. Mechanism of action
   a. Diloxanide, a dichloroacetamide derivative, is **amebicidal;** its mechanism of action is unknown. (Not available commercially but can be compounded by Panorama Compounding Pharmacy, Van Nuys, CA—per Medical Letter 8/04.)
   b. Metronidazole is a synthetic compound with direct **amebicidal** and **trichomonacidal** action; it works at both intestinal and extraintestinal sites. Its mechanism of action involves disruption of the helical structure of DNA.
   c. Nitazoxanide is designated by the U.S. Food and Drug Administration (FDA) as an orphan drug. Its antiprotozoal activity is believed to be the result of interference with the pyruvate: ferredoxin oxidoreductase (PFOR) enzyme-dependent electron transfer reaction essential for energy metabolism.
   d. Quinacrine is an acridine derivative that inhibits DNA metabolism.
   e. Iodoquinol is a luminal or contact amebicide that is effective against the trophozoites of *Entamoeba histolytica* located in the lumen of the large intestine.
   f. Paromomycin is a poorly absorbed amebicidal aminoglycoside whose mechanism of action parallels other aminoglycosides (i.e., protein synthesis inhibitor). It is also effective against enteric bacteria *Salmonella* and *Shigella.*
   g. Tinidazole precise mechanism of action is unknown.

2. Spectrum of activity and therapeutic uses
   a. Diloxanide
      (1) This drug is used to treat asymptomatic carriers of amebic and *Giardia* cysts.
      (2) Diloxanide is therapeutic for invasive and extraintestinal amebiasis (given in combination with a systemic or mixed amebicide).
      (3) Diloxanide is not effective as single-agent therapy for extraintestinal amebiasis.
   b. Metronidazole
      (1) This agent is the preferred drug in amebic dysentery, giardiasis, and trichomoniasis.
      (2) Metronidazole also is active against all anaerobic cocci and gram-negative anaerobic bacilli.
      (3) This agent is the treatment of choice by the CDC for the treatment of *C. difficile* colitis infections owing to the emerging use of broad-spectrum antibiotics. This therapy is cost-effective.
   c. Quinacrine is useful in the treatment of giardiasis and tapeworms (see VIII.H.2).
   d. Iodoquinol is indicated for treatment of intestinal amebiasis. It is active against the protozoa *E. histolytica.*
   e. Nitazoxanide is indicated for treatment of diarrhea caused by *Cryptosporidium parvum* and *Giardia lamblia* in children.
   f. Paromomycin is indicated for acute and chronic intestinal amebiasis; it is not useful for extraintestinal amebiasis because it is not absorbed. Paromomycin has been used for *Dientamoeba fragilis, Taenia saginata, Dipylidium caninum,* and *Hymenolepis nana.*
   g. Tinidazole is a second-generation synthetic nitroimidazole active against trichomoniasis, *Giardia duodenalis/G. lamblia, and E. histolytica.*

3. Precautions and monitoring effects
   a. Diloxanide rarely causes serious adverse effects. Vomiting, flatulence, and pruritus have been reported.
   b. Metronidazole
      (1) The most common adverse effects of this drug are nausea, epigastric distress, and diarrhea.
      (2) Metronidazole is carcinogenic in mice and should not be used unnecessarily.
      (3) Headache, vomiting, metallic taste, and stomatitis have been reported.

(4) Occasionally, neurological reactions (e.g., ataxia, peripheral neuropathy, seizures) develop.

(5) A disulfiram-type reaction may occur with concurrent ethanol use.

c. Quinacrine. See VIII.H.4.

(1) This drug frequently causes dizziness, headache, nausea, and vomiting. Nervousness and seizures also have been reported.

(2) Quinacrine should not be taken in combination with primaquine because this may increase primaquine toxicity.

(3) Quinacrine should be administered with extreme caution in patients with psoriasis because it may cause marked exacerbation of this disease.

d. Iodoquinol may produce optic neuritis or atrophy or peripheral neuropathy with high-dose, long-term use. Protein-bound iodine levels may be increased during treatment and may interfere with the results of thyroid tests for 6 months after treatment. Iodoquinol should not be used in patients who are hypersensitive to 8-hydroxy-quinolone (e.g., iodoquinol, iodochlorhydroxyquin) or iodine-containing agents or in patients with hepatic disorders.

e. Paromomycin may cause nausea, cramping, and diarrhea at high doses (> 3 g/day). Inadvertent absorption through ulcerative bowel lesions may result in ototoxicity or renal damage.

f. Nitazoxanide may cause abdominal pain, diarrhea, vomiting, headache, flatulence, fever, eye discoloration, rhinitis, and discolored urine.

g. Tinidazole may produce metallic taste, nausea, anorexia, dyspepsia, vomiting, weakness, dizziness, and headache.

D. Pentamidine isethionate (Pentam 300) is an aromatic diamide antiprotozoal agent. It can be administered intramuscularly, intravenously, or by inhalation.

1. Mechanism of action is not fully understood, but in vitro studies indicate interference with nuclear metabolism and inhibition of DNA, RNA, phospholipid, and protein synthesis.

2. Therapeutic uses

a. Pentamidine is indicated for the prevention and treatment of infections caused by *P. carinii.*

b. Unlabeled uses include treatment of trypanosomiasis, visceral leishmaniasis, and babesiosis.

3. Precautions and monitoring effects

a. Nephrotoxicity, bronchospasm, and cough are the most common effects produced by intravenous or inhaled pentamidine.

b. Severe hypotension may occur after a parenteral dose of pentamidine. Cardiorespiratory arrest can occur after a single rapid infusion of the drug.

c. Pain, erythema, and tenderness may occur after an IM administration of the drug. This can be minimized by using the Z-track technique of drug administration. Phlebitis may occur following IV administration.

d. Hypoglycemia may occur with initial administration of drug via the IV, IM, or inhalational route. After the patient has been on the drug for a period of time, hyperglycemia will result. The effect of the drug may actually induce a reversible insulin-dependent diabetes mellitus.

e. Leukopenia and thrombocytopenia, which can be severe, occur occasionally.

f. Pentamidine may result in elevated liver function tests, AST, and ALT.

g. GI effects can also occur, including nausea, vomiting, abdominal discomfort, pain, diarrhea, and dysgeusia.

h. Neurological effects can occur with parenteral administration and may include dizziness, tremors, confusion, anxiety, insomnia, and seizures.

i. Hypocalcemia and fever have also been reported and may be severe at times.

E. Atovaquone (Mepron) is a hydroxynaphthoquinone initially synthesized as an antimalarial drug.

1. Mechanism of action. Atovaquone blocks mitochondrial electron transport at complex III of the respiratory chain of protozoa, resulting in inhibition of pyrimidine synthesis.

2. Spectrum of activity. It is active against *P. carinii, T. gondii, C. parvum, P. falciparum, Isosporidia,* and *Microsporidia.*

3. **Therapeutic uses.** Atovaquone is used for second-line treatment of mild to moderate *P. carinii* pneumonia in patients intolerant of cotrimoxazole or other sulfonamides or who are nonresponsive to cotrimoxazole.

4. **Precautions and monitoring effects**
   a. Oral absorption significantly increases when administered with food (especially a high-fat meal).
   b. Rash, nausea, diarrhea, headache, fever, abdominal pain, dizziness, and elevated liver function tests commonly are reported.

5. **Significant interactions.** Atovaquone is highly bound to plasma protein. It should be used with caution when administered with other highly protein-bound drugs with a narrow therapeutic range.

F. **Eflornithine HCl (Ornidyl).** This is an IV antiprotozoal agent. Its activity has been attributed to the inhibition of the enzyme ornithine decarboxylase.

1. **Mechanism of action.** This is a specific, enzyme-activated, irreversible inhibitor of ornithine decarboxylase.

2. **Spectrum of activity and therapeutic uses.** Eflornithine is active in the treatment of the meningoencephalitic stage of *Trypanosoma brucei gambiense* (sleeping sickness).

3. **Precautions and monitoring effects**
   a. Myelosuppression is the most frequent serious side effect.
   b. Seizures occur in about 8% of treated patients.
   c. Cases of hearing impairment have been reported.

VI. Antitubercular Agents

A. **Definition and classification.** Drugs used to treat tuberculosis suppress or kill the slow-growing mycobacteria that cause this disease. Antitubercular agents fall into two main categories: first-line and second-line drugs. Because the causative organisms tend to develop resistance to any single drug, combination drug therapy has become standard in the treatment of tuberculosis.

1. The **incidence** of tuberculosis in the United States is increasing owing to shifts in populations considered to be endemic for tuberculosis, the rise in HIV-positive patients, and drug resistance.

2. Agents chosen for **therapy** must eradicate mycobacterium. First-line agents available include isoniazid, ethambutol, pyrazinamide, rifampin, rifabutin, and rifapentine. **Combination chemotherapy** is essential. Agents showing the lowest incidence of resistance (isoniazid, rifampin) are usually used in combination with pyrazinamide or ethambutol.

3. Choice of therapy depends on many patient and disease factors (e.g., duration of therapy needed, likelihood of drug resistance, and HIV status).

4. **Treatment choices based on CDC recommendations** (Table 44-4).

B. **First-line.** These drugs, isoniazid, ethambutol, rifampin, rifabutin, rifapentine, and pyrazinamide usually offer the greatest effectiveness with the least toxicity; they are successful in most tuberculosis patients. At least three to four drug combinations are recommended. The CDC recommends daily treatment with isoniazid, rifampin, pyrazinamide, and ethambutol for the initial phase of 2 months, followed by a continuation phase of isoniazid and rifampin for 4–5 months (Table 44-4).

1. **Ethambutol (Myambutol)** is a synthetic water-based compound.
   a. **Mechanism of action.** This drug is **bacteriostatic.** Its precise mechanism of action is unknown; however, it has demonstrated activity only against susceptible bacteria actively undergoing cell division.
   b. **Spectrum of activity and therapeutic uses.** Ethambutol is active against many *M. tuberculosis* strains as well as many other mycobacterial species. However, drug resistance develops fairly rapidly when it is used alone. In most cases, ethambutol is given adjunctively in combination with isoniazid or rifampin for tuberculosis. It is also useful in

Table 44-4. Treatment for Active Tuberculosis

		Initial Phase		Continuation Phase	
Rank	Agent	Dosage	Agent	Dosage	
1	INH RIF PZA EMB	7 days a week × 8 weeks *or* 5 days a week × 8 weeks	INH/RIF	7 days a week × 18 weeks *or* 5 days a week × 18 weeks	
2	INH RIF PZA EMP	7 days a week × 2 weeks, *then* 2 times a week × 6 weeks *or* 5 days a week × 2 weeks, *then* 2 times a week × 6 weeks	INH/RIF	2 times a week × 18 weeks	
3	INH RIF PZA EMB	3 times a week × 8 weeks	INH/RIF	3 times a week × 19 weeks	
4	INH RIF EMP	7 days a week × 8 weeks *or* 5 days a week × 8 weeks	INH/RIF	7 days a week × 31 weeks *or* 5 days a week × 31 weeks *or* 2 times a week × 31 weeks	

EMB, ethambutol; *INH,* isoniazid; *PZA,* pyrazinamide; *RIF,* rifampin.
Adapted with permission from CDC guidelines for treatment of tuberculosis 2003. MMWR 2003; 52 (RR11); 1–77.

combination with other agents such as clarithromycin or azithromycin and rifabutin in treating MAC.

    c. Precautions and monitoring effects. Rarely, ethambutol causes such adverse effects as reversible dose-related (= 15 mg/kg/day) optic neuritis, drug fever, abdominal pain, headache, dizziness, and confusion. Liver function tests should be periodically monitored. Visual testing and renal function (reduce dose with impairment) should also be monitored.

2. Isoniazid (Nydrazid) is a hydrazide of isonicotinic acid. The mainstay of antitubercular therapy, this drug should be included (if tolerated) in all therapeutic regimens.

    a. Mechanism of action. Isoniazid is **bacteriostatic** for resting bacilli and **bactericidal** for rapidly dividing organisms. Its mechanism of action is not fully known; the drug probably disrupts bacterial cell wall synthesis by inhibiting mycolic acid synthesis.

    b. Spectrum of activity. Isoniazid has activity only against organisms in the genus *Mycobacterium.* More specifically, it has demonstrated activity against *M. tuberculosis, Mycobacterium bovis,* and select strains of *Mycobacterium kansasii.*

    c. Therapeutic uses

        (1) The most widely used antitubercular agent, isoniazid should be given in combination with other antitubercular drugs (such as rifampin, ethambutol, and pyrazinamide) to prevent drug resistance in tuberculosis.

        (2) Treatment of latent infection (previously referred to as preventive therapy of chemoprophylaxis). Isoniazid may be administered alone for up to 1 year in adults or children who have a positive tuberculin test result but lack active lesions.

    d. Precautions and monitoring effects

        (1) The most common adverse effects of isoniazid are skin rash, fever, jaundice, and peripheral neuritis.

        (2) Hepatitis, an occasional reaction, can be severe and, in some cases, fatal. The risk of hepatitis increases with the patient's age and rises with alcohol abuse. Monitor liver function tests.

        (3) Blood dyscrasias (e.g., agranulocytosis, aplastic or hemolytic anemia, thrombocytopenia) may occur. Monitor complete blood count (CBC) routinely.

        (4) Adverse GI effects include nausea, vomiting, and epigastric distress.

        (5) CNS toxicity may result from pyridoxine deficiency. Signs and symptoms include insomnia, restlessness, hyperreflexia, and convulsions. Pyridoxine 15–50 mg/day should be administered to patients taking isoniazid to minimize the peripheral neuropathy associated with its use (especially in patients with diabetes, HIV, uremia, alcoholism, malnutrition, pregnancy, or seizure disorder).

   e. Significant interactions

     (1) With concurrent **phenytoin** therapy, blood levels of both phenytoin and isoniazid may increase, possibly causing toxicity.

     (2) **Aluminum-containing antacids** may reduce isoniazid absorption.

     (3) Concurrent **carbamazepine** therapy may increase the risk of hepatitis.

     (4) Use of isoniazid with other antitubercular agents, such as cycloserine or ethionamide, may cause additive nervous system effects.

     (5) There is the potential for the serotonin syndrome to exist when isoniazid is used in combination with selective serotonin reuptake inhibitors or in patients taking meperidine. Isoniazid has been shown to have some monoamine oxidase (MAO) inhibiting activity.

3. Rifampin (Rimactane) is a complex macrocyclic agent.

   a. Mechanism of action. This drug is **bactericidal;** it impairs bacterial RNA synthesis by binding to DNA-dependent RNA polymerase.

   b. Spectrum of activity. Rifampin has activity against most mycobacterial strains. In addition, rifampin has activity against many other organisms, including *N. meningitidis, S. aureus, H. influenzae, Legionella pneumophila,* and *C. trachomatis.*

   c. Therapeutic uses

     (1) In recommended combinations for treatment of active tuberculosis

     (2) Prophylactic rifampin is effective when administered to carriers of *N. meningitidis* disease and chemoprophylaxis of patients with *H. influenzae* type b organisms.

     (3) Rifampin may be used in combination with dapsone for the treatment of leprosy.

   d. Precautions and monitoring effects

     (1) Serious hepatotoxicity may result from rifampin therapy. Liver function tests should be routinely conducted.

     (2) In rare cases, this drug induces an influenza-like syndrome.

     (3) Other adverse effects include skin rash, drowsiness, headache, fatigue, confusion, nausea, vomiting, and abdominal pain.

     (4) Rifampin colors urine, sweat, tears, saliva, and feces orange red.

   e. Significant interactions

     (1) Rifampin induces hepatic microsomal cytochrome P450 isoenzymes and thus may decrease the therapeutic effectiveness of **corticosteroids, warfarin, oral contraceptives, quinidine, digitoxin, protease inhibitors (PIs), nonnucleoside reverse transcriptase inhibitors, ketoconazole, verapamil, methadone, oral antidiabetic agents, cyclosporine, dapsone, chloramphenicol,** and **barbiturates.**

     (2) **Probenecid** may increase blood levels of rifampin.

     (3) **Aminosalicylic acid** may impair absorption of rifampin secondary to bentonite, an excipient used in preparation of aminosalicylic granules.

   f. The newer rifamycins, **rifabutin (Mycobutin)** and **rifapentine (Priftin)** may be substituted for rifampin in speciali situations, e.g., intolerance or serious drug interactions.

4. Rifabutin (Mycobutin) is an antimycobacterial agent that is similar to rifampin, with activity against both tubercular and nontubercular mycobacterial, and offers no clear advantage over rifampin.

   a. Mechanism of action. In addition to its antimycobacterial activity against tubercular and nontubercular mycobacterial, rifabutin has been reported to inhibit reverse transcriptase and block the in vitro infectivity and replication of HIV.

   b. Therapeutic uses. Rifabutin is indicated for the prevention of disseminated MAI complex disease in patients with advanced HIV infections.

   c. Precautions and monitoring effects. The use of rifabutin has resulted in mild elevation of liver enzymes and thrombocytopenia.

   d. Significant interactions

     (1) Rifabutin antagonizes and potentially negates the immune response mediated by the bacillus Calmette-Guérin (BCG) vaccine.

     (2) Rifabutin may increase the clearance of drugs by inducing hepatic microsomal enzymes, but does so to a lesser extent than rifampin. The concentrations of the following drugs may be reduced while taking rifabutin: **cyclosporine, zidovudine,**

prednisone, digitoxin, quinidine, ketoconazole, protease inhibitors, propranolol, phenytoin, sulfonylureas, and warfarin. Serum cyclosporine levels should be monitored in patients receiving both agents.

5. **Rifapentine (Priftin)** is a long-acting rifamycin-derivative and has a similar profile of microbiological activity to rifampin. It is usually administered once or twice weekly.
   a. **Mechanism of action.** Rifapentine is bactericidal against intracellular and extracellular *M. tuberculosis* at therapeutic levels.
   b. **Spectrum of activity and therapeutic uses.** Indicated for treatment of primary tuberculosis. Rifapentine should always be used in conjunction with ≥ 1 other antituberculosis drug to which the isolate is susceptible.
   c. **Precautions and monitoring effects.** Rifapentine induces cytochrome P450 isoenzymes 3A4 and 2C8/9 responsible for inactivation of certain calcium channel blocking agents (verapamil, diltiazem, nifedipine), antifungals (ketoconazole, fluconazole, itraconazole), sulfonylurea antidiabetic agents, methadone, corticosteroids, cardiac glycosides, certain antiarrhythmic agents (disopyramide, mexiletine, quinidine, tocainide), quinine, dapsone, chloramphenicol, clarithromycin, doxycycline, fluoroquinolones, transcriptase inhibitor cyclosporin, tacrolimus, and warfarin. Concomitant use of rifapentine with these drugs may decrease plasma concentrations and dosage adjustments may be required.

6. **Pyrazinamide** is a pyrazine analog of nicotinamide.
   a. **Mechanism of action.** This drug is **bactericidal** and/or **bacteriostatic,** depending on the cell concentration achieved.
   b. **Spectrum of activity and therapeutic uses.** Pyrazinamide is a highly specific agent and has activity only against *M. tuberculosis.* Pyrazinamide is used as a primary agent with isoniazid and rifampin for at least 2 months, followed by isoniazid and rifampin.
   c. **Precautions and monitoring effects.** This agent may result in hepatotoxicity and, rarely, hepatic necrosis resulting in death. Anorexia, nausea, vomiting, malaise, and fever have been reported. Hyperuricemia may result in gouty exacerbations. Both liver function tests and uric acid levels should routinely be monitored.

C. **Second-line agents.** These agents include aminosalicylic acid **(Paser)**, capreomycin **(Capastat)**, cycloserine **(Seromycin)**, ethionamide **(Trecator-SC)**, quinolones (ciprofloxacin, ofloxacin, levofloxacin, sparfloxacin), streptomycin and kanamycin. Second-line drugs are mainly substituted or added to preferred therapy owing to intolerance or drug resistance. These agents are less effective, more toxic, and are used in combination with primary agents.

1. **Mechanism of action**
   a. **Aminosalicylic acid** is **bacteriostatic;** it probably inhibits the enzymes responsible for folic acid synthesis.
   b. **Cycloserine** can be **bacteriostatic** or **bactericidal,** depending on its concentration at the infection site; it impairs amino acid use, thereby inhibiting bacterial cell wall synthesis.
   c. The mechanism of action of capreomycin (**bacteriostatic**), ethionamide (**bactericidal**), and pyrazinamide (**bactericidal**) is unknown.

2. **Spectrum of activity and therapeutic uses.** Second-line antitubercular agents are active against various microorganisms, including *M. tuberculosis.* These agents generally are reserved for patients with extensive extrapulmonary or drug-resistant disease or for patients who need retreatment. These drugs are almost always administered in combination.

3. **Precautions and monitoring effects**
   a. Adverse effects of **aminosalicylic acid** include leukopenia, agranulocytopenia, thrombocytopenia, hemolytic anemia, mononucleosis-like syndrome, malaise, joint pain, fever, and skin rash.
   b. **Capreomycin** and **streptomycin** are ototoxic and nephrotoxic; they should not be administered together.
   c. **Cycloserine** may cause adverse CNS effects, including headache, suicidal and psychotic tendencies, hyperirritability, confusion, paranoia, and nervousness.
   d. **Ethionamide** may induce nausea, vomiting, orthostatic hypotension, metallic taste, epigastric distress, and peripheral neuropathy.
   e. **Streptomycin.** See II.B.3.

D. Alternative agents

1. **Rifater.** A combination of rifampin 120 mg, isoniazid 50 mg, and pyrazinamide 300 mg in one tablet is used in patients expected to have low compliance with tuberculosis drug therapy. One **disadvantage** is that many patients are required to take as many as 5–6 tablets daily, which may reduce compliance.

2. **Quinolones.** Ciprofloxacin and levofloxacin are used in tuberculosis therapy. Levofloxacin is preferred owing to increased serum concentrations. Levofloxacin is usually used in combination with other tuberculosis agents for active treatment. For prophylaxis, levofloxacin is combined with pyrazinamide.

3. **Macrolides.** Clarithromycin and azithromycin have shown limited activity against *M. tuberculosis.*

VII. Antiviral Agents

A. Definition. These drugs treat viral infections by affecting viral replication. Because viruses lack independent metabolic activity and can replicate only within living host cells, antiviral agents tend to injure host as well as viral cells. Although most antiviral drugs are active against either DNA or RNA viruses, some (e.g., adefovir, ribavirin) are active against both.

B. DNA viruses. Currently approved antiviral therapies against the *Herpesviridae* family of DNA viruses—herpes simplex virus 1 and 2 (HSV-1, HSV-2), varicella-zoster virus (VZV), cytomegalovirus (CMV)—are **virustatic** and arrest DNA synthesis by inhibiting viral DNA polymerase. Many of these agents are prodrugs and require viral and host cellular enzymes (e.g., thymidine, deoxyguanosine kinase) to phosphorylate them into the active triphosphate form before exerting their antiviral activity. Hence, a common mechanism of resistance is a deficiency or structural alteration in viral thymidine kinase (Table 44-5). Some of these agents also demonstrate activity against RNA viruses, including hepatitis C and HIV.

1. **Acyclovir** (Zovirax) is a synthetic acyclic analog of guanosine with activity against various herpes viruses.
   a. **Mechanism of action.** Acyclovir monophosphate is phosphorylated to the triphosphate, where it becomes incorporated into viral DNA and inhibits viral replication.
   b. **Spectrum of activity.** This agent is active against herpes viruses, particularly HSV-1, HSV-2, VZV, and chickenpox (varicella).
   c. **Therapeutic uses**
      (1) Acyclovir is used to treat initial and recurrent HSV-1 and HSV-2 infections and for acute treatment of herpes zoster (shingles) and chickenpox.
      (2) This agent is available in topical, oral, and IV forms. Topical acyclovir is applied directly on herpes lesions in recurrent herpes labialis (cold sores). It is not recommended for use on genital herpes lesions due to poor efficacy.

Table 44-5. Activity of Various Anti-DNA Viral Agents

Agent	HSV-1	HSV-2	VZV	CMV	Influenza A	Influenza B
Acyclovir[a]	+	+	+	—	—	—
Amantadine	—	—	—	—	+	—
Cidofovir	—	—	—	+	—	—
Famciclovir	+	+	+	—	—	—
Foscarnet	+	+	+	+	—	—
Ganciclovir[a]	—	—	—	+	—	—
Oseltamivir	—	—	—	—	+	+
Rimantadine	—	—	—	—	+	—
Valacyclovir[a]	+	+	+	—	—	—
Valganciclovir[a]	—	—	—	+	—	—
Zanamivir	—	—	—	—	+	+

HSV, herpes simplex virus, *VZV,* varicella-zoster virus; *CMV,* cytomegalovirus.
[a]Requires activation into triphosphate form.

(3) Acyclovir may be administered intravenously in the treatment of initial and recurrent mucocutaneous HSV infection and VZV infection in immunocompromised patients, as well as in the treatment of HSV infections of the central nervous system.

  d. Precautions and monitoring effects

    (1) Oral acyclovir may induce nausea, vomiting, diarrhea, and headache.

    (2) IV administration may cause dose-dependent renal impairment, crystalline nephropathy, neurological effects (e.g., lethargy, confusion, tremors, agitation, seizures, coma, obtundation), hypotension, rash, itching, and phlebitis at the injection site.

    (3) Local discomfort and pruritus may result from topical administration.

    (4) Acyclovir is removed by hemodialysis. Doses should be adjusted in renal impairment and hemodialysis.

  e. Significant interactions. Probenecid reduces the renal clearance of acyclovir, resulting in increases in acyclovir half-life and serum concentration.

2. Adefovir dipivoxil (Hepsera) is a phosphonate nucleoside analog with activity against various DNA and RNA viruses.

  a. Mechanism of action. Adefovir is phosphorylated to the active diphosphate form by cellular kinases. It is then incorporated into viral DNA, resulting in termination of replication.

  b. Spectrum of activity and therapeutic uses

    (1) Adefovir is active against hepatitis B virus (including lamivudine-resistant strains), herpes viruses, and HIV.

    (2) However, adefovir is approved for use only for treatment of chronic hepatitis B infection in adults with evidence of active viral replication with persistently elevated liver function tests or histologically active disease.

  c. Precautions and monitoring effects

    (1) Severe acute hepatitis exacerbations have occurred in patients who discontinue therapy (**black box warning**). If therapy is discontinued, liver function tests must be monitored closely.

    (2) Nephrotoxicity has been reported with adefovir, especially in patients with underlying renal dysfunction or those taking concomitant nephrotoxins (**black box warning**).

    (3) Other adverse effects include rash, GI disturbances, headache, and weakness.

    (4) Dose adjustment is required for renal insufficiency.

3. Amantadine (Symmetrel) is a synthetic tricyclic amine with a unique chemical structure similar to rimantadine. It is effective against influenza A viral infection.

  a. Mechanism of action. Amantadine inhibits replication of the influenza A virus by interfering with viral attachment and uncoating.

  b. Spectrum of activity and therapeutic uses

    (1) Amantadine is effective in the prophylaxis and treatment of influenza A virus strains only (not influenza B virus). However, an annual influenza virus vaccine is considered first line for prophylactic therapy.

    (2) Clinicians recommend that all nonimmunized high-risk patients receive this drug at the first sign of community influenza A activity.

    (3) Suppressive therapy should continue for 24–48 hr after influenza symptoms disappear or, if necessary, up to 90 days for repeated exposure to the virus.

    (4) This drug may also be used to treat parkinsonism as well as drug-induced extrapyramidal symptoms.

  c. Precautions and monitoring effects

    (1) The most pronounced adverse effects of amantadine are ataxia, nightmares, and insomnia. Other CNS effects include depression, confusion, dizziness, fatigue, anxiety, and headache. Elderly patients may be at increased risk of CNS adverse reactions. Patients with a history of seizures or psychiatric disorders should be monitored closely during therapy.

    (2) Anticholinergic reactions (e.g., dry mouth, blurred vision) have been reported.

    (3) Dosage adjustment is needed for patients with impaired renal function.

4. Cidofovir (Vistide) is a synthetic acyclic purine nucleoside phosphonate derivative.

  a. Mechanism of action. Cidofovir diphosphate suppresses CMV replication by selective inhibition of viral DNA synthesis.

b. Spectrum of activity. In vitro activity has been demonstrated against CMV, VZV, Epstein-Barr virus (EBV), and HSV-1 and HSV-2. Controlled clinical studies are limited to patients with AIDS and CMV retinitis.

c. Therapeutic use includes the treatment, but not the cure of, CMV retinitis in patients with AIDS.

d. Precautions and monitoring effects

(1) Avoid using this drug in patients with serum creatinine > 1.5 mg/dL or creatinine clearance (CrCl) < 55 mL/min.

(2) Cidofovir is contraindicated in patients with a history of severe hypersensitivity to probenecid or sulfa-containing medications.

(3) The dose-limiting toxicity of cidofovir is **nephrotoxicity;** neutropenia, peripheral neuropathy, and diarrhea are common adverse effects.

(4) Probenecid must be administered before and after each cidofovir dose. The patient must be hydrated with 1 L of normal saline before infusing. Cidofovir is available only in IV form.

5. Entecavir (Baraclude) is a carbocyclic analog of guanosine used for treatment of chronic hepatitis B infection.

a. Mechanism of action. Once phosphorylated to the active triphosphate form, entecavir inhibits hepatitis B viral polymerase and ultimately halts hepatitis B DNA synthesis.

b. Spectrum of activity. Entecavir exhibits activity against hepatitis B virus, including lamivudine-resistant strains. It does not demonstrate activity against HIV.

c. Therapeutic uses

(1) Entecavir is approved for treatment of chronic hepatitis B infection in adults with evidence of active viral replication and persistent elevations in liver function tests or histologically active disease.

(2) It is effective for patients who have failed treatment with lamivudine owing to resistance development.

d. Precautions and monitoring effects

(1) Severe acute exacerbations of hepatitis B have been observed in patients who discontinue therapy, necessitating close monitoring (**black box warning**).

(2) Common adverse effects include dizziness, fatigue, headache, and nausea.

(3) Dose adjustment is required for renal insufficiency.

(4) Counsel patients to take entecavir on an empty stomach.

6. Famciclovir (Famvir) is a prodrug of the antiviral agent penciclovir.

a. Mechanism of action. Famciclovir is rapidly phosphorylated in virus-infected cells by viral thymidine kinase to penciclovir monophosphate. Penciclovir is a competitive inhibitor of viral DNA polymerase and prevents viral replication by inhibition of herpes virus DNA synthesis.

b. Spectrum of activity and therapeutic uses

(1) Famciclovir has activity against HSV-1, HSV-2, and VZV. The drug is indicated for management of acute herpes zoster (shingles) and oral and genital herpes.

(2) Therapy must be promptly initiated as soon as herpes zoster or genital herpes is diagnosed (within 48–72 hr), at a dose of 500 mg every 8 hr for 7 days. Treatment is for 5–7 days only.

c. Precautions and monitoring effects

(1) **Common adverse events** include fatigue, GI complaints (nausea, diarrhea, vomiting, constipation), and anorexia. Headache is also commonly reported.

(2) Dose adjustment is necessary in patients with renal dysfunction. Famciclovir is removed by hemodialysis.

7. Foscarnet (Foscavir) is a synthetic pyrophosphate analog that directly inhibits enzymes involved in viral DNA synthesis without incorporation into viral DNA. It is a broad-spectrum antiviral agent and is the drug of choice in cases of acyclovir or ganciclovir resistance.

a. Mechanism of action

(1) Viral DNA replication requires the addition of deoxynucleoside triphosphates at the end of the DNA strand by DNA polymerase and the subsequent cleavage of pyrophosphate from the newly attached nucleotide. Foscarnet binds noncompetitively to DNA polymerase to form an inactive complex and prevents pyrophosphate cleavage. Viral DNA chain elongation is thus terminated.

(2) Foscarnet is also active against HIV. It is a noncompetitive, reversible inhibitor of HIV reverse transcriptase, the enzyme responsible for converting viral RNA to viral DNA.

b. Spectrum of activity and therapeutic uses. Foscarnet has in vitro activity against HSV-1 and HSV-2, CMV, VZV, EBV DNA polymerases, influenza polymerase, and HIV reverse transcriptase. Therapeutically, the drug is used to treat CMV disease as well as acyclovir-resistant HSV and VZV infections.

   (1) Foscarnet is an alternative to ganciclovir and valganciclovir for treatment of CMV infection in immunocompromised patients. Foscarnet causes less hematologic toxicity than ganciclovir in patients who have received allogeneic stem cell transplants. An initial induction therapy lasts 2–3 weeks. Maintenance therapy within 1 month after induction may be needed to prevent relapse.

   (2) Foscarnet is indicated for the treatment of acyclovir-resistant mucocutaneous HSV in immunocompromised patients. It is not, however, a cure for HSV infections.

   (3) Foscarnet is able to cross the blood–brain barrier.

c. Precautions and monitoring effects

   (1) IV foscarnet is highly **nephrotoxic**, causing acute tubular necrosis. The incidence of acute renal failure can be markedly reduced if adequate hydration and daily monitoring of serum creatinine and BUN are maintained throughout therapy.

   (2) Other common adverse effects include electrolyte abnormalities (e.g., hypocalcemia, hypomagnesemia, hypophosphatemia and hyperphosphatemia, hypokalemia), anemia, fever, headache, and seizures.

   (3) Dose adjustment for renal dysfunction is required. Foscarnet is removed by hemodialysis.

   (4) Foscarnet must be administered using an infusion pump over at least 1–2 hr. Do not administer the drug as an IV bolus.

d. Significant interactions

   (1) Concomitant **cyclosporine** increases the risk of renal toxicity.

   (2) Foscarnet is exclusively eliminated by glomerular filtration; concurrent nephrotoxic agents should be avoided whenever possible.

8. Ganciclovir (Cytovene) is a synthetic purine nucleoside analog that is approved for the treatment and prophylaxis of CMV infections in immunocompromised patients (e.g., HIV-positive patients, transplant recipients).

a. Mechanism of action. After conversion to ganciclovir triphosphate, ganciclovir is incorporated into viral DNA, which inhibits viral DNA polymerase, thereby terminating viral replication.

b. Spectrum of activity. Ganciclovir has in vitro activity against HSV-1 and HSV-2, VZV, EBV, and CMV (owing to its enhanced ability to penetrate host cells).

c. Therapeutic uses. It is indicated for treatment of CMV infections, such as colitis, pneumonia, esophagitis, and retinitis. It is also indicated for prophylaxis of CMV infection in HIV-positive patients (secondary prophylaxis) and transplant recipients.

   (1) Conversion into the triphosphate form is greater in infected host cells, even though drug penetration occurs in both uninfected and infected cells.

   (2) Inhibitory concentrations for the viral DNA polymerase are lower than those for the host cellular polymerase.

   (3) It is available in oral and IV formulations as well as an intraocular implant. Although the oral formulation is approved for prevention and maintenance treatment of CMV, its poor bioavailability has limited its use. Valganciclovir has become the drug of choice for these indications, owing to its markedly improved bioavailability.

d. Precautions and monitoring effects

   (1) Ganciclovir has **black box warnings** concerning increased potential for neutropenia, anemia, and thrombocytopenia. It is also teratogenic, carcinogenic, and mutagenic.

   (2) Adverse effects commonly include fever, rash, and GI disturbances. Phlebitis and pain may occur at the site of infusion.

   (3) Because ganciclovir is cleared by glomerular filtration and tubular secretion, renal function and adequate hydration should be monitored. Doses should be adjusted in cases of renal impairment and hemodialysis.

   (4) Solutions of ganciclovir are extremely alkaline. Avoid direct contact with skin.

  e. Significant interactions
  (1) Probenecid may increase ganciclovir concentrations and possibly toxicity.
  (2) Use of **zidovudine, azathioprine,** or **mycophenolate mofetil** in combination with ganciclovir may result in neutropenia; careful monitoring of neutrophil count is required when these are taken concurrently with ganciclovir.
  (3) Imipenem–cilastatin in combination with ganciclovir may increase the potential for seizures.

9. Oseltamivir (Tamiflu) is pharmacologically similar to zanamivir but structurally different. Both of these agents are in a class known as the neuraminidase inhibitors and have a unique mechanism of action.
  a. Mechanism of action. Oseltamivir is a prodrug that must be hydrolyzed to oseltamivir carboxylate in vivo to exert its antiviral activity. It is a potent selective inhibitor of the influenza virus enzyme, neuraminidase. Inhibition of this enzyme prevents viral replication and spread to other host cells.
  b. Spectrum of activity. This agent is active against both influenza A and B viruses.
  c. Therapeutic uses
  (1) It is approved for the symptomatic treatment of influenza A and B infections in adults who present with symptoms within 48 hr.
  (2) Oseltamivir has been shown to decrease the duration of symptoms by 1 day if taken within 48 hr of onset of viral symptoms.
  (3) It is also approved for the prophylaxis of influenza infections in patients 13 years of age and older. *Note:* The influenza virus vaccine is still the gold standard for prophylaxis.
  (4) Oseltamivir demonstrates some activity against strains of avian influenza, making it a possible option for treatment and prophylaxis.
  d. Precautions and monitoring effects
  (1) The most common adverse effects are nausea and vomiting, followed by vertigo and insomnia.
  (2) Dosage adjustments are required for patients with impaired renal function.
  (3) Cross-resistance between oseltamivir and zanamivir has been reported.

10. Ribavirin (Rebetol) is a synthetic nucleoside analog.
  a. Mechanism of action. Ribavirin may inhibit RNA and DNA synthesis by depleting intracellular nucleotide reserves.
  b. Spectrum of activity. This agent is active in vitro against a broad spectrum of DNA and RNA viruses, including influenza A and B, RSV, herpes simplex, and hepatitis C virus.
  c. Therapeutic uses. The aerosolized form of ribavirin is no longer recommended for treatment of RSV in infants and children, owing to inconsistent clinical benefits observed in clinical trials. Combination therapy with oral ribavirin and subcutaneous interferon-α is effective in treatment of chronic hepatitis C.
  d. Precautions and monitoring effects
  (1) Common adverse effects of oral ribavirin include anemia and GI disturbances. Hemoglobin and hematocrit should be monitored carefully, especially during the first 4 weeks of treatment.
  (2) Ribavirin is teratogenic; its use is contraindicated in pregnancy.
  (3) Ribavirin should be avoided in patients with a CrCl < 50 mL/min.
  (4) Ribavirin should never be used as monotherapy in treatment of chronic hepatitis C.

11. Rimantadine (Flumadine) is a synthetic antiviral agent and an α-methyl derivative of amantadine that blocks the early step in the replication of the influenza A virus.
  a. Mechanism of action. Rimantadine inhibits the early viral replication cycle, possibly inhibiting the uncoating of the virus. It has the same mechanism of action and spectrum of activity as amantadine.
  b. Spectrum of activity and therapeutic uses
  (1) Rimantadine is safe and effective in the prophylaxis and treatment of infections caused by various strains of influenza A virus in adults and for prophylaxis in adults and children > 1 year old.
  (2) The method of choice for prophylaxis against influenza is vaccination; however, in some cases, vaccine is contraindicated or not available.

(3) Rimantadine therapy should be considered for people who develop flu-like symptoms during influenza A season. Therapy should be initiated within 48 hr of onset of symptoms.

c. Precautions and monitoring effects

(1) Rimantadine may increase the incidence of seizure in patients with seizure disorder.

(2) The most frequent adverse reactions include GI disturbance (e.g., nausea, vomiting, anorexia) and CNS toxicity (e.g., insomnia, dizziness, headache), which are less than those observed with amantadine.

(3) Dose reductions are recommended in patients with hepatic or renal dysfunction.

12. Valacyclovir (Valcyte) is the L-valyl ester prodrug of the antiviral agent acyclovir.

a. Mechanism of action. Valacyclovir is rapidly converted to acyclovir. Acyclovir is selective for the thymidine kinase enzyme, beginning the conversion of acyclovir to acyclovir triphosphate, stopping the replication of herpes viral DNA.

b. Spectrum of activity and therapeutic uses

(1) Valacyclovir is active against HSV-1, HSV-2, and VZV.

(2) This agent is used for the acute treatment of herpes zoster (shingles), herpes labialis (cold sores), and genital herpes in immunocompetent adults. It is also effective for suppression of recurrent episodes of genital herpes as well as reduction of transmission of genital herpes.

(3) Advantages over acyclovir include oral dosing of only once to three times daily and attainment of higher plasma concentrations than oral acyclovir. A disadvantage is that there is no IV form available.

c. Precautions and monitoring effects

(1) Valacyclovir is not indicated for use in immunocompromised individuals (e.g., advanced HIV disease, transplant recipients) owing to the occurrence of thrombotic thrombocytopenic purpura/hemolytic uremic syndrome.

(2) Begin therapy within 72 hr of herpes zoster rash onset.

(3) Most commonly reported adverse reactions are mild and include nausea, headache, and vomiting. Dosage adjustment is needed in patients with renal dysfunction.

13. Valganciclovir (Valcyte) is the L-valyl ester prodrug of the antiviral agent ganciclovir.

a. Mechanism of action. Valganciclovir is converted in vivo to ganciclovir. After conversion to the active form, ganciclovir triphosphate, ganciclovir is incorporated into viral DNA, which inhibits viral DNA polymerase, thereby terminating viral replication.

b. Spectrum of activity and therapeutic uses

(1) For in vitro activity, see VII.B.8.b.

(2) Valganciclovir is indicated for the treatment of CMV retinitis in patients with AIDS and for prevention of CMV after transplantation.

(3) The markedly improved bioavailability of valganciclovir over oral ganciclovir has resulted in the widespread use of valganciclovir for treatment and prevention of CMV disease.

c. Precautions and monitoring effects

(1) Same **black box warnings** as for ganciclovir.

(2) Doses should be adjusted in cases of renal impairment. Do not use in hemodialysis patients; ganciclovir must be used.

(3) Only available orally. Do not substitute doses of oral valganciclovir 1:1 for oral ganciclovir; they are not equivalent.

(4) A potential carcinogen and teratogen; common adverse effects are the same as for ganciclovir.

(5) If the tablet is broken, avoid contact with skin owing to teratogenic and carcinogenic potential.

(6) Be aware of the potential for errors as a result of the look-alike and sound-alike names of valganciclovir and valacyclovir.

d. Significant interactions. Same as for ganciclovir; see VII.B.8.e.

14. Zanamivir (Relenza) is the first of a class of antiviral agents called neuraminidase inhibitors approved by the FDA for the treatment of influenza A and B infections in adults and children at least 7 years of age.

a. Mechanism of action. Zanamivir inhibits replication of the influenza A and B viruses by selective inhibition of the influenza virus neuraminidase enzyme.

    b. Spectrum of activity. This agent is active against both the influenza A and B viruses.

    c. Therapeutic uses

        (1) It is approved for the treatment of uncomplicated influenza A and B infection for patients who have been symptomatic for < 48 hr.

        (2) Zanamivir is approved for oral inhalation use only, using the Diskhaler device provided by the manufacturer.

        (3) Use for prophylaxis of influenza A or B is effective but has not been approved by the FDA.

        (4) Shown to decrease duration of symptoms by approximately 1.5 days if taken within 48 hr of onset of viral symptoms.

    d. Precautions and monitoring effects

        (1) The use of zanamivir is generally not recommended in patients with a history of asthma or chronic obstructive pulmonary disease, owing to the risk of bronchospasm and acute decline in lung function.

        (2) The most common adverse effects were mild and included diarrhea, nausea, and vomiting. The incidence of these was no different than placebo.

        (3) Do not puncture the Rotadisk blister until immediately before administering the dose to ensure full dosage. Manual dexterity required for this device.

C. RNA viruses (HIV)

  1. Currently, four classes of antiretroviral agents are approved. These drugs are active against HIV and include the nucleoside reverse transcriptase inhibitors (NRTIs) **abacavir, didanosine, emtricitabine, lamivudine, stavudine, zalcitabine,** and **zidovudine;** the nucleotide reverse transcriptase inhibitor (NtRTI) **tenofovir disoproxil fumarate;** the nonnucleoside reverse transcriptase inhibitors (NNRTIs) **delavirdine, efavirenz,** and **nevirapine;** the fusion inhibitor **enfuvirtide;** and the PIs **amprenavir, atazanavir, darunavir fosamprenavir, indinavir, lopinavir/ritonavir, nelfinavir, ritonavir, saquinavir,** and **tipranavir.**

  2. These agents are virustatic and require lifelong therapy. They are currently approved for use in various combinations known as potent combination antiretroviral therapy.

    a. Appropriate combinations include those that have demonstrated efficacy and safety in controlled clinical trials (Table 44-6).

    b. Monotherapy with any single antiretroviral agent is unacceptable in the treatment of HIV infection owing to rapid development of viral resistance.

    c. Before designing a treatment plan, a minimum of two CD4$^+$ cell counts and one HIV RNA level (viral load) should be obtained to confirm the initial measurements and determine if treatment should be initiated. After starting therapy, repeat these measurements in 2–8 weeks, followed by every 3–4 months thereafter.

    d. A minimum of 1.0-$\log_{10}$ copies/mL decline in HIV RNA levels should be seen after the first 2–8 weeks of therapy for clinical response; a subsequent decrease to undetectable levels should be achieved by 16–24 weeks.

  3. Reverse transcriptase inhibitors are classified as either nucleosides or nucleotides. These agents are competitive inhibitors of reverse transcriptase, which leads to chain termination when incorporated into the viral DNA chain. They are inactive until phosphorylated by this reference refers to this description of mechanism of action.human cellular kinases into the active triphosphate metabolite. Each agent has a corresponding three-letter acronym as well as a brand name. With the exception of abacavir, each agent in this class of antiretrovirals requires dosage adjustment in patients with renal dysfunction. **All agents in the nucleoside class have a black box warning concerning the potential for development of lactic acidosis and severe hepatomegaly with steatosis.**

    a. Abacavir (ABC; Ziagen) is a synthetic carbocyclic nucleoside analog indicated for the treatment of both adult and pediatric patients with HIV.

        (1) Mechanism of action. See VII.C.3.

        (2) Spectrum of activity and therapeutic uses. Abacavir is approved for use in adults and children ≥ 3 months of age only in combination with other antiretroviral agents.

            (a) Abacavir is available alone or co-formulated as a combination tablet with lamivudine and zidovudine (Trizivir) which is dosed twice daily.

            (b) Abacavir is also available in a combination tablet with lamivudine (Epzicom) which is dosed once daily.

        (3) Precautions and monitoring effects. Abacavir has a **black box warning** for a life-threatening hypersensitivity reaction that can lead to death. It occurs in approxi-

Table 44-6. Department of Health and Human Services Guidelines for the Use of Antiviral Agents in HIV-1-Infected Adults and Adolescents

When to begin treatment

Treat any symptomatic patient (severe symptoms or AIDS)

Treat any asymptomatic or AIDS patients with CD4$^+$ cell count < 200/mm^3 and any value of plasma HIV RNA (viral load)

Offer treatment if asymptomatic patient with CD4$^+$ cell count > 200/mm^3 but < 350/mm^3 and any value of HIV RNA (Most clinicians recommend deferring treatment in asymptomatic patients with CD4$^+$ cell count > 350/mm^3 and HIV RNA ≥ 100,000; some clinicians will offer treatment)

Defer treatment of asymptomatic patients with CD4$^+$ cell count > 350/mm^3 and HIV RNA < 100,000

Regimen selection

Selection of a treatment regimen should be individualized for each patient based on adverse effect profiles, drug interactions, comorbidities, pill burden, etc. Preferred and alternative treatment regimens in previously untreated patients are as follows:

Preferred Regimens		Alternative Regimens	
NNRTI based	Efavirenz[a] + (lamivudine or emtricitabine) + (zidovudine or tenofovir)	NNRTI based	Efavirenz[a] + (lamivudine or emtricitabine) + (abacavir or didanosine or stavudine) Nevirapine[b] + (lamivudine or emtricitabine) + (zidovudine or stavudine or didanosine or abacavir or tenofovir)
PI based	Lopinavir/ritonavir + (lamivudine or emtricitabine) + zidovudine	PI based	Atazanavir + (lamivudine or emtricitabine) + (zidovudine or stavudine or abacavir or didanosine) or (tenofovir + ritonavir 100 mg/day) Fosamprenavir + (lamivudine or emtricitabine) + (zidovudine or stavudine or abacavir or tenofovir or didanosine) Fosamprenavir/ritonavir + (lamivudine or emtricitabine) + (zidovudine or stavudine or abacavir or tenofovir or didanosine) Indinavir/ritonavir + (lamivudine or emtricitabine) + (zidovudine or stavudine or abacavir or tenofovir or didanosine) Lopinavir/ritonavir + (lamivudine or emtricitabine) + (stavudine or abacavir or tenofovir or didanosine) Nelfinavir + (lamivudine or emtricitabine) + (zidovudine or stavudine or abacavir or tenofovir or didanosine) Saquinavir (any formulation)/ritonavir + (lamivudine or emtricitabine) + (zidovudine or stavudine or abacavir or tenofovir or didanosine)
		Triple NRTI based	Abacavir + zidovudine + lamivudine

(Continued on next page)

Table 44-6. Continued.

Agents or combinations that should not be offered at any time

All monotherapies
2-NRTI regimens
Abacavir + tenofovir + (lamivudine or emtricitabine) as a triple NRTI regimen
Tenofovir + didanosine + (lamivudine or emtricitabine) as a triple NRTI regimen
Ritonavir + nelfinavir
Saquinavir (hard gel capsule) as the sole PI in a PI-based regimen
Zalcitabine plus any of the following: didanosine, lamivudine, stavudine
Zidovudine + stavudine
Didanosine + stavudine
Lamivudine + emtricitabine
Atazanavir + indinavir

Monitoring

Before initiating drug therapy, must obtain CD4$^+$ cell count and plasma HIV RNA levels plus
  complete blood count, chemistry, lipid profile, and liver enzymes
If HIV RNA does not reach undetectable levels (< 50 copies/mL) by 16–24 weeks, perform
  resistance testing, compliance assessment, and consider a regimen change

NNRTI, nonnucleoside reverse transcriptase inhibitor; *NRTI,* nucleoside reverse transcriptase inhibitor; *PI,* protease
inhibitor.
[a]Cannot be used in the first trimester of pregnancy or in women who wish to conceive or are not using effective
contraception.
[b]Should not be initiated in women with pre-nevirapine CD4$^+$ cell counts > 250/mm^3 or men with pre-nevirapine
CD4$^+$ cell counts > 400/mm^3 owing to high incidence of hepatic adverse effects.

mately 5% of patients taking this drug, typically within the first 6 weeks of therapy.
This reaction involves respiratory symptoms, fever, rash, and GI complaints. Reex-
posure following these symptoms can mimic anaphylaxis and may result in death.
Therefore, rechallenge is contraindicated.

  (4) Significant interactions. Alcohol increases abacavir's AUC by 41%.
  b. **Didanosine (ddl; Videx),** a synthetic purine analog, inhibits HIV replication and has a
  longer intracellular half-life (> 20 hr) than zidovudine (7 hr).
    (1) Mechanism of action. See VII.C.3.
    (2) Spectrum of activity and therapeutic uses. Didanosine is approved for the treatment
    of adults and children only in combination with other antiretroviral agents.
    (3) Precautions and monitoring effects
      (a) Didanosine can cause reversible peripheral neuropathy and acute, potentially
      lethal pancreatitis (**black box warning**). Serum triglycerides should be moni-
      tored, and didanosine should be withheld when initiating potential pancreatitis-
      inducing agents (e.g., IV pentamidine, sulfonamides). Transiently elevated
      serum amylase may not reflect pancreatitis.
      (b) Other adverse effects include headaches, diarrhea, nausea, and hyperuricemia
      (because didanosine is catalyzed to uric acid).
      (c) Didanosine is available in an enteric coated capsule or buffered oral tablet
      formulation to prevent degradation at acidic pH. It must be taken on an empty
      stomach.
      (d) Do not use in combination with stavudine or zalcitabine because of additive
      potential for toxicity.
      (e) Do not use the combination regimen of didanosine, tenofovir, and NNRTIs
      owing to high rates of early virologic failure.
    (4) Significant interactions. Pancreatitis-inducing drugs, such as **cimetidine, ranitid-
    ine, sulfonamides, pentamidine,** and **alcohol** and **those known to cause peripheral
    neuropathy** should not be used with didanosine.
  c. **Emtricitabine (FTC; Emtriva)** is a synthetic nucleoside analog structurally related to
  lamivudine with activity against HIV infection.
    (1) Mechanism of action. See VII.C.3.
    (2) Spectrum of activity and therapeutic uses. Emtricitabine is indicated for use in
    HIV-infected adults in combination with other antiretroviral agents. It is available by

itself or as a combination tablet with tenofovir (Truvada) and as a combination tablet with tenofovir and efavirenz (Atripla). Although it demonstrates activity against hepatitis B virus, it is not approved for use in treatment of this infection.

(3) Precautions and monitoring effects

(a) Adverse effects most commonly observed in clinical trials were mild-moderate and include headache, rash, diarrhea, and nausea. Hyperpigmentation of the palms or soles may occur.

(b) Serious acute exacerbations of hepatitis B have been documented in HIV/hepatitis B co-infected patients who discontinued therapy with emtricitabine (**black box warning**); therefore, liver function tests should be monitored for several months after discontinuation.

(4) Significant interactions. None have been identified.

d. Lamivudine (3TC; Epivir) is a synthetic nucleoside analog with activity against HIV and hepatitis B virus.

(1) Mechanism of action. See VII.C.3.

(2) Spectrum of activity and therapeutic uses. Lamivudine is indicated for use in HIV-positive adults and children > 3 months of age in combination with other antiretroviral agents. It is also used in a lower dosage for the treatment of chronic hepatitis B in patients with active liver inflammation and evidence of hepatitis B viral replication.

(a) Lamivudine is available alone or within a twice daily combination tablet containing lamivudine, zidovudine and abacavir (Trizivir).

(b) Lamivudine is also available as a combination tablet with abacavir (Epzicom) and zidovudine (Combivir).

(3) Precautions and monitoring effects

(a) Reported adverse reactions are minor and include headache, fatigue, and GI reactions such as nausea, vomiting, and diarrhea. CNS toxicity includes neuropathy, dizziness, and insomnia. Lab test abnormalities such as neutropenia and elevations in liver enzymes have also been reported.

(b) Do not use in combination with zalcitabine owing to antagonism of effects and overlapping toxicities.

(4) Significant interactions. Co-administration with **cotrimoxazole** results in increased lamivudine levels. No dose adjustment is required.

e. Stavudine (d4T; Zerit) is a synthetic thymidine nucleoside analog that is active against HIV infection.

(1) Mechanism of action. See VII.C.3.

(2) Spectrum of activity and therapeutic uses. Stavudine is indicated for use in combination with other antiretroviral agents in adults and children of all ages.

(3) Precautions and monitoring effects

(a) The major toxicity with stavudine is a dose related but reversible peripheral neuropathy occurring in up to 21% of patients.

(b) Other adverse effects include headache, rash, diarrhea, nausea, and vomiting.

(c) Fatal episodes of pancreatitis have been reported.

(4) Significant interactions. Do not use in combination with zidovudine or zalcitabine.

f. Tenofovir disoproxil fumarate (TDF; Viread) is an acyclic nucleoside phosphonate diester analog (**nucleotide**) with antiviral activity against HIV and hepatitis B virus.

(1) Mechanism of action. Tenofovir (a prodrug) is rapidly hydrolyzed by plasma esterases to tenofovir, with subsequent conversion to the active tenofovir diphosphate. *Note:* NtRTIs are active as the diphosphate, unlike the NRTIs, which require conversion to the triphosphate.

(2) Spectrum of activity and therapeutic uses. Tenofovir is approved for use in combination with other antiretroviral agents for the treatment of HIV in adults. It is also available as a once daily combination tablet containing tenofovir and emtricitabine (Truvada) and tenofovir, emtricitabine, and efavirenz (Atripla).

(3) Precautions and monitoring effects

(a) Minor adverse effects have been reported in clinical trials. These include complaints of diarrhea, vomiting, and nausea.

(b) Additional adverse effects observed during postmarketing surveillance include acute renal failure and decreases in bone mineral density.

 (c) Tenofovir has the same **black box warning** that emtricitabine has for patients with concomitant hepatitis B (see VII.C.3.c).

 (d) Dose adjustment is required for renal insufficiency.

 (4) **Significant interactions**

 (a) Tenofovir increases **didanosine** serum concentrations, necessitating a dose reduction of didanosine.

 (b) Tenofovir decreases serum concentrations of **atazanavir.** When these 2 agents are used together, ritonavir must be added to the regimen.

g. **Zalcitabine (ddC; Hivid)** is a synthetic pyrimidine nucleoside analogue that is active against HIV.

 (1) **Mechanism of action.** See VII.C.3.

 (2) **Spectrum of activity and therapeutic uses.** Zalcitabine is no longer recommended as a component of initial combination therapy of HIV owing to its severe adverse effect profile. The manufacturer is currently planning to discontinue its production.

 (3) **Precautions and monitoring effects**

 (a) The major clinical toxicity of zalcitabine is peripheral neuropathy, which occurs in up to 35% of patients and may be potentially disabling.

 (b) Other adverse effects include pancreatitis, stomatitis, cardiomyopathy, and hypersensitivity reactions.

 (c) Do not use in combination with lamivudine, stavudine, or zidovudine.

 (4) **Significant interactions**

 (a) Drugs that have the potential to cause peripheral neuropathy should be avoided. These include **chloramphenicol, cisplatin, dapsone, didanosine, disulfiram, hydralazine, isoniazid, metronidazole, nitrofurantoin, phenytoin, ribavirin,** and **vincristine.**

 (b) Zalcitabine treatment should be interrupted when a drug with the potential to cause pancreatitis is initiated (i.e., **pentamidine**).

 (c) Do not take with magnesium-, calcium-, or aluminum-containing antacids.

 (d) **Cimetidine** and **probenecid** may increase zalcitabine levels, causing increased zalcitabine toxicity.

h. **Zidovudine (AZT; Retrovir)** is a synthetic thymidine analog. This agent was the first available drug for the treatment of HIV infection.

 (1) **Mechanism of action.** See VII.C.3.

 (2) **Spectrum of activity and therapeutic uses**

 (a) Zidovudine is indicated in the treatment of adults and children > 6 weeks of age for the treatment of HIV.

 (b) It is indicated for the prevention of maternal–fetal HIV transmission.

 (c) Zidovudine is available as oral capsules, tablets, and solution as well as an IV solution.

 (d) Oral zidovudine is also available as a co-formulation with lamivudine (Combivir) and with lamivudine and abacavir (Trizivir).

 (3) **Precautions and monitoring effects**

 (a) Zidovudine can cause severe bone marrow suppression, including macrocytic anemia and neutropenia after the first few weeks to months of therapy. The risk is increased in patients with preexisting bone marrow suppression or who are taking concomitant medications that cause bone marrow suppression.

 (b) Erythropoietin can be considered as an adjunctive therapy in patients with zidovudine-induced anemia, in cases for which it cannot be discontinued.

 (c) Other adverse effects include headache, malaise, seizures, anxiety, fever, and rash.

 (d) Prolonged use may lead to symptomatic myopathy.

 (4) **Significant interactions**

 (a) **Cotrimoxazole, atovaquone, valproic acid, methadone,** and **probenecid** may increase zidovudine concentrations, causing increased risk of zidovudine toxicity.

 (b) Other **cytotoxic drugs,** such as **ganciclovir, dapsone,** and **interferon-α,** can cause additive bone marrow suppression.

 (c) Acetaminophen, ribavirin, rifabutin, and rifampin may decrease levels of zidovudine.

4. **Nonnucleoside reverse transcriptase inhibitors.** The NNRTI class binds directly to and produces a noncompetitive inhibition of the HIV reverse transcriptase, leading to chain

termination. These agents are indicated for use in adults and pediatric patients in combination with either NRTIs or possibly PIs. Efavirenz is considered a preferred NNRTI, whereas the others are currently recommended as alternatives. NNRTI-based regimens provide potent antiviral activity with less pill burden than many PI-based regimens. All NNRTIs may cause **rash and hepatotoxicity;** patients should be monitored closely for these adverse effects.

a. Delavirdine (Rescriptor)

   (1) Mechanism of action. See VII.C.3.

   (2) Spectrum of activity and therapeutic uses. Delavirdine is approved for use in adults in the treatment of HIV in combination with other antiretroviral agents. Its use has fallen out of favor owing to its three times daily dosing schedule.

   (3) Precautions and monitoring effects

      (a) In clinical trials, 4.3% of patients discontinued delavirdine because of rash. Cases of Stevens-Johnson syndrome have been reported.

      (b) Other adverse effects include headache and nausea.

   (4) Significant interactions

      (a) The concentrations of the following medications are greatly increased by delavirdine and must be avoided: **alprazolam, midazolam, triazolam, simvastatin, lovastatin, rifabutin,** and **cisapride.**

      (b) Decreased delavirdine concentrations result when it is administered with **St. John's wort, carbamazepine, phenobarbital, phenytoin,** or **rifampin.** Concomitant use should be avoided.

      (c) Because delavirdine requires an acidic GI tract for optimal absorption, its use is contraindicated with **proton pump inhibitors** and H_2-**receptor antagonists**.

b. Efavirenz (Sustiva)

   (1) Mechanism of action. See VII.C.3.

   (2) Spectrum of activity and therapeutic uses. Efavirenz is approved for use in combination with other antiretroviral agents for the treatment of HIV infection in adults and pediatric patients (> 3 years of age). Its advantage over other NNRTIs is once-daily dosing. It is available alone or as a combination tablet with tenofovir and emtricitabine (Atripla).

   (3) Precautions and monitoring effects

      (a) Most common adverse effects are CNS (52%), including insomnia, dizziness, drowsiness, nightmares, and hallucinations, necessitating bedtime dosing to minimize these effects. These effects typically subside after 4 weeks of treatment.

      (b) Owing to its teratogenic effects, efavirenz should be avoided in the first trimester of pregnancy and in women of childbearing potential who wish to conceive.

      (c) Other adverse effects include rash, increased transaminases, and GI disturbances.

   (4) Significant interactions

      (a) Efavirenz induces and inhibits the cytochrome P450 3A4 isoenzyme system. It should not be used concomitantly with **cisapride, midazolam, triazolam,** or **ergot derivatives.**

      (b) **St. John's wort** decreases efavirenz concentrations and should be avoided.

      (c) Efavirenz decreases **methadone** concentrations by 60%; patients should be monitored for opiate withdrawal and have their doses titrated accordingly.

c. Nevirapine (Viramune) was the first NNRTI approved for use by the FDA for the treatment of HIV infection.

   (1) Mechanism of action. See VII.C.3.

   (2) Spectrum of activity and therapeutic uses. Nevirapine is indicated in combination with other antiretrovirals in adult and pediatric (> 2 months old) HIV patients.

   (3) Precautions and monitoring effects

      (a) Nevirapine has the highest incidence of Stevens-Johnson syndrome of all NNRTIs.

      (b) Symptomatic hepatitis, including fatal hepatic necrosis, has been observed with nevirapine (**black box warning**). The frequency of this adverse effect is increased in women with pre-nevirapine $CD4^+$ **counts > 250 cells/mm^3 and men with $CD4^+$ counts > 400 cells/mm^3. Nevirapine should not be initiated in these patients.**

      (c) Other adverse effects include fever, nausea, and headache.

      (d) To decrease the frequency of adverse effects, a 2-week dose escalation is required.

(4) Significant interactions
- **(a)** Nevirapine induces cytochrome P450 3A4, resulting in decreased concentrations of **caspofungin, ketoconazole, itraconazole, oral contraceptives,** and **protease inhibitors**.
- **(b)** Use of **rifampin** and **St. John's wort** should be avoided, as they decrease the serum concentrations of nevirapine.
- **(c)** **Methadone** concentrations decrease significantly with nevirapine, often necessitating a dose increase.

5. Protease inhibitors. The PIs competitively inhibit the viral protease enzyme, preventing the enzyme from cleaving the gag and gag-pol polyproteins necessary for virion production. PIs are used in combination with other antiretroviral agents, including other PIs, to suppress HIV replication. All of the PIs are cytochrome P450 inhibitors; ritonavir is the most potent inhibitor. All PIs are contraindicated with numerous drugs, including **simvastatin, lovastatin, rifampin, cisapride, pimozide, midazolam, triazolam, ergots,** and **St. John's wort**. Concomitant therapy with antiepileptic drugs, erectile dysfunction drugs, and azole antifungals must be undertaken with caution. Owing to the wide array of drug interactions with PIs, always assess medication profiles carefully for drug interactions before initiation.

a. Amprenavir (Agenerase)
- **(1) Mechanism of action.** See VII.C.5.
- **(2) Spectrum of activity and therapeutic uses.** Amprenavir is no longer recommended for use in initial treatment regimens for HIV owing to the high pill burden associated with its use.
- **(3) Precautions and monitoring effects.**
  - **(a)** Use of the oral solution in pregnant women, children < 4 years old, and patients with hepatic or renal insufficiency is contraindicated owing to the propylene glycol vehicle (**black box warning**).
  - **(b)** Because amprenavir is a sulfonamide, the potential for cross-sensitivity to other sulfonamides exists.
  - **(c)** Adverse effects include hyperlipidemia, hyperglycemia, fat maldistribution, rash, and GI disturbances.
  - **(d)** Dosage adjustment is required for hepatic insufficiency.
- **(4) Significant interactions** (see VII.C.5). Amprenavir decreases **methadone** concentrations, possibly requiring a methadone dose increase to prevent withdrawal.

b. Atazanavir (Reyataz)
- **(1) Mechanism of action.** See VII.C.5.
- **(2) Spectrum of activity and therapeutic uses.** Atazanavir is a component of alternative PI-based regimens for HIV. It is dosed once daily.
- **(3) Precautions and monitoring effects.**
  - **(a)** Atazanavir may prolong the PR interval and possibly cause first-degree AV block. Electrocardiogram (ECG) should be monitored.
  - **(b)** Other adverse effects include fat maldistribution, hyperglycemia, and indirect hyperbilirubinemia. In contrast to the other PIs, atazanavir appears to be devoid of effects on lipids.
  - **(c)** Dose adjustment is required for hepatic insufficiency.
- **(4) Significant interactions** (see VII.C.5). Atazanavir is the most problematic of all PIs in terms of drug interactions.
  - **(a)** If used in combination with **efavirenz or tenofovir,** low-dose ritonavir must be administered concomitantly.
  - **(b)** Because atazanavir requires an acidic GI tract for optimal absorption, concomitant use of **proton pump inhibitors** is contraindicated. If other acid suppressants are used with atazanavir, the doses must be separated by as much time as possible (up to 12 hr apart).

c. Darunavir (Prezista)
- **(1) Mechanism of action.** See VII.C.5
- **(2) Spectrum of activity and therapeutic uses.** Darunavir is the newest PI to receive FDA approval for the treatment of HIV. Its use is limited to highly treatment-experienced patients or patients with HIV resistance mutations.
- **(3) Precautions and monitoring effects**
  - **(a)** Darunavir must be co-administered with ritonavir
  - **(b)** Because darunavir contains a sulfonamide moiety, cross-reactivity may occur in sulfa-allergic patients.

(c) Adverse effects include nausea, increased amylase, hyperlipidemia, hyperglycemia, and rash.

(4) Significant interactions. See VII.C.5.

d. **Fosamprenavir (Lexiva)**

(1) Mechanism of action. See VII.C.5. Fosamprenavir is the prodrug of amprenavir.

(2) Spectrum of activity and therapeutic uses. Fosamprenavir has largely replaced
amprenavir because of its improved dosing convenience. It is recommended as an
alternative in PI-based regimens for initial treatment of HIV.

(3) Precautions and monitoring effects

(a) Fosamprenavir may be dosed once daily in treatment naive patients. PI-experi-
enced patients require twice daily dosing.

(b) Adverse effects are the same as those with amprenavir (see VII.C.5.a.(3).b–d).

(4) Significant interactions (see VII.C.3). If used in combination with **efavirenz,** fosamprenavir must be administered with a booster dose of ritonavir.

e. **Indinavir (Crixivan)**

(1) Mechanism of action. See VII.C.5.

(2) Spectrum of activity and therapeutic uses. Indinavir, in combination with ritonavir,
is recommended as part of an alternative PI-based regimen for patients receiving
initial treatment for HIV.

(3) Precautions and monitoring effects

(a) Because indinavir may cause **nephrolithiasis** (kidney stones), patients should
be instructed to drink at least 1.5 L of water daily to prevent this adverse effect.

(b) Indinavir can cause **indirect hyperbilirubinemia.** Combination therapy with
atazanavir is not recommended owing to the potential for additive effects.

(c) Other adverse effects include hyperglycemia, hyperlipidemia, fat maldistribution, headache, and GI intolerance.

(d) Dose adjustment is required for hepatic insufficiency.

(4) Significant interactions (see VII.C.5). Vitamin C in doses > 1 g daily decreases
indinavir concentrations. Caution patients not to exceed the recommended daily
allowance for vitamin C.

f. **Lopinavir/ritonavir (Kaletra)**

(1) Mechanism of action. See VII.C.5.

(2) Spectrum of activity and therapeutic uses. This product is available as a co-formulation of lopinavir with a "booster" dose of ritonavir, which inhibits lopinavir metabolism and results in higher serum concentrations. Lopinavir/ritonavir is the preferred
PI used in initial PI-based regimens owing to its potency and convenient dosing.

(3) Precautions and monitoring effects

(a) Lopinavir/ritonavir was recently reformulated as a film-coated tablet that does
not require refrigeration.

(b) Adverse effects include GI intolerance, hyperlipidemia, hyperglycemia, fat maldistribution, and pancreatitis.

(4) Significant interactions. See VII.C.5.

(a) Lopinavir/ritonavir decreases **methadone** concentrations, possibly necessitating
a methadone dose increase to prevent opiate withdrawal.

(b) Concomitant administration with **bupropion or zolpidem** is contraindicated
because of the risk of toxicity.

g. **Nelfinavir (Viracept)**

(1) Mechanism of action. See VII.C.5.

(2) Spectrum of activity and therapeutic uses. Nelfinavir is a component of an alternative PI-based regimen for initial treatment of adults with HIV infection. Unlike the
other PIs, it is never used in combination with ritonavir.

(3) Precautions and monitoring effects

(a) Diarrhea is commonly reported with nelfinavir. This can often be managed
with antidiarrheals.

(b) Other adverse effects are similar to those with lopinavir/ritonavir.

(c) Use caution with look-alike, sound-alike names (nelfinavir and nevirapine).

(4) Significant interactions (see VII.C.5.) Nelfinavir decreases **methadone** concentrations, necessitating increased monitoring and dose adjustment if indicated.

h. **Ritonavir (Norvir)**

(1) Mechanism of action. See VII.C.5.

(2) Spectrum of activity and therapeutic uses. Ritonavir is rarely used as the sole PI
in a PI-based regimen owing to its poor tolerability and high pill burden when

administered in full doses. Alternatively, it is used in low doses as a pharmacokinetic boosting agent with other PIs. Because it is such a potent cytochrome 450 enzyme inhibitor, ritonavir markedly increases the serum concentrations of other PIs, resulting in higher concentrations with improved viral suppression.

(3) Precautions and monitoring effects

    (a) Capsules should be refrigerated before dispensing. Capsules then may be stored at room temperature for up to 30 days.

    (b) Adverse effects include GI intolerance, circumoral paresthesias, hyperlipidemia, hyperglycemia, fat maldistribution, increased liver function tests, and taste perversion.

(4) Significant interactions (see VII.C.5). Many drug interactions occur with ritonavir because it is such a potent inhibitor of so many cytochrome P450 isoenzymes. Always refer to proper resources to assess for drug interactions.

i. Saquinavir (Invirase, Fortovase)

    (1) Mechanism of action. See VII.C.5.

    (2) Spectrum of activity and therapeutic uses. Use of saquinavir without booster doses of ritonavir is not recommended because of the poor bioavailability of saquinavir.

    (3) Precautions and monitoring effects

        (a) Saquinavir is available as a hard gel capsule and tablet (Invirase) and a soft gel capsule (Fortovase). The various dosage forms are **not bioequivalent** and cannot be used interchangeably.

        (b) The soft gel capsule formulation is no longer manufactured (effective February 2006).

        (c) Adverse effects are similar to lopinavir/ritonavir.

    (4) Significant interactions. See VII.C.5.

j. Tipranavir (Aptivus)

    (1) Mechanism of action. See VII.C.5.

    (2) Spectrum of activity and therapeutic uses. The use of tipranavir is limited to highly treatment-experienced patients with HIV who are resistant to other PIs as well as to other classes of antiretrovirals.

    (3) Precautions and monitoring effects.

        (a) Owing to the poor bioavailability of tipranavir, it must be co-administered with ritonavir.

        (b) Capsules must be refrigerated. Once dispensed, they are stable at room temperature for up to 60 days.

        (c) Tipranavir has been associated with clinical hepatitis and fatal hepatic decompensation (**black box warning**). Liver function tests should be monitored closely, especially in patients with underlying liver disease.

        (d) Because the structure of tipranavir contains a **sulfonamide** moiety, cross-reactivity may occur in sulfa-allergic patients.

        (e) Other adverse effects include rash, hyperlipidemia, hyperglycemia, and fat maldistribution.

    (4) Significant interactions (see VII.C.5). Loperamide may decrease tipranavir concentrations.

6. Fusion inhibitors. Enfuvirtide (T-20; Fuzeon) is the first and only member of this class of antiretrovirals.

  a. Mechanism of action. Enfuvirtide inhibits the entry of HIV into CD4$^+$ **cells by interfering with the fusion of viral and cellular membranes.**

  b. Spectrum of activity and therapeutic uses. Enfuvirtide is primarily used in highly treatment-experienced patients with extensive viral resistance. It is not recommended for use as initial therapy in treatment-naive patients, as it has not been studied in this population.

  c. Precautions and monitoring effects

    (1) Enfuvirtide is injected subcutaneously twice daily. Local injection site reactions occur in almost all patients, including pain, redness, pruritus, and nodules.

    (2) Other adverse effects include hypersensitivity reactions and increased rate of bacterial pneumonia.

    (3) No dose adjustment is necessary for renal impairment.

  d. Significant interactions. There are no significant drug interactions with enfuvirtide.

VIII. Anthelmintics

A. **Definition.** These drugs are used to rid the body of worms (**helminths**). These agents may act locally to rid the GI tract of worms or work systemically to eradicate worms that are invading organs or tissues.

B. **Mebendazole (Vermox)** is a synthetic benzimidazole-derivative anthelmintic.

1. **Mechanism of action.** Mebendazole interferes with reproduction and survival of helminths by inhibiting the formation of microtubules and irreversibly blocking glucose uptake, thereby depleting glycogen stores in the helminth.

2. **Spectrum of activity.** Mebendazole is active against various nematodes that are pathogenic to humans, including *Ancylostoma duodenale* (common hookworm), *Ascaris lumbricoides* (roundworm), *Capillaria philippinensis* (Philippine threadworm), *Enterobius vermicularis* (pinworm), *Necator americanus* (American hookworm), and *Trichuris trichiura* (whipworm).

3. **Therapeutic uses.** Mebendazole is used for the treatment of single or mixed infections with the helminths listed in VIII.B.2. Immobilization and subsequent death of helminths are slow, with complete GI clearance up to 3 days after therapy.

4. **Precautions and monitoring effects**
   a. In cases of massive infection, abdominal pain, nausea, and diarrhea associated with expulsion of organisms may result.
   b. Myelosuppression (neutropenia and thrombocytopenia) can occur with high doses (40–50 mg/kg/day).
   c. If the patient is not cured in 3 weeks, retreatment is necessary.

5. **Significant interactions.** Agents that may reduce the serum concentrations and subsequent efficacy of mebendazole include carbamazepine and phenytoin.

C. **Albendazole (Albenza)** is a synthetic benzimidazole-derivative anthelmintic.

1. **Mechanism of action.** See VIII.B.1.

2. **Spectrum of activity.** Albendazole is active against *Taenia solium* (pork tapeworm) and *Echinococcus granulosus* (dog tapeworm).

3. **Therapeutic uses.** Albendazole is used to treat parenchymal neurocysticercosis in combination with corticosteroids as well as cystic hydatid disease (before and after surgical removal of the disease).

4. **Precautions and monitoring effects**
   a. The drug should be administered with a fatty meal to achieve optimal absorption.
   b. Hepatotoxicity occurs in 16% of patients; liver function tests every 2 weeks are recommended while taking albendazole.
   c. Rarely, leukopenia, thrombocytopenia, granulocytopenia, pancytopenia, and agranulocytosis occur. A CBC should be checked every 2 weeks while taking albendazole.

D. **Diethylcarbamazine citrate (Hetrazan)**

1. **Mechanism of action.** Diethylcarbamazine citrate is a synthetic organic compound highly specific for several common parasites.

2. **Spectrum of activity.** This agent is active against *Wuchereria bancrofti, Onchocerca volvulus, Brugia malayi, Mansonella perstans, Mansonella ozzardi, Ascaris lumbricoides,* and *Loa loa.*

3. **Therapeutic uses.** Diethylcarbamazine citrate is used for the treatment of Bancroft's filariasis, onchocerciasis, ascariasis, and loiasis. It is available directly from the manufacturer for compassionate use only.

4. **Precautions and monitoring effects**
   a. Patients treated for *W. bancrofti* infection often present with headache and general malaise. Severe allergic phenomena in conjunction with a skin rash have been reported.

b. Patients treated for onchocerciasis present with pruritus, facial edema, and systemic symptoms secondary to the inflammatory response caused by pathogen death (known as a **Mazzotti reaction**). Severe reactions may be noted after a single dose. For this reason, ivermectin is used to treat onchocerciasis.

c. Children who are undernourished or are suffering from debilitating ascariasis infection may experience giddiness, malaise, nausea, and vomiting after treatment. Other drugs are available to treat *Ascaris* (mebendazole and albendazole).

E. Pyrantel (Pin-Rid) is a pyrimidine-derivative anthelmintic.

1. Mechanism of action. Pyrantel is a depolarizing neuromuscular blocking agent that causes a spastic paralysis of the helminth.

2. Spectrum of activity. Pyrantel is active against *A. lumbricoides* (roundworm), *E. vermicularis* (pinworm), *A. duodenale* (hookworm), *N. americanus* (hookworm), and *Trichostrongylus orientalis* (hairworm).

3. Therapeutic uses. Pyrantel is used for the treatment of roundworm, pinworm, and hookworm infections.

4. Precautions and monitoring effects
  a. Most commonly reported reactions include anorexia, nausea, vomiting, diarrhea, headache, and rash.
  b. A single dose may be mixed with food, milk, juice, or taken on an empty stomach.

F. Thiabendazole (Mintezol), a pyrazinoisoquinoline derivative, is a synthetic heterocyclic anthelmintic.

1. Mechanism of action is not known precisely. Thiabendazole is shown to inhibit the helminth-specific enzyme, fumarate reductase. Thiabendazole also demonstrates anti-inflammatory, antipyretic, and analgesic effects.

2. Spectrum of activity. It is active against most intestinal nematodes, including *Ancylostoma braziliense* (dog and cat hookworm), *A. duodenale* (hookworm), *A. lumbricoides* (roundworm), *E. vermicularis* (pinworm), *N. americanus* (hookworm), *Strongyloides stercoralis* (threadworm), *T. trichiura* (whipworm), *T. spiralis,* and *Toxocara canis* and *Toxocara cati* (dog and cat roundworms).

3. Therapeutic uses. Thiabendazole is used for the treatment of strongyloidiasis (threadworm infection), cutaneous larva migrans (creeping eruption), and visceral larva migrans. It is used for the treatment of uncinariasis (hookworm), *N. americanus, A. duodenale,* trichuriasis (whipworm), and ascariasis (large roundworm) when more specific therapy is unavailable or further treatment is required with a second agent.

4. Precautions and monitoring effects
  a. Adverse effects of thiabendazole are usually mild and transient, occurring 3–4 hr after the drug has been administered and lasting for 2–8 hr.
  b. Most common reactions include anorexia, nausea, vomiting, and dizziness.
  c. Giddiness, seizures, vertigo, paresthesias, and psychic disturbances may also occur, but less frequently.
  d. If hypersensitivity develops, the drug should be discontinued. Erythema multiforme (including Stevens-Johnson syndrome) has been reported.

5. Significant interactions. Serum **xanthine** levels (theophylline and caffeine) may increase.

G. Ivermectin (Stromectol)

1. Mechanism of action. Ivermectin potentiates the inhibitory effects of γ-aminobutyric acid (GABA) in various nematodes and arthropods, resulting in paralysis and death of the organisms.

2. Spectrum of activity. This agent is active against *S. stercoralis* (intestinal forms only) and *O. volvulus* (immature forms only). It is also useful for treatment of infections with *A. lumbricoides, E. vermicularis, M. ozzardi, T. trichiura,* and *W. bancrofti.*

3. **Therapeutic uses**
   a. Ivermectin is useful for treatment of infections with the parasites listed in VIII.G.2.
   b. Two studies demonstrated that ivermectin was more effective than albendazole for treatment of strongyloidiasis.
   c. Ivermectin is often favored over diethylcarbamazine citrate owing to its less severe adverse effect profile.

4. **Precautions and monitoring effects,**
   a. May cause a **Mazzotti reaction** (see VIII.D.4.b) that is less severe than with diethylcarbamazine citrate.
   b. Reports of serious and possibly fatal encephalopathy have occurred in patients with concomitant *L. loa* infection
   c. Other adverse effects include edema, dizziness, headache, rash, and GI disturbances.
   d. Counsel patients to take ivermectin with water.

H. **Praziquantel (Bitricide)**

1. **Mechanism of action.** Praziquantel increases cell membrane permeability in susceptible helminths, with loss of intracellular calcium and paralysis of their musculature. Vacuolization and disintegration of the schistosome tegument result, followed by attachment of phagocytes to the parasite and death.

2. **Spectrum of activity.** Praziquantel is active against trematodes (flukes), including all *Schistosoma* spp. and *Clonorchis sinensis, Opisthorchis viverrini, Fasciola hepatica* (liver flukes), *Paragonimus uterobilateralis, Paragonimus westermani* (lung flukes), *Metagonimus yokogawai, Fasciolopsis buski,* and *Heterophyes heterophyes* (intestinal flukes).

3. **Therapeutic uses.** Praziquantel is active in treating all types of schistosomiasis that are pathogenic to humans; clonorchiasis and opisthorchiasis (Chinese and southeast Asian liver flukes); many other types of infections involving intestinal, liver, and lung flukes; and cestodiasis (tapeworm) infections.

4. **Precautions and monitoring effects**
   a. Treatment of ocular cysticercosis is contraindicated because parasite destruction within the eyes may cause irreparable lesions.
   b. In general, adverse effects are generally mild and well tolerated. It is difficult to differentiate between effects caused by the praziquantel versus effects demonstrated by dying parasites.
   c. The most common side effects are transient and may include malaise, headache, dizziness, and abdominal discomfort.
   d. Praziquantel may impair activities that require mental alertness.

STUDY QUESTIONS

Directions for questions 1–12: Each of the questions, statements, or incomplete statements in this section can be correctly answered or completed by **one** of the suggested answers or phrases. Choose the **best** answer.

1. Isoniazid is a primary antitubercular agent that

(A) requires pyridoxine supplementation.
(B) may discolor the tears, saliva, urine, or feces orange red.
(C) causes ocular complications that are reversible if the drug is discontinued.
(D) may be ototoxic and nephrotoxic.
(E) should never be used because of hepatotoxic potential.

2. All of the following factors may increase the risk of nephrotoxicity from gentamicin therapy *except* which one?

(A) age > 70 years
(B) prolonged courses of gentamicin therapy
(C) concurrent amphotericin B therapy
(D) trough gentamicin levels < 2 mg/mL
(E) concurrent cisplatin therapy

3. In which of the following groups do all four drugs warrant careful monitoring for drug-related seizures in high-risk patients?

(A) penicillin G, imipenem, amphotericin B, metronidazole
(B) penicillin G, chloramphenicol, tetracycline, vancomycin
(C) imipenem, tetracycline, vancomycin, sulfadiazine
(D) cycloserine, metronidazole, vancomycin, sulfadiazine
(E) metronidazole, imipenem, doxycycline, erythromycin

4. AC is a 34-year-old male admitted with a diagnosis of peritonitis. Cultures are positive for *Bacteroides fragilis, Enterococcus faecalis,* and *Staphylococcus aureus.* Which of the following would be the best initial therapy to recommend?

(A) telithromycin
(B) quinupristin/dalfopristin
(C) tigecycline
(D) trimethoprim/sulfamethoxazole
(E) kanamycin

5. TJ is a 45-year-old female presenting with an *Enterobacter aerogenes* bacteremia with a low-grade fever (101.6°F). The most appropriate management of her fever would be to

(A) give acetaminophen 1000 mg orally every 6 hr.
(B) give aspirin 650 mg orally every 4 hr.
(C) give alternating doses of aspirin and acetaminophen every 4 hr.
(D) withhold antipyretics and use the fever curve to monitor her response to antibiotic therapy.
(E) use tepid water baths to reduce the fever.

6. BC has an upper respiratory infection. Two years ago, she experienced an episode of bronchospasm after penicillin therapy. Current cultures are positive for a strain of *Streptococcus pneumoniae* that is sensitive to all of the following drugs. Which of these drugs would be the best choice for this patient?

(A) amoxicillin/clavulanate
(B) telithromycin
(C) ampicillin
(D) cefaclor
(E) loracarbef

7. All of the following drugs are appropriate therapies for a lower urinary tract infection owing to *Pseudomonas aeruginosa except*

(A) norfloxacin.
(B) trimethoprim–sulfamethoxazole.
(C) ciprofloxacin.
(D) tobramycin.
(E) methenamine mandelate.

8. BT is a 43-year-old female seen by her primary-care physician for a mild staphylococcal cellulitis on the arm. Which of the following regimens would be appropriate oral therapy?

(A) dicloxacillin 125 mg every 6 hr
(B) vancomycin 250 mg every 6 hr
(C) methicillin 500 mg every 6 hr
(D) cefazolin 1 g every 8 hr
(E) penicillin V 500 mg every 6 hr

9. RC is a 33-year-old male with a history of HIV for 10 years who now presents with *Mycobacterium avium-intracellulare* (MAI). Which of the following drugs has demonstrated in vitro activity against MAI?

(A) daptomycin
(B) clarithromycin
(C) erythromycin base
(D) cloxacillin
(E) minocycline

10. All of the following statements regarding pentamidine isethionate are true *except* which one?

(A) It is indicated for treatment or prophylaxis of infection owing to *Pneumocystis carinii*.
(B) It may be administered intramuscularly, intravenously, or by inhalation.
(C) It has no clinically significant effect on serum glucose.
(D) It is effective in the treatment of leishmaniasis.

11. RE is a 23-year-old male with a history of influenza A infections. An outbreak of influenza A has just been reported in his community, and he is exhibiting initial symptoms of the infection. Which agent would be the most useful to treat RE?

(A) cidofovir
(B) famciclovir
(C) rimantadine
(D) foscarnet
(E) ribavirin

12. Dr. Jones requests your help in prescribing a protease inhibitor for his patient. He has heard that not all agents are the same and asks for your recommendation as to which agent would be least likely to cause the patient's cholesterol to increase. Which agent would you recommend?

(A) saquinavir
(B) ritonavir
(C) indinavir
(D) nelfinavir
(E) atazanavir

Directions for questions 13–14: The questions and incomplete statements in this section can be correctly answered or completed by **one or more** of the suggested answers. Choose the answer, **A–E.**

A	if **I only** is correct
B	if **III only** is correct
C	if **I and II** are correct
D	if **II and III** are correct
E	if **I, II, and III** are correct

13. Drugs usually active against penicillinase-producing *Staphylococcus aureus* include which of the following?

(I) piperacillin–tazobactam
(II) amoxicillin–clavulanate
(III) nafcillin

14. Antiviral agents that are active against cytomegalovirus (CMV) include which of the following?

(I) ganciclovir
(II) foscarnet
(III) acyclovir

Directions for questions 15–17: Each description listed in this section is most closely associated with **one** of the following drugs. The drugs may be used more than once or not at all. Choose the **best** answer, **A–E.**

A	clofazimine
B	itraconazole
C	lomefloxacin
D	neomycin

15. It may be administered once per day for the treatment of urinary tract infections.

16. It may cause pink to brownish skin pigmentation within a few weeks of initiation of therapy.

17. Co-administration with astemizole or terfenadine may lead to life-threatening cardiac dysrhythmias.

ANSWERS AND EXPLANATIONS

1. The answer is A *[see V.B.2.d.(5)].*
Isoniazid increases the excretion of pyridoxine, which can lead to peripheral neuritis, particularly in poorly nourished patients. Pyridoxine (a form of vitamin B₆) deficiency may cause convulsions as well as the neuritis, involving synovial tenderness and swelling. Treatment with the vitamin can reverse the neuritis and prevent or cure the seizures.

2. The answer is D *[see II.B.4.b].*
Trough serum levels < 2 mg/mL are considered appropriate for gentamicin and are recommended to minimize the risk of toxicity from this aminoglycoside. Because aminoglycosides accumulate in the proximal tubule of the kidney, nephrotoxicity can occur.

3. The answer is A *[see II.E.1.e.(2); II.J.5.d.(2); III.B.4.b; IV.C.3.c].*
Seizures have been attributed to the use of penicillin G, imipenem, amphotericin B, and metronidazole. Seizures are especially likely with high doses in patients with a history of seizures and in patients with impaired drug elimination.

4. The answer is C *[see II.K.13].*
Although active against various gram-positive and negative organisms, tigecycline is only agent approved for the treatment of intra-abdominal infections caused by these organisms.

5. The answer is D *[see I.H.1].*
The fever curve is useful for monitoring a patient's response to antimicrobial therapy. Antipyretics can be used to reduce high fever in patients at risk for complications (e.g., seizures) or, in some cases, to make the patient more comfortable.

6. The answer is B *[see II.K.12].*
Amoxicillin and ampicillin are all penicillins and should be avoided in patients with histories of hypersensitivity to other penicillin compounds. Although the risk of cross-reactivity with cephalosporins (e.g., cefaclor, loracarbef) is now considered low, most clinicians avoid the use of these agents in patients with histories of type I hypersensitivity reactions (e.g., anaphylaxis, bronchospasm, giant hives).

7. The answer is B *[see II.E.4; II.H.3.a–b; II.I.2.a; II.I.3.a; II.J.7].*
Norfloxacin, ciprofloxacin, tobramycin, and methenamine mandelate achieve urine concentrations high enough to treat urinary tract infections caused by *P. aeruginosa.* Trimethoprim-sulfamethoxazole is not useful for treating infection caused by this organism, although the combination is useful for treating certain other urinary tract infections.

8. The answer is A *[see II.C; II.E.1.c.(3); II.E.2.b; II.J.8].*
Although vancomycin, methicillin, and cefazolin have excellent activity against staphylococci, they are not effective orally for systemic infections. Vancomycin is prescribed orally for infections limited to the gastrointestinal tract, but because it is poorly absorbed orally, it is not effective for systemic infections. Most hospital- and community-acquired staphylococci are currently resistant to penicillin. Thus of the drugs listed, the most appropriate drug for oral therapy of staphylococcal cellulitis is dicloxacillin.

9. The answer is B *[see II.D.6.a–b].*
Clarithromycin, an alternative to erythromycin, has demonstrated in vitro activity against MAI. Clarithromycin is also used against *Toxoplasma gondii* and *Cryptosporidium* spp., and it is more active than erythromycin against staphylococci and streptococci. Vancomycin and cloxacillin are used to treat staphylococci and streptococci, but has no demonstrated activity versus MAI.

10. The answer is C *[see IV.D].*
Pentamidine isethionate is indicated for both treatment and prophylaxis of infection from *P. carinii.* It can be administered intramuscularly, intravenously, or by inhalation. Inhalation may produce bronchospasm. Blood glucose should be carefully monitored because pentamidine may produce either hyperglycemia or hypoglycemia.

11. The answer is C *[see VII.B.7].*
Cidofovir, famciclovir, and foscarnet have little or no in vivo activity against influenza A. Ribavirin has some activity but is a second-line agent for influenza A and is mainly indicated for treatment of RSV. Rimantadine is a derivative of amantadine with excellent activity against influenza A. It is indicated for the prophylaxis and treatment of influenza A viral infections.

12. The answer is E *[see VII.C.4.b.(3).(b)].*
The majority of protease inhibitors cause hyperlipidemia. Atazanavir does not cause this adverse effect and may be preferred in certain clinical situations.

13. The answer is E *(I, II, III) [see II.E.2–4].*
Piperacillin and amoxicillin each include a β-lactamase inhibitor. These combinations offer activity against *S. aureus* similar to that of the penicillinase-resistant penicillins, such as nafcillin.

14. The answer is C *(I and II) [see VII.B.1; VII.B.7–8].*
Only ganciclovir and foscarnet are active against CMV infections. These agents are virustatic and arrest DNA synthesis by inhibiting viral DNA polymerase. Foscarnet is a broad-spectrum antiviral agent and is used in patients with ganciclovir resistance. Acyclovir is not clinically useful for the treatment of CMV infections because CMV is relatively resistant to acyclovir in vitro.

15. The answer is C *[see II.H.3.c].*
Lomefloxacin may be administered daily for treating urinary tract infections. Enoxacin is another fluoroquinolone used to treat urinary tract infections. Compared to other fluoroquinolones, neither lomefloxacin nor enoxacin improves the spectrum of activity.

16. The answer is A *[see II.J.9].*
Because clofazimine contains phenazine dye, it can cause pink to brown skin pigmentation. This change in pigmentation occurs in 75%–100% of patients taking clofazimine, and it occurs within a few weeks of the initiation of therapy. The discoloration of skin has reportedly led to severe depression and even suicide in some patients. Clofazimine is used in the treatment of leprosy and several atypical *Mycobacterium* infections.

17. The answer is B *[see III.E.5.d].*
Administration of itraconazole or ketoconazole with astemizole or terfenadine may increase the level of astemizole or terfenadine, which can lead to life-threatening dysrhythmias and death. Itraconazole, which is an imidazole, is a fungistatic agent. Specifically, itraconazole can be taken orally to treat aspergillosis infections and other deep fungal infections, such as blastomycosis, coccidioidomycosis, cryptococcosis, and histoplasmosis.

I. INTRODUCTION

A. Definitions

1. **Seizures** are characterized by an excessive, hypersynchronous discharge of cortical neuron activity, which can be measured by the electroencephalogram (EEG). In addition, there may be disturbances in consciousness, sensory motor systems, subjective well-being, and objective behavior; seizures are usually brief, with a beginning and an end, and may produce postseizure impairment.

2. **Epilepsy** is defined as a chronic seizure disorder, or group of disorders, characterized by seizures that usually recur unpredictably in the absence of a consistent provoking factor. The term *epilepsy* is derived from the Greek word meaning "to seize upon" or "taking hold of." It was first described by Hughlings Jackson in the 19th century as an intermittent derangement of the nervous system due to a sudden, excessive, disorderly discharge of cerebral neurons.

3. **Convulsions** are violent, involuntary contractions of the voluntary muscles. A patient may have epilepsy or a seizure disorder without convulsions.

B. Classification.
An alternative seizure classification is being developed that is purely symptom based. This consists of four categories: sensorial (auras), consciousness, autonomic, and motor. Also, the international league against epilepsy is establishing a four-level descriptive seizure classification based on symptoms, apathophysiological seizure, an epileptic syndrome, and functional disability. At present, there are two systems of classification of seizure disorder: one is based on the seizure type and characteristics (Table 45-1), and the other is based on the

---

Table 45-1. International Classification of Epileptic Seizures

I. Partial seizures (seizures beginning locally)

  A. Simple partial seizures (consciousness not impaired)
    1. With motor symptoms
    2. With somatosensory or special sensory symptoms
    3. With autonomic symptoms
    4. With behavioral symptoms

  B. Complex partial seizures (with impairment of consciousness)
    1. Beginning as simple partial seizures and progressing to impairment of consciousness
      a. Without automatisms
      b. With automatisms
    2. With impairment of consciousness at onset
      a. With no other features
      b. With features of simple partial seizures
      c. With automatisms

  C. Partial seizures (simple or complex), secondarily generalized

II. Generalized seizures (bilaterally symmetric, without localized onset)

  A. Absence seizures
    1. **True absence seizures (petit mal)**
    2. **Atypical absence seizures**
  B. Myoclonic seizures
  C. Clonic seizures
  D. Tonic seizures
  E. Tonic–clonic seizures (grand mal)
  F. Atonic seizures

III. Unclassified seizures

Reprinted from Commission on Classification and Terminology of the International League against Epilepsy. Proposal for classification of epilepsies and epileptic syndromes. Epilepsia 1985;26:268–278.

characteristics of the epilepsy (including age at onset, etiological factors, and frequency) and characteristics of the seizure (Table 45-2).

1. **Partial seizures** are the most common seizure type, occurring in approximately 80% of patients with epilepsy.

Table 45-2. Classification of Epilepsies and Epileptic Syndromes

I. **Localized-related (focal, local, partial) epilepsies and syndromes**
  A. **Idiopathic** (with age-related onset)
    1. Benign childhood epilepsy with centrotemporal spikes (rolandic epilepsy)
    2. Childhood epilepsy with occipital paroxysms
  B. **Symptomatic**
    1. Chronic progressive epilepsia partialis continua of childhood
    2. Syndromes characterized by specific modes of precipitation
    3. Temporal lobe epilepsies
    4. Frontal lobe epilepsies
    5. Parietal lobe epilepsies
    6. Occipital lobe epilepsies
  C. **Cryptogenic**

II. **Generalized epilepsies and syndromes**
  A. **Idiopathic** (with age-related onset)
    1. Benign neonatal familial convulsions
    2. Benign neonatal convulsions
    3. Benign myoclonic epilepsy in infancy
    4. Childhood absence epilepsy (pyknolepsy)
    5. Juvenile absence epilepsy
    6. Juvenile myoclonic epilepsy
    7. Epilepsy with generalized tonic–clonic seizures on awakening
    8. Other generalized idiopathic epilepsies not defined above
    9. Epilepsies with seizures precipitated by specific modes of activation
  B. **Cryptogenic or symptomatic** (in order of age)
    1. West syndrome (infantile spasms)
    2. Lennox-Gastaut syndrome
    3. Epilepsy with myoclonic–astatic seizures
    4. Epilepsy with myoclonic absences
  C. **Symptomatic**
    1. **Nonspecific etiology**
      a. Early myoclonic encephalopathy
      b. Early infantile epileptic encephalopathy with suppression burst
      c. Other symptomatic generalized epilepsies not defined above
    2. **Specific syndromes and generalized seizures complicating other disease states**

III. **Epilepsies and syndromes undetermined whether focal or generalized**
  A. **With both focal and generalized seizures**
    1. Neonatal seizures
    2. Severe myoclonic epilepsy in infancy
    3. Epilepsy with continuous spike waves during slow-wave sleep
    4. Acquired epileptic aphasia (Landau-Kleffner syndrome)[a]
    5. Other undetermined epilepsies not defined above
  B. **Without unequivocal generalized or focal features**

IV. **Special situations**
  A. Febrile convulsions
  B. Isolated seizures or isolated status epilepticus
  C. Seizures occurring only when there is an acute metabolic or toxic event due to such factors as alcohol, drugs, eclampsia, and nonketotic hyperglycemia

[a]Believed to be a localized-related epilepsy.
Reprinted with permission from Bleck TP. Convulsive disorders: the use of anticonvulsant drugs. Clin Neuropharmacol 1990;1:198–209.

a. Clinical and EEG changes indicate initial activation of a system of neurons limited to part of one cerebral hemisphere that may spread to other or all brain areas. Manifestations of the seizures depend on the site of the epileptogenic focus in the brain.

b. Partial seizures are subclassified as **simple** (usually unilateral involvement) or **complex** (usually bilateral involvement). Impairment of consciousness is a feature of complex seizures. Consciousness is defined as the degree of awareness and responsiveness of the patient to externally applied stimuli.

   (1) Simple partial seizures generally do not cause loss of consciousness. **Signs and symptoms** of simple partial seizures may be primarily motor, sensory, somatosensory, autonomic, or behavioral. These signs and symptoms may help pinpoint the site of the abnormal brain discharge, for example, localized numbness or tingling reflects a dysfunction in the sensory cortex, located in the parietal lobe.

   (a) Motor signs include convulsive jerking, chewing motions, and lip smacking.

   (b) Sensory and somatosensory manifestations include paresthesias and auras.

   (c) Autonomic signs include sweating, flushing, and pupil dilation.

   (d) Behavioral manifestations, which are sometimes accompanied by impaired consciousness, include déjà vu experiences, structured hallucinations, and dysphasia.

   (2) Complex partial seizures are accompanied by impaired consciousness; however, in some cases, the impairment precedes or follows the seizure. These seizures have variable manifestations.

   (a) Purposeless behavior is common.

   (b) The affected person may have a glassy stare, may wander about aimlessly, and may speak unintelligibly.

   (c) Psychomotor (temporal lobe) epilepsy may lead to aggressive behavior (e.g., outbursts of rage or violence).

   (d) Postictal confusion usually persists for 1–2 min after the seizure ends.

   (e) Automatism (e.g., picking at clothes) is common and may follow visual, auditory, or olfactory hallucinations.

2. Generalized seizures are diffuse, affecting both cerebral hemispheres.

   a. Clinical and EEG changes indicate initial involvement of both hemispheres.

   (1) Consciousness may be impaired, and this impairment may be the initial manifestation.

   (2) Motor manifestations are bilateral.

   (3) The ictal EEG patterns initially are bilateral and presumably reflect neuronal discharge, which is widespread in both hemispheres.

   b. There are three **types** of generalized seizures.

   (1) Idiopathic epilepsies have an age-related onset, typical clinical and EEG characteristics, and a presumed genetic origin.

   (2) Symptomatic epilepsies are considered the consequence of a known or suspected underlying disorder of the central nervous system (CNS).

   (3) Cryptogenic epilepsy refers to a disorder for which the cause is hidden or occult; it is presumed to be symptomatic, but the causal factors are unknown. It is age related, but often does not have well-defined clinical and EEG characteristics.

   c. Signs and symptoms of generalized seizures may be minor or major.

   (1) Absence (petit mal) seizures present as alterations of consciousness (absences) lasting 10–30 sec.

   (a) Staring (with occasional eye blinking) and loss or reduction in postural tone are typical. If the seizure takes place during conversation, the individual may break off in midsentence.

   (b) Enuresis and other autonomic components may occur during absence seizures.

   (c) Some patients experience 100 or more absences daily.

   (d) Onset of this seizure type occurs from age 3 to 16 years; in most patients, absence seizures disappear by age 40.

   (2) Myoclonic (bilateral massive epileptic myoclonus) seizures present as involuntary jerking of the facial, limb, or trunk muscles, possibly in a rhythmic manner.

   (3) Clonic seizures are characterized by sustained muscle contractions alternating with relaxation.

      (4) Tonic seizures involve sustained tonic muscle extension (stiffening).

      (5) Generalized (grand mal) tonic–clonic seizures cause sudden loss of consciousness.

        (a) The individual becomes rigid and falls to the ground. Respirations are interrupted. The legs extend, and the back arches; contraction of the diaphragm may induce grunting. This tonic phase lasts for about 1 min.

        (b) A clonic phase follows, marked by rapid bilateral muscle jerking, muscle flaccidity, and hyperventilation. Incontinence, tongue biting, tachycardia, and heavy salivation sometimes occur.

        (c) During the postictal phase, the individual may experience headache, confusion, disorientation, nausea, drowsiness, and muscle soreness. This phase may last for hours.

        (d) Some patients with epilepsy have serial grand mal seizures, regaining consciousness briefly between attacks. In some cases, grand mal seizures occur repeatedly with no recovery of consciousness between attacks (**status epilepticus**); this disorder is discussed in III.A.

      (6) Atonic seizures (drop attacks) are characterized by a sudden loss of postural tone so that the individual falls to the ground. They occur primarily in children.

C. Epidemiology

    1. Most common neurological disorder

    2. Epilepsy has a prevalence of approximately 1% (i.e., 500,000 cases per 50 million persons worldwide).

    3. In the United States, the prevalence of epilepsy is 6.42 cases per 1000 people.

    4. The onset of seizures is greatest during the 1st year of life; this probability decreases each decade after the 1st year until age 60. Approximately 1 of 50 children and 1 of 100 adults are affected.

    5. Approximately 70% of people with epilepsy have only one seizure type; the remainder have two or more seizure types.

D. Cause. Some seizures arise secondary to other conditions. However, in most cases, the cause of the seizure is unknown.

    1. Primary (idiopathic) seizures have no identifiable cause.

      a. This type of seizure affects about 75% of people with epilepsy.

      b. The onset of primary seizures typically occurs before age 20.

      c. Birth trauma, hereditary factors, and unexplained metabolic disturbances have been proposed as possible causes.

    2. Secondary seizures (symptomatic or acquired seizures) occur secondary to an identifiable cause.

      a. Disorders that may lead to secondary seizures include

        (1) Intracranial neoplasms

        (2) Infectious diseases, such as meningitis, influenza, toxoplasmosis, mumps, measles, and syphilis

        (3) High fever (in children)

        (4) Head trauma

        (5) Congenital diseases

        (6) Metabolic disorders, such as hypoglycemia and hypocalcemia

        (7) Alcohol or drug withdrawal

        (8) Lipid storage disorders

        (9) Developmental abnormalities

      b. Age at seizure onset is associated with specific causes (Table 45-3).

E. Pathophysiology. Seizures reflect a sudden, abnormal, excessive neuronal discharge in the cerebral cortex. Any abnormal neuronal discharge could precipitate a seizure (Figure 45-1).

    1. Normal firing of neurons, which usually originate from the gray matter of one or more cortical or subcortical areas, requires the following elements:

      a. Voltage-dependent ion channels are involved in action-potential propagation or burst generation.

Table 45-3. Probable Causes of Recurrent Seizures by Age Group

Age at Seizure Onset	Probable Cause of Seizure
Birth–1 month	Birth injury or anoxia, congenital hereditary diseases, and metabolic disorders
1–6 months	As above, plus infantile spasms
6 months–2 years	Infantile spasms, febrile convulsions, birth injury or anoxia, meningitis, and head trauma
3–10 years	Birth injury or anoxia, meningitis, cerebral vessel thrombosis, and idiopathic epilepsy
10–18 years	Idiopathic epilepsy and head trauma
18–25 years	Idiopathic epilepsy, trauma, neoplasm, and withdrawal from alcohol or drugs
35–60 years	Trauma, neoplasm, vascular disease, and withdrawal from alcohol or drugs
> 60 years	Vascular disease, neoplasm, degenerative disease, and trauma

  b. Neurotransmitters control neuronal firing, including excitatory neurotransmitters, acetylcholine, norepinephrine, histamine, corticotropin-releasing factors (CRFs), inhibitory neurotransmitters, γ-aminobutyric acid (GABA), and dopamine; therefore, normal neuronal activity requires adequate ions (e.g., sodium, potassium, calcium); excitatory and inhibitory neurotransmitters; and glucose, oxygen, amino acids, and adequate systemic pH.
  c. People with epilepsy may be **genetically** predisposed to a **lower seizure threshold.**
  d. A diencephalic nerve group that normally suppresses excessive brain discharge may be deafferentated, hypersensitive, and vulnerable to activation by various stimuli in individuals with epilepsy.

Figure 45-1. Gross anatomy of the brain. Clinical manifestation of seizures depends on the area of the cortex that is affected and its function, the degree of irritability, and the identity of the impulse.

e. During seizures, there is an increased use of energy, oxygen, and, consequently, an increased production of carbon dioxide. Because of the limited capacity to increase the blood flow to the brain, the blood supply may be **oxygen deficient.** The ratio of supply to demand decreases when the seizure episode is prolonged, leading to increased ischemia and neuronal destruction. Thus it is crucial to diagnose seizures and treat them as soon as possible.

2. **Abnormal electrical brain activity** occurring during a seizure usually produces **characteristic changes on the EEG.** Each part of the cortical area has its own function, and the clinical presentation of a seizure depends on the site, the degree of irritability of the area, and the intensity of the impulse.

3. Seizure activity may include three major **phases.**
   a. **A prodrome** may precede the seizure by hours or days.
      (1) Changes in behavior or mood typically occur during the prodrome.
      (2) This phase may include an aura—a subjective sensation, such as an unusual smell or flashing light.
   b. The **ictal phase** is the seizure itself. In some cases, its onset is heralded by a scream or cry.
   c. The **postictal phase** takes place immediately after the seizure.
      (1) Extensor plantar reflexes may appear.
      (2) The patient typically exhibits lethargy, confusion, and behavioral changes.

F. **Clinical evaluation**

1. **History** includes an evaluation of the seizure, including interviews of the patient's family and eyewitness accounts to establish
   a. The frequency and duration of the episodes
   b. Precipitating factors
   c. The times at which episodes occur
   d. The presence or absence of an aura
   e. Ictal activity
   f. Postictal state

2. **Physical and neurological examinations** are the tools with which to identify an underlying cause to rule out diseases that manifest as seizures (Table 45-4).

3. **Laboratory tests** may also identify an underlying cause.
   a. Liver and kidney function tests, complete blood count (CBC), urinalysis, and serum drug levels (e.g., antidepressants and amphetamines may precipitate seizures) are necessary.
   b. Lumbar puncture may be required for evidence of cerebrospinal fluid (CSF) infection for patients with a fever who have seizures.

Table 45-4. Disorders That Mimic Epilepsy

Gastroesophageal reflux	Movement disorders
Breath-holding spells	Shuddering attacks
Migraine	Paroxysmal choreoathetosis
Confusional	Nonepileptic myoclonus
Basilar	Tics and habit spasms
With recurrent abdominal pain and cyclic vomiting	Psychological disorders
Sleep disorders (especially parasomnias)	Panic disorder
Cardiovascular events	Hyperventilation attacks
Pallid infantile syncope	Pseudoseizures
Vasovagal attacks	Rage attacks
Vasomotor syncope	
Arrhythmias	

Reprinted with permission from Scheurer ML, Pedley TA: The evaluation and treatment of seizures. N Engl J Med 1990;323:1469. Copyright © 1990 Massachusetts Medical Society. All rights reserved.

4. **Neurological imaging studies,** including MRI and/or CT, complement electrophysiological studies and can identify structural brain disorders (anatomical abnormalities).

    a. An MRI can detect cerebral lesions related to epilepsy and should be used in all cases, especially in patients with partial seizure, to exclude brain abnormalities.

    b. Positron-emission tomography (PET), single-photon emission CT (SPECT), and stable xenon-enhanced x-ray CT offer functional views of the brain to detect hypometabolism or relative hypoperfusion. PET and SPECT scans are not available in all institutions.

    c. EEG studies measure the electrical activity of the brain. These studies help identify functional cerebral changes underlying structural abnormalities and are useful with MRI for patients considered for epilepsy surgery.

        (1) An EEG is useful for classifying the seizure or as an additional diagnostic tool, but the EEG by itself cannot rule seizures in or out, because some patients with normal interictal EEGs have seizure disorders.

        (2) The best time to obtain an EEG is *during* a seizure episode. EEG recordings done while the patient is asleep can often record the abnormal activity; therefore, EEGs performed during a sleep-induced state under normal conditions or in a sleep-deprived state can be more sensitive for making a diagnosis.

G. Treatment objectives

1. To prevent or suppress seizures or reduce their frequency through drug therapy

2. To control or eliminate the factors that cause or precipitate seizures

3. To prevent serious consequences of seizures, such as anoxia, airway occlusion, or injury, by protecting the tongue and placing a pillow under the victim's head

4. To encourage a normal lifestyle and prevent the patient from feeling like or being treated as an invalid

5. Short- and long-term side effects

6. Drug interactions

II. THERAPY

A. Principles of drug therapy

1. Seizure control. Approximately 50% of patients with epilepsy achieve complete seizure control through drug therapy. In another 25%, drugs reduce the frequency of seizures. People with epilepsy generally require continuous drug therapy for at least 2 seizure-free years before the drug discontinuation can be considered.

2. Initial treatment

    a. Before anticonvulsive drug treatment is instituted, treatable underlying causes of the seizure activity should be excluded.

    b. A single primary drug that is most appropriate for the seizure type must be selected. If there is more than one appropriate primary drug, then age, sex, and compliance of the patient must be considered.

    c. For patients with newly diagnosed epilepsy, administer low doses for a few days. Patients may respond to a dosage that is lower than that traditionally prescribed initially by their physicians, and this may have important implications in terms of limiting adverse effects. The incidence of adverse effects increases with increasing drug levels, even when the plasma concentrations are maintained within the so-called therapeutic or optimal range.

    d. Between one fourth and one third of the maintenance dose of a single medication is used to begin therapy; it is then increased over 3–4 weeks. The exceptions are phenytoin and phenobarbital, which can be started with the loading or maintenance dose. The dose should be titrated until seizure control or intolerable side effects occur.

    e. With the initiation of therapy, blood concentrations of medications should be measured:

        (1) To establish therapeutic ranges and dosage regimens based on symptomatic toxicity or seizure frequency

        (2) To assess the patient's compliance with therapy

        (3) To control the correlation among the dose, blood levels, and clinical therapeutic levels or toxicity

            (a) Phenytoin follows nonlinear kinetics, as drug levels increase dramatically (more than onefold) with only a small increase in the dose. However, before this twofold increase in drug level with a small increase in dose, there is a predictable linear increase with dose increases; for this reason, it is recommended to increase the dose in small increments to be able to predict when the drug follows the nonlinear kinetic. When this happens, that means the maximum rate of hepatic enzyme clearance is reached and the body can no longer clear the drug as it is introduced into the body.

- **(b)** If physical examination reveals a new onset of nystagmus (except with phenytoin, in which nystagmus develops before clinical intoxication), ataxia, and unsteady wide gait, the next dose increase should be minimal.
- **(c)** There is no justification for increasing drug dosage when a patient's seizures are fully controlled, even if the plasma concentration is below the lower limit of the therapeutic range. If the patient continues to have seizures without any evidence of adverse effects at a plasma concentration near the toxic range, there are two approaches:
  - **(i)** Some clinicians increase the dosage according to clinical response up to the highest tolerated limit.
  - **(ii)** Some clinicians do not increase the dosage because of the likelihood of producing adverse effects.
- **(d)** Carbamazepine has an autoinduction metabolism property, which means that if the dose is increased twofold, blood levels increase less than twofold because of increased metabolism.
- **(4)** To determine the free drug level, which is helpful in patients who are in the therapeutic range but have side effects or no response. The plasma protein binding may be altered in these patients by some other disease state or medication. Because of this alteration, there is more free drug available in the system than the total level shows, especially with phenytoin, valproic acid, and carbamazepine.

3. **Paradoxical intoxication** occurs when a high concentration of a single drug causes an increased frequency of seizures without classical adverse events. This is common with hydantoins and carbamazepine. The proposed reason is that their effect on the cerebellum is blocked at high concentrations. Management usually requires no more than withholding enough doses of the drug to allow the concentration to drift down.

4. When seizures cannot be controlled, there are two options.
   - **a.** The initial drug can be substituted with another agent. This is accomplished by gradually discontinuing the initial drug while simultaneously increasing the dosage of the second agent. Then the dosage of the second agent is titrated up to the maintenance level as the initial agent is gradually discontinued. There are three main advantages of gradual substitution:
     - **(1)** It allows evaluation of the effects of individual drugs
     - **(2)** It reduces the risk of toxicity
     - **(3)** It reduces the risk of adverse drug interactions
   - **b.** A second drug can be added. Combination therapy is reserved for patients with severe epilepsy to rapidly control the seizures. Rapid control can be important for psychosocial reasons as well as for the possibility of a more favorable prognosis.

5. **Long-term drug treatment.** Most physicians review the patient's condition when the patient has been seizure free for 2 years. This has important implications in children because early termination of treatment has better remission rates compared with adults. It is recommended to gradually decrease the dose, over at least 6 months. The age of onset of epilepsy, the presence of an underlying neurological condition, and any abnormal EEGs should be considered.

6. **Diseases and conditions that alter antiepileptic drug–protein bindings**
   - **a.** Liver disease
   - **b.** Hypoalbuminemia
   - **c.** Burns
   - **d.** Pregnancy
   - **e.** High protein-binding drugs or antiepileptic agents. (Most important interactions are discussed under individual agents.)

7. **Medications.** Some medications decrease levels of phenytoin, carbamazepine, phenobarbital, and primidone by enhancing their metabolism. These drugs also cause false decreases in thyroid function tests.

    a. Oral contraceptives
    b. Oral hypoglycemics
    c. Glucocorticoids
    d. Tricyclic antidepressants
    e. Azathioprine
    f. Cyclosporine
    g. Quinidine
    h. Theophylline
    i. Warfarin
    j. Doxycycline
    k. Levodopa

8. Overview of drug therapy in seizure disorder
    a. Monotherapy. Start the drug therapy as single agent.
    b. Dosage treatment. Use a low dose for a few days. Patients with newly diagnosed epilepsy may respond to dosages that are lower than those prescribed initially by their physicians, and this may have important implications in terms of adverse effects. The incidence of adverse effects increases with increasing drug dosage, even when the plasma concentration is maintained within the so-called therapeutic or optimal range.
    c. Drug monitoring. There is no justification for increasing drug dosage when a patient is fully controlled, even if the plasma concentration is below the lower limit of the therapeutic range. If the patient continues to have seizures without any evidence of adverse effects at a plasma concentration near the toxic range, there are two approaches:
        (1) Some clinicians increase the dosage according to clinical response up to the highest tolerated limit.
        (2) Some clinicians do not increase the dosage because of the likelihood of producing adverse events.

9. Adverse effects of anticonvulsive drugs
    a. Alternation in cognition and mentation
        (1) Sedation and depression are the most common symptoms of overdose of anticonvulsive drugs, but they are difficult to assess. For example, barbiturates commonly cause depression, with primidone being the worst offender; diazepam and clorazepate are less likely to cause depression. Barbiturates, clonazepam, and trimethadione commonly cause cognitive impairment, ranging from sensation to confusion.
        (2) Excitation can be a paradoxical effect of barbiturates with younger children and the elderly. For example, felbamate can cause restlessness and hyperactivity.
    b. Deterioration of motor performance and primary coordination includes trembling hands, staggering when rounding corners, and mild limb ataxia. Drugs associated with these effects include hydantoins, methsuximide, carbamazepine, and primidone. These effects are less common with barbiturates and lamotrigine and are rarely seen with gabapentin.
    c. Gastrointestinal symptoms include nausea and vomiting. Two purposed mechanisms include
        (1) A local effect on the stomach, as in the case of valproic acid; divalproex acid, however, has less incidence compared with valproic acid. These symptoms decrease in incidence if the drug is given with meals.
        (2) A brainstem effect, as in the cases of felbamate and carbamazepine. Nausea and vomiting caused by these drugs are associated with brainstem involvement; therefore, drug levels play a role in these symptoms. Administration in smaller, more frequent doses decreases the incidence of these symptoms by lowering the transient peak concentration.
    d. Appetite and body weight. Few anticonvulsants affect appetite separate from nausea and vomiting, including anorexia or increased appetite.
        (1) Drugs that cause anorexia are felbamate, and to a lesser extent, carbamazepine, ethosuximide, and valproic acid.
        (2) Drugs that cause increased appetite are valproic acid, and to a lesser extent, carbamazepine.
    e. Headache and dizziness
        (1) Diffuse headaches may be caused by ethosuximide and, to a lesser extent, by methsuximide and felbamate.

(2) Dizziness seen in association with anticonvulsants is caused by a combination of ataxia and loss of eye movement coordination, which is part of motor coordination symptoms.

B. Specific antiseizure agents. Table 45-5 lists the uses of antiepileptic medications based on seizure type. Table 45-6 lists classifications of anticonvulsive drugs. Table 45-7 lists dosage characteristics of antiepileptic medications.

1. Carbamazepine (Tegretol)
   a. Mechanisms of action. Carbamazepine is chemically related to tricyclic antidepressants. Its mechanism of action is unknown in the treatment of seizure disorders, but it is thought to act by reducing polysynaptic responses and blocking the posttetanic potentiation.
   b. Administration and dosage (Table 45-7)
   (1) Adults and children > 12 years of age receive an initial oral dose of 200 mg twice daily. This may be increased gradually to 800–2000 mg daily (usually given in divided doses).
   (2) Children < 12 usually receive 10–20 mg/kg daily in two or three divided doses.
   c. Precautions and monitoring effects
   (1) Carbamazepine should be used with caution in patients with bone marrow depression. A CBC should be obtained and platelets measured to determine baseline levels before therapy, and levels should be monitored during therapy. Aplastic anemia and agranulocytosis have been reported.
   (2) Tricyclic antidepressants should be avoided if there is a history of hypersensitivity to tricyclics. Monoamine oxidase (MAO) inhibitors should be discontinued 2 weeks before carbamazepine therapy.
   (3) Carbamazepine should be used cautiously in patients with glaucoma because of its mild anticholinergic effects.
   (4) Carbamazepine is an enzyme inducer; therefore, the half-life ($t_{1/2}$) decreases over 3–4 weeks ($t_{1/2}$ 18–54 hr; $t_{1/2}$ 10–25 hr); for maximal enzyme induction, levels should be rechecked to avoid breakthrough seizures.
   (5) Carbamazepine is metabolized in the liver to 10-11 epoxide, which also has anticonvulsant activity; carbamazepine may induce its own metabolism.
   (6) Adverse effects. The physician should be notified if any of the following adverse effects occur: jaundice, abdominal pain, pale stool, darkened urine, unusual bruising and bleeding, fever, sore throat, or an ulcer in the mouth. The most common side effects are dizziness, drowsiness, unsteadiness, nausea, and vomiting.

Table 45-5. Uses of Antiepileptic Medications Based on Seizure Type

Seizure Type	Drug Therapy			
	Choice 1	Choice 2	Choice 3	Choice 4
Simple partial	Carbamazepine (alone or combination)	Phenytoin	Primidone Lamotrigine Oxcarbazepine	Gabapentin, levetiracetam Zonisamide
Complex partial	Carbamazepine Lamotrigine	Phenytoin	Phenobarbital Zonisamide Oxcarbazepine	Valproic acid Primidone Topiramate Tiagabine
Primary generalized Tonic–clonic	Valproic acid Lamotrigine	Carbamazepine	Phenytoin Valproic acid	Phenobarbital Topiramate Tiagabine
Absence	Lamotrigine,[a] ethosuximide	Zonisamide, valproic acid		
Myoclonic atonic	Valproic acid Valproic acid	Clonazepam Clonazepam	Zonisamide[a]	Felbamate[a] (alone or in combination)
Status epilepticus	Diazepam	Phenytoin	Phenobarbital	
Psychomotor	Phenytoin			

[a]Also indicated for treatment of Lennox-Gastaut syndrome in children.

Table 45-6. Anticonvulsive Drug Classification

Barbiturates	Hydantoins	Succinimides	Sulfonamides	Oxazolidinediones	Benzodiazepine	Miscellaneous
Phenobarbital	Phenytoin	Ethosuximide	Zonisamide	Paramethadione	Clonazepam	Lamotrigine
Primidone	Mephenytoin	Methsuximide	Trimethadione	Diazepam	Felbamate	Gabapentin
Mephobarbital	Ethotoin	Phensuximide		Lorazepam	Clorazepate dipotassium	Pregabalin
	Fosphenytoin				Carbamazepine	Oxcarbazepine
					Valproic acid	
					Topiramate	
					Tiagabine	
					Levetiracetam	

Table 45-7. Dosages Characteristic of Antiepileptic Medications

Drug	Loading Dose	Usual Adult Dose (mg/day)	Half-life (hr)	Therapeutic Range of Total Plasma Concentration (µg/mL)	Major Mode of Elimination	Protein-Binding Level (%)
Carbamazepine	No	800–2000	11[a]–22	4–12	Hepatic	75–80
Phenytoin	Yes	300–700	22–72 1–2 (free)	5–20	Hepatic	90
Phenobarbital	Yes	90–300	100	15–40	Hepatic > renal	40–60
Primidone	No	750–3000	15[a,b]	5–12	Hepatic	20–25
Valproic acid	Yes	1000–3000	15–20	50–150	Hepatic	75–90
Ethosuximide	No	750–1000	30–60[c]	40–100	Hepatic > renal	0
Felbamate	No	2400	20–23	30–100	Hepatic > renal	22–25
Gabapentin	Yes	900–1000	5–7	5–7	Renal	<3
Lamotrigine	No	200–400	25 12.6[d] 70[e]	2–6	Hepatic > renal	55
Topiramate	No	200–400	21	n/a	Renal > hepatic	9–15
Tiagabine	No	32–56	6–8	n/a	Hepatic	96
Levetiracetam	Yes	500–3000	7	n/a	Renal	<10
Zonisamide	No	100–600	63	n/a	Hepatic	40–60
Oxcarbazepine	No	900–1800	8'10	n/a	Hepatic	40–60

[a]The half-life decreases autometabolism after chronic use.
[b]Metabolized in part to phenobarbital.
[c]Lower range in children and higher range in adults.
[d]Receiving other enzyme-inducing drugs.
[e]Valproic acid slows the metabolism.

- **(a) CNS effects.** These include dizziness, ataxia, and diplopia. If diplopia and ataxia are common and occur after a dose, the schedule could be adjusted to include more frequent administration or a larger proportion of the dose at night. CNS side effects may decrease with chronic administration.
- **(b) Gastrointestinal (GI) effects.** These most commonly include nausea, vomiting, and anorexia.
- **(c) Metabolic effects.** Hyponatremia occurs after several weeks to months of therapy, and the incidence increases with age. The antidiuretic hormone (ADH) level may be low. Levels of 125–135 mEq/L without symptoms should be monitored. Fluid restriction should be instituted when levels decrease to < 125 mEq/L with or without symptoms. Another agent should be used if fluid dose reduction does not help or the seizures recur.
- **(d) Hematopoietic effects.** Aplastic anemia is rare. Thrombocytopenia and anemia have a 5% incidence, and they respond to a cessation of drug therapy. Leukopenia is the most common hematopoietic side effect: 10% of cases are transient, and about 2% of patients have persistent leukopenia but do not seem to have increased infections even with white blood cell (WBC) counts of 3000/mL.
- **(e) Dermatological effects.** Pruritic and erythematous rashes, the Stevens-Johnson syndrome, and lupus erythematosus have been reported.

d. Significant interactions
- **(1) Antiepileptic drugs,** such as **phenytoin, primidone,** and **phenobarbital,** decrease the level of carbamazepine (increase metabolism).
- **(2) Valproic acid** increases the level of carbamazepine (decreases metabolism).
- **(3)** Other medications such as **erythromycin, isoniazid, cimetidine, propoxyphene, diltiazem,** and **verapamil** increase the level of carbamazepine (decrease metabolism).
- **(4)** Carbamazepine decreases levels of **calcium channel blockers,** increasing its own level.
- **(5)** Carbamazepine decreases the effect of warfarin.
- **(6)** Antibiotics increase the level of carbamazepine.
- **(7)** Carbamazepine decreases tricyclic antidepressant levels.

2. Phenytoin (Dilantin)

a. Mechanism of action
- **(1)** Phenytoin inhibits the spread of seizures at the motor cortex and blocks posttetanic potentiation by influencing synaptic transmission. There is an alternation of ion fluxes in depolarization, repolarization, and membrane stability phase and alternating calcium uptake in presynaptic terminals.
- **(2)** Phenytoin is effective for the treatment of generalized tonic–clonic (grand mal) seizures and for partial seizures, both simple and complex. It is not effective for absence seizures.

b. Administration and dosage (Table 45-7)
- **(1)** The usual daily dose for **adults** is 300–700 mg, with adjustments made as needed.
  - **(a)** Regular daily doses above 500 mg are poorly tolerated.
  - **(b)** A loading dose of 900 mg to 1.5 g may be given intravenously (IV). The infusion rate should not exceed 50 mg/min. (Alternatively, an oral loading dose may be given.)
- **(2)** The usual daily dose for **children** is 4–7 mg/kg divided every 12 hr. An IV loading dose of 15 mg/kg may be given.
- **(3)** Phenytoin sodium is available as capsules and parenteral solution. Phenytoin is available as tablets and oral suspension.

c. Precautions and monitoring effects
- **(1)** IV phenytoin should not be used in patients with sinus bradycardia, sinoatrial block, second- and third-degree atrioventricular (AV) block, or Adams-Stokes syndrome.
- **(2)** Phenytoin should be used cautiously in patients with myocardial insufficiency and hypotension.
- **(3)** Elimination of phenytoin converts from first-order elimination (proportional to its concentration) to zero-order elimination (a fixed amount per unit time), usually at high therapeutic levels. The daily dose of phenytoin can be increased 100 mg daily until therapeutic blood levels are attained, after which increases of 30–50 mg will avoid twofold to threefold increases in blood levels.

(4) It is necessary to measure free drug levels or correct the total level when aluminum levels are abnormal or the patient has renal failure.

(5) **Adverse effects.** The physician should be notified if any of the following adverse effects occur: swollen or tender gums, skin rash, nausea and vomiting, swollen glands, bleeding, jaundice, fever, or sore throat (i.e., signs of infection or bleeding).

    (a) **CNS effects** include ataxia (limiting side effect), dysarthria, and insomnia. Transient hyperkinesia may follow IV phenytoin infusion. Alcoholic beverages should be avoided while on this medication.

    (b) **GI effects** most commonly include nausea and vomiting. Phenytoin should be taken with food to enhance absorption and decrease GI upset.

    (c) **Dermatological effects** include maculopapular rashes sometimes with fever, Stevens-Johnson syndrome, and lupus erythematosus. Gingival hyperplasia may be reduced by frequent brushing and appropriate oral care.

    (d) **Connective tissue disorders** include a coarsening of the facial features.

    (e) **Hematopoietic effects** include thrombocytopenia, leukopenia, and granulocytopenia.

    (f) **Miscellaneous effects** include hyperglycemia and increased body hair.

d. Significant interactions

(1) **Antiepileptic drugs,** such as **carbamazepine, valproic acid, clonazepam,** and **phenobarbital,** decrease the level of phenytoin (increase metabolism).

(2) Phenytoin increases the **conversion of primidone to phenobarbital** (increases metabolism).

(3) Other medications such as **disulfiram, isoniazid, chloramphenicol,** and **propoxyphene** increase the level of phenytoin (decrease metabolism).

(4) Drugs whose efficacy is impaired by phenytoin include **corticosteroids, digitoxin, doxycycline, estrogens, furosemide, oral contraceptives, quinidine, rifampin, theophylline, vitamin D,** and **enteral nutritional therapy.**

(5) **Coumarin** and **warfarin** anticoagulants increase the serum phenytoin levels and prolong the serum half-life of phenytoin by inhibiting its metabolism.

(6) Phenytoin decreases **tricyclic antidepressant** levels.

(7) Phenytoin interacts with **diabetes and arthritis medications.**

3. Fosphenytoin (Cerebyx)

a. Mechanism of action

(1) Water-soluble prodrug of phenytoin. It is converted to phenytoin by the bloodstream phosphatases, with a half-life of about 8 min in both adults and children.

(2) It is indicated for patients who cannot take oral drugs, and in the acute treatment for status epilepticus.

(3) Administered via IV or intramuscular (IM) injection

(4) A dose conversion table should be used to convert the phenytoin dose to fosphenytoin.

(5) Characteristics similar to phenytoin

(6) **Advantages**

    (a) Fosphenytoin is an aqueous solution, unlike phenytoin, which is an alkaline solution; therefore, there is no need to add propylene glycol and ethanol to the solution.

    (b) Fosphenytoin causes less soft-tissue injury at the site of injection. When administered by IM injection, it is completely absorbed and has more predictable serum concentration than IM-injected phenytoin.

4. Valproic acid (Depakote)

a. Mechanism of action

(1) Increases levels of GABA

(2) Potentiates a postsynaptic GABA response by inhibiting the enzymatic response for the catabolism of GABA

(3) Affects the potassium channel, creating a direct membrane-stabilizing effect

b. Administration and dosage (Table 45-7)

(1) For **adults,** valproic acid is administered orally in a usual dose of 1000–3000 mg daily in divided doses.

    (2) For **children,** valproic acid is administered orally in a dose of 15–60 mg/kg daily, divided into two or three doses.

    (3) Medication should be taken with food to reduce GI upset.

    (4) Tablets or capsules should be swallowed, not chewed, to avoid irritation of the mouth and throat.

c. Precautions and monitoring effects. There are some reports of hepatotoxicity and increased liver function tests, which are mostly reversible. The severity and incidence of hepatotoxicity increase when the patient is younger than 2 years of age.

d. Adverse effects. Contact the physician if abdominal pain, nausea, vomiting, or anoxia occurs; these could be symptoms of pancreatitis.

    (1) CNS effects include tremor, ataxia, diplopia, lethargy, drowsiness, behavioral changes, and depression.

    (2) GI effects include nausea and increased appetite. Enteric-coated divalproex sodium may reduce these side effects.

    (3) Dermatological effects include alopecia and petechiae.

    (4) Hematopoietic effects include thrombocytopenia, bruising, hematoma, and bleeding.

    (5) Hepatic effects include minor elevations of aspartate aminotransferase (AST), alanine aminotransferase (ALT), and lactate dehydrogenase (LDH).

    (6) Endocrine effects include decreased levels of prolactin, resulting in irregular menses, and secondary amenorrhea.

    (7) Pancreatic effects include acute pancreatitis.

    (8) Metabolic effects include hyperammonemia owing to renal origin. Discontinuation may be considered if lethargy develops.

e. Significant interactions

    (1) Antiepileptic drugs

        (a) Primidone decreases valproic acid clearance (increases metabolism).

        (b) Phenobarbital and **phenytoin** displace protein binding, resulting in an increased total phenytoin level and an increase or no change of free phenytoin.

        (c) Clonazepam increases CNS toxicity in patients on valproic acid.

    (2) Other medications

        (a) Aspirin increases the level of valproic acid.

        (b) Warfarin inhibits the secondary phase of platelet aggregation.

        (c) Antacids increase the level of valproic acid.

    (3) Laboratory tests

        (a) False-positive urine ketone tests may result in patients taking valproic acid; thus patients with diabetes must use caution when using urine tests.

        (b) Thyroid function tests may be altered by antiepileptic drugs.

5. Phenobarbital (Luminal)

a. Mechanism of action. Phenobarbital increases the seizure threshold by decreasing postsynaptic excitation by stimulating postsynaptic GABA-A receptor inhibitor responses as a CNS depressant.

b. Administration and dosage (Table 45-7)

    (1) For **adults,** phenobarbital is administered orally at 90–300 mg daily (in three divided doses or as a single dose at bedtime).

    (2) Children typically receive 3–6 mg/kg daily in two divided doses. Adjustment is made as needed.

c. Precautions and monitoring effects

    (1) Phenobarbital produces respiratory depression, especially with parenteral administration.

    (2) Phenobarbital should be used with caution in patients with hepatic disease who may need dose adjustments.

    (3) Phenobarbital has sedative effects in adults and produces hyperactivity in children.

    (4) Abrupt discontinuation of phenobarbital produces withdrawal convulsions. If the drug must be discontinued, another GABA-A agonist (e.g., benzodiazepine, paraldehyde) should be substituted.

    (5) Adverse effects. The physician should be notified if any of the following adverse effects occur: sore throat, mouth sores, easy bruising or bleeding, and any signs of infection.

(a) **CNS effects** include agitation, confusion, lethargy, and drowsiness. Patients should avoid alcohol and other CNS depressants.

(b) **Respiratory effects** include hypoventilation and apnea.

(c) **Cardiovascular effects** include bradycardia and hypotension.

(d) **GI effects** include nausea, diarrhea, and constipation. If GI upset is experienced, phenobarbital should be taken with food.

(e) **Hematological effects** include megaloblastic anemia after chronic use (a rare side effect).

(f) **Miscellaneous effects** include osteomalacia and Stevens-Johnson syndrome, both of which are rare.

d. Significant interactions

(1) **Antiepileptic drugs,** such as **valproic acid** and **phenytoin,** increase the level of phenobarbital (decrease metabolism).

(2) Other drugs such as **acetazolamide, chloramphenicol, cimetidine,** and **furosemide** increase the level of phenobarbital (decrease metabolism).

(3) **Rifampin, pyridoxine,** and **ethanol** decrease the level of phenobarbital (increase metabolism).

6. Primidone (Mysoline)

a. Mechanism of action. Primidone is a metabolite of phenobarbital and phenylethylmalonamide (PEMA), which has some anticonvulsive effects. It has drug characteristics similar to phenobarbital, with some differences in dose and half-life.

b. Administration and dosage (Table 45-7)

(1) Primidone has a short half-life of 7 hr, which may require three-times daily dosing.

(2) Primidone is tolerated better if started at 50 mg at night for 3 days until the target daily dose is reached.

7. Ethosuximide (Zarontin)

a. Mechanism of action

(1) Ethosuximide may inhibit the sodium–potassium adenosine triphosphatase (Na^+/K^+ ATPase) system and the reduced form of nicotinamide adenine dinucleotide phosphate (NADPH) linked aldehyde reductase (which is necessary for the formation of γ-hydroxybutyrate, which is associated with the induction of absence seizures).

(2) Ethosuximide reduces or eliminates the EEG abnormality; however, absence seizures are the only seizures in which the normal EEG has clinical value (i.e., when the EEG abnormality is corrected, the seizures are also controlled).

(3) Ethosuximide is a relatively benign anticonvulsant with minimum protein binding.

b. Administration and dosage (Table 45-7). Ethosuximide is usually given orally in an initial dose of 500 mg daily in **adults and older children** and 250 mg daily in **children ages 3–6 years**. The dose may be raised by 250 mg every week to a maximum of 1.5 g daily in adults.

c. Precautions and monitoring effects

(1) Blood dyscrasias have been reported, making periodic blood counts necessary.

(2) There have been reports of hepatic and renal toxicity; thus periodic renal and liver function monitoring is necessary.

(3) Cases of systemic lupus erythematosus have been reported.

d. Adverse effects

(1) **GI effects** include nausea and vomiting. Small doses may lessen these effects. Ethosuximide should be taken with food if GI upset occurs.

(2) **Hematopoietic effects** include eosinophilia, granulocytopenia, leukopenia, and lupus.

(3) **CNS effects** include drowsiness, blurred vision, fatigue, lethargy, hiccups, and headaches. Alcoholic beverages should be avoided with this medication.

(4) **Psychiatric–psychological** effects include confusion and emotional instability.

(5) **Dermatological effects include** pruritus, photosensitivity, urticaria, and Stevens-Johnson syndrome.

(6) **Genitourinary effects include** increased frequency of urination, vaginal bleeding, renal damage, and hematuria.

(7) **Miscellaneous effects include** periorbital edema and muscle weakness. Patients should also be advised of the risks of exposure to sunlight and ultraviolet light.

e. Significant interactions.

(1) Antiepileptic drugs, such as **carbamazepine,** decrease the level of ethosuximide (increases metabolism).

(2) Valproic acid increases the level of ethosuximide (decreases metabolism).

8. Clonazepam (Klonopin)

a. Mechanism of action. Clonazepam is a potent GABA-A agonist, but its efficacy decreases over several months of treatment.

b. Administration and dosage

(1) For **adults,** clonazepam is an oral agent that may be given in an initial dose of 1.5 mg daily divided two or three times. The dose may be increased to a maximum of 20 mg daily.

(2) Children should receive 0.01–0.03 mg daily in two or three doses. The dosage may be increased to a maximum of 0.2 mg/kg daily.

c. Precautions and monitoring effects

(1) Patients with psychoses, acute narrow-angle glaucoma, and significant liver disease should use this medicine cautiously.

(2) Adverse effects

(a) CNS effects include drowsiness, ataxia, and behavior disturbances in children; these may be corrected by dose reduction.

(b) Respiratory effects include hypersalivation and bronchial hypersecretion.

(c) Miscellaneous effects include anemia, leukopenia, thrombocytopenia, respiratory depression, anorexia, and weight loss.

d. Significant interactions

(1) Antiepileptic drugs, such as **phenytoin,** increase the level of clonazepam (decrease metabolism).

(2) Other drugs. Clonazepam decreases the efficacy of **levodopa** and increases the serum level of **digoxin.**

9. Felbamate (Felbatol)

a. Mechanism of action. A proposed mechanism of action is that the drug interacts with glycine modulatory site on *N*-methyl-D-aspartate (NMDA) receptors. Blockade of NMDA may contribute to neuroprotective effects of felbamate. Felbamate is used as monotherapy or adjunctive therapy or without secondary generalization in adults and generalized seizures associated with Lennox-Gastaut syndrome in children. The U.S. Food and Drug Administration (FDA) recommended that use of felbamate be restricted to only those patients who are refractory to other medications and in whom the risk–benefit relationship warrants its use, because of severe hepatotoxicity.

b. Administration and dosage (Table 45-7)

(1) Adults and children > 14 years of age

(2) Monotherapy, initially 1.2 g in three to four doses daily. The dosage may be increased in 600-mg increments every 2 weeks to 2.4 g daily based on clinical response and, thereafter, 3.6 g daily if necessary.

(3) Adjunctive therapy, 1.2 g in three to four doses daily, with reduction of the dosage of other antiepileptic drugs by 20%–33%. The dosage of felbamate may be increased in increments of 1.2 g at weekly intervals to a maximum of 3.6 g daily.

(4) Conversion to monotherapy initially 1.2 g daily in three to four doses, with reduction of the dosage of other antiepileptic drugs by 33% at week 3. The felbamate dosage may be increased to 3.6 g daily, and other antiepileptic drugs discontinued or dosage further reduced in stepwise fashion.

(5) Children 2–14 years of age with Lennox-Gastaut syndrome, as adjunctive therapy, initially 15 mg/kg daily in three to four doses. The dosage of other antiepileptic drugs is reduced by 20%. The amount of felbamate may be increased in increments of 15 mg/kg at weekly intervals to 45 mg/kg daily. Further reduction in the dosage of other antiepileptic drugs may be necessary.

c. Precaution and monitoring effects. There are two very serious toxic effects, aplastic anemia and liver failure, which lead to death for some patients.

(1) For aplastic anemia, the onset range from 5 to 30 weeks of initiation of therapy. Weekly or biweekly CBCs are recommended initially.

(2) For liver, toxicity time between initiation of treatment and diagnosis of these cases ranges from 14 to 257 days. It is recommended that liver function tests be performed before initiation of therapy to identify patients who have evidence of preexisting liver damage. Liver function tests should also be performed weekly or biweekly. The FDA recommends that this drug be used only in patients who are refractory to other medications and in whom the risk–benefit relationship warrants its use.

(3) Photoallergy or phototoxicity may occur; patients should take protective measures against exposure to ultraviolet light or sunlight.

(4) Instruct patients to store medication in its own tightly closed container at room temperature away from excessive heat, direct sunlight, and moisture.

(5) **Adverse effects.** Contact the physician if signs of infection (e.g., bleeding or bruising) occur.

(a) This drug has the potential to cause aplastic anemia (bone marrow).

(b) The patient should be monitored for these toxicities by CBCs and liver function tests weekly or biweekly until discontinuation of any sign of these toxicities occurs.

(c) **CNS effects** are insomnia, headache, anxiety, hyperactivity, and fatigue.

(d) **Cardiovascular effects** are peripheral edema, vasodilation, hypotension, and hypertension.

(e) **Ocular** effects are diplopia and blurred vision.

(f) **GI effects** are anorexia, weight decrease, and nausea.

(g) **Hematological effects** may include lymphadenopathy, leukopenia, and thrombocytopenia.

(h) **Metabolic/nutrition effects** may include hypokalemia and hyponatremia.

d. **Significant interactions**

(1) **Felbamate and phenytoin.** Felbamate causes an increase in phenytoin plasma concentration. Phenytoin doubles felbamate clearance, resulting in 45% decrease in felbamate levels.

(2) **Felbamate and carbamazepine.** Felbamate causes a decrease in carbamazepine levels and an increase in carbamazepine metabolites. In addition, carbamazepine causes a 50% increase in felbamate clearance, resulting in a 40% decrease in steady-state trough levels.

(3) **Felbamate and valproic acid.** Felbamate causes an increase in valproic acid levels, but valproic acid does not affect felbamate levels.

(4) **Adverse effects.** Signs and symptoms associated with increased plasma level and toxicity are anorexia, nausea, vomiting, insomnia, and headache.

10. **Gabapentin (Neurontin)**

a. **Mechanism of action.** It is an analog of GABA. It increases GABA turnover, but it does not bind to GABA or any other established neurotransmitter receptor. Its mechanism of action is currently unknown, although it binds to a specific receptor in the brain and inhibits voltage-dependent sodium currents. It has been shown to be effective as an add-on drug in patients with partial seizure with or without secondary generalization.

b. **Administration and dosage** (Table 45-7)

(1) Patients **> 12 years** receive 900 mg to 1.8 g daily, administered as adjunctive therapy in three divided doses. Titrating to an effective dose normally can be achieved within 3 days by initiating therapy with 300 mg and then increasing the dose in 300-mg increments over the next 2 days to establish a dosage of 900 mg daily in three doses. If necessary, the dosage may be increased to 1.8 g daily. To minimize potential side effects, especially somnolence, dizziness, or fatigue, the first dose on day 1 may be administered at bedtime.

(2) Patients 3–12 years of age should receive 10–15 mg/kg/day in 3 divided doses up to 25–50 mg/kg/day.

(3) The drug is primarily excreted renally; therefore, the dosage should be adjusted for patients who have compromised renal function.

(4) The drug does not bind to plasma protein. There are no significant pharmacokinetic interactions with other commonly used antiepileptic drugs.

(5) If gabapentin is discontinued or an alternate anticonvulsant medication is added, it should be done gradually over a minimum of 1 week.

c. **Precautions and monitoring effects**

(1) The value of monitoring blood concentration has not been established and would not alter blood concentration of other antiepileptic drugs when used together.

(2) It has a low level of toxic side effects, which include somnolence, dizziness, ataxia, and minimal interaction with other drugs.

(3) Gabapentin is useful in patients who are taking other medications for epilepsy or other chronic diseases. It may be especially useful for elderly patients.

(4) Gabapentin is well absorbed orally; it can be taken with or without food. However, patients who have GI problems might have problems with absorption.

(5) Adverse effects. Common side effects are somnolence, dizziness, ataxia, fatigue, weight gain and nystagmus.

    (a) CNS effects are somnolence, dizziness, ataxia, and fatigue.

    (b) GI effects include dyspepsia, dryness of mouth, constipation, and increased appetite.

    (c) Ocular effects are diplopia, blurred vision, and nystagmus.

d. Significant interactions

(1) Antacids and gabapentin. Antacids reduce the bioavailability of gabapentin by 20%; gabapentin could be taken 2 hr after antacid use.

(2) Cimetidine and gabapentin. Cimetidine decreases the renal excretion of gabapentin by 14% and consequently increases gabapentin plasma levels (however, this amount is not clinically significant).

(3) Oral contraceptives and gabapentin. Oral contraceptives increase the level of norethindrone by 13%; this amount may not be clinically significant.

11. Lamotrigine (Lamictal)

a. Mechanism of action. Its antiepileptic effect is similar to that of phenytoin. Its effect may be the result of inhibition of voltage-dependent sodium currents and reduction of sustained repetitive neuronal activity. It is indicated for the treatment of partial seizures and secondary generalized tonic–clonic seizures that are not controlled with other drugs. It is also used to treat Lennox-Gastaut syndrome. Lamotrigine is broad spectrum, as well tolerated as monotherapy, and probably the least teratogenic of the first-line agents. It may aggravate severe myoclonic epilepsy.

b. Administration and dosage (Table 45-7)

(1) Adults (> 16 years), initially 50 mg/day in two divided doses (patients taking valproic acid should be given 25 mg every other day), up to 100 mg/day (up to 25 mg daily with valproic acid treatment).

(2) Children 2–12 years 0.6 mg/kg/day in two divided dosed (0.15 mg/kg/day on valproic acid treatment), up to 1.2 mg/kg/day (up to 0.3 mg/kg/day with valproic acid treatment).

(3) The smallest available chewable dispersible tablet is 5 mg. Then, after 2 weeks, increase by 0.3 mg/kg/day in one to two divided doses, up to 200 mg/day.

(4) Swallow chewable dispersible tablet whole, chewed, or in dispersing water or diluted fruit juice. If chewed, consume a small amount of water or dilute fruit juice to aid in swallowing. To disperse, add the chewable dispersible tablet to a small amount of liquid (1 teaspoon or enough to cover the medication). Approximately 1 min later, when the tablet is completely dispersed, swirl the solution and consume the entire quantity immediately.

(5) For patients taking valproic acid, the initial dose is 50 mg daily for 2 weeks, followed by maintenance doses of 100–200 mg daily in two divided doses.

(6) Reduced clearance in the elderly necessitates dosage reduction.

(7) Patients with hepatic impairment may require dosage reduction because of reduction in metabolism.

c. Precautions and monitoring effects

(1) The value of monitoring plasma concentration has not been established.

(2) Caution should be used for patients taking this drug. It may adversely affect the patient's metabolism or complicate the elimination of the drug because of renal, hepatic, or cardiac impairment.

(3) Lamotrigine binds to melanin and can accumulate in melanin-rich tissue over time. Periodic ophthalmological monitoring is recommended.

(4) Photosensitization (photoallergy and phototoxicity) patients should take protective measures against exposure to ultraviolet light or sunlight.

(5) Serious rashes requiring hospitalization have been reported. The incidence of rashes, including Stevens-Johnson syndrome, is approximally 1% in patients < 16 years old and 0.3% in adults. Rare cases of toxic epidermal necrolysis or rash-related death have occurred. Most rashes occur within 2–8 weeks of initial treatment.

(6) **Adverse effects.** The most common side effects are dizziness, diplopia, ataxia, blurred vision, nausea, dose-related rash and vomiting.

   (a) **CNS effects** are headache, dizziness, and ataxia.

   (b) **GI effects** are nausea, vomiting, diarrhea, and dyspepsia.

   (c) **Ocular effects** are diplopia, blurred vision, and vision abnormality.

   (d) **Dermatological effects** are pruritus, and a rash may form similar to that found when using phenytoin and carbamazepine. In many cases, the rash disappears during continued therapy, but 1%–2% of patients with the rash represent a more serious allergic reaction. Occasionally, patients have developed the Stevens-Johnson syndrome. Concomitant use with valproic acid may increase the likelihood of serious rash. The occurrences of life-threatening rash that were reported developed within 2–8 weeks following therapy; other cases of rash have been reported developing up to 6 months after therapy. The incidence of rash is higher in children than in adults.

   (e) Monotherapy during pregnancy found no teratogenic effect.

d. **Significant interactions**

   (1) Carbamazepine decreases lamotrigine concentration by 70% and increases carbamazepine levels.

   (2) Phenobarbital or primidone decreases lamotrigine concentration by 40%.

   (3) Valproic acid decreases the metabolism of lamotrigine and extends its half-life to 60 hr, which necessitates a dose reduction.

12. **Topiramate (Topamax)**

   a. **Mechanism of action.** Topiramate is a derivative of fructose. It decreases rapid hippocampal neuronal firing, possibly because of sodium- or calcium-channel inhibition. It is also a weak carbonic anhydrase inhibitor and a sodium-channel blocking agent. Topiramate potentiates the activity of GABA. It has been shown to be effective adjunctive therapy for partial seizure treatment in adults, tonic–clonic seizure, infantile spasms, and Lennox-Gastaut syndrome.

   b. **Administration and dosage** (Table 45-7)

      (1) **Adults** 17 years and older, 25–50 mg/day, up to 400 mg/day in two divided doses. **Children** 2–16 years, 1–3 mg/kg/day, up to 5–9 mg/kg/day in two divided doses.

      (2) Topiramate is 80% bioavailable, and food does not affect its bioavailability.

      (3) Dose adjustment is necessary for patients with renal or hepatic impairments.

      (4) Enzyme-inducing anticonvulsive drugs can decrease topiramate levels, but topiramate has a significant effect on metabolism of other anticonvulsive drugs.

      (5) Initial treatment is 50 mg daily, followed by titration to an effective dosage. More than 400 mg daily has not been shown to improve response.

   c. **Precaution and monitoring effects**

      (1) Increased incidence of kidney stones (renal calculus) in older patients who received this drug. Patients should be advised to increase intake of fluids while taking topiramate.

      (2) Paresthesia is a common side effect of anhydrase inhibitors.

      (3) **Adverse effects**

         (a) The physician should be notified if any of the following adverse effects occur:

            (i) Breast pain in females

            (ii) Nausea or tremor, which are dose-related side effects.

            (iii) Back pain, chest pain, dyspepsia, or leg pain

         (b) **CNS effects** include psychomotor slowing, difficulty with concentration and speech, somnolence, fatigue, asthenia, weight loss, cognitive disturbances and difficulties, tremors, dizziness, ataxia, and headache.

         (c) **GI effects** include upset, such as nausea, vomiting, and gastroenteritis.

         (d) **Genitourinary effects** include renal calculi.

         (e) **Cardiovascular effects** include chest pain, palpitation, and vasodilation.

         (f) **Ocular effects** include abnormal vision, eye pain, and diplopia.

         (g) **Hematological effects** include anemia, epistaxis, leukopenia, and aplastic anemia.

   d. **Significant interactions**

      (1) Phenytoin and carbamazepine will increase clearance.

      (2) Topiramate increases the clearance of other drugs that are cleared by cytochrome P450.

13. Tiagabine (Gabitril)

a. **Mechanism of action.** Tiagabine is designed to act on the inhibitory action of GABA by blocking its uptake, thereby prolonging its action after synaptic release. It is indicated as adjunctive therapy for partial seizures and secondary generalized tonic–clonic seizures.

b. **Administration and dosage** (Table 45-7)

(1) Starting dose of 4 mg daily for 2 weeks may be increased 4–8 mg weekly thereafter, to a maintenance dose of 32–56 mg daily.

(2) Maximum recommended dosage for **children** is 32 mg daily; maximum recommended dosage for **adults** is 56 mg daily.

(3) A high-fat meal decreases the rate of tiagabine absorption but does not affect the extension of absorption. Tiagabine should be taken with food.

c. **Precautions and monitoring effects**

(1) Moderately severe to severe **generalized weakness** has been reported. It resolves in all cases after reduction in dose or discontinuation of therapy.

(2) **Ophthalmic effects,** as indicated by animal studies, include the possibility for residual binding to retina and melanin binding; this finding, however, has not been confirmed in human studies. Periodic ophthalmological monitoring is necessary.

(3) **Dermatological effects** include the possibility of severe rash to Stevens-Johnson syndrome, as reported in clinical studies.

(4) **Adverse effects**

(a) **CNS effects** are confusion, dizziness, and fatigue.

(b) **GI effects** are upset stomach, nausea, mouth ulceration, and anorexia.

d. **Significant interactions.** Phenobarbital, phenytoin, and carbamazepine will increase tiagabine clearance.

14. Zonisamide (Zonegran)

a. **Mechanism of action.** It is not well known. It may block the sensitive sodium channels and T-type calcium channels. It is an effective agent for refractory partial seizure, generalized seizure indicated for adjunct therapy for partial seizure for adults, infantile spasm, mixed seizure types of Lennox-Gastaut syndrome, myoclonic, and generalized tonic–clonic seizure.

b. **Administration and dosage** (Table 45-7)

(1) **Adults and children** > 16 years of age, 100 mg daily; within 2 weeks, increase to 200 mg/daily in 2-week bases, up to 600 mg daily.

(2) Can be taken with or without food.

c. **Precautions and monitoring effects**

(1) May increase mean concentration of serum creatinine and blood, urea, nitrogen; renal function should be monitored periodically.

(2) May increase serum alkaline phosphatase.

(3) May produce drowsiness.

(4) **Side effects.** The physician should be contacted if sudden pain or abdominal pain occurs or if blood in urine is detected; these symptoms could indicate a **kidney stone.** Increase fluid intake to decrease the risk of stone formation. Also, contact the physician if fever, sore throat, oral ulcer, or easy bruising is seen; these symptoms could be the result of a **hematological complication.**

(5) Most commonly reported adverse events are **somnolence, anorexia, dizziness, headache, nausea, allergic reactions,** and **agitation.**

(a) **CNS effects** are ataxia, confusion, tremor, and abnormal thinking.

(b) **Cardiovascular effects** are palpitation, tachycardia, and vascular insufficiency.

(c) **Dermatologic effects** are maculopapular rash, and acne alopecia.

(d) **Other effects** are bladder calculus and leukopenia.

d. **Significant interactions**

(1) Zonisamide induces **liver enzymes** by increasing metabolism and through clearance of zonisamide and decreases half-life.

(2) **Food** will delay absorption but will not affect the bioavailability of the drug.

15. Levetiracetam (Keppra)

a. **Mechanism of action.** It is a pyrrolidone derivative and is chemically unrelated to other antiepileptic drugs. It displays inhibitory properties in the kindling model in rats. It is used as adjunctive therapy in the treatment of partial seizure in adult patients.

b. **Administration and dosage** (Table 45-7). Starting dose of 1000 mg/day given in two divided doses may be increased every 2 weeks, to a maximum of 3000 mg/day.

c. **Precautions and monitoring effects**
   (1) **Hematological effects** are minor, but there is a statistically significant decrease compared to placebo in total mean RBC count, mean hemoglobulin, and mean hematocrit.
   (2) Decrease in WBC count and neurophil count
   (3) It also causes drowsiness.
   (4) **Side effects.** Most commonly reported adverse events are **somnolence, weakness (asthenia), infection,** and **dizziness.**
      (a) **CNS effects** are somnolence, dizziness, depression, and nervousness.
      (b) **Cardiovascular effects** are palpitation, tachycardia, and vascular insufficiency.
      (c) **Respiratory effects** are pharyngitis, rhinitis, and increased cough.
      (d) **Miscellaneous effects** are weakness, headache, and infection.
   e. **Significant interactions.** Levetiracetam does not influence the **plasma concentration** of existing antiepileptic drugs, and other **antiepileptic drugs** do not influence the pharmacokinetic effects of levetiracetam.

16. **Oxcarbazepine (Trileptal)**
   a. **Mechanism of action.** This drug produces blockade of voltage-sensitive sodium channels, resulting in stabilization of hyperexcited neural membranes, inhibition of repetitive neuronal firing, and diminution of propagation of synaptic impulses. These actions are thought to be important in the prevention of seizure spread in the intact brain. In addition, increased potassium conductance and modulation of high-voltage activated calcium channels may contribute to the anticonvulsant effects of the drug.
   b. **Administration and dosage** (Table 45-7)
      (1) **Children** 4–16 years, 8–10 mg/kg/day to 600 mg/day as adjunctive therapy and 8–10mg/kgday as monotherapy.
      (2) **Adults,** 600mg/day as adjunctive therapy and 1200mg/day as monotherapy. A dosage adjustment is needed for patients with renal failure; no dosage adjustment is needed for patients with mild to moderate hepatic impairment.
      (3) Can be taken with or without food.
   c. **Precaution and monitoring effects**
      (1) Clinically significant **hyponatremia** (sodium < 125 mmol/L) can develop during therapy.
      (2) **Side effects**
         (a) Use of this product have been associated with **CNS effects** such as cognitive symptoms (psychomotor slowing, difficult concentrating).
         (b) May reduce the efficacy of oral contraceptive.
      (3) **Adverse effects**
         (a) **CNS effects** are dizziness, somnolence, headache, ataxia, fatigue, and vertigo.
         (b) **GI effects** are vomiting, nausea, and abdominal pain.
         (c) **Neuromuscular and skeletal effects are** abnormal gait and tremor.
         (d) **Ocular effects** are Diplopia, nystagmus, and abnormal vision.
         (e) **Endocrine and metabolic effects** include hyponatremia (low level of sodium in the blood).
   d. **Significant interactions**
      (1) Oxcarbazepine inhibits **cytochrome P450 2C19** and induces **cytochrome P450 3A4/5** with potentially important effects on plasma concentrations of other drugs.
      (2) Serum concentrations of **phenytoin** and **phenobarbital** are increased.
      (3) It decreases **oral contraceptive** effects, benzodiazepine, and calcium channel blockers.
      (4) Cross-sensitivity with **carbamazepine** (25%–30%).

17. **Less common drugs** are listed in Table 45-8.

18. **Vagus nerve stimulation (VNS)**
   a. It is used as adjunctive therapy for adults and children >r 12 years of age whose partial seizures are refractory to antiepileptic medications.
   b. A programmable signal generator that is implanted in the patient's left upper chest has a bipolar VNS lead that connects the generator to the left vagus nerve in the neck, a programming wand that uses radio-frequency signals to communicate noninvasively with the generator, and handheld magnets used by the patient or caregiver to manually turn the stimulator on or off.

Table 45-8. Less Common Drugs Used in Practice

Drug	Labeled Indication	Half-Life (hr)	Total Plasma Concentration (mg/L)	Therapeutic Range of Adult Dose (mg/day)	Usual Mode of Elimination	Major Protein Binding Level
Mephobarbital	• Grand mal • Petit mal • Gets converted to phenobarbital • Indicated when phenobarbital must be decreased because of excessive drowsiness • Hyperexcitability • Mood disturbances	11–67	n/a	400–600	Liver	40–60
Mephenytoin	• Tonic–clonic • Psychomotor • Status epilepticus • Used with phenytoin; together more sedative compared to phenytoin alone	95 (active metabolite)	n/a	200–600	Liver > renal	90
Ethotoin	• Tonic–clonic • Psychomotor • Used as second-line therapy; less toxic and less effective than phenytoin (alone or combined)	3–9[a]	15–50	2000–3000	Liver	N/A
Methsuximide	• Absence • Does not precipitate tonic–clonic (compared to other succinimides)	2–40[b]	n/a	1200	Liver	n/a
Phensuximide	• Absence • Less toxic and less effective compared to other succinimides	8[b]	n/a	1000–3000	Urine, bile	n/a
Paramethadione[c]	• Absence • Useful when other seizures exist with absence seizure • *Note:* Do not use with mephenytoin	n/a	n/a	900–2400	Liver > renal	n/a
Trimethadione[c]	• Absence • Useful when other seizures exist with absence seizure • *Note:* Do not use with mephenytoin	6–13 days	n/a	≥ 700	Liver	0
Pregabalin	• Simple partial seizure	6	n/a	150–600	Renal	0

[a]At high doses, nonlinear kinetic like phenytoin.
[b]Active metabolite.
[c]Possible fetal malformation if used during pregnancy.

c. The implantation procedure usually lasts 1 hr under general anesthesia. Once programmed, the generator will deliver intermittent stimulation at the desired setting until any additional programming is entered.

C. **Surgery.** If seizures do not respond to drug therapy, surgery may be performed to remove the epileptogenic brain region. The most common is cortical excision (lobectomy). Between 70% and 80% of patients who have anterior temporal lobectomy have fewer seizures. Between 30% and 40% patients who have frontal lobectomy have fewer seizures.

1. **Indications** for surgery are intractable or disabling seizures recurring for 6–12 months. Should be considered for patients with medically refractory seizures.

2. In **stereotaxic surgery,** the surgeon uses three-dimensional coordinates to guide a needle through a hole drilled in the skull, then destroys abnormal pathways via small intracerebral incisions.

3. **Other surgical approaches** include temporal lobe resection, removal of the temporal lobe tip, and cerebral hemispherectomy.

III. Complications

A. **Convulsive status epilepticus.** This disorder is characterized by rapid repetition of generalized tonic–clonic seizures with no recovery of consciousness between seizures. This life-threatening condition may persist for hours or even days; if it lasts longer than 1 hr, severe permanent brain damage may result.

1. **Causes** of status epilepticus include poor therapeutic compliance, intracranial infection or neoplasm, alcohol withdrawal, drug overdose, and metabolic imbalance.

2. **Management**
   a. A patent airway must be maintained.
   b. If the cause of the condition is unknown, dextrose 50% in water (25–30 mL) is given via IV in case hypoglycemia is the cause.
   c. If the seizures persist, **diazepam** (10 mg) is administered via IV at a rate not exceeding 2 mg/min until the seizures stop or 20 mg has been given.
   d. **Phenytoin or fosphenytoin** is then administered via IV no faster than 50 mg/min to a maximum dose of 11–18 mg/kg. Blood pressure is monitored to detect hypotension.
   e. If these measures do not stop the seizures, one of the following drugs is given.
      (1) **Diazepam** is given as an IV drip of 50–100 mg diluted in 500 mL dextrose 5% in water, infused at 40 mL/hr until the seizures stop.
      (2) **Phenobarbital** is given as an IV infusion of 8–20 mg/kg no faster than 100 mg/min.
   f. If seizures continue despite these measures, one of the following steps is then taken.
      (1) **Paraldehyde** is given via IV in a dosage of 0.10–0.15 mL/kg diluted to a 4% solution in normal saline solution.
      (2) **Lidocaine** is given in an IV loading dose of 50–100 mg, followed by an infusion of 1–2 mg/min.
      (3) **General anesthesia** is induced with ventilatory assistance and neuromuscular junction blockade.

B. **Nonconvulsive status epilepticus.** This condition presents as repeated absence seizures or complex partial seizures. The patient's mental state fluctuates; confusion, impaired responses, and automatisms are prominent. **Initial management** typically involves intravenous diazepam. Complex partial status epilepticus may also necessitate administration of such drugs as phenytoin or phenobarbital.

IV. Seizure Disorder and Pregnancy

A. **Epidemiology.** About 0.5% of all pregnancies occur in women with epilepsy.

B. **Preconception counseling.** The risks for mother and fetus should be discussed, including the risks of fetal malformation associated with antiepileptic drugs and other genetic factors.

C. Drug therapy

1. If the patient is seizure free for at least 2 years, withdrawal of the drug should be considered. If antiepileptic drug therapy is necessary, a switch to monotherapy should be made if possible.

2. Five antiepileptic medications have been used or studied in pregnant patients: carbamazepine, phenobarbital, phenytoin, primidone, and valproic acid. Monotherapy of lamotrigine during pregnancy found no teratogenic effect. Congenital malformations associated with these drugs include craniofacial abnormalities, cardiac defects, and neuronal tube defects. Most of the studies did not consider paternal genetic factors, environmental factors, drug dosing, or combination therapy.

3. Antiepileptic drugs interfere with folate metabolism. Administration of folic acid, 4 mg daily, and multivitamins decreases the risk of malformation, especially of the neuronal tube.

4. Vitamin K, 10 mg per day for the last 1–2 months of gestation, will help prevent neonatal hemorrhage, especially in cases of phenytoin or phenobarbital use.

5. Seizure disorder and oral contraceptives. Gabapentin, lamotrigine, levetiracetam, ethosuximide, valproate, zonisamide and tiagabine do not affect the efficacy of oral contraceptives.

6. Seizure disorder and the elderly population. The new generation of antiepileptic drugs such as levetiracetam and gabapentin may be more useful owing to low levels of protein binding and safer side effects. Also, the newer agents have less potential for drug interactions than agents eliminated from the liver.

D. Monitoring

1. Free serum antiepileptic drug levels should be monitored monthly, immediately before the next dose; and the dose should be adjusted to the lowest dose providing adequate control.

2. Serum α-fetoprotein levels should be checked, and ultrasonography should be performed at 16 weeks of gestation to evaluate for fetal neuronal tube defects. An alternative to these tests is amniocentesis, especially if the mother is taking valproate or carbamazepine.

3. Comprehensive ultrasonography should be performed at 18 and 22 weeks of gestation for patients taking antiepileptic drugs that cause cardiac anomalies.

4. Intrapartum plans should include IV administration of a short-acting benzodiazepine. If there is concern about fetal or maternal respiratory depression, administering intravenous phenytoin or intramuscular phenobarbital should be considered. Clotting studies should be performed, and 1 mg vitamin K should be given to the infant. Nurses and physicians should be alerted for possible hemorrhage of the infant and apprised that the infant may experience antiepileptic drug withdrawal.

STUDY QUESTIONS

Directions: Each of the questions, statements, or incomplete statements in this section can be correctly answered or completed by **one** of the suggested answers or phrases. Choose the **best** answer.

1. Phenytoin is effective for the treatment of all of the following types of seizures *except*

   (A) generalized tonic–clonic.
   (B) simple partial.
   (C) complex partial.
   (D) absence.
   (E) grand mal.

2. Which of the following anticonvulsants is contraindicated in patients with a history of hypersensitivity to tricyclic antidepressants?

   (A) phenytoin
   (B) ethosuximide
   (C) acetazolamide
   (D) carbamazepine
   (E) phenobarbital

3. Which of the following antiepileptic drugs is primary metabolized by the kidney?

   (A) phenytoin
   (B) gabapentin
   (C) topiramate
   (D) levetiracetam
   (E) B, C, and D

4. Which anticonvulsive drug treatment has a higher incidence of kidney stones?

   (A) phenytoin
   (B) carbamazepine
   (C) topiramate
   (D) tiagabine

5. What are the most common adverse effects of anticonvulsive drugs?

   (A) headache and dizziness
   (B) gastrointestinal symptoms
   (C) alternation of cognition and mentation
   (D) adverse effects on appetite and body weight
   (E) all of the above

6. Which antiepileptic drug has the least effect on the efficacy of oral contraceptives?

   (A) phenytoin
   (B) tiagabine
   (C) gabapentin
   (D) lamotrigine
   (E) C and D

7. Which of the following drugs could cause hyponatremia?

   (A) carbamazepine
   (B) phenytoin
   (C) oxcarbazepine
   (D) felbamate
   (E) topiramate
   (F) A, C, and D

ANSWERS AND EXPLANATIONS

1. The answer is D *[see I.B.2.c.(1)].*
Phenytoin (diphenylhydantoin) is the most commonly prescribed hydantoin for seizure disorders. It is one of the preferred drugs for generalized tonic–clonic (grand mal) seizures and for partial seizures, both simple and complex. However, phenytoin is not effective for absence (petit mal) seizures.

2. The answer is D *[see II.B.1.c.(2)].*
Carbamazepine is structurally related to the tricyclic antidepressants (e.g., amitriptyline, desipramine, imipramine, nortriptyline, protriptyline) and should not be administered to patients with hypersensitivity to any of the tricyclic antidepressants.

3. The answer is B *[see II.B.5–6].*
Primidone's antiseizure activity may be partly attributable to phenobarbital. In patients receiving primidone, serum levels of both primidone and phenobarbital should be measured.

4. The answer is C *[see II.B.12]*
There is a higher incidence of kidney stones (renal calculus) with topiramate administration.

5. The answer is E *[see I.B.1–9]*
Alternation in cognition and mentation, gastrointestinal symptoms, appetite and body weight, and headache and dizziness are all common adverse effects of anticonvulsive drugs.

6. The answer is E *[see IV.C.5]*
Gabapentin and lamotrigine do not increase the metabolism of oral contraceptives to a clinically significant level; therefore, they could be used with oral contraceptives.

7. The answer is F *[see II.B.1; II.B.9; II.B.16].*
Carbamazepine, oxcarbazepine, and felbamate all cause hyponatremia.

46
Parkinson Disease
Azita Razzaghi

I. DISEASE STATE AND PATHOLOGY

A. Definition. Parkinson disease is a slowly progressive degenerative neurological disease characterized by tremor, rigidity, bradykinesia (sluggish neuromuscular responsiveness), and postural instability. Parkinson disease was first described by Dr. James Parkinson in 1817 as "shaking palsy."

B. Incidence

1. It has a prevalence of 1–2 per 1000 of the general population and 2 per 100 among people > 65 years.

2. Onset generally occurs between age 50 and 65; it usually occurs in the 60s.

C. Pathogenesis. Parkinson disease is a neurodegenerative disease associated with **depigmentation of the substantia nigra** and the **loss of dopaminergic input to the basal ganglia** (extrapyramidal system); it is characterized by distinctive **motor disability.** The basal ganglia are responsible for initiating, sequencing, and modulating motor activity.

1. In healthy individuals, dopamine is produced by neurons that project from the substantia nigra to the neostriatum (which include caudate and putamen) and globus pallidus. In these areas, dopamine acts as an inhibitory neurotransmitter.

2. Lewy bodies are widespread but occur especially in the basal ganglia, brainstem, spinal cord, and sympathetic ganglia.

3. In Parkinson disease, the loss of dopamine-producing neurons in the substantia nigra results in an imbalance between dopamine, an inhibitory neurotransmitter, and the excitatory neurotransmitter acetylcholine. Alterations in the concentrations of other neurotransmitters, such as norepinephrine, serotonin, and γ-aminobutyric acid (GABA), are also involved in the pathophysiology of Parkinson disease (Figure 46-1).

D. Cause. Several forms of Parkinson disease have been recognized.

1. **Primary (idiopathic) Parkinson disease**
   a. This is also called classic Parkinson disease or **paralysis agitans.**
   b. The cause is unknown; and while treatment may be palliative, the disease is incurable.
   c. Most patients suffer from this type of parkinsonism.
   d. **Hypotheses of neuronal loss** in idiopathic Parkinson disease are as follows:
      (1) **Absorption of highly potent neurotoxins,** such as carbon monoxide, manganese, solvents, and N-methyl-4-phenyl-1,2,3,6-tetrahydropyridine (MPTP), which is a product of improper synthesis of a synthetic heroin-like compound. Exposure to these agents, alone or in combination with the neuronal loss of age, may be the cause of Parkinson disease.
      (2) **Exposure to the free radicals.** Normally, dopamine is catabolized by monoamine oxidase (MAO). Hydrogen peroxide and production of free radicals—both toxic to cells—are products of catabolism. Protective mechanisms, enzymes, and free radical scavengers, such as vitamins E and C, protect cells from damage. It is proposed that either a decrease in these protective mechanisms or an increase in the production of dopamine causes a destruction of the neurons by free radicals.

2. **Secondary parkinsonism—from a known cause**
   a. Only a small percentage of cases are secondary, and many of these are curable.
   b. Secondary parkinsonism may be caused by drugs, including dopamine antagonists, such as the following:

Figure 46-1. Extrapyramidal system involved in Parkinson disease. [Reprinted with permission from Netter F. Ciba Collection of Medical Illustrations. West Caldwell, NJ: Ciba Geigy Pharmaceuticals, 1983:69.]

(1) Phenothiazines (e.g., chlorpromazine, perphenazine)
(2) Butyrophenones (e.g., haloperidol)
(3) Reserpine
  c. Poisoning by chemicals or toxins may be the cause; these include
    (1) Carbon monoxide poisoning
    (2) Heavy-metal poisoning, such as that by manganese or mercury
    (3) MPTP, a commercial compound used in organic synthesis and found (as a side product) in an illegal meperidine analog
  d. Infectious causes include
    (1) Encephalitis (viral)
    (2) Syphilis
  e. Other causes include
    (1) Arteriosclerosis
    (2) Degenerative diseases of the central nervous system (CNS), such as progressive supranuclear palsy
    (3) Metabolic disorders, such as Wilson disease

E. Signs and symptoms

1. Tremor
  a. Tremor may be the initial complaint in some patients. It is most evident at rest (**resting tremor**) and with low-frequency movement. When the thumb and forefinger are involved, it is known as the **pill-rolling tremor.** Before pills were made by machine, pharmacists made tablets (pills) by hand, hence the name (Figure 46-2).
  b. Some patients experience **action tremor** (most evident during activity), which can exist with or before the resting tremor develops.

2. Limb rigidity is present in almost all patients. It is detected clinically when the arm responds with a ratchet-like (i.e., cogwheeling) movement when the limb is moved passively. This is owing to a tremor that is superimposed on the rigidity.

3. Akinesia or bradykinesia. Akinesia is characterized by difficulty in initiating movements, and bradykinesia is a slowness in performing common voluntary movements, including

Figure 46-2. Resting (or static) tremors. [Adapted from Bates B. A Guide to Physical Examination and History Taking. 5th ed. Philadelphia: Lippincott, 1991:197.]

Stare

Decreased
mobility

Figure 46-3. Masked face of Parkinson disease. [Adapted from Bates B. A Guide to Physical Examination and History Taking. 5th ed. Philadelphia: Lippincott, 1991:197.]

standing, walking, eating, writing, and talking. The lines of the patient's face are smooth, and the expression is fixed (**masked face**) with little evidence of spontaneous emotional responses (Figure 46-3).

4. Gait and postural difficulties. Characteristically, patients walk with a stooped, flexed posture; a short, shuffling stride; and a diminished arm swing in rhythm with the legs. There may be a tendency to accelerate or festinate (Figure 46-4).

5. Changes in mental status. Mental status changes, including depression (50%), dementia (25%), and psychosis, are associated with the disease and may be precipitated or worsened by drugs.

6. Unified Parkinson disease rating scale (UPDRS)
   a. To evaluate the clinical efficacy of antiparkinson drugs and **to monitor disease progression,** most investigators have used the UPDRS.
      (1) The disadvantages associated with the use of scales for rating the functional and motor disabilities of patients with Parkinson disease include the potential of interrater variability and imprecision because of the semiquantitative scoring.
      (2) The result of testing depends highly on the stage of the disease, whether the patient is being evaluated during an on or off period, and the relative distribution of the improvement across all the items evaluated.
   b. Part I of the UPDRS is an **evaluation of mentation, behavior,** and **mood.**
   c. Part II is a **self-reported evaluation of the activities of daily living (ADLs)** and includes speech, swallowing, handwriting, ability to cut food, dressing, hygiene, falling, salivating, turning in bed, and walking.
   d. Part III is a **clinician-scored motor evaluation.**
      (1) Patients are evaluated for speech, rest–tremor facial expression and mobility, action or postural tremor of hands, rigidity, finger taps, hand movements, rapid alternative pronation–supination movement of hands, leg agility, ease of arising from a chair, posture, postural stability, gait, and bradykinesia.

Figure 46-4. Characteristic walk of patients with Parkinson disease. [Adapted from Bates B. *A* Guide to Physical Examination and History Taking. 5th ed. Philadelphia: Lippincott, 1991:553.]

(2) Each item is evaluated on a scale of 0–4.
   (a) **A rating of 0** on the motor performance evaluation scale indicates **normal performance.**
   (b) **A rating of 4** on the motor performance evaluation scale indicates **severely impaired performance.**
  e. **Part IV** is the **Hoehn and Yahr** staging of severity of Parkinson disease (Table 46-1).
  f. **Part V** is the **Schwan and England ADL scale.**

Table 46-1. Stages of Parkinson Disease

Stage	Characteristics
0	No clinical signs evident
I	Unilateral involvement, including the major features of tremor, rigidity, or bradykinesia; minimal functional impairment
II	Bilateral involvement but no postural abnormalities
III	Mild to moderate bilateral disease, mild postural imbalance, but still ability to function independently
IV	Bilateral involvement with postural instability; patient requires substantial assistance
V	Severe disease; patient restricted to bed or wheelchair unless aided

Reprinted with permission from Hoehn MM, Yahr MD. Parkinsonism: Onset, progression, and mortality. Neurology 1967;17:427.

F. Diagnosis

1. Diagnosis depends on clinical findings.

2. Tests (including imaging) are most often used to rule out an origin of secondary Parkinson disease.

3. New technologies—for example, positron-emission tomography (PET) scan—are used to visualize dopamine uptake in the substantia nigra and basal ganglia. The PET scan measures the extent of neuronal loss in these areas.

4. A specific form of single-photon emission computed tomography (SPECT) can be helpful for diagnosis of parkinsonian syndromes and nonparkinsonism syndromes, particularly essential tremor.

5. Other diseases that are similar to Parkinson disease are multiple system atrophy (striatonigral degeneration, olivopontocerebellar atrophy, shy-dragger syndrome), corticobasal ganglionic degeneration, and progressive supranuclear palsy.

G. Treatment (Figure 46-5)

1. **Nondrug treatment**
   a. **Exercise** is an important adjunctive therapy and is most beneficial. Although exercise does not help with the symptoms of Parkinson disease, regular focused exercise, stretching, and strengthening activities can have a positive effect on mobility and mood.
   b. **Nutrition.** Patients with Parkinson disease are at increased risk of poor nutrition, weight loss, and reduced muscle mass. Examples of the beneficial effects of proper nutrition in this group of patients include the following:
      (1) Sufficient fiber and fluid intake help prevent constipation associated with Parkinson disease and the medications used to treat the disease.
      (2) Calcium supplementation helps maintain the existing bone structure.
      (3) Excessive dietary protein in the late stages of the disease causes erratic responses to levodopa therapy.
      (4) A large body of literature supports the pathophysiological role of antioxidants in the relief of oxidative stress in Parkinson disease. High doses of antioxidants and α-tocopherol or vitamin E are recommended in this group of patients.

2. **Drug therapy for symptomatic relief.** Treatment is divided into two generalized categories: symptomatic therapies and preventive or protective measures. Neuroprotective strategies are used to slow the development and progression of the disorder.

H. Neuroprotective treatment

1. MAO-B, such as selegiline and tocopherol (vitamin E), acts as a scavenger of free radicals.

2. Dopamine agonists serve as scavengers of free radicals and decrease dopamine turnover, which reduces oxidative stress. During early development of the disease, there are increases in oxidative stress. Four classes of drugs are available:
   a. Anticholinergics (for resting tremor)
   b. Precursor of dopamine (e.g., carbidopa/levodopa)
   c. Direct-acting dopamine agonists (e.g., bromocriptine, pergolide)
   d. Indirect-acting dopamine agonists
      (1) Decrease reuptake (e.g., amantadine)
      (2) Decrease metabolism (e.g., selegiline)

3. **Drug therapy for treating associated symptoms**
   a. **Tricyclic antidepressants** are used to treat **depression.** They exhibit some dopaminergic and anticholinergic effects.
   b. **β–Blockers,** especially **propranolol** with its high lipophilicity, **benzodiazepines,** and **primidone,** are medications used for **action tremor.** Usually, patients show a clinical response in low doses.
   c. **Antihistamines.** Diphenhydramine hydrochloride has some mild anticholinergic effects and is used for symptomatic release of mild tremor; because of its adverse reaction in the CNS, it should be used with caution in the elderly.

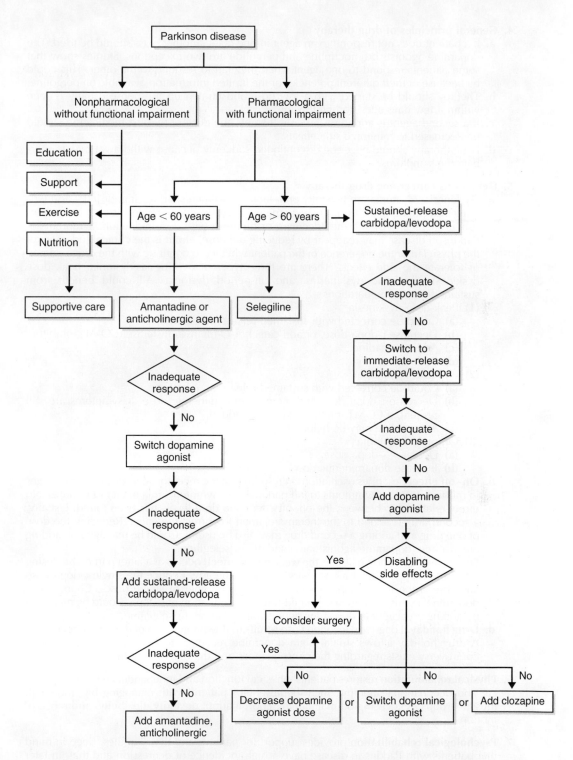

Figure 46-5. Management of Parkinson disease.

4. **General principles of drug therapy**
   a. If a patient does not respond to an agent in one class, another class should be tried. The dopamine agonists bromocriptine and pergolide are two exceptions. Studies show that some patients respond to one agent when they fail to respond to the other. This could be because of their different potencies or the limited information available on pergolide.
   b. Therapy should be started with a low dose and titrated up. Response usually is seen within a few days after starting therapy.
   c. If a second agent is added to the drug therapy, the dose of the first medication should be decreased to minimize side effects.
   d. Drug therapy should never be discontinued suddenly because withdrawal may exacerbate the symptoms.

5. **Definitions concerning drug therapy**
   a. **Dyskinesias/dystonia** are typically oral–facial movements, grimacing, or jerky and writhing movements of the trunk and extremities. They are always reversible with antiparkinsonian medications, and they decrease or diminish with dose reduction. Symptoms of Parkinson disease may reappear by reducing the dose, and it is the clinical judgment of the physician or the preference of the patient whether to continue with the drug regimen or tolerate the side effects. There are three types of dyskinesias/dystonia: peak dose dyskinesia, biphasic dyskinesias, and off-period dystonia. All could benefit from sustained-release preparations.
      (1) Peak-dose dyskinesia
         (a) Could be corrected with sustained-release preparations.
         (b) Decrease L-dopa dose, or add catechol-*O*-methyltransferase (COMT) inhibitor.
         (c) Add amantadine.
         (d) Perform surgery.
      (2) Biphasic dyskinesias
         (a) Could be corrected with sustained-release preparations.
         (b) Decrease L-dopa dose and increase dopaminergic dose. If symptoms are still present, a COMT inhibitor should be added.
         (c) Amantadine may be helpful.
      (3) Off-period dystonia
         (a) Decrease L-dopa dose.
         (b) Increase dopaminergic dose.
   b. **On–off effect** describes oscillations in response (at the receptor site) and sudden changes in mobility from no symptoms to full parkinsonian symptoms in a matter of minutes. No direct relationship between the on–off effect and drug levels has been found. Usually, a second drug is added to the therapy regimen to correct the effect. Reducing the dose of one drug and adding a second drug may also be useful. Could be managed by adding entacapone, dopamine agonist, amantadine, or selegiline.
   c. **End-dose effect,** known also as the **wearing-off effect,** occurs at a latter part of the dosing interval; it happens after a few years of L-dopa therapy. Reduce the single L-dopa dose and spread the total L-dopa dose over a larger number of single doses. Change to a dopamine agonist and use a sustained-release formulation of L-dopa. Could be managed by adding entacapone, dopamine agonist, amantadine, or selegiline.
   d. **Drug holiday.** Long-term levodopa use results in downregulation of dopamine receptors. A drug holiday allows striatal nigra dopamine receptors to be resensitized, although controversy exists regarding the consequences and the outcome of this holiday.

6. **Physical rehabilitation** restores patients' physical function and independence through physical and occupational therapy. Such therapy helps patients with managing big and small muscle groups by focusing on maintaining coordination, dexterity, flexibility, and range of motions.

7. **Psychological rehabilitation** provides support for patients and their families. Keep in mind that patients with Parkinson disease have a high incidence of depression and that, in later stages of the disease, they develop dementia (Table 46-2).

8. **Secondary effects of Parkinson disease include**
   a. **Cardiovascular effects,** including orthostatic hypotension and arrhythmia
   b. **Gastrointestinal effects,** including constipation and hypersalivation
   c. **Genitourinary effects,** including increased urinary frequency and impotence

Table 46-2. Overview of Parkinson Disease Management

Stage	Characteristics	Treatment Considerations	
		Physical	**Psychosocial**
Early	Fully functional May have unilateral tremor, rigidity	Preventive exercise program	Education Information
Early middle	Symptoms bilateral, bradykinesia, rigidity Mild speech impairment Axial rigidity, stooped posture, stiffness Gait impairment begins	Corrective exercise program	Counseling Support group Monitor for depression
Late middle	All symptoms worse but independent in ADLs May need minor assistance Balance problems	Compensatory and corrective exercise Speech therapy Occupational therapy	Caregiver issues (medications, mobility) Monitor for dementia
Late	Severely disabled, impaired Dependent with ADLs	Compensatory exercise Dietary concerns Skin care Hygiene Pulmonary function	Dementia Depression

ADLs, activities of daily living.
Reprinted with permission from Custin TM. Overview of Parkinson's disease management. Phys Ther 1995;75: 363–373. This material is copyrighted, and any further reproduction or distribution is prohibited.

    d. Central nervous system effects, including hallucinations, depression, and psychosis. Could be treated with reducing or eliminating amantadine, selegiline, anticholinergics, or dopamine agonists.

  9. Late disabilities of Parkinson disease can be divided into two groups.
    a. Levodopa-related disabilities, which include motor fluctuation, dyskinesia, neuropsychiatric toxicity, and reduced response
    b. Non-levodopa-related disabilities, which include cognitive impairment, instability resulting in more frequent falls, gait disturbance, incontinence, dysphagia, and speech disturbance
    c. Late disabilities management therapies include the following:
      (1) Motor fluctuation. Altering the levodopa dosage and timing, using alternative means of levodopa administration, delivery, and absorption; using direct-acting dopamine agonists or experimental agonists; altering metabolism of dopamine and levodopa parental agonists; using glutamate antagonists; and performing functional neurosurgery
      (2) Miscellaneous late disabilities and management therapies include
        (a) Urinary urgency: oxybutynin
        (b) Urinary retention: apomorphine
        (c) Constipation: fiber, polyethylene glycols
        (d) Tenesmus: clonazepam, apomorphine
        (e) Hypersalivation: antihistamine, anticholinergic
        (f) Dysphagia: liquid levodopa
        (g) Sweating crises: β-blockers, anticholinergic agents
        (h) Daytime sleepiness: selegiline
        (i) Nightmares: amitriptyline, clonazepam
        (j) Panic attacks and depression: liquid levodopa, amitriptyline
        (k) Orthostatic hypotension: domperidone, desmopressin
        (l) Dysphonia: reduce levodopa dosage, speech therapy
        (m) Pain: amitriptyline, fluvoxamine

II. INDIVIDUAL DRUGS

A. **Anticholinergic agents** are used for mild symptoms, predominantly tremors.

1. **Mechanism of action.** This class of drugs blocks the excitatory neurotransmitter cholinergic influence in the basal ganglia. These drugs are more effective for tremor and rigidity than for bradykinesia and less effective for postural imbalance.

2. **Administration and dosage** (Table 46-3)

3. **Precautions and monitoring effects**
   a. Anticholinergics should be used with caution in patients with obstructed gastrointestinal (GI) or genitourinary (GU) tracts, narrow-angle glaucoma, or severe cardiac disease. Physicians should be notified if a rapid heartbeat or eye pain are experienced. (Frequent ophthalmological visits are recommended.)
   b. The sedative side effects of antihistamines may be beneficial in some patients.
   c. Alcohol and other CNS depressants should be used with caution.
   d. **Adverse effects** of anticholinergic therapy include the following:
      (1) **Peripheral anticholinergic effects** include dry mouth (hard candies may be helpful); decreased sweating, resulting in decreased tolerance to heat; urinary retention; constipation (stool softeners may be helpful); increased intraocular tension; and nausea. Because of patients' decreased tolerance to heat, these agents should be used with caution in hot weather. They should also be taken with food to minimize GI upset.
      (2) **CNS effects** include dizziness, delirium, disorientation, anxiety, agitation, hallucinations, and impaired memory. The incidence of CNS effects increases in elderly individuals.
      (3) **Cardiovascular effects** include hypotension and orthostatic hypotension.

4. **Significant interactions**
   a. Side effects may be potentiated by other drugs with anticholinergic activity such as **antihistamines, antidepressants,** and **phenothiazines.**

Table 46-3. Dosage Range and Characteristics of Drug Treatment

Drug	Time to Peak Concentration (hr)	Half-Life (hr)	Daily Dosage Range (mg/day)
Anticholinergic agents			
Benztropine	n/a	n/a	1–6
Biperiden	1–1.5	18.4–24.3	2–8
Procyclidine	1.1–2	11.5–12.6	6–20
Trihexyphenidyl	1–1.3	5.6–10.2	2–15
Ethopropazine	n/a	n/a	50–400
Dopamine agents			
Carbidopa/levodopa	1	1–1.75	10/100–200/2000
Carbidopa/levodopa, sustained-release	2	> standard treatment	10/400–25/1000, in 2–3 divided doses
Amantadine	4–8	9.7–14.5	100–400
Bromocriptine	1–3	3–8	2.5–40
Pergolide	2	27	0.1–5
Selegiline	0.5–2	2–20.5	5–108
Non-ergot dopamine agents			
Pramipexole	1–2 (3–4[a])	8–12[b]	1.5–4.5, in 3 divided doses
Ropinirole	1–2 (3–4[a])	6	3–24, in 3 divided doses
COMT inhibitor	0.5–4	70	0.5–6
Tolcapone	2	2–3	300–600
Entacapone	1	2–3	200–1600

[a]With food.
[b]Over 65 years of age.
COMT, catechol-*O*-methyltransferase; *n/a,* not available.

  b. Anticholinergic agents increase **digoxin** levels.
  c. When anticholinergic agents are taken with **haloperidol,** the following occurs:
    (1) Schizophrenic symptoms may increase.
    (2) Haloperidol levels may decrease.
    (3) The severity of (not the risk of) tardive dyskinesia may increase.
  d. When **phenothiazines** are taken with anticholinergic drugs, the effects of the phenothiazines decrease and the anticholinergic symptoms increase.
  e. Patients on high doses of anticholinergics combined with **levodopa** should be watched for decreased levodopa activity because of a delayed gastric emptying time.

B. Dopamine precursor. Levodopa/carbidopa is the most effective drug for managing Parkinson disease; however, prolonged use decreases its therapeutic effects (there is a decline in efficacy after 3–5 years) and increases adverse drug reactions. Dopamine does not cross the blood–brain barrier; therefore, a precursor is used. Peripheral conversion of levodopa to dopamine causes adverse reactions like nausea, vomiting, cardiac arrhythmias, and postural hypotension. To decrease the peripheral conversion and peripheral adverse effects, a peripheral dopa decarboxylase inhibitor (carbidopa) is added to levodopa.

  1. Mechanism of action
    a. Levodopa is converted to dopamine by the enzyme dopa decarboxylase, which elevates CNS levels of dopamine.
    b. The sustained-release formulation is designed to release the drug over 4–6 hr, thereby inhibiting variation in plasma concentration and decreasing motor fluctuation "off" time or improving overall dose response in patients with advanced disease.

  2. Administration and dosage (Table 46-3)
    a. It is necessary to give at least 100 mg daily of carbidopa to decrease the incidence of the peripheral conversion of levodopa and GI side effects (e.g., nausea) and increase the bioavailability of levodopa for the CNS.
    b. If carbidopa is given in a separate dosage form, the dose of levodopa can be decreased by 75%.
    c. If patients still complain of GI side effects after combination levodopa/carbidopa, plain carbidopa can be given.
    d. Sustained-release preparations are approximately 30% less bioavailable as compared with levodopa/carbidopa. Because of this lower bioavailability, the daily dosage should be higher. If a patient is receiving a standard preparation and needs to be converted to the sustained-release dose, approximately 10% more levodopa should initially be added to the daily dosage and at least 3 days should pass between increased dosages; then gradually increase the levodopa dose up to 30% of standard preparation.
    e. With the sustained-release preparation, the peak plasma concentration is lower and the trough plasma concentration is higher.
    f. The sustained-release preparation could be divided in half at the scored point only. The tablet should not be chewed or crushed.
    g. When carbidopa is given to patients being treated with levodopa, give the two drugs at the same time, starting with no more than 20%–25% of the previous daily dosage of levodopa and initiating therapy with carbidopa and levodopa.
    h. Long-term treatment could lead to motor fluctuation and dyskinesias, especially at high doses.

  3. Precautions and monitoring effects
    a. Levodopa must be used with caution in patients with narrow-angle glaucoma.
    b. Levodopa may activate a malignant melanoma in patients with suspicious undiagnosed skin lesions or a history of melanoma.
    c. The efficacy of levodopa declines with long-term therapy by desensitizing the receptors or because of the decreased number of receptors, resulting from the progression of the disease.
    d. Adverse drug reactions
      (1) GI effects include anorexia, nausea and vomiting, and abdominal distress. Levodopa should be taken with food to minimize stomach upset.
      (2) Cardiovascular effects include postural hypotension and tachycardia.
      (3) Musculoskeletal effects include dystonia or choreiform muscle movement.

    (4) CNS effects include confusion, memory changes, depression, hallucinations, and psychosis. Physicians should be notified if any of these symptoms occur.

    (5) Hematological effects include hemolytic anemia, leukopenia, and agranulocytosis (rare).

4. Significant interactions

    a. Antacids cause rapid and complete intestinal levodopa absorption (by decreasing gastric emptying time).

    b. Hydantoin decreases the effectiveness of levodopa.

    c. Methionine increases the clinical signs of Parkinson disease.

    d. Metoclopramide increases the bioavailability of levodopa, which decreases the effects of metoclopramide on gastric emptying and on lower esophageal pressure. As a dopamine blocker, it may also precipitate parkinsonian symptoms.

    e. False-positive results are seen with the Coombs test.

    f. The uric acid test increases with the calorimetric method but not with the uricase method.

    g. Hypertensive reactions may occur if levodopa is administered to patients receiving **MAO inhibitors** and **furazolidone.** MAO inhibitors must be discontinued 2 weeks before starting levodopa.

    h. Administering **papaverine** may decrease the effect of levodopa.

    i. Tricyclic antidepressants decrease the rate and extent of absorption of levodopa; hypertensive episodes have been reported when levodopa is combined with tricyclic antidepressants.

    j. Food decreases the rate and extent of absorption and transport to the CNS across the blood–brain barrier. A **protein-restricted diet** may also help minimize the "fluctuations" (i.e., the decreased response to levodopa) at the end of each day or at various times of the day.

C. Direct-acting dopamine agonists are classified as ergot derivatives (such as bromocriptine and pergolide) and non-ergolines (such as pramipexole and ropinirole).

1. These agents mimic dopamine agonist and reduce motor fluctuations.

2. Drugs in this class have a range of half-lives, and the half-life of any particular drug can vary among patients.

3. These drugs are not metabolized by the oxidative pathway and do not produce free-radical metabolites.

4. Dopamine agonists may have a direct antioxidative effect.

5. They take longer than L-dopa to reach effective doses and require supplementary L-dopa for relief of symptoms after a varying period of time.

6. Common side effects are nausea and psychiatric side effects similar to L-dopa such as hallucinations and delusions; dyskinesias are less common.

7. Other adverse effects are headache, nasal congestion, erythromelalgia, pleural and retroperitoneal fibrosis, pulmonary infiltrates, and vasospasm (except with the new, non-ergot derivatives such as ropinirole).

8. Annual chest radiographs have been recommended for patients on high-dose therapy with bromocriptine or pergolide to detect pleuropulmonary changes.

9. New dopaminergic agonists (non-ergot derivatives) cause postural hypotension, sleep disturbances, peripheral edema, constipation, nausea, dyskinesias, and confusion.

10. Bromocriptine (Parlodel)

    a. Mechanism of action. Bromocriptine is responsible for directly stimulating postsynaptic dopamine receptors; it is most commonly used as an adjunct to levodopa therapy in patients:

      (1) With a deteriorating response to levodopa

      (2) With a limited clinical response to levodopa secondary to an inability to tolerate higher doses

      (3) Who are experiencing fluctuations in response to levodopa

b. Administration and dosage (Table 46-3)
   (1) Initially, patients are given one half of a tablet twice daily, which is then increased to one tablet twice daily every 2–3 days.
   (2) Patients' responses are extremely variable. Many patients show a dopamine antagonist response at both low and high doses, with the desirable agonist response in the midrange.
   (3) Because postural hypotension may result from the first few doses of bromocriptine, the first dose should be administered with the patient lying down, and sudden changes in posture should be avoided.

c. Precautions and monitoring effects
   (1) Bromocriptine may cause a first-dose phenomenon that can trigger sudden cardiovascular collapse. It should be used with caution in patients with a history of myocardial infarction or arrhythmias.
   (2) Early in therapy, dizziness, drowsiness, and fainting may occur, so patients should be cautious about driving or operating machinery. A physician should be notified if these symptoms appear.
   (3) Cardiac dysrhythmias. Patients on bromocriptine were found to have significantly more episodes of atrial premature contractions and sinus tachycardia.
   (4) Other adverse effects
      (a) GI effects, including anorexia, nausea, vomiting, and abdominal distress, may be decreased by taking bromocriptine with food.
      (b) Cardiovascular effects include postural hypotension (to which tolerance develops) and tachycardia. Blood pressure must be monitored, particularly for patients taking antihypertensive medication.
      (c) Pulmonary effects, including reversible infiltrations, pleural effusions, and pleural thickening, may develop after long-term treatment, so pulmonary function should be monitored in patients treated longer than 6 months.
      (d) CNS effects, including confusion, memory changes, depression, and hallucinations, as well as psychosis may be exacerbated by bromocriptine; thus patients with psychiatric illnesses must be monitored.

d. Significant interactions
   (1) A combination of **antihypertensive drugs** and bromocriptine could decrease blood pressure.
   (2) Dopamine antagonists increase the effect of bromocriptine.

11. Pergolide (Permax)
   a. Mechanism of action. Pergolide is a semisynthetic ergosine derivative. In Parkinson disease, it exerts its effect by directly stimulating postsynaptic dopamine receptors in the nigrostriatal system.
      (1) It is 1000 times more potent than bromocriptine on a milligram basis.
      (2) It inhibits the secretion of prolactin, increases the serum concentration of growth hormone, and decreases the serum concentration of luteinizing hormone.
      (3) It is most commonly used as adjunctive treatment to levodopa/carbidopa.
   b. Administration and dosage (Table 46-3)
   c. Precautions and monitoring effects
      (1) Hypersensitivity reactions to pergolide and other ergot derivatives can occur.
      (2) Caution must be used with patients who are at high risk for ventricular arrhythmia, especially when doses higher than 3 mg/day are used.
      (3) Cardiac dysrhythmias. Adverse effects are similar to those experienced with bromocriptine (see II.C.10.c.(3)).
      (4) CNS effects include dyskinesia, hallucinations, somnolence, and insomnia.
      (5) GI effects include nausea, constipation, diarrhea, and dyspepsia.
      (6) Cardiovascular effects include premature atrial contractions and sinus tachycardia (alone or in combination with levodopa).
      (7) Miscellaneous effects include transient elevations of aspartate aminotransferase, alanine aminotransferase, and alkaline phosphatase, and pleural thickening.
   d. Significant interactions
      (1) Because pergolide is 90% protein bound, it must be used with caution with other highly **protein-bound drugs.**
      (2) Antipsychotic agents (e.g., phenothiazines, haloperidol, metoclopramide) combined with dopamine agonists decrease the dopamine action and decrease the therapeutic action of the antipsychotic agent.

D. Indirect-acting dopamine agonists

   1. Selegiline (Eldepryl)
   a. Mechanism of action
   (1) MAO catabolizes various catecholamines (e.g., dopamine, norepinephrine, epinephrine), serotonin, and various exogenous amines (e.g., tyramines) found in foods (e.g., aged cheese, beer, wine, smoked meat) and drugs. Lack of MAO in the intestinal tract causes absorption of these amines, creating a hypertensive crisis. MAO type A is predominantly found in the intestinal tract, and MAO type B in the brain. They differ in their substrate specificity and tissue distribution. This specificity decreases with selegiline as the dose increases. Most patients experience side effects at doses of selegiline higher than 30–40 mg/day.
   (2) Selegiline is a selective inhibitor of MAO-B, which prevents the breakdown of dopamine selectively in the brain at recommended doses.
   (3) Selegiline is most commonly used as an adjunct with levodopa/carbidopa when patients experience a "wearing-off" phenomenon; it decreases the amount of off time and decreases the dose needed of levodopa/carbidopa by 10%–30%.
   (4) Results of some studies show that selegiline delays the time before treatment with a more potent dopaminergic drug like levodopa is needed; the proposed mechanism of action is that an oxidation mechanism contributes to the emergence and progression of Parkinson disease.
   b. Administration and dosage (Table 46-3). Exceeding the recommended dose of 10 mg/day increases the risk of losing MAO selectivity. The precise selectivity dose is unknown but seems to be above 30–40 mg/day.
   c. Precautions and monitoring effects
   (1) **Hypertensive crisis** (see II.D.1.a.(1)).
   (2) Levodopa-associated side effects may be increased because the increased amounts of dopamine react with supersensitive postsynaptic receptors. Reducing the dose of levodopa/carbidopa by 10%–30% may decrease levodopa side effects.
   (3) Patients should be educated about foods and drugs containing tyramine and the signs and symptoms of hypertensive reactions.
   (4) **CNS effects** include dizziness, confusion, headache, hallucinations, vivid dreams, dyskinesias, behavioral and mood changes, and depression. Patients who experience insomnia should avoid taking the drug late in the day.
   (5) **Cardiovascular effects** include orthostatic hypotension, hypertension, arrhythmia, palpitations, sinus bradycardia, and syncope.
   (6) **GI effects** include nausea and abdominal pain and **lead to GI bleeding,** weight loss, poor appetite, and dysphagia.
   (7) **GU effects** include slow urination, transient nocturia, and prostatic hypertrophy.
   (8) **Dermatological effects** include increased sweating, diaphoresis, and photosensitivity.
   (9) **Hepatic effects** include mild and transient elevations in liver function tests.
   d. Significant interactions. MAO inhibitors are contraindicated with **meperidine** and other opioids. Because the mechanism of action is unknown, administration with opioids should be avoided.
   e. Death has occurred after initiation of selegiline shortly after discontinuation of fluoxetine. At least 5 weeks should elapse between discontinuation of fluoxetine and initiation of selegiline.

   2. Amantadine (Symmetrel)
   a. Mechanism of action. Amantadine is an antiviral agent (used to prevent influenza).
   (1) Amantadine increases dopamine levels at postsynaptic receptor sites by decreasing presynaptic reuptake and enhancing dopamine synthesis and release.
   (2) It may also have some anticholinergic effects. It decreases tremor, rigidity, and bradykinesia.
   (3) It can be given in combination with levodopa as Parkinson disease progresses.
   (4) Clinical effects of amantadine can be seen within the first few weeks of therapy, unlike the other antiparkinsonian medications (e.g., carbidopa/levodopa), which need weeks to months to show their full clinical effects.
   b. Administration and dosage (Table 46-3)
   (1) Amantadine should be started at 100 mg/day. This may be increased to 200–300 mg/day as a maintenance dose.

(2) Patients experiencing a decline in response may benefit from the following:
  (a) Discontinuing the drug for a few weeks, then restarting it
  (b) Using the drug episodically, only when the patient's condition most needs a therapeutic boost
(3) Amantadine is also available in liquid form for patients with dysphagia.

c. Precautions and monitoring effects
  (1) Amantadine should be used with caution in patients with renal disease, congestive heart failure (CHF), peripheral edema, history of seizures, and mental status changes. It may be necessary to modify dosages in patients with renal failure.
  (2) Tolerance usually develops within 6–12 months. If tolerance occurs, another drug from a different class can be added, or the dose may be increased.
  (3) Patients should be informed about the side-effect profile.
    (a) **Peripheral anticholinergic effects** include those mentioned in II.A.3.d.(1).
    (b) **CNS effects** include seizures as well as those mentioned in II.A.3.d.(2).
    (c) **Cardiovascular effects.** Patients may develop CHF. Periodic blood pressure monitoring and electrocardiograms (ECGs) are necessary in patients with myocardial infarction or arrhythmias.
    (d) **Dermatological effects** include **livedo reticularis,** a diffuse rose-color mottling of the skin, which is reversible on discontinuation of the drug.
    (e) **Hematological effects.** Periodic complete blood counts (CBCs) should be done for patients with long-term therapy.
  (4) **Renal function impairment.** Dose adjustment is necessary in patients with renal function impairment.

d. Significant interactions
  (1) Amantadine increases the anticholinergic effects of **anticholinergic drugs,** requiring a decrease in the dosage of the anticholinergic drug.
  (2) **Hydrochlorothiazide** plus **triamterene** decreases the urinary excretion of amantadine and increases its plasma concentration.

E. Non-ergot dopamine agonists

  1. Pramipexole and ropinirole are indicated for both early and advanced stages of Parkinson disease.

  2. Both selectively bind to dopamine receptors and activate the D_2-receptor but have little or no affinity to the D_1-receptor. They have greater affinity for the D_3-receptor than for the D_2-receptor. The incidence of adverse events (such as pleuropulmonary fibrosis and retroperitoneal fibrosis, coronary vasoconstriction, erythromelalgia, and Raynaud phenomenon), is low compared to nonselective dopamine agonists.

  3. **Non-ergot dopamine agonists** have a low potential for the development of motor fluctuations and dyskinesia.
    a. Pramipexole (Mirapex)
      (1) **Mechanism of action**
        (a) **D_2 subfamily of dopamine receptors.** Pramipexole fully stimulates the dopamine receptors to which it binds. Its action may be related to its capacity to function as an antioxidant and oxygen free-radical scavenger.
        (b) Pramipexole also has antidepressant activity in moderate depression, which may be related to its preferential binding to the dopamine D_1-receptor subtype.
        (c) Long-acting dopamine agonists appear to have a lower risk of inducing abnormal movements. Their use as initial treatment in early Parkinson disease seems warranted, particularly for those with disease onset at a younger age.
      (2) **Administration and dosage**
        (a) Initial treatment: starting dose of 0.375 mg daily given in three divided doses.
        (b) Do not increase more frequently than every 5–7 days.
        (c) Maintenance treatment: 1.5–4.5 mg daily in three divided doses with or without levodopa.
        (d) When given in combination with levodopa, consider reduction of levodopa dose by an average of 27% from baseline.
        (e) Titrate slowly to balance benefits and side effects, such as dyskinesia, hallucinations, somnolence, and dry mouth.
        (f) May be taken with food to reduce the occurrence of nausea. Food decreases the rate of absorption but not the extent of absorption.

(g) Dosage adjustment is necessary in patients with renal function impairment.

(h) Weak protein bound 15%

  (i) Not extensively metabolized; > 90% of the dose is excreted unchanged in urine.

(j) Dose needs to be decreased by 25% in the elderly.

(3) Precautions and monitoring effects

  (a) Dose reduction necessary in patients > 65 years, and in patients with renal function impairment or failure

  (b) Symptomatic hypotension

   (i) Dopaminergic agents appear to impair the systemic regulation of blood pressure, which results in orthostatic hypotension.

   (ii) Monitoring and education of the patient is necessary, especially during dose-escalation periods.

  (c) Hallucinatory effects are increased in patients > 65 years of age with early or advanced stages of Parkinson disease.

  (d) Other effects include nausea, insomnia, constipation, dizziness, somnolence, GI side effects, and visual hallucinations.

(4) Significant interactions

  (a) Cimetidine reduces renal clearance of pramipexole.

  (b) No interaction with selegiline, probenecid, or domperidone.

  (c) When combined with levodopa, the dosage of levodopa must be decreased by 27%.

b. Ropinirole (Requip)

(1) Mechanism of action is similar to pramipexole.

(2) Administration and dosage

  (a) Initial treatment: 0.25 mg three times daily

  (b) Titrate weekly increments.

  (c) After week 4, if necessary, daily dosage may be increased by 1.5 mg/day on a weekly basis up to 9 mg/day, to a total of 24 mg/day.

  (d) Discontinue gradually over a 7-day period. Decrease the frequency of administration from three times to two times daily for 4 days, and then once daily for the remainder of the week.

  (e) When given in combination with levodopa, consider reduction of levodopa dose.

  (f) May be taken with food to reduce the occurrence of nausea. Food decreases the rate of absorption, but not the extent of absorption.

  (g) Metabolized by the liver (cytochrome P450 1A2), and first-pass effect.

  (h) Smoking induces the liver metabolism.

  (i) Between 30% and 40% protein bound

(3) Precautions and monitoring effects

  (a) Syncope. Bradycardia is observed in patients treated with ropinirole. Most cases occur within the first 4 weeks of therapy and are usually associated with a recent increase of dose.

  (b) Binds to melanin-containing tissues like the eyes and skin.

  (c) Symptomatic hypotension

   (i) Dopaminergic agents appear to impair the systemic regulation of blood pressure, which results in orthostatic hypotension.

   (ii) Monitoring and education of the patient is necessary, especially during dose-escalation periods.

  (d) Hallucinatory effects are increased in patients > 65 years of age with early or advanced stages of Parkinson disease.

  (e) Other side effects include nausea, dizziness, somnolence, headache, fatigue, and abnormal vision.

(4) Significant interactions

  (a) Smoking induces the liver metabolism, but the affect of smoking on clearance of ropinirole has not been studied.

  (b) There is no interaction between levodopa, theophylline, digoxin, or domperidone.

  (c) Estrogens decrease the clearance of ropinirole by approximately 36%.

  (d) Ciprofloxacin increases ropinirole area under the curve (AUC) by 84% and maximum plasma concentration by 60%.

4. COMT inhibitors
  a. Tolcapone (Tasmar)
    (1) Mechanism of action
      (a) Tolcapone is a selective and reversible inhibitor of COMT and is used as an adjunct to levodopa/carbidopa therapy.
      (b) Tolcapone inhibits COMT both peripheral and centrally.
      (c) COMT is the main enzyme responsible for peripheral and central metabolism of catecholamines, including levodopa. Addition of a COMT inhibitor results in the doubling of the elimination half-life of levodopa and in increased oral bioavailability of levodopa by 40%–50%.
      (d) Tolcapone is indicated as an adjunct therapy to carbidopa/levodopa therapy.
    (2) Administration and dosage
      (a) Starting dose of 100–200 mg, three times daily
      (b) Usual daily dose of 200 mg, three times daily
      (c) If patient fails to show expected benefit after 3 weeks of treatment, discontinue drug because of associated risk of liver failure. Rapid withdrawal or abrupt reduction dose could lead to hyperpyrexia and confusion symptoms such as high fever and severe rigidity similar to those in neuroleptic malignant syndrome.
    (3) Precautions and monitoring
      (a) Liver toxicity. High risk of fatal liver failure has been reported with tolcapone. Discontinue use if substantial benefit is not seen within 3 weeks of commencement of therapy.
      (b) Do not use in patients with liver disease or in patients who have two alanine aminotransferase (ALT) or aspartate aminotransferase (AST) values greater than the upper limit of normal.
      (c) Advise patient regarding self-monitoring for liver disease (i.e., clay-colored stool, jaundice, fatigue, appetite loss, or lethargy).
      (d) Monitor AST and ALT every 2 weeks for the first year, then every 4 weeks for the next 6 months and every 8 weeks thereafter.
      (e) MAO and COMT are two major enzyme systems involved in the metabolism of catecholamines; combination of tolcapone with a non-selective MAO inhibitor will result in inhibition of the pathway responsible for normal catecholamine metabolism.
      (f) Tolcapone can be taken concomitantly with a selective MAO-B inhibitor, such as selegiline.
    (4) Other side effects
      (a) Orthostatic hypotension. Tolcapone enhances levodopa bioavailability and, therefore, may increase the occurrence of orthostatic hypotension.
      (b) Diarrhea usually manifests within 6–12 weeks after administration of tolcapone, but can develop as early as 2 weeks after administration. Diarrhea normally resolves after discontinuation of the drug.
      (c) Hallucinations are sometimes accompanied by confusion, insomnia, and excessive dreaming. Hallucinatory effects usually occur after initiation of tolcapone and are usually resolved by decreasing the dose of levodopa.
      (d) Tolcapone may potentiate the dopaminergic side effect of levodopa and may cause or exacerbate preexisting dyskinesia. Decreased doses of levodopa may or may not alleviate the symptoms.
      (e) Severe cases of rhabdomyolysis have been reported, which present as fever, alternation of consciousness, and muscular rigidity.
      (f) Others. Dyspepsia, abdominal cramping, mild paresthesia of the legs, and temporary discoloration of urine have also been noted but are not considered clinically important.
      (g) Drug interactions. Although no drug interaction studies have been conducted, concurrent use of tolcapone and drugs that are metabolized by the COMT system (i.e., methyldopa, dobutamine, apomorphine) should be monitored. Tolcapone also has affinity for the cytochrome P450 2C9 isoenzyme, similar to warfarin. Coagulation parameters should be monitored when tolcapone is administered with warfarin.
  b. Entacapone (Comtan)
    (1) Mechanism of action
      (a) Entacapone is a selective and reversible inhibitor of COMT and permits additional levodopa to reach the brain. It does not have any anti-Parkinson effect of its own.

(b) It acts only peripherally by inhibiting COMT.

(c) It improves the duration of on time and decreases the duration of off time.

(d) It is indicated as an adjunct to those on levodopa/carbidopa therapy who experience the signs and symptoms of end-of-dose wearing-off.

(2) Administration and dosage

(a) Dosage: 200 mg with each dose of L-dopa up to 8 times daily with a maximum dose of 1600 mg daily.

(b) Rapid withdrawal could lead to emergency signs and symptoms of Parkinson disease such as hyperpyrexia and confusion (symptoms resembling neuroleptic malignant syndrome).

(3) Precautions and monitoring effects

(a) MAO. COMT and MAO are two major enzymes in the metabolism of catecholamines. Do not use together.

(b) Drugs metabolized by COMT. Drugs that are metabolized by this pathway, such as isoproterenol, epinephrine, norepinephrine, dopamine, and dobutamine, as well as methyldopa, may interact and may result in increased heart rate, arrhythmias, and an excessive increase in blood pressure.

(c) Hepatic function impairment. The majority of the drug is metabolized by the liver; therefore, use caution in patients who have liver function abnormalities.

(d) Fibrotic complication. Cases of retroperitoneal fibrosis, pulmonary infiltrates, pleural effusion, and pleural thickening have been reported. These complications may resolve when the drug is discontinued, but complete resolution may not always occur.

(e) Biliary excretion. Entacapone is excreted by bile; therefore, use caution with drugs known to interfere with biliary excretion, such as probenecid, erythromycin, and ampicillin.

(4) Other side effects. Dyskinesia/hyperkinesia, nausea, urine discoloration (brownish orange), diarrhea, and abdominal pain

(5) Drug interactions. May interact with drugs that are metabolized by the liver cytochrome P450.

III. SURGICAL TREATMENT.

All surgeries require needle insertion into the brain, which in turn increases the risk of hemorrhage.

A. Globus pallidus internus (Gpi) pallidotomy

1. Definition. A pallidotomy entails the surgical resection of parts of the globus pallidus.

2. Advantages. Improves contralateral dyskinesia

3. Disadvantages. Increased risk of damage to other parts of the brain, including optic nerve and internal capsule, and risk of emotional, behavioral, and cognitive deficits

B. Deep-brain stimulation

1. Definition. High-frequency stimulation that induces functional inhibition of target regions of the brain by implanting an electrode into a target site and connecting the lead to a subcutaneously placed pacemaker.

2. Advantages. No destructive lesion is formed. Stimulation parameters can be readjusted at any time to improve efficacy or decrease adverse events.

3. Disadvantages. Side effects associated with equipment (such as lead breaks, infection, skin erosion, mechanical malfunction, and need for battery replacement). Other side effects include paresthesia limb dystonia, ataxia, intracerebral hemorrhage, seizure, and confusion.

C. Fetal nigral transplantation

1. Definition. Implantation of embryonic dopaminergic cells into the denervated striatum to replace degenerated neuronal cells.

2. Advantages. Implanted cells all survive, and innervation of the striatum is accomplished in an organotypic manner. Does not necessitate making a destructive lesion.

3. Disadvantages. Optimal transplant variables and target site not defined.

STUDY QUESTIONS

Directions: Each of the questions, statements, or incomplete statements in this section can be correctly answered or completed by **one** of the suggested answers or phrases. Choose the **best** answer.

1. Which of the following drugs is a catechol-*O*-methyltransferase (COMT) inhibitor and has reports of fatal liver toxicity with it?

   (A) tolcapone
   (B) entacapone
   (C) pergolide
   (D) selegiline

2. Levodopa is associated with which of the following problems?

   (A) gastrointestinal side effects
   (B) involuntary movements
   (C) decline in efficacy after 3–5 years
   (D) All of the above

3. Amantadine has which of the following advantages over levodopa?

   (A) more rapid relief over symptoms
   (B) higher success rate
   (C) better long-term effects

4. Which drug is a non-ergot dopamine agonist and has a side-effect profile different from the rest of the dopaminergic agents?

   (A) pergolide
   (B) levodopa/carbidopa
   (C) ropinirole
   (D) selegiline

5. Which of the following medications is indicated as an adjunct to carbidopa/levodopa therapy?

   (A) pramipexole
   (B) bromocriptine
   (C) amantadine
   (D) tolcapone

ANSWERS AND EXPLANATIONS

1. The answer is A *[see II.E.4.a.(3).(a)].*
Severe cases of hepatocellular injury—including fulminant liver failure, which causes death—have been reported. Patients should be monitored and instructed to look for signs of liver disease such as clay-colored stool, jaundice, fatigue, loss of appetite, and lethargy.

2. The answer is D *[see II.B.3.c–d].*
Levodopa can cause GI side effects such as nausea and vomiting, particularly when starting treatment. Bowel irregularity and gastrointestinal bleeding can also occur. With long-term levodopa therapy, involuntary choreiform movements can develop, and the efficacy of the drug declines. Other unwanted effects of levodopa include tachycardia and cardiac arrhythmias, postural hypotension, and psychiatric disturbances such as confusion or depression.

3. The answer is A *[see II.D.2.a.(4), II.D.2.c–d].*
Amantadine is most efficacious within the first few weeks, whereas benefits from levodopa may not be seen for weeks to months. Amantadine is more beneficial than the anticholinergics but is less effective than levodopa. Unfortunately, the efficacy of amantadine declines after 6–12 months of therapy. The efficacy of levodopa declines after 3–5 years of therapy.

4. The answer is C *[see II.E.3.a–b].*
Non-ergot dopamine agonists, sucha s ropinirole, are indicated for both early and advanced stages of Parkinson disease. These drugs selectively bind to dopamine receptors and activate the D_2-recepto, but have little or no affinity for the D_1-receptor. They have a greater affinity for the D_3-receptor than for the D_2-receptor. The incidence of adverse events (e.g., pleuropulmonary fibrosis and retroperitoneal fibrosis, coronary vasoconstriction, erythromelalgia, and Raynaud phenomenon) is low compared to nonselective dopamine agonists. Non-ergot dopamine agonists have a low potential for the devolment of motor fluctuations and dyskinesis.

5. The answer is D *[see II.E.4.a.(1).(d)].*
Tolcapone is an inhibitor of COMT enzyme used to metabolize catecholamines, including levodopa. It is indicated as an adjunct therapy to carbidopa/levodopa therapy.

47
Schizophrenia
Rebekah R. Arthur

I. INTRODUCTION

A. **Schizophrenia** is a major psychological disorder affecting approximately 1% of the population.

B. It is a disease that can markedly affect social and occupational functioning, interpersonal relationships, morbidity, and mortality.

   1. As many as 45% of the homeless population in the United States suffer from schizophrenia.

   2. Mortality rates of patients with schizophrenia are two to four times higher than the general population.

   3. Suicide attempt rates for patients suffering from schizophrenia range from 20% to 42%, with a success rate of 10%.

C. The cost of schizophrenia on the U.S. economy is estimated to be $62.7 billion per year. One half of this cost is the result of indirect losses, such as lost work.

II. PATHOPHYSIOLOGY.
The actual cause of schizophrenia is uncertain, however multiple theories exist, each of which provide partial explanations. These include genetic theories, the dopamine theory, the neurodevelopmental theory, and psychosocial theories.

A. **Genetic theories.** A strong genetic link exists for the development of schizophrenia.

   1. Schizophrenia occurs in 1% of the general population; however, this increases to 10% if a first-degree relative has a history of schizophrenia.

   2. The risk of developing schizophrenia further increases to 40% when both parents have a history of schizophrenia.

   3. Monozygotic twins have demonstrated a 48% risk of both twins developing schizophrenia if one twin has the disease.

   4. Studies are ongoing to locate specific genes linked to the development of schizophrenia.

B. **Dopamine theory.** This theory postulates that dopamine hyperactivity in the brain is responsible for psychotic symptoms present in schizophrenia.

   1. While dopamine hyperactivity is present in the mesolimbic pathway, other areas of the brain, such as the prefrontal, frontal, and temporal cortices, have decreased dopamine activity during acute psychosis.
      a. Typical antipsychotics block dopamine activity in the brain. Blockade of dopamine with these agents has not resulted in a response for all patients.
      b. The dopamine theory has not been found to be a complete explanation for schizophrenia.

   2. Other neurotransmitters thought to be involved in schizophrenia include **5-hydroxytryptamine (serotonin; 5-HT)** and **glutamate.**
      a. The role of 5-HT is largely evidenced by the blockade of 5-HT with the newer atypical antipsychotics.
      b. The role of glutamate is also being evaluated because one of its major functions is to regulate dopamine activity. Glutamate deficiency has been found to cause similar effects to that of dopamine hyperactivity.

C. **Neurodevelopmental theory.** This theory suggests that schizophrenia occurs as a result of an in utero disturbance during pregnancy. Potential causes of this disturbance include upper-respiratory infections, obstetric complications, and neonatal hypoxia. Studies exist that link these prenatal conditions with an increased risk of development of schizophrenia; however, this theory continues to be evaluated.

   D. Psychosocial theories. These theories propose that situations such as stress, poor interpersonal skills, conflicting family communication, and various socioeconomic influences are linked to the development of schizophrenia. While these theories have been unproved, such situations can serve as triggers for the development of the disease in people with a predisposition.

III. DIAGNOSIS AND CLINICAL FEATURES

   A. Schizophrenia is **diagnosed** based on *Diagnostic and Statistical Manual of Mental Disorders,* 4th ed. (DSM-IV-TR) criteria.

   1. A patient must have at least two of the following symptoms: delusions, hallucinations, disorganized speech, disorganized or catatonic behavior, and negative symptoms.

   2. The symptoms should be present for at least 1 month, with at least 6 months of continuous prodromal or residual symptoms.

   3. At least one area of the patient's social or occupational functioning should be significantly affected.

   4. Other conditions causing similar symptoms such as schizoaffective disorder, mood disorders, substance abuse, and general medical conditions should be ruled out.

   B. Five **types** of schizophrenia exist (Table 47-1).

   C. The clinical features of schizophrenia are categorized as **positive, negative,** or **disorganized** symptoms (Table 47-2). The most common symptoms are **hallucinations** and **delusions.**

   1. An **hallucination** is a perception disturbance in sensory experiences of the environment. Hallucinations can be auditory, visual, olfactory, or tactile. Auditory hallucinations are most common.

Table 47-1. Types of Schizophrenia

Type	Presentation
Catatonic	Motor symptoms are most notable. The patient may either demonstrate rigid immobility or excessive purposeless movement. The patient may be silent and withdrawn or may become loud and shout. Bizarre voluntary movements such as posturing may also occur. The patient may fluctuate between the two extremes.
Disorganized	The patient tends to have disorganized speech and behavior with a flat affect. Hallucinations and delusions are not well formed and fragmented. The patient may also have bizarre mannerisms and grimacing.
Paranoid	The most common type of schizophrenia. Patients are usually preoccupied with paranoid delusions or auditory hallucinations. Cognitive function is usually preserved; if thought disorder is present, it does not prevent description of delusions or hallucinations.
Residual	The patient does not have acute psychosis, but some symptoms of schizophrenia remain. Largely negative symptoms are seen, such as flat affect, social withdrawal, and loose associations. Prominent delusions or hallucinations are not present.
Undifferentiated	The patient meets the criteria for a diagnosis of schizophrenia but does not meet the criteria for a specific type, or the patient may meet the criteria for multiple types of schizophrenia. No one type appears to be dominant.

Table 47-2. Symptoms of Schizophrenia

Positive Symptoms	Negative Symptoms	Disorganized Symptoms
Delusions	Affective flattening	Disorganized speech
Hallucinations	Alogia	Thought disorder
Combativeness	Anhedonia	Disorganized behavior
Insomnia	Amotivation	Poor attention
	Apathy	
	Asocial behavior	

   2. A **delusion** is an incorrect or false belief. Delusions can be religious, paranoid/persecutory, grandiose, somatic, influential, or sexual. Persecutory or paranoid delusions are the most common.

IV. RISK FACTORS. Risk factors for the development of schizophrenia include a family history of schizophrenia, any potential cause of fetal hypoxic brain damage, history of birth complications, advanced age of mother during pregnancy, birth during winter months, substance abuse, single marital status, lower socioeconomic class, urban environment, and environmental stress.

V. TREATMENT GOALS AND OBJECTIVES. There is currently no known cure for schizophrenia. Treatment options include **psychotherapy** as well as **pharmacotherapy.** The goals and objectives of treatment are as follows:

   A. Minimize symptoms of schizophrenia

   B. Improve quality of life and social/occupational functioning

   C. Prevent relapse and hospitalization

   D. Minimize adverse effects of medications

   E. Prevent suicide attempts or self-harm

VI. PHARMACOTHERAPY: ANTIPSYCHOTIC MEDICATIONS

   A. Two generations of antipsychotic medications are available for treatment: **first-generation or typical antipsychotics** and **second-generation or atypical antipsychotics.**

      1. The choice of an appropriate antipsychotic agent depends on the patient's previous experiences with antipsychotic medications, adverse effects, the patient's concomitant medical conditions, medication interactions, and the patient's preference.

      2. Current American Psychiatric Association (APA) guidelines recommend using an atypical antipsychotic first, owing to less risk for extrapyramidal symptoms (EPS). Patients who prefer or have a history of response to typical antipsychotics may first use typical antipsychotics.

      3. Response to medications is not immediate, and maximal treatment response may take 6 months or longer to be seen.

      4. After a treatment response is seen, patients should be maintained on the current therapy for a minimum of 6 months. Most patients will require chronic therapy, because 80% of first-episode patients who do not receive antipsychotic treatment will relapse within 5 years.

Table 47-3. Properties of Typical Antipsychotics

Agent	CPZ[a] Equivalent	Dose Range[a] (mg/day)	Sedation	EPS	Anticholinergic Side Effects	Orthostatic Hypotension
Chlorpromazine (Thorazine)	100	300–1000	+ + +	+ +	+ +	+ + +
Trifluoperazine (Stelazine)	5	5–15	+	+ + +	+	+
Thioridazine (Mellaril)	100	300–800	+ + +	+	+ + +	+ + +
Perphenazine (Trilafon)	10	16–64	+ +	+ +	+	+
Fluphenazine (Prolixin)	2	5–20	+	+ + +	+	+
Thiothixene (Navane)	5	15–50	+	+ + +	+	+ +
Haloperidol (Haldol)	2	5–20	+	+ + +	+	+
Molindone (Moban)	10	30–100	+ +	+ +	+	+
Loxapine (Loxitane)	10	30–100	+	+ +	+	+

[a]Data from Lehman AF, Lieberman JA, Dixon LB, et al. Practice guideline for treatment of patients with schizophrenia, 2nd ed. Am J Psych 2004;161:1–56.
CPZ, chlorpromazine; *EPS,* extrapyramidal symptoms; + + +, high; + +, moderate; +, low.

B. Typical antipsychotic medications (Table 47-3)

1. **Mechanism of action.** The antipsychotic effect of these medications is primarily mediated through the blockade of dopamine receptors. These agents also have activity at histamine, muscarinic, and α-receptors, although these receptors are not responsible for desired therapeutic activity.

2. **Potency.** Typical antipsychotic agents are classified by their potency for the dopamine receptor into high-, moderate-, and low-potency antipsychotics. High-potency agents have a higher affinity for the dopamine receptor and are associated with higher risk for the development of EPS. Low-potency agents have less affinity for dopamine receptors; and although they have less risk for causing EPS, they are associated with more adverse effects from their activity at histamine, muscarinic, and α-receptors.

3. **Efficacy.** When dosed in equivalent doses, the various typical antipsychotics have similar efficacy. Equivalent doses are described using **chlorpromazine (CPZ) equivalents** (Table 47-3). Typical antipsychotics are thought to be as effective as atypical antipsychotics for positive symptoms but are less effective for negative symptoms.

4. **Adverse effects.** Typical antipsychotics are associated with several adverse effects (Tables 47-3 and 47-4).
   a. The activity of the various typical antipsychotics at the dopamine, α-, muscarinic, and histamine receptors are responsible for many of the adverse effects of these medications (Table 47-5).
   b. **Extrapyramidal side effects** can occur with all the typical antipsychotics, especially with high-potency typical antipsychotics. Four types of extrapyramidal side effects have been described: acute dystonia, akathisia, pseudoparkinsonism, and tardive dyskinesia.
      (1) **Acute dystonia** describes sudden muscle spasms that primarily occur in the eye, neck, face, and throat muscles.
         (a) Types of acute dystonia include torticollis (a muscle spasm of the neck causing the head to be twisted to the side), retrocollis (a muscle spasm of the neck causing the head to be pulled back), trismus (a muscle spasm of the mouth causing the jaw to be clenched), and oculogyric crisis (a spasm of the eye muscles causing one or both eyes to become fixed in a upward gaze).

Table 47-4. General Adverse Effects of Antipsychotics

Typical Antipsychotics	Atypical Antipsychotics
Sedation	Sedation
Anticholinergic effects	Anticholinergic effects (clozapine, olanzapine)
Blurred vision	Orthostatic hypotension
Constipation	Moderate to severe weight gain
Dry mouth	Diabetes mellitus
Urinary retention	Hypercholesterolemia
Extrapyramidal symptoms	Hyperprolactinemia (risperidone)
Lowered seizure threshold	Lowered seizure threshold
Orthostatic hypotension	QT prolongation
Hyperprolactinemia	Neuroleptic malignant syndrome
Moderate weight gain	Extrapyramidal symptoms
QT prolongation	Sexual dysfunction
Photosensitivity	
Temperature dysregulation	
Neuroleptic malignant syndrome	
Sexual dysfunction	
Elevated liver enzymes	

(b) Acute dystonias can occur within hours of initiating the medication or increasing the dose. This is most common in young men and in patients using high doses of high-potency typical antipsychotics.

(c) Management includes the use of anticholinergic agents like benztropine and diphenhydramine; if ineffective, benzodiazepines can also be used. Prevention of future reactions may be achieved by decreasing the dose of antipsychotic, using oral anticholinergics, or changing therapy to an atypical antipsychotic.

(2) Akathisia is described as motor restlessness associated with internal agitation and feelings of having to move.

(a) Patients with akathisia may pace or be unable to sit still. This may occur within days to a few months after the initiation of therapy or increase in dose.

(b) Treatment of akathisia includes dose reduction of the antipsychotic, lipophilic β-blockers, benzodiazepines, or anticholinergics. Therapy may also be changed to an atypical antipsychotic.

(3) Pseudoparkinsonism clinically appears similar to idiopathic Parkinson disease, and includes symptoms like shuffling gait, mask-like face, cogwheel rigidity, and resting or pill-rolling tremor.

(a) This can occur within 1–3 months after starting therapy or increasing the dose of the antipsychotic agent.

(b) This is treated by changing to an atypical antipsychotic, decreasing the dose, and/or adding an anticholinergic agent.

Table 47-5. Adverse Effects by Receptor Affinities

Receptor Antagonized	Adverse Effects
Histamine	Sedation
	Weight gain
Dopamine	Extrapyramidal symptoms
	Hyperprolactinemia
Muscarinic	Anticholinergic adverse effects
	Cognitive impairment
	Tachycardia
Alpha	Orthostatic hypotension
	Reflex tachycardia
Serotonin	Weight gain

    (4) Tardive dyskinesia (TD) usually does not occur until the patient has been taking antipsychotics for a year or more. It is a movement disorder that can occur in various locations of the body, including the face, tongue, hips, and extremities.

        (a) Movements can be dystonic (fixed) or choreoathetoid (rhythmic). Common movement disorders include tongue chewing, lip smacking, and rhythmic movements of the trunk.

        (b) TD may be irreversible, so patients taking antipsychotics should be monitored closely for the appearance of any movement disorders.

        (c) Tools such as the Abnormal Involuntary Movement Scale (AIMS) or Dyskinesia Identification System Condensed User Scale (DISCUS) are available to assist in monitoring patients.

        (d) Treatment should include stopping the antipsychotic. Multiple agents have been used to attempt to treat TD, although none has been definitively proven to be effective. These include vitamin E, benzodiazepines, baclofen, and reserpine.

  c. Neuroleptic malignant syndrome (NMS) is an uncommon but potentially fatal adverse effect of antipsychotics. Signs and symptoms include fever, severe rigidity, altered mental status, unstable blood pressure, tachycardia, incontinence, elevated creatine kinase, and increased white blood count.

    (1) NMS has a sudden onset, and should prompt immediate discontinuation of all antipsychotics.

    (2) Treatment includes supportive care and the use of bromocriptine and/or dantrolene.

C. Atypical antipsychotic medications (Table 47-6)

  1. Six atypical antipsychotics are currently on the U.S. market: clozapine (Clozaril), risperidone (Risperdal), olanzapine (Zyprexa), quetiapine (Seroquel), ziprasidone (Geodon), and aripiprazole (Abilify).

  2. The **mechanism of action** for atypical antipsychotics is different from that of the typical antipsychotics. With the exception of aripiprazole, the atypical antipsychotics are dopamine antagonists but also block $5\text{-}HT_{2A}$-receptors. They block 5-HT to a greater extent than dopamine. Aripiprazole is a partial dopamine and $5\text{-}HT_{1A}$-agonist and a $5\text{-}HT_{2A}$-antagonist.

  3. Receptor affinity differs for the various atypical antipsychotics. All atypical antipsychotics have activity at the $5\text{-}HT_{2A}$-receptor and dopamine receptor. Different agents have different activity for histamine, α-, and muscarinic receptors (Table 47-6).

  4. Atypical antipsychotics have increased efficacy for negative symptoms compared to typical antipsychotics. With the exception of clozapine, all antipsychotics are thought to have similar efficacy for positive symptoms. Clozapine has demonstrated efficacy for treatment-refractory schizophrenia.

  5. Adverse effects. Atypical antipsychotics differ from typical antipsychotics in their adverse effect profile (Table 47-4). Owing to their higher affinity for 5-HT-receptors compared to dopamine receptors, they are associated with less EPS and hyperprolactinemia than typical antipsychotics. However, they have problematic adverse effects, which limit their use (Table 47-6).

  a. Atypical antipsychotics have been linked with weight gain, hyperlipidemia, and hyperglycemia. The risk for the development of these metabolic adverse effects differs among agents.

  b. A recent meta-analysis of the atypical antipsychotics demonstrated an increased risk of death in patients with dementia. Atypical antipsychotics now carry a **black box warning** cautioning providers **against the use of atypical antipsychotics in the treatment of dementia-related psychosis.** For more information, refer to Schneider LS, Dagerman KS, Insel P. Risk of death with atypical antipsychotic drug treatment for dementia. JAMA 2005;294:1934–1943.

  6. Clozapine was the first atypical antipsychotic to be marketed in the United States, is the only antipsychotic with no risk of EPS or TD and is the only antipsychotic with proven efficacy for treatment-refractory schizophrenia. However, clozapine is indicated only in patients who have failed two to three antipsychotics (including typical and atypical antipsychotics) because of its risk of agranulocytosis. Complete blood count (CBC) must be monitored at baseline, every week for the first 6 months of therapy, every other week for the next 6 months, and then every month thereafter. Clozapine may also lower seizure threshold in

Table 47-6. Properties of Atypical Antipsychotics

Medication	Dose Range[a] (mg/day)	Receptor Affinity[a]	Sedation	EPS	Anticholinergic Effects	Orthostatic Hypotension	Weight Gain
Clozapine	150–600	D, 5-HT, M, H$_1$, α	+++	0	+++	+++	+++
Risperidone	2–8	D, 5-HT, H$_1$, α	+	+ to ++	0	+	++
Olanzapine	10–30	D, 5-HT, M, H$_1$, α	++	+	++	+	+++
Quetiapine	300–800	D, 5-HT, H$_1$, α	++	+	0	++	++
Ziprasidone	120–200	D, 5-HT, H$_1$, α	0	+	0	0	0
Aripiprazole	10–30	D, 5-HT, H$_1$, α	+	+	0	0	0

[a]Data from Lehman AF, Lieberman JA, Dixon LB, et al. Practice guideline for treatment of patients with schizophrenia, 2nd ed. Am J Psych 2004;161:1–56.
5-HT, 5-hydroxytryptamine (serotonin); α, alpha; D, dopamine; EPS, extrapyramidal symptoms; H$_1$, histamine; M, muscarinic; +++, high; ++, moderate; +, low.

patients, especially with higher doses. Clozapine should be used with caution in patients at risk for seizures or with a history of a seizure disorder.

7. Unique formulations of atypical antipsychotics are available for patients.
   a. **Orally disintegrating tablets.** Risperidone and olanzapine both are available as orally disintegrating tablets, and are manufactured as Risperdal M tablets and Zyprexa Zydis tablets.
   b. **Parenteral formulations.** Ziprasidone and olanzapine are available in parenteral formulations for use in acutely agitated patients with schizophrenia.
      (1) Ziprasidone may be given as 10 or 20 mg intramuscularly. The 10-mg dose may be repeated in 2 hr, and the 20 mg dose may be repeated in 4 hr. The maximum daily dose is 40 mg.
      (2) Olanzapine may be given as 10 mg intramuscularly. The 10-mg dose may be repeated every 2 hr, up to a maximum of 30 mg daily.

D. **Rapid tranquilization** is used for acutely psychotic patients with aggression or who are severely agitated. Parenteral typical or atypical agents may be used in these patients. Typical agents available in a parenteral form include chlorpromazine (Thorazine), fluphenazine (Prolixin), and haloperidol (Haldol). As described earlier, available atypical agents include ziprasidone and olanzapine.

E. **Noncompliant patients.** Those patients with a history of noncompliance or who have frequent hospitalizations secondary to noncompliance may be candidates for a long-acting intramuscular formulation of antipsychotic. Currently three options exist: haloperidol decanoate, fluphenazine decanoate, and long-acting risperidone (Risperdal Consta).

   1. **Haloperidol decanoate** is given intramuscularly every 3–4 weeks. The starting dose should be 10–15 times the total daily dose of oral haloperidol . This equation is only a rough conversion, and the lowest effective dose should be given. The first dose should not exceed 100 mg, and subsequent doses should not exceed 450 mg.

   2. **Fluphenazine decanoate** is administered intramuscularly every 2–3 weeks. The starting dose is 1.2–1.6 times the total daily dose of oral fluphenazine. The maximum dose of fluphenazine decanoate is 100 mg at any one time. The lowest effective dose of this formulation should be used.

   3. **Long-acting risperidone** is administered intramuscularly every 2 weeks. An effective dose of oral risperidone should first be identified before changing to the long-acting formulation. Patients should be started at 25 mg every 2 weeks and covered with oral medications for 3 weeks after initiation. Doses may be increased to a maximum of 50 mg every 2 weeks.

F. **Antipsychotic agents** may be switched for several reasons, such as lack of efficacy and adverse effects. When switching antipsychotic agents, the original agent should be titrated down while the new agent is titrated up. If changing from a typical antipsychotic to an atypical antipsychotic secondary to EPS, anticholinergic agents may be continued until the typical agent is completely discontinued unless the new agent is clozapine. Clozapine has high anticholinergic effects, thus additional anticholinergic agents would not be indicated.

G. **Adjunctive therapy.** In patients with partial or no response to therapy after an adequate trial of an antipsychotic, a second antipsychotic should be tried. After the failure of two to three antipsychotics, the patient meets the criteria for clozapine, and its use should be considered. Augmentation is an option for those patients unable to take clozapine or with partial/no response. Clozapine has been studied in combination with typical and atypical antipsychotics. Other options for augmentation include mood stabilizers, such as lithium, valproic acid, and carbamazepine. Antidepressants have also been used in patients suffering from depressive symptoms. Electroconvulsive therapy (ECT) has also been used as an adjunctive therapy in patients with partial or no response to antipsychotics.

STUDY QUESTIONS

Directions: Each of the questions, statements, or incomplete statements in this section can be correctly answered or completed by **one** of the suggested answers or phrases. Choose the **best** answer.

For questions 1–5: DG is a 23-year-old female committed to the inpatient psychiatric ward by her parents. They state that she has recently been under a large amount of stress from college, and they have noticed over the past year that she has become more withdrawn from her friends and social activities. They also state that she angers more easily than she used to as a child, and this morning they found her with a knife trying to slit her wrists. DG states that the voices keep telling her she is bad and that she should kill herself. She does not admit to any visual hallucinations but describes multiple voices (male and female) talking to her continuously telling her that she should harm herself or that people are out to get her. She keeps telling you that her parents are trying to get rid of her, and she wants to leave. She appears to be a healthy young woman although noticeably agitated. Her medical history is significant only for smoking one pack/day since age 16. DG is diagnosed with schizophrenia.

1. Which type of schizophrenia is DG likely experiencing based upon her presenting signs and symptoms?

(A) catatonic
(B) disorganized
(C) paranoid
(D) residual

2. Which of the following of DG's symptoms is best described as a negative symptom of schizophrenia?

(A) social withdrawal
(B) auditory hallucinations
(C) delusions
(D) agitation

3. The medical team decides to initiate treatment for DG. Which of the following antipsychotic medications is the best initial treatment for this patient?

(A) haloperidol
(B) risperidone
(C) thioridazine
(D) clozapine

4. Which of the following is *not* a potential adverse effect of the medication selected for DG in question 3?

(A) weight gain
(B) pseudoparkinsonism
(C) sedation
(D) urinary retention

5. DG is stabilized on the medication prescribed and is discharged home. DG is readmitted into the psychiatric ward 1 year later for auditory *and* visual hallucinations secondary to noncompliance on her current treatment regimen. Which of the following treatment options is most appropriate for DG at this time?

(A) haloperidol decanoate
(B) long-acting risperidone
(C) clozapine monotherapy
(D) adjunctive clozapine with haloperidol

For questions 6–8: TW is a 52-year-old female with a history of schizophrenia and diabetes mellitus type 2. She has been treated for many years with haloperidol with good response; however, she has recently developed lip smacking and tongue chewing.

6. What type of adverse effect is TW experiencing?

(A) akathisia
(B) acute dystonia
(C) pseudoparkinsonism
(D) tardive dyskinesia

7. Which of the following medications has been used to treat the adverse effect described in question 6?

(A) vitamin E
(B) propranolol
(C) diphenhydramine
(D) amantadine

8. Now that TW is experiencing this reaction, her healthcare providers want to change her therapy to a different antipsychotic. Which of the following antipsychotics is the best treatment option for her?

(A) olanzapine
(B) risperidone
(C) quetiapine
(D) fluphenazine

9. Which of the following atypical antipsychotics would be the least likely to cause weight gain?

(A) risperidone
(B) olanzapine
(C) quetiapine
(D) aripiprazole

10. Which of the following statements does not describe a way in which atypical antipsychotics differ from typical antipsychotics?

(A) Atypical antipsychotics have a higher affinity for serotonin receptors than dopamine receptors.
(B) Atypical antipsychotics are more efficacious for positive symptoms than typical antipsychotics.
(C) Atypical antipsychotics are more likely to cause weight gain and hyperlipidemia than typical antipsychotics.
(D) Atypical antipsychotics are less likely to cause extrapyramidal symptoms (EPS) than typical antipsychotics.

ANSWERS AND EXPLANATIONS

1. The answer is C *[see Table 47-1]*.
DG's prominent symptoms include well-formed hallucinations and delusions. These hallucinations and delusions are characteristic of paranoid schizophrenia. DG also does not meet the criteria for any other type of schizophrenia.

2. The answer is A *[see Table 47-2]*.
Social withdrawal or asocial behavior is a negative symptom of schizophrenia. Hallucinations, delusions, and agitation are all positive symptoms of schizophrenia.

3. The answer is B *[see VI.A.2; VI.C.1; VI.C.6]*.
The American Psychiatric Association currently recommends using atypical antipsychotics first over typical antipsychotics, unless the patient has a preference. Haloperidol and thioridazine are typical antipsychotics. Clozapine should be used only for treatment refractory patients because of its adverse effect profile.

4. The answer is D *[see Table 47-4; Table 47-6]*.
Risperidone has been associated with moderate weight gain, low to moderate risk of EPS, and low risk of sedation. It has not been associated with anticholinergics effects such as urinary retention.

5. The answer is B *[see VI.A.1–2, VI.E.1–3]*.
DG has a history of response with risperidone; however, she is experiencing a relapse of symptoms owing to noncompliance. A long-acting formulation is indicated to assist with medication compliance. As she has not failed multiple antipsychotics, DG is not a candidate for clozapine or adjunctive clozapine. Long-acting risperidone is preferred in this patient over haloperidol decanoate owing to the patient's response history and its preferable adverse effect profile.

6. The answer is D *[see VI.B.4.b.(1)–(4)]*.
TW is experiencing lip smacking and tongue chewing of a late onset, which is best described as tardive dyskinesia.

7. The answer is A *[see VI.B.4.b.(4).(d)]*.
Vitamin E, benzodiazepines, baclofen, and reserpine have all been used in the treatment of tardive dyskinesia, although none has been definitively proven to be effective.

8. The answer is C *[see Table 47-3; Table 47-6]*.
Because TW is experiencing tardive dyskinesia, her therapy should be changed to an atypical antipsychotic. Her medical history is significant for type 2 diabetes mellitus. Olanzapine is associated with a high risk of causing weight gain, and other metabolic symptoms and should not be used in this patient. Risperidone has a low to moderate risk of EPS. Other atypical antipsychotics, such as quetiapine, that carry a lower risk of EPS would be preferable.

9. The answer is D *[see Table 47-6]*.
Olanzapine has a high risk of causing weight gain. Risperidone and quetiapine have a moderate risk of causing weight gain. Aripiprazole is associated with a low risk of weight gain.

10. The answer is B *[see VI.C.2–5.a; Table 47-4]*.
Atypical antipsychotics have a higher affinity for serotonin receptors than dopamine receptors, whereas typical antipsychotics have no activity at serotonin receptors. Atypical and typical antipsychotics have similar efficacy for positive symptoms of schizophrenia; however, atypical antipsychotics have increased efficacy against negative symptoms. Atypical antipsychotics are more likely to cause significant weight gain and hyperlipidemia and less likely to cause EPS than typical antipsychotics.

48
Mood Disorders
Rebekah R. Arthur

I. **DEFINITION.** **Mood disorders** are described as an elevation or depression in mood that persists over a period of time and affects the ability of the person to function. These disorders are associated with significant morbidity, mortality, and financial cost. Mood disorders can cause a 10- to 20-fold increase in suicide rates and impair social and occupational functioning. Two common types of mood disorders are **major depression** and **bipolar disorder.**

II. **MAJOR DEPRESSION**

A. **Major depressive disorder** is defined as a mood disorder in which the patient has one or more episodes of major depression but has no history of mania, mixed, or hypomania episodes. Major depressive episodes are described in II.D.

B. **Epidemiology**

1. Depression occurs in 16.2% of the United States population. Results from recent studies indicate that 6.6% of the population has experienced an episode in the prior 12 months.

2. Depression occurs more frequently in women than men, with women having a lifetime risk of 1.7–2.7 times higher than men.

3. The highest risk of depression occurs in adults between the **ages of 25 to 44 years,** although depression may occur at any age.

C. **Pathophysiology.** The pathophysiology of depression is not completely known, however several theories exist: genetic theories, the biogenic amine theory, and the dysregulation theory.

1. As with many psychiatric disorders, a **genetic link** exists for depression. People who have a parent or sibling with a history of depression have a 1.5–3 times greater risk for developing depression than the general population. Between 8% and 18% of patients with major depression have a parent or sibling with a history of depression.

2. The **biogenic amine theory** was originally described in the 1950s and is the basis for past and current pharmacological treatment options. This theory suggests that depression is associated with **decreased levels of norepinephrine (NE), 5-hydroxytryptamine (serotonin; 5-HT), and dopamine (DA) in the brain**.

3. The **dysregulation theory** was developed after the biogenic amine theory and suggests that **impaired homeostasis of NE, 5-HT, and DA in the brain** is associated with depression rather than absolute levels of these neurotransmitters. This theory in part attempts to explain the changes in neurotransmitter receptor sensitivities witnessed in the first few weeks of pharmacotherapy.

D. **Diagnosis and clinical features**

1. Major depressive episodes are diagnosed using the *Diagnostic and Statistical Manual of Mental Disorders,* 4th ed. (DSM-IV-TR) criteria. To meet the criteria for a major depressive episode, patients should experience at least five or more persistent symptoms for at least 2 weeks. These symptoms include depressed mood, loss of interest or pleasure in activities, change in appetite, unintentional weight gain or loss, insomnia or excess sedation, psychomotor agitation or retardation, decreased energy or fatigue, feelings of worthlessness or inappropriate guilt, decreased ability to concentrate, and recurrent thoughts of suicide, death, or suicide attempt.[1]

---

[1] American Psychiatric Association. Practice guideline for the treatment of patients with bipolar disorder. Am J Psych 2002;159(4 Suppl):1–50.

2. Symptoms should impair social or occupational functioning and should not be related to a general medical condition or substance abuse.

3. Patients presenting with excessive sedation (hypersomnia), increased appetite, weight gain, and agitation are classified as experiencing atypical depression.

E. **Treatment options.** Three treatment options exist for the treatment of depression: **pharmacotherapy**, **psychotherapy**, and **electroconvulsive therapy (ECT).** The choice of which treatment option or combination of treatment options to use should be patient specific and influenced by the severity of symptoms and patient preference.

1. **Pharmacotherapy options (antidepressants).** Pharmacotherapy can be used for mild to severe major depression and produces a response in 40%–70% of patients. Antidepressants have similar efficacy; however, they differ in adverse effects, mechanism of action, medication interactions, and cost. Therefore, selection of pharmacologic agents for patients should be based on the specific symptoms the patient is experiencing, adverse effects of the medications, medication interactions, patient preference, and ability of patient to afford the medication. Patients with a history of response to a particular agent may restart that agent if desired.

   a. **Monoamine oxidase inhibitors (MAOIs)** (Table 48-1)

      (1) **Indications.** MOAIs have numerous adverse effects and medication interactions and are indicated only in patients refractory to other antidepressants. These agents also have a role in patients presenting with atypical depression.

      (2) **Mechanism of action.** MOAIs inhibit monoamine oxidase, which is responsible for the breakdown of neurotransmitters such as DA, 5-HT, and NE. By blocking this enzyme, levels of these amines increase in the brain.

      (3) **Adverse effects.** MAOIs have numerous adverse effects that limit their use. These include hypertensive crises, serotonin syndrome, orthostatic hypotension, peripheral edema, weight gain, and sexual dysfunction.

         (a) **Hypertensive crises** can occur when increased levels of sympathetic amines, such as NE, build up in the body, which can be the result of ingestion of tyramine-containing foods like wine and cheese or the administration of sympathomimetic agents (e.g., decongestants). Patients should be counseled regarding the risk for drug and food interactions when taking MAOIs.

         (b) **Serotonin syndrome** can occur when levels of 5-HT become too high, usually as the result of the use of multiple serotonergic agents. MAOIs in combination with selective serotonin-reuptake inhibitors, tricyclic amines, serotonin and norepinephrine reuptake inhibitors, and any other agent with serotonergic activity can lead to serotonin syndrome. The clinical manifestations of serotonin syndrome are given in Table 48-2.

   b. Many **tricyclic amines (TCAs)** are commercially available in the United States and can be classified as tertiary and secondary (Table 48-3).

      (1) **Indications.** Owing to their numerous adverse effects, TCAs are not usually indicated first-line for the treatment of depression.

         (a) TCAs may be considered for patients with a history of response to TCAs, patients refractory to other medications, or patients with co-morbidities that might benefit from TCAs, such as neuropathic pain and migraines.

         (b) TCAs should not be used in patients with suicidal ideations and should probably be avoided in patients with cardiovascular conditions, closed angle glaucoma, urinary retention, or severe prostate hypertrophy.

Table 48-1. Monoamine Oxidase Inhibitors

Agent	Starting Dose (mg/day)	Dose Range[a] (mg/day)	Anticholinergic Effects	Sedation	Weight Gain
Phenelzine (Nardil)	10	15–90	+ +	+ +	+ + +
Isocarboxazid (Marplan)	20	20–40	+ +	+ +	+ +
Tranylcypromine (Parnate)	10	10–40	+ +	+	+ +

[a]For normal adults. Doses may need to be adjusted for elderly patients or those with impaired renal or hepatic function.
+ + +, high; + +, moderate; +, slight.

Table 48-2. Signs and Symptoms of Serotonin Syndrome

Cognitive-Behavioral Dysfunction	Autonomic Nervous System Dysfunction	Neuromuscular Dysfunction
Confusion	Diarrhea	Myoclonus
Hypomania	Shivering	Hyperreflexia
Agitation	Fever	Tremor
	Diaphoresis	Seizure
	Change in blood pressure	Death
	Nausea and vomiting	

    (2) Mechanism of action. TCAs produce their antidepressant effect by inhibiting the reuptake of 5-HT and NE. TCAs also have effect at α-adrenergic, histamine, and cholinergic receptors. Individual TCAs have different affinities for these receptors.

    (3) Adverse effects. Several adverse effects exist for TCAs and may differ between agents, depending on their affinity for α-adrenergic, cholinergic, and histamine receptors (Table 48-3).

        (a) Tertiary TCAs have been associated with a higher risk of causing anticholinergic adverse effects (blurred vision, constipation, urinary retention, dry mouth), sedation, weight gain, and orthostatic hypotension than secondary TCAs.

        (b) Additional adverse effects include tachycardia, QT prolongation, cardiac conduction abnormalities, decreased seizure threshold, and sexual dysfunction. TCAs may be lethal when taken as an overdose.

        (c) Owing to their activity on serotonin, TCAs have the potential for causing serotonin syndrome when used in combination with other serotonergic agents.

    (4) Medication interactions. TCAs are substrates of various cytochrome P450 enzymes and levels can be affected by enzyme inhibitors and inducers.

  c. Selective serotonin reuptake inhibitors (SSRIs). Five SSRIs are currently available in the United States for the treatment of depression (Table 48-4): fluoxetine (Prozac), paroxetine (Paxil), sertraline (Zoloft), citalopram (Celexa), and escitalopram (Lexapro). These medications are considered to be first line for the treatment of depression, and many are also

Table 48-3. Tricyclic Amines

Agent	Dose Range[a] (mg/day)	Anticholinergic Effects	Sedation	Orthostatic Hypotension	Cardiac Effects	Weight Gain
Tertiary amine						
Amitriptyline (Elavil)	50–300	+ + + +	+ + + +	+ + + +	+ + +	+ + + +
Doxepin (Sinequan)	50–300	+ + +	+ + + +	+ +	+ +	+ + + +
Imipramine (Tofranil)	50–300	+ + +	+ + +	+ + + +	+ + +	+ + + +
Trimipramine (Surmontil)	50–300	+ + + +	+ + + +	+ + +	+ + +	+ + + +
Secondary amine						
Nortriptyline (Pamelor)	25–150	+ +	+ +	+	+ +	+
Desipramine (Norpramin)	50–300	+	+ +	+ +	+ +	+
Protriptyline (Vivactil)	10–60	+ +	+	+ +	+ + +	+

[a]For normal adults. Doses may need to be adjusted for elderly patients or those with impaired renal or hepatic function.

+ + + +, very high; + + +, high; + +, moderate; +, slight.

Table 48-4. Selective Serotonin Reuptake Inhibitors and Serotonin and Norepinephrine Reuptake Inhibitors

Agent	Starting Dose (mg/day)	Dose Range (mg/day)	Half-Life	CYP450 Isoenzyme Inhibition
Fluoxetine (Prozac)	10–20	20–80; 90 mg weekly[a]	7–9 days[b]	2D6, 2C9/19 (potent); 3A4 (mild)
Paroxetine (Paxil)	10–20	20–60	21 hr	2D6 (potent)
Sertraline (Zoloft)	25–50	50–200	24 hr	2D6 (mild)
Citalopram (Celexa)	10–20	20–60	35 hr	2D6 (mild)
Escitalopram (Lexapro)	5–10	10–20	27–32 hr	2D6 (mild)
Venlafaxine (Effexor)	75	150–375	11 hr	2D6 (mild)
Duloxetine (Cymbalta)	40	40–60	9–19 hr	2D6 (moderate)

[a]Fluoxetine can be given in a once-weekly formulation in patients stabilized on fluoxetine 20 mg daily; should be started 1 week after the last dose of fluoxetine.
[b]Norfluoxetine is an active metabolite of fluoxetine and has a half-life of 7–9 days. The half-life of fluoxetine alone is 2–3 days.
CYP450, cytochrome P450.

indicated for anxiety, panic disorder, post-traumatic stress disorder, and obsessive–compulsive disorder.

  (1) **Mechanism of action.** SSRIs exert their antidepressant effect by blocking the reuptake of serotonin.
  (2) **Adverse effects**
    (a) SSRIs have been associated with nausea, vomiting, insomnia, sedation, sexual dysfunction, headache, agitation, and tremor.
    (b) Paroxetine has also been associated with anticholinergic adverse effects, such as blurred vision, dry mouth, constipation, and urinary retention.
    (c) These agents have been associated with serotonin syndrome when used in combination with other serotonergic agents.
  (3) Many SSRIs are substrates and inhibitors of the cytochrome P450 system and may interact with other medications.
  (4) Abrupt discontinuation of SSRIs has been associated with **withdrawal symptoms,** such as nightmares, vivid dreams, tremor, anxiety, nausea, and poor concentration. Fluoxetine has little risk of causing syndrome upon discontinuation, likely because of its long half-life. With the exception of fluoxetine, SSRIs should be slowly tapered when discontinued to prevent this syndrome.

 d. **Serotonin and norepinephrine reuptake inhibitors (SNRIs)** (Table 48-4). Two SNRIs are currently available for the treatment of depression: venlafaxine (Effexor) and duloxetine (Cymbalta). Data have shown these medications to have efficacy for the treatment not only of depression but also of painful peripheral neuropathies. Duloxetine carries a U.S. Food and Drug Administration (FDA) indication for the treatment of pain in diabetic neuropathy.

  (1) **Mechanism of action.** SNRIs inhibit the reuptake of 5-HT and NE, thereby increasing their levels. These medications differ from TCAs in that they have little activity for α-adrenergic, cholinergic, or histamine receptors.
  (2) **Adverse effects.** SNRIs have an adverse effect profile similar to that of the SSRIs. Common adverse effects include nausea, headache, somnolence, dry mouth, dizziness, sexual dysfunction, and insomnia. Venlafaxine and duloxetine have also been associated with elevations of diastolic blood pressure, particularly with higher doses.
  (3) **Medication interactions.** Venlafaxine and duloxetine are both substrates for the cytochrome P450 isoenzyme system and are mild to moderate inhibitors of the isoenzyme 2D6 (Table 48-4). SNRIs should not be used with MAOIs or other serotonergic agents owing to risk of serotonin syndrome.

 e. **Bupropion (Wellbutrin)** (Table 48-5).
  (1) The **mechanism of action** for bupropion is not completely understood. Bupropion is known to inhibit the reuptake of dopamine and to a smaller extent the reuptake of serotonin and norepinephrine.

Table 48-5. Miscellaneous Antidepressants

Agent	Starting Dose (mg/day)	Dose Range (mg/day)	Cytochrome P450 Isoenzyme Inhibition
Bupropion (Wellbutrin)	75–150	200–450	2D6
Mirtazapine (Remeron)	15	30–45	Does not inhibit
Trazodone (Desyrel)	50–100	150–600	Does not inhibit

      (2) In addition to its indication for depression, bupropion is also indicated for smoking cessation.

      (3) Common **adverse effects** associated with the use of bupropion include nausea, vomiting, and insomnia.

        (a) Bupropion has been associated with less sexual dysfunction than many other antidepressant medications, such as SSRIs.

        (b) Bupropion has been associated with an increased risk for seizures and is contraindicated in patients at risk for seizures. This includes patients with the following medical disorders: seizure disorder, history of anorexia or bulimia, or using or withdrawing from medications such as alcohol or benzodiazepines. Doses > 450 mg should not be used, and dose increases should be gradual.

  f. Mirtazapine (Remeron) (Table 48-5).

      (1) Mirtazapine antagonizes α-adrenergic and 5HT$_{2,3}$-receptors, causing an increase in levels of NE and 5-HT. In addition, mirtazapine has activity at histamine (H) receptors.

      (2) **Adverse effects** for mirtazapine include sedation, weight gain, constipation, dry mouth, and increased appetite. Sedation, increased appetite, and weight gain can be problematic, particularly at lower doses. Mirtazapine has a lower risk for causing sexual dysfunction as compared to SSRIs.

  g. Trazodone (Desyrel) (Table 48-5).

      (1) The **mechanism of action** for trazodone is not completely understood, but is thought to be owing an increase in 5-HT.

      (2) Trazodone is indicated for the treatment of depression, although it is not frequently used because of sedation. It is more frequently used in low doses as adjunctive treatment for insomnia in depressed patients.

      (3) The most common **adverse effects** of trazodone include sedation, nausea, and orthostatic hypotension. Trazodone has rarely been associated priapism and QT prolongation.

  h. Nefazodone (Serzone). Nefazodone is a medication structurally similar to trazodone. It was considered to be first line for treatment of depression; however, recent reports of hepatotoxicity have limited its use and led to a **black box warning** for possible liver failure leading to death.

      (1) Nefazodone inhibits 5-HT$_2$-receptors and blocks the reuptake of NE and 5-HT.

      (2) **Adverse effects.** Common adverse effects for nefazodone include dry mouth, nausea, constipation, orthostatic hypotension, and sedation. The most severe adverse effect associated with nefazodone is hepatic failure.

        (a) Reported rates by the FDA estimate 1 case of liver failure resulting in death or transplant per 250,000–350,000 patient-years.

        (b) No known predicators for the development of liver failure are available. If nefazodone is used, liver function enzymes should be monitored routinely.

        (c) The generic product is still available, although brand name nefazodone was withdrawn from the U.S. market in 2004.

      (3) Nefazodone is highly protein bound and is an inhibitor of cytochrome P450 isoenzyme 3A4, leading to the potential for multiple drug–drug interactions.

  2. Duration of treatment. Treatment is divided into three phases: acute phase, continuation phase, and maintenance phase.

    a. The **acute phase** begins with the initiation of therapy until remission is reached, typically lasting between 6 and 12 weeks.

    b. The **continuation phase** begins after remission is reached and typically lasts between 6 and 9 months. Medication from the acute phase is continued during this phase to prevent relapse of depression.

    c. A **maintenance phase** is used in patients with a high risk of recurrence of depression, such as those with a history of multiple episodes of depression, history of suicidal thoughts, and severe depression. These patients should receive maintenance treatment for 2–3 years, and many may receive life-long therapy.

3. Administration and dosage

    (a) Antidepressants are usually started at low doses and slowly titrated up to reach target doses over a period of a few weeks to prevent adverse reactions. Clinical response determines if the dose should be further titrated. While full effects may not be seen for 4–6 weeks, often some signs and symptoms of depression such as insomnia may resolve more rapidly. Patients must receive maximum tolerated doses for 4–6 weeks without response to be classified as ineffective.

    (b) If patients receive only a partial or no response, other antidepressants may be considered. When changing to another antidepressant agent, caution should be used to prevent serotonin syndrome. These guidelines should be followed if changing to or from a MAOI:

    (1) A 2-week washout period should be observed when changing to a MAOI from an antidepressant without a long half-life and when changing from a MAOI to another antidepressant.

    (2) A 5-week washout period should be observed when changing to a MAOI from an antidepressant with a long half-life, such as fluoxetine.

4. Augmentation of therapy. When patients fail to fully or partially respond to two or more medications, augmentation of antidepressant therapy with another agent may be considered.

    (a) Lithium and thyroid hormone have been used for augmentation of antidepressant medications. Lithium augmentation is currently preferred over thyroid augmentation.

    (b) Dual antidepressant augmentation has also been used. Agents that have been used include bupropion, TCAs, and mirtazapine.

5. Suicide risk. Risk of suicide is always a concern in patients suffering from a major depressive episode. In adolescents and children, recent studies have shown a link between antidepressant use and risk of increased suicidal thoughts and actions. Because of this increased risk, the FDA has now issued a **black box warning** for all antidepressants that an increase in suicidal thoughts and actions may occur with therapy and that adolescents and children receiving this therapy should be closely monitored.

III. BIPOLAR DISORDER

A. Definition. Bipolar disorder or manic depression is a syndrome in which patients suffer from episodes of mania and depression. Mania is an unusually elevated mood and is described in greater detail in III.D.1.

B. Epidemiology

1. Bipolar I and II disorders affect 3.7%–3.9% of the U.S. population. In patients presenting with depression, 21%–49% of patients have bipolar disorder.

2. Bipolar I disorder occurs equally in men and women although bipolar II disorder tends to occur more commonly in women.

3. Although patients may present with bipolar disorder at any age, most patients have an average age of onset of 21 years, with peak onset occurring between the ages of **15 and 24 years**.

4. Suicide occurs in 10%–15% of patients with bipolar I disorder.

C. Pathophysiology. As with many psychiatric disorders, the pathophysiology for bipolar disorder is not completely understood, although many theories exist.

1. A positive family history is present in 80%–90% of patients with bipolar disorder. Therefore, **genetics** is believed to play a role in its pathophysiology, although a direct genetic link has not been discovered.

2. Like major depression, bipolar disorder is believed to be caused by an **imbalance of neuro-transmitters.** However, in bipolar disorder, the neurotransmitter levels fluctuate and may be similar or reversed, depending on the patient's current clinical presentation.

   a. A manic episode is believed to result from elevations in NE.

   b. Depression has been associated with a decrease in NE.

3. A dysregulation of **γ-aminobutyric acid (GABA)** may play a role in bipolar disorder. A deficiency in GABA, an inhibitory neurotransmitter, may lead to mania caused by unopposed excitatory neurotransmitters, such as DA and NE.

4. Increased and decreased levels of **calcium** in the cerebrospinal fluid (CSF) have been detected in depressed and manic individuals, respectively. Changes in the extracellular and intracellular calcium levels, which can affect the excitability of neurons, may be a factor in emotional variations and switches from depression to mania.

5. Recent research has focused on **G proteins** and their effects on mood stabilization. G proteins are involved in signal transduction and activation of second messenger systems for various neurotransmitters, like NE, 5-HT, and DA.

   a. The current theory proposes that hyperactive G proteins cause mood instability; and by normalizing G proteins, mood stability will occur.

   b. G proteins and glutamate may also play a role in the long-term potentiation and cycling of mood disorders.

      (1) Glutamate binding to G proteins linked to *N*-methyl-D-aspartate (NMDA) receptors may be involved in long-term potentiation.

      (2) Serotonin and NE are involved in bipolar illness, but the cycling and long-term potentiation may be mediated by glutamate and the medications that affect the glutamate system.

6. **Psychosocial and physical stressors** have been proposed to trigger early episodes of bipolar disorder, although these stressors may or may not trigger later episodes. These later episodes and cyclic episodes are thought to be caused by increased sensitivity or electrophysiologic kindling of the brain.

D. **Diagnosis.** Bipolar disorder is diagnosed using DSM-IV-TR criteria. The symptoms should impair social or occupational functioning and should not be related to a general medical condition or use of a substance.

1. **Mania** is described as at least a 1-week period of a continuously elevated or irritable mood, although shorter durations of symptoms are acceptable if the patient is hospitalized. In addition to elevated mood, the patient should experience at least three of the following symptoms: elevated self-esteem or grandiose ideations, reduced need for sleep, pressured speech, racing thoughts or flight of ideas, easily distracted, psychomotor agitation, and excessive involvement in high risk activities.[2]

2. **Hypomania** has similar symptoms to that of mania; however, symptoms are not as severe. Hypomania is diagnosed by an elevated mood present for at least 4 days, with at least three of the same symptoms as described for mania. These symptoms should not interfere with social or occupational functioning and should not cause hospitalization.

2. A **mixed disorder** is diagnosed when the criteria for both mania and a major depressive episode are met every day for nearly 1 week, affects social and occupational functioning, and is not caused by a general medical condition or substance.

3. Bipolar disorder may be classified into bipolar I disorder, bipolar II disorder, cyclothymia, and rapid cycling.

   a. **Bipolar I disorder.** Patients are classified with bipolar I disorder with a history of at least one mixed or manic episode and at least one major depressive episode.

   b. **Bipolar II disorder.** Patients are classified with bipolar II disorder with a history of at least one episode of hypomania and one major depressive episode but have never experienced mania or a mixed episode.

---

[2]American Psychiatric Association. Practice guideline for the treatment of patients with bipolar disorder. Am J Psych 2002;159(4 Suppl):1–50.

   c. **Cyclothymic disorder.** Patients are classified with cyclothymic disorder with at least a 2-year history of multiple episodes of hypomania and depressive symptoms. These patients have never met full criteria for a major depressive or manic episode.

   d. **Rapid cycling.** Patients that experience at least four depressive, manic, hypomanic, or mixed episodes within a 12-month period of time are described as rapid cycling.

E. **Clinical course.** The course of bipolar disorder is variable and patient specific.

   1. Patients frequently present with episodes of depression. Patients presenting with depression should always be questioned for a history of signs and symptoms of mania.

   2. Episodes vary in length and severity; however, they may last from days to months if untreated.

   3. The duration of time between episodes varies. Commonly, 4 years or more may separate the first and second episode but subsequent episodes are more frequent. Untreated patients may experience 10 or more episodes during their life.

   4. The management of this disorder can be complicated by mixed episodes, rapid cycling, and substance abuse.

F. **Treatment options**

   1. **Pharmacotherapeutic options.** Mood stabilizers have historically been the mainstays of therapy for bipolar disorder. Agents include lithium (Eskalith, Lithonate, Lithobid), valproic acid (Depakene, Depakote), and carbamazepine (Tegretol, Carbatrol, Equetro). Recent literature has supported the use of atypical antipsychotics as monotherapy or adjunctive treatments in bipolar mania. Agents for the treatment of depressive episodes in patients with bipolar remains more limited, with recent data emerging for lamotrigine (Lamictal), quetiapine (Seroquel), and olanzapine-fluoxetine (Symbyax). The 2005 Texas Implementation of Medication Algorithms update for the treatment of bipolar I disorder is summarized in Table 48-6.

      a. **Lithium** is a first-line agent for the acute and maintenance treatment of mania and hypomania. It is also first-line for the maintenance treatment of mixed episodes and is useful as adjunctive treatment in depressive episodes.

         (1) Lithium is available as lithium carbonate and lithium citrate. Lithium carbonate is available as regular (Eskalith), controlled-release (Eskalith CR), or extended release (Lithobid) tablets and lithium citrate (Lithonate) is available as syrup.

         (2) **Pharmacokinetics**

            (a) Between 60% and 100% of lithium is absorbed from the gastrointestinal tract. The extent of absorption is not affected by food. The rate of absorption varies, depending on the formulation.

               (i) Lithium citrate syrup reaches peak concentrations in 15–60 min.

               (ii) Immediate-release tablets and capsules peak in 1–3 hr.

               (iii) Extended-release tablets have peak concentrations in 4–12 hr.

            (b) Lithium is distributed into total body water and penetrates many body tissues, such as the thyroid, bone, and brain. Lithium is not highly protein bound.

Table 48-6. Algorithms for Treatment of Bipolar I Disorder

Type of Episode	Monotherapy Options First-Line	Monotherapy Options Second-Line
Acute mania	Lithium, VPA, aripiprazole, quetiapine, risperidone, ziprasidone	Olanzapine, CBZ
Acute mixed	VPA, aripiprazole, quetiapine, risperidone, ziprasidone	Olanzapine, CBZ
Acute depressive	Lamotrigine or lamotrigine plus anti-manic	Quetiapine, olanzapine-fluoxetine
Maintenance mania or mixed	Lithium, VPA, or lamotrigine	Olanzapine
Depression	Lamotrigine plus anti-manic or lamotrigine	

CBZ, carbamazepine; *VPA,* valproic acid.
Adapted from Suppes T, Dennehy EB, Hirschfeld RM, et al. The Texas implementation of medication algorithms: Update to the algorithm for treatment of bipolar I disorder. J Clin Psychiatry 2005;66:870–886.

    (c) Lithium is eliminated primarily through the kidneys. It is filtered by the glomeruli in the kidneys and is also cleared by renal tubular reabsorption. Changes in renal function can significantly affect the clearance of lithium.

(3) The **mechanism of action** for lithium is currently unknown, although several theories exist.

    (a) Lithium is thought to help correct desynchronized biological rhythms in patients with bipolar disorder.

    (b) Lithium may affect membrane stabilization.

    (c) Lithium may augment homeostasis by enhancing the function of secondary messenger systems, especially cyclic adenosine monophosphate (cAMP), cyclic guanosine monophosphate (cGMP), and phosphatidylinositol.

    (d) Lithium can inhibit NE release and accelerate its metabolism.

    (e) Lithium may decrease receptor sensitivity and increase presynaptic reuptake of NE and 5-HT.

(4) Lithium has a **narrow therapeutic index,** with a therapeutic range of 0.5–1.2 mEq/L. Toxicity is associated with levels > 1.5 mEq/L. Patients presenting with acute mania generally require levels in the higher end of the therapeutic range than those on maintenance therapy.

    (a) Patients are generally started on 300 mg two to three times daily of lithium and titrated up by 300 mg increments as needed to achieve therapeutic effects and minimize toxicity.

    (b) Patient-specific factors should be considered when deciding the appropriate initial dose of lithium, such as age, weight, and renal function.

    (c) Serum concentrations may be monitored 3 days after initiation therapy or changing doses. Levels should be obtained 12 hr after the dose, usually in the morning before the first dose of the day.

(5) **Clinical response.** Clinical response may be seen within 2 weeks after lithium initiation for the treatment of acute mania. When used in depression, responses may not occur for 4–6 weeks.

(6) **Precautions and adverse effects**

    (a) Lithium has an absolute contraindication in patients experiencing acute renal failure or women in their first trimester of pregnancy.

    (b) Lithium has the following relative contraindications: renal impairment, cardiovascular disease, dehydration, pregnancy, seizure disorder, and thyroid disease.

    (c) Lithium has numerous **adverse effects** (Table 48-7). Certain adverse effects indicate toxicity. If toxicity occurs, lithium should be immediately discontinued, the patient should be properly hydrated, stomach contents should be emptied with gastric lavage, and if severe toxicity occurs (level ≥ 3 mEq/L), hemodialysis may be indicated.

(7) Many medications and disease states may affect lithium levels in the body (Table 48-8).

    (a) Use of lithium with antipsychotics or benzodiazepines may increase the risk for CNS toxicity, especially if used together long term.

    (b) Use of lithium with medications that can increase 5- HT may cause serotonin syndrome.

Table 48-7. Adverse Effects of Lithium

Early Onset	Long-Term Use	Toxicity
Gastrointestinal upset	Weight gain	Severe drowsiness
Nausea	Altered taste	Course hand tremor
Polydipsia	Decreased libido	Muscle twitching
Nocturia	Hypothyroidism	Seizures
Dry mouth	Rash	Choreoathetosis
Hand tremor	Acne	Vomiting
Leukocytosis	Psoriasis	Confusion
Polyuria	Alopecia	Vertigo

Table 48-8. Factors That Change Lithium Concentrations[a]

Increase Lithium Levels	Decrease Lithium Levels
Angiotensin-converting enzyme inhibitors	Acetazolamide
Angiotensin II receptor blockers	Methylxanthines (e.g., theophylline, caffeine)
Nonsteroidal anti-inflammatory drugs	Osmotic diuretics
Thiazides	Pregnancy (third trimester)
Dehydration	Sodium supplements
Renal dysfunction	Urine alkalinizers (ex. sodium bicarbonate)
Sodium loss	
Fluoxetine	

[a]Not an all-inclusive list.

b. Valproic acid (VPA) is indicated in the acute and chronic treatment of mania, hypomania, mixed disorders, and rapid cycling. It is also used as adjunctive treatment in depressive episodes (Table 48-6).
  (1) Mechanism of action. The mechanism of action for VPA is not entirely known. Efficacy for VPA is thought to be related to its ability to increase levels of GABA.
  (2) Many formulations exist for VPA. VPA is formulated as valproic acid (Depakene) in capsules and syrup, as divalproex in delayed-release tablets (Depakote) and extended-release tablets (Depakote ER), and as valproate in intravenous solution (Depacon).
  (3) VPA is generally initiated at doses of 20 mg/kg/day given in divided doses for inpatients and 250 mg three times daily for outpatients. The current therapeutic range (50–125 μg/mL) was originally described for the treatment of seizure disorders and has not been established for efficacy in bipolar disorder. However, this range can still be useful to minimize toxicities and assess compliance.
    (a) Levels may be first obtained after 4–5 days of therapy. These values should be representative of trough values and are frequently obtained in the mornings before the first dose of medication.
    (b) Patients that are treated for 4–6 weeks with VPA concentrations of 80–120 μg/mL without clinical response may be classified as failures of VPA therapy.
  (4) Adverse effects. Common adverse effects of VPA include nausea, vomiting, dyspepsia, sedation, elevated liver enzymes, hair loss, and tremor. Less frequent adverse effects include thrombocytopenia, leukopenia, pancreatitis, weight gain, and liver failure. VPA has also been associated with polycystic ovarian syndrome in women of child-bearing age.
    (a) Gastrointestinal adverse effects may be minimized by lowering the dose or by using divalproex formulations instead of valproic acid or sodium valproate.
    (b) Liver function tests and complete blood counts should be monitored at baseline, every month for the first 2 months of therapy, and then every 6–12 months thereafter.
  (5) Medication interactions. VPA has the potential for multiple drug interactions. VPA is highly protein bound in the body, thus levels can increase in the presence of another medication that is highly protein bound. VPA is also a substrate and inhibitor of the cytochrome P450 isoenzyme 2C9 and can potentially elevate levels of other medications that are metabolized via this isoenzyme.
c. Carbamazepine (CBZ) is indicated in the treatment of bipolar disorder and is considered to be a second-line agent owing to its numerous adverse effects and medication interactions (Table 48-6).
  (1) The **mechanism of action** for CBZ is not completely known; however, its efficacy in bipolar disorder is thought to be the result of its effects on GABA and G protein-linked second messenger systems, such as cAMP.
  (2) CBZ should be initiated at doses of 200–600 mg/day given in divided doses and increased by 200 mg/day to usual doses of 800–1000 mg/day.

      (a) A therapeutic range of 4–12 μg/mL has been described for seizure disorders. While correlation between this range and efficacy have not been fully established for bipolar disorder, it is used to minimize adverse effects.

      (b) Levels may be obtained 5–7 days after initiating therapy. Levels should continued to be obtained in the following few weeks because CBZ concentrations will decrease in the body once autoinduction occurs.

      (c) Patients who are treated for 4–6 weeks with CBZ concentrations of 6–12 μg/mL without clinical response may be classified as failures of CBZ therapy.

   (3) Adverse effects. CBZ is associated with numerous adverse effects, many of which are dose related.

      (a) Frequent adverse effects include dizziness, drowsiness, ataxia, fatigue, blurred vision, diplopia, nystagmus, confusion, headache, nausea, vomiting, diarrhea, and dyspepsia. The gastrointestinal adverse effects of CBZ are often dose related.

      (b) Additional adverse effects include rash, leukopenia, thrombocytopenia, hyponatremia, elevation in liver enzymes, and weight gain.

      (c) Severe idiosyncratic reactions may also occur, including agranulocytosis, aplastic anemia, severe thrombocytopenia, liver failure, Stevens-Johnson syndrome, and pancreatitis.

      (d) Complete blood counts, liver function tests, thyroid tests, and electrolytes should be monitored at baseline and every 3–6 months.

   (4) Medication interactions. CBZ is an inducer of many hepatic enzymes responsible for metabolism of medications and, therefore, has numerous medication interactions. Oral contraceptive levels in the body can be decreased in patients taking CBZ. Alternative forms of contraception should be used in patients taking CBZ. CBZ can also induce its own metabolism (autoinduction). Decreases in CBZ levels in the body may be seen after 3–30 days of therapy. CBZ levels should be monitored and adjusted accordingly.

  d. Lamotrigine is indicated in the treatment of bipolar disorder, primarily in patients presenting with depression (Table 48-6).

   (1) The **mechanism of action** for lamotrigine is not completely understood. It is currently thought to be related to its ability to decrease release of glutamate and aspartate by blocking sodium channels.

   (2) Owing to the risk of rash, lamotrigine should be initiated at low doses (25 mg/day) and slowly increased by 25 mg every 1–2 weeks. Lamotrigine should be administered twice daily in doses > 50 mg. Patients who are taking lamotrigine with VPA should decrease the dose by half owing to a significant medication interaction.

   (3) Common **adverse effects** include dizziness, diplopia, nausea, vomiting, rash, photosensitivity, ataxia, headache, and blurred vision. Rashes may be severe and life-threatening such as Stevens-Johnson rash, and patients should immediately discontinue the medication if a rash appears.

  e. Atypical antipsychotics have recently been the subject of multiple studies in the treatment of bipolar disorder. These medications are indicated in the treatment of bipolar disorder (Table 48-6). For information regarding dosing, adverse effects, and mechanism of action see Chapter 47. Olanzapine is available in a formulation with fluoxetine (Symbyax) and is approved for depressive episodes in bipolar disorder.

  f. Additional anticonvulsants

   (1) Gabapentin has been evaluated in two trials for its use in acute mania and has not been shown at this time to improve symptoms. It is not indicated for monotherapy in bipolar disorder but may be used as adjunctive therapy to assist with symptoms such as anxiety.

   (2) Oxcarbazepine is a medication structurally similar to carbamazepine but with fewer adverse effects. It is postulated to have similar therapeutic effects in bipolar disorder to carbamazepine; however, studies demonstrating its efficacy are limited. It currently is recommended only in combination with other mood stabilizers.

  g. Antidepressants should be used cautiously in patients with bipolar disorder because of the risk of inducing mania. When possible, patients should be receiving mood stabilizers at goal doses before initiating antidepressants and should be cautiously monitored. Bupropion and paroxetine have been associated with less risk of inducing mania than other antidepressants and may be preferable.

2. Treatment duration/phases. The treatment of bipolar disorder is structured similarly to that of depression with acute, continuation, and maintenance phases. Maintenance treatment is strongly recommended for all patients with bipolar disorder, especially those with a family history.

3. **Treatment augmentation**
   a. Patients with no or partial response to monotherapy may receive combination therapy with two agents. Agents that can be combined include lithium; VPA; and the atypical antipsychotics olanzapine, quetiapine, risperidone, and ziprasidone. Atypical antipsychotics, if used, should be combined with either VPA or lithium and not combined with another atypical antipsychotic.
   b. For depressive episodes, lamotrigine may be combined with another mood stabilizer as first-line therapy and the olanzapine-fluoxetine combination product is a second-line option.

4. **Treatment options in pregnancy**
   a. Multiple agents used in the treatment of bipolar disorder have been associated with birth defects.
      (1) Lithium, VPA, and CBZ are pregnancy category D medications.
      (2) Lithium has been associated with birth defects, primarily in the first trimester.
      (3) VPA and CBZ should be used during pregnancy only if the benefits outweigh the risks. If the decision is made to use these medications during pregnancy, folic acid should be given to minimize the risk of defects.
      (4) Lamotrigine and oxcarbazepine are pregnancy category C medications.

STUDY QUESTIONS

Directions: Each of the questions, statements, or incomplete statements in this section can be correctly answered or completed by **one** of the suggested answers or phrases. Choose the **best** answer.

1. Which of the following statements about depression is true?

(A) The incidence of depression is greater in men than in women.
(B) Depression occurs most frequently in adults between the ages of 60 and 85 years.
(C) Depression has no genetic link.
(D) Depression is diagnosed using the DSM-IV-TR criteria.

2. A patient with major depression should receive antidepressant therapy for at least

(A) 2 weeks.
(B) 6 weeks.
(C) 2 months.
(D) 6 months.

For questions 3–4: A 36-year-old woman presents with a 2-month history of depressed mood, anhedonia, increased appetite, weight gain, hypersomnolence, and suicidal ideation. This is the patient's first episode of major depression.

3. Which of the following antidepressants would be most appropriate in the treatment of this patient?

(A) amitriptyline
(B) sertraline
(C) phenelzine
(D) mirtazapine

4. Which of the following is *not* a potential adverse effect of the medication selected for the patient in question 3?

(A) sexual dysfunction
(B) nausea
(C) urinary retention
(D) insomnia

5. Which of the following medications would most likely exacerbate a preexisting seizure disorder?

(A) venlafaxine
(B) trazodone
(C) bupropion
(D) paroxetine

6. A patient who has received citalopram 40 mg/day for 2 weeks for the treatment of major depression complains that the medication is not working and would like to be switched to another agent. What is the appropriate recommendation?

(A) Provide the patient with some information on monoamine oxidase inhibitors (MAOIs) and call the physician to recommend switching the patient to phenelzine.
(B) Encourage the patient to continue with the current regimen, and inform him or her that it may take 4–6 weeks before the full response is evident.
(C) Recommend adding lithium to augment the current regimen.
(D) Recommend switching to mirtazapine because of therapeutic failure with citalopram.

7. A patient diagnosed with depression was unsuccessfully treated with fluoxetine. Fluoxetine was discontinued, and 14 days later, the patient started therapy with phenelzine. Then, 3 days after phenelzine was started, the patient presented with hyperreflexia, fever, elevated blood pressure, confusion, and diarrhea. What is the most likely cause of this clinical presentation?

(A) serotonin syndrome
(B) serotonin withdrawal syndrome
(C) hypertensive crisis
(D) neuroleptic malignant syndrome

8. A patient presents with pressured speech, inability to sleep for 72 hr, bizarre dress, inappropriate makeup, and grandiose delusions that interfere with social functioning. Which of the following is the most likely diagnosis?

(A) depression
(B) euthymia
(C) hypomania
(D) mania

9. Which of the following medications would be considered first-line monotherapy for an acute episode of mania?

(A) gabapentin
(B) lithium
(C) lamotrigine
(D) haloperidol

10. Which of the following is the appropriate therapeutic range for lithium in the treatment of mania?

(A) 0.4–0.6 mEq/L
(B) 0.6–1.5 mEq/L
(C) 1.0–2.0 mEq/L
(D) 0.5–1.2 mEq/L

11. Which of the following mood stabilizers would be most appropriate in a patient with liver disease?

(A) lithium
(B) valproic acid
(C) carbamazepine
(D) none of the above

12. A 32-year-old, 70-kg man diagnosed with bipolar I disorder is being treated with valproic acid (VPA). Which of the following is a reasonable loading dose for VPA in this patient?

(A) 250 mg twice a day
(B) 500 mg twice a day
(C) 250 mg three times a day
(D) 500 mg three times a day

13. Which of the following factors may increase lithium concentration?

(A) caffeine
(B) osmotic diuretics
(C) increased fluid intake
(D) nonsteroidal anti-inflammatory drugs

ANSWERS AND EXPLANATIONS

1. The answer is D   *[see II.B–D].*
The DSM-IV-TR criteria provide the diagnostic guidelines for psychiatric disorders. Depression occurs more often in women than in men and in adults between the ages of 25 and 44. A higher incidence of depression occurs among patients with a positive family history, supporting a genetic link.

2. The answer is D   *[see II.E.2].*
Patients should receive antidepressant therapy through the continuation phase, which is generally 6–9 months.

3. The answer is B   *[see II.E.1.a–c; II.E.1.f; Table 48-1; Table 48-3].*
Sertraline, an SSRI, is a good first-line agent, particularly in patients who would benefit from the stimulatory side effects. Amitriptyline and mirtazapine would not be good alternatives because of this patient's hypersomnolence and weight gain. In addition, a TCA (amitriptyline) is not recommended in patients at risk for suicide. Although some aspects of this patient's depression may be considered atypical, an MAOI would not be selected as first-line therapy, given that it is the patient's first episode of depression.

4. The answer is C   *[see II.E.1.c.(2)].*
Sertraline has been associated with nausea, sexual dysfunction, and insomnia. Sertraline does not express anticholinergic activity and would, therefore, not cause urinary retention. Of the SSRIs, only paroxetine has been associated with causing anticholinergic adverse effects.

5. The answer is C   *[see II.E.1.e.(3)(b)].*
Although all antidepressants can lower the seizure threshold, bupropion is contraindicated in patients with seizure disorder. Bupropion is specifically contraindicated in patients with a seizure disorder. Paroxetine was associated with a 0.1% incidence of seizures during clinical trials. Seizure associated with venlafaxine occurs infrequently (1/100 to 1/1000 patients). The overdosage of trazodone may be associated with seizures; but at normal doses, trazodone is not thought to alter the seizure threshold.

6. The answer is B   *[see II.E.3.a–b].*
An antidepressant must be given at the maximum tolerated dose for 4–6 weeks before it is considered a therapeutic failure; therefore, the best recommendation is to continue with the current regimen for at least 2 more weeks. MAOIs are reserved for refractory depressed patients and are not indicated in this patient scenario. Lithium is an appropriate augmentative agent but is not indicated until the patient has failed two or three different antidepressant trials.

7. The answer is A   *[see II.E.3.b; Table 48-2].*
Serotonin syndrome may result when starting an MAOI immediately after another agent that increases serotonin levels. Generally, a 2-week washout period is recommended; however, fluoxetine requires a 5-week washout period because of norfluoxetine (active metabolite).

8. The answer is D   *[see III.D.1].*
The clinical presentation described is consistent with mania. Hypomania generally does not impair functioning. Euthymia implies normal mood, whereas depression typically involves more neurovegetative symptoms.

9. The answer is B   *[see Table 48-6].*
Lithium is considered to be first-line monotherapy for euphoric mania. Gabapentin has demonstrated utility as a mood stabilizer but is considered only an adjunctive therapy. Lamotrigine is an anticonvulsant that currently has data supporting its use in depressive episodes of bipolar disorder, but not as first-line monotherapy for mania. Haloperidol is a traditional antipsychotic that may be used parenterally to manage acute agitation but is not appropriate as first-line monotherapy.

10. The answer is D   *[see III.F.1.a.(4)].*
The therapeutic range of lithium is 0.5–1.2 mEq/L. When using lithium in the treatment of acute mania, the upper end of the therapeutic range is typically used.

11. The answer is A   *[see III.F.1.a.(6)–(7); III.F.1.b.(4); III.F.1.c.(3).(b); Table 48-7].*
Lithium is not known to cause hepatic dysfunction, nor is it metabolized via the liver. However, both valproic acid and carbamazepine can impair liver function.

12. The answer is D   *[see III.F.1.b.(3)].*
The appropriate loading dose for VPA in acute mania is 20 mg/kg/day; therefore, in this patient, the appropriate loading dose is 1400 mg/day. This equation approximates the need for the patient, and it is appropriate to round up to available dosage forms.

13. The answer is D   *[see Table 48-8].*
Caffeine, osmotic diuretics, and increased fluid intake all decrease lithium concentrations. Nonsteroidal anti-inflammatory drugs decrease renal blood flow and decrease lithium clearance, resulting in increased lithium concentrations.

49

Asthma and Chronic Obstructive Pulmonary Disease

Roy A. Pleasants[1]

I. ASTHMA

A. **Definition.** Asthma is a chronic inflammatory disorder of the airways. It involves complex interactions between many cells (e.g. eosinophils, mast cells) and inflammatory mediators (e.g. interleukins, leukotrienes) that result in inflammation, obstruction (partially or completely reversible after treatment or resolves spontaneously), increased airway responsiveness (i.e., hyperresponsiveness), and episodic asthma symptoms (see I.G.1).

B. **Classification.** Asthma severity classifications were revised by the National Institutes of Health (NIH) in the second expert panel report of the Heart, Lung, and Blood Institute to include **mild intermittent asthma** in addition to **mild, moderate,** and **severe persistent asthma** (Table 49-1). A patient's severity classification plays an important role in determining the most appropriate pharmacotherapeutic approach and is determined by:

1. Symptoms (daytime and nocturnal)

2. Treatment requirements

3. Objective measurements of lung function, including diurnal variations

C. **Incidence.** In 1999, approximately 16.9 million American adults reported having been told by a healthcare professional that they had asthma.

1. It has been estimated that 7.8 million children age 18 years and younger have asthma.

2. Asthma improves in many children as they age; 50% appear to have "outgrown" asthma by their mid-teens. However, it is incorrect to consider that these individuals no longer have asthma, because many eventually have a return of symptoms.

3. In 1999, there were 10.8 million office and outpatient visits for asthma, and 2.0 million asthma-related visits to emergency departments.

4. Although death from asthma remains uncommon, death rates had been increasing in recent years but appear to have reached a plateau. In 1999, there were 4657 deaths attributed to asthma. The most common cause of death is believed to be inadequate assessment of the severity of airway obstruction by either practitioner or patient, leading to suboptimal therapy.

5. The cost to society of asthma is substantial. In 2000 alone, it is estimated that direct costs related to asthma exceeded $8.1 billion. These costs include $2.4 billion for medications and $3.5 billion for hospitalizations. Indirect costs of asthma are estimated at $4.6 billion. Acute care visits (e.g., hospitalizations) account for the majority of healthcare costs for asthma.

D. **Cause.** Precipitating factors of an acute asthma exacerbation may include the following:

1. Allergens (e.g., pollen, house dust mite, animal dander, mold, cockroaches, food)
   a. Concurrent predisposition to allergy is highly prevalent in patients with asthma, especially children.
   b. For example, allergic rhinitis is reported in 45% of patients with asthma compared to 20% of the general population.

---

[1]The author acknowledges the work of Mona G. Tsourkleris and Brian G. Katona, the authors of this chapter in the 5th ed. of this text. The current chapter has been updated but is largely based on their work.

Table 49-1. Classification of Asthma Severity[a]

Classification	Characteristics[b]	Nighttime of Occurrence Symptoms	Lung Function
Severe persistent (step 4)	Continual symptoms; limited physical activity; frequent exacerbations	Frequent	FEV$_1$/PEF ($\leq$ 60%) predicted; PEF variability > 30%
Moderate persistent (step 3)	Daily symptoms; daily use of inhaled short-acting β-agonist; exacerbations affect activity; exacerbations $\geq$ 2 times a week and may last days	> 1 night a week	FEV$_1$/PEF (> 60%–80%) predicted; PEF variability > 30%
Mild persistent (step 2)	Symptoms > 2 times a week but not every day; exacerbations may affect activity	> 2 nights a month	FEV$_1$/PEF ($\geq$ 80%) predicted; PEF variability 20%–30%
Mild intermittent (step 1)	Symptoms $\leq$ 2 times a week; asymptomatic between exacerbations; Exacerbations brief (from a few hours to a few days); intensity of exacerbations may vary	$\leq$ 2 times a month	FEV$_1$/PEF $\geq$ 80% predicted; PEF variability < 20%; PEF normal between exacerbations

[a]The characteristics listed in this table are general and may overlap because asthma is highly variable. The presence of any one of the features of severity is sufficient to place a patient in that category. An individual should be assigned to the most severe grade in which any feature occurs.
[b]Patients at any level of severity can have mild, moderate, or severe exacerbations. For example, some patients with intermittent asthma experience severe, life-threatening exacerbations separated by long periods of normal lung function and no symptoms.
FEV$_1$, forced expiratory volume in 1 sec; *PEF*, peak expiratory flow.
Adapted from National Institutes of Health, National Heart, Lung, and Blood Institute. National Asthma Education and Prevention Program expert panel report 2: Guidelines for the diagnosis and management of asthma [NIH Publication 97-4051]. July 1997.

2. Occupational exposures (e.g., chemical irritants, flour, wood, textile dusts)

3. Viral respiratory tract infections

4. Exercise

5. Emotions (e.g., anxiety, stress, hard laughter or crying)

6. Exposure to irritants (e.g., strong odors, chemicals, fumes)

7. Environmental exposures (e.g., weather changes, cold air, sulfur dioxide, cigarette smoke)

8. Drugs
   a. Reactions to drugs may occur as a result of hypersensitivity or as an extension of the pharmacological effect.
   b. Problematic drugs include
      (1) Aspirin and other nonsteroidal anti-inflammatory drugs such as ibuprofen (note: cyclooxygenase 2 inhibitors are not recommended for use in aspirin-sensitive asthma patients)
      (2) Antiadrenergic and cholinergic drugs (e.g., β-adrenergic blockers, bethanechol)
      (3) Medications (or foods) that contain tartrazine, sulfites, benzalkonium chloride, and other preservatives

E. Pathology. On postmortem examination of patients with asthma, the following characteristics have been identified:

1. Hypertrophy of smooth muscle

2. Airways containing plugs consisting of inflammatory cells and their debris, proteins, and mucus

3. Inflammatory cellular infiltrate with vasodilation, denuded airway epithelium, and microvascular leakage

4. Vasodilation of the vasculature

5. Denuded airway epithelium

6. Microvascular leakage

7. Collagen deposition in basement membranes

F. Pathophysiology (Figure 49-1)

1. **Major contributing processes**
   a. **Inflammatory cells** (i.e., mast cells, eosinophils, activated T cells, macrophages, and epithelial cells) secrete mediators and influence the airways directly or via neural mechanisms.
   b. **Airway obstruction** is responsible for many of the clinical manifestations of asthma.
      (1) Severity of obstruction is variable and believed to be a result of bronchoconstriction, airway wall edema, mucus plug formation, airway remodeling, smooth muscle hypertrophy, and hyperplasia.
      (2) Airway obstruction reduces ventilation to some lung regions, which causes a ventilation/perfusion (V/Q) imbalance that leads to hypoxemia. This is reflected by a reduc-

Figure 49-1. The pathophysiology of asthma.

tion in the partial pressure of arterial oxygen (Pa_{O_2}) observed in moderate to severe exacerbations.

c. **Hyperresponsiveness,** an exaggerated response to certain stimuli, is an important feature of asthma and appears to correlate with clinical severity and medication requirements. Increased levels of inflammatory mediators and infiltration by inflammatory cells are thought to be the primary mechanisms responsible for airway hyperresponsiveness.

d. **Airway inflammation** is crucial to development of asthma and contributes to airway hyperresponsiveness, airflow obstruction, respiratory symptoms, and disease chronicity. Inflammatory cells and their mediators are responsible for altered mucociliary function, epithelial disruption ranging from minor ciliary loss to severely denuded epithelium, increased airway permeability (to inhaled allergens, irritants, and inflammatory mediators), and reduced clearance of inflammatory mediators.

(1) Acute inflammation is associated with early recruitment of cells to the airway.

(2) Subacute inflammation is associated with recruited and resident cell activation, resulting in more persistent inflammation.

(3) Chronic inflammation is associated with persistent cell damage and ongoing repair, resulting in airway abnormalities that may become permanent.

e. Alteration in **autonomic neural control** also contributes to obstruction.

(1) Elevated parasympathetic tone and reflex bronchoconstriction may occur as a result of increased cholinergic sensitivity or a change in muscarinic receptor function.

(2) Increased smooth muscle responsiveness may be the result of smooth muscle hypertrophy. Exposure of the nerve endings, caused by inflammation, may also contribute.

f. **Airway remodeling** can result from persistent inflammation when asthma is poorly controlled. The resulting damage can yield permanent airway abnormalities because of sub-basement membrane collagen deposition and fibrosis. Hypertrophy of the airway smooth muscle is another form of tissue remodeling in asthma. These events may occur even in the face of mild disease but does not necessarily occur in all asthma patients.

2. **Sequencing of events in asthma.** There are five main events that occur in asthma.

a. **Triggering. In an allergic asthma patient,** after exposure to an allergic trigger, the antigen binds to immunoglobulin E (IgE), which is attached to activated mast cells. Nonallergic factors (e.g., aspirin, viral infections) may also function as triggers.

b. Early and late responses

(1) The **early asthmatic response** begins within 30 min of trigger exposure (usually only several minutes after exposure) and resolves within 2 hr. This results in constriction of the airway smooth muscles, bronchospasm, and subsequently asthma symptoms. This response can be blocked by the administration of short-acting β-agonists (albuterol [Ventolin, Proventil], bitolterol [Maxair] or levalbuterol [Xopenex]) .

(2) The **late asthmatic response** involves a second decline in lung function typically 4–8 hr after the initial trigger exposure. The early asthma response does not necessarily progress into the late asthmatic response. The late asthmatic response, principally an inflammatory response, is characterized by persistent airflow obstruction, airway inflammation, and bronchial hyperresponsiveness. The response may last several days, and bronchial hyperreactivity may persist for several weeks. This response can be blocked by the administration of corticosteroids—inhaled steroids such as budesonide (Pulmicort) and leukotriene modifiers such as montelukast (Singulair) or cromones (i.e., cromolyn sodium (Intal) or nedocromil (Tilade).

G. **Clinical evaluation**

1. **Physical findings**

a. **Acute exacerbations** may have a sudden or gradual onset. Symptoms are frequently nocturnal or occur in the early morning hours.

(1) Common findings in an acute exacerbation include

(a) Shortness of breath

(b) Wheezing (usually occurs at the end of exhalation but may be heard throughout inspiration and exhalation in more severe asthma)

(c) Chest tightness

(d) Cough

(e) Tachypnea and tachycardia (moderate to severe exacerbations)

(f) Pulsus paradoxus (severe exacerbations)

(2) Between acute asthma exacerbations, the patient may be asymptomatic.

Table 49-2. Stages of Severity of an Acute Asthmatic Attack

Stage	Symptoms	FEV₁ or FVC	Arterial pH	Pao₂	Paco₂
I Mild	Mild dyspnea and wheezing	50%– 80% of normal	Normal or ↑	Normal or ↓	Normal or ↓
II Moderate	Respiratory distress at rest and marked wheezing	50% of normal	↑	↓	↓
III Severe	Marked respiratory distress, loud wheezing, coughing difficulty speaking, accessory chest muscle use, and chest hyperinflation	< 50% of normal	Normal or ↓	↓	Normal or ↑
IV Respiratory failure	Severe respiratory distress, confusion, lethargy, cyanosis, disappearance of breath sounds, and pulsus paradoxus >12 mm Hg	< 25% of normal	↓↓	↓	↑↑

FEV₁, forced expiratory volume in 1 sec; *FVC,* forced vital capacity; *Pao₂*; partial pressure of arterial oxygen; *Paco₂*; partial pressure of arterial carbon dioxide; ↑, increased; ↓, decreased; ↑↑, markedly increased; ↓↓, markedly decreased.

    b. Patients with **chronic, poorly controlled, severe asthma** may have evidence of chronic hyperinflation, including barrel chest and decreased diaphragmatic excursion, similar to chronic obstructive pulmonary disease

    c. Physical findings depend on the severity of the underlying disease and the severity of the exacerbation. Regardless of the underlying disease severity, patients can have mild, moderate, or severe exacerbations (Table 49-2).

  2. Diagnostic test results

    a. Pulmonary function tests determine the degree of airway obstruction and may be normal between exacerbations. These include spirometry and peak flow meter testing.

      (1) Forced expiratory volume in 1 second (FEV₁) and forced vital capacity (FVC) both decrease during an acute exacerbation. The spirometer is used to generate the FEV₁ and FVC.

      (2) Residual volume (RV) and total lung capacity (TLC) may increase in asthma because of **air trapping** and subsequent **lung hyperinflation.**

      (3) Peak expiratory flow rate (PEFR), obtained through the patient forcefully breathing out into a **peak flow meter,** correlates well with FEV₁. However, PEFR measurement is not used in making the diagnosis of asthma.

        (a) Uses of PEFR monitoring at home include assessment of therapy, trigger identification, and assessment of the need for referral to emergency care.

        (b) PEFR monitoring at home is recommended for patients who have had severe exacerbations, who are poor perceivers of asthma symptoms, and who have moderate to severe disease.

        (c) PEFR is best measured in early morning, before medication administration. More frequent monitoring over a few weeks may also be indicated to identify specific patterns and to identify a patient's personal best PEFR measurement. In this case, measurements are taken before medications are taken in the morning (i.e., on awakening) and again at midday (i.e., after taking a short-acting β-agonist). **Diurnal variation** of > 20% in PEFR measured during the day suggests airway hyperresponsiveness and less-than-adequate asthma control.

      (4) Provocation testing with **histamine or methacholine challenge** may be performed to assess hyperresponsiveness and to rule out asthma in a patient who has had normal pulmonary function test results but in whom asthma is still suspected.

b. **Blood analysis, although not typically undertaken in asthma,** typically shows a slightly increased white blood cell (WBC) count during an acute exacerbation; eosinophilia also may be present. Leukocytosis may be present because of WBC demargination that occurs when patients receive systemic corticosteroids.

c. **Pulse oximetry** is a noninvasive means of assessing the degree of hypoxemia during an acute exacerbation. The oximeter measures oxygen saturation in arterial blood (SaO_2) and pulse.

d. **Arterial blood gas measurements** may be required to help gauge the severity of the asthma exacerbation (Table 49-2).

(1) In the early stages of an asthma exacerbation, **hyperventilation** results in a decrease in the partial pressure of arterial carbon dioxide ($PaCO_2$). If the exacerbation progresses and the airways remain narrowed, respiratory muscles may fatigue and the $PaCO_2$ level increases.

(2) **Respiratory acidosis** is a poor prognostic sign. It develops if hypoxemia worsens and the patient's respiratory rate is not maintained owing to respiratory fatigue. This results in a rising $PaCO_2$ level.

e. An **electrocardiogram (ECG)** may show sinus tachycardia. An ECG may be particularly useful in an older patient.

f. A **chest radiograph** may be normal or could detect accompanying pneumothorax, atelectasis, or pneumonia. Evidence of hyperinflation may be present in acute asthma and in chronic, poorly controlled asthma. A chest radiograph may also be needed to exclude other causes of the patient's symptoms.

3. **Signs of respiratory distress** include
   a. Use of accessory muscles
   b. Inability to speak in sentences or ambulate owing to dyspnea
   c. Declining mental status
   d. PEFR > 50% of predicted (or personal best)
   e. Cyanosis
   f. Suprasternal retractions
   g. Absence of respiratory sounds
   h. Increasing $PaCO_2$
   i. Unable to sleep for extended time because of shortness of breath

4. Patients with **potentially fatal asthma** should be quickly identified and aggressively managed. These patients have the following characteristics:
   a. History of severe exacerbations, particularly exacerbations that develop suddenly
   b. Poor self-perception of asthma symptoms and severity
   c. History of intubation or intensive care unit (ICU) admission for asthma
   d. Two or more hospitalizations or three or more visits to the emergency department for asthma within 1 year
   e. Hospitalization or treatment in the emergency department for asthma within the last month
   f. Frequent β-agonist use (i.e., more than two canisters per month), current systemic steroid treatment, or recent systemic steroid withdrawal
   g. Concurrent conditions (e.g., cardiovascular or psychiatric disease, substance abuse, low socioeconomic status [particularly in urban areas])

H. Therapy

1. **Treatment objectives**
   a. The goal of therapy is to provide symptomatic control with normalization of lifestyle and to return pulmonary function as close to normal as possible.
   b. The treatment goals listed in the 2002 NIH's expert panel update report include the following:
      (1) Minimal or no chronic symptoms day or night
      (2) Peak expiratory flow rate > 80% of personal best
      (3) No limitations of activities, no work/school missed
      (4) Minimal or no exacerbations
      (5) Minimal use of short-acting inhaled β_2-agonist (< 1 time daily; < 1 canister/ month)
      (6) Minimal or no adverse effects from medications

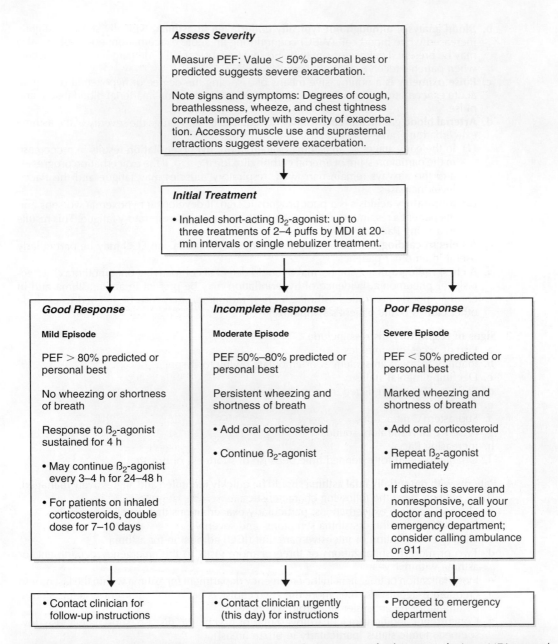

Figure 49-2. The NIH treatment algorithm for the home-based management of asthma exacerbations. *MDI*, metered dose inhaler; *PEF*, peak expiratory flow. From NIH highlights of the expert panel report 2: Guidelines for the diagnosis and management of asthma [NIH Publication No. 97-4051A]. May 1997:41, Fig. 3-8.]

2. **Management of acute asthma exacerbations**
   a. **Home-based** treatment of an acute asthma exacerbation (Figure 49-2)
   b. Treatment of an acute asthma exacerbation in the **hospital or emergency department** (Figure 49-3)

3. **Management of persistent asthma**
   a. A stepped approach based on severity of disease is used to manage persistent asthma (Table 49-3). Gaining control of asthma may be achieved with either a step-up or step-

Figure 49-3. NIH treatment algorithm for management of asthma exacerbations in the emergency department and hospital. *FEV$_1$*, forced expiratory volume in 1 sec; *PEF*, peak expiratory flow; *PCO_2*, partial pressure of carbon dioxide. [From NIH highlights of the expert panel report 2: Guidelines for the diagnosis and management of asthma [NIH Publication No. 97-4051A]. May 1997:46, Fig. 3-11.]

down approach (determined by severity of disease); however, the more aggressive step-down approach is advocated by the NIH expert panel.

   (1) **The step-down approach** starts with treatment one step above the patient's assessed asthma severity to give rapid disease control. For example, for step 2 asthma, start with the step 3 drug regimen, then review treatment every 1–6 months. Gradual stepwise reduction in treatment may be possible based on the patient's response to therapy.

   (2) **The step-up approach** begins with a treatment regimen at the same step as the patient's severity. The regimen is adjusted upward if the patient fails to respond to treatment.

Table 49-3. Stepwise Approach for Managing Asthma in Adults and Children > 5 Years of Age

Classify Severity: Clinical Features

Step	Symptoms $\frac{\text{Day}}{\text{Night}}$	$\frac{\text{PEF or FEV}_1}{\text{PEF Variability}}$	Daily Medications Required to Maintain Long-Term Control

4 Severe persistent	$\frac{\text{Continual}}{\text{Frequent}}$	$\frac{\leq 60\%}{>30\%}$	Preferred treatment
			  High-dose inhaled corticosteroids AND
			  Long-acting inhaled β_2-agonists AND (if needed)
			  Corticosteroid tablets or syrup long term (2 mg/kg/day; generally not to exceed 60 mg/day). Make repeated attempts to reduce systemic corticosteroids and maintain control with high-dose inhaled corticosteroids

3 Moderate persistent	$\frac{\text{Daily}}{>1 \text{ night/week}}$	$\frac{>60\%-<80\%}{>30\%}$	Preferred treatment
			  Low- to medium-dose inhaled corticosteroids AND
			  Long-acting inhaled β_2-agonists
			Alternative treatment
			  Increase inhaled corticosteroids in medium-dose range AND
			  Add either leukotriene modifier or theophylline (here listed alphabetically)

2 Mild persistent	$\frac{>2\text{/week but 1} \times\text{/day}}{>2 \text{ nights/month}}$	$\frac{\geq 80\%}{20\%-30\%}$	Preferred treatment Low-dose inhaled corticosteroids Alternative treatment (here listed alphabetically). Cromolyn, leukotriene modifier, nedocromil, or sustained-release theophylline to serum concentration of 5–15 µg/mL
1 Mild intermittent	$\frac{\leq 2 \text{ days/week}}{\leq 2 \text{ nights/week}}$	$\frac{\geq 80\%}{<20\%}$	No daily medication needed Severe exacerbations may occur, separated by long periods of normal lung function and no symptoms; a course of systemic corticosteroids is recommended
All patients			Short-acting bronchodilator: 2–4 puffs of a short-acting inhaled β_2-agonist as needed for symptoms Intensity of treatment depends on severity of exacerbation; up to 3 treatments at 20-min intervals or a single nebulizer treatment as needed; course of systemic corticosteroids may be needed Use of a short-acting inhaled β_2-agonist on a daily basis, or increasing use, indicates the need to initiate or increase long-term control therapy

(Continued on next page)

Table 49-3. Continued

		Notes
➤ **Step down**		The stepwise approach is meant to assist, not replace, the clinical decision making required to meet individual patient needs
Review treatment every 1–6 months; a gradual stepwise reduction in treatment may be possible		
➤ **Step up**		Classify severity; assign patient to most severe step in which any feature occurs (PEF is percent of personal best; FEV_1 is percent predicted)
If control is not maintained, consider step up; first review patient medication technique, adherence, and environmental control		
Minimal or no chronic symptoms day or night	PEF > 80% of personal best	Gain control as quickly as possible (consider a short course of systemic corticosteroids); then step down to the lest medication necessary to maintain control
Minimal or no exacerbations	Minimal use of short-acting inhaled β_2-agonist (< 1 × per day; < 1 canister per month)	Provide education on self-management and controlling environmental factors that make asthma worse (e.g., allergens and irritants)
No limitations on activities; no school/work missed	Minimal or no adverse effects from medications	Refer to an asthma specialist if there are difficulties controlling asthma or if step 4 care is required; referral may be considered if step 3 care is required

FEV_1, forced expiratory volume in 1 sec; *PEF,* peak expiratory flow.
Modified from National Asthma Education and Prevention Program expert panel report guidelines for the diagnosis and management of asthma—Update on selected topics 2002 [NIH Publication No. 02-5075]. June 2002.

Consider the step-up approach if control is not maintained and after reviewing adherence to therapy, medication administration technique, and environmental control actions.

b. At each step, patients should control their environment to avoid or control factors, when possible, that make their asthma worse (e.g., allergens, irritants). This requires specific diagnosis and education.

c. Inhaled β-agonists such as albuterol and levalbuterol are used as needed for acute symptoms for all levels of severity.

   (1) Daily or increasing use of a short-acting inhaled β_2-agonist suggests the need for additional long-term controller (i.e., anti-inflammatory) therapy.

   (2) Pretreatment with either an inhaled β-agonist, cromolyn sodium, or nedocromil may be used before exercise or allergen exposure.

d. A rescue course of systemic corticosteroid (e.g., prednisone) may be needed at any time and at any step.

4. Prevention and treatment of exercise-induced bronchospasm (EIB)

  a. Steps to prevent EIB should be implemented in all patients with asthma.

  b. Patients should be advised that a warmup period might be helpful in preventing EIB.

  c. EIB can usually be prevented with one of the following options.

    (1) Short-acting β-agonists (e.g., albuterol) should be administered 15 min before exercise. These are considered the drug of choice for EIB.

    (2) Long-acting β-agonists—salmeterol (Serevent) and formoterol (Foradil)—should be administered 30–60 min before exercise. When salmeterol is used chronically for EIB, some patients may lose protection toward the end of the 12-hr dosing interval. Because of its rapid onset, formoterol may be dosed 15 min before exercise. Generally, short-acting agents are preferred over long-acting β-agonists.

    (3) Cromolyn sodium and nedocromil may be used to prevent EIB and exacerbations related to exposure to other asthma triggers. Cromolyn and nedocromil should be administered no more than 1 hr before exercise or exposure.

    (4) Leukotriene modifiers given daily help with EIB but should not be used on a as-needed bases just before exercise, as done with short-acting β_2-agonists.

d. Regardless of the prophylactic approach, all patients who experience EIB should have a short-acting β-agonist available for treatment of breakthrough symptoms.

5. Concurrent diseases

a. Allergic rhinitis, sinusitis, and **gastroesophageal reflux disease** frequently coexist with asthma.

b. GERD is frequent in persons with obstructive lung disease. Management of GERD with proton pump inhibitors (PPIs), such as pantoprazole (Protonix) can improve asthma symptoms and in some patients breathing tests. H_2-antagonists, such as ranitidine (Zantac) are less effective than PPIs in this situation.

c. Asthma control has been shown to improve if these conditions are adequately controlled.

I. Therapeutic agents

1. **β-Agonists**—albuterol, formoterol, levalbuterol, metaproterenol (Metaprel), pirbuterol, salmeterol

   a. Short-acting β-agonists are best reserved for worsening symptoms, treatment of acute exacerbations, and prophylaxis for EIB. Assessing the frequency of short-acting β-agonist use for rescue therapy can help determine the patient's level of asthma control. Those requiring regular use (e.g., four times a day), of short-acting β-agonists have uncontrolled disease and should receive more aggressive controller therapy.

   b. Indications for long-acting β-agonists

   (1) Maintenance treatment of moderate and severe persistent asthma in combination with inhaled corticosteroids, particularly for patients with frequent nocturnal symptoms.

   (a) Long-acting β_2-agonists should not be used as sole therapy for an acute asthma exacerbation in lieu of short-acting agents.

   (b) Research indicates that rather than increasing the dose of the inhaled corticosteroid in uncontrolled chronic asthma, adding a long-acting β-agonist results in a greater improvement in symptoms and breathing tests.

   (c) Recent warnings have been placed in the package inserts for long-acting β_2-agonists regarding an increased risk of asthma death.

   (2) Prophylaxis of EIB

   (3) Patients with chronic obstructive pulmonary disease (COPD)

   c. Therapeutic effects. These sympathomimetic agents relieve bronchoconstriction during acute asthma exacerbations as well as during chronic therapy and prevent exacerbations from occurring during exercise.

   d. Mechanism of action

   (1) β_2-Agonists stimulate β_2-receptors, activating adenyl cyclase, which increases intracellular production of cyclic adenosine monophosphate (cAMP).

   (a) Increased intracellular cAMP and activation of cAMP result in bronchodilation, improved mucociliary clearance, and reduced inflammatory cell mediator release.

   (b) Stimulation of β_2-receptors in skeletal muscle accounts for tremor.

   (2) β-Agonists differ in their affinity for the β_1- and β_2-receptors. Agents with greater β_1-receptor affinity are more likely to cause cardiac effects.

   e. Administration and dosage

   (1) Whenever possible, agents should be administered via **inhalation** to minimize systemic exposure and adverse reactions. **Systemic** administration should be reserved for patients who cannot use inhalation therapy.

   (2) Regimens with long-acting β_2-agonists should also include a concurrent inhaled corticosteroid, unless it is being used only to prevent EIB. All regimens containing long-acting agents should also include a short-acting agent for treatment of acute symptoms.

   (3) Dosage information is provided in Table 49-4.

   f. Precautions and monitoring effects

   (1) Common adverse effects of β-agonists include tremor, palpitation, tachycardia, nervousness, and headache. Leg cramps may occur with high doses owing to hypokalemia.

Table 49-4. β-Adrenergic Agonists Used in the Treatment of Asthma or COPD

Agent	Severe Acute		Chronic		Site of Action	Duration of Action	Comments
	Pediatric	Adult	Pediatric	Adult			
Albuterol							
NEB: 0.5% (5 mg/mL)	ET: 0.15 mg/kg (minimum 2.5 mg) q 20 min × 3 doses, then 0.15–0.30 mg/kg up to 10 mg q 1–4 hr prn or 0.5 mg/kg/hr continuously QR: 0.05 mg/kg (minimum 1.25 mg; maximum 2.5 mg) in 2–3 mL saline q 4–6 hr	ET: 2.5–5.0 mg q 20 min × 3 doses, then 2.5–10.0 mg q 1–4 hr prn or 10–15 mg/hr continuously QR: 1.25–5.00 mg in 2–3 mL saline q 4–8 hr	Not currently recommended	Not currently recommended	β_1-receptors + β_2-receptors + + + +	3–8 hr inhalation 4–8 hr oral	May mix with cromolyn or ipratropium NEB May double dose for mild exacerbations
MDI: 0.09 mg/puff	ET: 4–8 puffs q 20 min × 3 doses, then q 1–4 hr with spacer QR: 2 puffs t.i.d.–q.i.d. prn PT: 1–2 puffs 5 min before exercise	ET: 4–8 puffs q 20 min up to 4 hr, then q 1–4 hr prn QR: 2 puffs t.i.d.–q.i.d. prn PT: 2 puffs 5 min before exercise	Not currently recommended	Not currently recommended			
Rotahaler: 0.2 mg/capsule	QR: 1 capsule q 4–6 hr prn PT: 1 capsule before exercise	QR: 1–2 capsules q 4–6 hr prn PT: 1–2 capsules before exercise	Not currently recommended	Not currently recommended			
Oral: 4-mg sustained release	Not currently recommended	Not currently recommended	0.3–0.6 mg/kg/day (maximum 8 mg/day)	4 mg q 12 hr			

(Continued on next page)

Table 49-4. Continued

Agent	Severe Acute		Chronic		Site of Action	Duration of Action	Comments
	Pediatric	Adult	Pediatric	Adult			
Bitolterol NEB: 0.2% (2 mg/mL)	ET: 0.15 mg/kg (minimum 2.5 mg) q 20 min × 3 doses, then 0.15–0.30 mg/kg q 1–4 hr prn or 0.5 mg/kg/hr continuously	ET: 2.5–5.0 mg q 20 min × 3 doses, then 2.5–10.0 mg q 1–4 hr prn or 10–15 mg/hr continuously QR: 0.5–3.5 mg in 2–3 mL saline q 4–8 hr	Not currently recommended	Not currently recommended	β_1-receptors + β_2-receptors + + + +	6–8 hr	Dilute NEB with 2–3 ML normal saline Do not mix NEB with other NEB solutions Thought to be about half as potent as albuterol on a milligram basis
MDI: 0.37 mg/puff	ET: 4–8 puffs q 20 min × 3 doses, then q 1–4 hr with spacer QR: 2 puffs t.i.d.–q.i.d. prn PT: 1–2 puffs 5 min before exercise	ET: 4–8 puffs q 20 min up to 4 hr, then q 1–4 hr prn QR: 2 puffs t.i.d.–q.i.d. prn PT: 2 puffs 5 min before exercise	Not currently recommended	Not currently recommended			
Epinephrine SC: 1:1000 (1 mg/mL)	ET: 0.01 mg/kg/dose up to 0.3–0.5 mg q 20 min × 3 doses	ET: 0.3–0.5 mg/dose q 20 min × 3 doses	Not currently recommended	Not currently recommended	α-receptors + + + β_1-receptors + + + β_2-receptors + + +	1–4 hr SC; 1–3 hr inhalation	
Formoterol DPI: 12 μg/ caps for inhalation	Not currently recommended	Not currently recommended	≥ 5 years: 1 capsule q 12 h	1 capsule q 12 h	β_1-receptors + β_2-receptors + + + +	10–12 hr	Approved for chronic treatment in children > 5 years old and for prevention of EIB in children > 12 years old Use at least 15 min before exercise for EIB prophylaxis

Medication					Selectivity	Duration	Comments
Levalbuterol NEB: 0.63 mg, 1.25 mg	6–11 years: QR: 0.31 mg t.i.d. prn; >11 years: 0.63–1.25 mg t.i.d. prn	QR: 0.63 mg t.i.d. (q 6–8 hr) up to 1.25 mg t.i.d. (q 6–8 hr)	Not currently recommended	Not currently recommended	β_1-receptors +; β_2-receptors ++++	6–8 hr	Thought to be about half as potent as albuterol on a milligram basis
Pirbuterol MDI: 0.2 mg/puff	ET: 4–8 puffs q 20 min × 3 doses, then q 1–4 hr with spacer; QR: 2 puffs t.i.d.–q.i.d. prn; PT: 1–2 puffs 5 min before exercise	ET: 4–8 puffs q 20 min up to 4 hr, then q 1–4 hr prn; QR: 2 puffs t.i.d.–q.i.d. prn; PT: 2 puffs 5 min before exercise	Not currently recommended	Not currently recommended	β_1-receptors +; β_2-receptors ++++	5 hr	
Salmeterol MDI: 0.025 mg/puff	Not currently recommended	Not currently recommended	>4 years: 1–2 puffs q 12 hr	2 puffs q 12 hr	β_1-receptors +	10–12 hr	Not indicated for acute exacerbations; Take 30–60 min before exercise for EIB prophylaxis
DPI: 0.05 mg/inhalation	Not currently recommended	Not currently recommended	>4 years:1 inhalation q 12 hr	1 inhalation q12 hr	β_2-receptors ++++		
Terbutaline MDI: 0.2 mg/puff	QR: 2 puffs t.i.d.–q.i.d. prn; PT: 1–2 puffs 5 min before exercise	QR: 2 puffs t.i.d.–q.i.d. prn; PT: 2 puffs 5 min before exercise; ET: 0.25 mg q 20 min × 3 doses	Not currently recommended	Not currently recommended	β_1-receptors +; β_2-receptors ++++	3–6 hr inhalation; 1.5–4 hr parenteral; 4–8 hr oral	Parenteral solution not FDA-approved for nebulization
SC: 0.1% (1 mg/mL)	ET: 0.01 mg/kg q 20 min × 3 doses, then q 2–6 hr prn		Not currently recommended	Not currently recommended			

DPI, dry-power inhaler; *ET*, emergency treatment; *FDA*, U.S. Food and Drug Administration; *MDI*, metered dose inhaler; *NEB*, solution for nebulizer; *QR*, quick relief; *PT*, prophylactic treatment; *SC*, subcutaneous.

Adapted from National Institutes of Health, National Heart, Lung, and Blood Institute. National Asthma Education and Prevention Program expert panel report 2: Guidelines for the diagnosis and management of asthma [NIH Publication 97-4051]. July 1997:91, Figure 3-5d (NIH ERR-2, Fig. 3–5d).

(2) Nonselective β-agonists (e.g., isoproterenol (Isuprel) may induce myocardial ischemia, myocardial necrosis, and arrhythmias because of excessive cardiac stimulation. Use of β_2-selective agents (e.g., albuterol, bitolterol) is preferred.

(3) Tachyphylaxis (form of tolerance) can occur with regular use of inhaled or oral β-agonists. Suggested mechanisms include

   (a) A decrease in the number of active β-receptors owing to movement of receptors from the cell surface into the cell (**downregulation**)

   (b) A decreased sensitivity in the β-receptors to stimuli, making them unable to activate adenyl cyclase

   (i) The clinical significance of this effect is unclear with normal doses of β-agonists.

   (ii) This effect may be lessened by adding corticosteroids to the regimen.

(4) Hypokalemia may occur in some patients, particularly those receiving concurrent medications that cause hypokalemia (e.g., diuretics, amphotericin) and high doses, including inhaled agents.

(5) Paradoxical bronchoconstriction found with β-agonists may be the result of a "cold-Freon effect" or the use of additives such as benzalkonium chloride in the formulation.

(6) Unlike albuterol, which is a racemic mixture of albuterol's R- and S-isomers, levalbuterol HCl (Xopenex) is composed of the active R-enantiomer.

(7) Systemic adverse reactions when the recommended starting dose of levalbuterol is used appear to be similar to or *slightly less frequent* than the effects of albuterol. When the dose of levalbuterol is increased to 1.25 mg, however, the incidence of adverse reactions is similar to the corresponding dose of albuterol.

(8) It is important to be aware of **significant drug–drug interactions.**

   (a) Concomitant use of systemic β-agonists with **monoamine oxidase inhibitors, tricyclic antidepressants,** or **methyldopa** may infrequently lead to severe hypertension. The risk with aerosolized agents may be smaller.

   (b) β-Adrenergic blockers (especially nonselective agents as propranolol) precipitate bronchospasm and increase the dose of β-agonist necessary to achieve bronchodilation. The risk of bronchospasm should be weighed against the potential benefits of β-blockers. β_1-Selective agents such as metoprolol (Toprol XL) may be used carefully (e.g., in the hospital), in asthma patients when the risk–benefit ratio indicates such, as in an acute myocardial infarction.

   (c) β-Agonists should not be combined with other sympathomimetic agents because of additive cardiovascular effects. Vasoconstrictor and vasopressor effects of epinephrine are antagonized by **β-adrenergic blocking agents** (e.g., phentolamine).

(9) The effects of β-agonists should be closely monitored in the elderly and in patients with a history of hyperthyroidism, diabetes, seizures, arrhythmias, and coronary artery disease.

2. Corticosteroids

   a. Therapeutic effects. Corticosteroids suppress the inflammatory response and decrease airway hyperresponsiveness.

   b. Mechanism of action. Corticosteroids bind to glucocorticoid receptors on the cytoplasm of cells. The activated receptor **regulates transcription** of target genes.

   (1) Corticosteroids reduce inflammation via:

   (a) Inhibition of transcription and release of inflammatory genes

   (b) Increased transcription of anti-inflammatory genes that produce proteins that participate in or suppress the inflammatory process

   (2) Clinical effects include

   (a) Reduced production of inflammatory mediators

   (b) Enhanced β-adrenergic receptor expression (thus making the β_2-agonist work better)

   (c) Decreased mucus production

   (d) Prevention of endothelial and vascular leakage

   (e) Partial reversal of tissue-remodeling

   c. Administration and dosage

   (1) There is no significant difference in the clinical efficacy of the corticosteroid agents currently available. The **route of administration** is determined by the condition of the patient.

(2) Systemic corticosteroids are used for rapid response during an exacerbation. Improvement in pulmonary function may begin within 1–3 hr; however, the maximum effect is not achieved until 6–9 hr, or longer, after administration. Supplemental doses should be administered to patients who are already taking systemic corticosteroids when they experience an exacerbation, even if the exacerbation is mild.

(3) Intravenous corticosteroids (e.g., methylprednisolone (Solu-Medrol) are administered to patients who are unable to take oral medications in severe exacerbations. Large doses (e.g. methylprednisolone 60 mg or 125 mg intravenously [IV]) can be quickly administered; however, patients can usually be switched to oral therapy as soon as they show clinical improvement and can tolerate oral medication.

(4) Oral corticosteroids are acceptable as emergency treatment if the patient can tolerate the oral route and is not believed to be in imminent danger of respiratory arrest. **Prednisone** and **prednisolone (Prelone)** are the most frequently used oral corticosteroids.

  (a) Prednisone and prednisolone are frequently administered in short "bursts" over 3–10 days [see I.I.2.c.(2).(b)] to treat acute exacerbations in the outpatient setting and in the emergency department. This type of regimen may also be used to rapidly achieve asthma control.

  (b) During burst therapy, these agents may be administered for 3–10 days in one or two daily doses and then discontinued. When used in this fashion, tapering is not usually necessary, but is often done by physicians. However, if a patient's condition appears to worsen after the last dose has been administered, it is reasonable to reinstitute the corticosteroid and then begin a tapering regimen.

(5) Because **inhaled corticosteroids** are least likely to produce adverse reactions, the inhaled route should be used whenever possible for chronic treatment.

  (a) Inhaled corticosteroids should not be used alone to treat serious acute exacerbations.

  (b) In milder outpatient flares, doses of the inhaled steroids may be increased temporarily.

  (c) The number of corticosteroids available for inhalation therapy is increasing. The two most recent additions are budesonide and fluticasone propionate (Flovent).

  (d) Dosages of inhaled corticosteroids are provided in Table 49-5. When asthma control is achieved, attempts should be made to use the lowest effective dose to maintain control (step-down therapy). Side effects of inhaled steroids (and systemic steroids) are dose dependent.

  (e) Inhaled corticosteroids are considered first-line anti-inflammatory therapy for mild to severe persistent asthma in both adults and children.

(2) Treatment of asthma exacerbation in adults

  (a) For treatment of a severe exacerbation, prednisone may be given at a dose of 2 mg/kg (maximum of 60 mg/day). For intravenous treatment, methylprednisolone is given at a dosage of 120–180 mg/day in three or four divided doses for 48 hr or until the patient can tolerate oral medications. The dosage is then reduced to 60–80 mg/day until PEFR reaches 70% predicted (or personal best).

  (b) For outpatient burst therapy, the dosage of prednisone is 1–2 mg/kg/day (maximum of 60 mg/day) in one or two divided doses for 3–10 days.

(3) Treatment of asthma exacerbation in children

  (a) For inpatient treatment of a severe exacerbation, prednisone, methylprednisolone, or prednisolone is given at a dosage of 1 mg/kg every 6 hr for 48 hr. The dosage is then reduced to 1–2 mg/kg/day (maximum of 60 mg/day) in two divided doses until PEFR is 70% predicted (or personal best).

  (b) For outpatient burst therapy, the dosage of prednisone is 1–2 mg/kg/day (maximum of 60 mg/day) in one or two divided doses for 3–10 days.

d. Precautions and monitoring effects

  (1) Systemic corticosteroids

    (a) Careful monitoring is necessary in patients with diabetes (steroids commonly increase blood sugar), hypertension, adrenal suppression, congestive heart failure (fluid retention owing to mineralocorticoid effects), peptic ulcer disease, candidiasis, immunosuppression, osteoporosis, chronic infections, cataracts, glaucoma, myasthenia gravis, and psychiatric diseases (e.g., depression, psychosis). Some of these side-effects begin shortly after beginning systemic steroids (e.g.,

Table 49-5. Estimated Comparative Daily Dosages for Inhaled Corticosteroids[a]

Drug	Low Daily Dose		Medium Daily Dose		High Daily Dose	
	Adult	**Child**	**Adult**	**Child**	**Adult**	**Child**
Beclomethasone						
CFC: 42 or 84 µg/puff	168–504 µg	84–336 µg	504–840 µg	336–672 µg	> 840 µg	>672 µg
HFA: 40 or 80 µg/puff	80–240 µg	80–160 µg	240–480 µg	160–320 µg	>480 µg	>320 µg
Budesonide						
DPI: 200 µg/inhalation	200–600 µg	200–400 µg	600–1200 µg	400–800 µg	>1200 µg	>800 µg
Inhalation suspension for nebulization (child dose)		0.5 mg		1.0 mg		2.0 mg
Flunisolide						
250 µg/puff	500–1000 µg	500–750 µg	1000–2000 µg	1000–1250 µg	>2000 µg	>1250 µg
Fluticasone						
MDI:[b] 44, 110, or 220 µg/puff	88–264 µg	88–176 µg	264–660 µg	176–440 µg	>660 µg	>440 µg
DPI: 50, 100, or 250 µg/inhalation	100–300 µg	100–200 µg	300–600 µg	200–400 µg	>7600 µg	>400 µg
Triamcinolone						
100 µg/puff	400–1000 µg	400–800 µg	1000–2000 µg	800–1200 µg	>2000 µg	>1200 µg

[a]In all cases, the lowest dose to maintain control should be used. Some doses are outside package labeling.
[b]MDI doses are actuator doses (i.e., amount leaving actuator).
CFC, chlorofluorocarbons; *DPI,* dry-powder inhaler; HFA, hydrofluoroalkanes; *MDI,* metered dose inhaler.
Modified from National Asthma Education and Prevention Program expert panel report guidelines for the diagnosis and management of asthma—Update on selected topics 2002 [NIH Publication No. 02-5075]. June 2002.

hyperglycemia), whereas others (e.g., osteoporosis) only occurs with long-term use.

(b) If a prolonged course of systemic therapy is necessary to maintain asthma control, interference with the hypothalamic-pituitary-adrenal axis is lessened by a single morning dose (i.e., 6–8 A.M.) or alternate-day therapy. For alternate-day therapy, the dose is twice that of the single morning dose.

(c) Patients on regular systemic therapy should be closely monitored and should receive regular ophthalmological evaluations and osteoporosis screening, and preventative therapy (e.g., calcium, vitamin D, bisphosphonates) if indicated.

(2) Inhaled corticosteroids

(a) Local effects associated with inhaled corticosteroids include dry mouth, hoarseness (dysphonia), and fungal infection of the mouth and throat. Local side effects can be lessened through mouth rinsing, use of a spacer, and use of certain inhaled steroid products.

(b) The U.S. Food and Drug Administration (FDA) recently revised the warning labels on inhaled corticosteroid products to include dose-related slowing of growth velocity in children (approximately one third in. per year). Shortly after the labeling was revised, two major publications demonstrated short-term growth suppression of approximately 1 cm in the 1st year of budesonide treatment, but without long-term effects on final adult height. However, children should be treated with the lowest effective dose and should be reminded that poorly controlled asthma also slows growth.

(c) Large doses of inhaled corticosteroids may result in systemic effects, such as reduced bone density, changes in adrenal function, skin changes, adrenal suppression, and cataract formation. Further study is needed to fully understand these effects and to determine their clinical significance. However, patients receiving high doses of inhaled corticosteroids should be closely monitored and should receive regular ophthalmological evaluations and osteoporosis screening and treatment (e.g., calcium, vitamin D) if indicated.

(d) Spacers (e.g. AeroChamber) are generally prescribed for patients who receive moderate to high doses of inhaled corticosteroids via metered dose inhalers (MDIs). Patients should also gargle, rinse their mouth and throat, and expectorate after administration. Both of these interventions minimize oropharyngeal drug deposition, local adverse reactions, and gastrointestinal absorption.

  (i) Inhaled steroids in dry-powder inhalers (Pulmicort Turbuhaler) generally have a lower incidence of local side effects.

  (ii) A new form of beclomethasone (Qvar) MDI also has a low incidence of local side effects.

(3) Significant interactions

  (a) Concurrent use of **hepatic microsomal enzyme inducers** (e.g., rifampin, barbiturates, hydantoins) causes enhanced corticosteroid metabolism, reducing therapeutic efficacy.

  (b) Concurrent use of **estrogens, oral contraceptives, itraconazole (Sporanox),** or **macrolide antibiotics** (e.g., erythromycin, clarithromycin [Biaxin]) may decrease corticosteroid clearance.

  (c) **Cyclosporine** may increase the plasma concentration of corticosteroids.

  (d) Administration of **potassium-depleting diuretics** (e.g., thiazides, furosemide) or other potassium-depleting drugs (e.g., amphotericin) with corticosteroids causes enhanced hypokalemia. Serum potassium should be closely monitored, especially in patients on **digitalis glycosides.**

3. Leukotriene modifiers are the newest agents with anti-inflammatory properties to be approved for use in asthma. Leukotrienes are important participants in asthma pathophysiology. Cellular effects of leukotrienes include enhanced migration of eosinophils and neutrophils, increased adhesion of leukocytes, and increased monocyte and neutrophil aggregation. Leukotrienes also increase capillary permeability and cause smooth muscle contraction.

  a. Leukotriene receptor antagonists currently available in the United States include montelukast and zafirlukast (Accolate).

  (1) Therapeutic effects

   (a) Leukotriene receptor antagonists have anti-inflammatory and bronchodilator activity. They may allow reduction in corticosteroid doses in some patients.

   (b) Because they may be less effective anti-inflammatory agents than inhaled corticosteroids, they are considered second-line agents.

   (c) In children, for whom administration of inhaled drugs is challenging, oral leukotriene receptor antagonists may be particularly useful.

   (d) They may be useful in patients with concurrent allergic rhinitis and asthma.

  (2) Mechanism of action. The leukotriene receptor antagonists are selective cysteinyl leukotriene 1 (cys-LT-1) receptor antagonists; therefore, they prevent leukotrienes from interacting with their receptors.

  (3) Administration and dosage

   (a) The dosage of **zafirlukast** in children > 12 years and adults is 20 mg twice daily. Food reduces bioavailability, so zafirlukast should be taken at least 1 hr before or 2 hr after meals. Children 5–11 years of age should receive 10 mg twice daily.

   (b) The dosage of **montelukast** in adolescents 15 years of age or older and adults is one 10-mg tablet once every evening. The dosage for children 6–14 years of age is one 5-mg chewable tablet once every evening. Children ages 2–5 should receive one 4-mg chewable tablet once every evening. Food does not appear to change bioavailability.

  (4) Precautions and monitoring effects

   (a) Adverse reactions to montelukast are uncommon and include headache, dizziness, and dyspepsia.

   (b) Adverse reactions associated with zafirlukast include headache, dizziness, nausea, and diarrhea.

   (c) **Churg-Strauss syndrome,** a form of eosinophilic vasculitis, has rarely been associated with zafirlukast, montelukast, and pranlukast (available in Japan). It has usually, but not always, occurred in patients whose chronic steroid regimens were tapered and discontinued. At-risk patients should be monitored for vasculitic rash, eosinophilia, and increasing pulmonary, cardiac, and neuropathic symptoms.

(d) Significant drug–drug interactions may occur.
  (i) Aspirin increases zafirlukast levels.
  (ii) Erythromycin, theophylline, and **terfenadine** decrease zafirlukast concentrations.
  (iii) Zafirlukast may increase the anticoagulant effect of **warfarin** and levels of dofetilide.
  (iv) Drug interactions appear to be less significant with montelukast. Patients who are receiving montelukast with **hepatic enzyme inducers** (e.g., rifampin, phenobarbital) should be monitored closely.
  (v) The chewable forms of montelukast (4- and 5-mg tablets) contain aspartame and should be avoided in patients with **phenylketonuria.**

b. The only **lipoxygenase inhibitor** approved by the FDA is **zileuton (Zyflo).** Zileuton may allow reduction in corticosteroid doses in some patients.
  (1) Therapeutic effects. Lipoxygenase inhibitors have anti-inflammatory and bronchodilator activity.
  (2) Mechanism of action. Lipoxygenase inhibitors prevent the formation of leukotrienes. Zileuton blocks 5-lipoxygenase, the enzyme responsible for leukotriene formation.
  (3) Administration and dosage. In adults and children 12 years of age and older, the dosage of zileuton is 600 mg four times daily. It may be taken without regard to meals.
  (4) Precautions and monitoring effects
    (a) Zileuton is contraindicated in patients with hepatic function impairment and should be monitored closely in patients who drink large quantities of alcohol.
    (b) Adverse effects include headache, abdominal pain, asthenia, nausea, dyspepsia, and myalgia. Drug therapy was discontinued in almost 10% of patients owing to side effects, although this was similar to placebo.
    (c) Significant drug–drug interactions may occur.
      (i) Zileuton increases concentrations of **propranolol, terfenadine,** and **theophylline.**
      (ii) The anticoagulant effect of **warfarin** is increased by zileuton.
    (d) Hepatic enzymes (e.g., alanine aminotransferase [ALT]) may become elevated during therapy, with most occurrences during the first several months of therapy. Symptomatic hepatitis has been reported. Therefore, the manufacturer recommends that serum ALT be checked before initiation of treatment, monthly for 3 months, and every 2–3 months for the rest of the first year. ALT should be checked periodically thereafter.
      (i) Patients should be monitored closely for signs or symptoms of liver dysfunction (e.g., right upper quadrant abdominal pain, flu-like symptoms, fatigue, nausea, lethargy, itching, jaundice).
      (ii) If ALT increases to more than five times the upper limit of normal, therapy should be discontinued and the patient should be monitored until enzymes normalize.

4. Cromolyn sodium and nedocromil sodium
  a. Therapeutic effects. Cromolyn sodium and nedocromil sodium are nonsteroidal drugs with anti-inflammatory properties. These medications are less effective in their anti-inflammatory properties than the inhaled corticosteroids; however, because of their excellent safety profile, they are sometimes used in children.
    (1) When used prophylactically, cromolyn sodium and nedocromil sodium prevent the early and late response of asthma.
    (2) When used as maintenance therapy for asthma, these medications suppress nonspecific airway reactivity.
  b. Mechanism of action. Cromolyn sodium and nedocromil sodium are believed to act locally by stabilizing mast cells and thereby inhibiting mast cell degranulation.
  c. Administration and dosage
    (1) Cromolyn sodium is available as an MDI (800 mg per inhalation), and a nebulizer solution (20 mg/2 mL). The required dosage is two puffs of the MDI or 20 mg of

nebulizer solution. Because of the dosage needed to achieve asthma control, the nebulizer is preferred.

(2) **Nedocromil sodium** is available as an MDI (1.75 mg per inhalation). The required dosage is two inhalations four times a day.

(3) When used for prophylaxis of EIB, cromolyn sodium and nedocromil sodium should be administered 1 hr before exercise.

(4) After administration, initial improvement is seen within 1–2 weeks; however, the maximum effect may take longer.

d. **Precautions and monitoring effects**

(1) Cromolyn sodium and nedocromil sodium are **not effective during an acute asthma exacerbation.** They should be used only for maintenance therapy of persistent asthma or for prevention of EIB.

(2) Both drugs are well-tolerated, although paradoxical bronchospasm, wheezing, coughing, nasal congestion, and irritation or dryness of the throat may occur.

5. **Theophylline compounds (methylxanthines)**
   a. **Indications**

(1) Theophylline compounds may be considered if β-agonists and corticosteroids fail to control an acute asthma exacerbation.

(2) Theophylline is an alternative to long-acting β-agonists in the treatment of persistent asthma.

(3) Theophylline is most beneficial as an adjuvant to inhaled corticosteroids in patients with nocturnal or early morning symptoms.

   b. **Therapeutic effects**

(1) Theophylline compounds produce bronchodilation to a lesser extent than β-agonists.

(2) Nonbronchodilator effects include reduced mucus secretion, enhanced mucociliary transport, improved diaphragmatic contractility, and possibly reduced fatigability.

(3) There may also be notable degree of anti-inflammatory activity

   c. **Mechanism of action.** Theophylline-induced phosphodiesterase inhibition results in increased levels of cAMP.

   d. **Administration and dosage**

(1) **Oral therapy** (e.g., sustained-release theophyllines) allows for a longer dosing interval and improves compliance. Compliance to oral theophylline also may be better than that of inhaled bronchodilators and corticosteroids.

   (a) Because theophylline does not distribute well into fatty tissue, dosages should be calculated using lean body weight.

   (b) The initial dose of theophylline for adults and children > age 1 is 10 mg/kg/day (maximum of 300 mg/day) given in divided doses. Usual dosage should be adjusted to achieve serum theophylline concentration of 5–15 μg/mL (5–10 μg/mL acceptable).

   (c) The dosage can be titrated slowly upward and the serum level monitored until a therapeutic level is obtained.

   (d) The usual maximal daily dose in adults is 800 mg/day.

   (e) The maximum recommended dosage in children < age 1 is 0.2 × (age in weeks) + 5 = mg/kg/day and in children ≥ 1 year is 16 mg/kg/day, given in divided doses.

   (e) (f) In addition to theophylline, other methylxanthine compounds are available (e.g., oxtriphylline, dyphylline) but infrequently used. Dosing of these compounds is based on theophylline content (Table 49-6).

(2) **Intravenous therapy.** Although frequently used in the past, IV administration is now uncommon. IV administration is generally used only in hospitalized patients for whom oral therapy is not possible (e.g., vomiting, nothing by mouth).

   (a) The usual **loading dose** for adults and children not previously receiving a methylxanthine is 5 mg/kg of theophylline administered over 20–30 min at a rate not exceeding 25 mg/min.

   (b) The usual **maintenance infusion** rate of theophylline in healthy nonsmoking adults on no interacting drugs is 0.4 mg/kg/hr. This rate should be adjusted for factors that affect theophylline metabolism and serum levels (see Table 49-7).

   d. **Precautions and monitoring effects**

(1) Theophyllines are contraindicated in patients with hypersensitivity to xanthine compounds and should be used cautiously in patients with a history of peptic ulcer or untreated seizure disorder.

Table 49-6. Theophylline Content of Theophylline-Containing Products

Preparation	Theophylline Content (%)	Equivalent Dose (mg)
Theophylline anhydrous (most oral solids)	100	100
Theophylline monohydrate (oral solutions)	91	110
Aminophylline anhydrous	86	116
Aminophylline hydrous	79	127
Oxtriphylline	64	156

(2) Adverse effects include nausea, vomiting, diarrhea, anorexia, palpitations, dizziness, restlessness, nervousness, insomnia, seizures, reduced lower esophageal sphincter tone, and reduced control of gastroesophageal reflux disease. Patients who experience adverse gastrointestinal effects should be evaluated to rule out theophylline toxicity versus local gastrointestinal effect.

(3) Theophylline clearance can be altered by several factors and drug interactions (Table 49-7). Close drug-level monitoring is required for patients with factors that alter theophylline clearance.

Table 49-7. Factors That Alter Theophylline Clearance

Factors that increase theophylline clearance (decrease levels)
Age 1–9 years
Drugs
    Carbamazepine
    Phenobarbital
    Phenytoin
    Rifampin
Fever
Food (may delay or reduce absorption of some sustained-release products)
High-protein diet
Smoking (marijuana and tobacco)

Factors that decrease theophylline clearance (increase levels)
Age
    Elderly
    Premature neonates
    Term infants < 6 months
Cor pulmonale
Congestive heart failure, decompensated
Drugs
    Allopurinol
    β-Blockers (nonselective)
    Calcium channel blockers
    Cimetidine
    Fluoroquinolones (e.g., ciprofloxacin)
    Influenza virus vaccine
    Macrolides (e.g., clarithromycin, erythromycin)
    Oral contraceptives
    Ticlopidine
    Zafirlukast
Fever/viral illness
Fatty foods (may increase rate of absorption of some products)
High-carbohydrate diet
Liver dysfunction (e.g., cirrhosis)

(4) Careful monitoring is required in patients with hepatic disease, hypoxemia, hypertension, congestive heart failure, alcoholism, and in the elderly. Because of developmental changes in the neonate and child, dosing must be carefully established and monitored in these populations as well.

(5) Therapeutic drug monitoring of serum levels, adverse reactions, and concomitant drug use is essential for long-term therapy owing to theophylline's age- and condition-specific clearance.

(a) Therapeutic effect is achieved and toxicity minimized by keeping drug concentrations at 5–15 μg/mL.

(b) Drug levels should be assessed at steady state (typical half-life 8 hr, up to 24 hr in severe heart and liver failure),

(c) During oral therapy, trough drug levels should be obtained at steady state.

(d) Dyphylline serum levels should be monitored during therapy because serum theophylline levels will not measure dyphylline. The minimal effective therapeutic concentration of dyphylline is 12 μg/mL.

6. Anticholinergics. Bronchodilation occurs when these drugs block postganglionic muscarinic receptors in the airway. Response to anticholinergics is most pronounced in patients with fixed airway obstruction (e.g., COPD).

a. Ipratropium bromide (Atrovent is a quaternary ammonium compound.)

(1) Indications

(a) Ipratropium bromide is recommended for use in combination with β-agonists for the treatment of an acute asthma exacerbation in the emergency department or hospital settings. However, benefits in the chronic management of asthma have not been established.

(b) Ipratropium bromide may be particularly useful in older patients and patients with coexisting COPD.

(c) Ipratropium should not be used alone to treat an asthma exacerbation.

(d) Ipratropium bromide is an alternative bronchodilator in some patients who cannot tolerate β-agonists and in patients who present with bronchospasm induced by a β-blocker.

(2) Administration and dosage

(a) Closed-mouth MDI technique or the use of a spacer is recommended for patients receiving anticholinergic therapy via MDI.

(b) The starting dose of the MDI is two inhalations four times a day. When administered via nebulizer, the dose is 500 μg (2.5 mL) four times a day.

(3) Precautions and monitoring effects

(a) If the anticholinergic spray contacts the eye, intraocular pressure may increase.

(b) The onset of action (approximately 15 min) and peak effect (1–2 hr) are more delayed than for β-agonists.

b. Aerosolized **atropine** is used rarely now that ipratropium bromide nebulization solution is available owing to atropine's high incidence of systemic adverse effects.

7. Antihistamines are useful for patients with coexisting allergic rhinitis; however, their role in the treatment of asthma remains unclear. Antihistamines compete with histamine for H_1-receptor sites on effector cells and thus help prevent the histamine-mediated responses that influence asthma.

8. Antibiotics are generally not used for the treatment of asthma, unless other signs of infection are present.

9. Magnesium sulfate, administered intravenously, may be useful in some patients because of its modest ability to cause bronchodilation. When administered intravenously, it also improves respiratory muscle strength in hypomagnesemic patients. Research has suggested that magnesium may reduce admission rate and improve FEV_1 in severe, acute asthma exacerbations and in stable, chronic asthma.

10. Immunotherapy (allergy shots) improves asthma control in some patients and is ineffective in others. A recent meta-analysis demonstrated that immunotherapy may improve lung function, reduce symptoms, and decrease medication requirements in a significant number of patients.

11. **Mucus** may contribute to airway obstruction in asthma. However, because some mucolytics such as acetylcysteine may precipitate bronchospasm, they should not be used for the treatment of patients with asthma.

J. Drug delivery options

1. **MDIs**

   a. When administered with good technique and a spacer, the efficacy of MDIs is similar to that of nebulizers, despite the lower doses administered with an MDI and spacer. The only MDI that comes with a built-in spacer is the Azmacort (triamcinolone) inhaler.

   b. For small children to be able to use an MDI, a spacer with a face mask must be used.

   c. MDIs can be difficult to use. Steps for properly using an MDI are outlined in Table 49-8.

   d. MDIs can be administered to patients on mechanical ventilation with the use of an attachment device designed for the mechanical ventilator circuit. Higher doses of the β_2-agonist are often used in this setting.

   e. Breath-actuated MDIs (e.g., Maxair Autohaler) require the patient to use a closed-mouth technique. When inhalation is begun, the medication is released automatically. This type of inhaler is useful for a patient who is having problems coordinating actuation and inhalation.

2. **Spacers and holding chambers** (e.g., AeroChamber, AeroVent Ellipse, InspirEase, OptiChamber)

   a. Spacers and holding chambers reduce the amount of drug deposited in the oral cavity.

   b. The use of spacers and holding chambers may minimize local and systemic adverse reactions.

   c. Addition of a spacer in a patient with poor MDI technique may improve pulmonary delivery of the agent.

   d. Spacers should be considered in all patients who are receiving medium to high doses of inhaled corticosteroids.

   e. They are especially beneficial for patients with poor hand–lung coordination, such as very young and old.

   f. Devices vary in construction and efficacy. The presence of a one-way mouthpiece valve, inhalation rate whistle, size, and durability are all factors that should be considered when selecting a particular spacer for a patient.

3. **Nebulizers**

   a. Compared to MDI and spacer administration, nebulizers require less patient coordination during administration of multiple inhalations.

   b. Disadvantages of nebulizers include cost, preparation and administration time, size of the device, and drug delivery inconsistencies among devices.

   c. Despite the disadvantages, nebulization is recommended for delivery of high-dose β-agonists and anticholinergics in severe exacerbations and for delivery of cromolyn sodium to children.

Table 49-8. Procedure for the Proper Use of Metered Dose Inhalers (MDIs)

Assemble MDI, if necessary.
Remove cap and inspect mouthpiece for foreign objects.
Attach MDI to spacer (if applicable).
Shake MDI (with spacer).
Tilt head back slightly and exhale normally.
Position inhaler:
  Wrap lips around spacer mouthpiece.
  Position inhaler 1–2 in. from open mouth.
  Wrap lips around inhaler mouthpiece.
Just as you begin to inhale, depress canister once to release medication.
Continue inhaling slowly (over 3–5 sec) until lungs are full.
Hold breath for 10 sec.
Wait 1 min before repeating steps to deliver additional puffs.

---

4. Dry-powder inhalers

  a. Dry-powder inhalers (DPIs) are coming to the market as a result of the international move to avoid the use of chlorofluorocarbon (CFC) propellants. They are also being used more frequently because many patients find them easier to use than an MDI.

  b. Dry-powder inhalers require the user to:
  (1) First load the dose into the delivery chamber
  (2) Inhale rapidly or slowly, depending on the device (versus only slow inhalation required for MDI administration)
  (3) Use the closed-mouth technique
  (4) Avoid exhaling into the mouthpiece before inhalation.

  c. Spacers are not used with dry-powder inhalers.

  d. Patients should be advised to keep these devices away from moisture.

K. Nonpharmacological treatment

1. **Humidified oxygen** is administered to all patients with severe, acute asthma to reverse hypoxemia. Although the fraction of inspired oxygen (FIo_2) administered is based on the patient's arterial blood gas status, 1–3 L/min is generally given via face mask or nasal cannula. The goal is to keep the $Sao_2 > 90\%$ ($> 95\%$ if the patient is pregnant or has heart disease).

2. **Heliox** is a mixture of helium and oxygen that has a lower density than air. Because of its decreased airflow resistance, heliox may increase ventilation during acute asthma exacerbations. Because conflicting information has been published in studies using heliox, its role in asthma is unclear.

3. **Intravenous fluids** and electrolytes may be required if the patient is volume depleted.

4. **Environmental control** and allergen avoidance are important in the management of a patient with asthma.

  a. Available data suggest that avoidance of known allergens can improve asthma control.

  b. Some measures include use of allergen-resistant mattress and pillow encasements, use of high-filtration vacuum cleaners, removal of carpets and draperies, and avoidance of furry pets.

5. **Vaccines** (e.g., influenza virus, polyvalent pneumococcals) are recommended to prevent infection, which may precipitate an exacerbation.

II. CHRONIC OBSTRUCTIVE PULMONARY DISEASE

A. Definitions.
The 2001 National Heart, Lung, and Blood Institute/World Health Organization (NHLBI/WHO) Global Initiative for Chronic Obstructive Lung Disease (GOLD) definition of COPD is "a disease state characterized by airflow limitation that is not fully reversible. The airflow limitation is usually both progressive and associated with an abnormal inflammatory response of the lungs to noxious particles or gases." The American Thoracic Society definition is similar: a disease state characterized by the presence of airflow limitation owing to chronic bronchitis or emphysema; the airflow obstruction is generally progressive, may be accompanied by airway hyperreactivity, and may be partially reversible. The two major forms of COPD—**chronic bronchitis** and **emphysema**—frequently coexist. COPD also coexists with asthma.

1. **Chronic bronchitis** is characterized by excessive mucus production by the tracheobronchial tree, which results in airway obstruction as a result of edema and bronchial inflammation. Bronchitis is considered chronic when the patient has a cough producing more than 30 mL of sputum in 24 hr for at least 3 months of the year for 2 consecutive years and other causes of chronic cough have been excluded.

2. **Emphysema** is marked by permanent alveolar enlargement distal to the terminal bronchioles and destructive changes of the alveolar walls. There is a lack of uniformity in airspace enlargement, resulting in loss of alveolar surface area. The collapse of these small airways results in airflow limitation that is independent of exertion.

B. Incidence.
Approximately 17 million Americans have COPD. COPD is the fourth leading cause of death in the United States and the leading cause of hospitalization in the older population.

It is most commonly diagnosed in older men; however, the incidence is increasing in women owing to an increasing population of women smokers.

C. **Cause.** Various factors have been implicated in the development of COPD, including the following:

1. **Cigarette smoking** is the primary causal factor for the development of COPD, present in > 90% of patients.
   a. One mechanism suggests that pulmonary hyperreactivity secondary to smoking results in persistent airway obstruction.
   b. There is also an increased risk of COPD in people who have α_1-antitrypsin (AAT) deficiency. One in three people with genetic AAT deficiency develop emphysema, usually as young adults.
      (1) AAT is a serine protease inhibitor, and it is also an acute-phase reactive protein. The major physiological function of AAT is inhibition of neutrophil elastase.
      (2) AAT deficiency should be suspected when emphysema develops early in the absence of a significant smoking history.

2. Exposure to irritants such as sulfur dioxide (as in polluted air), noxious gases, and organic or inorganic dusts

3. A history of respiratory infections or bronchial hyperreactivity

4. Social, economic, and hereditary factors

D. **Pathophysiology**

1. **Chronic bronchitis**
   a. **Respiratory tissue inflammation** results in vasodilation, congestion, mucosal edema, and goblet cell hypertrophy. These events trigger goblet cells to produce excessive amounts of mucus.
   b. **Changes in tissue** include increased smooth muscle, cartilage atrophy, infiltration of neutrophils and other cells, and impairment of cilia.
   c. Airways become blocked by thick, tenacious mucous secretions, which trigger a productive cough.
   d. Normally sterile airways can become colonized with *Streptococcus pneumoniae, Haemophilus influenzae, Moraxella catarrhalis, Staphylococcus aureus,* and *Pseudomonas aeruginosa* species. Recurrent lung infections (viral and bacterial) reduce ciliary and phagocytic activity, increase mucus accumulation, weaken the body's defenses, and further destroy small bronchioles.
   e. As the **airways degenerate,** overall gas exchange is impaired, causing **exertional dyspnea.**
   f. Hypoxemia results from a V/Q imbalance and is reflected in an increasing arterial carbon dioxide tension (i.e., increasing $Paco_2$).
   g. Sustained hypercapnia (increased $Paco_2$) desensitizes the brain's respiratory control center and central chemoreceptors. As a result, compensatory action to correct hypoxemia and hypercapnia (i.e., a respiratory rate or depth increase) does not occur. Instead, hypoxemia serves as the stimulus for breathing. Use of narcotics or benzodiazepines, especially in combination, should be done cautiously in these patients to avoid respiratory failure.

2. **Emphysema**
   a. **Anatomical changes** are the result of loss of tissue elasticity.
      (1) **Inflammation** and **excessive mucus secretion** (as from long-standing chronic bronchitis) cause air trapping in the alveoli. This contributes to breakdown of the bronchioles, alveolar walls, and connective tissue.
      (2) As clusters of alveoli merge, the number of alveoli diminishes, leading to increased space available for air trapping.
      (3) Destruction of alveolar walls causes collapse of small airways on exhalation and disruption of the pulmonary capillary beds.
      (4) These changes result in V/Q abnormalities; blood is shunted away from destroyed areas to maintain a constant V/Q ratio, unlike the case in chronic bronchitis.
      (5) Hypercapnia and respiratory acidosis are uncommon in emphysema because V/Q imbalance is compensated for by an increased respiratory rate.
   b. There are **specific regions of the lung** in which characteristic anatomical changes of emphysema occur.

(1) In **centrilobular** (centriacinar) emphysema associated with cigarette smoking, destruction is central, selectively involving respiratory bronchioles. Typically, bronchioles and alveolar ducts become dilated and merge.

(2) In **panlobular** (panacinar) emphysema, all lung segments are involved. The alveoli enlarge and atrophy, and the pulmonary vascular bed is destroyed. This form of emphysema is associated with AAT deficiency.

(3) In **paraseptal** emphysema, the lung periphery adjacent to fibrotic regions is the site of alveolar distention and alveolar wall destruction. This is associated with spontaneous pneumothorax.

E. Clinical evaluation

1. Physical findings

a. Predominant chronic bronchitis typically has an insidious onset after age 45.

(1) A **chronic productive cough** is the hallmark of chronic bronchitis. It occurs first in winter, then progresses to year-round. It is usually worse in the morning. Smoking cessation can help lessen the productive cough.

(2) **Exertional dyspnea,** the most common presenting symptom, is progressive. However, the severity of this symptom may not reflect the severity of the disease.

(3) Other common findings include obesity, rhonchi and wheezes on auscultation, prolonged expiration, and a normal respiratory rate. As the disease progresses, right ventricular failure is common, which presents as jugular venous distention, peripheral edema, hepatomegaly, and cardiomegaly. Because patients tend to develop cyanosis, the term *blue bloater* is sometimes used to describe patients with chronic bronchitis.

b. Predominant emphysema has an insidious onset, and symptoms occur after age 55.

(1) The **cough** is chronic but less productive than in chronic bronchitis.

(2) **Exertional dyspnea** is progressive, constant, severe, more characteristic of emphysema than chronic bronchitis.

(3) Other common findings include weight loss, tachypnea, pursed-lip breathing, prolonged expiration, accessory chest muscle use, hyperresonance on percussion, diaphragmatic excursion, and diminished breath sounds. Because patients are able to maintain reasonably good oxygenation because of their tachypnea, the term *pink puffer* is sometimes used to describe patients with emphysema. Note however, that the pink puffer and blue bloater presentations are not specific for the respective diseases.

c. Patients may have elements and physical findings from each of these diseases simultaneously.

2. Diagnostic test results

a. COPD patients with characteristic symptoms of cough, dyspnea, sputum production, and/ or exposure to known risk factors (e.g., smoking) should be evaluated for a COPD diagnosis. If the patient has $FEV_1/FVC < 70\%$ and a postbronchodilator $FEV_1 < 80\%$ predicted, he or she has airflow limitation that is not fully reversible. Patients with a smoking history (e.g. > 20 pack year history and > 45 years old) should be considered for the diagnosis. Spirometry can be used to help make the diagnosis.

b. Chronic bronchitis

(1) Blood analysis usually reveals polycythemia as a result of to erythropoiesis secondary to hypoxemia. With bacterial infection, the WBC count may be increased.

(2) Sputum inspection reveals thick purulent or mucopurulent sputum tinged yellow, white, green, or gray; an acute change in color and/or quantity suggests infection.

(3) Arterial blood gas studies may show a markedly decreased Pao_2 level (45–60 mm Hg), reflecting hypoxemia, and a $Paco_2$ level that is normal or elevated (50–60 mm Hg), reflecting hypercapnia.

(4) Pulmonary function tests may be normal in the early disease stages. Later, they show a reduced FEV_1/FVC ratio, increased residual lung volume, a decreased vital capacity, and a decreased FEV_1. Unlike emphysema, chronic bronchitis patients tend to have normal diffusing capacity, normal static lung compliance, and normal total lung capacity.

(5) Chest radiograph typically identifies lung hyperinflation, a barrel chest, and increased bronchovascular markings.

(6) An ECG may reveal right ventricular hypertrophy and changes consistent with cor pulmonale.

   c. Emphysema

     (1) Sputum inspection reveals scanty sputum that is clear or mucoid. Infections are less frequent than in chronic bronchitis.

     (2) Arterial blood gas studies typically indicate a reduced or normal Pa_{O_2} level (65–75 mm Hg) and, in late disease stages, an increased Pa_{CO_2} level (50–60 mm Hg).

     (3) Pulmonary function tests show a reduced FEV_1/FVC ratio, normal or increased static lung compliance, reduced FEV_1 and diffusing capacity, and increased TLC and RV.

     (4) Chest radiograph usually reveals bullae, blebs, a flattened diaphragm, lung hyperinflation, vertical heart, enlarged anteroposterior chest diameter, decreased vascular markings in the lung periphery, and a large retrosternal air space.

F. Treatment objectives endorsed by GOLD include the following

   1. Prevent disease progression (smoking cessation)

   2. Relieve symptoms and improve exercise tolerance (enable the patient to perform normal daily activities)

   3. Improve health status

   4. Prevent and treat exacerbations

   5. Prevent and treat complications

   6. Reduce mortality

G. Therapy

   1. Pharmacological treatment. Therapy is based on disease staging, which is determined by spirometry (Table 49-9).

     a. Short-acting anticholinergics and β-agonists, alone or in combination, are the most commonly used initial agents. Long-acting bronchodilators, such as salmeterol, formoterol, tiotropium (Spiriva), and theophylline are added to the short-acting agents. Methylxanthines are usually added when the response to other agents is inadequate. In addition to bronchodilation, these agents can decrease dyspnea, improve exercise capacity, improve quality of life, and decrease the frequency and severity of exacerbations, especially tiotropium.

     b. Bronchodilators are the most important therapy for symptoms in COPD. Figure 49-4 indicates a strategy of use.

     c. Inhaled corticosteroids, such as fluticasone and budesonide, have shown small benefits in FEV_1; the majority of their benefit occurs in reducing the severity of exacerbations, not the number of exacerbations.

     d. Anticholinergics (e.g., ipratropium bromide, tiotropium bromide, atropine)

       (1) Indications. Anticholinergics may be used as first-line bronchodilators or in conjunction with β-agonists in the treatment of COPD because these agents are the most potent bronchodilators for the condition.

       (2) Mechanism of action. Ipratropium bromide, tiotropium bromide, and atropine produce bronchodilation by competitively inhibiting cholinergic responses. Ipratropium bromide and tiotropium bromide also reduce sputum volume without altering viscosity. Some studies have shown an increased response to these agents in COPD when they are combined with β-agonists. Tiotropium has greater affinity for cholinergic receptors than ipratropium.

       (3) Administration and dosage

         (a) Ipratropium bromide is three to five times more potent and has significantly fewer side effects than atropine, which is rarely used today since the development of nebulized ipratropium.

         (b) Initial MDI dosing of ipratropium bromide is two inhalations (40 μg) four times daily, but dosing can be increased to six inhalations four times daily without significant risk. These higher doses are often required to achieve therapeutic benefit. Administration should be via MDI with spacer or MDI alone using a closed-mouth technique.

Table 49-9. Therapy at Each Stage of COPD

	0: At Risk	I: Mild	IIA / II: Moderate	IIB / II: Severe	III: Severe / IV: Very Severe
Old	0: At Risk	I: Mild		II: Moderate	III: Severe
New	0: At Risk	I: Mild	II: Moderate	II: Severe	IV: Very Severe
Characteristics	Chronic symptoms Exposure to risk factors Normal spirometry	$FEV_1/FBC < 70\%$ $FEV_1 \geq 80\%$ With or without symptoms	$FEV_1/FVC < 70\%$ $50\% \leq FEV_1 < 80\%$ With or without symptoms	$FEV_1/FVC < 70\%$ $30\% \leq FEV_1 < 50\%$ With or without symptoms	$FEV_1/FVC < 70\%$ $FEV_1 < 30\%$ or $FEV_1 < 50\%$ predicted plus chronic respiratory failure
	Avoidance of risk factor(s); influenza vaccination				
		Add short-acting bronchodilator when needed			
			Add regular treatment with one or more long-acting bronchodilators *Add rehabilitation*		
				Add inhaled glucocorticosteroids if repeated exacerbations	
					Add long-term oxygen if chronic respiratory failure *Consider surgical treatments*

FEV₁, forced expiratory volume in 1 sec; *FVC*, forced vital capacity.
Reprinted with permission from Global Initiative for Chronic Obstructive Lung Disease (GOLD). Global Strategy for the Diagnosis, Management, and Prevention of Chronic Obstructive Pulmonary Disease. Updated 2005. www.goldcopd.org.

Figure 49-4. Stepped care approach to bronchodilators in COPD. *AC,* anticholinergic; *LA,* long acting; *PDE,* phosphodiesterase; *SA,* short acting.

(c) Dosing of ipratropium bromide solution is 500 μg/2.5 mL (1 unit dose vial) or more via nebulizer four times daily.

(d) Tiotropium bromide capsules contain 22.5 μg tiotropium bromide monohydrate, equivalent to 18 μg tiotropium.

　(i) Tiotropium is an inhalation powder contained in a hard capsule. It should be administered once daily only via a HandiHaler device, which delivers 10 μg tiotropium.

　(ii) Patients should generally not be placed on both ipratropium and tiotropium because of the increased risk of anticholinergic side effects, and no additional bronchodilation is likely achieved by adding ipratropium. For example, if a COPD patient is currently on ipratropium/albuterol (Combivent, DuoNeb), and tiotropium is started, the albuterol should be continued as the short-acting bronchodilator and ipratropium discontinued.

e. β-Agonists (see I.I.1; Table 49-4)

(1) Indications. β_2-Agonists may be used as first-line bronchodilators or in conjunction with anticholinergic agents in the maintenance treatment of COPD. Short-acting agents are used regularly or on an as-needed basis for symptoms. Some patients may respond clinically to the prolonged treatment with β_2-agonists even after demonstrating lack of acute reversibility (spirometry testing showing < 12% or < 200-mL increase in FEV_1) to short-acting agents.

(2) Mechanism of action. β_2-Agonists relieve dyspnea caused by airway obstruction, although the response is usually not as significant as in patients with asthma. These agents may also increase mucociliary clearance by stimulating ciliary activity (helps patients expectorate sputum).

(3) Administration and dosage

(a) β_2-Agonists are administered via inhalation (e.g., dry-powder inhaler, nebulizer, MDI with or without a spacer), unless the patient cannot use the drug properly; then an oral agent is used cautiously.

(b) β_2-Agonists of the same duration should not be used in combination because an adequate dose of a single agent provides peak bronchodilation. However, it is reasonable to administer a long-acting product (e.g., salmeterol, formoterol) on a regular basis with a short-acting agent reserved for as-needed or rescue therapy.

(c) Salmeterol and formoterol (long-acting β-agonists) are administered twice daily. They may also be used in combination with ipratropium bromide or tiotropium. Neither agent is used on an as-needed basis for rescue therapy, although formoterol does have a rapid onset of action.

(d) Inhaler devices that require a rapid inspiratory rate may result in suboptimal lung deposition in the COPD patient with limited inspiratory capacity. An MDI or nebulizer may be more optimal in this type of patient.

f. Theophylline (see I.I.5)

(1) Indications. Theophylline compounds typically are added to the drug regimen after an unsuccessful trial of ipratropium bromide and β-adrenergics. Theophylline appears to have a greater clinical role in COPD than in asthma. Other similar agents (phosphodiesterase inhibitors) are in development.

(2) Mechanism of action. In COPD, theophylline compounds are used because they increase mucociliary clearance, stimulate the respiratory drive, enhance diaphragmatic contractility, improve the ventricular ejection fraction, and stimulate renal diuresis. Their bronchodilator properties are modest, at best. Theophylline may be used in lieu of other long-acting bronchodilators or in combination.

(3) Administration and dosage. A trial of 1–2 months with the serum drug level maintained at 5–12 μg/mL and maximized

(a) Because of the nonbronchodilator effects of methylxanthines, they may be continued in the face of a clinical response, even in the absence of improved FEV_1.

(b) If no change occurs in the patient's clinical condition and/or FEV_1, theophylline therapy should be discontinued owing to the potential for side effects.

(4) Precautions and monitoring effects. Serum drug levels should be closely monitored in all patients, especially those with signs of toxicity (tachycardia, nausea, vomiting) as well as with liver impairment, congestive heart failure and/or cor pulmonale as a result of reduced theophylline metabolism. Potential drug interactions (e.g. with ciprofloxacin) may warrant blood testing.

g. Corticosteroids (see I.I.2; Table 49-5)

(1) Indications

(a) Systemic corticosteroids (preferably oral) are indicated in the treatment of acute COPD exacerbations and chronically in some severe patients.

(b) Inhaled corticosteroids play a less prominent role in COPD than in asthma.

(c) Candidates for prolonged use of inhaled corticosteroid therapy should

(i) Be symptomatic and have a documented spirometric response (i.e., an increase in FEV_1 of at least 15% and 200 mL after 6 weeks to 3 months of use)

(ii) Have an $FEV_1 < 50\%$ predicted, with a history of repeated exacerbations requiring systemic corticosteroids or antibiotics

(d) Long-term use of systemic steroids should be avoided if possible. Osteoporosis of the spine and ribs is especially common in COPD patients receiving frequent or maintenance systemic steroids.

(2) Administration and dosage

(a) For oral use in outpatient management of acute exacerbations, prednisone or prednisolone is administered at a dosage of 40 mg/day for 10 days.

(b) The dose of oral (e.g., prednisolone) or intravenous corticosteroids (e.g., methylprednisolone) for hospital management of acute COPD exacerbations is not established. However, doses and duration of therapy should be limited (e.g., 30–40 mg/day of prednisolone for 10–14 days) to avoid significant adverse effects.

(c) The role of inhaled corticosteroids for chronic management of COPD is also limited (see II.G.1.d.(1).(c)).

(d) In appropriate patients, corticosteroids may be administered via dry-powder inhaler or MDI with spacer.

(e) Response to oral corticosteroids does predict response to inhaled corticosteroids.

(f) Medium doses of inhaled corticosteroids are recommended for COPD (e.g., Flovent 110 μg 2 puffs twice a day or the combination of Advair 250 μg 1 puff twice a day).

(g) Inhaler devices that require a rapid inspiratory rate (e.g., Pulmicort Turbuhaler) are generally not desirable in COPD patients.

h. Antibiotics

(1) Indications

(a) Antibiotics are used to treat exacerbations with suspected infection as evidenced by an increase in volume or change in color or viscosity of the sputum, along with dyspnea.

(b) Prevention of infection with chronic antibiotic therapy is controversial and should be considered only in patients with multiple exacerbations annually (i.e., more than two per year).

(2) Antibiotic therapy

(a) Ambulatory antibiotic treatment of exacerbations in patients with COPD is recommended when there is evidence of worsening dyspnea and cough with purulent sputum and increased sputum volume.

    (i) Hospital or laboratory antibiograms should be reviewed when selecting an appropriate agent for *S. pneumoniae, M. catarrhalis,* and *H. influenzae.*

    (ii) Agents may include either a second-generation cephalosporin (e.g., cefuroxime, cefaclor), trimethoprim-sulfamethoxazole, a β-lactam with or without a β-lactamase inhibitor (e.g., amoxicillin, amoxicillin-clavulanate), macrolides (azithromycin [Zithromax]), ketolides (telithromycin [Ketek]), or an oral fluoroquinolone (ciprofloxacin [Cipro], gatifloxacin [Tequin]).

    (iii) If infection with *M. pneumoniae* or *Legionella pneumophila* is a concern, although uncommon in COPD flares, a macrolide or fluoroquinolone may be added.

(b) Antibiotic treatment of pneumonia in hospitalized patients with COPD includes either a second- or third-generation cephalosporin (e.g., cefuroxime, ceftriaxone, cefotaxime) or a β-lactam with or without a β-lactamase inhibitor (e.g., amoxicillin-clavulanate – [Augmentin], piperacillin-tazobactam [Zosyn]), a macrolide, or fluoroquinolone.

(c) COPD exacerbations are treated for 3–10 days, depending on the agent used (e.g., moxifloxacin 400 mg × 5 days) and the patient.

i. Mucolytics (e.g., iodinated glycerol) may improve sputum clearance and disrupt mucus plugs.

j. Expectorants (e.g., guaifenesin) may be used. Potassium iodide should be avoided because of side effects associated with iodine therapy.

k. Antioxidants (e.g., *N*-acetylcysteine) may reduce exacerbation frequency. However, routine use cannot be recommended based on currently available data.

l. Influenza virus vaccine is recommended because of its ability to reduce death and serious illness by almost 50%.

2. Nonpharmacological Therapy

a. Vaccinations

(1) Influenza vaccination administered each Fall/Winter. **Polyvalent pneumococcal** vaccine is recommended by the American Thoracic Society

b. Oxygen Therapy

(1) Recommended for hypoxemia chronically or during exacerbations. Currently recommended to administer oxygen at least 15 hours/day.

(2) Reverses hypoxemia (particularly at night and during exercise).

(3) Indications for home oxygen treatment include

(a) $PaO_2 < 55$ mm Hg or $SaO_2 < 88\%$

(b) PaO_2 of 55–60 mm Hg or $SaO_2 < 89\%$ with evidence of cor pulmonale, pulmonary hypertension, or polycythemia (hematocrit > 55%).

(4) Patients hospitalized for COPD exacerbations should receive controlled oxygen to keep $PaO_2 > 60$ mm Hg or $SaO_2 > 90\%$. Arterial blood gas (ABG) tests may be performed 30 min after placing the patient on oxygen to identify and minimize CO_2 retention.

c. Chest physiotherapy loosens secretions, helps reexpand the lungs, and increases the efficacy of respiratory muscle use. Techniques include postural drainage, chest percussion and vibration, coughing, and deep breathing. These efforts may help patients with lobar atelectasis or who produce large quantities (i.e., > 25 mL/day) of sputum.

d. Physical rehabilitation improves the patient's exercise tolerance and quality of life. A pulmonary rehabilitation program usually includes physical conditioning and social, psychological, and nutritional interventions. This can be an effective intervention.

   e. **Smoking cessation** and avoidance of other irritants has been shown to slow the rate of decline in FEV_1 in COPD patients. It is obviously one of the most important interventions. Nicotine gum, patches, inhalers, lozenges, bupropion, vareniciline (Chantix), and clonidine may be useful in smoking cessation. Behavior intervention significantly enhances the effectiveness of pharmacological therapy in smoking cessation.

   f. **Surgery.** There is a growing body of evidence that lung volume reduction surgery may be beneficial to patients with severe emphysema. Clinical trials have now delineated proper patient selection for this type of surgery. Lung transplantation is also done in selected patients.

H. Complications of COPD

1. **Pulmonary hypertension.** With decreased pulmonary vascular bed space (owing to lung congestion), pulmonary arterial pressure increases. In some cases, pressure increases enough to cause **cor pulmonale** (right ventricular hypertrophy) with consequent heart failure.

2. **Acute respiratory failure.** In advanced stages of COPD, the brain's respiratory center may become seriously compromised, leading to poor cerebral oxygenation and an increased Pa_{CO_2} level. Hypoxia and respiratory acidosis may ensue. If the condition progresses, respiratory failure occurs.

3. **Infection.** In chronic bronchitis, trapping of excessive mucus, air, and bacteria in the tracheobronchial tree sets the stage for infection. In addition, impairment of coughing and deep breathing, which normally cleanses the lungs, leads to destruction of respiratory cilia. Once an infection sets in, reinfection can easily occur.

4. **Polycythemia.** An increase in red blood cells infrequently can lead to hypercoagulable states, embolism, and stroke.

STUDY QUESTIONS

Directions for questions 1–7: Each of the questions, statements, or incomplete statements in this section can be correctly answered or completed by **one** of the suggested answers or phrases. Choose the **best** answer.

1. The symptoms of allergen-mediated asthma result from which of the following?

(A) increased release of mediators from mast cells
(B) increased adrenergic responsiveness of the airways
(C) increased vascular permeability of bronchial tissue
(D) decreased calcium influx into the mast cells
(E) decreased prostaglandin production

2. Acute exacerbations of asthma can be triggered by all of the following *except*

(A) bacterial or viral pneumonia.
(B) hypersensitivity reaction to penicillin.
(C) discontinuation of asthma medication.
(D) hot, dry weather.
(E) stressful emotional events.

3. A 45-year-old male with a history of asthma has a peak expiratory flow rate (PEFR) of 65%, nocturnal wheezing once a month, and daytime wheezing usually less than twice a week. According to the National Institutes of Health (NIH) guidelines for the treatment of asthma, he has which type?

(A) mild intermittent
(B) mild persistent
(C) moderate persistent
(D) severe persistent

4. The patient in question 3 should be treated with which *two* agents?

(A) inhaled steroid and ipratropium
(B) inhaled steroid and albuterol MDI (as needed)
(C) inhaled steroid and aspirin

5. A 15-year-old female is brought to the emergency department. She is breathing 30 times per minute, is unable to speak in full sentences, and has a peak expiratory flow rate (PEFR) < 50% predicted. The preferred first-line therapy for her asthma exacerbation is

(A) theophylline
(B) a β-agonist
(C) a corticosteroid
(D) cromolyn sodium
(E) a and b
(F) b and c

6. The primary goals of asthma therapy include all of the following *except*

(A) maintain normal activity levels.
(B) maintain control of symptoms.
(C) avoid adverse effects of asthma medications.
(D) prevent acute exacerbations and chronic symptoms.
(E) prevent destruction of lung tissue.

7. Which of the following tests is used at home to assess therapy and determine if a patient with asthma should seek emergency care?

(A) forced expiratory volume in one second (FEV_1)
(B) forced vital capacity (FVC)
(C) total lung capacity (TLC)
(D) peak expiratory flow rate (PEFR)
(E) residual volume (RV)

Directions for question 8: The incomplete statement in this section can be correctly answered or completed by **one or more** of the suggested answers. Choose the answer, **A–E.**

> A   if **I only** is correct
> B   if **III only** is correct
> C   if **I and II** are correct
> D   if **II and III** are correct
> E   if **I, II, and III** are correct

8. The disease process of chronic bronchitis is characterized by

   I. the destruction of central and peripheral portions of the acinus.
  II. an increased number of mucous glands and goblet cells.
 III. edema and inflammation of the bronchioles.

Directions for questions 9–11: Each description in this section is most closely associated with **one** of the following agents. The agents may be used more than once or not at all. Choose the **best** answer, **A–E.**

> A   cimetidine
> B   albuterol
> C   ipratropium bromide
> D   epinephrine
> E   atropine

9. Decreases theophylline clearance

10. Has anticholinergic activity with few side effects

11. Has high β_2-adrenergic selectivity

ANSWERS AND EXPLANATIONS

1. The answer is A *[see I.D.4.(a); Figure 49-1].*
In asthma, airborne antigen binds to the mast cell, activating the IgE-mediated process. Mediators (e.g., histamine, leukotrienes, prostaglandins) are then released, causing bronchoconstriction and tissue edema.

2. The answer is D *[see I.D; Figure 49-1].*
Exacerbations of asthma can be triggered by allergens, respiratory infections, occupational stimuli (e.g., fumes from gasoline or paint), emotions, and environmental factors. Studies have shown that cold air can cause release of mast cell mediators by an undetermined mechanism. Hot, dry air does not cause this release.

3. The answer is C *[see Table 49-3].*
The patient has moderate persistent asthma. All three parameters are consistent with mild persistent asthma. If any one of the three parameters indicated moderate persistent asthma, then the patient would be classified as moderate asthma (PEFR = 65%)

4. The answer is B *[see Figure 49-3].*
Inhaled steroids are the anti-inflammatory drug of choice owing to proven efficacy. All patients should be prescribed a short-acting β_2-agonist to use as rescue therapy for worsening symptoms. If chronic symptoms worsen, a long-acting β_2-agonist can be added (e.g., Adavir). Remember that increasing the dose of the inhaled steroid may not improve symptoms, a long-acting bronchodilator is more likely to do so.

5. The answer is F *[see Figure 49-3].*
Patient is obviously in respiratory distress. Aggressive treatment with oxygen, systemic steroids, and short-acting bronchodilators is indicated. Ipratropium could also be added to the albuterol in the acute setting.

6. The answer is E *[see I.F, I.H.1; II.D].*
Asthma is characterized by reversible airway obstruction in response to specific stimuli. Mast cells release mediators, which trigger bronchoconstriction. After an acute attack, in most cases symptoms are minimal, and pathological changes are not permanent. Unlike asthma, chronic obstructive pulmonary disease does cause progressive airway destruction, chronic bronchitis by excessive mucus production and other changes, and emphysema by destruction of the acinus.

7. The answer is D *[see I.G.2.a.(3)].*
For home monitoring, PEFR is the best test for assessment of therapy, trigger identification, and the need for referral to emergency care. It is recommended for patients who have had severe exacerbations of asthma, who are poor perceivers of asthma symptoms, and those with moderate to severe disease.

8. The answer is D *(II, III) [see II.D.1–2].*
Chronic bronchitis is characterized by an increase in the number of mucous and goblet cells owing to bronchial irritation. This results in increased mucus production. Other changes include edema and inflammation of the bronchioles and changes in smooth muscle and cartilage. Emphysema is a permanent destruction of the central and peripheral portions of the acinus distal to the bronchioles. In this disease, adequate oxygen reaches the alveolar duct, owing to increased rate of breathing, but perfusion is abnormal.

9. The answer is A *[see Table 49-8].*

10. The answer is C *[see II.G.1.a].*

11. The answer is B *[see Table 49-4].*
Cimetidine, an H_2-receptor antagonist, decreases theophylline clearance by inhibiting hepatic microsomal mixed-function oxidase metabolism, thus increasing serum theophylline concentrations. Theophylline clearance can be decreased by 40% during the first 24 hr of concurrent therapy. Anticholinergic agents such as atropine and ipratropium bromide produce bronchodilation by competitively inhibiting cholinergic receptors. The disadvantages of atropine include dry mouth, tachycardia, and urinary retention. Ipratropium bromide is three to five times more potent than atropine and does not have these side effects. Albuterol is one of the most β_2-selective adrenergic agents available. Other such agents include terbutaline, bitolterol, and pirbuterol. Agents with β_2-selectivity dilate bronchioles without causing side effects related to β_1-stimulation (e.g., increased heart rate).

50

Osteoarthritis and Rheumatoid Arthritis

Tina Harrison Thornhill

I. DEFINITION AND CAUSE

A. Osteoarthritis (OA) is a common chronic condition of cartilage degeneration. Secondary changes can occur in the bone, leading to pain, decreased functioning, and even disability. OA affects nearly 21 million middle-aged and elderly Americans. It is the most common form of arthritis. Although not always symptomatic, most people over the age of 55 years have radiological evidence of the disease. Until age 55 years, OA affects men more frequently than women, but after age 55, women are more likely to have the disease.

B. Rheumatoid arthritis (RA) is a chronic, systemic autoimmune disease that involves inflammation in the membrane lining of the joints and often affects internal organs. Most patients exhibit a chronic fluctuating course of disease that can result in progressive joint destruction, deformity, and disability. RA affects 1% of the U.S. population. It occurs two to three times more often in women, and the peak onset occurs between the 4th and 6th decades of life.

II. NORMAL JOINT ANATOMY AND PHYSIOLOGY

A. The **synovial joint** consists of two bone ends covered by articular cartilage. The roles of articular cartilage include

1. Enabling frictionless movement of the joint

2. Distributing the load across the joint (shock absorber), to prevent damage

3. Promoting stability during use

B. Cartilage is avascular and aneural. It is metabolically active and undergoes continual internal remodeling. It is composed primarily of water but is also made from chondrocytes and extracellular matrix.

C. Chondrocytes control the synthesis and degradation of the matrix. They produce proteoglycans and collagen in the extracellular matrix to maintain the integrity of the matrix in healthy cartilage.

D. The **joint capsule** is a fibrous outer layer that encapsulates the joint. The joint capsule is lined by **synovium,** a membrane that produces a viscous fluid that lubricates the joint.

E. The **synovial fluid** is composed, in part, of hyaluronic acid. Glucosamine is a component of hyaluronic acid. The role of hyaluronic acid is to maintain functional and structural characteristics of the extracellular matrix.

F. Bursae are small sacs that are lined with synovial membrane and filled with fluid to provide cushioning and lubrication for the movement of the joint.

III. OSTEOARTHRITIS

A. Pathophysiology. The disease is not a normal part of the aging process; however, there are many age-related changes that contribute to the development of OA.

1. The strength of tendons, ligaments, and muscles declines with advancing age and may contribute to the development of the disease.

2. The number of chondrocytes declines owing to apoptosis (cell death), decreased proliferation, or both.

3. The synthesis of normal proteoglycans is reduced.

4. Chondrocytes lose the ability to promote healing and cartilage remodeling, resulting in cartilage matrix degradation. Proteoglycans are depleted.

5. Matrix metalloproteinases (MMPs) and proinflammatory cytokines promote cartilage degradation.

6. Interleukin 1 (IL-1) has several roles in the development of OA:
  a. Responsible for the induction of chondrocytes and synovial cells to synthesize MMPs
  b. Inhibits the synthesis of type II collagen and proteoglycans, preventing collagen from repairing itself
  c. Enhances nitric oxide production and induces chondrocyte apoptosis

7. Pain occurs as a result of
  a. Osteophytes (spurs of cartilage and bone at the joint)
  b. Synovitis
  c. Bursitis
  d. Tendonitis

B. Risk factors for OA include advanced age, female gender, muscle weakness, obesity, joint trauma, heredity, congenital or developmental anatomical defects, and repetitive stress.

C. Clinical presentation. OA is characterized by a deep, localized ache in a joint. Pain and stiffness usually occurs with rest or immobility and lasts < 30 min. Inflammation, if present, is mild. Patients will often complain of crepitus, a popping or cracking noise, heard in the joint upon moving. OA most commonly affects the hips, knees, neck, and hands.

D. DIAGNOSIS

1. Physical examination. Joint tenderness, diminished range of motion, crepitus, abnormalities in joint shape.

2. Laboratory tests. No specific lab tests are diagnostic for OA; however, if arthrocentesis is performed, synovial fluid will reveal mild leukocytosis with predominance of mononuclear lymphocytes.

3. Radiography. Narrowing of joint space (owing to loss of cartilage), subchondral sclerosis, and osteophytes are seen.

4. The American College of Rheumatology (ACR) has defined **criteria for OA of the hip, knee, and hand:**
  a. OA of the hip is characterized by hip pain and at least two of the following:
    (1) Erythrocyte sedimentation rate (ESR) < 20 mm/hr
    (2) Radiographic evidence of femoral or acetabular osteophytes
    (3) Radiographic evidence of joint space narrowing
  b. OA of the knee is characterized by knee pain, radiographic evidence of osteophytes, and at least one of the following:
    (1) Age > 50 years
    (2) Morning stiffness that lasts < 30 min
    (3) Articular crepitus on motion
  c. OA of the hand is characterized by hand pain, aching, or stiffness and at least three of the following:
    (1) Hard tissue enlargement of ≥ 2 distal interphalangeal (DIP) joints
    (2) Hard-tissue enlargement of ≥ 2 selected joints (2nd and 3rd DIP and/or proximal interphalangeal [PIP], and the 1st carpometacarpal joints of both hands)
    (3) Fewer than three swollen metacarpophalangeal (MCP) joints
    (4) Deformity of at least one of ten selected joints

E. Treatment

1. **Goals**
   a. Control pain and other symptoms
   b. Maintain or improve joint mobility
   c. Correct or minimize functional limitations and disability

2. **Nonpharmacological treatments**
   a. Patient education may include tips on joint protection, community exercise programs, and support groups.
   b. **Weight loss** (if overweight) has been shown to decrease pain and symptoms of OA.
   c. **Aerobic exercise programs;** bedrest and immobility are not necessary with OA.
   d. **Physical therapy** for range-of-motion exercises and strengthening.
   e. **Assistive devices** (e.g., canes, walkers, crutches) may help decrease the load on a joint; however, patients should be instructed on their proper use for safety.
   f. **Acupuncture** leads to improvements in pain and function after 26 weeks, compared to placebo or arthritis education in patients with mild knee OA.
   g. **Wedge insoles** can help reduce mechanical stress in persons with medial knee OA.
   h. **Thermal therapy** (e.g., hot shower or tub, ice pack) may be of benefit for some patients with OA.

3. **Pharmacological treatment**
   a. **Acetaminophen** (APAP) is considered first-line therapy by the ACR for OA of the hip or knee. It has excellent analgesic and antipyretic activity, but no anti-inflammatory effects.
      (1) A dose of $\leq$ 4 g/day is recommended to avoid toxicity. Concomitant use of other medications with acetaminophen should be evaluated closely to avoid overdose.
      (2) Hepatotoxicity can occur in patients taking > 4 g acetaminophen a day. Symptoms can include nausea, vomiting, abdominal pain, malaise, and diaphoresis. In patients with chronic stable liver disease, doses of up to 4 g/day did not cause any evidence of hepatotoxicity.
      (3) Because there is little, if any, inflammation in the OA joint, APAP has been shown to be equally efficacious as ibuprofen and naproxen in patients with mild to moderate OA pain.
   b. **Nonsteroidal anti-inflammatory drugs (NSAIDs)** and **cyclooxygenase 2 (COX-2) specific inhibitors** are indicated in OA treatment when the response to APAP is inadequate (Table 50-1).
      (1) **Mechanism of action.** NSAIDs are nonselective inhibitors of COX-1 and -2 as well as thromboxane synthetase.
      (2) **Analgesia** is seen with a short treatment duration and at lower doses (e.g., ibuprofen $\leq$ 1200 mg/day).
      (3) **Anti-inflammatory** response is seen with higher doses and usually requires several days of therapy to achieve anti-inflammatory affect.

Table 50-1. Selected Anti-Inflammatory Drugs

Generic (Brand)	Initial Daily Dose	Maximum Daily Dose
Nonacetylated salicylates		
Salsalate (Disalcid)	500 mg three times a day	3000 mg
Nonsteroidal anti-inflammatory drugs		
Aspirin (various)	650 mg every 4 hr	6000 mg
Diclofenac (Voltaren)	75 mg twice a day	200 mg
Ibuprofen (Motrin, Advil)	400 mg three times a day	3200 mg
Naproxen (Naprosyn, Aleve)	500 mg twice a day	1250 mg
Nabumetone (Relafen)	500 mg twice a day	2000 mg
Sulindac (Clinoril)	150 mg twice a day	400 mg
Tolmetin (Tolectin)	400 mg three times a day	1800 mg
Cyclooxygenase 2 inhibitors		
Celecoxib (Celebrex)	100 mg twice a day	400 mg

(4) Adverse effects

    (a) Gastrointestinal (GI) toxicity is caused by direct mucosal injury and inhibition of prostaglandins. Symptoms include dyspepsia, ulceration, and bleeding.

        (i) COX-2 inhibitors may be an option for patients with a history of peptic ulcer disease; however, the GI safety of these agents has not been demonstrated long term.

        (ii) People at risk for GI toxicity include the elderly and those with a history of peptic ulcer disease, chronic alcohol use, high-dose or multiple NSAID use, concomitant corticosteroid use, and NSAID treatment of < 3 months.

    (b) Renal toxicity results from the inhibition of prostaglandins. While the risks are low (~ 5%), it does not appear to be dose dependent and is usually reversible.

        (i) Effects can include hyperkalemia, hyponatremia, increased serum creatinine, sodium and water retention, and acute renal failure.

        (ii) People at risk for renal toxicity include the elderly and those with preexisting renal disease, hypertension, diabetes mellitus, congestive heart failure, cirrhosis, and volume depletion (e.g., hemorrhage, sepsis, diuretics, diarrhea).

    (c) Hematological effects are the result of decreased platelet aggregation.

    (d) Hepatic toxicity, although not common, can include elevated liver enzymes. Patients at risk include those with a history of hepatitis, alcoholism, and congestive heart failure.

    (e) CNS effects can include sedation, confusion, and mental status changes and are primarily seen in the elderly.

    (f) Allergic reactions, such as asthma, urticaria, and photosensitivity, may be seen. Cross-sensitivity has been seen in patients allergic to aspirin.

    (g) Cardiovascular (CV) effects (e.g., myocardial infarction, stroke, and heart failure) have been reported. Rofecoxib and valdecoxib were voluntarily withdrawn from the market in 2005 owing to their association with CV disease and mortality. Studies of celecoxib have shown a dose-related increase in CV events in patients with a history of colorectal neoplasia who were at risk of recurrent adenomatous polyps. The U.S. Food and Drug Administration (FDA) recommends using celecoxib at the lowest possible dose for least time possible. Hypertension has also been reported with the use of these agents and can increase the risk of CV disease.

c. Other oral analgesics

    (1) Tramadol (Ultram). Considered a good choice when the patient's pain is unrelieved by NSAIDs, when the patient cannot take NSAIDs, or when the patient experiences breakthrough pain while taking NSAIDs.

        (a) Mechanism of action. Centrally acting analgesic that inhibits the reuptake of norepinephrine and serotonin and mildly binds to the μ-receptor.

        (b) Dose. 50–100 mg every 4–6 hr, not to exceed 400 mg/day. In patients with impaired renal function (creatinine clearance [CrCl] < 30 mL/min), the dosage interval should be every 12 hr, with a maximum dose of 200 mg.

        (c) Adverse effects. Although it is not an opioid analgesic, its side effects are similar: nausea, constipation, rash, dizziness, somnolence, and orthostatic hypotension.

        (d) Drug interactions. Carbamazepine can decrease the effects of tramadol. Increased toxicity can occur with the concomitant use of quinidine, cimetidine, and selective serotonin reuptake inhibitors (SSRIs; e.g., paroxetine, sertraline, fluoxetine).

    (2) Opiate analgesics (codeine, oxycodone) are usually reserved for patients who fail single- or multiple-analgesic therapy. They may also be useful for acute exacerbations of pain. Side effects can include constipation, sedation, nausea, respiratory depression, and confusion.

    (3) Propoxyphene. The use of propoxyphene is controversial, as it has demonstrated efficacy similar to acetaminophen. The clinician must also consider the acetaminophen content (650 mg) of propoxyphene/acetaminophen (e.g., Darvocet-N 100 mg) and the potential for overdose. Propoxyphene should be avoided in the elderly.

    (4) Topical analgesics (e.g., capsaicin) are effective in relieving OA pain in some patients. Topical therapy can be used in conjunction with oral therapy or as monotherapy. Capsaicin is derived from hot chili peppers and with chronic use (> 2 weeks) works by depleting stores of substance P. Patients should be counseled to wash hands thoroughly after application to avoid contact with other skin to avoid burning and stinging.

(5) Intra-articular injections

(a) Corticosteroids may be useful in knee OA when inflammation is present but are not routinely recommended in hip OA owing to administration difficulties. Duration of action is up to 4 weeks. Because of adverse effects on the bone, injections should be limited to three or four per year. Long-term benefits and safety have not been established definitively.

(b) Hyaluronic acid derivatives. Indicated for the treatment of knee OA when treatment failure to other therapies occurs. Intended to improve elasticity and viscosity of synovial fluid. **Sodium hyaluronate (Hyalgan;** 2 mL weekly for 5 weeks) and **hylan polymers (Synvisc;** 2 mL weekly for 3 weeks) are the two agents currently available. Most benefits are seen after the last dose; effects are superior to placebo and comparable to corticosteroid injections. These agents should be used with caution in patients with allergies to avian proteins, feathers, and egg products. Patients should be counseled to avoid strenuous or prolonged (> 1 hr) weight-bearing activities within 48 hr after treatment.

(6) Adjunctive treatments

(a) Glucosamine acts as a substrate for and promotes the synthesis of the glycosaminoglycans.

(i) The dose is 500 mg three times a day.

(ii) Side effects may include GI discomfort, fatigue, and skin rash.

(b) Chondroitin helps protect against the breakdown of collagen and proteoglycans. It is usually found in combination with glucosamine, but the added benefits are not clear.

(i) The dose is 1200 mg/day.

(ii) Side effects can include prolonged bleeding time and nausea.

(c) The mechanism of **S-adenosylmethionine (SAMe)** is unclear; however, it does play a role in maintaining cartilage. The dose is 600 mg/day for 2 weeks, then 400 mg/day.

(7) Surgical interventions (e.g., arthroscopy, joint replacement) are considered when pain is severe and not responding to medical treatment or when disability interferes with daily activities.

IV. RHEUMATOID ARTHRITIS

A. Etiology and pathogenesis. The cause of RA is not fully understood but appears to be multifactorial. It is considered an autoimmune disease, in which the body loses its ability to distinguish between synovial and foreign tissue. Other factors involved in RA are as follows:

1. **Environmental influences,** such as bacterial and viral infections, are thought to play a role in the development of RA.

2. **Genetic markers,** such as human leukocyte antigen DR4 (HLA-DR4), have been associated with triggering the inflammatory process in RA. However, such markers are not considered diagnostic because as up to 30% of people with HLA-DR4 never develop RA.

3. **Tumor necrosis factor** α (TNF-α), **IL-1, IL-6,** and **growth factors** propagate the inflammatory process, and agents found to alter these cytokines show promise in reducing pain and deformity.

4. **Inflamed synovium** is a hallmark of the pathophysiology of RA. Synovium proliferates abnormally, growing into the joint space and into the bone, forming a pannus. The pannus migrates to the articular cartilage and into the subchondral bone. Through stimulation by the cytokines, the cells of the pannus produce proteolytic enzymes, which degrade cartilage. These same cytokines activate osteoclasts, which causes the demineralization of bone.

B. Clinical manifestations

1. The onset of RA is insidious. In early disease, symptoms include malaise and anorexia, accompanied by symmetrically tender and swollen joints. Pain in the joints is common and aggravated by movement.

2. Most commonly, the joints first affected by RA include the MCP and PIP joints of the hands, the metatarsophalangeal (MTP) joints, and the wrists. Other areas affected by RA include the spine, shoulder, ankle, and hip.

C. Clinical course. The severity of the disease is variable.

1. Within 4 months of diagnosis, irreversible joint damage is detectable on radiographic images. The rate at which joint damage occurs is greatest during the 1st year.

2. Prognosis is poorest with an early onset of the disease, significant functional disability during the 1st year, involvement of 20 or more joints, the presence of rheumatoid nodules, or extra-articular involvement.

3. Extra-articular manifestations can include rheumatoid nodules, anemia, peripheral neuropathy, kidney disease, CV effects, and pulmonary disease.

4. Osteoporosis may occur secondary to RA in patients receiving treatment with corticosteroids.

D. Diagnosis and clinical evaluation. The ACR classifies RA by having at least four of the following seven criteria, and the first four criteria must have been present for at least 6 weeks:

1. Morning stiffness for 1 hr

2. Arthritis of three or more joint areas of the hand, wrist, elbow, knee, ankle, or foot

3. Arthritis of hand joints—swelling in at least one area in a wrist, MCP, or PIP joint

4. Symmetrical arthritis—simultaneous involvement of the same joint areas on both sides of the body

5. Rheumatoid nodules—observable subcutaneous nodules, over bony prominences or extensor surfaces

6. Serum rheumatoid factor (see VIII.E.1)

7. Radiological changes (see VIII.F)

E. Laboratory assessment

1. **Rheumatoid factor (RF)** is found in $> 60\%$ of patients with RA; however, as many as 5% of healthy individuals will also have elevated titers of RF. If initially negative, the test can be repeated in 6–12 months. The most commonly found rheumatoid factors are IgM and IgG. IgA is also a good indicator because it correlates well with the ESR. RF is not an accurate measure of disease progression.

2. **ESR and C-reactive protein (CRP)** are markers of inflammation and are usually elevated in patients with RA. They can also help indicate the activity of the disease.

3. Because anemia is a common feature of RA, a **complete blood count (CBC)** should be regularly obtained. Anemia associated with RA tends to be hypochromic in 50%–100% of RA cases, and mild leukocytosis is evident in 25% of cases.

4. The **antinuclear antibody (ANA)** test is positive in 15% of patient with RA.

F. Radiographic examination. Baseline evaluations of the feet and hands are important to ascertain structural damage. As the disease progresses, evidence of periarticular osteopenia becomes apparent. The radiograph is a good indicator of the extent of bone erosion and cartilage loss. An MRI study detects the proliferative pannus.

G. Treatment objectives. The goals in the management of RA are

1. To prevent or control joint damage

2. To prevent loss of function

3. To decrease pain

4. To maintain the patient's quality of life

5. To avoid or minimize adverse effects of treatment

H. Prognosis. Poor prognosis is suggested by a high RF titer, elevated ESR, > 20 joints involved, onset of disease at an early age, and extra-articular involvement.

I. **Therapy**

1. **Nonpharmacological.** Optimal therapy involves both drug- and nondrug therapy. Patients should be instructed on joint protection and range-of-motion exercises. Regularly scheduled rest periods are important to reduce physical stress on the joints. Physical therapy and occupational therapy may help patients maintain their activities of daily living. Arthritis support groups may help with psychological well-being.

2. **Pharmacological.** Drug therapy for RA involves the treatment of symptoms and disease modifying agents. Drugs with anti-inflammatory activity are the agents of choice for the symptomatic relief of RA.

   a. **Salicylates, NSAIDs, and COX-2 inhibitors** reduce joint pain and swelling, but they do not alter the course of the disease or prevent joint destruction (Table 50-1).

   b. **Corticosteroids.** Low-dose systemic corticosteroids (e.g., prednisone, methylprednisolone) can work well either orally or parenterally. They have excellent anti-inflammatory activity and are immunosuppressants. The lowest effective dose should be used because of adverse effects (e.g., hyperglycemia, GI toxicity, osteoporosis). These agents have shown to slow joint damage; however, they are often used to "bridge" therapy as patients start on disease-modifying antirheumatic drugs or during an acute attack.

   c. **Disease-modifying antirheumatic drugs (DMARDs)** (Table 50-2). The objective of DMARD therapy is to reduce or prevent joint damage and preserve joint function.

      (1) The 2002 ACR guidelines recommend that DMARD therapy be initiated within 3 months of diagnosis, despite good control with NSAIDs.

      (2) The onset for most of these agents is prolonged; therefore, anti-inflammatory drugs are usually given concurrently as a bridge until therapeutic effects occur.

      (3) Factors such as cost, toxicity, compliance, and onset of action influence the selection of a DMARD.

      (4) Inflammatory markers (e.g., ESR, CRP) are reduced significantly by DMARDs, but not by NSAIDs.

         (a) **Methotrexate (MTX; Rheumatrex)** works by inhibiting dihydrofolate reductase and is considered standard therapy for RA. It is approved as monotherapy for RA.

         (b) **Leflunomide (Arava)** inhibits pyrimidine synthesis and is indicated as monotherapy for RA or can be used in combination with MTX.

            (i) Liver toxicity can develop within 6 months of use. Liver function tests should be performed as recommended by the manufacturer.

            (ii) In the event of serious adverse drug reactions, the use of cholestyramine is recommended to aid in the elimination of leflunomide because elimination can take up to 2 years without a binding agent.

            (iii) The average wholesale **cost of therapy** per year is $4500.

         (c) **Etanercept (Enbrel)** binds to TNF-α and -β, inhibiting the inflammatory response mediated by immune cells. It is indicated as monotherapy or in conjunction with methotrexate.

            (i) Immunosuppression occurs with the use of etanercept. Activation of tuberculosis has been reported. Lymphoma has been associated with its use; however, a clear cause and effect relationship has not been established.

            (ii) The average wholesale **cost of therapy** per year is $24,000.

         (d) **Infliximab (Remicade)** and **adalimumab (Humira)** bind to TNF-α. Infliximab is FDA-approved only in combination with methotrexate, but adalimumab can be used as monotherapy.

            (i) Like etanercept, **immunosuppression** is the most serious adverse effect. Tuberculosis has been associated with their use. Patients receiving concomitant therapy with other immunosuppressants should be closely monitored.

            (ii) The average wholesale **cost of therapy** per year is $15,000 plus infusion charges.

         (e) **Anakinra (Kineret)** is an IL-1 receptor antagonist. It is used as monotherapy or in conjunction with methotrexate.

            (i) **Immunosuppression** is the most serious adverse effect. Neutrophil counts should be monitored at baseline and monthly for 3 months, and quarterly

Table 50-2. Disease-Modifying Antirheumatic Drugs (DMARDs)

Agent (Brand)	Time to Effect (months)	Starting Dosing	Adverse Effects	Monitoring Parameters	Some Drug Interactions
More commonly used DMARDs					
Hydroxychloroquine (Plaquenil)	2–6	200–300 mg PO b.i.d.	Ocular toxicity, nausea, rash, myopathy	Eye exam, SrCr, CBC, LFTs	Cimetidine
Sulfasalazine (Azulfidine)	1–3	500 mg PO b.i.d; gradually increase to 2–3 g/day in 2–4 divided doses	Nausea, diarrhea, rash, photosensitivity	CBC, LFTs, SrCr	Iron, digoxin, warfarin
Methotrexate (Rheumatrex)	0.5–6	7.5–15 mg PO weekly	Nausea, diarrhea, mouth ulcers, hepatotoxicity, pulmonary toxicity, myelosuppression	LFTs, SrCr, CBC, chest x-ray	Penicillin, cyclosporine, NSAIDs
Less frequently used DMARDs					
Azathioprine (Imuran)	2–3	50–150 mg/day	Chills, fever, N/V, diarrhea, leukopenia, thrombocytopenia	CBC, LFTs	Allopurinol
Cyclosporine (Neoral)	2–4	3–10 mg/kg/day	HTN, HA, nausea, paresthesia, tremor, leukopenia	BP, SrCr, LFTs, serum drug levels	Cytochrome P450 3A3/4 inhibitors, glucocorticoids, MTX, digoxin, allopurinol
Gold salts (IM) (Aurolate)	3–6	25–50 mg IM every 2–4 weeks	Itching, rash, conjunctivitis, stomatitis, proteinuria	CBC with differential, renal function, urinalysis	Penicillamine
D-penicillamine (Cuprimine)	3–6	125–250 mg PO daily; increase gradually to 250 mg t.i.d.	Nausea, rash, photosensitivity, myelosuppression	urinalysis, CBC, SrCr	Gold, antimalarials, immunosuppressants, digoxin, iron, zinc, antacids
Newer DMARDs					
Leflunomide (Arava)	1–4	100 mg/day PO × 3 days (load), then 10–20 mg/day	Diarrhea, nausea, infection, rash, HTN, alopecia, liver toxicity	LFTs, CBC, SrCr, hepatitis B and C serology	MTX, rifampin, warfarin
Etanercept (Enbrel)	0.25–3	50 mg SC weekly or 25 mg SC twice a week	Abdominal pain, HA, injection site reactions, infections	PPD	Cyclophosphamide

(Continued on next page)

Table 50-2. Continued.

Agent (Brand)	Time to Effect (months)	Starting Dosing	Adverse Effects	Monitoring Parameters	Some Drug Interactions
Infliximab (Remicade)	0.5	3 mg/kg IV over 2 hr at weeks 0, 2, and 6; then every 8 weeks (maximum 10 mg/kg)	Nausea, HA, abdominal pain, dizziness, hematologic, hepatic, infections	PPD	None known
Adalimumab (Humira)	0.25–1	40 mg SC every 2 weeks	Injection site reactions, infection, HA, rash	PPD	None known
Anakinra (Kineret)	0.25–1	100 mg/day SQ	HA, injection site reactions, infections	CBC with neutrophil counts	Etanercept, thalidomide
Abatacept (Orencia)	n/d	10 mg/kg IV at day 0; then 2 weeks, 4 weeks, and continuing every 4 weeks	Injection site reactions, infections, HA, nausea, HTN, nasopharyngitis	PPD	None known

BP, blood pressure; *CBC,* complete blood count; *HA,* headache; *HTN,* hypertension; *IM,* intramuscularly; *IV,* intravenously; *LFTs,* liver function tests; *MTX,* methotrexate; *n/d,* no data available; *N/V,* nausea and vomiting; *NSAIDs,* nonsteroidal anti-inflammatory drugs; *PO,* by mouth; *PPD,* tuberculosis skin test; *SC,* subcutaneously; *SrCr,* serum creatinine.

for 1 year after initiation of therapy. The manufacturer cautions about the use of other immunosuppressants concurrently.

(ii) The average wholesale **cost of therapy** per year is $4000.

(f) **Abatacept (Orencia)** is the newest agent approved for the treatment of RA. Abatacept is the first selective modulator of a co-stimulatory signal required for full T cell activation. It is FDA approved for reducing the signs and symptoms of RA, inducing major clinical response, slowing the progression of structural damage, and improving physical function in adult patients with moderate to severe RA who have had an inadequate response to one or more DMARDs. It can be used as monotherapy or concomitantly with DMARDs; however, concurrent administration with TNF antagonists or anakinra is not recommended.

(i) **Immunosuppression** is the most serious adverse effect. Patients with a diagnosis of chronic obstructive pulmonary disease should be monitored closely for worsening respiratory status.

d. **Combination therapy.** Concurrent use of several DMARD agents has been studied. Patients with new symptoms or whose current DMARD therapy has failed have benefited from combination DMARD therapy. It is unclear when combination therapy should be initiated; however, instead of using a step-up approach to care, some evidence suggests using triple therapy (e.g., MTX, hydroxychloroquine, and sulfasalazine) and using a step-down approach. Careful monitoring for adverse effects should be maintained.

3. **Surgical treatment** (e.g., carpal tunnel release, total joint arthroplasty, joint fusion) may be considered when pain is severe, range of motion is lost, or joint function is poor owing to joint damage. Patients with good preoperative functional status generally have a relatively fast rate of recovery.

STUDY QUESTIONS

Directions for questions 1–3: The questions in this section can be correctly answered or completed by **one or more** of the suggested answers. Choose the answer, **A–E.**

A	if **I only** is correct
B	if **III only** is correct
C	if **I and II** are correct
D	if **II and III** are correct
E	if **I, II, and III** are correct

1. Which of the following statements best characterizes osteoarthritis (OA)?

(I) OA is a systemic disease that is characterized by profound, diffuse inflammation, resulting in joint destruction, deformity, and disability.

(II) OA is a common disorder characterized by cartilage degeneration that can cause joint pain, decreased functioning, and disability.

(III) OA, the most common form of arthritis, can result from age-related changes in the joint, loss of function of the chondrocytes, and proteoglycan depletion.

For questions 2–3: Betty is 65 years old; is obese; and has Type 2 diabetes mellitus, diabetic nephropathy, renal insufficiency, and hypertension. She works as a seamstress. She was active as a younger woman, played several sports and skied. She injured her right knee in a skiing accident. She complains of hand pain and stiffness and right knee pain and stiffness. Morning stiffness lasts < 30 min. No crepitus is heard on joint manipulation.

2. All of the following nonpharmacological treatments should be recommended for Betty *except*

(I) lose weight

(II) engage in aerobic exercise programs

(III) limit activity to ≤ 30 min at one time and rest the joint as often as possible

3. Which of the following pharmacological agents are relatively contraindicated for the treatment of Betty's osteoarthritis (OA)?

(I) oxycodone

(II) acetaminophen

(III) diclofenac

Directions for questions 4–8: Each of the questions, statements, or incomplete statements in this section can be correctly answered or completed by **one** of the suggested answers or phrases. Choose the **best** answer.

4. Which set of factors is associated with a poor prognosis of rheumatoid arthritis (RA)?

(A) absence of rheumatoid factor (RF), minimal inflammation, limited joint involvement at the onset

(B) age of disease onset ≥ 60 years, family history of the disease, high erythrocyte sedimentation rate (ESR)

(C) involvement of internal organs, poor response to aspirin, age of onset ≥ 60 years

(D) good response to methotrexate, presence of rheumatoid factor, low ESR

(E) high RF titer, elevated ESR, age of onset ≤ 25 years

5. All of the following statements are true about the use of hyaluronic acid derivatives *except* which one?

(A) Injections must be given in weekly intervals, and optimal effects are seen after the last dose.

(B) These are viable options for patients with osteoarthritis (OA) of the hip.

(C) Patients should avoid strenuous activities for 2 days after treatment.

(D) Use caution when prescribing these products to patients with allergy to eggs or feathers.

(E) These are considered second-line therapy when other treatments have failed.

6. Which of the following agents necessitates an ophthalmic examination to monitor for toxicity?

(A) penicillamine
(B) methotrexate
(C) hydroxychloroquine
(D) cyclosporine
(E) auranofin

7. Which of the following disease-modifying antirheumatic drugs (DMARDs) has the shorter onset of action?

(A) penicillamine
(B) hydroxychloroquine
(C) etanercept
(D) cyclosporine
(E) auranofin

8. Osteoporosis is associated with the use of which of the following drugs used in rheumatoid arthritis (RA)?

(A) leflunomide
(B) prednisone
(C) methotrexate
(D) penicillamine
(E) hydroxychloroquine

ANSWERS AND EXPLANATIONS

1. The answer is D *(I, II) [see IA; III.A.1–7].*
Osteoarthritis is not considered a disease of inflammation. Although there are times of minor inflammation (e.g., OA flare), it is localized to the affected joint(s).

2. The answer is B *(III) [see III.E.2].*
Nonpharmacological treatment should include aerobic exercise, physical therapy, joint protection, thermal therapy, and weight loss (if the patient is overweight).

3. The answer is B *(III) [see III.E.4.b.(ii)].*
Patients at higher risk of renal toxicity include the elderly; patients with hypertension, diabetes, congestive heart failure, or cirrhosis; patients who are volume depleted; and patients who have preexisting renal disease.

4. The answer is E *[see IV.H].*
Factors associated with a poor prognosis for RA include > 20 joints involved, extra-articular involvement, onset of the disease at an early age, high RF titers, and an elevated ESR.

5. The answer is B *[see III.E.3.c;5.b.].*
Hyaluronic acid derivatives are indicated only for OA of the knee.

6. The answer is C *[see Table 50-2].*
An ophthalmic exam is recommended when patients are receiving hydroxychloroquine.

7. The answer is C *[see Table 50-2].*
All DMARDs have a fairly long onset of action; however, etanercept and infliximab are associated with the shortest onset of action.

8. The answer is B *[see IV.I.2.b.].*
Steroid (e.g., prednisone) use can lead to osteoporosis; therefore, patients taking prednisone should consider therapy with calcium and a bisphosphonate.

51
Hyperuricemia and Gout

Larry N. Swanson

I. INTRODUCTION

A. Definitions

1. **Hyperuricemia** refers to a serum uric acid level that is elevated more than two standard deviations above the population mean. In most laboratories, the upper limit of normal is 7 mg/dL (uricase method). However, the level varies with the laboratory method used; the upper limit of normal is about 1 mg/dL lower for women than for men.

2. **Gout** is a disease that is characterized by recurrent acute attacks of urate crystal-induced arthritis. It may include **tophi**—deposits of monosodium urate—in and around the joints and cartilage and in the kidneys, as well as uric acid nephrolithiasis.

B. General information

1. The prevalence of gout is believed to be 8.4 per 1000 individuals in the United States but this estimate is based on patient self-reporting; thus this figure may overestimate the true prevalence.

2. Most gout victims are men (approximately 95% of cases); most women with the disease are postmenopausal.

3. The mean age at disease onset is 47 years.

4. The risk of developing gout increases as the serum uric acid level rises. Virtually all gout patients have a serum uric acid level > 7 mg/dL.

5. Research shows that among patients with a serum uric acid level above 9 mg/dL, the cumulative incidence of gout reached 22% after 5 years.

6. Gout has a familial tendency; 10%–60% of cases occur in family members of patients with the disease.

7. Obesity, hypertension, hyperlipidemia, atherosclerosis, and alcohol abuse are often associated with hyperuricemia and gout. Certain nutritional strategies (i.e., achieving ideal body weight or limitation of alcohol intake) can treat both the hyperuricemia and the associated conditions.

C. Uric acid production and excretion

1. Uric acid, an end product of **purine metabolism,** is produced from both dietary and endogenous sources. Its formation results from the conversion of adenine and guanine moieties of nucleoproteins and nucleotides (Figure 51-1).

2. **Xanthine oxidase** catalyzes the reaction that occurs as the final step in the degradation of purines to uric acid.

3. The body ultimately excretes uric acid via the kidneys (300–600 mg/day; two thirds of total uric acid) and via the gastrointestinal (GI) tract (100–300 mg/day; one third of the total uric acid).

4. Uric acid has no known biological function.

5. The body has a total uric acid content of 1.0–1.2 g; the daily turnover rate is 600–800 mg.

6. At a pH of 4.0–5.0 (i.e., in urine), uric acid exists as a poorly soluble free acid; at physiological pH, it exists primarily as **monosodium urate salt.**

7. Uric acid filtration, reabsorption, and secretion sites are shown in Figure 51-2.

Figure 51-1. Uric acid formation. *HGPRT,* hypoxanthine–guanine phosphoribosyltransferase; *PRPP,* phosphoribosyl-1-pyrophosphate. [Adapted with permission from DiPiro J, Talbert R, Yee G, et al. Pharmacotherapy—A Pathophysiologic Approach, 5th ed. The McGraw-Hill companies, 2002:1660.]

D. Cause. Hyperuricemia and gout may be primary or secondary.

  1. Primary hyperuricemia and **gout** apparently result from an innate **defect in purine metabolism** or **uric acid excretion.** The exact cause of the defect usually is unknown.
    a. Hyperuricemia may result from **uric acid overproduction, impaired renal clearance of uric acid,** or a **combination** of these.
    b. Some patients with primary hyperuricemia and gout have a known enzymatic defect, such as hypoxanthine–guanine phosphoribosyltransferase (HGPRT) deficiency or phosphoribosyl-1-pyrophosphate (PRPP) synthetase excess (Figure 51-1).
    c. Principally for therapeutic purposes, patients with primary hyperuricemia and gout can be classified as **overproducers** or **underexcretors** of uric acid.
      (1) Overproducers (about 10% of patients) synthesize abnormally large amounts of uric acid and excrete excessive amounts: > 800–1000 mg daily on an unrestricted diet

Figure 51-2. Uric acid filtration, reabsorption, and secretion sites. At the glomerulus, uric acid is filtered and enters the proximal tubule. There, approximately 99% of uric acid is reabsorbed into the bloodstream. At the distal tubule, uric acid is secreted; subsequently, about 75% of the amount secreted is reabsorbed. Therefore, almost all urinary uric acid is excreted at the distal tubule.

or > 600 mg daily on a purine-restricted diet. These individuals generally have a markedly increased miscible urate pool (> 2.5 g).

    (2) Underexcretors (about 90% of patients) generally produce normal or nearly normal amounts of uric acid but excrete < 600 mg daily on a purine-restricted diet. They generally have only a slightly increased miscible urate pool. Some underexcretors are also overproducers.

  2. Secondary hyperuricemia and **gout** develop during the course of another disease or as a result of drug therapy.

    a. Hematological causes of hyperuricemia and gout (associated with increased nucleic acid turnover and breakdown to uric acid)

      (1) Lymphoproliferative disorders

      (2) Myeloproliferative disorders

      (3) Certain hemolytic anemias and hemoglobinopathies

    b. Chronic renal failure. In this condition, reduced renal clearance of uric acid can lead to hyperuricemia.

    c. Drug-induced disease

      (1) Aspirin and **other salicylates** inhibit tubular secretion of uric acid when given in low doses (e.g., < 2 g/day of aspirin). At high doses, these agents frequently cause uricosuria.

      (2) Cytotoxic drugs increase uric acid concentrations by enhancing nucleic acid turnover and excretion.

      (3) Diuretics (except spironolactone) may cause hyperuricemia; most likely, this occurs either via volume depletion, which, in turn, increases proximal tubular reabsorption, or via impaired tubular secretion of uric acid.

      (4) Ethambutol and **nicotinic acid** increase uric acid concentrations by competing with urate for tubular secretion sites, thereby decreasing uric acid excretion.

(5) **Cyclosporine** decreases renal urate clearance, as do pyrazinamide and levodopa.

(6) **Ethanol** alters uric acid metabolism both by **increasing uric acid production** through an increase in adenine nucleotide catabolism and by **suppressing renal uric acid excretion** as a result of lactate inhibition of renal tubular uric acid secretion.

  d. **Miscellaneous disorders.** Diabetic ketoacidosis, psoriasis, and chronic lead poisoning are examples of conditions that may cause hyperuricemia.

E. **Pathophysiology**

1. Gouty arthritis develops when **monosodium urate crystals** are deposited in the synovium of involved joints.

2. An **inflammatory response** to monosodium urate crystals leads to an attack of acute gouty arthritis; painful joint swelling is characterized by redness, warmth, and tenderness. A systemic reaction may accompany joint symptoms.

3. If gout progresses untreated, **tophi,** or **tophaceous deposits** (deposits of monosodium urate crystals) eventually lead to joint deformity and disability; kidney involvement may lead to renal impairment. However, these developments are uncommon in the general gout population and represent late complications of hyperuricemia.

4. **Renal complications** of hyperuricemia and gout can have serious consequences.
  a. **Acute tubular obstruction**
    (1) This complication may develop secondary to uric acid precipitation in the collecting tubules and ureters, with subsequent blockage and renal failure. It is most common in patients with gout secondary to myeloproliferative or lymphoproliferative disorders, particularly after chemotherapy when allopurinol is omitted.
    (2) Another agent, **urate oxidase** (Rasburicase), may be used in the prophylaxis and treatment of hyperuricemia in pediatric patients with leukemia, lymphoma, and solid-tumor malignancies who are receiving anticancer therapy. This agent works by converting uric acid into allantoin, which is five times more soluble in urine than uric acid.
  b. **Urolithiasis.** Occurring in about 20% of gout patients, urolithiasis is characterized by formation of uric acid stones in the urinary tract. Low urine pH seems to be a contributing factor. The risk of urolithiasis rises as serum and urinary uric acid levels increase.
  c. **Chronic urate nephropathy.** In this complication, urate deposits arise in the renal interstitium. Most clinicians agree, however, that chronic hyperuricemia rarely, if ever, leads to clinically significant nephropathy. The presence of concomitant disease (e.g., diabetes mellitus, hypertension) may explain the finding of nephropathy in gout patients.

F. **Clinical presentation.** Clinical evaluation and the need for intervention depend on the clinical presentation.

1. **Asymptomatic hyperuricemia**

2. **Acute gouty arthritis**

3. **Intercritical gout**

4. **Chronic tophaceous gout**

II. ASYMPTOMATIC HYPERURICEMIA is characterized by an elevated serum uric acid level but has no signs or symptoms of deposition disease (arthritis, tophi, or urolithiasis).

A. **Clinical presentation.** No definitive evidence indicates that asymptomatic hyperuricemia is harmful. Serum urate levels of up to 13 mg/dL in men and 10 mg/L in women have not been shown to cause a deterioration in renal function. Clinicians cannot predict which asymptomatic patients will develop gout symptoms or hyperuricemia-related complications. However, the risk of symptom development and complications increases as the serum uric acid level rises.

B. **Therapy.** Asymptomatic hyperuricemia does not have any adverse effects before the development of gout. Therefore, **drug treatment is not required,** although it is prudent to determine the causes of the hyperuricemia and correct them, if possible. **Supportive interventions** may include maintenance of adequate urine output (to prevent uric acid stone formation), avoidance of high purine foods, and regular medical appointments to monitor the serum uric acid level and check for clinical evidence of deposition disease.

III. ACUTE GOUTY ARTHRITIS. This clinical presentation of gout is characterized by **painful arthritic attacks** of sudden onset.

   A. Pathogenesis. Monosodium urate crystals form in articular tissues; this process sets off an inflammatory reaction. Trauma, exposure to cold, or another triggering event may be involved in the development of the acute attack.

   B. Signs and symptoms

      1. The **initial attack** is abrupt, usually occurring at night or in the early morning as synovial fluid is reabsorbed. This severe arthritic pain progressively worsens and generally involves only one or a few joints.

         a. The **affected joints** typically become hot, swollen, and extremely tender. Seventeenth-century British physician Thomas Sydenham described his personal experience with gout this way: "Now it is a violent stretching and tearing of the ligaments—now, it is a gnawing pain and now a pressure and tightening. So exquisite and lively . . . is the feeling of the part affected, that it cannot bear the weight of bedclothes nor the jar of a person walking in the room."

         b. The **most common site** of the initial attack is the **first metatarsophalangeal joint;** an attack there is known as **podagra.** Other sites that may be affected include the instep, ankle, heel, knee, wrist, elbow, and fingers.

      2. The first few untreated attacks typically last 3–14 days. Later attacks may affect more joints and take several weeks to resolve.

      3. During recovery, as edema subsides, local desquamation and pruritus may occur.

      4. Systemic symptoms during an acute attack may include fever, chills, and malaise.

   C. Diagnostic criteria

      1. Definitive diagnosis of gouty arthritis can be made by demonstration of **monosodium urate crystals** in the synovial fluid of affected joints. These needle-shaped crystals are termed negatively birefringent when viewed through a polarized light microscope.

      2. Serum analysis usually reveals an above-normal uric acid level: however, this finding is not specific for acute gout. Other **common serum findings** include leukocytosis and a moderately elevated erythrocyte sedimentation rate.

      3. A **dramatic therapeutic response to colchicine** may be helpful in establishing the diagnosis, but this is not absolute because other causes of acute arthritis may respond as well.

      4. When fluid cannot be aspirated from the affected joint, a **diagnosis of gout is supported by:**

         a. A prior **history of acute monarticular arthritis** (especially of the **big toe**) followed by a **symptom-free period**

         b. The presence of **hyperuricemia**

         c. Rapid **resolution of symptoms after colchicine** therapy

      5. Other conditions that may **mimic** gout include pseudogout (calcium pyrophosphate dihydrate crystal disease) or septic arthritis.

   D. Treatment goals

      1. To relieve pain and inflammation

      2. To terminate the acute attack

      3. To restore normal function to the affected joints

   E. Therapy

      1. General therapeutic principles

         a. The affected joint (or joints) should be immobilized.

         b. Anti-inflammatory drug therapy should begin immediately. For maximal therapeutic effectiveness, these drugs should be kept on hand so that the patient may begin therapy as soon as a subsequent attack begins.

c. Urate-lowering drugs **should not be given until the acute attack is controlled,** as these drugs may prolong the attack by causing a change in uric acid equilibrium.

2. Specific drugs. Any of the following agents may be used:

a. Nonsteroidal anti-inflammatory drugs (NSAIDs)

(1) Indications. Most physicians consider these drugs the agents of choice, especially the newer NSAIDs. These drugs may be preferred when treatment is delayed significantly after symptom onset or when the patient cannot tolerate the adverse GI effects of colchicine.

(a) Indomethacin (Indocin) is usually given in a dose of 50 mg three times daily until pain is tolerable; then the dose is rapidly reduced to complete cessation of the drug. Definite relief of pain usually occurs within 2–4 hr. Tenderness and heat usually subside in 24–36 hr, and swelling gradually disappears in 3–5 days. Do not use the sustained-release dosage form.

(b) Specific NSAIDs—such as **naproxen** (Naprosyn) 750 mg followed by 250 mg every 8 hr until the attack subsides or **sulindac** (Clinoril) 200 mg twice a day to start, reducing the dose with satisfactory response (7 days of therapy are usually adequate)—are specifically approved for this indication, but many other NSAIDs have been used successfully. There is no evidence that any particular NSAID is more effective than others in the treatment of an acute gouty attack. Some have also used selective cyclooxygenase 2 (COX-2) inhibitors for these attacks.

(2) Precautions and monitoring effects

(a) Adverse effects of indomethacin are usually dose related. These effects occur in 10%–60% of patients and may warrant drug discontinuation. They primarily include GI complaints of nausea and abdominal discomfort and central nervous system (CNS) effects of headaches and dizziness. Indomethacin should be taken with food or milk to minimize gastric mucosal irritation.

(b) Precautions. NSAIDs, in general, require cautious use in patients with a history of hypertension, congestive heart failure (CHF), peptic ulcer disease, or mild to moderate renal failure.

b. Colchicine. The traditional drug for relieving pain and inflammation and ending the acute attack, colchicine is most effective when initiated 12–36 hr after symptoms begin (the period of maximal leukocyte migration). Some would use this agent only if the patient is intolerant to NSAIDs or for those who have used colchicine successfully in the past.

(1) Mechanism of action. Colchicine apparently **impairs leukocyte migration** to inflamed areas and disrupts urate deposition and the subsequent inflammatory response.

(2) Dosage and administration

(a) Oral regimen

(i) The effective dose of colchicine in patients with acute gout is close to that which causes GI symptoms. The drug usually is administered orally in a dose of 1.2 mg initially, followed by 0.6 mg every 2 hr until pain relief occurs or abdominal discomfort or diarrhea develops or a total dose of 8 mg has been administered. Except in patients who have renal or hepatic dysfunction or are elderly and frail, colchicine given in this way is safe, although it entails some discomfort for the patient.

(ii) Most patients have some pain relief by 18 hr and diarrhea by 24 hr; joint inflammation subsides gradually within 48 hr for 75%–80% of patients.

(iii) During **subsequent attacks,** patients may receive half of the total dose administered for the initial attack, then receive the remaining half as 0.6 mg every 1–2 hr.

(b) Intravenous (IV) regimen. This route is used rarely now when NSAIDs are contraindicated or when patients cannot take oral medications.

(i) A single dose of 2 mg usually is given in 30 mL of normal saline solution and infused slowly over 5 min. Two additional doses of 1 mg each may be given at 6-hr intervals, but the total dose should **never exceed 4 mg.** The doses should be reduced by at least 50% in patients with hepatic or renal disease or in elderly patients. Because it causes tissue irritation, colchicine should **never be given intramuscularly or subcutaneously.**

(ii) IV administration may relieve acute gouty arthritis more rapidly than oral administration. However, severe toxicity may occur without warning because the early signs of toxicity (e.g., GI hypermobility) may not occur.

(3) Precautions and monitoring effects
  (a) GI distress (e.g., nausea, abdominal cramps, diarrhea) occurs in up to 80% of patients receiving oral colchicine. This dosage form should be avoided in patients with peptic ulcer disease and other GI disorders.
  (b) Local extravasation (causing local pain and necrosis) can occur with administration of IV colchicine. This risk can be reduced by use of a secure IV line.
  (c) Colchicine therapy may cause bone marrow depression. This rare effect develops mainly in patients who receive excessive doses or who have underlying renal or hepatic disease. Excessively high acute doses (especially given intravenously) or long-term therapy may result in neurological, renal, hepatic, or other toxicity.
c. Corticosteroids
  (1) Intra-articular injections of a corticosteroid are usually very effective in patients with acute monarticular gout, and their use is becoming more widespread as experience with the diagnostic aspiration of joints increases. Aspiration alone can sometimes greatly reduce the pain of gout. The appropriate dose of corticosteroids is related to the size of the joint: An intra-articular dose of **triamcinolone hexacetonide** (e.g., Aristospan intra-articular) 20–40 mg for a large joint such as the knee and lower doses for smaller joints
  (2) Systemic corticosteroid therapy is administered usually only when NSAIDs and colchicine have been ineffective or are contraindicated. There are reports of good responses, without a rebound effect, to **oral prednisone** (30–50 mg per day initially, with the dose tapered during a period of 7–10 days). **IV glucocorticoids** or **subcutaneous ACTH** are options if patients can't receive oral prednisone. One approach is to give 40-80 USP units of adrenocorticotropic hormone (ACTH) twice daily for 2 days and then once daily for several additional days as needed. Others have used 40 U as a single injection.

IV. INTERCRITICAL GOUT is the symptom-free period after the first attack. This phase may be interrupted by the recurrence of acute attacks.

A. Onset of subsequent attacks varies. In most patients, the second attack occurs within 1 year of the first, but in some it may be delayed for 5–10 years. A small percentage of patients never experience a second attack. If hyperuricemia is insufficiently treated, subsequent attacks may become progressively longer and more severe and may involve more than one joint.

B. Treatment goals

1. To reduce the frequency and severity of recurrent attacks

2. To minimize urate deposition in body tissues, thereby preventing progression to chronic tophaceous gout

C. Therapy. Gout can be prevented by identifying and correcting the cause of hyperuricemia or by administering drugs that inhibit the synthesis of urate or increase its excretion.

1. Nondrug urate-reducing measures. Potentially reversible factors that contribute to increased urate production include a high-purine diet (e.g., all meats, including organ meats, seafood, beans, peas, asparagus), obesity, and regular alcohol consumption. The purine content of the diet does not usually contribute more than 1.0 mg/dL to the serum urate concentration, but moderation in dietary purine consumption should be considered. Weight reduction sometimes reduces the serum uric acid level slightly; however, crash diets should be avoided. Drinking two or more beers increased the risk of gout by 2.5-fold in one study vs. a 1.6-fold increase for other spirits. Wine was not associated with an increased risk of gout.

2. Prophylaxis after resolution of an acute gout attack may consist of **low-dose colchicine,** 0.6 mg twice daily in the patient with normal renal function.
  a. Adverse effects from colchicine at these doses are usually uncommon. In patients, particularly the elderly, who develop loose or diarrheal stools, 0.6 mg daily or every other day might suffice.
  b. Low-dose NSAIDs may also be used, but the incidence of side effects is typically higher than with low doses of colchicine.

c. Generally, prophylaxis is administered for 6 months after normal serum uric acid levels are achieved. Prolonged use of these agents may prevent recurrent episodes of gouty arthritis, but they do not prevent the development of silent bony erosions and tophi deposits.

3. Urate-reducing drug therapy. Gout may be prevented by reducing serum urate concentrations to values < 6.0 mg/dL. A reduction to < 5.0 mg/dL may be required for the resorption of tophi. The decision to begin drug therapy should be carefully considered, as urate-lowering drug treatment should be lifelong. Urate-reducing drugs include **uricosurics,** which increase renal uric acid excretion, and the xanthine oxidase inhibitor, **allopurinol,** which reduces uric acid production.

   a. Indications for therapy with a drug that lowers serum urate concentrations should be considered when **all** of the following criteria are met:

   (1) The cause of the hyperuricemia cannot be corrected or, if corrected, does not lower the serum urate concentration to < 7.0 mg/dL.

   (2) The patient has had two or three definite attacks of gout or has tophi.

   (3) The patient is convinced of the need to take medication regularly and permanently.

   b. Specific drugs

   (1) Uricosurics include **probenecid** (Benemid) and **sulfinpyrazone** (Anturane). These drugs are preferred for underexcretors. Long-term uricosuric therapy reduces the incidence of gouty arthritis attacks, prevents formation of new tophi, and helps resolve existing tophi.

   (a) Mechanism of action. Probenecid and sulfinpyrazone block uric acid reabsorption at the proximal convoluted tubule, thereby increasing the rate of uric acid excretion (Figure 51-2).

   (b) Indications. Uricosurics generally are used to reduce hyperuricemia in patients who excrete < 600 mg of uric acid per day.

   (c) Dosage and administration

   (i) Probenecid is given initially in two daily oral doses of 250 mg for 1 week, then increased to 500 mg twice daily every 1–2 weeks until the serum uric acid level drops below 6 mg/dL. Most patients respond to a dose of 1.5 g/day or less.

   (ii) Sulfinpyrazone is given initially in two daily oral doses of 50 mg, then increased by 100 mg weekly. Most patients respond to a dose of 200 mg/day or less.

   (d) Precautions and monitoring effects

   (i) Uricosuric therapy **should not be initiated during an acute gout attack.** During the first 6–12 months of therapy, these drugs may increase the frequency, severity, and duration of acute attacks (by changing the equilibrium of body urate). Therefore, some clinicians administer prophylactic colchicine concomitantly during the early months of uricosuric therapy.

   (ii) The **risk** is **minimized** by concurrently **administering prophylactic drugs** (see IV.C.2), delaying urate-lowering therapy until several weeks after the last attack of gout, and starting therapy with a low dose of the drug that is chosen. When used concurrently with urate-lowering drugs, colchicine may be discontinued after the serum urate level becomes normal and is stable for 6 months.

   (iii) Patients should maintain a **high fluid intake** (at least 2 L/day) and a high urine output during uricosuric therapy to decrease renal urate precipitation. The **greatest potential risks** of therapy with uricosuric drugs are the formation of **uric acid crystals** in urine and the deposition of **uric acid** in the **renal tubules, pelvis,** or **ureter,** causing renal colic or the deterioration of renal function. These risks can be reduced by initiating therapy with a low dose and increasing the dose slowly and by maintaining a high urine volume. Alkalinization of the urine is usually not necessary (but can be achieved with 1 g of sodium bicarbonate taken 3–4 times daily; plus a high fluid intake of at least 2 L/day).

   (iv) Uricosurics are **contraindicated** in patients with urinary tract stones.

   (v) These drugs generally are ineffective in patients with creatinine clearances below 50–60 ml/min.

- **(vi)** **Aspirin** and **other salicylates** antagonize the action of uricosurics. **Daily low dose aspirin** for antiplatelet function **probably does not have this effect**. In a small study, the addition of low dose aspirin to probenecid therapy did not alter the daily excretion of uric acid nor the serum uric acid level.
- **(vii)** **Probenecid** is well tolerated by most patients, but it occasionally causes **adverse effects**—for example, GI distress (8%) and hypersensitivity reactions (5%).
- **(viii)** **Sulfinpyrazone** causes GI distress in 10%–15% of patients. Hypersensitivity reactions occur rarely. Sulfinpyrazone reduces platelet adhesiveness and may cause blood dyscrasias; periodic blood counts should be done.

(2) The only **xanthine oxidase inhibitor** available on the U.S. market is **allopurinol.**

- **(a)** **Mechanism of action.** Allopurinol and its long-acting metabolite, **oxypurinol,** block the final steps in uric acid synthesis by inhibiting xanthine oxidase, an enzyme that converts xanthine to uric acid (Figure 51-1). Thus the drug reduces the serum uric acid level while increasing the renal excretion of the more soluble oxypurine precursors; this decreases the risk of uric acid stones and nephropathy.
- **(b)** **Indications.** Allopurinol is considered by many to be the drug of choice for lowering uric acid levels because of its effectiveness in both underexcretors and overproducers, but it is specifically the preferred urate-reducing agent for patients in the following categories:
  - **(i)** Patients who are clearly overproducers (overexcretors) of uric acid
  - **(ii)** Patients with recurrent tophaceous deposits or uric acid stones
  - **(iii)** Patients with renal impairment (but dose needs to be decreased)
- **(c)** **Dosage and administration.** Allopurinol is given initially in a daily dose of 100–300 mg (preferably as a single dose), then increased in weekly increments if needed. Typically, the uric acid level starts to fall after 1–2 days with maximal effect for a given dose in 7–10 days. A dose of 300 mg/day reduces serum urate concentrations to normal values in 85% of patients with gout. The normal dose of 300 mg/day is for a patient with normal renal function; the dose should be decreased to 200 mg/day for a patient with a creatinine clearance (CrCl) of 60 mL/min and to 100 mg/day for a patient with a CrCl of 30 mL/min.
- **(d)** **Precautions and monitoring effects.** Allopurinol is generally well tolerated.
  - **(i)** A **rash** develops in approximately 2% of patients treated with allopurinol and in approximately 20% of those receiving both allopurinol and ampicillin. The rash usually subsides after the allopurinol has been discontinued and may not recur if therapy is resumed with a lower dose.
  - **(ii)** The most serious side effect of allopurinol, which occurs in < 1 in 1000 cases, is **exfoliative dermatitis,** often with vasculitis, fever, liver dysfunction, eosinophilia, and acute interstitial nephritis. Up to 20% of patients with this type of reaction become very sick. It is more likely to occur in patients with renal disease or those receiving diuretic therapy. Prednisone seems to be effective in such patients, but the discontinuation of allopurinol and the use of supportive therapy may be sufficient in cases that are not severe.
  - **(iii)** Allopurinol may induce more frequent acute gout attacks. This risk can be minimized by administration of low doses and concurrent colchicine therapy.

(3) **Other drugs that increase uric acid excretion**

- **(a)** **Losartan** (Cozaar)**,** an angiotensin II receptor blocker (ARB), might be a useful antihypertensive agent in the patient who has **both hyperuricemia and hypertension** because this agent can lower serum uric acid levels by inhibiting the uptake of uric acid by the urate anion exchange transporter in the proximal tubule. This effect is minimal or not seen in other ARBs.
- **(b)** **Fenofibrate** (TriCor) is a fibric acid agent used to treat elevated cholesterol and triglyceride levels. It has been shown to decrease serum uric levels by increasing renal uric acid clearance and would be a useful agent in the patient with **both hyperlipidemia and hyperuricemia.**
- **(c)** **Febuxostat,** a non-purine-base analog xanthine oxidase inhibitor, is an investigational agent that may eventually reach the U.S. market.

V. CHRONIC TOPHACEOUS GOUT.
This rare clinical presentation may develop if hyperuricemia and gout remain untreated for many years.

A. **Pathogenesis.** Persistent hyperuricemia leads to the development of tophi in the synovia, olecranon bursae, and various periarticular locations. Eventually, articular cartilage may be destroyed, resulting in joint deformities, bone erosions, deposition of tophi within tissues, and renal disease.

B. **Clinical evaluation**

1. Patients may develop large subcutaneous tophi in the pinna of the external ear (the classic site) as well as in other locations.

2. Typically, the urate pool is many times the normal size.

C. **Therapy.** Allopurinol and probenecid may be given in combination to treat severe cases.

STUDY QUESTIONS

Directions for questions 1–3: Each of the questions, statements, or incomplete statements in this section can be correctly answered or completed by **one** of the suggested answers or phrases. Choose the **best** answer.

1. All of the following statements concerning an acute gouty arthritis attack are correct *except* which one?

(A) The diagnosis of gout is ensured by a good therapeutic response to colchicine because no other form of arthritis responds to this drug.

(B) To be ensured of the diagnosis, monosodium urate crystals must be identified in the synovial fluid of the affected joint.

(C) Attacks frequently occur in the middle of the night.

(D) An untreated attack may last up to 2 weeks.

(E) The first attack usually involves only one joint, most frequently the big toe (first metatarsophalangeal joint).

2. A 42-year-old obese man has been diagnosed with gout. He has had three acute attacks this year, and his uric acid level is presently 11.5 mg/dL (upper limit of normal is 7 mg/dL). He has no other diseases. Rational treatment of this patient during the interval period between gouty attacks might include any of the following *except*

(A) acetaminophen or aspirin 650 mg as needed for joint pain.

(B) probenecid.

(C) colchicine.

(D) allopurinol.

(E) a decrease in caloric intake.

3. A 45-year-old man is admitted to the hospital with the diagnosis of an acute attack of gout. His serum uric acid is 10.5 mg/dL (normal is 3–7 mg/dL). Which of the following would be the most effective initial treatment plan?

(A) Before treating this patient, immobilize the affected joint and obtain a 24-hr urinary uric acid level to determine which drug, either allopurinol or probenecid, would be the best agent to initiate therapy.

(B) Begin oral colchicine 1.2 mg initially, followed by 0.6 mg every 2 hr until relief is obtained, gastrointestinal distress occurs, or a maximum of 8 mg has been taken; also, begin probenecid 250 mg twice a day concurrently.

(C) Administer oral indomethacin 50 mg three times a day for 2 days; then gradually taper the dose over the next few days.

(D) Administer oral naproxen 750 mg, followed by 250 mg every 8 hr for 3 weeks.

(E) Give colchicine 0.5 mg intramuscularly followed by 1 mg intravenous piggyback every 12 hr for 2 weeks.

Directions for question 4: The question in this section can be correctly answered or completed by **one or more** of the suggested answers. Choose the answer, **A–E.**

A	if **I only** is correct
B	if **III only** is correct
C	if **I and II** are correct
D	if **II and III** are correct
E	if **I, II, and III** are correct

4. Allopurinol is recommended instead of probenecid in the treatment of hyperuricemia in which of the following situations?

(I) when the patient has several large tophi on the elbows and knees
(II) when the patient has an estimated creatinine clearance of 15 mL/min
(III) when the patient has leukemia and there is concern regarding renal precipitation of urate

Directions for question 5: The incomplete statement in this section can be correctly answered or completed by **one** of the suggested answers or phrases. Choose the **best** answer.

5. In a patient who has had documented gouty arthritis and hyperuricemia and who also has hypertension, a preferred antihypertensive agent would be

(A) hydrochlorothiazide
(B) losartan
(C) clonidine
(D) lisinopril
(E) irbesartan

ANSWERS AND EXPLANATIONS

1. The answer is A *[see III.B.1–2; III.C.1; III.C.3].*
Other forms of acute arthritis may respond to colchicine, so that the diagnosis of gout cannot be established unequivocally by a good response to this agent. A definitive diagnosis requires the presence of urate crystals in the affected joint, although the presence of other symptoms or laboratory findings may suggest a probable diagnosis of gout.

2. The answer is A *[see I.D.2.c.(1); IV.C].*
Aspirin in doses < 2 g/day can inhibit uric acid secretion. Weight reduction, allopurinol or probenecid to lower the serum uric acid levels, and prophylactic colchicine are all appropriate interventions in the interval phase to reduce the incidence of acute gouty attacks.

3. The answer is C *[see III.E.1.c; III.E.2.a; III.E.3.b.(1).(d).(i); IV.C].*
Of the selections, the most effective initial plan in treating an acute attack of gout is to administer indomethacin orally, giving 50 mg three times a day for 2–3 days, then gradually tapering the dosage over the next few days. Even though joint immobilization is an appropriate initial step, drugs for pain relief should be administered as soon as possible. Uric acid modification therapy (allopurinol or probenecid) should not be initiated until the acute attack is under control. Initiating therapy with probenecid at this point may prolong the resolution of an acute attack of gouty arthritis, which can usually be accomplished within 7 days of NSAID therapy. Colchicine should never be given intramuscularly because it causes tissue irritation.

4. The answer is E *(I, II, III) [see IV.C].*
In the treatment of hyperuricemia, allopurinol is indicated rather than probenecid when large tophi are present, when the creatinine clearance is < 50–60 mL/min (probenecid would be ineffective, but the allopurinol dosage would have to be decreased), when the patient is an overproducer of uric acid, and when there is a need to prevent the formation of large amounts of uric acid (e.g., when conditions such as leukemia are present).

5. The answer is B *[see IV.C.3.b.(3).(a)]*
Losartan, an angiotensin II receptor blocker has been shown to increase urinary uric acid secretion and can, therefore, lower serum uric acid levels. Hydrochlorothiazide actually decreases urinary uric acid excretion and must be used cautiously in gout patients, if at all. The other antihypertensive agents mentioned have minimal or no effects on the serum uric acid.

52

Peptic Ulcer Disease and Related Acid-Associated Disorders

Paul F. Souney

Anthony E. Zimmermann

I. INTRODUCTION

A. Definition

1. **Peptic ulcer disease** (PUD) refers to a group of disorders characterized by circumscribed lesions of the mucosa of the upper gastrointestinal (GI) tract (particularly the stomach and duodenum). The lesions occur in regions exposed to gastric juices.

2. **Gastroesophageal reflux disease (GERD)** refers to the retrograde movement of gastric contents from the stomach into the esophagus. Reflux may occur without consequences and thus be considered a normal physiological process, or it may lead to profound symptomatic or histological conditions (e.g., GERD). When reflux leads to inflammation (with or without erosions or ulcerations) of the esophagus, it is called **reflux (erosive) esophagitis.** Most patients (50%–70%) report typical symptoms but lack evidence of esophageal mucosal injury **(nonerosive reflux disease; NERD).**

3. **Dyspepsia** is defined as persistent or recurrent abdominal pain or abdominal discomfort centered in the upper abdomen.

B. Manifestations

1. **Duodenal ulcers** almost always develop in the duodenal bulb (the first few centimeters of the duodenum). A few, however, arise between the bulb and the ampulla.

2. **Gastric ulcers** form most commonly in the antrum or at the antral–fundal junction.

3. **Less common forms of peptic ulcer disease**
   a. **Stress ulcers** result from serious trauma or illness, major burns, coagulopathy not related to anticoagulant therapy, need for mechanical ventilation > 48 hr, or ongoing sepsis. The **most common site** of stress ulcer formation is the proximal portion of the stomach.
   b. **Zollinger-Ellison syndrome** is a severe form of peptic ulcer disease in which intractable ulcers are accompanied by extreme gastric hyperacidity and at least one gastrinoma (a non-β-islet cell tumor of the pancreas or another site).
   c. **Stomal ulcers** (also called marginal ulcers) may arise at the anastomosis or immediately distal to it in the small intestine in patients who have undergone ulcer surgery and have experienced subsequent ulcer recurrence after a symptom-free period.
   d. **Drug-associated ulcers** occur in patients who chronically ingest substances that damage the gastric mucosa, such as nonsteroidal anti-inflammatory drugs (NSAIDs).

4. **Reflux esophagitis** is most often recognized by the presence of recurrent symptoms (e.g., heartburn) or altered epithelial morphology visualized radiologically, endoscopically, or histologically.
   a. Heartburn is substernal burning or regurgitation that may radiate to the neck. Other symptoms include belching, water brash, chest pain, asthma, chronic cough, hoarseness, and laryngitis.
   b. Endoscopic evaluation detected **Barrett esophagus (BE)** in 6% of patients with frequent heartburn. Barrett's esophagus is a premalignant condition that may lead to adenocarcinoma of the esophagus or esophagogastric junction.

C. Epidemiology

1. **Incidence.** Peptic ulcer disease is the most common disorder of the upper GI tract.
   a. **Duodenal ulcers** affect 4%–10% of the U.S. population; **gastric ulcers** occur in 0.03%–0.05% of the population.
   b. Nearly 80% of peptic ulcers are duodenal; the others are gastric ulcers.
   c. Most duodenal ulcers appear in people between age 20 and 50; onset of gastric ulcers usually occurs between age 45 and 55.
   d. The 1-year point prevalence of active gastric or duodenal ulcer in the United States in men and women is about 1.8%; the lifetime prevalence of peptic ulcer ranges from 11% to 14% for men and 8% to 11% for women.
   e. Approximately 10%–20% of gastric ulcer patients also have a concurrent duodenal ulcer.
   f. In the United States, 44% of the adult population experience **heartburn** at least once a month; 14% take some type of "indigestion" medication at least twice a week. Of patients with GERD symptoms who have undergone endoscopy, 50%–65% have apparent esophagitis.
   g. The annual prevalence of dyspepsia in Western countries is approximately 25%; 2%–5% of primary-care consultations are for dyspepsia.

2. **Hospitalization**
   a. Hospitalization rates in the United States for peptic ulcers have been declining; these rates dropped from 25.2 per 10,000 in 1965 to 16.5 per 10,000 in 1981. This reflects a decrease in hospitalization for uncomplicated cases owing to increased outpatient diagnosis and treatment. There has been little change in hospitalization rates since then.
   b. There has been little or no decrease in duodenal ulcer perforations and only a slight decrease in hemorrhages.

3. **Mortality**
   a. The mortality rate for gastric ulcers declined between 1962 and 1979 from 3.5 per 100,000 to 1.1 per 100,000.
   b. For duodenal ulcer, the mortality rate declined from 3.1 per 100,000 to 0.9 per 100,000.
   c. Although death from GERD is uncommon, morbidity is not, because of the prevalence of the well-recognized complications such as esophageal ulceration (5%), stricture formation (4%–20%), and the development of Barrett columnar-lined esophagus (8%–20%).

D. Description

1. **Ulcer size.** The average duodenal ulcer typically has a diameter < 1 cm; most gastric ulcers are somewhat larger (1–2.5 cm in diameter).

2. Most ulcers are sharply demarcated and have a round, oval, or elliptical shape.

3. The mucosa surrounding the ulcer typically is inflamed and edematous.

4. Ulcers penetrate the **muscularis propria** and, in some cases, extend into the serosa or even into the pancreas.

5. Fibrous tissue, granulation tissue, and necrotic debris form the ulcer base. During ulcer healing, a scar forms as epithelium from the edges covers the ulcer surface.

6. Nearly all duodenal ulcers are benign; up to 10% of gastric ulcers are malignant.

E. Cause.
The two major observations regarding PUD are the causal relationship among NSAID intake; gastroduodenal mucosal injury; the pathogenesis of gastric ulcer and, to a lesser extent, duodenal ulcer; and the association of **Helicobacter pylori** infection in the pathogenesis of duodenal ulcer (and to a lesser extent, gastric ulcer).

1. *H. pylori* (formerly *Campylobacter pylori*) is a gram-negative microaerophilic, spiral bacterium with multiple flagella that lives and infects the gastric mucosa. This bacterium is able to survive in the acidic gastric environment by its ability to produce urease, which hydrolyzes urea into ammonia. Ammonia neutralizes gastric hydrochloric acid (HCl), creating a neutral cloud surrounding the organism.
   a. In the United States, the **prevalence** of *H. pylori* increases with age from approximately 10% at 20 years of age to approximately 50% at 60 years of age; approximately 17% of *H. pylori*–positive individuals will develop a duodenal ulcer. Prevalence is higher in developing countries.

    b. *H. pylori* is associated with several common GI disorders.

        (1) Always present in the setting of active chronic gastritis

        (2) Present in the vast majority of duodenal (> 90%) and gastric (60%–90%) ulcers. Recent studies indicate a decline in the prevalence of *H. pylori* in duodenal ulcer patients.

        (3) Sometimes present with nonulcer dyspepsia (probably in 50% of cases); eradication of *H. pylori,* when present, leads to symptom improvement in only about one half of treated patients.

        (4) In gastric cancer, 85%–95% (Although the association is strong, no causal relationship has yet been proven in gastric cancer. The World Health Organization has classified *H. pylori* as a Group 1 carcinogen.)

    c. *H. pylori* **eradication** can cure peptic ulcers and reduce ulcer recurrence; it can eliminate the need for maintenance therapy in many ulcer patients.

2. Genetic factors

    a. The lifetime prevalence of developing an ulcer in **first-degree relatives** of ulcer patients is about threefold greater than in the general population. This may be secondary to clustering of *H. pylori* within families.

    b. People with **blood type O** have an above-normal incidence of duodenal ulcers.

3. Smoking. Smokers have an increased risk of developing peptic ulcer disease. In addition, cigarette smoking delays ulcer healing and increases the risk and rapidity of relapse after the ulcer heals. Nicotine decreases biliary and pancreatic bicarbonate secretion. Smoking also accelerates the emptying of stomach acid into the duodenum.

4. NSAIDs. When ingested chronically, aspirin, indomethacin, and other NSAIDs promote gastric ulcer formation.

    a. These drugs may injure the gastric mucosa by allowing back-diffusion of hydrogen ions into the mucosa.

    b. NSAIDs also inhibit the synthesis of prostaglandins, which are substances with a cytoprotective effect on the mucosa.

    c. Selective cyclooxygenase 2 (COX-2) inhibitors, celecoxib or rofecoxib, are associated with fewer ulcers than nonselective NSAIDs, with rates comparable to placebo at 3 months. Questions regarding long-term safety of COX-2 inhibitors remain. With the recent documentation of increasing COX-2 expression with the progression of BE to cancer, trials have been initiated using COX-2 selective inhibitors in BE patients to prevent development of cancer.

5. Alcohol. A known mucosal irritant, alcohol causes marked irritation of the gastric mucosa if ingested in large quantities at concentrations of 20% or greater. The only association between ethanol intake and ulcer disease exists in patients with portal cirrhosis.

6. Coffee. Both regular and decaffeinated coffee contain peptides that stimulate release of gastrin, a hormone that triggers the flow of gastric juice. However, a direct link between coffee and peptic ulcer disease has not been proven.

7. Corticosteroids. Controversy over whether systemic corticosteroid therapy is associated with increased risk for the development of peptic ulcer disease has, for the most part, been resolved. Evidence for this direct association has always been weak in previous retrospective reviews/trials and reflected the concurrent use of an NSAID. Current data support no link between steroids and peptic ulcer disease in the absence of concurrent NSAID use.

8. Associated disorders. Peptic ulcer disease is more common in patients with hyperparathyroidism, emphysema, rheumatoid arthritis, and alcoholic cirrhosis.

9. Advanced age. Degeneration of the pylorus permits bile reflux into the stomach, creating an environment that favors ulcer formation.

10. Psychological factors. Once assigned key roles in the pathogenesis of PUD, stress and personality type now are viewed as relatively minor influences.

F. Pathophysiology. Ulcers develop when an imbalance exists between factors that protect gastric mucosa and factors that promote mucosal corrosion. Approximately 90% of patients with duodenal ulcer and 70% of patients with gastric ulcer have *H. pylori* infection.

1. **Protective factors**
   a. Normally, the mucosa secretes a thick mucus that serves as a barrier between luminal acid and epithelial cells. This barrier slows the inward movement of hydrogen ions and allows their neutralization by bicarbonate ions in fluids secreted by the stomach and duodenum.
   b. Alkaline and neutral pancreatic biliary juices also help buffer acid entering the duodenum from the stomach.
   c. An **intact mucosal barrier** prevents back-diffusion of gastric acids into mucosal cells. It also has the capacity to stimulate local blood flow, which brings nutrients and other substances to the area and removes toxic substances (e.g., hydrogen ions). Mucosal integrity also promotes cell growth and repair after local trauma.

2. **Corrosive factors.** Peptic ulcer disease reflects the inability of the gastric mucosa to resist corrosion by irritants, such as pepsin, HCl, and other gastric secretions.
   a. **Exposure to gastric acid** and **pepsin** is necessary for ulcer development.
   b. **Disrupted mucosal barrier integrity** allows gastric acids to diffuse from the lumen back into mucosal cells, where they cause injury.

3. **Physiological defects associated with peptic ulcer disease.** Researchers have identified various physiological defects in patients with duodenal and gastric ulcers.
   a. **Duodenal ulcer patients** may have the following defects:
      (1) Increased capacity for gastric acid secretion
         (a) Some duodenal ulcer patients have up to twice the normal number of parietal cells (which produce HCl).
         (b) Nearly 70% of duodenal ulcer patients have elevated serum levels of **pepsinogen I** and a corresponding increase in pepsin-secreting capacity.
      (2) Increased parietal cell responsiveness to gastrin
      (3) Above-normal postprandial gastrin secretion
      (4) Defective inhibition of gastrin release at low pH, possibly leading to failure to suppress postprandial acid secretion
      (5) Above-normal rate of gastric emptying, resulting in delivery of a greater acid load to the duodenum
   b. **Gastric ulcer patients** typically exhibit the following characteristics:
      (a) Deficient gastric mucosal resistance, direct mucosal injury, or both
      (b) Elevated serum gastrin levels (in acid hyposecretors)
      (c) Decreased pyloric pressure at rest and in response to acid or fat in the duodenum
      (d) Delayed gastric emptying
      (e) Increased reflux of bile and other duodenal contents
      (f) Subnormal mucosal levels of prostaglandins (these levels normalize once the ulcer heals)

4. **GERD** requires both initiation and perpetuation of the reflux of gastric contents. Esophagitis develops when noxious substances in the refluxate (i.e., acid, pepsin) are in contact with the esophageal mucosa long enough to cause irritation and inflammation.
   a. In patients with GERD, 65% of reflux events occur via transient relaxation (TLESR). The main difference between normal individuals and those with GERD is the frequency of TLESR. GERD patients have more frequent and prolonged TLESR. TLESR represents a decrease in lower esophageal sphincter (LES) pressure that is not associated with swallowing or peristalsis.
   b. Other mechanisms of LES incompetence are increased abdominal pressure and spontaneous reflux during periods of very low LES pressure.
   c. Such motility problems are permissive—that is, they allow reflux of acid and other noxious substances.

5. Many diseases cause dyspeptic symptoms, including PUD, GERD, gastric cancer, and biliary tract disease. However, in many cases, no clear pathological reason for a patient's symptoms can be determined. Dyspepsia in the absence of an identifiable organic cause is frequently described as "functional" or "nonulcer" dyspepsia.

G. **Clinical presentation.** Signs and symptoms of PUD vary with the patient's age and the location of the lesion. Only about 50% of patients experience classic ulcer symptoms. The remainder are asymptomatic or report vague or atypical symptoms.

1. **Pain.** Patients typically describe heartburn or a gnawing, burning, aching, or cramp-like pain. Some patients report abdominal soreness or hunger sensations. It is unclear whether peptic ulcer pain results from chemical stimulation or from spasm.

   a. **Duodenal ulcer pain** usually is restricted to a small, midepigastric area near the xiphoid. Pain may radiate below the costal margins into the back or the right shoulder. Pain from a duodenal ulcer frequently awakens the patient between midnight and 2 A.M.; it is almost never present before breakfast.

   b. **Gastric ulcer pain** is less localized. It may be referred to the left subcostal region. Gastric ulcer rarely produces nocturnal pain.

   c. **GERD** patients most commonly present with heartburn, belching, regurgitation, or water brash; **atypical presentations** include chest pain, hoarseness/laryngitis, loss of dental enamel, asthma, chronic cough, or dyspepsia. Complications of GERD include esophageal ulceration, strictures, BE, and adenocarcinoma of the esophagus or esophagogastric junction.

   d. **Dyspepsia** applies broadly to a range of symptoms, including abdominal or retrosternal pain and discomfort, heartburn, nausea, vomiting, and other symptoms referable to the proximal GI tract.

   e. **Food** usually relieves duodenal ulcer pain but may cause gastric ulcer pain. This finding may explain why duodenal ulcer patients tend to gain weight, whereas gastric ulcer patients may lose weight. Pain characteristically occurs 90 min to 3 hr after meals in duodenal ulcer patients, whereas pain in gastric ulcer patients is usually present 45–60 min after a meal. Food aggravates reflux disease.

2. **Nausea** and **vomiting** may occur with either ulcer type.

3. **Disease course.** Both duodenal and gastric ulcers tend to be chronic, with spontaneous remissions and exacerbations. Within a year of the initial symptoms, most patients experience a relapse.

   a. In many cases, relapse is seasonal, occurring more often in the spring and autumn.

   b. All patients with a confirmed duodenal or gastric ulcer should be tested for *H. pylori* infection. If the patient is *H. pylori*–positive, eradication therapy will reduce the recurrence rate significantly and preclude the need for maintenance medication.

   c. GERD is also a chronic disease; most patients with reflux esophagitis who are healed with antisecretory drug therapy will experience a recurrence within 6 months of discontinuation of the healing regimen. Maintenance therapy reduces the recurrence of esophagitis.

H. Clinical evaluation

1. **Physical findings.** Patients with peptic ulcer disease may exhibit superficial and deep epigastric tenderness and voluntary muscle guarding. With duodenal ulcer, patients also may show unilateral spasm over the duodenal bulb. Gastric ulcer patients may have weight loss.

2. **Diagnostic test results**

   a. **Blood tests** may show hypochromic anemia.

   b. **Stool tests** may detect occult blood if the ulcer is chronic.

   c. **Gastric secretion tests** may reveal hypersecretion of HCl in duodenal ulcer patients and normal or subnormal HCl secretion in gastric ulcer patients.

   d. **Upper GI series** (barium x-ray) reveals the ulcer crater in up to 80% of cases. Duodenal bulb deformity suggests a duodenal ulcer.

   e. **Upper GI endoscopy,** the most specific test, may be done if barium x-ray yields inconclusive results. This procedure confirms an ulcer in at least 95% of cases and may detect ulcers not demonstrable by radiography.

   f. **Biopsy** might be necessary to determine whether a gastric ulcer is malignant.

   g. *H. pylori* status is determined by noninvasive tests (not requiring endoscopy) or invasive methods (requiring endoscopy).

      (1) **Noninvasive.** Serology, the test of choice when endoscopy is not indicated, is inexpensive. Several office tests are available. Breath tests can also be used to detect the organism and are uniquely suited as noninvasive means of confirming eradication of *H. pylori* after therapy. False-negative breath tests may occur in patients receiving proton pump inhibitors, antibiotics, or bismuth compounds.

      (2) **Invasive.** These methods include histological visualization of *H. pylori* or measurement of urease activity, which require biopsy.

I. Treatment objectives

1. Relieve pain and other symptoms and promote healing

2. Prevent complications

3. Minimize recurrence (eradicate *H. pylori* in PUD)

4. Maintain adequate nutrition

5. Teach the patient about the disease to improve therapeutic compliance

6. Maintain the patient symptom free

II. THERAPY

A. **Drug therapy.** Peptic ulcer patients usually are treated with antacids, histamine 2– (H_2-) receptor antagonists, or proton pump inhibitors; other drugs are added as necessary. Drug regimens that suppress nocturnal acid secretion are found to result in the highest duodenal ulcer healing rates. Drug therapy typically provides prompt symptomatic relief and promotes ulcer healing within 4–6 weeks (Figure 52-1). GERD management requires more aggressive acid suppression regimens; the pharmacodynamic end point is to maintain the pH in the esophagus at 4 or more (Figure 52-2).

1. **Antacids.** These compounds, which neutralize gastric acid, are used to treat ulcer pain and heal the ulcer. Studies show antacids and H_2-receptor antagonists to be equally effective. Antacids are available as **magnesium, aluminum,** or **calcium.** The most widely used antacids are mixtures of aluminum hydroxide and magnesium hydroxide (Table 52-1). Duodenal ulcers rarely occur in the absence of acid or when the hourly maximum acid output is < 10 mEq. Peptic activity decreases as acidity decreases; experimental ulcer formation is inhibited by antacids; and acid-reducing operations cure ulcers.

   a. **Mechanism of action and therapeutic effects.** Antacids reduce the concentration and total load of acid in the gastric contents. By increasing gastric pH, antacids also inhibit pepsin activity. In addition, they strengthen the gastric mucosal barrier.

   b. **Choice of agent**

      (1) **Nonsystemic antacids** (e.g., magnesium or aluminum substances) are preferred to systemic antacids (e.g., sodium bicarbonate) for intensive ulcer therapy because they avoid the risk of alkalosis.

      (2) **Liquid antacid forms** have a greater buffering capacity than tablets. However, tablets are more convenient to carry. With either dosage form, the size and frequency of doses may limit patient compliance.

      (3) **Antacid mixtures** (e.g., aluminum hydroxide with magnesium hydroxide) provide more even, sustained action than single-agent antacids and permit a lower dosage of each compound. In addition, compounds in a mixture may interact so as to negate each other's untoward effects. For instance, the constipating effect of aluminum hydroxide may counter the diarrhea that magnesium hydroxide frequently produces.

      (4) **Calcium carbonate** usually is avoided because it causes acid rebound, may delay pain relief and ulcer healing, and induces constipation. Another potential adverse effect of this compound is hypercalcemia; the risk is increased if calcium carbonate is taken with milk or another alkaline substance. The milk–alkali syndrome (i.e., hypercalcemia, alkalosis, azotemia, nephrocalcinosis) can also occur.

   c. **Administration and dosage**

      (1) Antacids differ greatly in acid-neutralizing capacity (ANC), defined as the number of milliequivalents (mEq) of a 1 N solution of HCl that can be brought to a pH of 3.5 in 15 min. For most duodenal ulcer patients, approximately 50 mEq/hr of available antacid is needed for ongoing neutralization of gastric contents. Therefore, the required dosage depends on the ANC of the specific antacid.

      (2) In the fasting state, antacids have only a transient intragastric buffering effect (15–20 min). When ingested 1 hr after a meal, they have a much more prolonged effect, about 3–4 hr; therefore, they should optimally be taken 1 and 3 hr after meals and before sleep. Consequently, the typical antacid regimen calls for doses 1 and 3 hr after meals and at bedtime.

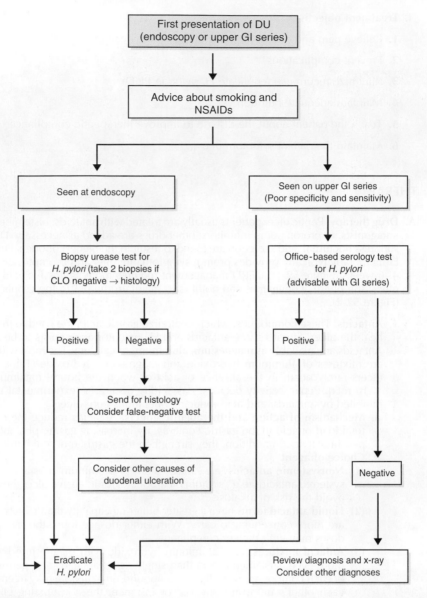

Figure 52-1. Treatment strategy for management of duodenal ulcer. *CLO, Campylobacter*-like organism; *DU,* duodenal ulcer; *GI,* gastrointestinal; *NSAIDs,* nonsteroidal anti-inflammatory drugs.

(3) Dosage

(a) Because the ANC of antacid products varies widely, no standard dosage can be given in terms of milliliters of suspension or number of tablets. However, patients with duodenal ulcers generally require individual dosages of 80–160 mEq of ANC (equivalent to 30–60 mL of Mylanta or Maalox). Thus the total daily dosage may be as much as 420 mL of Mylanta or Maalox if the standard seven-times–daily dosing regimen is used. Because of the large doses required, increase in adverse effects, need for frequent administration, and poor patient compliance, their role in the management of PUD is limited.

(b) Antacid therapy usually continues for 6–8 weeks.

d. Precautions and monitoring effects

(1) Calcium carbonate– and magnesium-containing antacids should be used cautiously in patients with severe renal disease.

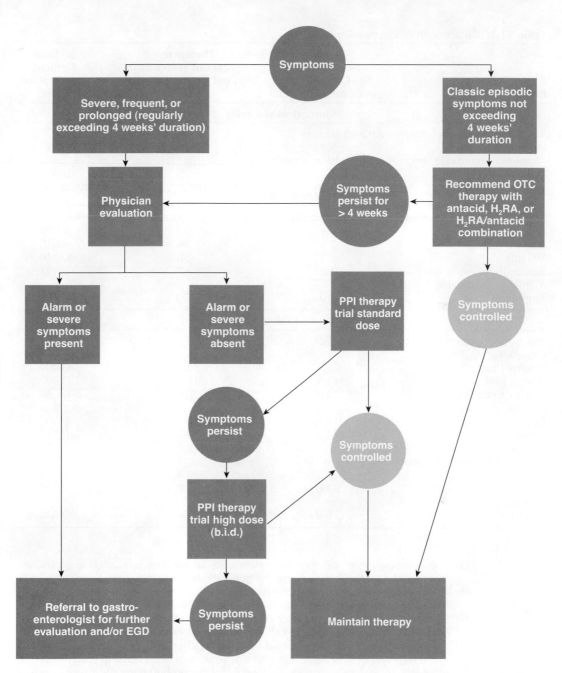

Figure 52-2. Treatment strategy for management of gastroesophageal reflux disease. *EGD,* esophagogastroduodenoscopy; *H₂RA,* histamine 2–receptor antagonist; *OTC,* over the counter; *PPI,* proton pump inhibitor. [Adapted with permission from Peterson WL. GERD evidence-based therapeutic strategies [AGA Consensus Development Panel], 2002. Available at www.gastro.org/user-assets/documents/GERDmonograph.pdf.

(2) Sodium bicarbonate is contraindicated in patients with hypertension, congestive heart failure (CHF), severe renal disease, and edema. It should not be used for ulcer therapy.
(3) All antacids should be used cautiously in elderly patients (particularly those with decreased GI motility) and renally impaired patients.
(4) Aluminum-containing antacids should be used cautiously in patients who suffer from dehydration or intestinal obstruction.

Table 52-1. Comparison of Common Antacids

Brand Name	Acid-Neutralizing Capacity (mEq/mL or tablet)	Therapeutic Amount (140 mEq) (mL or number of tablets)	Sodium Content (mg/5 mL or tablet)
Concentrated liquids			
Aluminum hydroxide, magnesium hydroxide			
Maalox TC	5.4	26	0.035
Aluminum hydroxide, magnesium hydroxide, simethicone			
Mylanta DS	5.0	28	0.050
Regular liquids			
Aluminum hydroxide, magnesium hydroxide, simethicone			
Gelusil	2.4	58	0.090
Maalox Plus	2.6	54	0.040
Mylanta	2.5	56	0.030
Riopan Plus	3.0	47	0.013
Aluminum hydroxide			
Amphojel	2.0	70	0.100
Tablets			
Aluminum hydroxide, magnesium hydroxide, simethicone			
Gelusil II	21	6.7	0.00
Maalox Plus	11.4	12.2	0.00
Riopan Plus	13.5	10.4	0.00
Maalox Extra Strength	23.4	6.0	0.040
Calcium carbonate			
Tums	10.0	14	0.00
Tums E-X	15.0	9.3	0.11
Titralac	7.5	18.7	0.00
Calcium carbonate and magnesium hydroxide			
Rolaids	8.5	16.5	0.040
Mylanta Max Strength	24.0	5.8	0.026
Aluminum hydroxide			
Amphojel	16.0	8.75	0.080

(5) The combination of calcium carbonate with an alkaline substance (e.g., sodium bicarbonate) and milk may cause the milk–alkali syndrome.

(6) Always check brand name extension products for major ingredient changes (i.e., Maalox Total Stomach Relief contains bismuth subsalicylate).

(7) Chronic administration of calcium carbonate–containing antacids should be avoided because of hypercalcemia and calcium ion stimulation of acid secretion.

(8) Aluminum or magnesium toxicity is unlikely in patients with normal renal function. The encephalopathy of tissue deposition of aluminum occurs only in dialysis patients receiving aluminum hydroxide for control of hyperphosphatemia. Chronic use of magnesium-containing antacids is not advisable in patients with renal insufficiency.

(9) Constipation can occur in patients using calcium carbonate– and aluminum-containing antacids.

(10) Diarrhea is a common adverse effect of magnesium-containing antacids. If diarrhea occurs, the patient may alternate the antacid mixture with aluminum hydroxide.

(11) Hypophosphatemia and osteomalacia can occur with long-term use of aluminum hydroxide, but these conditions can also occur with short-term use in severely malnourished patients, such as alcoholics.

e. **Significant interactions.** Because antacids alter gastric pH and affect absorption of ingested substances, they have a high potential for drug interactions. To ensure consistent absorption and therapeutic efficacy, orally administered drugs should be given 30–60 min before antacids.

      (1) Antacids bind with **tetracycline and fluoroquinolones,** inhibiting the absorption and reducing therapeutic efficacy.

      (2) Antacids may destroy the coating of **enteric-coated drugs,** leading to premature drug dissolution in the stomach.

      (3) Antacids may interfere with the absorption of many drugs, including **cimetidine, ranitidine, digoxin, isoniazid, anticholinergics, iron products,** and **phenothiazines** (see II.A.2.e.(3)).

      (4) Antacids may reduce the therapeutic effects of **sucralfate** (see II.A.3.d).

2. H$_2$-receptor antagonists. These drugs may be preferred to other antiulcer agents because of their convenience and lack of effect on GI motility. Although reasonably effective in treating mild to moderate GERD symptoms, H$_2$-receptor antagonists are less reliable for healing erosive esophagitis. All current choices require multiple, divided doses for GERD management.

    a. Mechanism of action and therapeutic effects. H$_2$-receptor antagonists competitively inhibit the action of histamine at parietal cell receptor sites, reducing the volume and hydrogen ion concentration of gastric acid secretions (Figure 52-3 and Table 52-2). These agonists accelerate the healing of most ulcers.

    b. Choice of agent. Cimetidine (Tagamet), ranitidine (Zantac), famotidine (Pepcid), or **nizatidine (Axid)** may be administered to treat peptic ulcers or hypersecretory states (e.g., Zollinger-Ellison syndrome).

      (1) Cimetidine, the first H$_2$-receptor antagonist approved for clinical use, reduces gastric acid secretion by approximately 50% (at a total daily dosage of 1000 mg).

      (2) Ranitidine, a more potent drug, causes a 70% reduction in gastric acid secretion (at a total daily dosage of 300 mg).

      (3) Famotidine is the most potent H$_2$-receptor antagonist. After a 40-mg dose, mean nocturnal gastric acid secretion is reduced by 94% for up to 10 hr.

      (4) Nizatidine, the newest H$_2$-receptor antagonist, may be used to treat and prevent recurrence of duodenal ulcers.

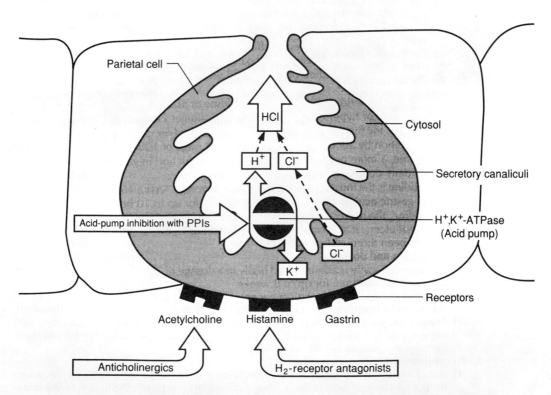

Figure 52-3. Sites of drug action in a parietal cell. *HCl,* hydrochloric acid; *PPIs,* proton pump inhibitors.

Table 52-2. H$_2$-Receptor Antagonists

Characteristic	Cimetidine (Tagamet)	Ranitidine (Zantac)	Famotidine (Pepcid)	Nizatidine (Axid)
Ring structure	Imidazole	Furan	Thiazole	Thiazole
Relative potency	1	4–10	4–10	20–50
Evening dose (mg)				
Active ulcer	800	300	40	300
Maintenance	400	150	20	150
Bioavailability (F) (%)	60–70	50–60	40–45	90–100
Peak time (t_{max}) (hr)	1–3	1–3	1–3.5	0.5–3
Volume of distribution (L/kg)	1	1.4	1.1–1.4	0.8–1.6
Protein binding (%)	20	15	15–22	32–35
Renal elimination (%)	60–75	30 oral; 70 intravenous	65–70	65–75
Half-life (hr)				
Normal	2	2–3	2.5–4	1.6
Anuric	4–5	4–10	20+	6–8.5
Clearance (L/h)	30–48	46	19–29	40–60

Reprinted with permission from Hurwitz A. Clinical pharmacology of agents for the treatment of acid-related disorders. In Zakim D, Dannenberg AJ, eds. Peptic Ulcer Disease and Other Acid-Related Disorders. New York, Academic Research Associates, 1991:343.

  c. Administration and dosage
    (1) Cimetidine usually is administered orally in a dosage of 300 mg four times daily (with meals and at bedtime) for up to 8 weeks.
      (a) Alternatively, duodenal ulcer patients may receive 400 mg twice daily or 800 mg at bedtime. An 800-mg bedtime dose is also effective in treating gastric ulcers.
      (b) Hospitalized patients may receive parenteral doses of 300 mg intravenously every 6 hr.
      (c) For duodenal ulcer prophylaxis, 400 mg may be given orally at bedtime. (However, in 20%–40% of patients, the ulcer recurs despite cimetidine prophylaxis.)
    (2) Ranitidine usually is given orally in a dosage of 150 mg twice daily. Duodenal ulcer patients may receive 300 mg at bedtime, alternatively. Therapy continues for up to 8 weeks.
      (a) Hospitalized patients may receive ranitidine by the intravenous or intramuscular route (50 mg every 6–8 hr).
      (b) Prophylactic therapy may be administered to reduce the risk of ulcer recurrence. The approved prophylactic dosage is 150 mg at bedtime.
      (c) Ranitidine 150 mg twice daily can be administered to maintain healing of erosive esophagitis; for this purpose, it is better than placebo but less effective than the proton pump inhibitors.
      (d) Ranitidine bismuth citrate, combined with antibiotics such as clarithromycin, is indicated for eradication of *H. pylori* in patients with duodenal ulcer.
    (3) Famotidine, administered to duodenal ulcer patients, is given in an oral dosage of 40 mg at bedtime for acute therapy for a maximum of 8 weeks. For prophylactic therapy, the dosage is 20 mg at bedtime.
      (a) Hospitalized patients may receive an intravenous injection of 20 mg every 12 hr.
      (b) As with cimetidine and ranitidine, the ulcer may recur after drug discontinuation.
    (4) Nizatidine, for the treatment of duodenal ulcers, is given orally in a dosage of 300 mg once daily at bedtime or 150 mg twice daily for up to 8 weeks. For prophylactic therapy, the dosage is 150 mg at bedtime.
  d. Precautions and monitoring effects
    (1) Ranitidine must be used cautiously in patients with hepatic impairment. Hepatotoxicity is unusual and occurs most often during intraveous administration. Cimetidine has also been associated with hepatotoxicity.

(2) Cimetidine may cause such hematological disorders as thrombocytopenia, agranulocytosis, and aplastic anemia.

(3) All of these agents may cause headache and dizziness. Cimetidine additionally may lead to confusion, particularly if patients are > 60 years of age or if the dosage is not adjusted for patients with decreased kidney or liver function. All agents require dosage reductions in patients with impaired renal function.

(4) Cimetidine has a weak androgenic effect, possibly resulting in male gynecomastia and impotence.

(5) Cimetidine and ranitidine rarely can cause bradycardia, which is reversible on discontinuation of therapy.

(6) Evaluate *H. pylori* status in any patient with confirmed ulcer disease; eradication of *H. pylori* reduces the need for maintenance therapy in patients with duodenal or gastric ulcers. Patients with complicated ulcer disease should continue maintenance therapy until the eradication of *H. pylori.*

(7) Tolerance develops frequently to histamine 2–receptor antagonists (H$_2$RAs) and may explain diminished responses to these agents over time.

e. Significant interactions

(1) Cimetidine binds the cytochrome P450 system of the liver and thus may interfere with the metabolism of such drugs as **phenytoin, theophylline, phenobarbital, lidocaine, warfarin, imipramine, diazepam,** and **propranolol.**

(2) Cimetidine decreases hepatic blood flow, possibly resulting in reduced clearance of **propranolol** and **lidocaine.**

(3) **Antacids** impair absorption of cimetidine and ranitidine and should be given 1 hr apart from these drugs.

(4) Cimetidine inhibits the excretion of procainamide by competing with the drug for the renal proximal tubular secretion site.

3. Sucralfate (Carafate). This mucosal protectant is a nonabsorbable disaccharide containing sucrose and aluminum.

a. Mechanism of action and therapeutic effects. Sucralfate adheres to the base of the ulcer crater, forming a protective barrier against gastric acids and bile salts.

(1) Sucralfate's ulcer-healing efficacy compares favorably to that of the H$_2$RAs.

(2) Duodenal ulcers respond better than gastric ulcers to sucralfate therapy.

b. Administration and dosage

(1) An oral agent, sucralfate usually is given in a dosage of 1 g four times daily (1 hr before meals) and at bedtime. Unless radiography or endoscopy documents earlier ulcer healing, therapy continues for 4–8 weeks.

(2) Continued sucralfate therapy after remission postpones ulcer relapse more effectively than does cimetidine therapy.

(3) There is no evidence that combining sucralfate with H$_2$RAs improves healing or reduces recurrence rates.

c. Precautions and monitoring effects. Constipation is the most common adverse effect of sucralfate.

d. Significant interactions

(1) **Antacids** may reduce mucosal binding of sucralfate, decreasing its therapeutic efficacy and thus should be given 30–60 min apart from sucralfate if used in combination ulcer therapy.

(2) Sucralfate may interfere with the absorption of orally administered **digoxin, tetracycline, phenytoin, iron, ciprofloxacin and other fluoroquinolones,** and **cimetidine** if doses are given simultaneously.

4. GI anticholinergics (e.g., belladonna leaf, atropine, propantheline) sometimes are used as adjunctive agents for relief of refractory duodenal ulcer pain. However, these agents have no proven value in ulcer healing.

a. Mechanism of action. Anticholinergics decrease basal and stimulated gastric acid and pepsin secretion.

(1) Given in combination with antacids, anticholinergics delay gastric emptying, thereby prolonging antacid retention. They are most effective when taken at night and in large doses.

(2) Anticholinergics occasionally are used in patients who do not respond to H$_2$-receptor antagonists alone.

b. Administration and dosage
 (1) Taken 30 min before food, anticholinergics inhibit meal-stimulated acid secretion by 30%–50% for a duration of 4–5 hr.
 (2) The optimal effective dose varies from patient to patient.
c. Precautions and monitoring effects
 (1) All anticholinergics have side effects to varying degrees, such as dry mouth, blurred vision, tachycardia, urinary retention, and constipation.
 (2) These drugs are contraindicated in patients with gastric ulcers because they prolong gastric emptying. They also are contraindicated in patients with narrow-angle glaucoma and urinary retention.

5. **Prostaglandins.** These agents suppress gastric acid secretion and may guard the gastric mucosa against damage from NSAIDs. **Misoprostol (Cytotec)** has been approved for use in the prevention of gastric ulcers caused by NSAIDs.
 a. Mechanism of action. Misoprostol has both antisecretory (inhibiting gastric acid secretion) and mucosal protective properties. NSAIDs inhibit prostaglandin synthesis, and a deficiency of prostaglandin within the gastric mucosa may lead to diminishing bicarbonate and mucus secretion, contributing to the mucosal damage caused by NSAIDs. Misoprostol increases bicarbonate and mucus production at doses of 200 μg and above—doses that can also be antisecretory. Misoprostol also maintains mucosal blood flow.
 b. Administration and dosage
  (1) Misoprostol is indicated for the prevention of NSAID-induced gastric ulcers in patients at high risk for complications from gastric ulcers (e.g., patients > 60 years of age, patients with concomitant debilitating disease, patients with a history of ulcers).
  (2) Misoprostol has not been shown to prevent duodenal ulcers in patients taking NSAIDs.
  (3) The recommended adult dosage is 200 μg four times daily with food; it must be taken for the duration of NSAID therapy. If this dose cannot be tolerated, 100 μg four times daily can be used.
  (4) Adjustment of dosage in renally impaired patients is not routinely needed.
 c. Precautions and monitoring effects
  (1) Misoprostol is contraindicated in pregnant women because of its abortifacient property. Patients must be advised of the abortifacient property and warned not to give the drug to others.
  (2) Misoprostol should not be used in women with childbearing potential unless the patient requires NSAID therapy and is at high risk of complications from gastric ulcers associated with use of the NSAIDs or is at high risk of developing gastric ulceration. In such a patient, misoprostol may be prescribed if the patient:
   (a) Is capable of complying with effective contraceptive measures
   (b) Has received both oral and written warnings of the hazards of misoprostol, the risk of possible contraception failure, and the danger to other women of childbearing potential should the drug be taken by mistake
   (c) Had a negative serum pregnancy test within 2 weeks before beginning therapy
   (d) Will begin misoprostol only on the 2nd or 3rd day of the next normal menstrual period
  (3) The most frequent adverse effects are diarrhea (14%–40%) and abdominal pain (13%–20%). Diarrhea is dose-related, usually develops early in the course (> 2 weeks), and is often self-limiting. Discontinuation of misoprostol is necessary in about 2% of patients. Administration with food minimizes the diarrhea.
 d. Significant interactions. None has been reported.

6. **Proton pump inhibitors (PPIs). Omeprazole (Prilosec)** was the first PPI available in the United States, followed by **lansoprazole (Prevacid), rabeprazole (Aciphex), pantoprazole (Protonix), and esomeprazole (Nexium)** (Table 52-3). The intravenous forms of esomeprazole, lansoprazole and pantoprazole have been approved by the U.S. Food and Drug Administration (FDA).
 a. Mechanism of action and therapeutic effects. The gastric proton pump H^+/K^+-ATPase has a sulfhydryl group near the potassium-binding site on the luminal side of the canalicular membrane. Omeprazole sulfonamide (the active form) forms a stable disulfide bond with this specific sulfhydryl, thereby inactivating the ATPase and shutting off acid secretion. All other PPIs exhibit a similar irreversible mechanism of action.

Table 52-3. Pharmacokinetics Proton Pump Inhibitors

Characteristic	Omeprazole (Prilosec)	Lansoprazole (Prevacid)	Rabeprazole (Aciphex)	Pantoprazole (Protonix)	Esomeprazole (Nexium)
Bioavailability (%)	30–40	80–85	52	77	64–89
Time to peak plasma concentration (hr)	0.5–3.5	1.7	2.0–5.0	1.1–3.1	1.56
Plasma elimination half-life (hrs	0.5–1	1.3–1.7	1.0–2.0	1.0–1.9	0.85–1.25
Protein binding (%)	95	97	96	98	97
Urinary excretion of oral dose (%)	77	14–23	30–35	71–80	80

(1) Because of the potency and marked reduction in gastric acidity, the PPIs are more rapidly effective than other approved agents in treating peptic ulcer disease (i.e., PPIs tend to control symptoms and heal ulcers more rapidly than other antiulcer drugs). PPIs provide effective healing of duodenal ulcers; healing rates at 4 weeks are similar to those reported for H_2-receptor antagonist therapy at 8 weeks.

(2) All PPIs are effective in healing erosive esophagitis, provide more rapid symptom relief and more consistent healing than H_2-receptor antagonists, and are also effective in maintenance of healing of erosive esophagitis.

(3) All PPIs except pantoprazole have been approved in various combinations of antibiotics for the eradication of *H. pylori* (Table 52-4).

Table 52-4. Food and Drug Administration–Approved Oral Regimens Used to Eradicate *Helicobacter pylori* and Reduce the Risk of Duodenal Ulcer Recurrence

Drug Combination	Dose and Frequency	Duration
Omeprazole	20 mg	Days 1–10
	20 mg every day b.i.d.	Days 11–28[a]
Clarithromycin	500 mg b.i.d.	Days 1–10
Amoxicillin	1 g b.i.d.	Days 1–10
Lansoprazole	30 mg b.i.d.	14 days
Amoxicillin	1 g tid	14 days
Clarithromycin	500 mg b.i.d.	14 days
Lansoprazole	30 mg b.i.d.	10 days
Amoxicillin	1 g b.i.d.	10 days
Clarithromycin	500 mg b.i.d.	10 days
Esomeprazole	40 mg every day	10 days
Amoxicillin	1 g b.i.d.	10 days
Clarithromycin	500 mg b.i.d.	10 days
Rabeprazole	20 mg b.i.d.	7 days
Amoxicillin	1 g b.i.d.	7 days
Clarithromycin	500 mg b.i.d.	7 days
Bismuth subsalicylate	525 mg q.i.d.	Days 1–14
Metronidazole	250 mg q.i.d.	Days 1–14
Tetracycline HCl	500 mg q.i.d.	Days 1–14
H_2RA of choice	Ulcer healing regimen	Days 1–28

[a]In patients with an ulcer present at the time of initiation of therapy, additional omeprazole treatment is recommended for ulcer healing and relief of symptoms.
H_2RA, H_2-receptor antagonist; *HCl*, hydrochloric acid.

(4) PPIs have resulted in significant improvement in patients with pathological hypersecretory conditions (e.g., Zollinger-Ellison syndrome) and GERD compared to H_2-receptor antagonists.

(5) Esomeprazole and lansoprazole have been approved by the FDA for healing and prevention of NSAID-induced gastric ulcers.

(6) Omeprazole and lansoprazole have been approved by the FDA for use in infants and children for the short-term treatment of GERD and erosive esophagitis. Omeprazole is approved for use in children ages 2–16 years, and lansoprazole is approved for use in children 1–11 years old.

b. Administration and dosage

(1) PPIs are more potent than H_2-blockers. In the usual dosage (omeprazole 20 mg daily), these agents inhibit > 90% of 24-hr acid secretion in most patients, rarely producing achlorhydria. Esomeprazole 40 mg daily provided significantly higher intragastric pH values above 4 during 24-hr monitoring compared to lansoprazole 30 mg, rabeprazole 20 mg, omeprazole 20 mg, and pantoprazole 40 mg.

(2) PPIs should optimally be taken in the morning 30-60 min before eating; food activates parietal cells, maximizing the effect of the PPI. Optimal binding to proton pumps occurs when the pumps are actively secreting.

(3) **Recommended adult dosages**

(a) Erosive esophagitis initially is healed with 20 mg omeprazole or equivalent doses of other PPIs for 8–12 weeks; only omeprazole has a demonstrated dose response in GERD patients (patients failing omeprazole 20 mg daily may benefit from higher doses; this has not been demonstrated with esomeprazole, lansoprazole, rabeprazole, or pantoprazole). In addition, esomeprazole 40 mg every day has been shown to produce significantly higher healing rates than omeprazole 20 mg or lansoprazole 30 mg across all grades of erosive esophagitis.

(b) Esomeprazole 20-40 mg, lansoprazole 30 mg, omeprazole 20 mg, rabeprazole 20 mg, and pantoprazole 40 mg may be used to manage GERD symptoms in patients who have failed previous therapy with H_2-receptor antagonist therapy.

(c) The recommended dosage to maintain healing of erosive esophagitis is esomeprazole 20 mg, omeprazole 20 mg, lansoprazole 15 mg, pantoprazole 40 mg, or rabeprazole 20 mg daily for as long as medically necessary.

(d) Duodenal ulcer healing requires omeprazole 20 mg, lansoprazole 15 mg, or rabeprazole 20 mg once daily. Most patients heal within 4 weeks.

(4) Esomeprazole, lansoprazole, and omeprazole are delayed-release capsules and should be taken before eating, can be used concomitantly with antacids, and should not be chewed or crushed. Capsule contents can be sprinkled on foods (i.e., applesauce) or mixed with acidic juices. Suspensions of omeprazole or lansoprazole in sodium bicarbonate have been used for administration to patients with nasogastric and jejunostomy tubes.

(5) Rabeprazole and pantoprazole are available as enteric-coated tablets that should not be crushed or chewed.

(6) Lansoprazole is available as the first orally disintegrating tablet formulation. It is placed on the tongue, with or without water, until dissolved. However, it needs to be swallowed to be absorbed.

(7) Omeprazole in sodium bicarbonate powder for suspension (Zegerid) is the first PPI approved by the FDA for reduction in the risk of upper GI bleeding in critically ill patients. It has a peach/mint flavor that is tolerable. It is dosed at 40 mg every 6 hr times two doses (as a loading dose), then 40 mg daily.

(8) No dosing adjustments are necessary in patients with impaired renal or hepatic function or in the elderly.

(9) Intravenous pantoprazole is indicated for management of erosive esophagitis and treatment of Zollinger-Ellison syndrome. Esomeprazole, lansoprazole, and pantoprazole are currently being widely used for the treatment of acute bleeding gastric ulcers, though not FDA approved.

(10) Intravenous esomeprazole (20-40 mg daily) and lansoprazole (30 mg daily) are FDA approved for the short-term use in patients with GERD with a history of erosive esophagus unable to take oral medications.

(11) In patients with nocturnal signs and symptoms of GERD, twice daily PPIs have been effective when taken appropriately. The addition of an H_2RA to the twice-daily PPI has shown little added benefit and is not recommended.

c. Precautions and monitoring effects
   (1) Headache, diarrhea, abdominal pain, nausea and vomiting, and flatulence have been reported in > 1% of patients.
   (2) Fever, fatigue, malaise, elevated liver enzymes, dizziness, vertigo, skin rash, and itching have been reported in < 1% of patients.

d. Significant interactions
   (1) Omeprazole interferes with the hepatic microsomal enzyme metabolism (cytochrome P450) of **diazepam, warfarin,** and **phenytoin, although clinically significant interactions are infrequent.**
   (2) Lansoprazole may increase clearance of theophylline by approximately 10%.
   (3) Because gastric pH plays a role in the bioavailability of **ketoconazole, ampicillin esters,** and **iron salts,** prolonged gastric acid inhibition with PPIs may decrease the absorption of these agents.
   (4) Antacids may be used concomitantly with all PPIs.
   (5) No clinically significant drug interactions have been reported to date with esomeprazole, rabeprazole, or pantoprazole.
   (6) Food may reduce the bioavailability of esomeprazole and lansoprazole by 50%; food does not reduce the bioavailability of omeprazole or rabeprazole.

7. Bismuth compounds. In the United States, bismuth subsalicylate (Pepto-Bismol) is the only available bismuth product.
   a. Mechanism of action. Bismuth prevents adhesion of *H. pylori* to gastric mucosa, decreases resistance when used with other anti–*H. pylori* agents, inhibits release of proteolytic enzymes, and suppresses *H. pylori* growth.
   b. Administration and dosage
      (1) Bismuth subsalicylate is highly effective when combined with PPIs and/or antibiotics. Eradication rates with these combinations are > 80% (Table 52-4).
      (2) Preferred regimen with bismuth: bismuth subsalicylate 525 mg four times a day, metronidazole 250 mg four times a day, tetracycline 500 mg four times a day plus PPI (omeprazole 20 mg every day or lansoprazole 30 mg every day) for 2 weeks total. This regimen provides consistently high eradication rates (> 90%) and may be useful for patients who have failed previous therapy. This regimen is not currently FDA approved.
   c. Precautions and monitoring effects
      (1) CNS toxicity with higher doses, including neurotoxicity
      (2) Tinnitus, hyperpyrexia, tachycardia, and confusion (salicylism) from high doses of bismuth subsalicylate
   d. Reversible proton pump inhibitors are currently under development by a number of pharmaceutical companies (AstraZeneca and Altana). When compared with the currently available irreversible proton pump inhibitors, these agents are expected to offer more rapid symptom resolution, control pH more quickly, achieve higher pH levels, and sustain these more aggressive pH levels consistently over a 24-hr period.

8. Prokinetic agents. Cisapride (Propulsid) is currently the only approved agent in this class; however, the manufacturer (Janssen Pharmaceutica) has **discontinued marketing** of cisapride in the United States owing to the agent's highly arrhythmogenic potential. The manufacturer will supply cisapride through a limited-access program for those who meet specific eligibility criteria and for whom other therapies are not effective. Metoclopramide and erythromycin have well-studied prokinetic effects, and prucalopride is still under review by the FDA.
   a. Mechanism of action. Cisapride produces release of acetylcholine from the myenteric plexus and thereby may increase gastric emptying and LES pressure; cisapride does not affect TLESR. It does not increase or decrease gastric acid secretion.
   b. Administration and dosage. Cisapride is indicated for the relief of nocturnal symptoms of reflux; it is administered in doses of 10–20 mg four times a day.
   c. Precautions and monitoring
      (1) The **most common** side effects are diarrhea, abdominal pain, and headache. Other less common effects include bronchospasm, angioedema, and depression.
      (2) Cisapride is contraindicated in patients with a history of ischemic heart disease, respiratory failure, congestive heart failure, renal failure, severe dehydration, arrhythmias, or medications that prolong the QT interval. Serious cardiac arrhythmias, including ventricular tachycardia and torsades de pointes, have been reported.

d. Significant interactions

(1) **Ketoconazole** potently inhibits the metabolism of cisapride, resulting in an eightfold increase in the area under the curve (AUC) of cisapride. Co-administration of cisapride and ketoconazole can result in prolongation of the QT interval on the electrocardiogram (ECG). Co-administration of itraconazole, fluconazole, or intravenous miconazole is similarly contraindicated.

(2) The following oral or intravenous drugs are contraindicated with cisapride. These may lead to elevated cisapride blood levels and increased potential for arrhythmias.
   a. Antibiotics: erythromycin, clarithromycin, sparfloxacin
   b. Protease inhibitors: indinavir, ritonavir
   c. Antiarrhythmics: quinidine, procainamide, sotalol

(3) The acceleration of gastric emptying by cisapride could affect the rate of absorption of other drugs. Patients receiving narrow therapeutic drugs or other drugs that require careful titration should be monitored closely.

(4) Coagulation times in patients receiving oral anticoagulants have increased in some cases.

(5) Cimetidine may increase peak plasma concentration and AUC of cisapride.

e. γ-Aminobutyric acid B (GABA$_B$) agonists (i.e., baclofen) have been shown to significantly reduce reflux episodes in healthy volunteers and GERD patients. Several compounds are under development that have greater peripheral specificity and are expected to provide fewer CNS-related adverse effects, while providing effective normalization of TRLES.

f. Tegaserod (Zelnorm), a selective 5-hydroxytryptamine 4 (5-HT4) receptor agonist, is a promotility drug currently approved for irritable bowel syndrome. Early studies have demonstrated that tegaserod reduces esophageal acid exposure by enhancing esophageal acid clearance and gastric emptying and/or reducing TRLES but more definitive studies are needed. Initial studies in patients with heartburn have shown a decrease in esophageal pain.

9. Sedatives are useful adjuncts in promoting rest for highly anxious ulcer patients.

B. Other therapeutic measures

1. Modification of diet and social habits

a. Previously emphasized in ulcer therapy, strict dietary limitations now are considered largely unnecessary.

(1) Bland or milk-based diets formerly were recommended; however, research indicates that these diets do not speed ulcer healing. In fact, most experts now advise ulcer patients to **avoid milk** because recent studies show that milk increases gastric acid secretion. Also, because milk leaves the stomach quickly, it lacks an extended buffering action.

(2) Small, frequent meals, also previously recommended, can worsen ulcer pain by causing acid rebound 2–4 hr after eating.

b. **Current dietary guidelines** emphasize avoiding foods and beverages known to exacerbate gastric discomfort or promote acid secretion. This category typically includes coffee, caffeinated beverages, and alcohol.

c. **Smoking.** Patients who smoke should be encouraged to quit because smoking markedly slows ulcer healing, even during optimal ulcer therapy.

d. **NSAIDs** should be avoided by ulcer patients.

2. Surgery. An ulcer patient who develops complications may require surgery—sometimes on an emergency basis (see III). Incapacitating recurrent ulcers also may warrant surgery.

a. **Types of surgical procedures** for ulcer disease include antrectomy and truncal vagotomy (Billroth I procedure), partial gastrectomy and truncal vagotomy (Billroth II procedure), highly selective (proximal gastric) vagotomy, and total gastrectomy (the treatment of choice for Zollinger-Ellison syndrome that is unresponsive to medical management).

(1) A **vagotomy** severs a branch of the vagus nerve, thereby decreasing HCl secretion.

(2) An **antrectomy,** by removing the antrum, eliminates some acid-secreting mucosa as well as the major source of gastrin.

b. The general indications for antireflux surgery are failure of medical therapy to heal or prevent relapse of erosive esophagitis, inability of medical therapy to prevent recurrence of stricture, or a patient whose lifestyle is adversely affected by the need for medical therapy. **Laparoscopic fundoplication** is currently the gold standard for GERD and successfully relieves symptoms and heals lesions in approximately 85% of patients. However, recent studies have demonstrated that most patients require continued medical therapy after fundoplication.

3. **Emerging endoscopic therapies.** Three endoscopic techniques to treat GERD have recently been introduced.
   a. Augmentation of LES pressure may be achieved by delivery of radiofrequency energy to the muscle of the gastroesophageal junction (Stretta procedure). The radiofrequency is delivered by means of a flexible catheter made up of a bougie tip, a balloon-basket combination, and four-needle delivery sheaths.
   b. Another endoscopic procedure, the EndoCinch, augments the LES by suturing of the mucosa.
   c. The third endoscopic/endoluminal treatment is by use of Enteryx injection.
   d. Early studies have demonstrated good feasibility in performing these procedures and an overall satisfactory safety profile. Further studies are necessary to assess long-term failure rate, early versus late complications, and success rate in the different GERD groups.

III. **COMPLICATIONS** of peptic ulcer disease cause approximately 7000 deaths in the United States annually.

A. **Hemorrhage.** This life-threatening condition develops from widespread gastric mucosal irritation or ulceration with acute bleeding.

1. **Clinical features.** The patient may vomit fresh blood or a coffee grounds–like substance. Other signs include passage of bloody or tarry stools, diaphoresis, and syncope. With major blood loss, manifestations of **hypovolemic shock** may appear: The pulse rate may exceed 110, or systolic blood pressure may drop below 100.

2. **Management**
   a. Patient stabilization, bleeding cessation, and measures to prevent further bleeding are crucial.
      (1) Airway, breathing, and circulation must be ensured.
      (2) Intravenous crystalloids and colloids (e.g., hetastarch) should be infused as needed.
      (3) The patient's electrolyte status must be monitored and any imbalances corrected promptly.
   b. **Gastric lavage** may be performed via a nasogastric or orogastric tube; iced saline solution is instilled until the aspirate returns free of blood.
   c. Vasoconstrictors or continuous infusion proton pump inhibitors have been administered with good response.
      (1) Decrease rebleeding rates were found when the continuous infusion PPI maintained the gastric pH to 6 or above. The doses required were much higher than normal doses (e.g. pantoprazole 80 mg bolus plus 8 mg/hr or lansoprazole 90 mg bolus plus 9 mg/hr). However, none of the intravenous PPIs are currently FDA approved for this indication.
      (2) **Vasopressin,** an agent that causes contraction of the GI smooth muscle, may be given to constrict vessels and control bleeding but only in patients with hemorrhagic gastritis.
   d. **Emergency surgery** usually is indicated if the patient does not respond to medical management.

B. **Perforation.** Penetration of a peptic ulcer through the gastric or duodenal wall results in this acute emergency. Perforation most commonly occurs with ulcers located in the anterior duodenal wall.

1. **Clinical features.** Sudden acute upper abdominal pain, rigidity, guarding, rebound tenderness, and absent or diminished bowel sounds are typical manifestations. Several hours after onset, symptoms may abate somewhat; this apparent remission is dangerously misleading because peritonitis and shock may ensue.

2. **Management.** Emergency surgery is almost always necessary.

C. **Obstruction.** Inflammatory edema, spasm, and scarring may lead to obstruction of the duodenal or gastric outlet. The pylorus and proximal duodenum are the most common obstruction sites.

1. **Clinical features.** Typical patient complaints include postprandial vomiting or bloating, appetite and weight loss, and abdominal distention. Tympany and a succussion splash may be audible on physical examination. Gastric aspiration after an overnight fast typically yields more than 200 mL of food residue or clear fluid contents. (Gastric cancer must be ruled out as the cause of obstruction.)

2. **Management**
   a. **Conservative measures** (as in routine ulcer therapy) are indicated in most cases of obstruction.
   b. Patients with marked obstruction may require **continuous gastric suction** with careful monitoring of fluid and electrolyte status. A **saline load test** may be performed after 72 hr of continuous suction to test the degree of residual obstruction.
   c. If < 200 mL of gastric contents are aspirated, liquid feedings can begin. **Aspiration** is performed at least daily for the next few days to monitor for retention and to guide dietary modifications as the patient progresses to a full regular diet.
   d. **Surgery** is indicated if medical management fails.

D. **Postsurgical complications**

1. **Dumping syndrome.** Affecting about 10% of patients who have undergone partial gastrectomy, this disorder is characterized by rapid gastric emptying.
   a. **Causes.** The mechanism underlying dumping syndrome is poorly defined. However, intestinal exposure to hypertonic chyme may play a key role by triggering rapid shifts of fluid from the plasma to the intestinal lumen.
   b. **Clinical features.** The patient may experience weakness, dizziness, anxiety, tachycardia, flushing, sweating, abdominal cramps, nausea, vomiting, and diarrhea.
      (1) Manifestations may develop 15–30 min after a meal (early dumping syndrome) or 90–120 min after a meal (late dumping syndrome).
      (2) Reactive hypoglycemia may partly account for some cases of late dumping syndrome.
   c. **Management.** The patient usually is advised to eat six small meals of high protein and fat content and low carbohydrate content. Fluids should be ingested 1 hr before or after a meal but never with a meal. **Anticholinergics** may be given to slow food passage into the intestine.

2. **Other postsurgical complications** include reflux gastritis, afferent blind loop syndrome, stomal ulceration, diarrhea, malabsorption, early satiety, and iron-deficiency anemia.

E. **Refractory ulcers.** Ulcers that fail to heal on a prolonged course of drug treatment should not be confused with ulcers that recur after therapy is stopped. It is difficult to predict which patients will have a refractory ulcer.

1. **Differential diagnosis.** Any compliant patient who continues to have dyspeptic symptoms after 8 weeks of therapy should have gastroscopy and biopsy to exclude rare causes of ulceration in the duodenum, such as Crohn disease, tuberculosis, lymphoma, pulmonary or secondary carcinoma, and cytomegalovirus (CMV) infection in immunodeficient patients. Fasting plasma gastrin concentration should be measured to exclude Zollinger-Ellison syndrome.

2. **Treatment**
   a. Available data indicate that only maximum acid inhibition, with a regimen such as omeprazole (20 mg twice a day) or lansoprazole (30 mg twice a day), offers advantages over continued therapy with standard antiulcer regimens.
   b. Eradication of *H. pylori* infection, when present, is likely to facilitate healing and alter the natural history of refractory ulcers.
   c. Every effort should be made to discover and reduce or eliminate NSAID use.
   d. Perform surgery.

F. **Maintenance regimens**

1. Despite healing after withdrawal of therapy, 70% of ulcers recur in 1 year, and 90% in 2 years. Similarly, erosive esophagitis will recur in more than 80% of individuals within 1 year after discontinuation of antisecretory therapy.

2. Candidates for long-term maintenance therapy include patients with serious concomitant diseases; four relapses per year; or a combination of risk factors, producing a more severe

natural history of peptic disease (e.g., old age, male sex, a long history of aspirin or NSAID use, heavy alcohol intake, cigarette smoking, a history of peptic ulcer disease in an immediate relative, high maximal acid output, and a history of ulcer complications).

3. Patients with confirmed ulcer disease should be evaluated for presence of *H. pylori*. Eradication of *H. pylori* minimizes the recurrence of ulcer disease. Patients with a history of complicated ulcer disease should have *H. pylori* eradication confirmed.

STUDY QUESTIONS

Directions for questions 1–6: Each of the questions, statements, or incomplete statements in this section can be correctly answered or completed by **one** of the suggested answers or phrases. Choose the **best** answer.

1. ZZ is a 43-year-old female with a chief complaint of hematemesis and abdominal pain. Serology is positive for *H. pylori*. Which of the following would be the best regimens to treat ZZ?

(A) omeprazole 20 mg daily plus clarithromycin 500 mg b.i.d. × 14 days

(B) lansoprazole 30 mg b.i.d. plus tetracycline 500 mg q.i.d. × 14 days

(C) rabeprazole 20 mg b.i.d. plus amoxicillin 1g b.i.d. plus clarithromycin 500 mg b.i.d. × 7 days

(D) esomeprazole 40 mg b.i.d. plus amoxicillin 500 mg b.i.d. plus clarithromycin 500 mg b.i.d. × 7 days

(E) pantoprazole 40 mg b.i.d. plus amoxicillin 1g b.i.d. plus clarithromycin 500 mg t.i.d. × 10 days

2. All of the following statements concerning antacid therapy used in the treatment of duodenal or gastric ulcers are correct *except* which one?

(A) Antacids may be used to heal the ulcer but are ineffective in controlling ulcer pain.

(B) Antacids neutralize acid and decrease the activity of pepsin.

(C) If used alone for ulcer therapy, antacids should be administered 1 hr and 3 hr after meals and before bedtime.

(D) If diarrhea occurs, the patient may alternate the antacid product with aluminum hydroxide.

(E) Calcium carbonate should be avoided because it causes acid rebound and induces constipation.

3. As part of a comprehensive management strategy to treat peptic ulcer disease, patients should be encouraged to do all of the following *except*

(A) decrease caffeine ingestion.

(B) eat only bland foods.

(C) stop smoking.

(D) avoid alcohol.

(E) avoid the use of milk as a treatment modality.

4. A gastric ulcer patient requires close follow-up to document complete ulcer healing because

(A) perforation into the intestine is common.

(B) spontaneous healing of the ulcer may occur in 30%–50% of cases.

(C) there is the risk of the ulcer being cancerous.

(D) symptoms tend to be chronic and recur.

(E) weight loss may be severe in gastric ulcer patients.

5. IT is a 58-year-old male admitted to the intensive care unit with acute respiratory failure and thrombocytopenia. He is at high risk for an upper gastrointestinal bleed. Which of the following agents are approved by the U.S. Food and Drug Administration (FDA) for the prevention of this type of bleed?

(A) sucralfate

(B) famotidine

(C) esomeprazole

(D) lansoprazole

(E) omeprazole

6. All of the following provide acid suppression similar to omeprazole 20 mg every day *except*

(A) lansoprazole 30 mg every day.

(B) pantoprazole 40 mg every day.

(C) rabeprazole 20 mg every day.

(D) famotidine 20 mg twice a day.

(E) all provide equivalent acid suppression.

Directions for questions 7–8: The questions and incomplete statements in this section can be correctly answered or completed by **one or more** of the suggested answers. Choose the answer, **A–E.**

A   if **I only** is correct
B   if **III only** is correct
C   if **I and II** are correct
D   if **II and III** are correct
E   if **I, II, and III** are correct

7. Correct statements concerning cigarette smoking and ulcer disease include which of the following?

(I)   Smoking delays healing of gastric and duodenal ulcers.
(II) Nicotine decreases biliary and pancreatic bicarbonate secretion.
(III) Smoking accelerates the emptying of stomach acid into the duodenum.

8. When administered at the same time, antacids can decrease the therapeutic efficacy of which of the following drugs?

(I)   sucralfate
(II) ranitidine
(III) cimetidine

Directions for questions 9–13: Each description in this section is most closely associated with **one** of the following agents. Each agent is used only **once**. Choose the **best** answer, **A–E.**

A   sodium bicarbonate
B   aluminum hydroxide
C   calcium carbonate
D   magnesium hydroxide
E   propantheline

9. may cause diarrhea

10. cannot be used by patients with heart failure

11. if used with milk and an alkaline substance can cause milk–alkali syndrome

12. may cause dry mouth

13. can be alternated with an antacid mixture to control diarrhea.

ANSWERS AND EXPLANATIONS

1. The answer is C *[see Table 52-4].*
Though all agents are useful in the treatment of *Helicobacter pylori,* only the combination of rabeprazole with amoxicillin and clarithromycin for 7 days is correct. The other doses and duration of therapy are incorrect.

2. The answer is A *[see II.A.1].*
Antacids have been shown to heal peptic ulcers, and their main use in modern therapy is to control ulcer pain. Antacids should be taken 1 hr and 3 hr after meals because the meal prolongs the acid-buffering effect of the antacid. If diarrhea becomes a problem with antacid use, an aluminum hydroxide product can be alternated with the antacid mixture; this takes advantage of the constipating property of aluminum. Because calcium carbonate causes acid rebound and constipation, its use should be avoided.

3. The answer is B *[see II.B.1.a.(1)].*
Bland food diets are no longer recommended in the treatment of ulcer disease because research indicates that bland or milk-based diets do not accelerate ulcer healing. Studies show that patients can eat almost anything; however, they should avoid foods that aggravate their ulcer symptoms.

4. The answer is C *[see I.D.6].*
Between 5% and 10% of gastric ulcers may be the result of cancer. The ulcer may respond to therapy; however, failure of the ulcer to decrease satisfactorily in size and to heal with therapy may suggest cancer. Close follow-up is necessary to document complete ulcer healing.

5. The answer is E *[see II.6.B].*
Though all of these agents have been used with success in the prevention of GI bleeds in critically ill patients, only omeprazole (as a powder for oral suspension) has been FDA approved for this indication.

6. The answer is D *[see II.A.6.b.(1)].*
Doses of omeprazole 20 mg, lansoprazole 30 mg, pantoprazole 40 mg, and rabeprazole 20 mg administered once daily provide similar levels of acid suppression. All provide significantly better acid inhibition than famotidine, even at doses of 20 mg twice a day or more.

7. The answer is E *(I, II, III) [see I.E.3; II.B.1.c].*
Clinical studies have shown that smoking increases susceptibility to ulcer disease, impairs spontaneous and drug-induced healing, and increases the risk and rapidity of recurrence of the ulcer. These findings may result in part from nicotine's ability to decrease biliary and pancreatic bicarbonate secretion, thus decreasing the body's ability to neutralize acid in the duodenum. Also, the accelerated emptying of stomach acid into the duodenum may predispose to duodenal ulcer and may decrease healing rates.

8. The answer is E *(I, II, III) [see II.A.1.e.(3); II.A.3.d].*
The mean peak blood concentration of cimetidine and the area under the 4-hr cimetidine blood concentration curve were both reduced significantly when cimetidine was administered at the same time as an antacid. The absorption of ranitidine is also reduced when it is taken concurrently with an aluminum magnesium hydroxide antacid mixture. To avoid this interaction, the antacid should be administered 1 hr before or 2 hr after the administration of cimetidine or ranitidine. Antacids may reduce mucosal binding of sucralfate, decreasing its therapeutic efficacy. Antacids should, therefore, be given 30–60 min before or after sucralfate.

9. The answer is D *[see II.A.1.b.(3)].*

10. The answer is A *[see II.A.1.d.(2)].*

11. The answer is C *[see II.A.1.d.(5)].*

12. The answer is E *[see II.A.4.c.(1)].*

13. The answer is B *[see II.A.1.b.(3)].*
Magnesium-containing products tend to cause diarrhea, possibly because of magnesium's ability to stimulate the secretion of bile acids by the gallbladder. Because of its sodium content, sodium bicarbonate is contraindicated in patients with CHF, hypertension, severe renal disease, and edema. Sodium bicarbonate is no longer used in peptic ulcer therapy. In addition to causing acid rebound, calcium carbonate, if taken with milk and an alkaline substance for long periods, may cause milk-alkali syndrome. It also may cause adverse effects such as hypercalcemia, alkalosis, azotemia, and nephrocalcinosis. Propantheline, like other anticholinergic agents, may cause dry mouth, blurred vision, urinary retention, and constipation. These agents sometimes are used as adjuncts to relieve duodenal ulcer pain. They are contraindicated in gastric ulcer because they delay gastric emptying. Aluminum hydroxide is constipating and can be alternated with the patient's current antacid when that antacid product is causing diarrhea.

53
Diseases of the Bowel: Inflammatory Bowel Disease and Irritable Bowel Syndrome

Eric Coldiron

I. INTRODUCTION

A. Definition

1. **Inflammatory bowel disease (IBD)** is a designation commonly used to **describe** two idiopathic diseases of the gastrointestinal tract with closely related clinical presentations. These diseases are **ulcerative colitis (UC)** and **Crohn disease (CD).**

2. UC is a chronic inflammatory condition of the gastrointestinal tract mucosa and is primarily found in the rectum and colon.

3. CD is chronic transmural inflammation of the gastrointestinal mucosa and can be found throughout the gastrointestinal tract from the mouth to the anus. CD most commonly affects the small bowel and colon.

4. **Irritable bowel syndrome (IBS)** is a disorder that interferes with the normal motility functions of the gastrointestinal tract. The disorder is characterized by a group of symptoms that range from crampy abdominal pain, bloating, and constipation to diarrhea.

B. Manifestations

1. **IBD**
   a. **UC** onset is frequently insidious with increasing stool urgency and frequency. In addition to urgency, bloody stool and mucus in the stool can also gradually increase. The general course of UC can be generalized as bouts of varied disease intensity interspersed with asymptomatic periods.
   b. **CD** onset is typically insidious but can be as severe or fulminate disease. Despite similarities of CD presentation, there are patterns of symptoms that relate to disease location and type (e.g., inflammatory, fibrostenotic, fistulizing) that can be useful in determining therapy decisions.

2. **IBS**
   a. IBS can be characterized by pain relieved by defecation, alternating bowel habits, abdominal distention, mucus in the stool, and a sensation of incomplete defecation. IBS usually occurs as either constipation predominant or diarrhea predominant.
   b. **Constipation-predominant IBS** tends to present with pain and periodic constipation alternating with normal periods of bowel function. Pain has been described as colicky, periodic, and/or a continuous dull ache. Defecation may relieve the pain and eating can commonly trigger symptoms. Other common symptoms are bloating, nauseas, dyspepsia, flatulence, and heartburn.
   c. **Diarrhea-predominant IBS** is commonly characterized by precipitous diarrhea occurring immediately on rising or during meals or immediately postprandially. Nocturnal episodes are rare. Other common presenting complaints are pain, bloating, rectal urgency, and incontinence.
   d. IBS can also be alternating from constipation to diarrhea on a continual basis.

C. Epidemiology of IBD.
It has been estimated that approximately 1 million Americans have IBD. It is estimated that roughly half have UC and half have CD.

1. **UC incidence and prevalence rates** have remained relatively constant in North America and northern Europe and appear to be increasing in southern Europe and East Asia. UC historically has been more common than CD.

    a. UC incidence rates in North America are reported to be around 11 cases per 100,000 patients. Recent prevalence rates for UC in North America are reported to be 169–229 per 100,000 patients. Rates are comparable in northern European countries.

    b. UC incidence and prevalence rates are lower in southern Europe, Asia, and Latin America.

2. **CD incidence and prevalence rates** have seen a marked rise since the early 1950s. There is a great variance in published incidence rates of CD. Areas of higher CD incidence are generally similar to those of higher UC incidence. CD has recently become more common than UC in some areas.

    a. Reported CD incidence rate for North America is estimated to be 5 cases per 100,000 patients. CD prevalence rates in North America are estimated to be around 50 cases per 100,000 patients. CD rates for northern Europe are comparable to those in North America.

    b. Rates for southern Europe, Africa, and Asia have been reported to be lower than those seen in North America and northern Europe.

3. **Geographical-related components**

    a. Northern regions have historically reported higher rates of IBD than southern regions. Rates in southern Europe have recently seen increasing incidence rates compared to historical rates.

    b. CD rates have been reported to be higher in urban areas.

    c. UC rates have been reported to be higher in rural areas.

    d. IBD rates have historically been higher in developed countries compared to less-developed countries. This difference has been shown to decrease as less-developed areas are developed and a more Western diet is adopted.

4. **Ethnic, racial, and socioeconomic components**

    a. The risk for IBD and CD in particular is higher in Jews of European descent than in non-Jews. While IBD prevalence is reported to be higher in Jews compared to non-Jews there is considerable variation within Jewish populations from different geographical locations.

    b. Non-Jewish whites historically have been considered to be at higher risk for IBD compared to African Americans, but that difference has been questioned in recent reports. Blacks in Africa tend to be at less risk for IBD than either North American whites or African Americans.

    c. Asians appear to be at lower risk for developing IBD than whites. However, migrant Asians to the United Kingdom have been shown to be at higher risk for UC than non-migrants, nearly equaling the risk of developing CD as UK-born whites.

    d. Incidence rates of IBD have historically been reported to be higher in higher socioeconomic classes.

5. **Age- and sex-related components**

    a. IBD is more common in young adult patients than older patients.

    b. CD has historically demonstrated a bimodal distribution in regard to age of diagnosis; a large peak is seen in the 2nd and 3rd decades and a second, smaller peak appears in later decades.

    c. The average age of UC diagnosis is in the 4th decade.

    d. Men and women are at similar risk of developing IBD.

    e. Women are at increased risk of developing CD compared to men.

    f. Men are at slightly increased risk of developing UC compared to women, although the difference approaches unity.

6. **Other contributing factors**

    a. **Smoking** has been associated with a decrease in UC rates, but the risk factors to general health do not warrant forgoing counseling patients on the benefits of smoking cessation.

        (1) Former smokers are at increased risk of developing UC.

        (2) Smoking has been shown to be a risk factor for developing CD. CD patients who actively smoke also have increased morbidity compared to CD patients who stop smoking.

    b. **Appendectomy** has been shown to be protective in regard to development of UC.

    c. Use of **oral contraceptives** has been associated with increased risk of developing IBD.

7. **Genetic** predisposition to IBD is an area of recent research.

    a. Genetic predisposition to IBD is suggested by, among other factors, epidemiologic studies, studies of twins, family aggregation studies, and ethnic differences in disease patterns.

b. The nucleotide oligomerization domain 2 (*NOD2*)/caspase activation and recruitment domain 15 (*CARD15*) genetic mutation for example is seen more often in CD than in the general population. The mutation has been associated with altered immune response to bacteria. There are limitations to the usefulness of *NOD2/CARD15* in clinical practice; however, the identification of this mutation and others has opened the door for more work concerning genetic predisposition and possible disease mechanism, which, in turn, may lead to new modes of therapy.

D. Epidemiology of IBS

1. IBS is more common in women than men.

2. IBS usually presents in patients between 30 and 50 years of age.

3. There is a decrease in IBS frequency in elderly patients.

4. Prevalence seems to be equal in whites and blacks and lower in Hispanics. Overall prevalence rates are estimated at 2.9%.

5. IBS appears to be as common in Asia, South America, and India as in Western countries.

6. IBS usually presents between the ages of 30 and 50, with significant decreases at ages > 50.

E. Description

1. **IBD** is chronic inflammation of the gastrointestinal tract.

2. UC is chronic recurring mucosal inflammation of the colon.
   a. Proctitis. Inflammation of the rectum
   b. Proctosigmoiditis. Colitis affecting the rectum and sigmoid colon
   c. Left-sided colitis. Disease starting at the rectum and extending retrograde to the splenic flexure of the colon
   d. Pancolitis. Disease affecting the entire colon
   e. Backwash ileitis. Inflammation of the terminal ileum owing to retrograde flow of colonic contents in pancolitis patients

3. CD is chronic recurring transmural inflammation of the gastrointestinal tract.
   a. Ileocolitis. The most common form of CD, affecting the ileum and colon
   b. Ileitis. CD affecting the ileum
   c. Gastroduodenal Crohn disease. CD affecting the stomach and duodenum
   d. Jejunoileitis. CD producing inflammation of the jejunum and ileum
   e. Crohn (granulomatous) colitis. CD affecting only the colon

4. IBS
   a. IBS is recognized as being part of **functional bowel disease.**
   b. IBS is characterized by symptoms of abdominal pain or discomfort that is associated with disturbed defecation patterns. IBS is typically of a constipation- or diarrhea-predominant type, and a minority of patients alternate between the two.

F. Cause

1. **IBD** is thought to be caused by a poorly understood compilation of environmental and genetic factors and possibly infectious agents. IBD is likely a result of multiple environmental factors that elicit an abnormal immune response in genetically susceptible individuals.
   a. There is significant overlap between the clinical presentations of UC and CD, the two main idiopathic inflammatory disease states that make up IBD. Thus a clear differential diagnosis between UC and CD is not always possible.
   b. There is clear evidence of immune system activation with subsequent infiltration of the tissue by lymphocytes, macrophages, and other cells. The exact trigger of this apparent poorly regulated immune response has yet to be defined.
   c. Possible mechanisms postulated for IBD disease initiation include virus or bacterial infection, dietary antigens or inappropriate immune response to normally nonantigenic microbes, and the possibility of an inappropriate immune response to intestinal autoantigens expressed on the intestinal epithelium.

    d. Regardless of cause, there appears to be failure of normal suppressor mechanisms with a resultant overly vigorous and abnormally long immune response to a disease trigger.

    e. IBD occurs 30–100 times more frequently in first-degree relatives of IBD patients compared to the general population

    f. Infectious colitis can mimic IBD. Differential diagnosis includes bacterial, protozoal, and viral pathogens (notably *Clostridium difficile,* fungal protozoal viral, and helminthic pathogens).

    g. Ischemic colitis and **neoplastic** diseases such as cecal adenocarcinoma, lymphoma, and metastatic cancers may also present like IBD.

    h. Microscopic colitis and other inflammatory diseases such as **celiac sprue,** and **eosinophilic colitis** can present in much the same manner as IBD.

    i. Drug-induced enterocolitis can induce IBD-like symptoms. The most commonly implicated classes of drugs are nonsteroidal anti-inflammatory drugs (NSAIDs), gold compounds, oral contraceptives, enteric potassium supplements, pancreatic enzymes, phosphosoda bowel preps, and thermal injury secondary to colostomy irrigation.

    j. Other possibly confounding diseases include **endometriosis** and **diverticular disease.**

2. IBS

    a. The exact cause of IBS is unknown, and no anatomic cause has yet to be elucidated.

    b. Possible comorbid factors—such as emotional health, diet, environment, concurrent drug therapy, and hormones—have been implicated in gastrointestinal (GI) dysmotility.

    c. Anxiety disorders, particularly panic disorder; major depressive disorder; and somatization disorder have also been implicated as possible initiating factors for IBS.

    d. Learned aberrant illness behavior, in which patients may tend to express emotional conflict as a GI complaint, usually abdominal pain, may also be a contributing disease state. The clinician evaluating patients with IBS, particularly those with refractory symptoms, should investigate for unresolved psychological issues, including the possibility of sexual or physical abuse.

G. Pathophysiology

1. IBD

    a. UC. Physiologic changes in UC begin with edema followed by loss of fine vascular pattern and increased mucosal friability. Ulceration, exudates, and pseudopolyps may also be present. With longer disease history, the colon may begin to become featureless and tubular in nature. UC tends to occur in a **contiguous** manner.

    b. CD. Inflammation and subsequent injury of tissue known as cryptitis leads to crypt abscess and subsequently focal aphthoid ulceration. The inflammatory process can progress with influx and proliferation of macrophages and other inflammatory cells. Transmural inflammation may lead to lymphedema and bowel wall thickening. This thickening can lead to fibrosis. Affected areas are usually sharply demarcated from normal adjacent tissue and give rise to the **skip lesion** appearance of CD.

2. IBS

    a. Abnormalities in intestinal motility in IBS appear to be related to underlying muscle dysfunction as well as hyperactive response to initiating factors, such as food or parasympathomimetic drugs.

    b. Abnormal increases in frequency and amplitude of contractions can lead to functional constipation, whereas diminished motor function of the underlying musculature can lead to diarrhea.

    c. Hypersensitivity to normal amounts of intraluminal distention exists, as does a heightened perception of pain in the presence of normal quantity and quality of intestinal gas.

    d. The pain of IBS may be caused by abnormally strong contraction of the intestinal smooth muscle or by increased sensitivity of the intestine to distention.

    e. Hypersensitivity to the hormones gastrin and cholecystokinin may also be present. However, hormonal fluctuations have not correlated with clinical symptoms.

    f. The caloric density of food intake may increase the magnitude and frequency of myoelectrical activity and gastric motility. Fat ingestion may cause a delayed peak of motor activity, which can be exaggerated in IBS.

    g. The first few days of menstruation can lead to transiently elevated prostaglandin E_2 (PGE_2), resulting in increased pain and diarrhea.

H. Clinical presentation

1. **UC.** Most patients will present with symptoms related to altered stool frequency, bowel sensation, and abdominal pain.
   a. Most UC cases begin as mild disease and worsens as the disease course progresses.
   b. UC usually follows a chronic intermittent course.
   c. Quiescent periods tend to be long, with interspersed acute attacks.
   d. Attacks or flares can last weeks to months.
   e. Some patients suffer from continuous disease.
   f. Severe UC can result in **toxic megacolon**, a life-threatening condition.
   g. Elderly patients can rarely present with constipation secondary to rectal spasm.
   h. **Typical presenting symptoms of UC are as follows:**
      (1) Increased stool frequency
      (2) Hematochezia
      (3) Tenesmus
      (4) Lower left quadrant pain
      (5) Nausea, vomiting, and weight loss (usually only in severe disease)
   i. **Extraintestinal manifestations of UC**
      (1) Arthralgias
      (2) Ankylosing spondylitis
      (3) Pyoderma gangrenosum, erythema nodosum
      (4) Aphthous ulcers
      (5) Iritis and uveitis

2. **CD.** Many patients present with acute symptoms mimicking appendicitis or intestinal obstruction. CD can be exacerbated by infections, smoking, and NSAID use. While not well correlated in controlled trials, stress is often implicated by patients and family members as a contributing factor.
   a. A significant number of patients have a history of perianal disease, especially fissures and fistulas, which are sometimes the most prominent or even initial complaint.
   b. Extraintestinal manifestations can be more prominent than GI symptoms in pediatric patients.
   c. **Typical presenting symptoms of CD are as follows:**
      (1) Abdominal pain
      (2) Diarrhea
      (3) Weight loss
      (5) Fever
   d. **Extraintestinal manifestations of CD**
      (1) Arthralgias
      (2) Acute peripheral arthritis
      (3) Ankylosing spondylitis, peripheral arthritis
      (4) Erythema nodosum, pyoderma gangrenosum, Sweet syndrome
      (5) Iridocyclitis, uveitis, and episcleritis

3. **IBS**
   a. IBS symptoms are frequent in patients with active disease.
   b. Symptoms are commonly classified with the **Rome II criteria** and center around bowel movement and abdominal pain.
      (1) Abdominal pain has been characterized as crampy, localized to the lower left abdomen and with variable intensity. Patient presentation is highly variable in regard to intensity, location, and duration of pain. Some women will have exacerbations coinciding with menstrual periods.
      (2) Alteration of bowel habits is the second major identifying symptom of IBS, including diarrhea, constipation, and alternating diarrhea and constipation.
      (3) IBS can also present with bloating, gas, belching, heartburn, reflux disease, achalasia, early feeling of fullness on eating, nausea, painful menstruation, sexual dysfunction, and frequent or urgent urination.
   c. IBS tends to wax and wane over the long term; patients have acute bouts of disease interspersed with periods of no disease. While total prevalence numbers remain relatively constant, studies of defined patient populations at various time periods show the same number of active patients but the individual patients may be different.

Table 53-1. Differences between Ulcerative Colitis (UC) and Crohn Disease (CD)

Characteristic	UC	CD
Abdominal pain	Infrequent	Frequent
Bloody diarrhea	Frequent	Occasional
Perianal involvement	Rare	Frequent
Perianal fistula	Rare	Frequent
Rectovaginal fistula	Rare	Common
Fever	Occasional	Frequent
Weight loss	Occasional	Frequent
Palpable mass	Rare	Common
Intra-abdominal abscess	Rare	Common
Bowel obstruction	Rare	Common
Antibiotic response	Rare	Frequent
Skip lesions	Rare	Frequent
Contiguous disease	Frequent	Infrequent
Effect of smoking	Often improves	Often worsens
Serologic markers		
ASCA positive	15%	65%
p-ANCA positive	70%	20%

ASCA, anti-*Saccharomyces cerevisiae* antibody; *p-ANCA,* perinuclear antineutrophil cytoplasmic antibody.

I. Clinical evaluation

1. **IBD** Differences in typical clinical presentation between UC and CD are summarized in Table 53-1.
    a. **UC**
       (1) Patient symptoms are usually the first signs of disease. Diarrhea, bleeding, tenesmus, mucus in the stool, and pain are the most common.
       (2) The severity of symptoms correlates with disease severity.
       (3) Acute disease can be associated with increased C-reactive protein, platelet count, erythrocyte sedimentation rate (ESR), and a decrease in hemoglobin.
       (4) Serum albumin can fall quickly in severe disease.
       (5) Sigmoidoscopy can be useful for assessing disease severity and extent before therapy. Care must be used in severe disease as risk of perforation is increased
    b. **UC disease classification** according to extent (distal vs. extensive) and severity is of use in determining therapy.
       (1) **Mild** UC has been defined as less than four stools per day with or without blood, normal ESR.
       (2) **Moderate** UC has been defined as more than four stools per day but minimal signs of toxicity (fever, tachycardia, anemia, or elevated ESR).
       (3) **Severe** UC has been defined as more than six bloody stools per day, evidence of toxicity as demonstrated by fever, tachycardia, anemia, or elevated ESR. (*Note:* Elevated ESR is not always present, even in the most severe UC.)
       (4) **Fulminate** UC has been defined as more than ten bowel movements, continuous bleeding, toxicity, abdominal tenderness and distension, need for blood transfusion, and colonic dilation (toxic megacolon).
       (5) In addition to classifying UC as mild to fulminate, it is useful to ascertain the effect the disease is having on patient activity with a global assessment approach, including extraintestinal manifestations (ocular, oral, joint, skin, moods), general health (laboratory evaluation for anemia, liver function tests), and quality of life (impairment at work or school, interpersonal relationships).
    b. **CD**
       (1) CD patients may present with elevated ESR; C-reactive protein; and, in more severe disease, with hypoalbuminemia, anemia, and leukocytosis.
       (2) CD can occur throughout the bowel; the site of disease affects the disease course and treatment choices.

(3) Ileocolitis is the most common form of CD. It has been characterized by right lower quadrant pain and diarrhea and can mimic acute appendicitis. Pain can be colicky and usually precedes defecation and is relieved by defecation.

(4) Jejunoileitis. Extensive inflammation can lead to loss of absorptive surfaces with resultant malabsorption and steatorrhea. This malabsorptive state can lead to dietary deficiency, hypoalbunemia, electrolyte imbalances, coagulopathy, and increased risk of bone fractures.

(5) Colitis patients tend to present with low-grade fever, diarrhea, vomiting, and epigastric pain.

(6) Perianal CD patients may present with incontinence, stricture, anorectal fistula, and perirectal abscess.

c. CD classification based on severity and location is useful for determining therapy.

(1) Mild to moderate disease has been used to define CD in patients who are ambulatory; who are able to take food orally; who have no symptoms of dehydration, no signs of toxicity (high fever, rigors, prostration), no abdominal tenderness, no painful mass, and no obstruction; or who have weight loss > 10%.

(2) Moderate to severe disease describes patients who have failed to respond to therapy for mild to moderate disease or those with more prominent symptoms of fever, significant weight loss, abdominal pain or tenderness, intermittent nausea or vomiting (without obstruction), or anemia.

(3) Severe to fulminant disease describes patients with persisting symptoms despite therapy with steroids as outpatients or patients with high fever, persistent vomiting, obstruction, rebound tenderness, cachexia, or evidence of abscess.

(4) Remission refers to patients who have responded to acute medical therapy or who have had surgical intervention and do not have gross evidence of residual CD. Patients who require steroids to maintain control of CD are considered **steroid dependant** and are not considered to be in remission.

(5) CD disease location is often classified as being ileocolic, small bowel, colonic, or anorectal. The **Vienna classification** of disease location and type of CD is also often used. CD type is known to change in regard to type and location during the disease course.

(a) Terminal ileum disease is CD in less than one third of the small bowel, with or without spillover into the cecum.

(b) Colon CD is colonic involvement anywhere from the cecum to the rectum, without small bowel or upper gastrointestinal disease.

(c) Ileocolon is CD of the terminal ileum and any location between the ascending colon and the rectum.

(d) Upper GI CD is disease in any location proximal to the terminal ileum, with or without involvement distal to the terminal ileum.

(e) The type of disease is described as **inflammatory, stricturing,** or **penetrating.**

(6) The **Crohn Disease Activity Index (CDAI)** is a validated measurement tool used to assess clinical improvement. The CDAI is a complete scoring system of subjective aspects and objective observations. It is not normally used in clinical practice but is extensively used in clinical research. CD severity, as defined by the CDAI, breaks down into the following stratifications:

(a) A score of ≤ 150 is considered clinical remission

(b) A score of < 150 and up to 450 is considered mild to moderate disease.

(c) A score of > 450 is considered severe disease.

2. IBS

a. Diagnosis of IBS commonly includes identifying positive symptoms by medical history with the Rome II criteria (Table 53-2).

(1) Physical examination is also done to exclude non-IBS disease (e.g., abdominal mass, palpable liver) because the majority of IBS patients do not have these physical abnormalities.

(2) Both patient history and physical exam are also needed to exclude IBD and microscopic and eosinophilic colitis, which can have similar symptoms to IBS.

b. Routine blood testing is normal in most suspected IBS patients and helps rule out other possible diagnosis.

Table 53-2. Rome II Diagnostic Criteria for Irritable Bowel Syndrome

Criteria	Features/Symptoms
At least 12 weeks, which need not be consecutive, in the preceding 12 months of abdominal discomfort or pain that has two of these three features	1. Relieved with defecation 2. Onset associated with a change in frequency of stool 3. Onset associated with a change in form (appearance) of stool
Supportive symptoms of the irritable bowel syndrome	1. Fewer than three bowel movements a week 2. More than three bowel movements per day 3. Hard or lumpy stools 4. Loose (mushy) or watery stools 5. Straining during a bowel movement 6. Urgency (having to rush to have a bowel movement) 7. Feeling of incomplete bowel movement 8. Passing mucus (white material) during a bowel movement 9. Abdominal fullness, bloating or swelling
Diarrhea predominant	1 or more of 2, 4, or 6; none of 1, 3, or 5
Constipation predominant	1 or more of symptoms 1, 3, or 5; none of 2, 4, or 6

Adapted with permission from Thompson WG, Longstreth GF, Drossman DA, et al. Functional bowel disorders and functional abdominal pain. Gut 1999;45:43–47.

    c. Sigmoidoscopy and colonoscopy are done to visualize the bowel when clinically appropriate to exclude other possible diagnoses.

J. Treatment objectives

  1. IBD
    a. Induce remission with control of acute inflammatory flare
    b. Maintain remission as long as possible
    d. Normalize bowel function when possible
    e. Maintain nutritional status
    f. Improve quality of life (QOL)

  2. IBS
    a. Alleviate discomfort
    b. Normalize bowel habits
    c. Minimize negative effect on patient QOL

II. THERAPY

  A. Agents used in IBD

    1. Aminosalicylates are generally considered to be effective therapy of UC and CD.
      a. Description. The commercially available agents all deliver the active 5-aminosalicilate moiety.
        (1) The oldest agent sulfasalazine (Azulfidine) contains a 5-aminosalicylic acid (5-ASA) molecule azo-bound to sulfapyridine. This bond is cleaved by intestinal flora to release the active 5-ASA moiety.
        (2) Newer agents have been developed to allow dosing without the sulfapyridine moiety, which has been implicated in many of the common adverse events and intolerances to sulfasalazine.

(3) Sulfasalazine is considered by many to be the first choice owing to its long history of use, convincing clinical trial data, and relatively low cost.

(4) Disadvantages of sulfasalazine are increased incidence of adverse events.

(5) Topical 5-ASA has been added to oral 5-ASA with improved response and time to response.

b. **Mechanism of action.** 5-ASA differs from salicylic acid by the addition of an amino group.

(1) 5-ASA drugs have variable effects on arachidonic acid metabolites, unlike the salicylates, which block prostaglandin synthesis by inhibiting cyclooxygenase 1 (COX-1) and COX-2 enzymes.

(2) At low concentrations, 5-ASA drugs increase prostaglandin production, and at higher concentrations they inhibit prostaglandins and prostacyclins.

c. **Administration and dosage.** There are currently several 5-ASA derivatives available (Table 53-3). Dosages in UC are based on disease location, severity, and overall patient condition.

d. **Precautions and adverse effects**

(1) **Sulfasalazine.**

(a) Most common adverse events: fever, dizziness, headache, itching, rash, photosensitivity, GI upset, nausea, vomiting, diarrhea, and reversible oligospermia.

(b) Less common: Stevens-Johnson syndrome, Lyell syndrome, granulocytopenia, leucopenia, thrombocytopenia, aplastic anemia, hemolytic anemia, and hepatitis.

(c) Intolerance of the sulfapyridine moiety of sulfasalazine is common and is implicated in many adverse events associated with sulfasalazine.

(2) **Mesalamine (Asacol).**

(a) Most common adverse events: diarrhea, headache, abdominal pain, cramps, flatulence, and gas.

(b) Less common: alopecia and skin rash.

(c) Rare: pericarditis and myocarditis.

(3) **Olsalazine (Dipentum).**

(a) Most common adverse events: diarrhea and loose stools.

(b) Less common: abdominal pain, rash, and itching.

(c) Rare but serious: pancreatitis, hepatotoxicity, interstitial nephritis, and bone marrow suppression.

Table 53-3. Aminosalicylates

Drug (Brand)	How Supplied	Formulation	Delivery Site
Oral agents			
Azo bond			
Balsalazide (Colazal)	750 mg	Aminobenzoyl-alanine carrier	Colon
Olsalazine (Dipentum)	250 mg	5-ASA dimer	Colon
Sulfasalazine (Azulfidine)	500 mg	Sulfapyridine carrier	Colon
Delayed release			
Mesalamine (Asacol)	400 mg	Eudragit S (pH 7)	Distal ileum, colon
Mesalamine (Claversal, Mesasal, Salofalk)	250 mg	Eudragit L (pH 6)	Ileum-colon
Sustained release			
Mesalamine (Pentasa)	250 mg, 500 mg	Ethylcellulose granules	Stomach, colon
Topical agents			
Mesalamine (Rowasa)	4 g	60-mL suppositories	Rectum, splenic flexure
Mesalamine (Canasa)	500 mg, 1000 mg	Suppositories	Rectum

5-ASA, 5-aminosalicylic acid

e. Significant interactions

(1) The **aminosalicylates** may increase risk of toxicity and leukopenia when given in combination with mercaptopurine by decreasing mercaptopurine clearance.

(1) The **5-ASA drugs** have also been associated rarely with exacerbation of IBD.

2. Steroids. Steroids are useful for patients refractory to 5-ASA and patients with severe symptoms requiring rapid control.

a. Systemic corticosteroids are effective treatment for acute UC and CD. Use as maintenance therapy for IBD is normally avoided as the risk of systemic adverse effects outweighs limited benefit. **Steroid dependency**—when a patient is unable to be tapered completely off of steroids—does occur and should not be confused with maintenance.

b. Topical and nonsystemic steroids in the form of enemas, suppositories, and ileal release formulations have been effective in treating IBD. The rectally delivered topical formulations of steroids are of particular use in left-sided disease. Budesonide (Entocort) is an oral steroid delivered in an ileal controlled-release formulation that acts in a topical manner secondary to very high first-pass metabolism by the liver. Budesonide has been shown to be effective in IBD when the targeted-release formulation is able to reach the site of disease.

c. Mechanism of action. The glucocorticoid and mineralocorticoid effects of the steroids used in IBD are wide ranging. The anti-inflammatory effects are likely the result of glucocorticoid suppression of proinflammatory cytokines.

d. Precautions and adverse effects. Therapy with oral and intravenous (IV) corticosteroids produce systemic affects, can effect multiple organ systems, and should be closely monitored for adverse events.

(1) Adverse effects of steroids in IBD therapy are related to dose and length of dosing and are the typical glucocorticoid and mineralocorticoid effects seen with exogenous steroid therapy.

(2) Systemic steroids are more prone to inducing adverse effects. Topical delivery and targeted delivery of low bioavailability steroids have been developed to reduce the risk of adverse effects.

(3) Minimizing duration of therapy as well as tapering patients off of systemic steroids are also methods of minimizing adverse effects as much as possible.

(4) Affects on bone mass may be of significant importance because IBD patients are often also at risk of nutritional deficit.

3. Azathioprine (Imuran) and 6-mercaptopurine (6-MP; Purinethol) are effective at inducing and maintaining remission in IBD. Response is slow and may take months to be fully effective. 6-MP or azathioprine is effective for patients who do not respond to oral steroids but are not so acutely ill so as to require IV therapy.

a. Mechanism of action. Azathioprine and 6-MP are purine antimetabolite drugs which interfere with DNA synthesis, disrupting the inflammatory response seen in IBD.

b. Dosing and administration. There is known metabolic differences in regard to **thiopurine methyltransferase (TPMT)** activity, which can lead to toxicity in patients with low or absent TPMT activity. Testing for TPMT phenotype can be useful in initial dosing.

(1) Consensus on the value of monitoring of metabolite levels during therapy has not been reached.

(2) Monitoring complete blood counts 4 weeks after starting therapy and then monthly during therapy should be done to monitor for toxicity.

(3) Azathioprine is 50% 6-MP by molecular weight and equivalent doses are twice that of 6-MP.

c. Precautions and adverse effects

(1) Bone marrow suppression

(2) Both azathioprine and 6-MP have been implicated in increased risk for Epstein Barr–related non-Hodgkin lymphoma. This risk appears to be small but is serious.

4. Methotrexate (Rheumatrex) given parenterally is an effective treatment for inducing remission, maintaining remission, and steroid sparing in CD. Oral methotrexate is also effective for maintaining remission in CD. Methotrexate appears to be of little use in UC.

a. Mechanism of action. Methotrexate is a folate analog and inhibits dihydrofolate reductase with multiple modes of anti-inflammatory effects.

 b. Dosing and administration.
   (1) Inducing remission of active CD: 25 mg intramuscularly (IM) weekly has been shown to be effective.
   (2) Maintaining remission and as steroid-sparing therapy: 15 mg IM weekly has been shown to be effective.
   (3) Oral methotrexate 12.5–25 mg per week does not appear to be as effective as parenteral dosing.
 c. Precautions and adverse effects
   (1) Methotrexate is a known teratogen and should be avoided or used with extreme caution in patients of child-bearing age (female and male) and only when all other therapies have been ineffective and the patients understand the risks involved.
   (2) The doses used in CD are lower than those used in oncology and the adverse events seen are generally less severe.
   (3) The most common risks are rash, nausea, pneumonitis or *Mycoplasma* pneumonia, and elevated serum transaminases.
   (4) IBD patients treated with methotrexate appear to be at low risk for hepatic toxicity.
   (5) It is important to avoid alcohol consumption because it can increase the risk of hepatic toxicity in IBD patients on methotrexate.

5. Cyclosporine (Neoral) and tacrolimus (Prograf) are potent immunosuppressive agents that have been shown to be effective in IBD. They are typically used for severe IBD because there are little data to support efficacy in mild disease to offset the potential toxicities of these agents.
 a. Mechanism of action. Both cyclosporine and tacrolimus are calcineurin inhibitors and are potent inhibitors of T lymphocyte activation.
 b. Dosing and administration. Before therapy is initiated patients should be screened for potential drug interactions, normal renal function, cholesterol levels, blood pressure, and electrolyte status to help avoid toxicity.
   (1) Cyclosporine is started at 2–4 mg/kg/day IV and titrated to levels of 250–350 ng/mL.
   (2) Tacrolimus is initiated at 0.1–0.15 mg/kg twice weekly and titrated to trough concentrations of 10 to 20 ng/mL.
   (3) Patients who respond are discharged on oral drug. Oral cyclosporine is dosed at twice the intravenous dose, divided twice a day.
   (4) Azathioprine or 6-MP is added as soon as possible and oral systemic steroids are often given concomitantly for 3–4 months.
   (5) Cyclosporine and tacrolimus are normally stopped at 3–4 months. A steroid taper is also started at 3–4 months and should be done over 48 weeks.
 c. Precautions and adverse events. Cyclosporine and tacrolimus both have short- and long-term adverse events that can be serious. The most commonly seen in IBD patients are paresthesias, hypertension, hypertrichosis, renal insufficiency, infection, gingival hyperplasia, and seizure.
   (1) Patients should be monitored for effects on blood pressure, electrolytes, renal function, and cholesterol.
   (2) Hypocholesterolemia and hypomagnesemia increase the risk of seizure.
 d. Significant interactions. Care must be used in concomitant dosing of these agents with other drugs that can adversely affect renal function such as NSAIDs. Cyclosporine has been noted to increase methotrexate and methotrexate metabolite concentrations.

6. Biologics. Infliximab (Remicade) is the main biologic therapy used in IBD.
   (1) Infliximab is an **anti–tumor necrosis factor (anti-TNF)** therapy. Infliximab is effective for inducing remission of CD, treating enterocutaneous fistulae, and maintaining remission of CD. Infliximab is also effective in UC.
   (2) Other biologic agents have shown mixed efficacy in IBD. Infliximab has also been shown to be effective for treating ankylosing spondylitis. Other biologics of note are listed in Table 53-4.
 a. Infliximab mechanism of action. TNF is a cytokine involved in multiple proinflammatory and proliferative pathways in IBD. Infliximab is a chimeric mouse–human monoclonal TNF antibody made up of human immunoglobulin G_1 (IgG_1) constant regions, human κ light chains, and monoclonal murine regions that recognize TNF. Infliximab binds TNF, preventing the cytokine from binding to cell surface receptors and subsequently

Table 53-4. Biologic Therapies of Note in Inflammatory Bowel Disease (IBD)

Agent (Brand)	Mechanism	Efficacy in IBD/Comments
Adalimumab (Humira)	Fully human IgG$_1$ monoclonal antibody to TNF	Appears to be effective in CD, place in therapy not yet fully elucidated
Infliximab (Remicade)	Chimeric (mouse/human) IgG$_1$ monoclonal antibody to TNF	Effective therapy in CD and UC; primary biologic therapy used in IBD
Natalizumab (Tysabri)	Humanized IgG$_4$ monoclonal antibody to α4 integrin, which selectively inhibits leukocyte adhesion	Removed from U.S. market in 2005 secondary to association with PML; currently under review to be made available again and may offer benefit to patients failing infliximab; place in therapy not yet fully elucidated.
Etanercept (Enbrel)	p75-Soluble TNF receptor FC fusion protein that binds TNF	Not of benefit

CD, Crohn disease; *IgG,* immunoglobulin G; *PML,* progressive multifocal leukoencephalopathy; *TNF,* tumor necrosis factor; *UC,* ulcerative colitis.

decreasing inflammatory cytokines and increasing apoptosis of activated T lymphocytes and monocytes.

b. Dosing and administration.
   (1) Initial dosing is 5 mg/kg in a three-dose induction regimen. A dose is given at 0, 2, and 6 weeks to help reduce **human antichimeric antibody (HACA)** formation.
   (2) Duration of therapeutic effect appears to be 8–10 weeks and dosing every 8 weeks has been advocated.
   (3) HACA formation and infusion-related adverse reactions can also be decreased with concomitant administration of azathioprine, 6-MP, or methotrexate.
   (4) These immunosuppressant drugs have not been shown to improve clinical disease control when given concomitantly with infliximab.
c. Precautions and adverse effects
   (1) Infliximab is generally considered safe in long-term therapy of CD.
   (2) Acute anaphylactoid infusion-related reactions occur in approximately 22% of patients. These reactions are more common in patients who test positive for antibody to infliximab and are less frequent in patients given concomitant immunosuppressive drugs. Severe anaphylactic reactions are rare.
   (3) Delayed hypersensitivity reactions, including myalgias, rash, fever, arthralgias, pruritus, edema, urticaria, sore throat, and dysphagia occur 3–12 days after infusion and are much less common, seen in approximately 2% of patients receiving maintenance infliximab therapy.

7. Antibiotics. No specific infectious agent as been identified in either UC or CD.
   a. Metronidazole (Flagyl) and **ciprofloxacin (Cipro)** are used widely by convention as maintenance therapy in CD but controlled trial results do not conclusively support this use.
   b. Use of broad-spectrum antibiotics in UC is limited to empiric treatment of fulminant disease or in patients with toxic megacolon for whom short-term use of these antibiotics can be justified owing to the increased risk of perforation or bacteremia. Metronidazole has been useful in patients suffering from **pouchitis** after bowel resection surgery that involves formation of a pouch.

8. Probiotic and prebiotic therapy. Probiotic therapy involves using exogenously administered bacteria such as *Lactobacillus* GG, *Saccharomyces boulardii,* and nonpathogenic *E. coli,* for example, in an attempt to normalize the intestinal environment flora and thus decrease inflammatory triggers.
   a. Controlled trials of probiotic therapy in IBD have yet to define clinical utility.
   b. Remission maintenance of pouchitis with VSL#3, a probiotic preparation of four lactobacilli strains, three *Bifidobacterium* strains, and one *Streptococcus* strain was shown to be of benefit.

c. Probiotics are orally administered substances like nondigested carbohydrates with the goal of facilitating growth of commensal gut flora to displace possible antigenic microorganisms.

d. There are currently little data to support the use of probiotics.

9. **Antispasmodics and antidiarrheals**. Cramping and abdominal IBS-like symptoms are often noted in IBD patients. Use of symptomatic therapies is not well defined in the published IBD literature because most research is aimed at the inflammatory process. Once active inflammation is controlled or ruled out, anticholinergic antispasmodics are frequently used judiciously to treat cramping or discomfort in IBD inflammation, as are antidiarrheals in mild or quiescent disease. All of these agents should be avoided in serious disease because they may further impair the colon and increase risk of toxic megacolon.

10. **Antidepressants and anxiolytics** have been used when specific patient symptoms warrant their use as adjuvant therapy.

11. **Analgesics.** There is rarely a need for pain control in UC as the disease is limited to the mucosa of the colon with limited involvement of tissue containing pain receptors. Narcotics are to be avoided in UC therapy outside of perioperative situations because they increase the risk of toxic megacolon and can mask signs of perforation. NSAID medications should be avoided because they have been implicated in inducing IBD flares.

12. **Surgery.** Surgical resection of the colon is considered curative in UC. Surgical resection of bowel in CD is not curative because the disease will often recur at the resection site as well as other sites.

    a. Surgery in UC is most commonly indicated for disease refractory to medical therapy, inability to wean the patient off of high corticosteroid dosages, serious drug side effects or intolerance, and occurrence of premalignant or malignant changes in the colon.

    b. Approximately one third of UC patients eventually undergo colectomy. Patients with extensive disease (pancolitis) undergo colectomy more than patients with less extensive (distal) disease and also usually require colectomy sooner than patients with less extensive disease.

    c. **UC surgery** can be divided into two types: those that preserve continence and those that do not and subsequently require appliances to collect the fecal material.

        (1) **Proctocolectomy with permanent ileostomy** is the oldest procedure and involves formation of an abdominal stoma connected to the ileum. An external appliance is used to collect fecal material.

        (2) **Proctocolectomy with continent ileostomy** involves creation of a pouch inside the abdomen using the terminal ileum. A small leakproof opening is created in the abdomen wall and the pouch is periodically drained.

        (3) **Colectomy with ileorectal anastomosis** involves removing diseased large bowel and reattaching the remaining small intestine to a preserved rectum. While bowel movements via the rectum are preserved, patients are at risk of relapse because the rectum is often involved in UC.

        (4) **Ileal pouch anal anastomosis (IPAA)** is the most common surgical procedure done for IBD. The large bowel and rectum are removed, with preservation of the anal sphincter. A tubular pouch is formed from the small intestine and attached to the preserved sphincter, which allows bowel movements without external bags or appliances. A temporary ileostomy is often used during healing.

    d. **CD surgery,** while not curative, is required in a very high percentage of patients. Surgical intervention can be limited to specific areas of diseased bowel or total ileostomy or colectomy. Surgery is most commonly indicated in CD refractory to medical therapy, medication side effects, or steroid dependency.

        (1) Small bowel resection is preferred in most patients with ileal or ileocolic CD. Primary anastomosis versus ileostomy (permanent or temporary) choice is based on patient status and CD severity.

        (2) Large bowel CD may require some degree of resection secondary to the typical CD disease course involving "skip lesions." Primary anastomosis of the preserved bowel may be preferred for patient QOL reasons but has been linked to earlier reoccurrence of CD.

        (3) Colectomy with ileorectal anastomosis, while increasing risk of earlier CD recurrence, is useful in young patients for whom ileostomy may adversely affect QOL.

(4) Proctocolectomy and ileostomy is preferred in patients with extensive perianal disease or pancolitis CD.

(5) Strictureplasty can also be useful in stricturing CD.

e. **Pouchitis** is the most common complication of continent ileostomy and IPAA. It has been characterized as a syndrome including acute nonspecific inflammation of the reservoir pouch formed during surgery with unknown cause.

(1) Idiopathic pouchitis must be differentiated from inflammation of the pouch owing to anastomotic stricture and infection as a result of known pathogens.

(2) Broad-spectrum antibiotics have been the main medical therapy used for pouchitis. Metronidazole and ciprofloxacin have both been effective for acute pouchitis and have also been used as maintenance therapy.

(3) Probiotic therapy with VSL#3 has also been of benefit.

(4) Pharmacologic therapy used in IBD has been shown to be of mixed efficacy in pouchitis. Surgical revision may be required in chronic pouchitis unresponsive to medical therapy.

13. **Other therapy**

a. **Nutritional** issues are important to consider in IBD. While conclusive evidence does not exist showing that particular foods cause IBD, special attention to diet in patients with IBD can be beneficial.

(1) Nutritional and hydration deficiencies can occur secondary to a poorly functioning GI tract and the chronic nature of IBD.

(2) Foods that are known to exacerbate an individual patient's IBD should be avoided, and a well-balanced diet should be encouraged to maintain nutritional status. Restrictive diets are not normally required. Simply limiting offending foods while encouraging a balanced diet is usually sufficient to maintain nutritional status.

(3) Parenteral feeding is seldom used long term in IBD but can be useful to improve or maintain nutritional status in severely ill patients.

c. **Emotional factors.** Owing to the chronic nature of IBD, many sufferers have need for emotional support during the course of their disease. While IBD does not appear to be directly affected by emotional state, the QOL experienced by these sufferers can be noticeably affected in a negative manner. Many will benefit greatly by support groups and continued open dialogue with their healthcare providers; sometimes formal counseling or pharmacologic therapy may be needed.

B. Drug Therapy for IBD and UC

1. Classifying UC based on anatomic disease extent is useful for determining medical therapy. Distal disease (below the splenic flexure) can be treated effectively with topical therapy. Extensive disease (extending proximal to the splenic flexure) normally requires systemic therapy. Severity of acute UC is also useful in determining medical therapy. Severity is generally defined as mild, moderate, severe, or fulminate.

2. **Management of mild to moderate UC distal disease.** Patients with mild to moderate distal UC respond well to oral and topical aminosalicylates or topical steroids for inducing remission (control of inflammation).

a. Topical mesalamine is superior to topical steroids or oral aminosalicylates.

b. Topical mesalamine plus oral aminosalicylate is superior to either alone.

c. Topical mesalamine may be effective in patients refractory to oral aminosalicylates or topical steroids.

d. Infrequently, oral corticosteroids may be needed in patients refractory to topical/oral aminosalicylates and topical steroids in maximal doses.

e. Therapy is largely determined by patient preference to therapy modality.

f. Oral 5-ASA doses for inducing remission in mild to moderate distal disease are as follows:

(1) Sulfasalazine 4–6 g per day in four divided doses

(2) Mesalamine 2–4.8 g per day in three divided doses

(3) Balsalazide 6.75 g per day in three divided doses

(4) Olsalazine 1.5–3 g per day in divided doses

g. The oral 5-ASA drugs tend to work in 2–4 weeks and are effective in a high percentage of patients.

h. Oral corticosteroids. Budesonide is an oral corticosteroid that offers relatively lower systemic exposure compared to prednisone secondary to high first-pass metabolism.

Budesonide has been effective in UC treatment but is limited to UC when the ileal release formulation can reach the location of disease.

i. Topical therapy generally induces remission more quickly than oral therapy, and it offers less frequent dosing than oral therapy. Suppositories reach the disease approximately 10 cm proximally. Hydrocortisone foam reaches the disease 15–20 cm proximally. Enemas reach the disease approximately to the splenic flexure (52–56 cm)

j. Topical 5-ASA for inducing and maintaining remission of UC
   (1) Mesalamine suppositories 500 mg twice a day (proctitis)
   (2) Mesalamine enemas 1–4 g per day (distal colitis proximally to the splenic flexure)

k. Topical corticosteroids for inducing remission of UC
   (1) Hydrocortisone enema 100 mg per day
   (2) Hydrocortisone foam, 10% 1 application every day to twice a day

l. Oral plus topical therapy consisting of oral mesalamine 2.4 g per day in divided doses plus mesalamine 4 g per day enema may induce remission of UC more quickly.

3. **Maintenance of distal disease**

   a. **5-ASA** preparation dosages for maintaining remission of distal disease
      (1) Balsalazide 3–6 g per day
      (2) Mesalamine Eudragrit-S 3.2 g per day
      (3) Mesalamine suppository 500 mg every day or twice a day
      (4) Mesalamine enema 2–4 g daily, every other day, or every third day
      (5) Olsalazine 1 g per day
      (6) Sulfasalazine 2 g per day
      (7) Mesalamine 1.6 g orally per day plus 4-g enemas twice weekly is also effective

   b. Corticosteroids, topical and oral, are not effective in maintaining UC remission and should not be used.

4. **Mild to moderate extensive or relapsing disease**

   a. **Oral 5-ASA**
      (1) Sulfasalazine 4–6 g per day in four divided doses. Doses > 2 g per day appear to offer little benefit.
      (2) Newer 5-ASA preparations are generally considered to be equal to sulfasalazine in regard to efficacy and are likely superior in regard to adverse events and tolerance; but they are more expensive. The dosages used are a minimum of 2 g per day of active 5-ASA moiety titrated up to a maximum of 4.8 g per day.

   b. **Oral steroids**
      (1) Prednisone 40–60 mg per day (modest efficacy gain with 60 mg compared to 40 mg) until significant clinical effect is seen followed by a dose taper of 5–10 mg weekly until a daily dose of 20 mg is reached. Tapering generally continues from here at 2.5 mg per week until the patient is weaned from oral steroids.
      (2) Higher doses for longer periods increase risk of corticosteroid-associated risk.
      (3) IBD patients receiving corticosteroids for > 3 months should be evaluated and may benefit from dual-energy x-ray absorptiometry (DEXA) bone testing and possibly preventative therapy with bisphosphonates, alendronate (Fosamax), risedronate (Actonel), and etidronate (Didrocal).
      (4) For patients on long-term corticosteroid therapy and who have significant risk factors, such as previous fractures, bisphosphonates, calcium supplementation at 1–1.5 g per day, and vitamin D supplementation at 800 mg per day should also be considered.
      (5) Corticosteroid-induced osteoporosis has also been shown to respond to treatment with bisphosphonates.

5. **Maintenance of mild to moderate relapsing disease.** Sulfasalazine is as effective as equivalent doses of newer 5-ASA agents and is less costly in long-term therapy. Systemic corticosteroids as a rule are not accepted as long-term therapy options owing to adverse events and questionable therapeutic effect. 6-MP or azathioprine has been useful as a steroid sparing agent and as a long-term option to wean patients off corticosteroids.

   a. **Oral 5 ASA therapy**
      (1) Balsalazide 3–6 g per day
      (2) Mesalamine 2–4 g per day
      (3) Olsalazine 1 g per day
      (4) Sulfasalazine 2–4 g per day

   b. 6-MP and azathioprine 100–250 mg per day, maximum of 2.5 mg/kg/day

6. **Moderate to severe disease**. UC patients with moderate to severe disease are able to be managed on an outpatient basis or may require hospitalization. Patients with severe disease who are refractory to maximal oral therapy and patients with signs of toxicity should be hospitalized. Infection with enteric pathogens should be ruled out. Failure to demonstrate significant improvement within 7–10 days is an indication for surgical resection or alternate intravenous therapy such as with cyclosporine.

   a. Intensive IV steroid therapy is indicated for patients with severe disease who are hospitalized. Doses with prednisolone (40–60 mg), hydrocortisone (300 mg), or methylprednisolone (32–48 mg per day in divided doses or as continuous infusion) have been shown to be effective. Higher doses are of limited benefit and increase the risks of steroid toxicity.

   b. Empiric broad-spectrum antibiotics are of little use in moderate to severe UC.

   c. When possible, patients should be maintained on oral feedings with a modified diet to reduce abdominal discomfort and diarrhea and bowel frequency. Total parenteral nutrition is used when oral feeds are not tolerated and can be especially useful in patients with severe nutritional depletion.

   d. In patients with signs of toxicity, narcotics, antidiarrheals, and anticholinergics should be avoided because they can increase the risk of worsening colonic dilation and perforation.

   e. 5-ASA should be stopped in the acute setting to avoid intolerance issues and the rare instances of 5-ASA exacerbating colitis.

   f. Topical steroids may provide benefit in patients with rectal urgency or tenesmus.

   g. Intravenous cyclosporine at 2–4 mg/kg per day and titrated to blood levels between 200 and 400 ng/mL has been effective in a high percentage of patients who do not respond to maximal parenteral steroids.

   h. Oral cyclosporine at twice the daily intravenous dose is given in divided doses (twice a day) with oral steroids once clinical remission is reached with intravenous cyclosporine.

   i. Relapse on 5-ASA therapy alone after remission induced with cyclosporine is frequent, and azathioprine or 6-MP can be beneficial when added for maintenance.

   j. Sulfamethoxazole/trimethoprim (Bactrim) should be added as prophylaxis against *Pneumocystis* pneumonia for patients on cyclosporine.

7. **Fulminant disease.** Patients with fulminant colitis or toxic megacolon should be treated as noted for severe disease and should not take anything by mouth. Broad-spectrum antibiotics are often used empirically owing to the high risk of perforation. Any worsening of disease as evidenced by radiologic, clinical, or laboratory changes while on medical therapy is an indication for immediate colectomy.

C. **Drug therapy for CD** depends on the disease location, disease severity and any complications.

1. **Mild to moderate CD**
   a. 5-ASA orally
      (1) Mesalamine 3.2–4 g per day
      (2) Sulfasalazine 3–6 g per day
      (3) Specific disease locations may dictate which preparation to use based on site of delivery
      (4) Sulfasalazine may be more effective than newer 5-ASAs. It also is less expensive but less well tolerated
   b. Oral broad-spectrum antibiotics have been used with limited controlled clinical data to support such use.
      (1) Added to 5-ASA therapy for failures
      (2) Metronidazole 750–1500 mg per day
      (3) Ciprofloxacin 1000 mg per day
   c. Budesonide orally
      (1) Targeted delivery to the ileum, works well in ileal or proximal colon disease.
      (2) Dose at 9 mg per day for 8–16 weeks
      (3) Tapered 3 mg per week over 2–4 weeks
   d. If these fail, the presentation can be considered refractory and treated as moderate to severe.

2. **Moderate to severe CD**
   a. **Systemic steroids**
      (1) Prednisone 40–60 mg per day
      (2) Hospitalization for intravenous corticosteroids may also be considered

b. Azathioprine, 6-MP, and methotrexate
   (1) Effective for steroid failure
   (2) Azathioprine 2–3 mg/kg/day or 6-MP 1–1.5 mg/kg/day
   (3) Methotrexate 25 mg/week IM, tapered to 15 mg/week IM after 16 weeks
   (4) Azathioprine, 6-MP, and methotrexate are all antimetabolite drugs and will take considerable time to reach full effect, up to 3–4 months may be required.
   (5) Concomitant use of oral 5-ASA or antibiotics with immunosuppressant therapy have not been shown to be of benefit in controlled trials.

c. Anti-TNF therapy, infliximab
   (1) For patients refractory to or who do not tolerate systemic steroids and immunosuppressant therapy
   (2) Infliximab is effective therapy for perianal fistulizing CD .
   (3) Infliximab 5 mg/kg at 0, 2, and 6 weeks
   (4) Relapse at 1 year is high if infliximab is stopped.
   (5) HACA formation is common in noncontinuous therapy and may decrease efficacy of future courses of therapy. HACA formation may be limited with concomitant dosing of azathioprine, 6-MP, or methotrexate.
   (6) Concomitant therapy with 5-ASA, steroids, or antibiotics is of little added benefit.

3. Severe or fulminant CD includes active disease of a severe nature, toxic enteritis or colitis, megacolon, small bowel obstruction, and abdominal abscess. Patients often require hospitalization because of the severity of the disease and risk of complications.
   a. Typical therapy may include
      (1) Intravenous fluids and bowel rest (parenteral nutrition)
      (2) Intravenous antibiotics with metronidazole, aminoglycosides, and broad-spectrum penicillin or third-generation cephalosporins empirically for possible abscess or infections.
      (3) Intravenous corticosteroids
   b. Anti-TNF therapy with infliximab may be useful for patients who do not respond to intravenous corticosteroids.
   c. Surgical intervention may be required in patients who do not respond to intravenous corticosteroids and infliximab.

4. Maintenance of remission strategies have been of questionable efficacy. Historically, long-term treatment with 5-ASA agents and broad-spectrum antibiotics has been advocated with a lack of convincing controlled clinical data to support these measures. Newer evidence-based approaches may change therapy strategies.
   a. 5-ASA
      (1) May be of benefit but clinical data are mixed
      (2) Mesalamine 2.4–4.8 g per day or sulfasalazine 2–4 g per day
   b. Budesonide
      (1) Doses of 6–9 mg per day have been used with positive effect.
      (2) Appears to be safe compared to long-term systemic steroids
   c. Immunosuppressants
      (1) Azathioprine , 6-MP, methotrexate, and anti-TNF therapy have been used in maintenance; but adverse events must be weighed carefully, especially in patients with mild disease.
      (2) Azathioprine , 6-MP, and methotrexate may be useful in patients unable to wean off systemic steroids.
      (3) The duration of benefit of anti-TNF therapy with infliximab appears to be 8–12 weeks with a single dose. Dosing every 8 weeks seems to maintain response and reduce loss of efficacy. Concomitant azathioprine, 6-MP, or methotrexate can also reduce HACA formation and may increase efficacy.
   d. Systemic steroids are normally avoided in long-term therapy secondary to systemic toxicity; convincing data to support their use are lacking.
   d. Antibiotics have not been shown in controlled clinical trials to be effective in maintaining medically induced remission.

D. IBS

1. The treatment of IBS is based on the nature and severity of symptoms, correlation of symptoms to food intake and/or defecation, degree of functional impairment, and the presence of psychosocial or psychiatric disorders. Treatment is highly personalized and can be generalized as follows.

2. **Mild IBS** is the most common disease presentation, and patients normally suffer from few psychosocial problems.
   a. Education about the disease and support can be of great benefit.
   b. Diet and lifestyle changes
      (1) Specific foods are usually not as important as the size of meals; smaller meals are preferable. Care should be used and restrictive diets should be avoided.
      (2) Decrease fatty foods, gas-producing foods
      (3) Decrease alcohol
      (4) Decrease caffeine
      (5) Avoid dairy in lactose-intolerant patients
      (6) Excess fiber can also increase IBS symptoms
      (7) Prepare strategies to handle stress

3. **Moderate IBS** symptoms are normally intermittent but can be disabling at times. These patients suffer from more symptom-related distress. Patient symptoms historically are also associated with more gut reactivity (worse with eating and better with defecation).
   a. Anticholinergics used as antispasmodics
      (1) Dicyclomine (Bentyl) 20 mg by mouth four times a day
      (2) Hyoscyamine (Anaspaz) 0.15–0.3 mg by mouth four times a day
      (3) Clidinium plus chlordiazepoxide (Librax) 2.5/5 mg 1–2 tabs by mouth before every meal and at bedtime
      (4) Hyoscyamine + scopolamine, atropine, phenobarbital (Donnatal) 1–2 tablets every 6–8 hr
   b. Antidiarrheals
      (1) Diphenoxylate plus atropine (Lomotil) 0.025/2.5 mg 2 tabs by mouth four times a day, maximum of 8 tablets per day
      (2) Loperamide (Imodium) 4 mg followed by 2 mg after each unformed bowel movement up to a maximum of 16 mg per day
   c. Tegaserod (Zelnorm) a 5-hydroxytryptamine 4 (5-HT$_4$) agonist for constipation predominant IBS in women and chronic idiopathic constipation in patients aged $\leq$ 65
      (1) IBS dosing (**women only**) is 6 mg by mouth twice a day before meals
      (2) Chronic constipation dosing is 6 mg by mouth twice a day before meals
   d. Alosetron (Lotronex) is a 5-HT$_3$ antagonist available in the United States through a manufacturer-sponsored access program; it is to be used only for diarrhea-predominant IBS in women. The dose for severe IBS in **women only** is 0.5–1 mg by mouth twice a day.
   e. Low-dose tricyclic antidepressants (TCAs) can be effective for pain control. The dosages typically used are below the effective doses used for clinical depression. TCA also may slow GI transit time and be useful in diarrhea-predominate patient cases.

4. **Severe IBS** is a very small proportion of the entire IBS population. GI complaints can be refractory and of continuous nature. Psychosocial and psychiatric comorbidities are common.
   a. Antidepressants, including the selective serotonin reuptake inhibitors, are often useful in severe IBS patients owing to the increase in psychosocial components to patient presentation.
   b. Anxiolytic drugs, including diazepam, are occasionally used for IBS when patients are experiencing acute anxiety that is worsening their symptoms. In light of the risk of dependency, these drugs should be taken for only short periods of time.

III. COMPLICATIONS

A. IBD

1. **UC and CD** have many similar presenting features as well as commonalities in complications. The majority of UC patients will have a chronic relapsing disease course. Length of disease is related to risk of colectomy and colorectal cancer. Mortality is similar to rates in non- UC populations. CD may impose a slight increase in mortality with long standing disease.

2. **Musculoskeletal** manifestations of IBD are the most common extraintestinal manifestations of the disease.
    a. Arthralgias in the absence of arthritis signs are the most common complaint.
    b. Between 5% and 20% of IBD patients experience peripheral arthritis pain that is self-limiting and coincides with IBD flares and resolves with successful treatment of IBD. Occurrence is nearly equal between males and females.
    c. Ankylosing spondylitis in IBD is less common, at approximately 5%, and is equal in UC and CD. Males are affected more than females and the course is usually not related to the course of IBD.

3. **CD fistulas and abscess.** Long-standing inflammation may progress into penetrating disease, abscess formation, and fistula formation. These penetrating communications can be from diseased organ to neighboring organ, peritoneum, and skin. Fistula types include perianal, enteroenteric, enterocutaneous, enterovesical, and rectovaginal.

4. **Hemorrhage** in the colon is relatively rare in UC but is serious. Acute hemorrhage accounts for a significant percentage of urgent colectomies in UC. Severe bleeding tends to occur early in the course of disease. Hemorrhage in CD is extremely rare.

5. **Strictures** or narrowing of the colon or rectum occurs in a small percentage of the UC population. It is important that nearly one third of such strictures may be related to malignancy and so should be carefully evaluated.

6. **Toxic megacolon** is a serious complication mainly seen in UC but occasionally in CD as well. It occurs when the inflammatory process causes the colon to dilate, with subsequent bowel wall thinning. This results in the bowel becoming more fragile. The major risk is bowel perforation. Bowel dilation that does not respond to therapy within 72 hr is considered an indication for surgical resection.

7. **Cancer.** Overall, UC patients are at higher risk of developing **colorectal cancer** compared to patients without IBD. The risk to individuals is variable and is related to duration and extent of UC as well as patient-specific risk factors. Risk is greatest in patients with pancolitis of long-standing duration. Colorectal cancer is also a risk in CD patients, especially if it is CD involving the colon. Risk of cancer of the small intestine has been noted in CD as well.

8. **Primary sclerosing cholangitis** (PSC) is the most common hepatobiliary complication of IBD. PSC affects men more than woman. PSC is more common in UC than in CD.

9. **Osteoporosis** as evidenced by increased fractures and diminished bone density has been shown in CD patients.

10. **Quality of life.** While most IBD patients are able to lead nearly normal lives, many do suffer significantly during active flares of disease. The chronic nature of disease also has a negative effect on patient QOL.

B. **IBS.** Although IBS has been shown to produce substantial physical discomfort and emotional distress, most patients with IBS do not develop serious or long-term health complications. Most patients learn to control their individual symptoms with diet and lifestyle modification or medical therapy as needed.

STUDY QUESTIONS

Directions: Each of the questions, statements, or incomplete statements in this section can be correctly answered or completed by **one** of the suggested answers or phrases. Choose the **best** answer.

For questions 1–2: A 35-year-old male presents to his physician with the primary complaints of abdominal pain and frequent bowel movements over the past few weeks. Upon examination and routine laboratory testing, he is found to have a low-grade fever and an elevated erythrocyte sedimentation rate (ESR). Further questioning reveals he is having four to five loose bowel movements each day. The patient is a past smoker. Stool antigen tests are negative for known gastrointestinal (GI) pathogens. Physical examination and colonoscopy reveal contiguous areas of inflammation of the rectum and most of the descending colon. The physician diagnoses moderately severe ulcerative colitis.

1. Which therapy would be the most effective for inducing remission?

(A) topical corticosteroids
(B) topical 5-aminosalicylic acid (5-ASA)
(C) oral budesonide
(D) topical 5-ASA plus oral 5-ASA

2. Once remission is achieved, which therapy is most appropriate for maintenance?

(A) sulfasalazine 2 g per day
(B) balsalazide 2 g per day
(C) olsalazine 4 g per day
(D) topical corticosteroids

For questions 3–4: An 18-year-old female with mild Crohn disease who is being treated with oral sulfasalazine 4 g per day presents to her physician because her symptoms have returned. She is ambulatory with no signs of toxicity or weight loss. Her disease is mainly of the ileum.

3. What would be a logical next step in therapy?

(A) intravenous corticosteroids
(B) budesonide 9 mg per day
(C) prednisone 40 mg orally per day
(D) azathioprine 1 mg/kg per day

4. The patient fails this next therapy and is determined to be refractory. Her symptoms are increasing and her schooling is beginning to suffer. She is also noted to have been intolerant of a trial of 2.5 mg/kg day of 6-mercaptopurine (6-MP) therapy. What would be a logical next step in therapy?

(A) azathioprine 1mg/kg per day
(B) metronidazole 750 mg per day
(C) surgical resection with ostomy
(D) infliximab 5 mg/kg at 0, 2, and 6 weeks

For question 5: A man with diarrhea-predominant IBS is experiencing interruption of his work as a truck driver because of frequent bouts of diarrhea. He states his symptoms are worse after eating, especially fried foods. His physician discusses the possible benefit of avoiding fat in his diet. The patient agrees to try but also asks for something to use in emergencies.

5. What would be the most appropriate therapy to use?

(A) alosetron 0.5 mg twice a day
(B) hyoscyamine 0.15 mg by mouth as needed
(C) loperamide 4 mg then 2 mg as needed up to 16 mg per day
(D) fluoxetine 40 mg every day

6. Which is most appropriate for a woman with constipation-predominant IBS?

(A) a restrictive bland diet
(B) tegaserod 6 mg by mouth twice a day
(C) alosetron 1 mg by mouth twice a day
(D) excess dietary fiber

7. Patients with ulcerative colitis and Crohn disease present in similar ways. There are several clinical differences between the diseases that can help differentiate them. Which of the following clinical features is more common in Crohn disease than in ulcerative colitis?

(A) abnormal bowel movements
(B) slow onset of disease
(C) joint pain
(D) fistula formation

ANSWERS AND EXPLANATIONS

1. The correct answer is D *[see II.B.2].*
Topical 5-ASA therapy plus oral 5-ASA therapy has been shown to be superior to either alone or topical steroids at inducing remission in mild to moderate UC. Budesonide ileal release will not likely reach the site of disease in this patient because he has left-sided disease.

2. The correct answer is A *[see II.B.3].*
The correct dose for balsalazide is 3–6 g per day and for olsalazine is 1 g per day. Topical steroids have no place in maintenance of UC.

3. The correct answer is B *[see II.C.1].*
This patient has not responded to 5-ASA therapy for inducing remission of her mild disease. The patient is not showing signs of severe disease or toxicity and as such neither intravenous or oral therapy with systemic corticosteroids is warranted at this time. A dose of 1 mg/kg per day of azathioprine is below the recommended dose for inducing remission. Azathioprine also may take several months to induce remission. Budesonide is an ileal-release therapy, and her disease is mainly confined to that area. Budesonide has been shown to be effective in mild and moderate CD.

4. The correct answer is D *[see II.C.2].*
This patient is intolerant to azathioprine and it should not be used. Broad-spectrum antibiotics are unlikely to be of any benefit in this patient and should not be used. While likely to be beneficial, surgery with a permanent ostomy would also be severely limiting to a young patient because of social and QOL concerns. Infliximab has been shown to be effective for refractory CD.

5. The correct answer is C *[see II.D.3].*
This patient is male and as such alosetron is not an appropriate option for him. Hyoscyamine is an effective antispasmodic but will likely do little for his diarrhea. The patient makes no complaint of serious affect on his life and does not show signs of severe disease. Full-dose antidepressant fluoxetine dosing is not warranted. Loperamide can be of use in managing mild to moderate symptoms of IBS.

6. The correct answer is B *[see II.D.3].*
Tegaserod 6 mg by mouth twice a day with meals is appropriate and effective therapy for women suffering from constipation-predominant IBS. Alosetron is effective in women with diarrhea-predominant IBS. Restrictive diets are not normally of benefit, and excess dietary fiber can increase IBS symptoms.

7. The correct answer is D *[see I.B.1].*
While the overlap of clinical presentation of these two diseases is substantial, fistula formation is extremely rare in ulcerative colitis.

54
Diabetes Mellitus
Peggy C. Yarborough

I. INTRODUCTION

A. Definition. Diabetes mellitus (DM) is a chronic, progressive, systemic disease characterized by dysfunction in the following:

1. Metabolism of fats, carbohydrates, protein, and insulin

2. Function and structure of blood vessels and nerves

B. Classification. There are four clinical classes of diabetes: type 1, type 2, gestational diabetes mellitus (GDM), and other specific types (secondary DM). Although *not* a type of diabetes, prediabetes is included with the classification of glucose abnormalities.

1. **Type 1.** Previously described as insulin-dependent diabetes mellitus (IDDM), juvenile-onset diabetes, or ketosis-prone diabetes. Results from β cell destruction, usually leading to absolute deficiency of insulin secretion. β cell destruction may be from immune or nonimmune factors.
   a. Most common in children and in adults > 30 years old, but may occur at any age
   b. **Immune mediated**. More than 90% of type 1 is immune mediated.
      (1) Markers of immune destruction of β cells are present. Also related to environmental factors that are still poorly defined.
      (2) Predisposed to **ketoacidosis,** accumulation of ketone bodies in body tissues and fluids (see II.B.1).
      (3) Depends on exogenous insulin-replacement therapy to prevent ketoacidosis and sustain life.
      (4) Patients are also **prone to other autoimmune disorders**—for example, Graves disease, Hashimoto thyroiditis, Addison disease, vitiligo, celiac sprue, autoimmune hepatitis, myasthenia gravis, and pernicious anemia.
      (5) Rate of β cell destruction is variable; rapid in some (mainly infants and children) and slow in others (mainly adults)
      (6) **Latent autoimmune diabetes in adults (LADA)**, also described as type 1.5 diabetes, slowly progressive type 1 diabetes, latent type 1 diabetes, youth-onset diabetes of maturity, and LADA-type 1 and LADA-type 2. Good glycemic control may be maintained for several years with sulfonylureas, but patient eventually becomes insulin dependent.
   c. **Idiopathic type 1 diabetes.** No known cause; < 10% of type 1 is idiopathic.
      (1) Strongly inherited, lacks immunological evidence for β cell autoimmunity, and is not human leukocyte antigen (HLA) associated.
      (2) May have permanent insulinopenia and be prone to ketoacidosis.
      (3) Or may have episodic ketoacidosis and exhibit some degree of insulin deficiency between episodes. An absolute requirement for insulin-replacement therapy may come and go.
      (4) Most are of African or Asian ancestry
   d. The essential difference between type 1 and type 2 DM is that insulin production and secretion in type 1 is destroyed; in type 2 DM, insulin production and secretion may be altered or reduced but is not totally lacking.

2. **Type 2.** Previously described as non-insulin-dependent diabetes mellitus (NIDDM) or adult-onset diabetes. Results from a progressive insulin secretory defect on the background of insulin resistance.
   a. Approximately **90%** of individuals with diabetes in the United States have type 2 diabetes, with a disproportionate representation among certain ethnic groups and the elderly.
   b. May present as predominantly **insulin resistance** with relative insulin deficiency to predominantly an insulin secretory defect with insulin resistance.

1147

    c. Most patients are **obese** at diagnosis (approximately 80%), either by traditional weight criteria or by increased percentage of body fat distributed predominantly in the abdominal region.

    d. Usually diagnosed in adults >30 years old, but may occur at any age. The incidence of type 2 DM in adolescents is increasing, apparently related to an increasing incidence of obesity in this age group, decreasing exercise/physical activity, and genetic and other lifestyle factors.

    e. Insulin resistance may improve by interventions (weight loss, exercise, medications), but **seldom returns to normal.**

    f. Endogenous insulin levels may appear normal, increased, or decreased, and the requirement for exogenous insulin is variable. Despite apparently "normal" or "increased" insulin levels, β cell dysfunction is manifest by a *relative insulin insufficiency* to maintain euglycemia, especially in the face of significant insulin resistance.

    g. Diminished incretin effects develop early or later into the disease

    h. Not prone to ketosis except during periods of severe physical stress such as infections, trauma, or surgery.

3. Gestational diabetes mellitus. Defined as any degree of glucose intolerance that has its onset or is first detected during pregnancy.

    a. Occurs in 2%–4% of pregnant women, generally during the second or third trimester.

    b. A follow-up glucose tolerance test should be performed at 6 weeks after pregnancy. Glucose regulation would then be reclassified as DM, impaired fasting glucose (IFG), impaired glucose tolerance (IGT), or normoglycemia. In the majority of cases, glucose regulation returns to normal postpregnancy.

    c. Occurrence of GDM increases future risk for developing type 2 diabetes.

4. Other specific types (secondary diabetes). Broad term used to classify patients who have unusual causes of diabetes owing to certain diseases of the pancreas, genetic defects, endocrinopathies, or drugs.

5. Prediabetes. Term used to refer to an intermediate metabolic stage between normal glucose homeostasis and diabetes. Prediabetes is a risk factor for future DM and cardiovascular disease (CVD).

C. Diabetes demographics and statistics

1. In the United States, an estimated **6.3%** of the population has DM, and nearly half as many individuals remain undiagnosed.

2. Type 1 DM accounts for approximately 10% of cases and type 2 for about 90%

3. DM is listed as the **sixth leading cause of death** in the United States;[1] but it likely contributes to other significant causes, such as heart disease (number one cause of death), cerebrovascular diseases (number three), and kidney disease (number nine).

D. Cause. Various factors contribute to the development of DM.

1. Type 1 DM. Genetic predisposition, environmental factors, and autoimmunity have been proposed.

    a. Genetics. Certain genetic markers in the HLA system have been strongly linked with type 1 DM, and the risk of developing diabetes is substantially increased in the offspring of individuals diagnosed with diabetes.

    b. Environment. Not all individuals at genetic risk for type 1 DM develop the disease. Some type of trigger, such as a virus (e.g., rubella) or toxic chemical, is needed for the expression of the genetic propensity for type 1 DM.

    c. Autoimmunity. An autoimmune component, perhaps stimulated by the environmental trigger, is involved in the development of type 1 diabetes. Anti-insulin or anti–β cell antibodies are present in the blood of most individuals at the time of diagnosis of type 1 DM.

---

[1]Centers for Disease Control and Prevention, National Center for Health Statistics. Deaths: Final data for 2003. Available at www.cdc.gov/nchs/products/pubs/pubd/hestats/finaldeaths03/finaldeaths03.htm.

2. **Type 2 DM.** Genetic factors, a β cell defect, and peripheral site defects have been implicated.
   a. **Genetics.** There is a greater than 90% concordance rate between monozygotic twins if one has type 2 diabetes. It has been estimated that offspring of individuals with type 2 diabetes have approximately a 15% chance of developing the disease.
   b. Diminished **β cell function** is postulated to cause abnormalities in insulin secretion, resulting in a relative deficiency of insulin.
   c. A **peripheral site defect** is postulated to lead to **insulin resistance** (tissue insensitivity to the biological activity of insulin). This condition is thought to result primarily from postbinding abnormalities.

3. **Secondary diabetes** may arise from such conditions as endocrine disorders (e.g., Cushing syndrome), pancreatic disease, and the use of drugs that antagonize insulin (e.g., thiazide diuretics, adrenocorticosteroids).

II. PATHOPHYSIOLOGY OF THE DIABETIC STATE

A. **Normal glucose regulation** requires the intricate balance of insulin, counterregulatory hormones, intestinal incretins, and amylin hormone. Alterations in these key components form the basis for medication selection for the diabetic state.

1. **Insulin** is responsible for a variety of effects throughout body tissues.
   a. Stimulates **glucose transport** across cell membranes and promotes the storage of glucose as glycogen in muscle and liver cells
   b. Enhances fat storage (**lipogenesis**) and prevents the mobilization of fat for energy (**lipolysis** and **ketogenesis**)
   c. Inhibits production of glucose from liver or muscle glycogen (**glycogenolysis**)
   d. Promotes incorporation of **amino acids into proteins**
   e. Inhibits the formation of glucose from amino acids (**gluconeogenesis**)
   f. **Decreases the breakdown of fatty acids** to ketone bodies

2. **Counterregulatory hormones** antagonize the glycemic effects of insulin.
   a. Glucagon (produced in the α cells of the pancreas)
   b. Epinephrine
   c. Norepinephrine
   d. Growth hormone
   e. Cortisol

3. **Intestinal hormones**, notably **glucagon-like peptide 1 (GLP-1)** and **glucose-dependent insulinotropic polypeptide (GIP),** Hormones secreted by the intestines, in response to ingestion of food, enhance the ability of orally administered glucose to stimulate pancreatic β cell secretion of insulin.
   a. These effects are referred to as "incretin effects." *Incretin* stands for intestinal (stimulators for) secretion of insulin.
   b. Incretins do not directly stimulate insulin secretion but instead enhance the ability of glucose to stimulate insulin secretion.
   c. **Postprandial secretion** of GLP-1 is **diminished** in DM. GLP-1 actions include
      (1) Reduced rate of gastric emptying
      (2) Inhibited glucagon secretion by pancreatic α cells
      (3) Inhibited appetite
      (4) Altered β cell biosynthesis, resulting in increased β cell mass and increased insulin secretory capacity
   d. GIP secretion is normal or increased in DM, but β cell **response is diminished.**

4. **Amylin.** A neurohormone normally co-secreted with insulin, by pancreatic β cells in response to food intake.
   a. Amylin secretion is diminished when there is β cell destruction or dysfunction.
   b. Amylin **lowers postprandial concentrations** by
      (1) Slowing gastric emptying on ingestion of food, thus reducing the rate of glucose influx into the bloodstream

    (2) Suppressing nutrient-stimulated secretion of glucagon, thus reducing hepatic glucose output after meals

    (3) Modulating appetite by enhancing satiety, resulting in decreased food intake

B. Abnormal glucose regulation/hyperglycemic emergencies associated with diabetes. In untreated type 1 and type 2 DM, the disease follows a predictable progression from initial abnormalities of glucose metabolism to life-threatening diabetic ketoacidosis or hyperglycemic hyperosmolar nonketotic syndrome.

  1. Diabetic ketoacidosis (DKA; type 1 DM)

    a. Insulin deficiency results in hyperglycemia.

      (1) Impaired glucose uptake in the peripheral tissues (primarily muscle)

      (2) Reduction in the conversion of glucose to glycogen (impaired **glycogenesis**), primarily in the liver

      (3) Impaired insulin-induced suppression of hepatic glucose production (**neoglucogenesis** and **glycogenolysis**)

    b. As blood glucose (BG) concentrations increase, the glucose reabsorptive capacity of the kidneys will be exceeded. This occurs at about 180 mg/dL, referred to as the **renal threshold for glucose.** Glucose is then excreted into the urine, resulting in an **osmotic diuresis** with subsequent **dehydration** and **electrolyte abnormalities.**

    c. Insufficient glucose uptake in the peripheral tissues (owing to insulin deficiency) causes the cells to use protein and fat as energy sources rather than glucose.

    d. Breakdown of protein yields carbohydrate/glucose moieties, but with insufficient insulin, the additional glucose worsens hyperglycemia rather than serving as an energy source.

    e. Breakdown of triglycerides (the stored form of fat) yields **free fatty acids** and **glycerol** through the process of **lipolysis.** Without the administration of insulin, type 1 DM will progress to ketonemia and ketoacidosis, as described below:

      (1) Increasing amounts of glycerol leads to enhanced hepatic glucose production, further worsening hyperglycemia.

      (2) Free fatty acids are broken down in the liver into **ketone bodies,** which are excreted by the kidneys (**ketonuria**). Acetoacetate (a ketone body) is converted in the liver to acetone, which is excreted through the lungs. This is associated with a fruity odor and can sometimes be detected on the breath of the patient.

      (3) As the utilization (breakdown) of adipose tissue continues, ketone production exceeds the capacity for excretion, leading to accumulation in the bloodstream (**ketonemia**).

      (4) Increasing levels of free fatty acids contribute to the development and worsening of **acidosis.**

      (5) Initially, there is compensation for acidosis by changes in breathing patterns (**Kussmaul breathing**) and by buffering systems of the blood (e.g., proteins, bicarbonate).

      (6) As acidosis continues, breathing compensation and bicarbonate stores are insufficient or depleted. A state of ketosis with acidosis (**ketoacidosis**) then exists.

      (7) If ketoacidosis is not promptly treated by insulin, coma and death will ensue in type 1 DM.

      (8) The total lack of insulin in type 1 DM is a predisposing factor for DKA. Patients with type 1 DM are described as **ketosis prone.**

  2. Hyperglycemic hyperosmolar nonketotic (HHS) syndrome (type 2 DM)

    a. Insulin deficiency, often with concomitant insulin resistance, results in hyperglycemia

      (1) Impaired glucose uptake in the peripheral tissues (primarily muscle)

      (2) Reduction in the conversion of glucose to glycogen (impaired **glycogenesis**), primarily in the liver

      (3) Impaired insulin-induced suppression of hepatic glucose production (**neoglucogenesis** and **glycogenolysis**)

    b. Increasing blood glucose concentrations exceed the glucose reabsorptive capacity of the kidneys (occurs at about 180 mg/dL, referred to as the **renal threshold for glucose**). Glucose is then excreted into the urine, resulting in an **osmotic diuresis** with subsequent **dehydration** and **electrolyte abnormalities.**

    c. Insufficient glucose uptake in the peripheral tissues (owing to insulin deficiency and/or insulin resistance) causes the cells to use protein as energy sources rather than glucose. Breakdown of protein yields carbohydrate/glucose moieties; however, with insufficient insulin, the additional glucose worsens hyperglycemia rather than serving as an energy source.

   d. In type 2 DM, the presence of even minimal blood levels of endogenous insulin usually prevents the breakdown of fats and subsequent ketonemia and ketoacidosis. Thus patients with type 2 DM are described as **ketosis resistant.**

   e. Although sufficient to suppress ketosis, endogenous insulin secretion in type 2 DM is insufficient for glycemic control. If insulin is not administered, profound dehydration with very high blood glucose levels may occur; this state is described as **HHS syndrome.** Coma and death may result.

III. CLINICAL EVALUATION

A. Physical findings

1. **Symptom severity and onset** help differentiate type 1 from type 2 DM.
   - **a.** Type 1 DM typically presents with an abrupt onset and an acute presentation.
   - **b.** Symptoms in individuals with type 2 DM generally develop gradually, with some patients being asymptomatic or having only mild symptoms upon diagnosis.

2. **Classic signs and symptoms** of DM include polydipsia (excessive thirst), polyuria (excessive urination), and polyphagia (excessive hunger). Other common findings include dry skin, fatigue, weakness, frequent skin and vaginal infections, weight alterations, and visual disturbances.

3. Individuals with type 1 DM may additionally present with unintentional weight loss, with or without signs and symptoms of ketoacidosis.

4. Some of the progressive changes of long-standing DM may be evident at the time of diagnosis of type 2 DM: deterioration in function or structure of the retina, kidneys, peripheral nervous system, and integumentary system.

B. Diagnostic testing or screening for diabetes[2]

1. **Diabetes in nonpregnant adults**
   - **a.** The preferred test to diagnose DM in nonpregnant adults is the fasting plasma glucose (**FPG**). The 75-g oral glucose tolerance test (**OGTT**) is more sensitive and more specific than FPG, but OGTT is rarely performed correctly in the outpatient setting. Because of ease of process, acceptability to patients, and lower cost, the FPG is the preferred diagnostic tool.
   - **b.** Three types of findings are accepted as the diagnosis of DM:
     - **(1)** A random (casual) plasma glucose (PG) level **> 200 mg/dL** with classic symptoms of DM, including polydipsia, polyuria, polyphagia, and weight loss.
     - **(2)** FPG level **> 126 mg/dL**
     - **(3)** A 2-hr plasma glucose **> 200 mg/dL** during an OGTT using 75 g anhydrous glucose dissolved in water.
   - **c.** In the absence of unequivocal hyperglycemia with acute decompensation, the above criteria should be **confirmed with repeat testing** on a different day.
   - **d.** Note that these criteria do not distinguish between type 1 and type 2 DM; rather, they only **identify the presence** of clinical diabetes.

2. **Gestational diabetes**
   - **a.** Risk assessment for GDM should be undertaken at the **first prenatal visit**. Marked obesity, personal history of GDM, glycosuria, or a strong family history of DM would constitute a high risk for GDM.
   - **b.** **High-risk women**
     - **(1)** Perform glucose testing as soon as possible
     - **(2)** A FPG **> 125 mg/dL** or casual PG **> 200 mg/dL,** confirmed on a subsequent day

[2]American Diabetes Association. Standards of medical care for patients with diabetes mellitus. Diabetes Care 2006; 29:S4–42.

unless unequivocal symptoms of hyperglycemia are present, constitutes a diagnosis of DM.

(3) High-risk women not found to have GDM at the initial screening should be tested **between 24 and 28 weeks** of gestation. Testing should follow one of two approaches:

(a) **One-step approach.** Perform a diagnostic 100-g OGTT.

(b) **Two-step approach**

(i) Initial screening of **50-g oral glucose load** (glucose challenge test; GCT). A 1-hr plasma or serum glucose threshold value of 140 mg/dL identifies ~ 80% of GDM and 130 mg/dL identifies 90% of GDM.

(ii) Perform a diagnostic 100-g OGTT on the subset of women exceeding the threshold values for the GCT. Diagnosis of GDM may be made if two values equal or exceed the following:

{a} Fasting: 95 mg/dL

{b} 1 hr: 180 mg/dL

{c} 2 hr: 155 mg/dL

{d} 3 hr: 140 mg/dL

(iii) Alternatively, a 75-g glucose load may be used; but that test is not as well validated for detection of GDM.

c. **Average-risk women.** Test between 24 and 28 weeks of gestation, using one of the two approaches described for high-risk women.

d. **Low-risk women.** Require no glucose testing, but this status is limited to individuals meeting *all* of the following criteria:

(1) Younger than 25 years of age

(2) Normal body weight before pregnancy

(3) Ethnic group with a low prevalence of GDM (e.g., *not* Hispanic, African American, Asian, or Native American)

(4) No first-degree relative with DM

(5) No history of poor obstetrical outcome

3. **Type 2 DM in children**

a. Glucose testing should be performed in children at **10 years of age** or at onset of puberty (if puberty occurs < 10 years of age) who exhibit the following risk factors for DM:

(1) **Overweight**, defined as: body mass index (BMI) > 85th percentile for age and sex, weight for height > 85th percentile, or weight > 120% of ideal for height.

(2) *Plus* any two of the following:

(a) Family history of type 2 DM in first- or second-degree relative

(b) Race/ethnicity (Native American, African American, Latino, Asian American, or Pacific Islander)

(c) Signs of insulin resistance or conditions associated with insulin resistance—for example, acanthosis nigricans, hypertension, dyslipidemia, polycystic ovary syndrome (PCOS)

(d) Maternal history of DM or GDM

b. Diagnostic criteria for DM are the same as listed for nonpregnant adults (see III.A.2).

c. **FPG** is the preferred test for children because of its ease of testing and reproducibility.

d. **Repeat every 2 years** if testing is negative for DM.

4. **Screening for DM or prediabetes**

a. Screening should be considered in individuals beginning at **age 45,** particularly in those with a **BMI > 25 kg/m²**.

b. Screening should also be considered in individuals < 45 years if they are overweight and have one or more risk factor for DM, such as

(1) Habitually physically inactive

(2) Have a first-degree relative with DM

(3) Member of a high-risk ethnic population (African American, Latino, Native American, Asian American, Pacific Islander)

(4) Given birth to a baby weighing 9 lb or has been diagnosed with GDM

(5) Hypertension

(6) High-density lipoprotein (HDL) cholesterol level < 35 mg/dL and/or a triglyceride level > 250 mg/dL

(7) PCOS

(8) On previous testing, had IGT or IFG

(9) Other clinical condition associated with insulin resistance (e.g., acanthosis nigricans)

(10) History of vascular disease

   c. A **FPG** test or 2-hr 75-g **OGTT** may be used for screening.

   d. If normal, repeat screening **every 3 years.**

   e. Diagnosis of prediabetes. Nonpregnant individuals not meeting the criteria for diabetes but with abnormal test results can be classified as having **IFT** or **IGT**. In 2002, IFG and IGT were officially termed **prediabetes.** Use of this term better communicates to individuals the seriousness of this abnormality in the context of progression to DM.

     (1) IFT. Fasting plasma glucose level > **110 mg/dL and** < **126 mg/dL**

     (2) IGT. A 2-hr OGTT plasma glucose > **140 mg/dL and** < **200 mg/dL**

IV. DESIRED OUTCOMES OF DIABETES MANAGEMENT would include, but are not limited to, the following (adapt for individual patient):

A. Mortality outcomes Avoid diabetes-related premature death. Life expectancy for American males is 74.8 years and for American females, 80.1 years[3]

B. Morbidity outcomes

   1. Retard progression of the disease

   2. Prevent or in a timely manner treat acute complications

   3. Prevent, detect early, or adequately treat vascular and neuropathic disease and prevent or treat risk factors associated with those diseases (e.g., hypertension, tobacco use, triglycerides, cholesterol, obesity)

   4. Prevent or minimize drug-related problems

     a. Side effects—adverse drug reactions (ADRs)

     b. Toxicity

     c. Drug interactions (drug–drug, drug–disease, drug–food, drug–laboratory)

C. Behavioral outcomes

   1. Annual eye exams

   2. Routine self-monitoring of blood glucose (SMBG)

   3. Development of a consistent support system

   4. Adherence to medication regimen

   5. Routine and timely medical examinations and laboratory tests

   6. Avoidance of life-style or other behaviors—for example, alcohol, caffeine, nicotine, certain over-the-counter (OTC) medications—that may increase the risk of diabetes-associated problems

D. Pharmacoeconomic outcomes

   1. Drug and treatment costs within patient resources

   2. Cost-effective and efficient use of healthcare resources

---

[3]Centers for Disease Control and Prevention, National Center for Health Statistics. Deaths.

E. Quality-of-life outcomes

1. Match, or only minimally change, patient lifestyle and activities with disease treatment

2. Patient satisfaction with pharmaceutical care and healthcare team

3. Positive but realistic outlook for the future

V. DESIRED THERAPEUTIC END POINTS FOR DIABETES MANAGEMENT include, but are not limited to, the following (adapt for the individual patient):

A. Nonpharmacological end points

1. Attain and/or maintain BMI < 27.

2. Cessation of alcohol intake, or limit to no more than 1 oz. per day

3. Nicotine/tobacco cessation

4. Moderate sodium reduction to at least 2300 mg/day[4]

5. At least 150 min/week of moderate-intensity aerobic physical activity, distributed over at least 3 days/week with no more than 2 consecutive days without exercise.[5]

6. In the absence of contraindications, individuals with type 2 DM should perform resistance exercise 3 times a week, targeting all major muscle groups, progressing to attain three sets of 8–10 repetitions at a weight that cannot be lifted more than 8–10 times.[6]

B. Pharmacological end points

1. Attain or maintain glycemic control.
   a. ADA glycemic goals[7]
      (1) Glycosylated hemoglobin AIC **(HbAIC) goal:** < **7%** (based on 6% as upper limit of normal), for patients in general. For an individual patient's goal, the HbAIC should be as close to normal as possible without significant hypoglycemia.
      (2) **Preprandial** capillary plasma glucose: 90–130 mg/dL
      (3) Peak 1–2 hr **postprandial** capillary plasma glucose: 180 mg/dL
   b. General experiential, clinical goals
      (1) SMBG standard deviation < 40, based on daily testing (at least once daily, alternating prebreakfast and presupper, with occasional 2-hr postprandial, largest meal)
      (2) SMBG values: 50% within target of 70–140 mg/dL; not more than 30% above 200 mg/dL
      (3) No more than one to two episodes of mild hypoglycemia per 1–2 weeks

2. Attain or maintain lipid profile within target range.[8]
   a. Low-density lipoprotein **(LDL)** < **100 mg/dL.** For individuals with overt CVD, a target of < 70 mg/dL should be considered
   b. **Triglycerides (TGs)** < **150 mg/dL.** When TGs exceed 200 mg/dL, a "non-HDL cholesterol" goal (total cholesterol minus HDL) of 130 mg/dL should be used.
   c. **HDL** > **40** mg/dL for males and > 50 mg/dL for females

3. **Blood pressure (BP)** < **130/80 mm Hg,** with minimal or no signs or symptoms of orthostatic hypotension

4. Minimal or no peripheral edema

---

[4]American Diabetes Association. Position statement: Hypertension management in adults with diabetes. Diabetes Care 2004;27:S65–67.
[5]American Diabetes Association. Standards of medical care.
[6]American Diabetes Association. Standards of medical care.
[7]American Diabetes Association. Standards of medical care.
[8]American Diabetes Association. Standards of medical care

5. Urinary albumin excretion < 30 **µg albumin/mg creatinine** in a spot collection (adjust end point based on results of initial microalbumin test)

6. Retention of recognition of hypoglycemia symptoms

VI. THERAPY OF PREDIABETES. Modest weight loss and regular physical activity have been shown to reduce the rate of progression of prediabetes to type 2 DM.[9] Other CVD risk factors such as tobacco use, hypertension, and dyslipidemia should also be aggressively managed. Selected patients may benefit by adjunct drug therapy. Metformin, acarbose, and orlistat[10] have also been shown to reduce progression to DM in single trials, but not as effectively as intensive lifestyle interventions.

VII. THERAPY OF DIABETES MELLITUS. Medical nutrition therapy, physical activity, pharmacotherapy, SMBG, and patient self-management education—especially concerning decision-making skills—are essential for successful management of the metabolic aspects of DM and for the prevention of diabetes-related conditions. Although some patients with "early" type 2 diabetes may not need pharmacotherapy for a while, the progressive nature of the disease ultimately results in the requirement of drug therapy.

    A. Medical nutrition therapy (MNT). MNT incorporates the principles of good nutrition applied to the individual's diabetes control goals, eating preferences and habits, and concurrent medical conditions. Successful MNT intervention is generally assessed by blood glucose and HbAIC level, LDL and HDL cholesterol and triglyceride levels, blood pressure, and body weight.

        1. An effective MNT plan will not be merely a "diet sheet" given to all people with diabetes. However, some of the common approaches to diabetes MNT include the following:

        2. Carbohydrate (CHO) counting. The individual is taught to identify and quantify the amounts of CHO foods consumed at each meal and throughout the day. Both the **amount (grams)** as well as the type of CHO (**glycemic index/glycemic load**) in a food influence blood glucose level. Usually CHO intake is 45%–60% of total calories, based on current diabetes control, TG levels, kidney function, and other medical concerns as well as patient choice.

            a. When DM therapy includes a premeal short-acting insulin dose (bolus), patients may be taught to adjust the bolus dose to match the CHO intake.

            b. Even when bolus insulin is not employed, patients need to be taught to maintain consistent CHO intake at designated meals and across the day to match the antidiabetes effects of oral medications or intermediate-acting insulins. *All patients with diabetes should be taught the principles of carbohydrate counting and identification.*

            c. Sugar and simple CHOs are be counted as part of the CHO intake for the meal.

        3. Fat intake and type of fat. Saturated and trans-fatty acids are the principal dietary determinant of plasma LDL cholesterol, the major risk factor for CVD. No studies have established the optimal percentages of dietary **saturated** and **trans-unsaturated fatty acids** (hydrogenated vegetable oils) or specific amounts of dietary cholesterol in patients with DM. However, individuals with DM are considered to be at similar risk as for individuals without

---

[9]Tuomilehto J, Lindstrom J, Eriksson JG, et al. Prevention of type 2 diabetes mellitus by changes in lifestyle among subjects with impaired glucose tolerance. N Engl J Med 2001;344:1343–1350. Pan XR, Li GW, Hu YH, et al. Effects of diet and exercise in preventing NIDDM in people with impaired glucose tolerance: The Da Qing IGT and Diabetes Study. Diabetes Care 1997;20:537–544. Diabetes Prevention Program Research Group. Reduction in the incidence of type 2 diabetes with lifestyle intervention or metformin. N Engl J Med 2002;346:393–403.

[10]Diabetes Prevention Program Research Group. Reduction in the incidence of type 2 diabetes. Chiasson JL, Josse RG, Gomis R, et al. Acarbose for prevention of type 2 diabetes mellitus: The STOP-NIDDM Randomized Trial. Lancet 2002;359:2072–2077. Torgerson JS, Hauptman J, Boldrin MN, Sjostrom L. XENical in the Prevention of Diabetes in Obese Subjects (XENDOS) study: A randomized study of orlistat as an adjunct to lifestyle changes for the prevention of type 2 diabetes in obese patients. Diabetes Care 2004;27:155–161; erratum in Diabetes Care 2004;27:856.

DM with a past history of CVD. Therefore, the recommendations for the latter group are generally applied for individuals with DM:[11]
   a. **Total fat: 25%–35%** of total calories
   b. **Saturated fat:** < **7%** of total calories
   c. Intake of **trans-fat should be minimized**

4. **Protein intake and type of protein.** Intake of protein in the range of 15%–20% of total calories (which is the average U.S. protein consumption) may be a risk factor for the development of diabetic nephropathy.[12] It is therefore recommended that diabetes patients limit protein intake to the RDA **(0.8 g high-quality protein/kg/day)**, which would be about **10% of total calories**.

5. **Fiber intake** (e.g., bran, beans, fruits, whole-grain products, vegetables) is to be encouraged; however, there is no evidence that people with diabetes need a greater amount of fiber than other Americans. Very large amounts of fiber may benefit glycemic control, hyperinsulinemia, and plasma lipids; but the palatability and gastrointestinal side effects of such amounts of fiber may be unacceptable to most people.

6. **Spaced intervals between meals** may be helpful for matching the hypoglycemic actions of insulin or insulin secretagogues or when postprandial glycemic normalization is delayed.

7. **Dietary adjustment algorithms.** Alteration of dietary intake based on factors that change the blood glucose level, such as stress, illness, or exercise. For example, consumption of additional carbohydrate and/or protein before vigorous exercise.

B. **Physical activity (exercise).** A carefully planned and consistent program of physical activity enhances glucose uptake to cells, thereby reducing the BG level. In addition, exercise may improve CHO metabolism and insulin sensitivity in patients with type 2 DM; may reduce levels of triglyceride-rich very low density lipoprotein (VLDL); may reduce blood pressure, especially in hyperinsulinemic subjects; may enhance weight loss and weight maintenance; may reduce risk of CVD; and may prevent progression of prediabetes to DM.

1. Physical activity has potential problems for individuals with diabetes.
   a. Patients with severe (proliferative) **retinopathy** must consult an ophthalmologist before beginning any type of exercise program. Strenuous activity may precipitate vitreous hemorrhage or traction retinal detachment in these patients. These individuals should avoid anaerobic exercise and physical activity that involves straining, jarring, or Valsalva-like maneuvers.
   b. Patients with **cardiovascular disease;** those > 35 years of age; and individuals with autonomic neuropathy, peripheral vascular disease, or microvascular disease should receive a cardiovascular evaluation and stress test before beginning an exercise program.
   c. Patients with significant **peripheral neuropathy** (with loss of protective sensation in the feet) should limit weight-bearing exercise. Repetitive exercise on insensitive feet can lead to ulceration and fractures. Treadmill exercises, jogging, prolonged walking, and step exercises are contraindicated; swimming, bicycling, rowing, chair exercises, arm exercises, and other non-weight-bearing exercise should be recommended.
   d. High-intensity or strenuous physical activity should probably be discouraged in individuals with **overt nephropathy** (albuminuria > 200 mg/min), unless blood pressure is carefully monitored during exercise.

[11]Expert Panel on Detection, Evaluation, and Treatment of High Blood Cholesterol in Adults. Executive summary of the third report of the National Cholesterol Education Program (NCEP) Expert Panel on Detection, Evaluation, and Treatment of High Blood Cholesterol in Adults (Adult Treatment Panel III). JAMA 2001;285:2486–2497. Krauss RM, Eckel RH, Howard B, et al. AHA dietary guidelines: Revision 2000: A statement for healthcare professionals from the Nutrition Committee of the American Heart Association. Circulation 2000;102:2284–2299. Pearson TA, Blair SN, Daniels SR, et al. AHA guidelines for primary prevention of cardiovascular disease and stroke: 2002. Update: Consensus panel guide to comprehensive risk reduction for adult patients without coronary or other atherosclerotic vascular diseases. American Heart Association Science Advisory and Coordinating Committee. Circulation 2002;106:388–391.
[12]Pijls LT, de Vries H, Donker AJ, van Eijik JT. The effect of protein restriction on albuminuria in patients with type 2 diabetes mellitus: A randomized trial. Nephrol Dial Transplant 1999;14:1445–1453.

2. **Aerobic activity** (e.g., swimming, walking, running) is the preferred type of exercise because of its desirable hypoglycemic effects (promotes utilization of glucose as fuel), as well as desirable effects on cardiovascular health, hypertension, lipid profiles, circulation, and weight-loss efforts. Recommendations:
   a. At least 150 min/week of moderate-intensity aerobic physical activity (50%–70% of maximum heart rate),
   b. And/or at least 90 min/week of vigorous aerobic exercise (< 70% of maximum heart rate).
   c. Distribute exercise over at least 3 days/week, with no more than 2 consecutive days without physical activity.

3. **Anaerobic activity** (e.g., weight lifting) should generally be avoided by people with diabetes unless it has been specifically approved by appropriate medical specialists such as a cardiologist (because it could have potential deleterious cardiovascular or blood pressure effects) or an ophthalmologist (because it could have potential deleterious effects upon underlying retinopathy). In the absence of contraindications, recommendations for people with type 2 diabetes include
   a. Perform resistance exercise three times a week, targeting all major muscle groups
   b. Progress to three sets of 8–10 repetitions at a weight that cannot be lifted more than 8–10 times

4. The physical activity plan should be consistent in regard to frequency (daily, or at least 3–4 days per week), intensity, and duration.

5. General guidelines that may prove helpful in regulating the glycemic response to physical activity include
   a. Assess metabolic control before physical activity. Avoid physical activity if glucose level is > 250 mg/dL and ketosis is present; use caution if glucose level is > 300 mg/dL with no ketosis. Ingest additional carbohydrate if glucose level is < 100 mg/dL.
   b. Monitor blood glucose before and after physical activity (up to several hours postexercise) to identify when/if changes in insulin or food intake are necessary and to learn individual glycemic responses to different physical activity conditions.
   c. Consume added carbohydrate as needed to avoid hypoglycemia; CHO-based food should be readily available during and after physical activity.

C. **Insulin and insulin analog**

   1. **Types of insulin.** Refers to onset and duration of insulin preparation (Table 54-1)
      a. **Rapid-acting** insulin. Lispro (Humalog), aspart (NovoLog), and glulisine (Apidra) insulins
      b. **Short-acting** insulin. Regular insulin (Humulin regular, Novolin regular)

Table 54-1. Types of Insulin—Onset, Peak, and Duration of Action[a]

Agent	Onset (hr)	Peak (hr)	Effective Duration (hr)	Variability in Absorption and Duration
Rapid acting				
Lispro (Humalog)	< 0.5	0.5–1.5	3–4	Minimal
Aspart (NovoLog)	< 0.5	0.7–1	3–5	Minimal
Glulisine (Apidra)	< 0.5	0.5–1.5	3–5	Minimal
Short-acting				
Regular	0.5–1	2–4	5–8	Moderate
Intermediate-acting				
NPH	2–4	6–10	10–16	High
Detemir	3–4	6–12	12–18	Minimal
Long-acting				
Glargine (Lantus)	5	n/a	20–24	Minimal-Moderate

[a]Approximate time action in nonpregnant adult, with normal renal function.
n/a, not applicable, *NPH,* neutral protamine Hagedorn

c. **Intermediate-acting** insulins. Isophane insulin suspension (neutral protamine Hagedorn; NPH) insulin and detemir (Levemir) insulin

d. **Long-acting** insulin. Glargine (Lantus) insulin.

e. **Premixed insulin products.** Each mixture gives a rapid- or short-acting insulin as a premeal bolus plus an intermediate-acting insulin to control later hyperglycemia or the subsequent meal.

   (1) 50/50 insulin: 50% protamine lispro insulin with 50% lispro insulin, or 50% regular insulin with 50% NPH insulin

   (2) 70/30 insulin: 70% insulin aspart protamine with 30% aspart insulin or 70% NPH with 30% regular insulin

   (3) 75/25 insulin: 75% protamine lispro insulin with 25% lispro insulin

f. **Extemporaneous mixtures.** Two insulins mixed in one syringe, before administration. Extemporaneous mixtures allow the ratio to be tailor made to match the patient's blood glucose reading, anticipated eating or physical activity, or other factors influencing the requirement for specific insulin action.

2. **Chemical sources** of commercial insulin available in the United States

a. **Biosynthetic human, also called human insulin.** Produced by recombinant DNA techniques

b. **Insulin analog.** Produced by chemical alteration of human insulin

3. **Concentration** of insulin products available in the United States

a. **U-100:** a concentration of 100 Units/mL

b. **U-500:** concentration of regular insulin of 500 Units/mL, for patients with insulin resistance. Because of its high concentration, bioactivity of U-500 regular insulin mimics an intermediate-acting insulin. U-500 insulin is a prescription item.

4. **Indications.** Insulin therapy is required for all patients with type 1 DM and for those with type 2 DM when oral antidiabetes therapy alone does not achieve the desired DM control. Insulin and insulin analogs may be used in combination with certain oral antidiabetes agents in type 1 or type 2 DM. When diet and physical activity fail to achieve glycemic control in GDM or when a woman with diabetes becomes pregnant, insulin therapy should be instituted rather than oral antidiabetes agents.

5. **Mechanism of action.** Insulin lowers blood glucose and contributes to glucose homeostasis by a variety of physiological actions, including

a. ↑Glucose uptake and utilization by peripheral tissues

b. ↑Glycogenesis (conversion of glucose to glycogen in liver and muscle)

c. ↓Glycogenolysis (production of glucose from glycogen)

d. ↓Gluconeogenesis (formation of glucose from noncarbohydrates, such as amino acids)

e. ↓Lipolysis and ketogenesis (breakdown of fats to ketone bodies)

f. ↑Formation of protein from amino acids

g. ↑Formation of adipose tissue from triglycerides and fatty acids

6. **Initial dosage of insulin.** Assuming a waking time in the morning, meals/snacks spaced consistently during the day and waking hours, and a late evening bedtime, *the following are examples only and do not include all insulin options.*

a. **Type 1 DM, without concomitant infection or physiologic stress condition.** A typical initial total daily dose (TDD) is estimated as 0.5 Units/kg/day, which is divided into three or four injections per day. Regimens employing only one or two injections per day do not achieve euglycemia in type 1 DM.

   (1) Three injections per day

     (a) Prebreakfast injection. Two thirds of TDD. 25%–35% of the total breakfast dose is given as lispro, aspart, glulisine, or regular insulin; 65%–75% of the total breakfast dose is given as NPH insulin (1:2 ratio). May be mixed extemporaneously or may be a commercial premixed product.

     (b) Presupper injection. Between 10% and 20% of TDD. Given as lispro, aspart, glulisine, or regular insulin

     (c) Bedtime (10 p.m.) injection. Between 10% and 25% of TDD. Given as NPH insulin

   (2) Four injections per day

     (a) Premeal injections (three injections). Total of 40%–50% of TDD. Total amount is divided between the three meals in a ratio proportional to the desired/usual ratio of CHO ingestion at those three meals. Given as lispro, aspart, glulisine, or regular insulin before each meal

(b) Bedtime injection. Between 50% and 60% of TDD, given as NPH, detemir, or glargine insulin. *Caveat:* If NPH or detemir insulin is used for the bedtime injection, the premeal insulin must be regular insulin.

(3) Insulin pump therapy (use of external pump to provide continuous subcutaneous insulin infusion)

(a) Premeal and presnack boluses. Dosage based on premeal BG level and anticipated CHO intake for the meal. Initial estimate would be similar to the initial estimate for the four-injection regimen (see VII.C.6.a.(2)). Given as lispro, aspart, or glulisine insulin

(b) Basal insulin. Programmed to be delivered continuously. Initial estimate is 50%–60% of TDD but may be subsequently altered to give differing basal infusions at certain times of the day. Initial rate is often 0.5–1.25 Units/hr, given as lispro, glulisine, or aspart insulin

b. Type 2 DM. Initial TDD is 0.15–0.4 Units/kg/day but will vary greatly, depending on degree of concomitant insulin resistance and degree of β cell dysfunction.

(1) One injection per day. Bedtime insulin only, 0.25 Units/kg/day, given as NPH or glargine insulin. Bedtime insulin is most often used in combination with one or more oral antidiabetes medication. Monotherapy bedtime insulin is possible in the early stages of type 2 DM, but rarely used.

(2) Two injections per day

(a) Prebreakfast injection. Two thirds of TDD, given as a premix insulin (70/30, 75/25, or 50/50; choice depends on anticipated CHO intake at breakfast and lunch)

(b) Presupper injection. One third of TDD, given as a premix insulin (70/30, 75/25, or 50/50; choice depends on anticipated CHO intake at supper)

(3) Three or four injections per day. Types, initial ratios, and regimens are similar to type 1 (see VII.C.6.a.).

c. Adjust initial doses and regimen based on ongoing SMBG, symptoms of hypoglycemia or hyperglycemia, and periodic AIC results.

7. Routes of insulin administration

a. Subcutaneous injection. For routine self-administration of insulin

(1) Successful insulin therapy requires predictable and consistent insulin absorption and insulin action from day to day.

(2) In many patients, absorption of regular insulin is fastest from the abdomen, followed by the arm, buttocks, and thigh.

(a) Upon initiation of insulin therapy, patients should carefully monitor and record their own variations in absorption. If it is determined that the variation is sufficiently great, then a given injection (e.g., presupper dose) should always be given in the same anatomical region (e.g., arms). Random rotation of injection regions should be avoided in these individuals.

(b) Physical exercise increases blood flow to the exercising area, thus accelerating absorption of insulin injected at that site. To a lesser extent, hot showers, baths, and massage may have a similar effect. Patients should be advised to avoid giving an injection into a limb that will be subsequently exercised or heated. The abdomen may be preferable for the preexercise injection because that area is the least likely to have significant increases in absorption.

(3) Within an anatomical region, the injection site should be rotated to avoid lipohypertrophy and fibrosis.

b. Continuous intravenous (insulin drip) administration of regular insulin, primarily in the hospital setting. Used for treatment of acute hyperglycemia, ketoacidosis, HHS syndrome, or during surgical procedures or delivery.

c. Continuous subcutaneous infusion (insulin pump therapy)

(1) Rapid-acting insulin is infused continuously during the day in a patient-specific pattern to deliver low doses of insulin (basal insulin) to offset the glycemic effects of daily patterns of counterregulatory hormones.

(2) Before each meal, the patient sets the pump to deliver a bolus dose of rapid-acting insulin to control the glycemic effects of the meal. The bolus dose is determined by algorithms that consider the premeal glucose level, anticipated dietary intake, and activity.

(3) Offers the potential for tighter glycemic control.

(4) Indicated for selected individuals with diabetes with widely fluctuating blood glucose levels; irregular or inconsistent work schedules, lifestyles, or meals; or who achieve less-than-desired control using frequent injection routines.

(5) Requires frequent SMBG; thorough training in the use of the infusion equipment; and an advanced understanding and application of exercise, dietary, and insulin adjustment protocols.

8. Alterations in insulin requirement

a. Infection, exacerbations of other medical problems, weight gain, puberty, inactivity, hyperthyroidism, and Cushing disease tend to increase insulin needs.

b. Renal failure, adrenal insufficiency, nutrient malabsorption, hypopituitarism, weight loss, and increased exercise tend to reduce insulin needs.

c. Drug–drug or drug–disease interactions may increase or decrease insulin requirements.

D. Insulin secretagogues (oral hypoglycemic agents)

1. Agents

a. Sulfonylureas

(1) Chlorpropamide (Diabinese)

(2) Glyburide (DiaBeta, Micronase, Glynase)

(3) Glipizide (Glucotrol)

(4) Glimepiride (Amaryl)

b. Meglitinides

(1) Repaglinide (Prandin)

(2) Nateglinide (Starlix)

2. Indications/contraindications

a. Use in type 2 DM predicated on

(1) Adequate control not attained by medical nutrition therapy and physical activity alone

(2) *Or* pharmacological intervention is required based on the presenting blood glucose levels and diabetes symptomatology

(3) *And* there are sufficient numbers of functioning β cells

(4) May be used as monotherapy or in combination with other oral antidiabetes drugs or insulin

b. Use in type 1 DM not indicated. Pharmacological action depends on functioning pancreatic β cells.

c. Insulin secretagogues

(1) Are not recommended for children, pregnant and lactating women

(2) Should not be used for metabolic control during stressful conditions such as severe infection, injury, or surgery (all of which stimulate the release of counterregulatory hormones), which increase the risk of hyperglycemia. Insulin therapy should be instituted during these conditions.

d. Sulfonylurea agents

(1) Are contraindicated in patients with allergy to sulfa agents.

(2) Have been associated with a possible increased risk of cardiovascular morbidity and mortality.

(3) Pose a risk of cholestatic jaundice

e. Certain agents should not be used in patients with severe renal or hepatic impairment.

3. Mechanisms of action

a. Predominant effect is to stimulate pancreatic secretion of insulin

b. Improve "first phase" release of insulin/increase sensitivity of β cells to glucose stimulus

c. Lessor effects

(1) Increase hepatic sensitivity to insulin

(2) Increase number and/or sensitivity of insulin receptors in muscle and adipose tissue

(3) Reduce postreceptor defect (transport defect) in muscle and adipose tissue

4. Choice of agent. The most clinically significant difference among sulfonylureas is duration of action (Table 54-2), which then affects frequency of dosing and potential compliance

Table 54-2. Oral Monotherapy: Type 2 Diabetes[a]

Agent	Initial dose	Maximum Dose / Comments
α-glucosidase inhibitors Acarbose (Precose) Miglitol (Glyset)	25 mg/day with first bite of meal Instruct patient to increase dosage as tolerated (GI distress) Anticipate weeks to reach maximal therapeutic effect Sometimes given with just largest meal or may be given before each meal	50-100 mg four times a day with meals. 50 mg four times a day if TBW < 60 kg Diarrhea, abdominal distress may limit dosing or rate of dosage increase; GI effects usually diminish with continued use Increase in liver enzymes may occur When used with a hypoglycemic agent (sulfonylurea or insulin), patient must be taught importance of treating hypoglycemia with glucose-based product
Insulin sensitizers Metformin (Glucophage, Glucophage XR, Riomet solution)	500 mg once or twice a day with meals Instruct patient to increase dosage as tolerated (usually weekly) Daily dose of 1500 mg will likely be needed for therapeutic effect Metformin extended release 500 mg daily taken with evening meal	Short-acting: 2550 mg/day (850 mg four times a day). *Note:* 1000 mg two times a day gives maximum therapeutic effect Long-acting: 2000 mg/day Nausea and diarrhea, which usually subside after 5–10 days, may limit rate of dosage increase Teach patient lactic acidosis issues—for example, muscle aches, weakness Contraindicated in renal or liver disease, ETOH abuse, severe cardiopulmonary disease
Pioglitazone (Actos)	15 or 30 mg/day without regard to meals	45 mg/day in one dose
Rosiglitazone (Avandia)	2 mg/day without regard to meals	8 mg/day in one or two doses
Sulfonylurea agents Glipizide (Glucotrol, Glucotrol XL)	Glucotrol 2.5 mg/day Glucotrol XL 5 mg/day	Short acting: 40 mg, give in two doses when dose reaches 15 mg Extended length: 20 mg, give in one or two doses
Glyburide (DiaBeta, Micronase, Glynase)	DiaBeta, Micronase 2.5 mg/day	
Glynase (glyburide microcrystalline) 1.5 mg/day	20 mg in one or two doses Microcrystalline: 12 mg	
Glimepiride (Amaryl)	2 mg/day	6 mg/day in one or two doses
Chlorpropamide (Diabinese)	100 mg/day	750 mg in one dose
Meglitinides Repaglinide (Prandin)	Not previously treated with hypoglycemic agent and HbA$_{Ic}$ < 8.0%: 0.5–1.0 mg with each meal Previously treated with hypoglycemic agent or HbA$_{Ic}$ > 8.0%: 1–2 mg with each meal	4 mg with each meal or 16 mg total daily dose
Nateglinide (Starlix)	120 mg four times a day, 1–30 min before each meal 60 mg four times a day for patients near target HbA$_{Ic}$	180 mg with each meal Uric acid levels may be elevated

[a]Consult package insert for detailed prescribing details. Dosage should be reduced if frequent hypoglycemia occurs without apparent cause (such as medication error; changes in diet, exercise, or timing of regimen). When dosage reaches the minimum for a therapeutic agent, an attempt should be made to control diabetes by diet and exercise alone.
ETOH, ethyl alcohol; *GI,* gastrointestinal; *HbA$_{Ic}$,* glycosylated hemoglobin A$_{Ic}$; *TBW,* total body weight.

issues. Other considerations include frequency and consistency of eating and exercise, additional patient-specific risk factors for severe hypoglycemia (e.g., hypoglycemia unawareness), patient-specific contraindications, and cost considerations.

   a. Glimepiride exhibits an insulin-sparing effect compared to other members of this class, reportedly by its relatively greater extrapancreatic effect.

   b. β Cell stimulation of insulin secretion is more glucose dependent with repaglinide and nateglinide than with sulfonylurea agents. This action, along with its very short action, may present a reduced risk of late postprandial hypoglycemia for selected individuals.

   c. Chlorpropamide has the longest duration of action and poses a risk to patients with renal or hepatic impairment. It also causes more severe and frequent side effects (including hypoglycemia and hyponatremia) than other sulfonylureas.

   d. Glyburide has been associated with severe or prolonged hypoglycemia in the elderly.

5. Administration and dosage (Table 54-2)

6. Patient education and other concerns

   a. Adverse effects include gastrointestinal (GI) disturbances (e.g., nausea, gastric discomfort, vomiting, constipation), tachycardia, headache, skin rash, and hematological problems (e.g., agranulocytosis, pancytopenia, hemolytic anemia)

   b. Best if taken 30–45 min before meals, but may take with meal if GI distress. *Except:* repaglinide or nateglinide *must* be taken 15–30 min before a meal.

   c. Notify prescriber if skin changes occur

   d. Teach patient prevention, recognition, treatment of hypoglycemia

   e. Sunburn precautions

   f. Notify prescriber if unexpected/unintended weight gain occurs

   g. Hypoglycemia and alcohol intolerance may occur with chlorpropamide. Alcohol intolerance is less common with other agents.

   h. Primary failure. The agent fails to control hyperglycemia within the first 4 weeks after initiation. This most likely represents insufficient numbers of functioning β cells.

   i. Secondary Failure. The drug controls hyperglycemia initially but fails to maintain control. Between 5% and 30% of initial responders experience secondary failure. In most instances, this represents progression of the DM, with a diminishing number of functioning β cells, rather than a drug failure.

E. Insulin sensitizers

1. Agents

   a. Biguanides: metformin (Glucophage, Riomet)

   b. Thiazolidinediones (TZD)
     (1) Pioglitazone (Actos)
     (2) Rosiglitazone (Avandia)

   c. Combination products
     (1) Metformin/glyburide (Glucovance)
     (2) Metformin/glipizide (Metaglip)
     (3) Metformin/rosiglitazone (Avandamet)
     (4) Metformin/pioglitazone (Actoplus met)

2. Indications/Contraindications

   a. Insulin sensitizers are indicated in individuals with a significant component of insulin resistance.

   b. Use in type 2 DM
     (1) Monotherapy use in type 2 DM predicated on
       (a) Adequate control not attained by medical nutrition therapy and physical activity alone
       (b) *Or* pharmacological intervention is required based on the presenting blood glucose levels and diabetes symptomatology
       (c) *And* patient has adequate endogenous insulin
     (2) Combination therapy, with other oral antidiabetes agents and/or insulin

   c. Use in type 1 DM. As adjunct to insulin; must not be used as monotherapy

   d. Metformin contraindications and cautions

(1) Situations with potential for increased risk of lactic acidosis. Lactic acidosis is a rare but serious complication and is fatal in 50% of cases
  (a) Renal dysfunction (serum creatinine [SCr] > 1.4 mg/dL in females and > 1.5 mg/dL in males). Confirm adequate renal function in the elderly, even in the face of "low" SCr levels.
  (b) Hypoperfusion (hypoxic states)—for example:
      (i) During surgery
      (ii) Severe cardiovascular/pulmonary dysfunction
      (iii) Acute myocardial infarction or heart failure
  (c) Radiographic procedures using intravenous iodinated contrast agents (potential for transient renal dysfunction). Discontinue metformin during the procedure; reinitiate when renal function is reestablished and confirmed.
  (d) Chronic or binge ingestion of ethanol
  (e) Liver disease (hepatic function important for clearance of blood lactate)
(2) Serum vitamin B_{12} levels may decline, usually without clinical manifestations.
(3) Follow labeled recommendations for monitoring liver function, renal function, and vitamin B_{12} status.
  d. TZD contraindications and cautions
  (1) Hepatic disease: idiosyncratic hepatic failure, a rare but serious event, has occurred during therapy with troglitazone, a thiazolidinedione removed from the U.S. market in 1999. Because of their structural similarity to troglitazone, pioglitazone and rosiglitazone should be used cautiously in patients with hepatic disease. Clinical data have not shown evidence of drug-induced hepatoxicity from pioglitazone or rosiglitazone.
  (2) Follow labeled guidelines for routine monitoring of liver function.
  (3) Warning for use in patients with severe heart failure—New York Heart Association (NYHA) class III or IV cardiac status—owing to possible increase in plasma volume (found in human studies) and heart enlargement (found in animal studies).
  (4) Safety in children or during pregnancy has not been established.
  (5) Do not use TZD at maximum labeled dose when combined with insulin.

3. Mechanisms of action
  a. These agents are pharmacologically antihyperglycemic agents rather than hypoglycemic agents.
  b. Increase hepatic sensitivity to insulin, thereby suppressing hepatic glucose production. Major action for metformin; secondary action for pioglitazone and rosiglitazone.
  c. Reduce postreceptor defect (transport defect) in muscle and adipose tissue; this defect appears to be the major component of naturally occurring insulin resistance. Major action for pioglitazone and rosiglitazone; secondary action for metformin.
  d. Increase number and/or sensitivity of insulin receptors in muscle and adipose tissue, thereby addressing the cell surface binding defect; this defect correlates most significantly with hyperinsulinemia. Major action for pioglitazone and rosiglitazone; secondary action for metformin.

4. Administration and dosage (Table 54-2)

5. Patient education and other concerns
  a. Metformin
  (1) Most notable subjective side effect: GI disturbances (loose stools or diarrhea), usually subsiding after 7–10 days
  (2) Take with meals to minimize GI upset.
  (3) Optimal BG effects not seen for 5–10 days
  (4) Hypoglycemia is not likely caused by metformin but may occur if used with insulin or insulin secretagogue,
  (5) Often associated with small weight loss
  (6) Metformin is excreted into breast milk.
  b. Thiazolidinediones (TZD)
  (1) Most notable subjective side effects: edema, weight gain, headache, fatigue
  (2) Hypoglycemia is not likely caused by TZD but may occur if used with insulin or secretagogue.
  (3) Optimal BG effects not seen for 6–10 weeks
  (4) Teach patient signs and symptoms of liver toxicity and to report to prescriber if noticed

(5) Watch for weight gain, shortness of breath, girth expansion

(6) Animal studies suggest that pioglitazone and rosiglitazone are secreted in breast milk, but it is not known if these drugs or metabolites are excreted in human milk.

(7) Premenopausal anovulatory women may resume ovulation during therapy, placing the patient at risk of pregnancy.

F. α-Glucosidase inhibitors

1. Agents

    a. Acarbose (Precose)

    b. Miglitol (Glyset)

2. Indications/contraindications

    a. Used in individuals with significant postprandial hyperglycemia. These drugs have minimal effect on preprandial or fasting blood glucose levels.

    b. Use in type 2 DM

        (1) Monotherapy use in type 2 DM predicated on

            (a) Adequate control (especially postprandial) not attained by medical nutrition therapy and physical activity alone

            (b) *Or* pharmacological intervention is required based on the presenting postprandial blood glucose levels and diabetes symptomatology

            (c) *And* patient has adequate endogenous or exogenous insulin.

        (2) Combination therapy, with insulin or other oral antidiabetes agents, notably insulin secretagogues

    c. Use in type 1 DM

        (1) As an adjunct to insulin therapy; may be useful in individuals with delayed absorption of subcutaneous insulin

        (2) Not to be used as monotherapy

    d. Contraindicated in inflammatory bowel disease, colonic ulceration, or obstructive bowel disorders; chronic intestinal disorders of digestion or absorption; or any medical condition that might deteriorate with increased intestinal gas formation.

    e. Contraindicated in cirrhosis of the liver.

    f. Not indicated during pregnancy, in breast-feeding women, or in children.

3. Mechanism of action

    a. Inhibits the intestinal enzyme α-glucosidase (a class of enzymes). Intestinal absorption of complex carbohydrates such as starch, dextrins, and disaccharides (e.g., sucrose, maltose) requires the action of intestinal α-glucosidase.

    b. Inhibition of α-glucosidase retards the degradation and thus the absorption of carbohydrates, resulting in a slower and smaller rise in blood glucose following the meal.

4. Administration and dosage (Table 54-2)

5. Patient education and other concerns

    a. Most notable subjective side effects: Gastrointestinal effects, occurring primarily at initiation of therapy or when dosage is increased: diarrhea, abdominal pain, and flatulence (about 30%, 10%–20%, and 42%–77%, respectively).

        (1) GI side effects are usually self-limiting and resolve in several weeks.

        (2) GI side effects can be minimized by starting with a low dose and then slowly titrating dosage upward.

    b. Take with first bite of meal. Medication will be ineffective more than 30–45 min after eating carbohydrates.

    c. Hypoglycemia not likely caused by this drug, but may occur if used with insulin or insulin secretagogue.

    d. Hypoglycemia *must* be treated with glucose, not complex carbohydrate.

    e. Follow labeled recommendations for routine liver function monitoring.

G. Incretin mimetics

1. Agent: Exenatide (Byetta)

2. Indications/contraindications

    a. Used as an adjunct to metformin and/or a sulfonylurea agent, to reduce postprandial hyperglycemia and to improve HbAIC in patients with type 2 DM who have not achieved desired glycemic control using metformin and/or sulfonylurea.

b. Exenatide is not recommended (has not been studied) in patients taking insulin, TZDs, meglitinides, or glucosidase inhibitors.

3. **Mechanisms of actions.** Reduces postprandial glucose rise; antihyperglycemic agent, not a hypoglycemic agent
   a. Stimulates glucose-mediated insulin secretion; improves/restores first phase of insulin release
   b. Inhibits postprandial glucagon release
   c. Delays gastric emptying
   d. Improves satiety and thus reduces dietary intake; progressive weight loss has occurred, even after 18 months
   e. Lowers postprandial BG but also lowers hyperglycemia if injected during fasting state

4. **Administration and dosage**
   a. Initial: twice a day 5 μg subcutaneously taken 30 min before breakfast and before supper, for 30 days.
   b. Maintenance: If 5-μg dose is tolerated, advance to 10 μg subcutaneously twice a day before meals thereafter.
   c. Dose should be omitted if that meal is skipped.
   d. If the patient is taking sulfonylurea, the dose of sulfonylurea should be reduced when exenatide is started. The dose of metformin (if taking) does not need to be changed.

5. **SMBG is an important component of dosage titration.**
   a. BG testing before meals and 2-hr postprandial breakfast and supper until dose is established and determined to be effective.
   b. Frequent SMBG is also important if dose of sulfonylurea agent has been adjusted.
   c. Once the doses of exenatide, sulfonylurea, and/or metformin are stable, test before meal and at bedtime plus occasional 2 hr after meal, depending on strip coverage.

6. **Patient education and other concerns**
   a. Inject no more than 1 hr before meal
   b. Inject in thigh, abdomen, or upper arm
   c. Available in prefilled syringes, each containing 60 doses.
      (1) Two sizes: 5 μg/dose and 10 μg/dose; premeasured dose requires no dosing choices
      (2) Pen needles must be purchased separately
      (3) Each pen must be primed before initial dose
      (4) Clear, colorless injection
      (5) Refrigerate, even after opening. Discard after 30 days
   d. Most common side effect: mild to moderate nausea, which dissipates over time. Increased occurrence of hypoglycemia, in patients taking sulfonylurea

H. Aymlin receptor agonist

1. **Agent: Pramlintide** (Symlin)

2. **Indications/contraindications**
   a. Used as an adjunct to insulin to reduce postprandial hyperglycemia and to improve HbAIC in patients with type 1 DM or insulin-requiring type 2 DM who have not achieved desired glycemic control using insulin.
   b. Patients *not* appropriate for pramlintide therapy (because of lack of studies, or potential harm):
      (1) Poor compliance with current insulin regimen or SMBG
      (2) HbAIC > 9%
      (3) History of recurrent severe hypoglycemia requiring assistance during the past 6 months
      (4) Hypoglycemia unawareness
      (5) Confirmed diagnosis of gastroparesis or using drugs that stimulate gastrointestinal motility
      (6) Pediatric patients and pregnant or nursing women

3. **Mechanisms of action**. Reduces postprandial glucose rise; antihyperglycemic agent not hypoglycemic agent
   a. Delays gastric emptying

    b. Suppresses glucose-stimulated secretion of glucagon

    c. Enhances satiety, resulting in decreased appetite and decreased food intake

4. Administration and dosage

  a. Dosing for type 1 DM

    (1) Step 1—initiation

      (a) Reduce premeal insulin dose (rapid-acting, short-acting, or fixed-mix) by 50%

      (b) Start pramlintide at a dose of 15 μg subcutaneously just before each major meal

      (c) Monitor blood glucose frequently (before and after meals and at bedtime)

    (2) Step 2—titration

      (a) Increase pramlintide in 15-μg increments to a maintenance dose of 30 μg or 60 μg, as tolerated

      (b) Increase dose to the next increment when no nausea for 3 days

      (c) If nausea persists at the 45 μg or 60 μg doses, reduce dose to 30 μg

      (d) If the 30 μg dose is not tolerated, consider discontinuation

    (3) Step 3—when a stable pramlintide regimen has been established, adjust insulin doses to optimize glycemic control.

    (4) Step 4—instruct patients to contact healthcare professional at least once a week until pramlintide dose is stable and well tolerated and BG levels are stable. Notify provider if nausea and/or hypoglycemia is ongoing, frequent, or increasingly severe.

  b. Dosing for type 2 DM

    (1) Step 1—initiation

      (a) Reduce premeal insulin dose (rapid-acting, short-acting, or fixed-mix) by 50%

      (b) Start pramlintide at a dose of 60 μg subcutaneously just before each major meal

      (c) Monitor blood glucose frequently (before and after meals and at bedtime)

    (2) Step 2—titration

      (a) Increase pramlintide to a maintenance dose of 120 μg when no nausea for 5–7 days

      (b) If nausea persists at the 120-μg dose, reduce dose to 60 μg

    (3) Step 3—when a stable pramlintide regimen has been established, adjust insulin doses to optimize glycemic control.

    (4) Step 4—instruct patients to contact healthcare professional at least once a week until pramlintide dose is stable and well tolerated and BG levels are stable. Notify provider if nausea and/or hypoglycemia is ongoing, frequent, or increasingly severe.

  c. Dose only when major meal is consumed, defined as > 250 kcal or > 30 g CHO

  d. Dose should be omitted if that meal is skipped.

5. SMBG is an important component of dosage titration.

  a. Conduct SMBG at least before and after meals and at bedtime.

  b. Frequent SMBG is essential, because the doses of insulin and pramlintide will need to be adjusted frequently as the proper doses are established and the patient is able to tolerate the maximum dose

  c. Once the doses of insulin and pramlintide are stable, test before meals and at bedtime plus occasional 2 hr after a meal, depending on strip coverage

6. Patient education and other concerns

  a. Most common side effects: nausea 30%–40% (usually transient), increased occurrence of hypoglycemia (particularly in patients with type 1 DM), loss of appetite, vomiting, and headache.

  b. Available in 5-mL vial containing 0.6 mg/mL, for use with a syringe

    (1) Symlin is labeled in milligrams per liter (mg/mL), not units, and is dosed in micrograms (μg).

      (a) The U-100 insulin syringes are usually used for dosing (preferably a 0.3-cc syringe); 6 μg = 1 U on the syringe

      (b) This labeling and the necessity for converting to volume for use in a U-100 insulin syringe may be confusing to patients.

      (c) The U-100 syringes are generally not available in other countries, which may further compound the dosing confusion for patients traveling abroad.

    (2) Patient education is critical to proper dosing.

  c. Inject in abdomen or thigh (not arm)

  d. The decision to dose before a given meal is based on the carbohydrate (or calories) content of the meal. Thus it is essential that the patient knows the basics of carbohydrate identification and quantification (carbohydrate counting).

    e. Do not mix Symlin injection (pH ~ 4) in the same syringe with insulin (pH ~ 7). Give at two separate injections, at least 2 in. apart.

    f. Clear, colorless injection

    g. Refrigerate until use. Opened vials may be kept in the refrigerator or at room temperature. After opening, discard any remainder after 28 days.

VIII. PATIENT EDUCATION AND SELF-CARE. Patient education about the disease and patient participation in medical care are the most important aspects of DM management. *Without patient involvement and participation, even the ideal pharmacotherapy, dietary, or other intervention will fail.* **Patient education** improves understanding of the disease; promotes optimal patient choices regarding diet, medication, and exercise; and facilitates decision-making skills. National, state, and local diabetes professional groups have published guidelines to ensure thorough and effective teaching content and methods. Examples of patient education topics include, but are not limited to, the following:

  A. Prevention, recognition, and treatment of acute hypoglycemic and hyperglycemic episodes.

  B. Reduction of modifiable risk factors for the development of chronic complications

    1. Achievement of HbAIC < 7% (based on upper limit of normal = 6%)

    2. Smoking cessation

    3. Normalization of blood pressure

    4. Normalization of blood lipid profile

    5. Reduction of weight to at least a BMI of 25, if applicable

    6. Routine assessment/screening for and early treatment of chronic complications

  C. Pattern control. Adjustment algorithms for diet, exercise, and/or medications based on trends in BG control.

  D. Implementation of **specific self-care measures**

    1. Foot care. Neuropathy, peripheral vascular disease, trauma, and infection increase the risk for lower-extremity complications and amputation, causing hospitalizations, disability, morbidity, and mortality.

      a. Inspect feet and interdigital areas daily, looking for changes in color or skin integrity.

      b. Inspect shoes daily before putting them on, to detect loose objects or rough shoe materials that may injure or irritate the skin.

      c. Clean feet daily, and dry thoroughly. Use forearm, elbow, or a thermometer to check water temperature if the patient has neuropathy-induced sensation loss.

      d. Moisturize dry skin with hand lotion or Vaseline. Avoid area between the toes.

      e. Cut toenails straight across, or follow the natural curve of the toe.

      f. Avoid self-treatment of corns, calluses, or ingrown toenails.

      g. Wear well-fitting shoes and soft cotton socks. Avoid going barefoot.

      h. Seek prompt medical attention for any problems identified (e.g., cuts, blisters, calluses, unhealing wounds, or signs of infections such as redness, swelling, drainage, pus, or fever).

    2. Skin care. Dry skin occurs frequently in individuals with DM owing to dehydration (secondary to hyperglycemia-induced diuresis) and/or anhidrosis (secondary to autonomic neuropathic condition, resulting in little or no perspiration). Elevated blood glucose levels and impaired circulation also increase the risk for the development of skin infections.

      a. Inspect skin daily for abrasions, pain, or swelling. Consult the healthcare provider promptly if problems are noted.

      b. Keep skin clean using a mild soap and warm (not hot) water.

      c. Use moisturizing lotion (alcohol free and not oiled based) on dry skin areas.

    d. Use sunscreen products throughout the year. As a physical stress, severe sunburn may raise BG.

    e. Avoid situations with potential for local trauma, especially to legs and feet. If injury occurs, the lesion should be covered with sterile gauze and first-aid measures applied.

3. Dental care. Periodontal disease is often accelerated in people with long-standing or poorly controlled diabetes.

    a. A yearly dental exam is recommended.

    b. Effective brushing and flossing are essential.

4. Eye care. Diabetes is a leading cause of vision impairment in the United States and the leading cause of blindness for individuals between the ages of 20 and 74 years of age. A yearly dilated eye exam is recommended, with more frequent follow-up guided by the severity of disease.

IX. ASSESSMENT OF GLYCEMIC CONTROL

A. Self-monitoring of blood glucose

1. Indicated for all individuals with diabetes. The frequency and time of testing vary according to type of diabetes, type of antidiabetes medication, and goals of therapy.

2. Involves the patient in the treatment process

3. Allows the patient and the healthcare provider to assess the individual's response to various factors (e.g., lifestyle modifications, nutritional alterations, medication adjustments, stress, illness, infection, trauma, changes in physical activity)

4. Gives immediate feedback and data for the patient to use in the application of diet, exercise, or insulin adjustment algorithms (decision-making skills)

5. A variety of testing products and product features are available. The use of meters with test memory functions and the capacity to download (via computer) SMBG results provides efficient access and analysis of SMBG trends.

B. Urine glucose testing. No longer recommended because it provides only retrospective information and does not reflect current blood glucose. Reserved only for individuals unable or unwilling to perform SMBG.

C. Urine ketone monitoring. An essential component of diabetes management, particularly under the following conditions:

1. During illness in all patients with diabetes because even those with type 2 DM can become ketotic during periods of severe stress, infection, or trauma

2. Patients with type 1 DM when blood glucose is consistently > 240 mg/dL

3. Pregnant women with diabetes (including gestational diabetes)

4. Individuals actively trying to lose weight by calorie restriction

D. Long-term monitoring of glycemic control

1. **HbAIC test**
   a. Reflects average blood glucose level over the preceding **2–3 months**.
   b. Based on an upper limit of normal being 6% for HbAIC; anHbAIC level of 7.0% or lower indicates good overall glycemic control, whereas > 7.0% reveals the need for additional intervention. For many individuals, a goal closer to normal may be desirable, provided it does not pose undue risk for hypoglycemia.
   c. Underlying hemoglobinopathies may cause anomalous values.
   d. In general, the frequency of HbAIC testing is at least **twice a year** in patients with stable glycemic control and at least quarterly in patients whose therapy has recently changed or who are in poor control.

2. Glycosylated fructosamine test
   a. Measures glycemic control over the preceding 2–3 weeks
   b. Useful for short-term follow-up of recently implemented interventions, when timely assessment of the intervention is important (e.g., changes in diabetes therapy during pregnancy).

X. ACUTE CHANGES IN GLYCEMIC CONTROL

A. Hyperglycemia

1. **Mild to moderate severity.** Rapid onset (within hours), no metabolic abnormalities
   a. Acute-onset hyperglycemia. Owing to unplanned event such as illness, emotional distress, or excessive caloric intake
   b. Hyperglycemia following prolonged or severe hypoglycemia. Somogyi effect or rebound hyperglycemia (notably type 1 DM)
   c. Hyperglycemia occurring as a pattern in the early morning.
      (1) Caused by counterregulatory hormones (i.e., dawn phenomenon)
      (2) Caused by nocturnal hepatic glucose production (notably type 2 DM)

2. **Moderate to severe severity** (BG > 250 mg/dL). Short duration (one to several days), with acidosis and ketosis—**diabetic ketoacidosis (DKA)** (see II.B.1)
   a. Often the presenting disorder in children with previously undiagnosed type 1 DM
   b. Precipitating factors include stress, infection, exercise, excessive alcohol consumption, improper insulin therapy, and dietary noncompliance.
   c. Physical findings include Kussmaul respirations, acetone breath odor, dehydration, dry skin, poor skin turgor, reduced level of consciousness (ranging from confusion to coma), and abdominal pain.
   d. Laboratory findings include hyperglycemia, ketosis, low arterial pH and carbon dioxide partial pressure (P_{CO_2}) values, and abnormal serum electrolyte values.
   e. Therapy involves fluid, intravenous insulin by continuous infusion, electrolyte replacement, and hospitalization. Without treatment, death ensues.

3. **Severe** (BG > 500 mg/dL). Intermediate duration (days to weeks), with profound dehydration, diminished central nervous system (CNS) function and increased serum osmolality, without ketosis or acidosis—**HHS** coma.
   a. Occurs primarily in type 2 DM
   b. Has a higher mortality rate than DKA
   c. Precipitating factors include illnesses and conditions that increase insulin requirements and predispose the patient to dehydration.
      (1) Examples include severe burns, GI bleeding, CNS injury, and acute myocardial infarction.
      (2) Use of glucogenic drugs (e.g., steroids, glucagon, thiazide diuretics, cimetidine, propranolol)
      (3) Medical procedures or hypertonic high-glucose products such as intravenous hyperalimentation, peritoneal dialysis, and enteral nutrition
   d. Physical findings include polyuria, polydipsia, dehydration, hypotension, rapid respirations, abdominal discomfort, nausea, vomiting, tachycardia, palpitations, and profound signs of neurological deficits (such as confusion, coma, generalized or focal seizures, myoclonic jerking, and hemiparesis).
   e. Laboratory findings include hyperglycemia (often substantially above 500 mg/dL), absence of ketosis, and serum osmolarity > 320 mOsm/kg. Calculated as follows:

$$2\left[\frac{(\text{sodium} + \text{glucose})}{18}\right]$$

   where sodium is measured in milliequivalents per liter and glucose is measured in milligrams per deciliter.

   f. Therapy involves fluid, insulin, and electrolyte replacement.

B. Hypoglycemia

1. **Mild hypoglycemia.** Primarily adrenergic symptoms (tachycardia, palpitations, shakiness) or cholinergic (sweating) symptoms, or effects of mild CNS glucopenia (inability to concen-

trate, dizziness, hunger, blurred vision), but symptoms are not severe enough to interfere with self-medication for the hypoglycemia.

2. **Moderate hypoglycemia.** The CNS is more markedly deprived of glucose, eliciting symptoms of confusion, inappropriate behavior, and impairment of motor function. The patient is minimally capable of self-treatment, and assistance is usually needed. The patient is *not* unconscious.

3. **Severe hypoglycemia.** Coma, seizure, and/or impairment of motor function to the extent that self-treatment is not possible.

4. **Pseudohypoglycemia.** Patient perceives hypoglycemic symptoms (usually adrenergic), but BG may be normal, or slightly above normal, and may be rapidly falling.

5. **Hypoglycemia unawareness.** Patient perceives no or minimal symptoms. Family or co-workers may notice neurological impairment or sweating. BG may be low to seriously low.

6. **Precipitating factors**
   a. Relative or absolute excess of insulin or oral hypoglycemic agent
   b. Delayed or insufficient food intake
   c. More exercise than usual
   d. Alcohol ingestion
   e. Drug interaction resulting in potentiation of hypoglycemic medication or a direct hypoglycemic effect
   f. **Subtle causes**
      (1) Hormonal changes (e.g., drop in progesterone level as part of menstrual cycle)
      (2) Patient switches to a new bottle of insulin and, unknown to the patient or physician, the previous bottle had lost some of its potency
      (3) Gastroparesis (delayed emptying of the stomach following a meal), an autonomic neuropathy complication of diabetes
      (4) Change in insulin injection sites, especially if injection was given at a subcutaneous site associated with muscles used for exercise (blood flow, and thus insulin absorption, is increased owing to the exercising muscle)
   g. **Treatment**
      (1) **Conscious patient.** Use **10–15 g** fast-acting (simple) oral carbohydrate, such as 4 oz. of fruit juice, milk, or regular soda; 2–4 glucose tablets or hard candy. Honey or a glucose gel product may be placed into the patient's mouth, if the person is too confused or unresponsive for self-treatment. Treatment may be repeated in 10–15 min if BG does not return to normal.
      (2) **Unconscious patient**
         (a) Intravenous glucose, using 10% or 50% dextrose solution
         (b) **Glucagon** injection. Between 0.5 and 1 mg given subcutaneously, intramuscularly, or intravenously

XI. LONG-TERM COMPLICATIONS

A. **Macrovascular complications (coronary artery, cerebrovascular and peripheral vascular disease)**

1. **Atherosclerosis** (coronary, cerebrovascular, and peripheral vessels) occurs at an earlier age than nondiabetic individuals. Women with diabetes lose their gender protection from atherosclerosis.

2. **Peripheral vascular disease** may lead to pain (intermittent claudication), chronic cold feet, or insufficient circulation to enable healing of distal lesions (ultimately leading to gangrene and amputation).

3. **Hypertension (HTN)**
   a. Co-existence of HTN and DM strikingly increases the risk of **cardiovascular disease,** doubles the risk of cardiovascular death, and increases incidence of **stroke** and **transient ischemic events** in DM individuals.
   b. Severity or lability of hypertension is determined by factors such as age, race, sex, greater body mass, duration of DM, and persistence of proteinuria.

    c. Associated with acceleration of retinopathy, nephropathy, and atherosclerosis

    d. Hyperinsulinemia and/or insulin resistance may be a significant factor in the development of DM hypertension.

4. Mortality from **coronary artery disease** (CAD) is twofold to fourfold greater in both men and women with diabetes than those without DM, and mortality from cerebrovascular disease is three to five times greater.

5. May present as atypical presentation of CAD, including **silent myocardial infarction** and lack of chest pain (owing to autonomic neuropathy). Symptoms may be limited to nausea, shortness of breath, sweating, and vomiting.

6. Modifiable risk factors include hyperglycemia, hypertension, dyslipidemia, tobacco use, obesity, nutrition, increased insulin levels, physical inactivity, and increased homocysteine levels.

7. Prevention and treatment strategies to slow the development and/or progression of disease.

    a. Aggressive management of hypertension, hyperlipidemia, and hyperglycemia

    b. Smoking cessation

    c. Increased physical activity

    d. Daily aspirin therapy for those individuals with no contraindications

    e. Drug therapy appropriate for the complication, including angiotensin-converting enzyme (ACE) inhibitor therapy as a component of HTN therapy and a cardioselective β-blocker agent for cardiac disease.

B. Eye diseases

1. Diabetic **retinopathy**

    a. A consequence of microvascular changes

    b. Most prevalent eye complication and is often detectable within 5 years after the diagnosis of DM. Present in > 90% of patients with type 1 and 55%–80% of patients with type 2 DM, after 15 years of diabetes.

    c. Leading cause of new blindness in the United States

    d. Categories of retinopathy

        (1) Nonproliferative (background) retinopathy. Vascular abnormalities include retinal microaneurysms (early, mild stage), blot hemorrhages, and retinal edema with or without "hard" exudates. May progress to macula edema.

        (2) Preproliferative retinopathy. With increasing abnormality of the tiny vessels, retinal ischemia occurs, giving rise to the appearance of white patches of oxygen-starved retina, known as soft or cotton wool spots.

        (3) Proliferative retinopathy

            (a) In response to the lack of oxygen, new but weak vessels begin to grow (neovascularization).

            (b) The new vessels grow (proliferate) out from the retinal surface, into the vitreous cavity. These vessels are fragile and may bleed into the vitreous. Hemorrhages into the vitreous can obscure vision, but they are usually reabsorbed in 1–3 months.

            (c) Traction retinal detachment. Scar tissue, and more new blood vessels, continue to grow onto the vitreous. The vitreous pulls (traction) on the retina and detaches it.

    e. Generally does not result in visual alterations until advanced stages are reached

    f. Treatment. Loss of vision can be reduced by 50% with laser photocoagulation if ocular changes are identified and treated in a timely manner.

2. Other ocular complications include cataracts, primary open-angled glaucoma, and ischemic optic neuropathy.

3. Modifiable risk factors include hyperglycemia, hypertension, dyslipidemia, and nicotine use.

4. Prevention strategies

    a. Aggressive management of hypertension, hyperlipidemia, and blood glucose

    b. Smoking cessation

    c. Routine ophthalmologic screening and follow-up, including an annual dilated eye exam

C. Diabetic nephropathy

1. DM is the most common single cause of end-stage renal disease (**ESRD**) in the United States and Europe.

2. Renal failure occurs in 30%–40% of individuals with type 1 DM within 30 years after diagnosis and 20%–30% of patients with type 2 DM.

3. Findings/progression
   a. First evidenced by the presence of urinary **microalbuminuria** (> 30 mg albumin/24 hr)
   b. Clinical or dipstick positive **albuminuria** (> 300 mg/24 hr)
   c. Proteinuria often associated with hypertension, which accelerates the rate of nephropathic changes
   d. Progressive decrease in glomerular filtration rate with rising serum creatinine until ESRD occurs.

4. **Modifiable risk factors** include hyperglycemia, hypertension, tobacco use, and excessive dietary protein intake.

5. **Prevention and treatment strategies** to slow the development and/or progression of disease.
   a. Aggressive management of HTN and blood glucose
   b. Initiation of ACE inhibitor therapy
   c. Smoking cessation
   d. Limit daily dietary protein intake to 0.8 g/kg of ideal body weight. Note that lower protein meal plans should be used with caution to avoid malnutrition and associated muscle weakness.
   e. Early identification and aggressive treatment of urinary tract infections
   f. Yearly assessment of kidney function, including urinalysis for detection of microalbuminuria
   g. For ESRD, fluid and electrolyte restriction as well as intermittent or chronic dialysis treatments, as indicated by severity of pathology, laboratory findings, and patient symptomatology
   h. For ESRD, patient and caregiver counseling to prepare them for the psychosocial, financial, physical, medical, and quality-of-life changes that accompany dialysis and possible kidney transplantation

D. Diabetic neuropathies

1. **Peripheral neuropathy**
   a. The sensorimotor nervous system is most often affected, but sympathetic or parasympathetic abnormalities may be present also.
   b. Sensory deficits and symptoms originate in the distal portions of the lower extremities and gradually progress to the upper extremities, creating a stocking–glove distribution of pain and diminished sensation.
   c. Signs and symptoms depend on the class and stage of nerve fiber loss.
      (1) Small-fiber involvement impairs perception of pain and temperature and may lead to numbness/tingling or loss of sensation.
      (2) Large-fiber involvement produces impaired balance and diminished proprioception.
      (3) Motor nerve damage results in muscle weakness/atrophy.
      (4) The majority of patients experience damage to more than one type of nerve.

2. **Autonomic neuropathy** involves multiple systems throughout the body.
   a. **Genitourinary impairment** may lead to neurogenic bladder and sexual dysfunction in both males (impotence, retrograde ejaculation) and females (diminished vaginal lubrication and orgasm frequency).
   b. **Gastrointestinal impairment** may lead to gastroparesis, nocturnal diarrhea, fecal incontinence, or chronic constipation.
   c. **Cardiovascular impairment** may lead to orthostatic hypotension or cardiac denervation syndrome.

3. **Modifiable risk factors** include hyperglycemia, alcohol use, tobacco use, and hypertension.

4. **Prevention strategies**
   a. Aggressive management of blood pressure and blood glucose.

   b. Smoking and alcohol cessation.

   c. Proper foot care to prevent development of lower-extremity complications in the presence of peripheral neuropathy and diminished circulation.

E. Foot, skin, and mucous membrane complications stem from vascular changes and peripheral neuropathy that cause alterations in the nerves that control blood flow and skin hydration.

   1. Individuals with DM are at increased risk for the development of skin infections caused by staphylococci, β-hemolytic streptococci, and fungus.

   2. Common infections include
      a. Cutaneous infections such as furunculosis and carbuncles
      b. *Candida* infections of the genitalia, upper thighs, and under the breasts
      c. Cellulitis and/or lower-extremity vascular ulcers

   3. Atrophic lesions (round painless lesions) and diabetic dermopathy (reddish brown papular spots) are common, especially on the lower extremities

   4. An ulcerating necrotic lesion called **necrobiosis lipoidica diabeticorum** may develop on the anterior leg surface or the dorsum of the ankle.

   5. Approximately 50% of patients with DM of 15 years' duration have peripheral neuropathy that may result in a loss of protective sensation and inability to detect even minor trauma. This places the patient at significant risk for the development of ulcers.

   6. Injury, infection, neuropathy, vascular disease, or ischemia may lead to gangrene, which is 20 times more common in people with DM.

   7. Prevention strategies
      a. Good glycemic control
      b. Proper foot care (see VIII.D.1) and early detection/intervention of identified problems.
      c. Proper skin care (see VIII.D.2)
      d. Sensory exam of feet using a 5.07 (10-g) monofilament to identify patients with loss of protective sensation
      e. Patient education concerning protective footwear (e.g., deep-soled shoes, individually molded shoes, orthotics) and avoidance of foot injury, especially when a loss of protective sensation is noted.

F. Importance of glycemic control as preventive of chronic complications

   1. The **Diabetes Control and Complications Trial** (DCCT; 1993) demonstrated that intensive treatment of type 1 diabetic patients delays the onset and progression of diabetic retinopathy, nephropathy, and neuropathy.

   2. The **United Kingdom Prospective Diabetes Study** (UKPDS; 1998) similarly demonstrated that the complications of type 2 DM may be reduced by strict glycemic control, regardless of the therapeutic agent chosen to attain that control.

   3. The findings of the DCCT and UKPDS have been confirmed by numerous other clinical studies. There is today no reason for doubt that glycemic control is a major strategy for the prevention of diabetes-related conditions, reduced healthcare and societal costs, and preservation of quality-of-life issues.

XII. SIGNIFICANT DRUG INTERACTIONS AFFECTING GLYCEMIC CONTROL. This is only a partial list of potential drug interactions that may affect glycemic control. Consult standard references or drug package inserts for more detailed information.

   A. Potential hyperglycemia, as a dose-dependent, direct glucogenic effect. Corticosteroids, nicotinic acid, phenytoin, pentamidine (long-term effect), protease inhibitors, sympathomimetics, isoniazid, furosemide, thiazide diuretics

   B. Potential hypoglycemia, as a direct hypoglycemic effect; monoamine oxidase (MAO) inhibitors, fluoxetine, salicylates (large doses), fenfluramine, alcohol, pentamidine (initial effect)

C. Prolonged hypoglycemia and masking of hypoglycemic symptoms. β-Blockers

D. Altered protein binding of, or other drug interaction with, sulfonylurea agents. Alcohol, salicylates, nonsteroidal anti-inflammatory drugs (NSAIDs), methyldopa, chloramphenicol, MAO inhibitors, clofibrate, probenecid

XIII. SPECIAL ISSUES IN DIABETES. These situations cause unique problems in the management of diabetes, but are beyond the scope of this chapter. Readers are encouraged to learn about these, as these issues arise during the course of pharmacy practice.

A. Pregnancy in DM (not GDM)

B. Pediatrics

C. Adolescence

D. Geriatrics

E. Surgery

F. DM management during hemodialysis or peritoneal dialysis

G. Kidney transplantation

H. Self-care issues (e.g., SMBG, injections) in the visually impaired or blind DM patient

I. DM patients in institutionalized facilities

J. Pancreas and islet cell transplantation

STUDY QUESTIONS

Directions: Each of the questions, statements, or incomplete statements in this section can be correctly answered or completed by **one** of the suggested answers or phrases. Choose the **best** answer.

1. Current criteria used in the diagnosis of diabetes mellitus (DM) include all of the following symptoms *except*

(A) fasting hyperglycemia.
(B) polyuria.
(C) polydipsia.
(D) tinnitus.
(E) weight loss.

2. The most useful glucose test used in monitoring diabetes mellitus (DM) therapy is

(A) urine monitoring.
(B) blood monitoring.
(C) renal function monitoring.
(D) cardiovascular monitoring.
(E) vascular monitoring.

3. Which of the following statements concerning insulin therapy is true?

(A) Commercial insulin products vary little with respect to time, course, and duration of hypoglycemic activity.
(B) Regular insulin cannot be mixed with neutral protamine Hagedorn (NPH; isophane insulin suspension).
(C) Regular insulin cannot be given intravenously.
(D) Regulating carbohydrate consumption is a necessity for all diabetic patients.
(E) Insulin therapy does not have to be monitored closely.

4. A mass of adipose tissue that develops at the injection site is usually the result of the patient's neglect to rotate the insulin injection site. This is known as

(A) lipoatrophy.
(B) hypertrophic degenerative adiposity.
(C) lipohypertrophy.
(D) atrophic skin lesion.
(E) dermatitis.

5. Sulfonylurea agents (as monotherapy or in combination) are a primary mode of therapy in the treatment of

(A) insulin-dependent (type 1) diabetes mellitus patients.
(B) diabetes patients experiencing severe hepatic or renal dysfunction.
(C) pregnant women with diabetes.
(D) patients with diabetic ketoacidosis.
(E) non-insulin-dependent (type 2) DM patients.

6. Patients taking chlorpropamide should avoid products containing

(A) acetaminophen.
(B) ethanol.
(C) vitamin A.
(D) penicillins.
(E) milk products.

7. The standard recommended dose of glyburide is

(A) 0.5–2 mg/day.
(B) 1.25–20 mg/day.
(C) 50–100 mg/day.
(D) 200 mg/day.
(E) 200–1000 mg/day.

For questions 8–12: A 20-year-old previously healthy man presents to the emergency room with a 2-week history of polyuria, polydipsia, and a 20-lb unintentional weight loss. He complains of weakness, fatigue, nausea, and abdominal pain. Physical examination reveals dry, parched mucous membranes. Blood pressure is 110/70 mm Hg and the pulse is 90 beats per minute (bpm) supine; blood pressure is 90/60 mm Hg, and pulse is 120 bpm upright. Temperature is 100°F (axillary); respiratory rate is 24 breaths per minute. General examination of the heart and lungs is unremarkable. No retinopathy is present. The abdomen is soft with mild tenderness but no rebound. Laboratory values are as follows:

Blood glucose	420 mg/dL
Sodium (Na)	130 mEq/L
Potassium (K)	3.7 mEq/L
Chloride (Cl)	97 mEq/L
Bicarbonate (HCO_3)	10 mEq/L
Arterial blood gas	7.20 (pH)
Urinalysis	+3 glucose and moderate ketones
Chest radiograph	Unremarkable
Abdominal radiography	Unremarkable

8. What is the most likely diagnosis in this patient?

(A) type 2 diabetes mellitus (DM) with hyperosmolar state
(B) type 1 DM with diabetic ketoacidosis
(C) type 2 DM without hyperosmolar state
(D) type 1 DM without diabetic ketoacidosis

9. Initial appropriate therapy includes

(A) intravenous fluids and a sulfonylurea agent
(B) intravenous fluids alone
(C) intravenous fluids, 10 U of subcutaneous regular insulin, and discharge to home
(D) intravenous fluids, intravenous regular insulin by continuous drip at 6 Units/hr, and hospital admission

10. After the acute illness has resolved, what therapy would be appropriate?

(A) None, observe only
(B) Start a second-generation sulfonylurea, plus dietary modification and physical activity regimen
(C) Daily administration of a regimen of neutral protamine Hagedorn (NPH; isophane insulin suspension) and regular insulin, plus dietary modification and physical activity regimen
(D) Dietary modification alone

11. Appropriate follow-up of the patient once discharged to home includes all of the following *except*

(A) periodic monitoring of hemoglobin AIC levels.
(B) periodic ophthalmologic examinations.
(C) home glucose monitoring with a glucose meter.
(D) weight-loss diet and an attempt to wean from insulin.

12. The patient is at high risk for developing all of the following complications *except*

(A) hypoglycemia.
(B) coronary artery disease.
(C) retinopathy.
(D) nonketotic hyperglycemia hyperosmolar state.

ANSWERS AND EXPLANATIONS

1. The answer is D *[see III.A–B].*
Frequent urination (polyuria), thirst (polydipsia), and weight loss are all common signs of diabetes. When these symptoms are present, it is necessary to have a fasting or random (casual) blood glucose level drawn to determine a diabetic state. A fasting blood glucose level > 125 mg/dL on more than one occasion is diagnostic of a diabetic state.

2. The answer is B *[see IX.A–B].*
Blood glucose monitoring is the most useful form of monitoring glucose levels. Urine monitoring provides only gross estimates of the current status and cannot rule out hypoglycemia. Renal function and cardiovascular functions provide evidence of long-standing disease and are not useful for monitoring daily progress.

3. The answer is D *[see VII.A.1; VII.C.7; Table 54-1].*
Many commercial insulin preparations vary with respect to duration of activity and time for peak plasma level. Regular insulin can be mixed with NPH and given intravenously. All insulin therapies should be monitored closely and on a daily basis. Careful regulation of carbohydrate intake is very important for all diabetic patients—carbohydrate consumption plays a major role in the balance of glucose metabolism and antagonizes the effects of insulin therapy.

4. The answer is C *[see VII.C.7.a.(3)].*
Lipohypertrophy consists of masses of adipose tissue that develop at the injection site, usually in patients who do not rotate the injection sites properly. The masses gradually disappear if injection in these sites is avoided.

5. The answer is E *[see VII.D.2; X.A.2].*
Sulfonylureas should not be used as primary therapy in insulin-dependent (type 1) diabetes mellitus patients, in those who have severe hepatic or renal dysfunction, or in those patients who are pregnant. DKA should never be treated with sulfonylureas; this condition must be treated with insulin, fluids, and electrolyte replacement. However, sulfonylureas help reduce blood glucose levels in type 2 DM that does not respond to diet alone.

6. The answer is B *[see VII.D.6.g].*
Acute ingestion of ethanol (alcohol) by patients who are taking any antidiabetic agent carries the risk of severe hypoglycemia particularly because of the potential hypoglycemic effects of ethanol (especially if consumed in the fasting state). In addition, the interaction of chlorpropamide and ethanol (disulfiram-like reaction) is notable with this agent.

7. The answer is B *[see Table 54-2].*
The standard recommended dose of glyburide is 1.25–20 mg/day. Doses > 20 mg are not recommended by the manufacturer. Patients may be started on a low dose (e.g., 1.25 mg/day) and titrated up to an effective oral dose, as clinically indicated.

8. The answer is B *[see II.B.1; X.A.2].*
Type 1 DM with DKA is the most likely diagnosis in the patient described in the question. The patient presented with high blood sugar, weight loss, acidosis, and positive urine ketones (high level). This is a typical presentation of DKA.

9. The answer is D *[see X.A.2.d].*
Type 1 DM always requires insulin therapy; it can never be left untreated or treated with diet or liquids alone and can never be treated with sulfonylurea agents. DKA requires hospitalization and should be treated with an insulin drip until the acidosis clears. Patients with DKA are dehydrated and must be given intravenous fluids.

10. The answer is C *[see VII.C.4].*

11. The answer is D *[see VII.C.4; VIII.D.4; IX.A; IX.D.1].*
All diabetic patients should be followed with periodic hemoglobin AIC measurements and ophthalmologic examination annually. Home glucose monitoring is the optimal way to follow a patient's level of control. Weight loss and an attempt to wean from insulin are appropriate only for type 2 DM. Those patients with type 1 diabetes cannot be weaned from insulin therapy.

12. The answer is D *[see II.B.2; X.A.3].*
Hypoglycemia is a possible complication of insulin therapy. All diabetic patients are at risk for coronary artery disease and retinopathy. Nonketotic hyperglycemic hyperosmolar coma is typically a complication of type 2 DM.

55
Thyroid Disease
John E. Janosik

I. PHYSIOLOGY

A. Thyroid hormone regulation

1. The thyroid gland synthesizes, stores, and secretes hormones that are important to growth, development, and the metabolic rate. These hormones are **thyroxine (T_4)** and **triiodothyronine (T_3).**

2. The thyroid gland also secretes **calcitonin,** which reduces blood calcium ion concentration.

3. Thyroid hormone secretion and transport are controlled by **thyroid-stimulating hormone (thyrotropin; TSH).** TSH is released by the anterior pituitary gland, which is triggered by **thyrotropin-releasing hormone (TRH),** secreted from the hypothalamus.
   a. The process produces increased levels of thyroid hormone (circulating free T_4 and free T_3), which, in turn, signals the pituitary to stop releasing TSH (**negative feedback**).
   b. Conversely, low blood levels of free hormone trigger pituitary release of TSH, which stimulates the thyroid gland to secrete T_4 and T_3 until free hormone levels return to normal. At this point, the pituitary gland ceases to release TSH, which completes the feedback loop (Figure 55-1).
   c. This homeostatic mechanism attempts to maintain the level of circulating thyroid hormone within a narrow range.

B. Biosynthesis (Figure 55-2)

1. Essential to synthesis of thyroid hormones is dietary iodine, reduced to **inorganic iodide,** which the thyroid actively extracts from the plasma through iodide trapping (**iodide pump**). Some of this iodide is stored within the colloid; some diffuses into the lumen of thyroid follicles.

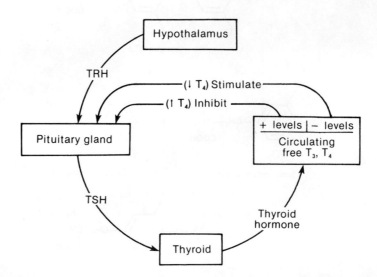

Figure 55-1. Thyroid hormone regulation loop. This carefully balanced hormone regulation system uses both positive (stimulating) and negative (inhibiting) feedback to maintain homeostasis. Disruption of any of these elements can produce serious consequences, such as myxedema crisis (under availability of thyroid hormone) or thyroid storm (overabundance of thyroid hormone). *T_3*, triiodothyronine; *T_4*, thyroxine; *TRH*, thyroid-releasing hormone; *TSH*, thyroid-stimulating hormone.

Figure 55-2. Biosynthesis of thyroid hormones. The major products are thyroxine (T$_4$) and triiodothyronine (T$_3$). These are formed in the follicle cells of the thyroid gland by iodination of tyrosine residues. Monoiodotyrosine and diiodotyrosine residues are formed first. These then react to form T$_3$ and T$_4$.

2. Iodide is oxidized by peroxidase and bound to tyrosyl residues within the thyroglobulin molecule in a process called **organification.**
   a. The synthesis begins with iodide binding to tyrosine, forming **monoiodotyrosine (MIT).**
   b. MIT then binds another iodide to form **diiodotyrosine (DIT).**
   c. Then, slowly, a coupling reaction binds MIT and DIT, producing T_3 and T_4.

C. Hormone transport

1. After TSH stimulation of the thyroid gland, T_3 and T_4 are cleaved from thyroglobulin and released into the circulation.

2. When in the circulation, thyroid hormone is transported bound to several plasma proteins, a process that
   a. Helps protect the hormone from premature metabolism and excretion
   b. Prolongs its half-life in the circulation
   c. Allows the thyroid hormone to reach its site of action

3. Most thyroid hormone is transported by **thyroxine-binding globulin (TBG). Prealbumin** and **albumin** also serve as carriers.

D. Hormone metabolism

1. Peripheral conversion of T_4 to T_3 occurs in the pituitary gland, liver, and kidneys and accounts for about 80% of T_3 generation.

2. Deiodination accounts for most hormone degradation. The major steps in this process are shown in Figure 55-3.

3. Deiodinated hormones are excreted in feces and urine.

4. Minor nondeiodination pathways of metabolism include conjugation with sulfate and glucuronide, deamination, and decarboxylation.

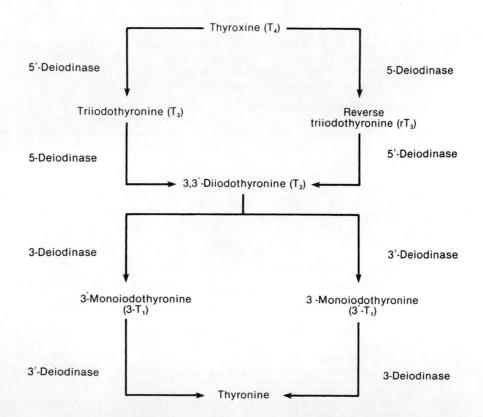

Figure 55-3. Thyroxine metabolism—major steps in the primary and alternative deiodination pathways.

E. Hormone function. Although the effects of thyroid hormones are known, the basic mechanisms producing these effects elude precise definition; however, they seem to activate the messenger RNA (mRNA) transcription process and can promote protein synthesis or (in excessive amounts) protein catabolism. **Thyroid hormones** affect the following:

1. Growth and development

2. Calorigenics by increasing the rate of basal metabolism

3. Cardiovascular system by increasing the metabolic rate, which increases blood flow, cardiac output, and heart rate (may be related in part to an increased tissue sensitivity to catecholamines)

4. The central nervous system (CNS) by increasing or diminishing cerebration

5. Musculature by causing a fine tremor

6. Sleep by inducing fatigued wakefulness with hyperthyroidism or somnolence with hypothyroidism

7. Lipid metabolism by stimulating lipid mobilization and degradation

F. Thyroid function studies (Table 55-1)

1. **Serum total thyroxine (TT$_4$)**
   a. This test provides the most direct reflection of thyroid function by indicating hormone availability to tissues. Total (free and bound) T$_4$ is determined by radioimmunoassay, which is sensitive and rapid.
   b. Changes in thyroid globulin concentration, particularly TBG, which increases during pregnancy, alter the total concentration of T$_4$ and may produce a misleading high or low test result.
   c. However, these changes in TBG do not affect the concentration of free T$_4$. Therefore, to clarify thyroid function, either protein-binding (T$_3$ uptake test) or free T$_4$ must be measured.
   d. An elevated TT$_4$ level indicates hyperthyroidism; a decreased TT$_4$ level, hypothyroidism. However, the TT$_4$ level in a euthyroid patient can be altered by other factors, such as pregnancy or febrile illnesses (which elevate the TT$_4$), nephrotic syndrome or cirrhosis (which lower it), and various drugs (Table 55-2).

2. **Serum total triiodothyronine (TT$_3$)**
   a. This sensitive and highly specific test measures total (free and bound) T$_3$.
   b. Serum T$_3$ and T$_4$ usually rise and fall together; however, hyperthyroidism commonly causes a disproportionate rise in T$_3$, and the TT$_3$ can rise before the TT$_4$ level. Therefore, TT$_3$ is useful for early detection or to rule out hyperthyroidism. Many of the symptoms associated with hyperthyroidism are the result of the elevated TT$_3$.
   c. This test may not be diagnostically significant for hypothyroidism, in which TT$_3$ levels may fall but stay within the normal range. The TT$_3$ may be low in only 50% of patients with hypothyroidism.

Table 55-1. Test Results in Thyroid Disorders

Thyroid Function Test	Hypothyroidism	Hyperthyroidism
Serum resin triiodothyronine uptake (RT$_3$U)	↓ (< 35%)	↑ (> 45%)
Serum total thyroxine (TT$_4$)	↓ (< 5 μg/dL)	↑ (> 12 μg/dLl)
Serum total triiodothyronine (TT$_3$)	↓ (< 80 ng/dL)	↑ (> 180 ng/dLl)
Free thyroxine index (FTI)	↓ (< 5.5)	↑ (< 10.5)
Serum thyrotropin (TSH) assay[a]	↑ (> 4.5 μU/mL)	↓ (< 0.4 μU/mL)[b]

↑, increased levels; ↓, decreased levels.
[a]In clinical practice the third-generation test is commonly used with sensitivity to detect 0.01–0.02 mIU/L.
[b]Fourth-generation assays detect 0.001–0.002 mIU/L.

Table 55-2. Effects of Drugs on Thyroid Function Tests

Drug	Serum T_4	Resin T_3 Uptake	Free Thyroxine Index	Serum T_3	Serum TSH	Comment
p-Aminosalicylic acid	↓	n/d	↓	n/d	↑[a]	Antithyroid effect, rarely, with long-term use
Aminoglutethimide (*Cytadren*)[b]	↑	n/d	n/d	n/d	↑	
Amiodarone[b]	↑	n/d	↓	↓	n/d	Inhibits peripheral conversion of T_4 to T_3
Anabolic steroids and androgens	↓	↑	0	↓[a]	n/d	Decreased serum TBG
Antithyroid drugs (propylthiouracil or methimazole)	↓	↓	↓	↓	0 or ↑	TSH may increase if patient becomes hypothyroid
Asparaginase (*Elspar*)	↓[c]	↑	n/d	↓[a]	↑[a]	Decreased serum TBG
Barbiturates	↓	n/d	↓	n/d	n/d	Stimulates T_4 metabolism
Calcium carbonate[d]	↓	n/d	n/d	0	↑	Subclinical signs of hypothyroidism; separate time of ingestion of calcium and levothyroxine
Ciprofloxacin[e]	↓	n/d	n/d	↓	↑	Clinical signs of hypothyroidism; separate administration by 6 hr.
Contraceptives, oral	↑	↓	0	↑	0	TBG usually increased
Corticosteroids	0 or ↓	0 or ↑	0 or ↓	↓	↓	Usual doses decrease TBG; high doses may increase TBG
Danazol (*Danocrine*)	↓	↑	0[p]	↓	0 or ↓	Decreased serum TBG
Estrogens and SERMs[g]	↑	↓	0	↑	0	Increased serum TBG
Ethionamide (*Trecator-SC*)	↑	n/d	↓[a]	n/d	↑[a]	Antithyroid effect
Fluorouracil (*Adrucil*)	↑	↓	n/d	↑	0	Patients clinically euthyroid; TBG increased
Heparin, IV	↑[h]	0 or ↑	↑[a]	0	n/d	FTI is increased with some measures
Hypoglycemics (sulfonylureas)	0[i]	0[i]	0[i]	n/d	n/d	
Iodides, inorganic	0	0	0	n/d	n/d	
Iodides, organic	0	0	0	n/d	n/d	
Levodopa and levodopa-carbidopa (*Sinemet*)	0	0	0	0	↓[j]	
Levothyroxine (*Levothroid*)	↑[s][k,l]	↑ or 0 or ↓[k,l]	0 or ↑[k,l]	↑ or 0[k,l]	↑ or 0[k]	
Liothyronine (*Cytomel*)	↓[k]	0 or ↓[k]	↓[k]	↑ or ↓[k,l]	0[k]	
Liotrix (*Thyrolar*)	0[k] or ↓[s]	0[k]	0[k]	0[k,l]	0[k]	

(Continued on next page)

Table 55-2. Continued.

Drug	Serum T4	Resin T3 Uptake	Free Thyroxine Index	Serum T3	Serum TSH	Comment
Lithium carbonate (Eskalith)	0 or ↓	0 or ↓	0 or ↓	0 or ↓	0 or ↑	Increased serum TBG
Methadone (Dolophine)	↑s	↓	0	↑	0	
Mitotane (Lysodren)	↓	0	0[a]	n/d	n/d	Clinical hypothyroidism
Nitroprusside (Nipride)	↓	n/d	n/d	n/d	n/d	
Oxyphenbutazone and phenylbutazone (Butazolidin)	0 or ↓	↑	↓	n/d	↑[a]	May compete with T4 for TBG binding, rarely, overt hypothyroidism and goiter may occur
Perphenazine (Trilafon)	↑	0 or ↑s	0 or ↓s	↑	0[a]	Stimulates T4 metabolism and may compete with T4 for TBG binding
Phenytoin (Dilantin)	↓	↑s		↓	0	
Propranolol (Inderal)	0 or ↑[m]	0[n]	n/d	↓[o]	0	
Raloxifene[g]	↑	↓	0	↑	0	Increased serum TBG
Resorcinol (excessive topical use)	↓	↑s		↑	↑	
Salicylates (large doses)	↓	↑s	↓[a]	↓	0[a]	Compete with T4 for TBG binding
Tamoxifene[g]	↑	↓	0	↑	0	Increased serum TBG

[a] Effect deduced, not based on reported clinical evidence.

[b] Data from Rae P, Farrar J, Beckett G, Toft A. Assessment of thyroid status in elderly people. Br Med J 1993;307:177–180.

[c] Patients requiring thyroid-replacement therapy have decreased serum thyroxine when barbiturates are given.

[d] Data from Singh N, Singh P, Hershman JM. Effect of calcium carbonate on the adsorption of levothyroxine. JAMA 2000;283:2822–2825.

[e] Data from Cooper JG, HarboeK, Frost SK, Skadberg O. Ciprofloxacin interacts with thyroid replacement therapy. Br Med J 2005;330:1002.

[f] May increase slightly but usually remains in the normal range.

[g] Data from Siraj ES, Gupta MK, Reddy SK. Raloxifene causing malabsorption of levothyroxine. Arch Intern Med 2003;163:1367–1370.

[h] T4 assay by competitive protein binding is spuriously increased, but T4 radioimmunoassay is probably not affected. Free thyroxine measured by dialysis may be increased.

[i] May occasionally decrease serum T4 and increase resin T3 uptake.

[j] Slight decrease in euthyroid patients; but in long-standing hypothyroid patients, levodopa considerably decreases the elevated TSH.

[k] In a patient on adequate doses for thyroid replacement.

[l] Increased T4, FTI, and T3 tend to return to normal after several months of therapy with levothyroxine. After liothyronine, T3 may be elevated 2 hr after a dose and depressed 24 hr after a dose.

[m] Increased T4 levels are reported in one study, but not in others.

[n] With short-term propranolol therapy.

[o] In euthyroid patients, the decreased serum T3 returns to normal with continued propranolol therapy.

[p] Free thyroxine index may increase slightly but usually remains in the normal range.

FTI, free thyroxine index; IV, intravenous; n/d, no data; s, slight effect; SC, subcutaneous; SERMs, selective estrogen receptor modulators; T3, triiodothyronine; T4, thyroxine; TBG, thyroxine-binding globulin; TSH, thyroid-stimulating hormone; 0, no effect; ↑, increased; ↓, decreased.

d. If there is an abnormality in binding proteins, this test can yield the same misleading results as the TT_4 readings. Other factors affecting test results include pregnancy (which increases TT_3 levels), malnutrition or hepatic or renal disease (which lower TT_3 levels), or various drugs (Table 55-2).

3. **Resin triiodothyronine uptake (RT_3U)**
   a. This test clarifies whether abnormal T_4 levels are the result of a thyroid disorder or to abnormalities in the binding proteins because it evaluates the binding capacity of TBG.
   b. If an abnormal amount (high or low) of thyroid hormone is present in the blood, the RT_3U results **change in the same direction** as the altered level—elevated in hyperthyroidism, decreased in hypothyroidism.
   c. However, if abnormalities in binding proteins underlie the abnormal levels of TT_4, TT_3, or both, the RT_3U results **change in the opposite direction**—decreasing as TBG increases, increasing as TBG decreases.
   d. Several drugs can cause spurious changes in the RT_3U (Table 55-2).

4. **Serum thyrotropin (TSH) assays**
   a. This test is the **most sensitive** test for detecting the hypothyroid state because the hypothalamic–pituitary axis compensates very quickly for even slight decreases in circulating free hormone by releasing more TSH. The TSH levels may be elevated even before low circulating levels of TT_4 are detectable by diagnostic testing.
   b. The early TSH assay used radioimmunoassay (RIA) methodology. The sensitivity of the assay has improved since, moving to the use of monoclonal antibodies in the late 1980s. Nomenclature established by the American Thyroid Association (ATA) has classified the improvement in sensitivity based on the lower limit of detection. The new classification follows a generational format, as shown in Table 55-3.
   c. The current (third-generation) serum TSH assay (level of detection 0.01–0.02 mIU/L) uses monoclonal antibodies referred to as immunoradiometric or immunometric (IMA) methodology (instead of the older radioimmunoassay techniques) and demonstrates greater sensitivity in the detection of thyroid disease than older tests.
   d. This assay is usually used to diagnose thyroid disease and monitor patients receiving replacement therapy to control overtreatment. (Overtreatment—TSH < 0.4 mIU/L—may contribute to excessive bone demineralization (reduced bone density), electrocardiogram [ECG] changes, atrial fibrillation, or elevation of liver function tests.)
   e. The IMA technique is very sensitive. The fourth-generation IMA can detect TSH levels in the range of 0.001–0.002 mIU/L.
   f. The third-generation IMA assays may also detect subclinical thyroid disease (TSH = 0.1–0.45 mIU/L). Treatment of subclinical hypothyroidism is controversial because there is insufficient evidence to indicate a benefit.
   g. TSH levels may also be influenced by psychiatric illness. Some studies of hospitalized patients have reported abnormally high or low TSH levels in otherwise euthyroid patients. Current findings in HIV-positive patients are uncertain; however, autoimmune thyroid disease appears to be more prevalent in these patients.
   h. Effects of drugs on the serum TSH are shown in Tables 55-2 and 55-4.

5. **Free thyroxine index (FTI)**
   a. This is not a separate test but rather an estimation of the free T_4 level through a mathematical interpretation of the relationship between RT_3U and serum T_4 levels.

$$FTI = \frac{TT_4 \times RT_3U}{\text{mean serum } RT_3U}$$

Table 55-3. Serum Thyroid-Stimulating Hormone Assay Nomenclature

Generation	Lower Level of Detection
First (RIA method)	1–2 mIU/L
Second	0.1–0.2 mIU/L
Third	0.01–0.02 mIU/L
Fourth	0.001–0.002 mIU/L

Table 55-4. Medications Influencing Thyroid-Stimulating Hormone (TSH) Levels

Agent	Mechanisms	Potential Clinical Thyroid Effect(s)	Effect on TSH	Effect on Other Thyroid Function Tests	Comments
Amiodarone	Iodine effects (see Iodine below) Direct inhibition of T_4 to T_3 conversion Direct toxic effects on thyroid Induction of thyroid autoimmunity	Clinical or subclinical hypothyroidism Hyperthyroidism	Usual pattern is mild elevation for first 8–12 weeks of therapy followed by normalization: marked elevation seen with hypothyroidism; suppression with hyperthyroidism	Increased total T_4 levels Increased free T_4 levels Increased reverse T_3 levels Decreased total and free T_3	Biochemical changes in thyroid function noted in a majority of patients on therapy, requiring frequent monitoring
Calcium carbonate	Adsorption of levothyroxine to calcium in acid environment	Subclinical hypothyroidism	Elevation	Decrease free T_4 and total T_4	
Ciprofloxacin	Decreases absorption of levothyroxine	Hypothyroidism	Elevation	Decreased thyroid hormone levels	Clinical hypothyroidism detected
Corticosteroids	Central suppression of TSH release Reduction of thyroid iodine uptake	Minimal or none	Suppression	Usually within normal range, although total T_4, free T_4, T_3 reduced, and reverse T_3 increased from baseline	Compensatory mechanisms lead to normalization of TSH levels with chronic exposure

Drug	Mechanism	Effect	TSH	Thyroid hormone levels	Comments
Dopamine and dopamine agonists	Inhibition of T_4 to T_3 conversion; Reduction of thyroid-binding globulin levels; Central suppression of TSH release	Minimal or none	Suppression	Normal or decreased hormone levels	Prolonged use of dopamine in high doses may potentiate the low thyroxine state of critical illness
Dopamine antagonists	Release of central TSH inhibition	Minimal or none	Elevation	Usually normal	Effects not well characterized
Iodine	Inhibition of iodine uptake and organification	Clinical or subclinical hypothyroidism	Elevation	Decreased thyroid hormone levels	Clinical hypothyroidism most common in those with underlying organification defects, such as autoimmune thyroiditis or previous radioiodine therapy; iodine-induced hyperthyroidism is generally confined to those with iodine deficiency or autoimmune thyroid disease
	Impairment of thyroid hormone; Inhibition of T_4 to T_3 conversion; Induction of thyroid autoimmunity	Hyperthyroidism	Suppression	Elevated thyroid hormone levels	

(Continued on next page)

Table 55-4. Continued.

Agent	Mechanisms	Potential Clinical Thyroid Effect(s)	Effect on TSH	Effect on Other Thyroid Function Tests	Comments
Interferon	Unclear; likely owing to immunomodulating properties and stimulation of autoimmunity	Hypothyroidism (silent thyroiditis, Graves disease)	Elevation	Decreased thyroid hormone levels	No apparent direct influence on TSH secretion; pretreatment detectable antimicrosomal antibodies may represent a risk factor for interferon-induced thyroid disease
		Hyperthyroidism (with or without autoantibodies)	Suppression	Increased thyroid hormone levels	
Lithium salts	Inhibition of iodothyronine biosynthesis; Reduction of thyroid iodine concentration; Suppression of thyroid hormone release; Induction of thyroid autoimmunity	Clinical or subclinical hypothyroidism	Elevation	Normal or decreased thyroid hormone levels	Some sources recommend thyroid function testing at 6-month intervals while on therapy
Radiographic contrast media	Iodine effects (See Iodine above); Direct inhibition of T_4 to T_3 conversion	Minimal or none	Elevation	Normal or decreased thyroid hormone levels; Elevation of reverse T_3 levels	Alterations are maximal 3–4 days after administration and may persist for up to 2 weeks
Raloxifene	Malabsorption; mechanism unknown	Hypothyroidism	Elevation	Decreased thyroid hormone levels	Clinical hypothyroidism detected
Somatostatin and analogs	Central suppression of TSH release	Minimal or none	Suppression	Usually normal	Effects not well characterized

T_3, triiodothyronine; T_4, thyroxine.

b. FTI values are elevated in hyperthyroidism, when TBG is low, and decreased in hypothyroidism, when TBG is elevated.

c. Effects of drugs on FTI are shown in Table 55-2.

G. **Strategies and cost considerations for testing**

1. The **most frequently** used and **least expensive** tests for screening are the TT_4 and the RT_3U, which are used to calculate the FTI. A serum TSH assay may also be used, but at an additional cost (Figure 55-4).

2. Thyroid disease screening for the otherwise generally healthy population has been shown to **not be cost-effective** based on the rate of detection and cost associated with massive screening. However, with increased use and improvements in technology, costs have been falling (Figure 55-5).

3. The most appropriate **target population** for screening includes elderly patients hospitalized for exacerbations of chronic diseases or who are coincidentally diagnosed with a chronic

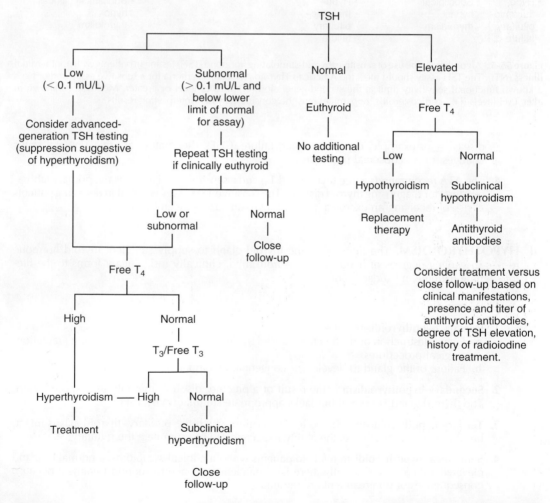

Figure 55-4. Algorithm for using a sensitive thyroid-stimulating hormone (TSH) assay as a single test of thyroid function. The algorithm assumes a clinically intact hypothalamic–pituitary axis, absence of medications known to influence TSH or other thyroid indices, and generally good physical and psychiatric health. The TSH assay should meet the American Thyroid Association criteria for a sensitive assay and/or have a known functional sensitivity limit at the second-generation (0.1 mIU/L) level or greater. *Close follow-up,* clinical observation for signs and symptoms of hyperthyroidism or hypothyroidism and repeated TSH determinations at intervals of 6 to 12 months. T_3, trirodothyronine; T_4, thyroxine.

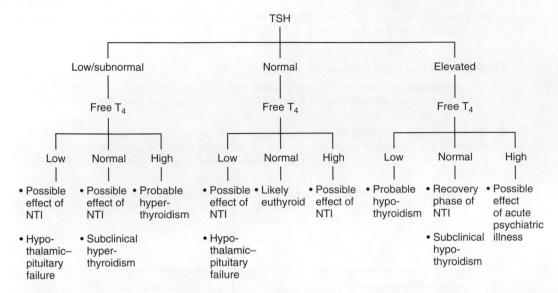

Figure 55-5. Algorithm for the use of sensitive thyroid-stimulating hormone (TSH) testing in patients with nonthyroidal illness (NTI). The TSH assay should meet the American Thyroid Association criteria for a sensitive assay and/or have a known functional sensitivity limit at the second-generation (0.1 mIU/L) level or greater. Medications known to alter TSH levels (i.e., corticosteroids, dopamine) must be considered when interpreting results.

disease—for example, congestive heart failure (CHF), rheumatoid arthritis—mental status changes, or psychosocial problems.

4. The ATA recommends a free thyroxine (FT_4) and a sensitive TSH assay as the primary laboratory tests for diagnosing thyroid disease. The sensitive TSH assay is useful in detecting patients at risk of receiving an excess amount of thyroxine as replacement therapy.

II. HYPOTHYROIDISM.
The inability of the thyroid gland to supply sufficient thyroid hormone results in varying degrees of hypothyroidism from mild, clinically insignificant forms to the life-threatening extreme, myxedema coma.

A. Classification

1. **Primary hypothyroidism** is the result of
   a. Gland destruction or dysfunction caused by disease or medical therapies (e.g., radiation, surgical procedures)
   b. Failure of the gland to develop or congenital incompetence (i.e., **cretinism**)

2. **Secondary hypothyroidism** is the result of a pituitary disorder that inhibits TSH secretion. The thyroid gland is normal but lacks appropriate stimulation by TSH.

3. **Tertiary hypothyroidism** refers to a condition in which the pituitary–thyroid axis is intact, but the hypothalamus lacks the ability to secrete TRH to stimulate the pituitary.

4. **Subclinical hypothyroidism** refers to patients without clinical symptoms, a normal FT_4, and elevated TSH levels. Currently there is insufficient evidence to support treatment because consequences of nontreatment are minimal.

B. Causes

1. **Hashimoto thyroiditis,** which is a chronic lymphocytic thyroiditis that is considered to be an autoimmune disorder

2. **Treatment of hyperthyroidism,** such as radioactive iodine therapy, subtotal thyroidectomy, or administration of antithyroid agents

3. **Surgical excision**

4. **Goiter** (enlargement of the thyroid gland)
   a. **Endemic goiter** results from inadequate intake of dietary iodine. This is common in regions with iodine-depleted soil and in areas of endemic malnutrition.
   b. **Sporadic goiter** can follow ingestion of certain drugs or foods containing **progoitrin** (L-5-vinyl-2-thiooxazolidone), which is inactive and converted by hydrolysis to goitrin.
      (1) Goitrins inhibit oxidation of iodine to iodide and prevent iodide from binding to thyroglobulin, thereby decreasing thyroid hormone production.
      (2) Progoitrin has been isolated in cabbage, kale, peanuts, brussels sprouts, mustard, rutabaga, kohlrabi, spinach, cauliflower, and horseradish.
      (3) **Goitrogenic drugs** include propylthiouracil (PTU), iodides, phenylbutazone, cobalt, and lithium.
   c. **Less common causes** include acute (usually traumatic) and subacute thyroiditis, nodules, nodular goiter, and thyroid cancer.

C. **Signs and symptoms**

   1. Early clinical features tend to be somewhat vague: lethargy, fatigue, forgetfulness, sensitivity to cold, unexplained weight gain, and constipation.

   2. Progressively, the characteristic features of myxedema emerge: dry, flaky, inelastic skin; coarse hair; slowed speech and thought; hoarseness; puffy face, hands, and feet; eyelid droop; hearing loss; menorrhagia; decreased libido; and slow return of deep tendon reflexes (especially in the Achilles tendon). If untreated, myxedema coma will develop.

D. **Laboratory findings** (Table 55-1)

E. **Treatment goal** is replacement therapy using oral agents (Table 55-5).

Table 55-5. Thyroid Replacement Preparations

Preparation (Trade Names)	Advantage	Disadvantage	Comments	Source
Desiccated thyroid (Thyroid USP, Thyroid Strong, Armour Thyroid, Thyrar, S-P-T)	Low cost	Some preparations have unpredictable results; inconsistent $T_3:T_4$ ratio T_3 increases adverse effects	Contains T_3; some brands are standardized by iodine content[a]	Porcine, bovine, or ovine thyroid glands
Liothyronine (Cytomel)	Predictable results; useful for myxedema crisis	Lacks T_4	Usually reserved for myxedema crisis	Synthetic
Liotrix (Thyrolar)	Standardized formulation	T_3 increases adverse effects; expensive	Fixed $T_3:T_4$ ratio of 1:4; metabolism of T_4 to T_3 renders T_3 component unnecessary	Synthetic
Levothyroxine[b] (Levothroid, Synthroid, Levoxyl)	Predictable results, intravenous preparation available	Expensive	Agent of choice; does not contain T_3; all preparations may be interchangeable	Synthetic

[a]Iodine content and $T_3:T_4$ ratio vary with species.
[b]Generic formulations manufactured by Pharmaceuticals Basics for Geneva Generics and Rugby have been shown to be bioequivalent to Synthroid and Levoxyl. (Dong BJ, Hauck WW, Gambertoglio JG, et al. Bioequivalence of generic and brand-name levothyroxine products in the treatment of hypothyroidism. JAMA 1997;277:1205–1213.)
T_3, triiodothyronine; T_4, thyroxine.

F. Therapeutic agents

1. Desiccated thyroid preparations

   a. At one time the agent of choice, desiccated thyroid (Armour Thyroid) has fallen out of favor since standardized synthetic levothyroxine preparations have become available.

   b. Desiccated thyroid preparations are not considered bioequivalent; they have evidenced varying amounts of active substances. Although they met established *United States Pharmacopeia (USP)* criteria for iodine content, variation in activity was noted. The content assay, while specific for iodine, was unable to specify the ratio of T_3 to T_4, and this ratio varies with the animal source. Porcine gland preparations have a higher T_3 to T_4 ratio than those from ovine and bovine sources.

2. Fixed-ratio liotrix (Thyrolar) preparations.
In an effort to standardize the T_3 to T_4 ratio, substances that mimic glandular content were developed. However, the T_3 component proved unnecessary (because T_4 is metabolized to T_3) and even disadvantageous because of T_3-induced **adverse effects** (e.g., tremor, headache, palpitations, diarrhea).

3. Levothyroxine

   a. Predictable results and lack of T_3-induced side effects have made levothyroxine (Levothroid, Synthroid, Levoxyl) the agent of choice.

   b. The **three major brands** of levothyroxine preparations (Levothroid, Synthroid, Levoxyl) have been compared for bioequivalence and were shown to be equivalent in patients with hypothyroidism.

   c. Recent studies in patients with hypothyroidism have compared brand and generic formulations of levothyroxine, which include Synthroid, Levoxyl, and generic formulations manufactured by Pharmaceutical Basics and sold by Geneva Generic and Rugby. Bioequivalence has been demonstrated with these formulations. However, when switching formulations, it is recommended to monitor the patient closely because there may be some individual patient variability among formulations (Figure 55-6).

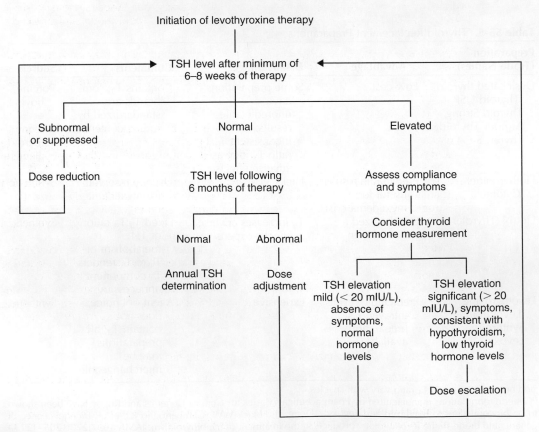

Figure 55-6. Algorithm for management of patients on levothyroxine therapy. *TSH,* tyroid-stimulating hormone.

    d. The **average adult maintenance** dose is 75–150 µg/day. The dose range has been shown to be 1.5–1.7 µg/kg/day or an average of 1.6 µg/kg/day for otherwise healthy adults.

    e. **Elderly** or **chronically ill patients** require an average dose of 50–100 µg/day, which is 25–50 µg/day less than otherwise healthy adults of the same height and weight.

    f. Thyroxine levels return to normal within a few weeks. Clinical improvement begins in 2 weeks with full resolution of signs and symptoms of hypothyroidism by 3–6 months of therapy.

    g. TSH levels begin to decrease after starting thyroid replacement. TSH remains elevated for some time after T_4 levels return to normal. Generally, TSH levels return to normal after a minimum of 6–8 weeks, but may continue to fall over 6–12 months (Figure 55-6).

G. Precautions and monitoring effects

  1. Adult patients with a history of cardiac disease and elderly patients should begin therapy with lower doses (e.g., 25 µg/day of levothyroxine). After 2–4 weeks, the dose should be increased gradually to an individually adjusted maintenance dose (usually < 100 µg daily).

  2. Patients should be observed on initiation of therapy for possible **cardiac complications,** such as angina, palpitations, or arrhythmias.

  3. Serum thyroid levels should be monitored, particularly T_4, sensitive TSH and RT_3U levels, and the FTI. Serum thyroxine tests remain elevated during the first few months of treatment even with the presence of clinical symptoms. Serum thyroxine tests do not predict the clinical state. Testing is unnecessary unless noncompliance is suspected.

  4. It is recommended to monitor the sensitive TSH test 2–6 months after the last dose change. However, this test continues to change for up to 1 year. Testing early may result in overtreatment. Refer to Figure 55-6 for the management of patients on levothyroxine therapy.

  5. Levothyroxine administration, particularly long-term therapy, can induce thyrotoxicosis; T_4 levels can rise even though the dosage remains unchanged. Monitor for clinical signs of thyroid disease.

  6. **Accelerated bone loss** has been associated with overtreatment. Patients receiving replacement therapy with low TSH values may have lower bone mineral density because excess hormone accelerates the rate of remodeling (rate of reporption > rate of formation) and may contribute to an increased incidence of nontraumatic fracture.

  7. **Drug interactions**

    a. **Cholestyramine (Questran) and colestipol (Colestid),** bile acid sequestrants, can contribute to a decrease in **thyroxine** bioavailability when administered concomitantly. Bile acid sequestrants should be administered at least 6 hr after oral thyroxine to reduce the potential for this clinically significant drug interaction.

    b. **Calcium carbonate** (Os-Cal, Tums) can reduce thyroxine bioavailability by adsorption in an acid environment. These should be administered separately to avoid interaction.

    c. **Estrogens** (Estrace, Premarin) and selective estrogen receptor modulators (SERMs) tamoxifen (Nolvadex) or raloxifene (Evista) may contribute to lower levels of FT_4 and elevated TSH levels, requiring an increase in levothyroxine dose.

    d. **Raloxifene** has been shown to cause malabsorption of levothyroxine when co-administered resulting in hypothyroidism. Absorption studies demonstrated that separating administration times by ~ 12 hr for the two medications prevents the interaction.

    e. **Ciprofloxacin** (Cipro) has been reported to interact with levothyroxine when given together, resulting in elevated TSH and reduced FT_4 and FT_3 levels. Administration of the drugs separately, with a 6-hr interval, resulted in rapid normalization of the thyroid function tests.

H. Myxedema coma is a life-threatening complication with a high mortality rate.

  1. It is **most common** in elderly patients with preexisting, although usually undiagnosed, hypothyroidism.

  2. **Precipitating factors** include alcohol, sedative, or narcotic use; overuse of antithyroid agents; abrupt discontinuation of thyroid hormone therapy; infection; exposure to cold temperatures; and iatrogenic insult owing to radiation therapy or thyroid surgery.

3. The patient usually declines from profound lethargy to coma, hypothermia, and a significant decrease in respiratory rate, potentially leading to respiratory failure as the crisis progresses. Hypometabolism produces a fluid and electrolyte imbalance that leads to fluid retention and hyponatremia. **Cardiac effects** include decreased heart rate and contractility, decreasing cardiac output.

4. **Treatment** consists of rapid restoration of T_3 and T_4 levels to normal.
   a. A loading dose of levothyroxine 400–500 μg is given as an intravenous (IV) bolus. Liothyronine (Cytomel), 25 μg, is then given orally every 6 hr.
   b. Treatment is continued until improvement is noted. Then liothyronine is discontinued, and levothyroxine is changed to the oral preparation. A maintenance dose is then determined (see II.G).

III. HYPERTHYROIDISM is the overabundance of thyroid hormone. Thyrotoxicosis is the general term applied to overactivity of the thyroid gland.

A. **Graves disease (diffuse toxic goiter)**

1. The **most common form** of hyperthyroidism, Graves disease occurs primarily, but not exclusively, in **young women.**

2. The basis of this disease is an **autoimmune disorder** in which antibodies bind to and activate TSH receptors, resulting in the overproduction of thyroid hormone.
   a. These antibodies are termed **long-acting thyroid stimulators (LATS)** because their duration of action extends beyond that of TSH. As TSH is only mimicked, not overabundant, neither testing for TSH nor attempts to influence it are productive.
   b. Antibody titers often are elevated in patients with Graves disease.

3. **Signs and symptoms** characteristic of Graves disease include
   a. Diffusely enlarged nontender goiter
   b. Nervousness, irritability, anxiety, and insomnia
   c. Heat intolerance and profuse sweating
   d. Weight loss despite increased appetite
   e. Tremor and muscle weakness
   f. Palpitations and tachycardia
   g. Exophthalmos, stare, and lid lag (slow upper lid closing)
   h. Diarrhea
   i. Thrill or bruit over the thyroid
   j. Periorbital edema

B. **Plummer disease (toxic nodular goiter)**

1. This **form of thyrotoxicosis** is less common than Graves disease. Its underlying cause remains unknown, but its incidence is highest in patients > 50 years of age, and it arises usually from a long-standing nontoxic goiter.

2. The thyrotoxicosis is a result of one or more adenomatous nodules autonomously secreting excessive thyroid hormone, which suppresses the rest of the gland. Scanning confirms the diagnosis if it indicates that activity and iodine uptake are confined to the nodular mass, unless TSH is introduced.

3. **Signs and symptoms** are essentially the same as for Graves disease except that one or more nodular masses are found, rather than diffuse glandular enlargement, and ophthalmopathy is usually absent. **Cardiac abnormalities** (e.g., CHF, tachyarrhythmias) are commonly seen with Plummer disease.

C. **Less common forms of hyperthyroidism**

1. **Jodbasedow phenomenon** is an overproduction of thyroid hormone following a sudden, large increase in iodine ingestion—through either a sudden reversal of an iodine-deficient diet or the introduction of iodide or iodine in contrast agents or drugs (e.g., the antiarrhythmic agent amiodarone).

2. **Factitious hyperthyroidism** occurs with abusive ingestion of thyroid-replacement agents, usually in a misguided effort to lose weight. Diagnosis is aided by the absence of glandular swelling and of exophthalmos and the lack of autoimmune activity found in Graves disease.

3. **Subclinical hyperthyroidism** refers to patients without clinical symptoms, a normal FT_4 and FT_3 and TSH levels below the lower limits of normal (<0.4 mIU/L). Currently there is insufficient evidence to support treatment because consequences of nontreatment are minimal.

D. **Laboratory findings** (Table 55-1)

E. **Treatment goal.** Symptomatic relief is provided until definitive treatment can be effected.

F. **Therapeutic agents**

1. β-Adrenergic blocking agents—propranolol
   a. Propranolol (Inderal) reduces some of the peripheral manifestations (e.g., tachycardia, sweating, severe tremor, nervousness) of hyperthyroidism.
   b. In addition to providing symptomatic relief, propranolol inhibits the peripheral conversion of T_4 to T_3.

2. **Antithyroid agents—propylthiouracil (PTU) and methimazole (Tapazole)**
   a. **Action.** These agents may help attain remission through direct interference with thyroid hormone synthesis. Both agents inhibit iodide oxidation and iodothiouracil coupling. In addition, PTU (but not methimazole) diminishes peripheral deiodination of T_4 to T_3.
   b. **Therapeutic uses** of these drugs include
      (1) **Definitive treatment** in which remission is achieved
      (2) **Adjunctive therapy** with radioactive iodine until the radiation takes effect
      (3) **Preoperative preparation** to establish and maintain a euthyroid state until definitive surgery can be performed
   c. **Dosages**
      (1) **Propylthiouracil**
         (a) For **adults,** the initial dose is 300–450 μg/day in three divided doses (i.e., 100–150 μg every 8 hr). Adult patients with severe disease may require as much as 600–1200 μg/day initially.
         (b) The initial dose is continued for about 2 months; then a maintenance dose of 100–150 μg/day is given, as a single dose or divided into two doses.
         (c) Maintenance therapy is continued for approximately 1 year, then gradually discontinued over 1–2 months while the patient is monitored for signs of recurrent hyperthyroidism. The patient may remain in remission for several years. A recurrent episode of hyperthyroidism is most likely to occur within 3–6 months of drug discontinuation.
         (d) If hyperthyroidism recurs after drug therapy is stopped, the agent should be restarted and alternative therapy should be considered (e.g., thyroid gland ablation or removal).
      (2) **Methimazole**
         (a) The initial dose range is 5–60 μg/day in three divided doses, depending on disease severity. After 2 months of therapy, a maintenance dose of 5–30 μg/day is initiated.
         (b) Maintenance therapy is continued for approximately 1 year at which time the drug is gradually discontinued, usually over 1–2 months.
   d. **Precautions and monitoring effects**
      (1) Serum thyroid levels and the FTI should be monitored for a return to normal.
      (2) Goiter size should decrease with reduced hormone output.
      (3) The incidence of **adverse effects** is < 1% with PTU and < 3% with methimazole. The adverse effects are similar for the two agents.
         (a) The most bothersome are **dermatologic reactions** (e.g., rash, urticaria, pruritus, hair loss, skin pigmentation). Others include headache, drowsiness, paresthesia, nausea, vomiting, vertigo, neuritis, loss of taste, arthralgia, and myalgia.
         (b) **Severe adverse effects**—agranulocytosis, granulocytopenia, thrombocytopenia, drug fever, hepatitis, and hypoprothrombinemia—occur less frequently. Patients receiving methimazole who are > 40 years old and are receiving doses above 40 μg/day are at increased risk of developing agranulocytosis. Patients receiving

PTU who are > 40 years old are at increased risk of developing agranulocytosis, but no dose association has been established.

3. Radioactive iodine (RAI)

a. Action. The thyroid gland picks up the radioactive element iodine-131 (^{131}I) as it would regular iodine. The radioactivity subsequently destroys some of the cells that would otherwise concentrate iodine and produce T_4, thus decreasing thyroid hormone production.

b. Advantages

(1) High cure rate—almost 100% for patients with Graves disease and only slightly less for patients with Plummer disease

(2) Avoids surgical risks—such as adverse reaction to anesthetics, hypoparathyroidism, nerve palsy, bleeding, and hoarseness

(3) Less expensive—avoids cost of hospitalization

c. Disadvantages

(1) Risk of delayed hypothyroidism

(2) Slight, though undocumented, risk of genetic damage

(3) Multiple doses, which may be required, may delay therapeutic efficacy for a long period (many months or a year).

d. Dosage. A dose of 80–100 mCi of ^{131}I per estimated gram of thyroid gland is recommended. Some protocols use lower dosages, but these may be less effective, requiring retreatment. When the dose is higher, there is a potential risk that hypothyroidism will develop.

e. Precautions and monitoring effects

(1) Radioiodine therapy generally is reserved for patients past the childbearing years because effects on future offspring are not known.

(2) Response to ^{131}I is hard to gauge, and patients must be monitored early for recurrence of hyperthyroidism, and later for hypothyroidism, which may develop even 20 years or more after therapy.

4. Subtotal thyroidectomy. Partial removal of the thyroid gland may be indicated if drug therapy fails or radioactive iodine is undesirable. This is a difficult procedure, but the success rate is high and the cure rapid. Risks include those mentioned in III.F.3.b.(2), precipitating thyroid storm, and permanent postoperative hypothyroidism. The risk of inducing thyroid storm can be minimized by obtaining a euthyroid state through use of antithyroid agents (see III.F.2) or propranolol (see III.F.1).

G. Complications

1. Hypothyroidism may occur iatrogenically or, it has been proposed, as a natural sequel to Graves disease.

2. Thyroid storm (thyrotoxic crisis) is a sudden exacerbation of hyperthyroidism caused by rapid release (leakage) of thyroid hormone. It is invariably fatal if not treated rapidly. In this crisis, unchecked hypermetabolism leads ultimately to dehydration, shock, and death.

a. Precipitating factors include thyroid trauma or surgery, RAI therapy, infection, and sudden discontinuation of antithyroid therapy.

b. Characteristics. It is characterized by a TT_4 level of 25–30 µg/dl, rapidly rising fever, tachycardia disproportionate to the fever, and unexplained, pronounced restlessness and tremor.

c. Treatment

(1) PTU, in doses of 150–250 µg orally every 6 hr, is the preferred agent because PTU blocks peripheral deiodination of T_4 to T_3, whereas methimazole does not. However, if necessary, **methimazole,** 15 mg orally every 6 hr, can be used instead.

(2) Propranolol, in doses of 20–200 mg orally every 6 hr or 1–3 mg intravenously every 4–6 hr, should be administered unless contraindicated (e.g., if the patient has CHF).

(3) Potassium iodide, in doses of 50–100 mg every 12 hr, is given (after PTU) to minimize intrathyroidal iodine uptake.

(4) Other supportive therapy includes rehydration, cooling, antibiotics, rest, and sedation.

STUDY QUESTIONS

Directions for questions 1–16: Each of the questions, statements, or incomplete statements in this section can be correctly answered or completed by **one** of the suggested answers or phrases. Choose the **best** answer.

1. What is the correct formula to use for calculating the free thyroxine index (FTI)?

 (A) $T_4 \times RT_3U$/mean serum RT_3U
 (B) $T_3 \times T_3$/mean serum RT_3U
 (C) $T_3 \times RT_3U$/mean serum RT_3U
 (D) $T_4 \times RT_3U \times$ mean serum RT_3U
 (E) $T_3 \times RT_3U \times$ mean serum RT_3U

2. What is the necessary precursor besides dietary iodine required for thyroxine biosynthesis?

 (A) triiodothyronine (T_3)
 (B) threonine
 (C) tyrosine
 (D) thyrotropin (thyroid-stimulating hormone)
 (E) thyroxine-binding globulin (TBG)

3. All of the following conditions are causes of hyperthyroidism *except*

 (A) Graves disease.
 (B) Hashimoto thyroiditis.
 (C) toxic multinodular goiter.
 (D) triiodothyronine toxicosis.
 (E) Plummer disease.

4. Which of the following preparations is used to attain remission of thyrotoxicosis?

 (A) propranolol
 (B) liotrix
 (C) levothyroxine
 (D) propylthiouracil
 (E) desiccated thyroid

5. The thyroid gland normally secretes which of the following substances into the serum?

 (A) thyrotropin-releasing hormone (TRH)
 (B) thyrotropin (thyroid-stimulating hormone)
 (C) diiodothyronine (DIT)
 (D) thyroglobulin
 (E) thyroxine (T_4)

6. All of the following conditions are causes of hypothyroidism *except*

 (A) endemic goiter.
 (B) surgical excision.
 (C) Hashimoto thyroiditis.
 (D) goitrin-induced iodine deficiency.
 (E) Graves disease.

7. Common tests to monitor patients receiving replacement therapy for hypothyroidism include all of the following *except*

 (A) thyrotropin (TSH) stimulation test.
 (B) serum TSH assay.
 (C) free thyroxine index (FTI).
 (D) resin triiodothyronine uptake (RT_3U).
 (E) total thyroxine (TT_4).

8. Which of the following pairs of preparations has been studied for bioequivalence?

 (A) Levoxyl—Thyrolar
 (B) thyroglobulin
 (C) Levothroid—Synthroid
 (D) Cytomel—Synthroid
 (E) desiccated thyroid—Armour Thyroid

9. The inhibition of pituitary thyrotropin secretion is controlled by which of the following?

 (A) free thyroxine (T_4)
 (B) thyroid-releasing hormone (TRH)
 (C) free thyroxine index (FTI)
 (D) reverse triiodothyronine (rT_3)
 (E) total thyroxine (TT_4)

10. Which of the following agents has been shown to interact with oral thyroxine (T_4) replacement therapy?

 (A) propylthiouracil
 (B) cholestyramine
 (C) thyrotropin
 (D) levothyroxine
 (E) lovastatin

11. What laboratory tests are currently recommended by the American Thyroid Association to diagnose thyroid disease?

(A) resin triiodothyronine uptake (RT$_3$U) and total thyroxine (TT$_4$)
(B) thyrotropin (TSH) and free thyroxine index (FTI)
(C) total thyroxine (TT$_4$) and sensitive TSH assay
(D) free T$_4$ and sensitive TSH assay
(E) free T$_4$ and RT$_3$U

12. What patient population should be screened for thyroid disease?

(A) hospitalized patients
(B) elderly patients with chronic disease
(C) elderly hospitalized patients
(D) college students
(E) women > 20 years old

13. What is the average replacement dose of levothyroxine for an otherwise healthy adult?

(A) 25–50 μg/day
(B) 50–100 μg/day
(C) 75–150 μg/day
(D) 100–200 μg/day
(E) 200–400 μg/day

14. What factors affect the optimal replacement dose of levothyroxine?

(A) age, height, and weight
(B) duration of hypothyroidism
(C) pretreatment thyroid-stimulating hormone (TSH) level
(D) presence of chronic illness
(E) All of the above

15. Which of the values represents the lower level of detection for the fourth-generation sensitive TSH assay as established by the American Thyroid Association?

(A) 0.5–5 mIU/L
(B) 1–2 mIU/L
(C) 0.01–0.02 mIU/L
(D) 0.001–0.002 mIU/L
(E) 0.0001–0.0002 mIU/L

16. In which of the following clinical presentations should the TSH assay be used?

(A) population screening for thyroid disease
(B) screening hospitalized patients
(C) patients receiving thyroid replacement after 6–8 weeks of therapy
(D) patients who are HIV positive
(E) screening patients with psychiatric illness

Directions for question 17: The question in this section can be correctly answered or completed by **one or more** of the suggested answers. Choose the answer, **A–E.**

A	if **I only** is correct
B	if **III only** is correct
C	if **I and II** are correct
D	if **II and III** are correct
E	if **I, II, and III** are correct

17. A 62-year-old women with a 5-year history of well managed hypothyroidism was recently started on raloxifene 60 mg daily in the morning for the prevention of postmenopausal osteoporosis. Her thyroid disease had been well controlled on 150 μg levothyroxine (Synthroid) daily in the morning. Her TSH has remained within the normal range while on treatment. Her most recent TSH of 2.5 mIU/L and normal FT$_4$ values where noted last year. She presents today with an elevated TSH 15.5 mIU/L after 4 months of raloxifene therapy and symptoms of hypothyroidism. What change in therapy would be best for this patient?

(I) repeat the TSH test and FT$_4$ Tests
(II) increase the dose of levothyroxine to 200 μg daily
(III) switch the dosing of the raloxifene to the evening

Directions for question 18: The question in this section can be correctly answered by **one** of the suggested answers. Choose the **best** answer.

18. A 69-year-old woman with hypertension and hypothyroidism is being treated for a wound infection In the past, she was maintained on 125 μg levothyroxine (Levoxyl) daily with a normal TSH of 2.0 mIU/L. After 6 weeks of treatment with oral ciprofloxacin (500 mg twice a day) she complains of fatigue and sensitivity to cold. Her serum TSH level was 14 mIU/L and FT_4 was below normal. What is the best management for this patient.

(A) increase the dose of levothyroxine
(B) switch the patient from Levoxyl to Synthroid
(C) discontinue levothyroxine until the wound is healed
(D) continue therapy without any changes
(E) separate the administration of ciprofloxacin and levothyroxine by at least 6 hr

Directions for question 19: The question in this section can be correctly answered or completed by **one or more** of the suggested answers. Choose the answer, **A–E.**

A	if **I only** is correct
B	if **IV only** is correct
C	if **I and IV** are correct
D	if **I, II, III, and IV** are correct
E	if **II, III, and V** are correct

19. Which of the following agents have been shown to interact with oral thyroxine (T_4) replacement therapy?

(I) atenolol
(II) calcium carbonate
(III) ciprofloxacin
(IV) levothyroxine
(V) raloxifene

ANSWERS AND EXPLANATIONS

1. The answer is A *[see I.F.15].*
The FTI is a mathematical interpretation of the relationship between the rRT_3U and T_4 levels, compared to the mean population value for RT_3U. The FTI is calculated using reported values for TT_4 and RT_3U. The normal FTI value in euthyroid patients is 5.5–12.

2. The answer is C *[see I.B].*
Biosynthesis of thyroid hormones begins with iodide binding to tyrosine, which forms MIT. MIT binds another iodide atom to form DIT. When MIT and DIT are formed, a coupling reaction occurs, which produces T_3, T_4, reverse triiodothyronine (rT_3), and other by-products.

3. The answer is B *[see II.B.1; III.A–B]*
Hashimoto thyroiditis (chronic lymphocytic thyroiditis) is a cause of hypothyroidism. The incidence of Hashimoto thyroiditis is 1%–2%, and it increases with age. It is more common in women than in men and more common in whites than in blacks. There may be a familial tendency. Patients with Hashimoto thyroiditis have elevated titers of antibodies to thyroglobulin: A titer < 1:32 is seen in > 85% of patients. Two variants of Hashimoto thyroiditis have been described: gland fibrosis and idiopathic thyroid atrophy, which is most likely an extension of Hashimoto thyroiditis.

4. The answer is D *[see III.F.1–2].*
In hyperthyroid patients, remission of thyrotoxicosis is achieved with PTU by two mechanisms: (1) interference of iodination of the tyrosyl residues, ultimately reducing production of T_4 and (2) inhibition of peripheral conversion of T_4 to T_3. Propranolol is commonly used as an adjunct to PTU for symptomatic management of hyperthyroidism.

5. The answer is E *[see I.A.1].*
The major compounds secreted by the thyroid gland, after its stimulation by thyrotropin, are T_3 and T_4. When released from the thyroid, T_3 and T_4 are transported by plasma proteins—namely TBG, thyroxine-binding prealbumin, and albumin.

6. The answer is E *[see II.B; III.A.1].*
Graves disease (diffuse toxic goiter) is the most common form of hyperthyroidism. It occurs most often in women in the 3rd and 4th decades of life. There is a genetic and familial predisposition. The cause is linked to an autoimmune reaction between immunoglobulin G (IgG) and the thyroid.

7. The answer is A *[see II.G.3].*
The TSH stimulation test measures thyroid tissue response to exogenous TSH. It is not commonly used to monitor thyroid-replacement therapy. It may be useful in the initial diagnosis of hypothyroidism.

8. The answer is C *[see II.F.3.b–c].*
Many brands of levothyroxine are currently available. Both generic and trade name preparations have been studied, with an emphasis on Levothroid and Synthroid. The importance of bioequivalence becomes apparent when patients have received different brands of levothyroxine and have exhibited changes in therapeutic response to equivalent replacement doses.

9. The answer is A *[see I.A.3.a].*
An increase in the blood level of thyroid hormone (see circulating free T_4 and free T_3) signals the pituitary to stop releasing TSH. The free fraction of T_4 is available to bind at the pituitary receptors.

10. The answer is B *[see II.G.7].*
Euthyroid patients receiving oral replacement therapy have become hypothyroid after concomitant administration of bile acid sequestrant therapy. It appears that bioavailability is reduced as a result of administering these agents at close dosing intervals. It is recommended that at least 6 hr pass before administration of a bile acid sequestrant. It would be preferable to select another nonbile acid sequestrant when clinically possible.

11. The answer is D *[see I.G.4].*
The free T_4 and the (third-generation) TSH assay should be used only for the diagnosis of patients most likely to have thyroid disease based on clinical presentation and relative risk (e.g., age, sex, family history), not for population screening. The third-generation TSH assay is also more commonly usee to monitor replacement therapy and to minimize overtreatment and the corresponding risk of accelerated bone loss.

12. The answer is B *[see I.G.3].*
Cost versus benefit is critical to the decision of choosing to screen entire populations. Because the frequency of detection has been proven to be higher in elderly patients (2%–5%) with chronic disease, the relative minor costs associated to obtain RT_3U and TT_4 to calculate a FTI are worth the cost. A serum TSH assay can be reserved for patients with an abnormal FTI. Another consideration is to use the sensitive TSH assay for diagnosis in place of the serum TSH assay at a higher cost but without the necessity of retesting. If patients admitted to the hospital for an acute illness were screened and the results were misleading, they may be prescribed inappropriate therapy because acute illness may be associated with the temporary effects causing abnormal test results.

13. The answer is C *[see II.F.3.d].*
The average adult maintenance dose is 75–150 μg/day, which has been shown to be 1.5–1.7 μg/kg/day. The dose is usually adjusted in increments of 25–50 μg/day every 4 weeks. The total daily dose used to be 100–200 μg/day, which resulted in overtreatment after the introduction of the sensitive TSH assay. Elderly or chronically ill patients require an average dose of 50–100 μg/day, which is 25–50 μg/day less than otherwise healthy adults of the same height and weight.

14. The answer is E *[see II.F.3.e].*
Elderly or chronically ill patients require an average dose of 50–100 μg/day, which is 25–50 μg/day less than otherwise healthy adults of the same height and weight. Because the average dose for replacement therapy is between 1.5 and 1.7 μg/kg/day, weight affects the total daily dose.

15. The answer is D *[see I.F.4.e–f].*
The American Thyroid Association has established standard nomenclature that indicates each technological improvement and the ability to detect lower levels of TSH using monoclonal antibodies. As the sensitivity of the assay improves, the lower level of detection is reported as a range in milli-International Units per liter. The most sensitive test is currently the fourth-generation IMA, with a reported lower level of detection of 0.001–0.002 mIU/L. In usual clinical practice the third-generation IMA is most commonly used, with sensitivity in the range of 0.01–0.02 mIU/L.

16. The answer is C *[see I.F.4.g; II.6; Figure 55-6].*
The current third-generation TSH assay is not indicated for use in hospitalized patients who are not suspected to have thyroid disease. Studies have indicated that abnormally high or low TSH levels are detected in euthyroid hospitalized patients. Psychiatric illness may also influence TSH levels.

17. The answer is B *(III) [see II.G.7; Tables 55-2 and 55-4]* .
The patient is most likely experiencing a drug interaction between raloxifene and levothyroxine. The best choice is to separate the medications by at least 12 hr. A repeat of the TSH assay will only confirm the results, which are significantly elevated. Increasing the dose of levothyroxine may result in overtreatment.

18. The answer is E *[see II.G.7; Tables 55-2 and 55-4]*
This patient is most likely experiencing a drug interaction between levothyroxine and ciprofloxacin when taken concomitantly. There is no benefit to switching to another brand of levothyroxine or increasing the dose. The best solution is to separate the doses of ciprofloxacin by 6 hr.

19. The answer is E *(I, III, V) [see II.G.7; Tables 55-2 and 55-4].*
Patients receiving oral replacement therapy who take calcium carbonate concomitantly have been shown to experience decreased free T_4 and total T_4 levels that resulted in an elevated TSH. The mechanism appears to be adsorption of levothyroxine to calcium carbonate at acid pH levels, which may reduce bioavailability. It is recommended to separate the time of ingestion of each product to reduce the chance of this interaction. Ciprofloxacin and Raloxifene have also been shown to interact with levothyroxine when administered together. Separate administration times by 6 hr for ciprofloxacin and by 12 hr for raloxifene.

56
Renal Failure
Donald F. Brophy

Andrew L. Wilson

I. ACUTE RENAL FAILURE

A. **Definition.** Acute renal failure (ARF) is the sudden, potentially reversible interruption of kidney function, resulting in retention of nitrogenous waste products in body fluids.

B. **Classification and etiology.** ARF is classified according to its cause.

1. **Prerenal ARF** stems from impaired renal perfusion, which may result from:
   a. Reduced arterial blood volume [e.g., dehydration, hemorrhage, vomiting, diarrhea, other gastrointestinal (GI) fluid loss]
   b. Urinary losses from excessive diuresis
   c. Decreased cardiac output [e.g., from congestive heart failure (CHF) or pericardial tamponade]
   d. Renal vascular obstruction (e.g., stenosis)
   e. Severe hypotension

2. **Intrarenal ARF (intrinsic or parenchymal ARF)** reflects structural kidney damage resulting from any of the following conditions.
   a. **Acute tubular necrosis (ATN),** the leading cause of ARF, may be associated with:
      (1) Exposure to nephrotoxic aminoglycosides, anesthetics, pesticides, organic metals, and radiopaque contrast materials
      (2) Ischemic injury (e.g., surgery, circulatory collapse, severe hypotension)
      (3) Pigment (e.g., hemolysis, myoglobinuria)
   b. Acute glomerulonephritis
   c. Tubular obstruction, as from hemolytic reactions or uric acid crystals
   d. Acute inflammation (e.g., acute tubulointerstitial nephritis, papillary necrosis)
   e. Renal vasculitis
   f. Malignant hypertension
   g. Radiation nephritis

3. **Postrenal ARF** results from obstruction of urine flow anywhere along the urinary tract. Causes of postrenal ARF include:
   a. Ureteral obstruction, as from calculi, uric acid crystals, or thrombi
   b. Bladder obstruction, as from calculi, thrombi, tumors, or infection
   c. Urethral obstruction, as from strictures, tumors, or prostatic hypertrophy
   d. Extrinsic obstruction, as from hematoma, inflammatory bowel disease, or accidental surgical ligation

C. **Pathophysiology.** ARF progresses in three phases.

1. **Initiating phase**
   a. The initiating phase is defined as the time between the renal insult and the point at which extrarenal factors no longer reverse the damage caused by the obstruction or other cause of ARF. This phase may not be well-defined clinically and may escape notice or diagnosis.
   b. **Urine output** may drop markedly to 400 mL/day or less **(oliguria).** In some patients, urine output falls below 100 mL/day **(anuria).** Oliguria may last only hours or as long as 4–6 weeks. However, it has been shown that 40%–50% of ARF patients are not oliguric or anuric.
   c. **Nitrogenous waste products** accumulate in the blood.
      (1) **Azotemia** reflects urea accumulation due to impaired glomerular filtration and concentrating capacity.
      (2) Serum creatinine concentration, sulfate, phosphate, and organic acid levels climb rapidly.
   d. The **serum sodium concentration** falls below normal from intracellular fluid shifting and dilution.

   e. Hyperkalemia occurs due to the accumulation of organic acids (metabolic acidosis). If potassium intake is not restricted or body potassium is not removed, hyperkalemia results. Without treatment, hyperkalemia may lead to neuromuscular depression and paralysis, impaired cardiac conduction, arrhythmias, respiratory muscle paralysis, cardiac arrest, and ultimately death.

2. Maintenance phase

   a. This phase begins when urine output rises above 500 mL/day—typically after several days of oliguria. A rise in urine output or a "diuretic response" may not be seen in non-oliguric patients. Increased urinary output does not signal recovery of renal function.

   b. Urine output rises in increments of several milliliters to 300–500 mL/day. Urine output may double from day to day in the initial recovery period.

   c. Azotemia and associated laboratory findings may persist until urine output reaches 1000–2000 mL/day.

   d. The maintenance phase carries a risk of fluid and electrolyte abnormalities, GI bleeding, infection, and respiratory failure.

3. Recovery phase. During the recovery phase, renal function gradually returns to normal. Most recovered renal function appears in the first 2 weeks; however, recovery of renal function may continue for a year. Residual impairment may persist indefinitely.

D. Clinical evaluation

1. Physical findings. Initially, ARF causes azotemia and, in 50%–60% of cases, oliguria. Later, electrolyte abnormalities and other severe systemic effects occur.

   a. Urine output typically is **low,** from 20–500 mL/day. Complete anuria is rare.

   b. Signs and **symptoms of hyperkalemia,** resulting from metabolic acidosis and reduced potassium excretion by impaired kidneys, include:

     (1) Neuromuscular depression (e.g., paresthesias, muscle weakness, paralysis)

     (2) Diarrhea and abdominal distention

     (3) Slow or irregular pulse

     (4) Electrocardiographic changes with potential cardiac arrest

   c. Uremia, caused by excessive nitrogenous waste retention, leads to nausea, vomiting, diarrhea, edema, confusion, fatigue, neuromuscular irritability, and coma.

   d. Metabolic acidosis, a common complication of ARF, is evidenced by:

     (1) Deterioration of mental status, obtundation, coma, and lethargy

     (2) Depressed cardiac contractility and decreased vascular resistance, leading to hypotension, pulmonary edema, and ventricular fibrillation

     (3) Nausea and vomiting

     (4) Respiratory abnormalities (e.g., hyperventilation, Kussmaul's respiration)

   e. Hyperphosphatemia arises from decreased phosphate excretion. It is generally not seen in ARF.

     (1) As serum phosphate rises, hypocalcemia results from the formation of insoluble calcium phosphate complexes.

     (2) The signs and symptoms relate to resultant hypocalcemia and metastatic soft-tissue calcification.

     (3) Manifestations of hypocalcemia include:

       (a) Neuromuscular irritability, cramps, spasms, and tetany

       (b) Hypotension

       (c) Soft-tissue calcification

       (d) Mental status changes (e.g., confusion, mood changes, loss of intellect and memory)

       (e) Hyperactive deep-tendon reflexes and Trousseau's and Chvostek's signs

       (f) Abdominal cramps

       (g) Stridor and dyspnea

   f. Hyponatremia results from dilution and intravascular fluid shifts during the diuretic phase of ARF. Physical findings include lethargy, weakness, seizures, cognitive impairment, and possible reduction in level of consciousness.

   g. Intravascular volume depletion, suggesting **prerenal failure,** may cause:

     (1) Flat jugular venous pulses when the patient lies supine

     (2) Orthostatic changes in blood pressure and pulse

     (3) Poor skin turgor and dry mucous membranes

h. **Other findings** suggesting **prerenal failure** include:
   (1) An abdominal bruit, possibly indicating renal artery stenosis
   (2) Increased paradoxus, suggesting pericardial tamponade
   (3) Increased jugular venous pressure, pulmonary rales, and a third heart sound, signaling CHF

i. **Postrenal failure** caused by obstructed urinary flow may manifest itself in:
   (1) A suprapubic or flank mass
   (2) Bladder distention
   (3) Costovertebral angle tenderness
   (4) Prostate enlargement

2. **Diagnostic test results**
   a. **Urinalysis** includes an examination of sediment; identification of proteins, glucose, ketones, blood, and nitrites; and measurement of urinary pH and urine-specific gravity (concentration) or osmolality (dilution). Prior administration of fluids, diuretics, and changes in urinary pH may confound accurate diagnosis, using urinalysis.
      (1) **Urinary sediment examination**
         (a) Few casts and formed elements are found in prerenal ARF.
         (b) Pigmented cellular casts and renal tubular epithelial cells appear with ATN.
         (c) Red blood cell and white blood cell casts generally reflect inflammatory disease.
         (d) Large numbers of broad white cell casts suggest chronic renal failure.
      (2) The presence of blood in the urine (**hematuria**) or proteins (**proteinuria**) indicates renal dysfunction.
      (3) **Urine-specific gravity** ranges from 1.010–1.016 in ARF.
      (4) **Urine osmolality** typically rises in prerenal ARF due to increased secretion of anti-diuretic hormone.
   b. **Measurement of urine sodium** and **creatinine levels** can help classify ARF.
      (1) In **prerenal** ARF, the urine creatinine concentration **increases,** and urine sodium level **decreases.**
      (2) In **intrarenal** ARF resulting from ATN, the urine creatinine concentration **decreases,** and the urine sodium level **increases.**
   c. **Creatinine clearance,** an index of the **glomerular filtration rate (GFR),** allows estimation of the number of functioning nephrons; decreased creatinine clearance indicates renal dysfunction. A timed urine collection should be used to calculate GFR in acute renal failure.
   d. **Blood chemistry** provides an index of renal excretory function and body chemistry status. Findings typical of ARF include:
      (1) Increased blood urea nitrogen (BUN)
      (2) Increased serum creatinine concentration
      (3) Possible increase in hemoglobin and hematocrit values due to dehydration
      (4) Abnormal serum electrolyte values
         (a) Serum potassium level above 5 mEq/L
         (b) Serum phosphate level above 2.6 mEq/L (4.8 mg/dl)
         (c) Serum calcium level below 4 mEq/L (8.5 mg/dl), reflecting hypocalcemia. (The serum calcium level must be correlated with the serum albumin level. Each rise or fall of 1 g/dl of serum albumin beyond its normal range is responsible for a corresponding increase or decrease in serum calcium of approximately 0.8 mg/dl. A below-normal serum albumin level may result in a deceptively low serum calcium level.)
         (d) Serum sodium level below 135 mEq/L, reflecting hyponatremia
      (5) Abnormal arterial blood gas values [pH below 7.35, bicarbonate concentration (HCO_3^-) below 22], reflecting metabolic acidosis
   e. **Renal failure index (RFI)** is the ratio of urine sodium concentration to the urine-to-serum creatinine ratio. The RFI helps determine the etiology of ARF. Typically, the RFI is less than 1 in prerenal ARF or acute glomerulonephritis (a cause of intrarenal ARF). The RFI is greater than 2 in postrenal ARF and in other intrarenal causes of ARF.
   f. **Electrocardiography (ECG)** may show evidence of hyperkalemia—that is, tall, peaked T waves; widening QRS complexes; prolonged PR interval, progressing to decreased amplitude and disappearing P waves; and, ultimately, ventricular fibrillation and cardiac arrest.

g. **Radiographic findings**
   (1) **Ultrasound** may detect upper urinary tract obstruction.
   (2) **Kidney, ureter,** or **bladder radiography** may reveal:
      (a) Urinary tract calculi
      (b) Enlarged kidneys, suggesting ATN
      (c) Asymmetrical kidneys, suggesting unilateral renal artery disease, ureteral obstruction, or chronic pyelonephritis
   (3) **Radionuclide scan** may reveal:
      (a) Bilateral differences in renal perfusion, suggesting serious renal disease
      (b) Bilateral differences in dye excretion, suggesting parenchymal disease or obstruction as the cause of ARF
      (c) Diffuse, slow, dense radionuclide uptake, suggesting ATN
      (d) Patchy or absent radionuclide uptake, possibly indicating severe, acute glomerulonephritis
   (4) **Computed tomography (CT) scan** may provide better visualization of an obstruction.
h. **Renal biopsy** may be performed in selected patients when other test results are inconclusive.

E. Treatment objectives

1. Correct reversible causes of ARF, preventing or minimizing further renal damage or complications.
   a. Discontinue nephrotoxic drugs; remove other nephrotoxins through dialysis or gastric lavage for poisonings.
   b. Treat underlying infection.
   c. Remove any urinary tract obstructions.
2. Correct and maintain proper fluid and electrolyte balance. Match fluid, electrolyte, and nitrogen intakes to urine output.
3. Treat body chemistry alterations, especially hyperkalemia and metabolic acidosis, when present. Treatment may include renal dialysis.
4. Improve urine output.
5. Treat systemic manifestations of ARF.

F. Therapy

1. **Conservative management** alone may suffice in uncomplicated ARF.
   a. **Fluid management**
      (1) Fluid intake should match fluid losses. **Sensible losses** (i.e., urine, stool, tube drainage) and **insensible losses** (i.e., skin, respiratory tract) of 500–1000 mL/day should be included in fluid balance calculations.
      (2) Volume overload should be avoided to minimize the risk of hypertension and CHF.
      (3) The patient should be weighed daily to determine fluid volume status.
   b. **Dietary measures**
      (1) Because catabolism accompanies renal failure, the patient should receive a **high-calorie, low-protein diet.** Such a diet helps to:
         (a) Reduce renal workload by decreasing production of end products of protein catabolism that the kidneys cannot excrete
         (b) Prevent ketoacidosis
         (c) Alleviate manifestations of uremia (e.g., nausea, vomiting, confusion, fatigue)
      (2) If edema or hypertension is present, sodium intake should be restricted.
      (3) Potassium intake must be limited in most patients. Fruits, vegetables, and salt substitutes containing potassium should be limited or avoided.
2. **Management of body chemistry alterations**
   a. **Treatment of hyperkalemia**
      (1) **Dialysis** may be used to treat acute, life-threatening hyperkalemia (see II.F.7).
      (2) **Calcium chloride or calcium gluconate**
         (a) **Mechanism of action and therapeutic effects.** Calcium chloride or calcium gluconate replaces and maintains body calcium, counteracting the cardiac effects of acute hyperkalemia.

(b) Administration and dosage. When used to reverse hyperkalemia-induced cardiotoxicity, calcium chloride is given intravenously, as 5–10 mL of a 10% solution (1.4 mEq Ca^{2+}/mL) administered over 2 minutes. Doses of up to 20 mL of a 10% solution are safe when given slowly. Another 10–20 mL of a 10% solution placed in a larger fluid volume and administered slowly may follow the initial dose. Calcium gluconate is administered as 10 mL of a 10% solution (1 g) over 2–5 minutes. This may be repeated a second time.

(c) Precautions and monitoring effects

   (i) Intravenous (IV) calcium is contraindicated in patients with ventricular fibrillation or renal calculi.

   (ii) The infusion rate should not exceed 0.5 mL/min. Patients should remain recumbent for about 15 minutes after infusion.

   (iii) The ECG should be monitored during calcium gluconate therapy.

   (iv) Calcium gluconate should not be mixed with solutions containing sodium bicarbonate because this can lead to precipitation.

   (v) Adverse effects include hypotension, tingling sensations, and renal calculus formation.

(d) Significant interactions. Calcium may cause increased digitalis toxicity when administered concurrently with digitalis preparations.

(3) Sodium bicarbonate may be given as an emergency measure for severe hyperkalemia or metabolic acidosis.

(a) Mechanism of action and therapeutic effect. IV sodium bicarbonate restores bicarbonate that the renal tubules cannot reabsorb from the glomerular filtrate and increases arterial pH. This results in a shift of potassium into cells and reduces serum potassium concentration.

(b) Onset of action is 15–30 minutes.

(c) Administration and dosage

   (i) Sodium bicarbonate is administered intravenously.

   (ii) The dosage is calculated as follows:

[50% of body weight (kg)] $\times$ [desired arterial bicarbonate (HCO_3^-) − actual HCO_3^-]

One ampule (50 mEq) may be given intravenously over 5 minutes.

(d) Precautions and monitoring effects

   (i) To avoid sodium and fluid overload, sodium bicarbonate must be given cautiously. Half of the patient's bicarbonate deficit is replaced over the first 12 hours of therapy.

   (ii) Sodium bicarbonate may precipitate calcium salts in IV solutions and should not be mixed in the same infusion fluid.

   (iii) Arterial blood gas values and serum electrolyte levels should be monitored closely during sodium bicarbonate therapy.

(4) Regular insulin with dextrose

(a) Mechanism of action and therapeutic effect. The insulin causes an intracellular shift of potassium. The combination of insulin with dextrose deposits potassium with glycogen in the liver, reducing the serum potassium.

(b) Onset of action is 15–30 minutes.

(c) Administration and dosage. Regular insulin (10 units in 500 mL of 10% dextrose) is administered intravenously over 60 minutes.

(d) Precautions and monitoring effects

   (i) The serum glucose level should be monitored during therapy.

   (ii) The patient should be assessed for signs and symptoms of fluid overload.

(5) Sodium polystyrene sulfonate (SPS)

(a) Mechanism of action. SPS is a potassium-removing resin that exchanges sodium ions for potassium ions in the intestine (1 g of SPS exchanges 0.5–1 mEq/L of potassium). The SPS is distributed throughout the intestines and excreted in the feces.

(b) Therapeutic effect. Administered as an adjunctive treatment for hyperkalemia, SPS reduces potassium levels in the serum and other body fluids.

(c) Onset of action of orally administered SPS is 2 hours; effects are seen in 1 hour when SPS is administered as a retention enema.

(d) Administration and dosage
- **(i)** SPS is usually administered orally, although it may be given through a nasogastric tube. The oral dose is 15–30 g in a suspension of 70% sorbitol, administered every 4–6 hours until the desired therapeutic effect is achieved.
- **(ii)** When oral or nasogastric administration is not possible due to nausea, vomiting, or paralytic ileus, SPS may be given by retention enema. The rectal dose is 30–50 g in 100 mL of sorbitol as a warm emulsion, administered deep into the sigmoid colon every 6 hours. Administration may be done with a rubber tube that is taped in place or via a Foley catheter with a balloon inflated distal to the anal sphincter.

(e) Precautions and monitoring effects
- **(i)** The patient's serum electrolyte levels should be monitored closely during SPS therapy. Sodium, chloride, bicarbonate, and pH should be monitored in addition to potassium.
- **(ii)** SPS therapy usually continues until the serum potassium level drops to between 4 and 5 mEq/L.
- **(iii)** The patient should be assessed regularly for signs of potassium depletion, including irritability, confusion, cardiac arrhythmias, ECG changes, and muscle weakness.
- **(iv)** SPS exchanges sodium for potassium, so sodium overload may occur during therapy. Patients with hypertension or CHF should be closely monitored.
- **(v)** For oral administration, SPS should be mixed only with water or sorbitol. Orange juice, which has a high potassium content, should not be used because it decreases the effectiveness of the SPS. For rectal administration, SPS should be mixed only with water and sorbitol, never with mineral oil.
- **(vi)** **Adverse effects** of SPS include constipation, fecal impaction with rectal administration, nausea, vomiting, and diarrhea.
- **(vii)** SPS should not be used as the sole agent in the treatment of severe hyperkalemia; other agents or therapies should be used in conjunction with this agent.

(f) Significant interactions. Magnesium hydroxide and other nonabsorbable cation-donating laxatives and antacids may decrease the effectiveness of potassium exchange by SPS and may cause systemic alkalosis.

b. Treatment of metabolic acidosis. Sodium bicarbonate may be given if the arterial pH is below 7.35 [see I.F.2.a.(3)].

c. Treatment of hyperphosphatemia
- **(1) IV calcium** is first-line therapy for severe life-threatening hyperphosphatemia. Calcium reduces the serum phosphorus concentration by chelation.
- **(2) Oral calcium salts** bind dietary phosphorus in the GI tract.
- **(3) Sevelamer** is a non-ionic polymer that binds dietary phosphorus in the GI tract.
- **(4) Dialysis** may be used to treat acute, life-threatening hyperphosphatemia accompanied by acute hypocalcemia (see II.F.7). It is also performed when volume overload is present.
- **(5) Aluminum hydroxide** (an aluminum-containing antacid)
  - **(a) Mechanism of action and therapeutic effect.** Aluminum binds excess phosphate in the intestine, thereby reducing phosphate concentration.
  - **(b) Onset of action** is 6–12 hours.
  - **(c) Administration and dosage.** Aluminum hydroxide is administered orally as a tablet or suspension. For the treatment of hyperphosphatemia, 0.5–2 or 15–30 mL of suspension is administered three or four times daily with meals.
  - **(d) Precautions and monitoring effects**
    - **(i)** Aluminum hydroxide may cause constipation and anorexia.
    - **(ii)** Serum phosphate levels should be monitored because aluminum hydroxide can cause phosphate depletion.
    - **(iii)** Aluminum hydroxide can cause calcium resorption and bone demineralization.

d. Treatment of hypocalcemia. Immediate treatment is necessary if the patient has severe hypocalcemia, as evidenced by tetany.
- **(1) Calcium gluconate** [see I.F.2.a.(2)]
  - **(a) Mechanism of action and therapeutic effect.** This drug replaces and maintains body calcium, raising the serum calcium level immediately.

   (b) Administration and dosage. When used to reverse hypocalcemia, calcium gluconate is administered intravenously in a dosage of 1–2 g over a period of 10 minutes, followed by a slow infusion (over 6–8 hours) of an additional 1 g.

   (c) Precautions, monitoring effects, and significant interactions [see I.F.2.a.(2).(c), (d)]

   (2) Oral calcium salts. Calcium carbonate, chloride, gluconate, or lactate may be given by mouth when oral intake is permitted or if the patient has relatively mild hypocalcemia. The usual adult dosage is 4–6 g/day given in three or four divided doses.

e. Treatment of hyponatremia

   (1) Moderate or asymptomatic hyponatremia may require only **fluid restriction.**

   (2) Sodium chloride may be given for severe symptomatic hyponatremia (i.e., a serum sodium level below 120 mEq/L).

   (a) Mechanism of action and therapeutic effect. Sodium chloride replaces and maintains sodium and chloride concentration, thereby increasing extracellular tonicity.

   (b) Administration and dosage

   (i) A 3% or 5% sodium chloride solution may be administered by slow IV infusion. The amount of solution needed is calculated from the following equation:

   (Normal serum sodium level − actual serum sodium level) × total body water

   (ii) Typically, 400 mL or less is administered.

   (c) Precautions and monitoring effects

   (i) Hypertonic sodium chloride must be administered very slowly to avoid circulatory overload, pulmonary edema, or central pontine demyelination.

   (ii) Serum electrolyte levels must be monitored frequently during therapy.

   (iii) Excessive infusion may cause hypernatremia and other serious electrolyte abnormalities and may worsen existing acidosis. Infusion rates should not exceed 0.5 mEq/kg/hr.

3. Management of systemic manifestations

a. Treatment of fluid overload and edema. As water and sodium accumulate in extracellular fluid during ARF, fluid overload and edema may occur. **Diuretics** and dopamine may be given to reduce fluid volume excess and edema. Treatment should be initiated as soon as possible after oliguria begins. **Mannitol** or a **loop diuretic** may be used; thiazide diuretics are avoided in renal failure because they are ineffective when creatinine clearance is less than 25 mL/min, and they may worsen the patient's clinical status.

   (1) Step 1. Loop (high-ceiling) diuretics. These agents include **furosemide, bumetanide, torsemide** and **ethacrynic acid.** Loop diuretics are more potent and faster-acting than thiazide diuretics.

   (a) Mechanism of action and therapeutic effects. Loop diuretics inhibit sodium and chloride reabsorption at the loop of Henle, promoting water excretion.

   (b) Onset of action for an oral dose is 1 hour; several minutes for an IV dose. Duration of action for an oral dose is 6–8 hours; 2–3 hours for an IV dose.

   (c) Administration and dosage

   (i) Furosemide, the **most commonly used** loop diuretic, usually is administered intravenously in patients with ARF to hasten the therapeutic effect. The dose is titrated to the patient's needs; the usual initial dose is 1–1.5 mg/kg. If the first dose does not produce a urine output of 10–15 mL within 20–30 minutes, a dose of 2–3 mg/kg is administered; if the desired response still does not occur, a dose of 3–6 mg/kg is administered 20–30 minutes after the second dose.

   (ii) Bumetanide may be given to patients who are unresponsive or allergic to furosemide. The usual dosage, administered intravenously or intramuscularly in the treatment of ARF, is 0.5–1 mg/day; however, some patients may require up to 20 mg/day. A second or third dose may be given at intervals of 2–3 hours. When bumetanide is given orally, the dosage is 0.5–2 mg/day, repeated up to two times, if necessary, at intervals of 2–3 hours.

   (iii) Ethacrynic acid is **less commonly used** to treat ARF because ototoxicity (sometimes irreversible) is associated with its use. It may be given intravenously (slowly over several minutes) in a dose of 50–100 mg. The usual oral dosage is 50–200 mg/day; some patients may require up to 200 mg twice daily. Ethacrynic acid can be safely given to patients who may have a sulfonamide allergy, which would preclude them from therapy with furosemide or torsemide.

  (iv) **Torsemide** may also be given to patients unresponsive to or allergic to furosemide. The usual dose is 20 mg, administered intravenously. Doses may be increased by doubling up to 200 mg; 10–20 mg of torsemide is equipotent to 40 mg of furosemide or 1 mg bumetanide. Torsemide offers better bioavailability compared to other loop diuretics; however, it is considerably more expensive.

(d) **Precautions and monitoring effects**

  (i) Loop diuretics must be used cautiously because they may cause overdiuresis leading to orthostatic hypotension, fluid and electrolyte abnormalities, including volume depletion and dehydration, hypocalcemia, hypokalemia, hypochloremia, hyponatremia, hypomagnesemia, and transient ototoxicity, especially with rapid IV injection.

  (ii) Serum electrolyte levels should be monitored frequently and the patient assessed regularly for signs and symptoms of electrolyte abnormalities.

  (iii) Blood pressure and pulse rate should be assessed during diuretic therapy.

  (iv) GI reactions include abdominal pain and discomfort, diarrhea (with furosemide and ethacrynic acid), and nausea (with bumetanide).

  (v) Blood glucose levels should be monitored in diabetic patients receiving loop diuretics because these agents may cause hyperglycemia and impaired glucose tolerance.

  (vi) Patients who are allergic to sulfonamides may be hypersensitive to bumetanide and furosemide.

  (vii) Furosemide and ethacrynic acid may cause agranulocytosis.

(e) **Significant interactions**

  (i) **Aminoglycoside antibiotics** may potentiate ototoxicity when administered with any loop diuretic.

  (ii) **Nonsteroidal anti-inflammatory drugs (NSAIDs)** may hamper the diuretic response to furosemide and bumetanide; **probenecid** may hamper the diuretic response to bumetanide.

  (iii) Ethacrynic acid may potentiate the anticoagulant effects of **warfarin.**

  (2) **Step 2. Mannitol,** an osmotic diuretic, is a non-reabsorbable polysaccharide.

(a) **Mechanism of action and therapeutic effect.** Mannitol increases the osmotic pressure of the glomerular filtrate; fluid from interstitial spaces is drawn into blood vessels, expanding plasma volume and maintaining or increasing the urine flow. This drug may be given to prevent ARF in high-risk patients, such as those undergoing surgery or suffering from severe trauma or hemolytic transfusion reactions.

(b) **Onset of action** is 15–30 minutes. Duration of action is 3–4 hours.

(c) **Administration and dosage.** Mannitol is available in solutions, ranging from 5%–25%. For the treatment of oliguric ARF or the prevention of ARF, the usual initial dose is 12.5–25 g, administered intravenously; the maximum daily dosage is 100 g, administered intravenously. The exact concentration of the solution is determined by the patient's fluid requirements.

(d) **Precautions and monitoring effects**

  (i) Mannitol is contraindicated in patients with anuria, pulmonary edema or congestion, severe dehydration, and intracranial hemorrhage (except during craniotomy).

  (ii) Mannitol may cause or worsen pulmonary edema and circulatory overload. If signs and symptoms of these problems develop, the infusion should be stopped.

  (iii) Other adverse effects of mannitol include fluid and electrolyte abnormalities, water intoxication, headache, confusion, blurred vision, thirst, nausea, and vomiting.

  (iv) Vital signs, urine output, daily weight, cardiopulmonary status, and serum and urine sodium and potassium levels should be monitored during mannitol therapy.

  (v) Mannitol solutions with undissolved crystals should not be administered.

4. **Dialysis.** If the above strategies fail, hemodialysis or peritoneal dialysis may be necessary in ARF patients who develop anuria, acute fluid overload, severe hyperkalemia, metabolic acidosis, or a BUN level above 100 mg/dl. For a discussion of dialysis, see II.F.7.

II. CHRONIC KIDNEY DISEASE

A. **Definition.** Chronic kidney disease (CKD) is the progressive, irreversible deterioration of renal function. Usually resulting from long-standing disease, CKD sometimes derives from ARF that does not respond to treatment.

B. **Classification and pathophysiology**

1. CKD is defined as kidney damage or GFR <60 mL/min/1.73 m^2 for ≥3 months. Kidney damage is defined as pathological abnormalities or markers of damage, including abnormalities in blood or urine tests or imaging studies. CKD has recently been reclassified as stages I–V to denote the severity of renal impairment. Generally, CKD, if left untreated, progresses at a predictable, steady rate from stage I through stage V.
   a. **Stage 1** is defined as kidney damage with a normal or increased GFR. The corresponding GFR in stage I CKD is usually >90 mL/min/1.73 m^2.
   b. **Stage 2** is defined as kidney damage or a mildly decreased GFR (60–89 mL/min/1.73 m^2).
   c. **Stage 3** signifies moderate reductions in GFR (30–59 mL/min/1.73 m^2).
   d. **Stage 4** connotes a GFR of 15–29 mL/min/1.73 m^2.
   e. **Stage 5** is kidney failure or a GFR of <15 mL/min/1.73 m^2.

2. As CKD progresses, nephron destruction worsens, leading to deterioration in the kidneys' filtration, reabsorption, and endocrine functions.

3. Renal function typically does not diminish until about 75% of kidney tissue is damaged. Ultimately, the kidneys become shrunken, fibrotic masses.

C. **Etiology. Causes of CKD in adults include:**

1. Diabetic nephropathy

2. Hypertension

3. Glomerulonephritis

4. Polycystic kidney disease

5. Long-standing vascular disease (e.g., renal artery stenosis)

6. Long-standing obstructive uropathy (e.g., renal calculi)

7. Exposure to nephrotoxic agents

D. **Clinical evaluation**

1. **Physical findings.** Signs and symptoms, which vary widely, do not appear until renal insufficiency progresses to renal failure.
   a. **Metabolic abnormalities** include loss of the ability to maintain sodium, potassium, and water homeostasis, leading to hyponatremia or hypernatremia, based on relative sodium or water intake. Hyperkalemia is uncommon until end-stage disease. Fluid overload, edema, and CHF may become a problem unless fluid intake is closely managed. As renal failure progresses, the inability to excrete acid and maintain buffer capacity leads to metabolic acidosis (see I.D.1.b, d, g, h). Calcium and phosphate metabolism is altered due to hyperparathyroidism.
   b. **Neurological manifestations** include short attention span, loss of memory, and listlessness. As CKD progresses, these advance to confusion, stupor, seizures, and coma. Neuromuscular findings include peripheral neuropathy; pain, itching, and a burning sensation, particularly in the feet and legs. Patients may appear intoxicated. If dialysis is not started after these abnormalities occur, motor involvement begins, including loss of deep-tendon reflexes, weakness, and finally, quadriplegia.
   c. **Cardiovascular problems** include arterial hypertension, peripheral edema, CHF, and pulmonary edema. Uremic pericarditis is now increasingly infrequent as a result of early dialysis.
   d. **GI manifestations** include hiccups, anorexia, nausea, vomiting, constipation, stomatitis, and an unpleasant taste in the mouth. CKD patients have an increased incidence of ulcers, pancreatitis, and diverticulosis.

e. **Respiratory problems** include dyspnea when CHF is present, pulmonary edema, pleuritic pain, and uremic pleuritis.
f. **Integumentary findings** typically include pale yellowish, dry, scaly skin; severe itching; uremic frost; ecchymoses; purpura; and brittle nails and hair.
g. **Musculoskeletal changes** range from muscle and bone pain to pathological fractures and calcifications in the brain, heart, eyes, joints, and vessels. Soft-tissue calcification and renal osteodystrophy may occur.
h. **Hematological disturbances** include anemia. The signs and symptoms of anemia arise from lack of erythropoietin and reduced life span of red blood cells, including:
   (1) Pallor of the skin, nail beds, palms, conjunctivae, and mucosa
   (2) Abnormal bruising or ecchymoses, and uremic bleeding due to platelet inactivation
   (3) Dyspnea and angina pectoris
   (4) Extreme fatigue

2. **Diagnostic test results**
   a. **Creatinine clearance** may range from 0–90 mL/min, reflecting renal impairment.
   b. **Blood tests** typically show:
      (1) Elevated BUN and serum creatinine concentration
      (2) Reduced arterial pH and bicarbonate concentration
      (3) Reduced serum calcium level
      (4) Increased serum potassium and phosphate levels
      (5) Possible reduction in the serum sodium level
      (6) Normochromic, normocytic anemia (hematocrit 20%–30%)
   c. **Urinalysis** may reveal glycosuria, proteinuria, erythrocytes, leukocytes, and casts. Specific gravity is fixed at 1.010.
   d. **Radiographic findings.** Kidney, ureter, and bladder radiography, IV pyelography, renal scan, renal arteriography, and nephrotomography may be performed. Typically, these tests reveal small kidneys (less than 8 cm in length).

E. **Treatment objectives**

1. Improve patient comfort and prolong life.

2. Treat systemic manifestations of CKD.

3. Correct body chemistry abnormalities.

F. **Therapy.** Management of the CKD patient is generally conservative. Dietary measures and fluid restriction relieve some symptoms of CKD and may increase patient comfort and prolong life until dialysis or renal transplantation is required or available (see I F 1 a, b).

1. **Treatment of edema. Angiotensin-converting enzyme (ACE) inhibitors** and **diuretics** may be given to manage edema and CHF and to increase urine output.
   a. **ACE inhibitors—captopril, enalapril, lisinopril, fosinopril—**are widely used to delay progression of CKD because they help preserve renal function and typically cause fewer adverse effects than other antihypertensive agents (see Chapter 39). They also decrease proteinuria and nephrotic syndrome.
   b. **Diuretics.** An osmotic diuretic, a loop diuretic, or a thiazide-like diuretic may be given.
      (1) **Osmotic and loop diuretics.** See I.F.3.a.(1), (2) for information on the use of these drugs in renal failure.
      (2) **Thiazide-like diuretics. Metolazone** is the most commonly used thiazide diuretic in CKD.
         (a) **Mechanism of action and therapeutic effect.** Metolazone reduces the body's fluid and sodium volume by decreasing sodium reabsorption in the distal convoluted tubule, thereby increasing urinary excretion of fluid and sodium.
         (b) **Administration and dosage.** Metolazone is given orally at 5–20 mg/day; the dose is titrated to the patient's needs. Due to its long half-life, metolazone may be given every other day. Furosemide and metolazone act synergistically. Combination use is common, and metolazone should be administered 30 minutes before furosemide to achieve the optimal diuretic effect.
         (c) **Precautions and monitoring effects**
            (i) Metolazone should not be given to patients with hypersensitivity to sulfonamide derivatives, including thiazides.

(ii) To avoid nocturia, the daily dose should be given in the morning.

(iii) Metolazone may cause hematological reactions, such as agranulocytosis, aplastic anemia, and thrombocytopenia.

(iv) Fluid volume depletion, hypokalemia, hyperuricemia, hyperglycemia, and impaired glucose tolerance may occur during metolazone therapy.

(v) Metolazone may cause hypersensitivity reactions, including vasculitis and pneumonitis.

(d) Significant interactions

(i) **Diazoxide** may potentiate the antihypertensive, hyperglycemic, and hyperuricemic effects of metolazone.

(ii) **Colestipol** and **cholestyramine** decrease the absorption of metolazone.

2. **Treatment of hypertension. Antihypertensive agents** may be needed if blood pressure becomes dangerously high as a result of edema and the high renin levels that occur in CKD. Antihypertensive therapy should be initiated in the lowest effective dose and titrated according to the patient's needs.

   a. **ACE inhibitors—captopril, enalapril, lisinopril, fosinopril**—as above in II.F.1.a (see also Chapter 39).

   b. **Dihydropyridine calcium-channel blockers,** including **amLodipine** and **felodipine,** have similar effects and may be used instead of ACE inhibitors.

   c. **β-Adrenergic blockers,** including **propranolol** and **atenolol,** reduce blood pressure through various mechanisms (see Chapter 39).

   d. **Other antihypertensive agents** are sometimes used in the treatment of CKD, including α-adrenergic drugs, **clonidine,** and vasodilators, such as **hydralazine** (see Chapter 39).

3. **Treatment of hyperphosphatemia** involves administration of a phosphate binder, such as aluminum hydroxide or calcium carbonate (see I.F.2.c).

4. **Treatment of hypocalcemia**

   a. **Oral calcium salts** [see I.F.2.d.(2)]

   b. **Vitamin D**

      (1) **Mechanism of action and therapeutic effect.** Vitamin D promotes intestinal calcium and phosphate absorption and utilization and, thus, increases the serum calcium concentration.

      (2) **Choice of agent.** For the treatment of hypocalcemia in CKD and other renal disorders, **calcitriol** (vitamin D_3, the active form of vitamin D) is the preferred vitamin D supplement because of its greater efficacy and relatively short duration of action. Other single-entity preparations include dihydrotachysterol, ergocalciferol, and calcifediol. Newer vitamin D analogues include doxercalciferol and paricalcitol.

      (3) **Administration and dosage.** Calcitriol is given orally or via IV; the dose is titrated to the patient's needs (0.5–1 mg/day may be effective).

      (4) **Precautions and monitoring effects**

         (a) Vitamin D administration may be dangerous in patients with renal failure and must be used with extreme caution.

         (b) Vitamin D toxicity may cause a wide range of signs and symptoms, including headache, dizziness, ataxia, convulsions, psychosis, soft-tissue calcification, conjunctivitis, photophobia, tinnitus, nausea, diarrhea, pruritus, and muscle and bone pain.

         (c) Vitamin D has a narrow therapeutic index, necessitating frequent measurement of BUN and serum urine calcium and potassium levels.

5. **Treatment of other systemic manifestations of CKD**

   a. **Treatment of anemia** includes administration of iron (e.g., ferrous sulfate), folate supplements, and erythropoietin.

      (1) Severe anemia may warrant transfusion with packed red blood cells.

      (2) Erythropoietin stimulates the production of red cell progenitors and the production of hemoglobin. It also accelerates the release of reticulocytes from the bone marrow.

         (a) An initial dose of erythropoietin is 50–100 U/kg intravenously or subcutaneously three times a week. The dose may be adjusted upward to elicit the desired response.

         (b) Erythropoietin works best in patients with a hematocrit below 30%. During the initial treatment, the hematocrit increases 1%–3.5% in a 2-week period. The target hematocrit is 33%–35%. Maintenance doses are titrated based on hematocrit after this level is reached.

(c) Erythropoietin therapy should be temporarily stopped if hematocrit exceeds 36%. Additional side effects include hypertension in up to 25% of patients. Headache and malaise have been reported.

(d) The effects of erythropoietin are dependent on a ready supply of iron for hemoglobin synthesis. Patients who do not respond should have iron stores checked. This includes serum iron, total iron-binding capacity, transferrin saturation, and serum ferritin. Iron supplementation should be increased as indicated.

(3) Darbepoeitin is a new erythropoietin analogue. Its advantage is a prolonged plasma half-life, thus allowing it to be administered once weekly or biweekly.

(4) Intravenous iron products may be given to replete iron stores. This route is preferred to oral supplementation due to low oral bioavailability and GI intolerance. Iron dextran is commonly used; however, it is associated with hypotension and anaphylaxis. Newer iron products include sodium ferric gluconate and iron sucrose, which are better tolerated and can be infused more rapidly compared to iron dextran. Patients with severe iron deficiency may receive up to a total of 1 g of an iron preparation over several days. The rate of infusion depends on the preparation used.

b. Treatment of GI disturbances

(1) Antiemetics help control nausea and vomiting.

(2) Docusate sodium or methylcellulose may be used to prevent constipation.

(3) Enemas may be given to remove blood from the GI tract.

c. Treatment of skin problems. An antipruritic agent, such as diphenhydramine, may be used to alleviate itching.

6. Management of body chemistry abnormalities (see I.F.2)

7. Dialysis. When CKD progresses to end-stage renal disease and no longer responds to conservative measures, long-term dialysis or renal transplantation is necessary to prolong life.

a. Hemodialysis is the preferred dialysis method for patients with a reduced peritoneal membrane, hypercatabolism, or acute hyperkalemia.

(1) This technique involves shunting of the patient's blood through a dialysis membrane-containing unit for diffusion, osmosis, and ultrafiltration. The blood is then returned to the patient's circulation.

(2) Vascular access may be obtained via an arteriovenous fistula or an external shunt.

(3) The procedure takes only 3–8 hours; most patients need three treatments a week. With proper training, patients can perform hemodialysis at home.

(4) The patient receives heparin during hemodialysis to prevent clotting.

(5) Various complications may arise, including clotting of the hemofilter, hemorrhage, hepatitis, anemia, septicemia, cardiovascular problems, air embolism, rapid shifts in fluid and electrolyte balance, itching, nausea, vomiting, headache, seizures, and aluminum osteodystrophy.

b. Peritoneal dialysis is the preferred dialysis method for patients with bleeding disorders and cardiovascular disease.

(1) The peritoneum is used as a semipermeable membrane. A plastic catheter inserted into the peritoneum provides access for the dialysate, which draws fluids, wastes, and electrolytes across the peritoneal membrane by osmosis and diffusion.

(2) Peritoneal dialysis can be carried out in three different modes.

(a) **Intermittent peritoneal dialysis** is an automatic cycling mode lasting 8–10 hours, performed three times a week. This mode allows nighttime treatment and is appropriate for working patients.

(b) **Continuous ambulatory peritoneal dialysis** is performed daily for 24 hours with four exchanges daily. The patient can remain active during the treatment.

(c) **Continuous cyclic peritoneal dialysis** may be used if the other two modes fail to improve creatinine clearance. Dialysis takes place at night; the last exchange is retained in the peritoneal cavity during the day, then drained that evening.

(3) **Advantages** of peritoneal dialysis include a lack of serious complications, retention of normal fluid and electrolyte balance, simplicity, reduced cost, patient independence, and a reduced need (or no need) for heparin administration.

(4) **Complications** of peritoneal dialysis include hyperglycemia, constipation, and inflammation or infection at the catheter site. Also, this method carries a high risk of peritonitis.

8. **Renal transplantation.** This surgical procedure allows some patients with end-stage renal disease to live normal and, in many cases, longer lives.

   a. **Histocompatibility** must be tested to minimize the risk of transplant rejection and failure. Human leukocyte antigen (HLA) type, mixed lymphocyte reactivity, and blood group types are determined to assess histocompatibility.

   b. Renal transplant material may be obtained from a living donor or a cadaver.

   c. **Three types of graft rejection** can occur.

      (1) **Hyperacute (immediate) rejection** results in graft loss within minutes to hours after transplantation.

         (a) Acute urine flow cessation and bluish or mottled kidney discoloration are intra-operative signs of hyperacute rejection.

         (b) Postoperative manifestations include kidney enlargement, fever, anuria, local pain, sodium retention, and hypertension.

         (c) Treatment for hyperacute rejection is immediate nephrectomy.

      (2) **Acute rejection** may occur 4–60 days after transplantation.

      (3) **Chronic rejection** occurs more than 60 days after transplantation.

         (a) Signs and symptoms include low-grade fever, increased proteinuria, azotemia, hypertension, oliguria, weight gain, and edema.

         (b) Treatment may include alkylating agents, cyclosporine, antilymphocyte globulin, and corticosteroids. In some cases, nephrectomy is necessary.

   d. **Complications** include:

      (1) Infection, diabetes, hepatitis, and leukopenia, resulting from immunosuppressive therapy

      (2) Hypertension, resulting from various causes

      (3) Cancer (e.g., lymphoma, cutaneous malignancies, head and neck cancer, leukemia, colon cancer)

      (4) Pancreatitis and mental and emotional disorders (e.g., suicidal tendencies, severe depression, brought on by steroid therapy)

STUDY QUESTIONS

Directions: Each of the numbered items or incomplete statements in this section is followed by answers or by completions of the statement. Select the **one** lettered answer or completion that is **best** in each case.

Questions 1–5 A 48-year-old black man has a history of mild to severe hypertension. His hypertension has been poorly controlled with enalapril and hydrochlorothiazide. On prior visits, his blood pressure control has varied and seems to correspond with a lack of compliance with his treatment regimen. The patient states that he occasionally forgets his pills or does not take them when he is feeling "okay." The patient's history does not include diabetes mellitus or heart disease. He completed a 14-day course of clarithromycin for an upper respiratory infection in the past month and has returned to the clinic for follow-up review of the infection and his hypertension therapy.

On this visit, the patient complains of dizziness, loss of energy, increased frequency of urination, and edema of the lower extremities. His physical examination reveals an overweight man with a standing blood pressure of 175/100 mm Hg moderate edema of the ankles, and a slight third heart sound. Laboratory results include blood urea nitrogen (BUN) of 45 mg/dl, serum creatinine concentration of 3.7 mg/dl, serum calcium of 5.3 mg/mL, serum potassium of 6.3 mg/mL, and a hematocrit of 25. Serum iron, total iron-binding capacity, transferrin saturation, and serum ferritin are normal. Microscopic urine and chemical analyses reveal mild proteinuria and a specific gravity of 1.010.

1. The history, physical examination, laboratory values, and current signs and symptoms suggest that the patient has which of the following conditions?

(A) Acute renal failure brought on by a nephrotoxic drug (clarithromycin, enalapril)

(B) Acute renal failure resulting from renal obstruction by a kidney stone

(C) Acute renal failure precipitated by severe dehydration

(D) Chronic renal failure resulting from hypertension

2. Treatment of the patient's fluid retention and edema should begin with all of the following EXCEPT

(A) restriction of fluid intake

(B) therapy with furosemide or metolazone

(C) treatment of hypertension using a β-blocker or angiotensin-converting enzyme inhibitor

(D) digitalis glycoside therapy if congestive heart failure is present

(E) hemodialysis

3. The most likely cause of the anemia seen in this patient is

(A) urinary blood loss

(B) vitamin B_{12} deficiency

(C) iron deficiency

(D) decreased red cell life span and a deficiency of erythropoietin

4. This patient's symptoms seemed to appear suddenly and may result from his history of uncontrolled hypertension. Which statement best describes hypertension?

(A) A major cause of chronic renal failure

(B) A major cause of acute renal failure

(C) A major cause of both chronic and acute renal failure

(D) Only seen in patients whose renal failure has caused excessive fluid retention

5. When should peritoneal dialysis or hemodialysis be considered to treat this patient's renal failure?

(A) As soon as possible to prevent further complications resulting from decreased renal function

(B) Only when renal function has decreased to a point where fluid and electrolyte status cannot be maintained using conservative measures

(C) On an intermittent basis as the situation demands

(D) Only if the patient is a kidney transplant candidate

6. Acute renal failure (ARF) may be caused by all of the following EXCEPT

(A) acute tubular necrosis (ATN) due to drug therapy (e.g., aminoglycosides, contrast media)

(B) severe hypotension or circulatory collapse

(C) decreased cardiac output, as from congestive heart failure

(D) hemolysis and myoglobinuria

(E) hyperkalemia

7. Life-threatening cardiac arrhythmias due to hyperkalemia should be treated with

(A) calcium chloride or calcium gluconate intravenously
(B) digoxin or other digitalis preparations
(C) loop diuretics to rapidly eliminate potassium
(D) sodium polystyrene sulfonate (SPS)

8. Aluminum hydroxide is used to treat hyperphosphatemia associated with renal failure. Chronic use of aluminum hydroxide may cause all of the following conditions EXCEPT

(A) phosphate depletion
(B) calcium resorption and bone demineralization
(C) anorexia and constipation
(D) fluid retention

9. The diuretic of choice for the initial treatment of a patient with either acute or chronic renal failure (ARF, CKD) whose creatinine clearance is below 25 mL/min is

(A) hydrochlorothiazide
(B) bumetanide
(C) furosemide
(D) ethacrynic acid

10. Erythropoietin is used commonly to treat the anemia associated with chronic renal failure (CKD). Which of the following conditions limits the effectiveness of erythropoietin?

(A) A patient's allergy to erythropoietin
(B) Depletion of iron stores, requiring oral or parenteral supplementation
(C) The ineffectiveness of erythropoietin, as 30% of patients do not respond
(D) The anemia of chronic renal failure is not due to a lack of erythropoietin, so erythropoietin will not ameliorate.

ANSWERS AND EXPLANATIONS

1. The answer is D *[II.D.1].*
The fluid and electrolyte status of the patient described in the case, combined with the urine-specific gravity, lack of crystals or casts in the urine, and the complaint of fatigue, suggest chronic renal failure resulting from uncontrolled hypertension or an unknown cause. The antibiotic therapy (clarithromycin) and antihypertensive drug (enalapril) are not nephrotoxic, and the patient's blood pressure and fluid status do not indicate a prerenal cause.

2. The answer is E *[II.F.1, 2].*
All of these measures are indicated as initial therapy for the treatment of edema and fluid retention due to chronic renal failure except hemodialysis, which should be reserved until more conservative measures are tried.

3. The answer is D *[II.D.1.h].*
There is no evidence of frank blood loss. The decreased hematocrit and the clinical signs indicate the anemia of chronic renal failure due to the shortened red blood cell life span. Decreased erythropoietin is the cause.

4. The answer is A *[II.C.2].*
Systemic long-standing high blood pressure is the second most common cause of chronic renal failure (CKD). Only malignant hypertension can cause acute renal failure (ARF), which is not common. High blood pressure is common after substantial renal damage has occurred in both CKD and ARF, but it does not occur as the first or only manifestation.

5. The answer is B *[II.F.7].*
Dialysis should be considered when the patient's renal function has decreased to a point where conservative measures are ineffective. Peritoneal dialysis and hemodialysis have associated complications and morbidity, so intermittent or early use of these therapies is not indicated. Patients can be maintained on dialysis for extended periods, so eligibility for transplant is not required.

6. The answer is E *[I.B.1–3].*
Hyperkalemia is a sign of acute and chronic renal failure, resulting from the decreased renal function and changes in acid–base balance.

7. The answer is A *[I.F.2.a].*
Intravenous calcium chloride or gluconate is used to treat potassium-induced arrhythmias. Digoxin is not indicated. Loop diuretics and sodium polystyrene sulfonate (SPS) do not have a significant enough effect on potassium in a short period to treat a life-threatening arrhythmia. SPS and loop diuretics, along with dialysis, may be considered to remove potassium in the short term, preventing the recurrence of arrhythmias.

8. The answer is D *[I.F.2.c.(5).(d).(i-iii].*
Common effects of the sustained use of aluminum-containing antacids include phosphate depletion, calcium resorption, bone demineralization, anorexia, and constipation. Fluid retention does not result from the use of antacids containing aluminum hydroxide.

9. The answer is C *[I.F.3.a.(1).(c)].*
Furosemide is the diuretic of choice for the initial treatment of a patient with either acute or chronic renal failure (ARF, CKD) whose creatinine clearance is below 25 mL/min. A thiazide diuretic has little effect at a creatinine clearance below 25 mL/min. Bumetanide, torsemide, and ethacrynic acid are appropriate only if the patient is allergic to furosemide or if repeated doses of furosemide are ineffective.

10. The answer is B *[II.F.5.a.(2).(d)].*
Erythropoietin is widely used and highly effective in treating the anemia associated with chronic renal failure (CKD). Few reports of patients refractory to erythropoietin therapy have appeared in medical literature. However, the depletion of iron stores will not allow the formation of red blood cells, even in the presence of appropriate amounts of erythropoietin. All CKD patients receiving erythropoietin require some iron supplementation, and most patients require parenteral iron to achieve sufficient supplies to continue developing hemoglobin over the term of their illness.

57
Cancer Chemotherapy

Judy Chase

Jamie Shapiro

I. PRINCIPLES OF ONCOLOGY. The term *cancer* refers to a heterogeneous group of diseases caused by an impairment of the normal functioning of genes, which leads to genetic damage.

A. Characteristics of cancer cells. Cancer cells are also referred to as tumors, or neoplasms. Tumors arise from a single abnormal cell, which continues to divide indefinitely. Uncontrolled growth, ability to invade local tissues, and ability to spread, or **metastasize,** are characteristics of cancer cells.

1. **Carcinogenesis.** The mechanism of how cancers occur is thought to be a multistage, multifactorial process that involves both genetic and environmental factors.
   a. **Initiation.** The first step involves the exposure of normal cells to a carcinogen, producing genetic damage to a cell.
   b. **Promotion.** The environment becomes altered to allow preferential growth of mutated cells over normal cells. The mutated cells become cancerous.
   c. **Progression.** Increased proliferation of cancer cells allows for invasion into local tissue and metastasis.

2. **Types of cancer.** Tumors can be benign or malignant. **Benign** tumors are generally slow growing, resemble normal cells, are localized, and are not harmful. **Malignant** tumors often proliferate more rapidly, have an atypical appearance, invade and destroy surrounding tissues, and are harmful if left untreated. Malignant cancers are further categorized by the location from where the tumor cells arise.
   a. **Solid tumors. Carcinomas** are tumors of epithelial cells. These include specific tissue cancers (e.g., lung, colon, breast). **Sarcomas** include tumors of connective tissue such as bone (e.g., osteosarcoma) or muscle (e.g., leiomyosarcoma).
   b. **Hematological malignancies. Lymphomas** are tumors of the lymphatic system and include Hodgkin and non-Hodgkin lymphomas. **Leukemias** are tumors of blood-forming elements and are classified as acute or chronic, myeloid or lymphoid.

B. Incidence. Cancer is the **second leading cause of death** in the United States. The lifetime probability of developing cancer is > 30%. The estimated incidences of new cancers and cancer-related deaths by site are given in Figure 57-1. The most common cancers are breast, prostate, lung, and colorectal. The leading cause of cancer death is lung cancer.

C. Cause. Many factors have been implicated in the origin of cancer. Some of these factors are as follows:.

1. **Viruses,** including Epstein-Barr virus (EBV), hepatitis B virus (HBV), and human papillomavirus (HPV)

2. **Environmental and occupational exposures,** such as ionizing and ultraviolet radiation and exposure to chemicals, including vinyl chloride, benzene, and asbestos

3. **Lifestyle factors,** such as high-fat, low-fiber diets and tobacco and ethanol use

4. **Medications,** including alkylating agents and immunosuppressants

5. **Genetic factors,** including inherited mutations, cancer-causing genes (oncogenes), and defective tumor-suppressor genes

D. Detection and **diagnosis** are critical for the appropriate treatment of cancer. Earlier detection may improve response to treatment.

Estimated new cases[a]

	Males			Females		
Prostate	232,090	33%		Breast	211,240	32%
Lung and bronchus	93,010	13%		Lung and bronchus	79,560	12%
Colon and rectum	71,820	10%		Colon and rectum	73,410	11%
Urinary bladder	47,010	7%		Uterine corpus	40,880	6%
Melanoma–skin	33,580	5%		Non-Hodgkin lymphoma	27,320	4%
Non-Hodgkin lymphoma	29,070	4%		Melanoma–skin	26,000	4%
Kidney and renal pelvis	22,490	3%		Ovary	22,220	3%
Leukemia	19,640	3%		Thyroid	19,190	3%
Oral cavity and pharynx	19,100	3%		Urinary bladder	16,200	2%
Pancreas	16,100	2%		Pancreas	15,780	2%
All sites	**710,040**	**100%**		**All sites**	**662,870**	**100%**

Estimated Deaths

	Males			Females		
Lung and bronchus	90,490	31%		Lung and bronchus	73,020	27%
Prostate	30,350	10%		Breast	40,410	15%
Colon and rectum	28,540	10%		Colon and rectum	25,750	10%
Pancreas	15,820	5%		Ovary	16,210	6%
Leukemia	12,540	4%		Pancreas	15,980	6%
Esophagus	10,530	4%		Leukemia	10,030	4%
Liver and intrahepatic bile duct	10,330	3%		Non-Hodgkin lymphoma	9,050	3%
Non-Hodgkin lymphoma	10,150	3%		Uterine corpus	7,310	3%
Urinary bladder	8,970	3%		Multiple myeloma	5,640	2%
Kidney and renal pelvis	8,020	3%		Brain and other nervous system	5,480	2%
All sites	**295,280**	**100%**		**All sites**	**275,000**	**100%**

Figure 57-1. Cancer incidence and deaths. Leading cancer sites for estimated new cases and deaths by gender in the United States, 2005 estimates. [a]Excludes basal and squamous cell skin cancers and in situ carcinomas except urinary bladder. [Adapted with permission from Jemal A, Murray T, Ward E, et al. Cancer statistics, 2005. CA Cancer J Clin 2005;55:10–30.]

1. **Warning signs** of cancer have been outlined by the American Cancer Society.
   a. **C**hange in bowel or bladder habits
   b. **A** sore that does not heal
   c. **U**nusual bleeding or discharge
   d. **T**hickening or lump in the breast or elsewhere
   e. **I**ndigestion or difficulty swallowing
   f. **O**bvious change in a wart or mole
   g. **N**agging cough or hoarseness

2. **Guidelines for screening** asymptomatic people for the presence of cancer have been established by the American Cancer Society, the National Cancer Institute, and the U.S. Preventive Health Services Task Force. Because many cancers do not produce signs or symptoms until they have become large, the goal of screening is to detect cancers early, when the disease is curable, and to reduce mortality. The different sets of guidelines vary slightly in their recommendations for age and frequency of screening procedures. Table 57-1 provides the American Cancer Society's recommendations for screening.

3. **Tumor markers** are biochemical indicators of the presence of neoplastic proliferation detected in serum, plasma, or other body fluids. These tumor markers may be used initially as screening tests, to reveal further information after abnormal test results, or to monitor the efficacy of therapy. Elevated levels of these markers are not definitive for the presence of

Table 57-1. American Cancer Society's Recommendations for the Early Detection of Cancer[a]

Cancer Site	Population	Starting Age	Tests or Procedures
Breast	Women	20+	Breast self-examination
		20+	Clinical breast examination
		40+	Mammography
Colorectal	Men and Women	50+	Fecal occult blood test or fecal immunochemical test
		50+	Flexible sigmoidoscopy
		50+	Colonoscopy
		50+	Double-contrast barium enema
Prostate	Men	50+	Digital rectal examination
		50+	Prostate-specific antigen
Cervix	Women	18+	Pap (Papanicolaou) test

[a]In average-risk, asymptomatic people.
Adapted with permission from Smith RA, Cokkinides V, Eyre HJ, et al. American Cancer Society guidelines for the early detection of cancer. CA Cancer J Clin 2005;55:31–44.

cancer because levels can be elevated in other benign and malignant conditions, and false-positive results do occur. Examples of some commonly used markers include

    a. Carcinoembryonic antigen (CEA) for colorectal cancer
    b. α-Fetoprotein (AFP) for hepatocellular carcinoma
    c. Prostate-specific antigen (PSA) for prostate cancer

  4. Tumor biopsy. The definitive test for the presence of cancerous cells is a biopsy and pathological examination of the biopsy specimen. Several types of procedures are used in the pathological analysis of tumors, including evaluating the morphological features (appearance) of the tissue and cells, looking for cell-surface markers, and cytogenetic evaluation for specific chromosomal abnormalities.

  5. Imaging studies, such as x-rays, CT scans, MRI, and positron-emission tomography (PET), may be used to aid in the diagnosis or location of a tumor and to monitor response to treatment.

  6. Other laboratory tests commonly used for cancer diagnosis include complete blood counts (CBCs) and blood chemistries.

E. Staging is the categorizing of patients according to the extent of their disease. The stage of the disease is used to determine prognosis and treatment. Two different staging systems are widely employed for the staging of neoplasms.

  1. TNM classification
    a. *T* indicates tumor size and is classified from 0 to 4, with 0 indicating the absence of tumor.
    b. *N* indicates the presence and extent of regional lymph node spread and is classified from 0 to 3, with 0 indicating no regional lymph node involvement and 3 indicating extensive involvement.
    c. *M* indicates the presence of distant metastases and is be classified as 0 (for absence) or 1 (for presence of distant metastases).
    d. For example, T2N1M0 indicates a moderate-size tumor with limited nodal disease and no distant metastases.

  2. AJCC staging, developed by the American Joint Committee on Cancer, classifies cancers as stages 0–IV. An assigned TNM translates into a stage. A high number indicates larger tumors with extensive nodal involvement and/or metastasis. Generally, high numbers also indicate a worse prognosis. There are specific staging criteria for each tumor type.

F. Survival depends on the tumor type, the extent of disease, and the therapy received. Although some patients are free of all detectable disease, not all patients are cured. Oncologists prefer to use the term **complete response** or **remission** to indicate a patient with no evidence of disease after treatment. This is not a synonym for *cure.* For some slow-growing tumors, these disease-free periods may extend for 10–15 years after the initial remission. However, a number of patients who have achieved complete remission may relapse.

II. CELL LIFE CYCLE. Knowledge of the cell life cycle and cell cycle kinetics is essential to the understanding of the activity of chemotherapy agents in the treatment of cancer (Figure 57-2).

A. Phases of the cell cycle

1. **M phase,** or **mitosis,** is the phase in which the cell divides into two daughter cells.

2. **G_1 phase,** or **postmitotic gap,** is when RNA and the proteins required for the specialized functions of the cell are synthesized in preparation for DNA synthesis.

3. **S phase** is the phase in which DNA synthesis and replication occurs.

4. **G_2 phase,** or the **premitotic** or **postsynthetic gap,** is the phase in which RNA and the enzymes topoisomerase I and II are produced to prepare for duplication of the cell.

5. **G_0 phase,** or **resting phase,** is the phase in which the cell is not committed to division. Cells in this phase are generally not sensitive to chemotherapy. Some of these cells may reenter the actively dividing cell cycle. In a process called **recruitment,** some chemotherapy regimens are designed to enhance this reentry by killing a large number of actively dividing cells.

B. Cell growth kinetics. Several terms describe cell growth kinetics.

1. **Cell growth fraction** is the proportion of cells in the tumor dividing or preparing to divide. As the tumor enlarges, the cell growth fraction decreases because a larger proportion of cells may not be able to obtain adequate nutrients and blood supply for replication.

2. **Cell cycle time** is the average time for a cell that has just completed mitosis to grow and again divide and again pass through mitosis. Cell cycle time is specific for each individual tumor.

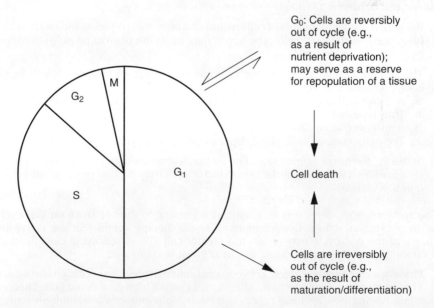

Figure 57-2. The cell cycle. The cell growth cycle, emphasizing the relationship between proliferating cell populations. [Reprinted with permission from Lenhard RE Jr., Osteen RT, Gansler T, et al., eds. The American Cancer Society's Clinical Oncology. Atlanta, American Cancer Society, 2001.]

Figure 57-3. The gompertzian growth curve. During the early stages of its development, a tumor grows exponentially. But as a tumor enlarges, its growth slows. By the time a tumor becomes large enough to cause symptoms and be clinically detectable, the majority of its growth has already occurred and is no longer exponential. [Reprinted with permission from Lenhard MJ Jr., et al., eds. The American Cancer Society's Clinical Oncology. Atlanta, American Cancer Society, 2001.]

3. **Tumor doubling time** is the time for the tumor to double in size. As the tumor gets larger, its doubling time gets longer because it contains a smaller proportion of actively dividing cells owing to restrictions of space, nutrient availability, and blood supply.

4. The **gompertzian growth curve** illustrates these cell growth concepts (Figure 57-3).

C. **Tumor cell burden** is the number of tumor cells in the body.

1. Because of the large number of cells required to produce symptoms and be clinically detectable (approximately 10^9 cells), the tumor may be in the plateau phase of the growth curve by the time it is detected.

2. The **cell kill hypothesis** states that a certain percentage of tumor cells will be killed with each course of cancer chemotherapy.
   a. As tumor cells are killed, cells in G_0 may be recruited into G_1, resulting in tumor regrowth.
   b. Thus repeated cycles of chemotherapy are required to achieve a complete response or remission (Figure 57-4).
   c. The percentage of cells killed depends on the chemotherapy dose.

3. In theory, the tumor burden would never reach absolute zero because only a percentage of cells are killed with each cycle. Less than 10^4 cells may depend on elimination by the host's immune system.

D. Chemotherapeutic agents may be classified according to their **reliance on cell cycle kinetics** for their cytotoxic effect. Combinations of chemotherapy agents that are active in different phases of the cell cycle may result in a greater cell kill. A cell cycle classification of some commonly used chemotherapeutic agents is given in II.D.1.a–d.

1. **Phase-specific agents** are most active against cells that are in a specific phase of the cell cycle. These agents are most effective against tumors with a high growth fraction. Theoretically, by administering these agents as continuous intravenous infusions or by multiple repeated doses, it may increase the likelihood of hitting the majority of cells in the specific phase at any one time. Therefore, these agents are also considered schedule-dependent agents. Examples are as follows:

Figure 57-4. Chemotherapy and tumor cell survival. Relationship between tumor cell survival and chemotherapy administration. The exponential relationship between chemotherapy drug dose and tumor cell survival dictates that a constant proportion, not number, of tumor cells is killed with each cycle of treatment. In this example, each cycle of drug administration results in 99.9% (3 log) cell kill, and 1 log of cell regrowth occurs between cycles. The broken line indicates what would occur if the last cycle of therapy were omitted. Despite complete clinical remission of disease, the tumor would ultimately recur. [Reprinted with permission from Lenhard MJ Jr., et al., eds. The American Cancer Society's Clinical Oncology. Atlanta, American Cancer Society, 2001.]

   a. M phase: mitotic inhibitors (e.g., vinca alkaloids, taxanes)
   b. G_1 phase: asparaginase, prednisone
   c. S phase: antimetabolites
   d. G_2 phase: bleomycin, etoposide

  2. Phase-nonspecific agents are effective while cells are in the active cycle but do not require that the cell be in a particular phase. These agents generally show more activity against slow-growing tumors. They may be administered as single bolus doses because their activity is independent of the cell cycle. These drugs are also considered dose-dependent agents. Examples are alkylating agents and antitumor antibiotics.

  3. Cell cycle–nonspecific agents are effective in all phases, including G_0. Examples are carmustine, lomustine, and radiation.

III. CHEMOTHERAPY

  A. Objectives of chemotherapy

    1. A **cure** may be sought with aggressive therapy for a prolonged period of time to eradicate all disease. For leukemias, this curative approach may consist of remission induction, attempting the maximal cell kill, followed by consolidation therapy to eradicate all clinically undetectable disease and to lower the tumor cell burden below 10^3, at which level host immunological defenses may keep the cells in control.

    2. If the goal is **palliation,** chemotherapy may be given to decrease tumor size, control growth, and reduce symptoms. Palliative therapy is usually given when complete eradication of the tumor is considered unlikely or the patient refuses aggressive therapy.

3. **Adjuvant** chemotherapy is given after more definitive therapy, such as surgery, to eliminate any remaining disease or undetected micrometastasis.

4. **Neoadjuvant** chemotherapy is given to decrease the tumor burden before definitive therapy, such as surgery or radiation.

5. **Salvage** chemotherapy is given as an attempt to get a patient into remission, after previous therapies have failed.

B. **Chemotherapy dosing** may be based on **body weight,** body surface area (**BSA**), or area under the concentration versus time curve (**AUC**). BSA is most frequently used because it provides an accurate comparison of activity and toxicity across species. In addition, BSA correlates with cardiac output, which determines renal and hepatic blood flow and thus affects drug elimination.

C. **Dosing adjustments** may be required for kidney or liver dysfunction to prevent toxicity.

D. **Combination chemotherapy** is usually more effective than single-agent therapy.

1. When combining chemotherapy agents, factors to consider include
   a. Antitumor activity
   b. Different mechanisms of action
   c. Minimally overlapping toxicities

2. The reasons for administering combination chemotherapy include:
   a. Overcoming or preventing resistance
   b. Cytotoxicity to resting and dividing cells
   c. Biochemical enhancement of effect
   d. Rescue of normal cells

3. **Dosing** and **scheduling** of combination regimens are important because they are designed to allow recovery of normal cells. These regimens generally are given as short courses of therapy in cycles.

4. **Acronyms** often are used to designate chemotherapy regimens. For example, CMF refers to a combination of cyclophosphamide, methotrexate, and fluorouracil used in the treatment of breast cancer.

E. **Administration**

1. **Routes** of administration vary, although intravenous (IV) administration is employed most commonly.

2. Other administration techniques include oral, subcutaneous, intrathecal, intra-arterial, intra-peritoneal, intravesical, continuous IV infusion, bolus IV infusion, and hepatic artery infusion.

3. Drugs that may be given **intrathecally** are methotrexate and cytarabine. Drugs should not be administered by the intrathecal route without specific information supporting intrathecal administration. Deaths have occurred when vincristine and other drugs have been administered by the intrathecal route. Caution should be used in the preparation and delivery of drugs to be used in this manner.

4. Products with different formulations, including liposomal or pegylated agents (e.g., liposomal doxorubicin, pegfilgrastim), are being used to decrease frequency of administration and/or reduce toxicities.

F. **Response to chemotherapy** is defined in a number of ways and does not always correlate with patient survival.

1. **Complete response (CR)** indicates disappearance of all clinical, gross, and microscopic disease.

2. **Partial response (PR)** indicates a > 50% reduction in tumor size, lasting a reasonable period of time. Some evidence of disease remains after therapy.

3. **Response rate (RR)** is defined as CR + PR.

4. **Stable disease** indicates tumor that neither grows nor shrinks significantly (< 25% change in size).

5. **Progression** or **no response** after therapy is defined by a > 25% increase in tumor size or the appearance of new lesions.

G. **Factors affecting response to chemotherapy**

1. **Tumor cell heterogeneity.** Large tumors have completed multiple cell divisions, resulting in several mutations and genetically diverse cells.

2. **Drug resistance.** The **Goldie-Coldman hypothesis** states that genetic changes are associated with drug resistance, and the probability of resistance increases as tumor size increases. The hypothesis assumes that at the time of diagnosis, most tumors possess resistant clones. The most well-studied mechanism of resistance involves the *mdr* (multidrug resistance) gene, which codes for membrane-bound P-glycoprotein. P-glycoprotein serves as a channel through which cellular toxins (i.e., chemotherapeutic agents) may be excreted from the cell.

3. **Dose intensity** is defined as a specific dose delivered over a specific period of time. Occasionally, the full dose cannot be given or a cycle is delayed owing to complications or toxicities. Suboptimal doses have resulted in reduced response rates and survival. **Dose density** involves shortening the usual interval between doses to maximize the drug effects on the tumor growth kinetics.

4. **Patient-specific factors** such as poor functional status, impaired organ function, or concomitant diseases may compromise how a chemotherapy regimen is given and affect how the patient responds to treatment.

IV. CLASSIFICATION OF CHEMOTHERAPEUTIC AGENTS

A. **Alkylating agents** were the first group of antineoplastic agents. The prototype of this class is mechlorethamine, or **nitrogen mustard,** which was researched as a chemical warfare agent. Alkylating agents cause cross-linking and abnormal base pairing of DNA strands, which inhibit replication of the DNA. This mechanism is known as **alkylation.** These are phase-nonspecific agents. Examples of alkylating agents and their toxicities are listed in Table 57-2.

B. Most of the **antitumor antibiotics** are obtained from organisms of the *Streptomyces* genus. These agents may act by either alkylation (mitomycin) or **intercalation.** Intercalation is the process by which the drug slides between DNA base pairs and inhibits DNA synthesis. These are phase-nonspecific agents. Examples of antitumor antibiotics and their toxicities are listed in Table 57-2.

C. **Antimetabolites** are structural analogs of naturally occurring substrates for biochemical reactions. They inhibit DNA synthesis by acting as false substitutions in the production of nucleic acids. These are S phase–specific agents. Examples of antimetabolites and their toxicities are listed in Table 57-2.

D. **Mitotic inhibitors.** The vinca alkaloids arrest cell division by preventing microtubule formation. The taxanes promote microtubule assembly and stabilization, thus prohibiting cell division. These are M phase–specific agents. Examples of these agents and their toxicities are listed in Table 57-2.

E. **Topoisomerase inhibitors** inhibit the enzymes topoisomerase I or II. The topoisomerases are necessary for DNA replication and RNA transcription. These are G_2 phase–specific agents. Examples of these agents and their toxicities are listed in Table 57-2.

F. **Enzymes.** Asparaginase is an enzyme that causes the degradation of the essential amino acid asparagine to aspartic acid and ammonia (Table 57-2). Unlike normal cells, tumor cells lack the ability to synthesize asparagine. This is a G_1 phase–specific agent.

G. **Protein tyrosine kinase inhibitors.** Imatinib mesylate is a selective tyrosine kinase inhibitor that causes apoptosis or arrest of growth in cells expressing the Bcr-Abl oncoprotein (Table 57-2). Bcr-Abl is the product of a specific chromosomal abnormality (Philadelphia chromosome), which is present in virtually all patients with chronic myelogenous leukemia (CML). It is the first approved antineoplastic agent designed to have targeted enzyme activity. Erlotinib is a

Table 57-2. Cancer Chemotherapeutic Agents by Mechanism of Action and Toxicities

Drug	Toxicities
Alkylating agents	
Altretamine (hexamethylmelamine)	Nausea and vomiting, myelosuppression, paresthesias, CNS toxicity
Busulfan	Myelosuppression, pulmonary fibrosis, aplastic anemia, skin hyperpigmentation
Carmustine (BCNU)	Delayed myelosuppression, nausea and vomiting, hepatotoxicity
Chlorambucil	Myelosuppression, pulmonary fibrosis, hyperuricemia
Carboplatin	Myelosuppression, nausea and vomiting, peripheral neuropathy, ototoxicity
Cisplatin	Nephrotoxicity, nausea and vomiting, peripheral neuropathy, myelosuppression, ototoxicity
Cyclophosphamide	Myelosuppression, hemorrhagic cystitis, immunosuppression, alopecia, stomatitis, SIADH
Dacarbazine (DTIC)	Myelosuppression, nausea and vomiting, flulike syndrome, hepatotoxicity, alopecia, flushing
Estramustine	Myelosuppression, ischemic heart disease, thrombophlebitis, hepatotoxicity, nausea and vomiting
Ifosfamide	Myelosuppression, hemorrhagic cystitis, somnolence, confusion
Lomustine (CCNU)	Delayed myelosuppression, nausea and vomiting, hepatotoxicity, neurotoxicity
Mechlorethamine	Myelosuppression, nausea and vomiting, phlebitis, gonadal dysfunction
Melphalan	Myelosuppression, anorexia, nausea and vomiting, gonadal dysfunction
Oxaliplatin	Sensory peripheral neuropathy, nausea and vomiting, diarrhea, mucositis, transaminase elevations, alopecia
Procarbazine	Myelosuppression, nausea and vomiting, lethargy, depression, paresthesias, headache, flulike syndrome
Streptozocin	Renal toxicity, nausea and vomiting, diarrhea, altered glucose metabolism, liver dysfunction
Temozolomide	Myelosuppression, nausea and vomiting, fatigue, headache, peripheral edema
Thiotepa	Myelosuppression, nausea and vomiting, mucositis, skin rashes
Antitumor antibiotics	
Bleomycin	Pneumonitis, pulmonary fibrosis, fever, anaphylaxis, hyperpigmentation, alopecia
Dactinomycin	Stomatitis, myelosuppression, anorexia, nausea and vomiting, diarrhea, alopecia
Daunorubicin	Myelosuppression, cardiotoxicity, stomatitis, alopecia, nausea and vomiting
Doxorubicin	Myelosuppression, cardiotoxicity, stomatitis, alopecia, nausea and vomiting
Epirubicin	Myelosuppression, nausea and vomiting, cardiotoxicity, alopecia
Idarubicin	Myelosuppression, nausea and vomiting, stomatitis, alopecia, cardiotoxicity
Mitomycin C	Myelosuppression, nausea and vomiting, anorexia, alopecia, stomatitis
Mitoxantrone	Myelosuppression, cardiotoxicity, alopecia, stomatitis, nausea and vomiting
Valrubicin	Urinary frequency, dysuria, hematuria, bladder spasm, incontinence, cystitis (For intravesical bladder administration)

(Continued on next page)

Table 57-2. Continued.

Drug	Toxicities
Antimetabolites	
Azacytidine	Myelosuppression, nausea and vomiting, diarrhea, constipation, injection site pain, muscle aches, fatigue, edema, dizziness
Capecitabine	Diarrhea, stomatitis, nausea and vomiting, hand–foot syndrome, myelosuppression
Cladribine (2Cda)	Myelosuppression, fever, rash
Cytarabine (Ara-C)	Myelosuppression, nausea and vomiting, diarrhea, stomatitis, hepatotoxicity, fever, conjunctivitis, CNS toxicity
Fludarabine	Myelosuppression, nausea and vomiting, fever, malaise, pulmonary infiltrates
Floxuridine	Hepatotoxicity, gastritis, mucositis
5-Fluorouracil	Stomatitis, myelosuppression, diarrhea, nausea and vomiting, cerebellar ataxia
Gemcitabine	Myelosuppression, fever, flu-like syndrome, rash, mild nausea and vomiting
Hydroxyurea	Myelosuppression, mild nausea and vomiting, rash
6-Mercaptopurine	Myelosuppression, nausea and vomiting, anorexia, diarrhea, cholestasis
Methotrexate	Mucositis, myelosuppression, pulmonary fibrosis, hepatotoxicity, nephrotoxicity, diarrhea, skin erythema
Pemetrexed	Myelosuppression, edema, fatigue, nausea and vomiting, diarrhea, mucositis, skin rash
Pentostatin	Nephrotoxicity, CNS depression, myelosuppression, nausea and vomiting, conjunctivitis
6-Thioguanine	Myelosuppression, hepatotoxicity, stomatitis
Mitotic inhibitors	
Docetaxel	Myelosuppression, fluid retention, hypersensitivity, paresthesias, rash alopecia
Paclitaxel	Myelosuppression, peripheral neuropathy, alopecia, mucositis, anaphylaxis, dyspnea
Vinblastine	Myelosuppression, paralytic ileus, alopecia, nausea, stomatitis
Vincristine	Peripheral neuropathy, paralytic ileus, SIADH
Vinorelbine	Peripheral neuropathy, myelosuppression, nausea and vomiting, hepatic dysfunction
Topoisomerase inhibitors	
Etoposide	Myelosuppression, nausea and vomiting, diarrhea, fever, hypotension with infusion, alopecia
Irinotecan	Myelosuppression, diarrhea, nausea and vomiting, anorexia
Teniposide	Myelosuppression, nausea and vomiting, alopecia, hepatotoxicity, hypotension with infusion
Topotecan	Myelosuppression, fever, flulike syndrome, nausea and vomiting
Enzymes	
Asparaginase	Allergic reactions, nausea and vomiting, liver dysfunction, CNS depression, hyperglycemia
Pegasparaginase	Hypersensitivity reactions, hepatotoxicity, fever, nausea and vomiting
Protein tyrosine kinase inhibitors	
Erlotinib (OSI-774)	Acneiform rash, diarrhea, nausea, pruritus, fatigue, eye irritation
Imatinib mesylate (STI-571)	Myelosuppression, hepatotoxicity, fluid retention, nausea, diarrhea

(*Continued on next page*)

Table 57-2. Continued.

Drug	Toxicities
Miscellaneous	
Tretinoin (all-trans retinoic acid, ATRA)	Leukocytosis, arrhythmias, headache, nausea and vomiting, scaling of skin, ATRA syndrome (fever, dyspnea, weight gain, pulmonary infiltrates)
Arsenic trioxide	Arrhythmias, hyperleukocytosis, nausea and vomiting, diarrhea, abdominal pain, APL differentiation syndrome (fever, dyspnea, weight gain, pulmonary infiltrates)
Bexarotene (Targretin R)	Hyperlipidemia, pancreatitis, hypothyroidism, hypercalcemia, leukopenia, peripheral edema, rash
Bortezomib (Velcade R)	Fatigue, peripheral neuropathy, myelosuppression, hypotension, arthralgias, diarrhea, nausea and vomiting, headache, fever
Thalidomide	Fatigue; headache; numbness in hands, feet, arms, and legs; constipation; increased risk for thrombotic events
Hormonal agents	
Adrenocorticoids Dexamethasone Methylprednisolone Prednisone	Fluid retention, hyperglycemia, hypertension, infection
Estrogens Diethylstilbestrol Estradiol	Fluid retention, feminization, uterine bleeding, nausea and vomiting, thrombophlebitis
Progestins Medroxyprogesterone Megestrol acetate	Weight gain, fluid retention, feminization, cardiovascular effects
Antiestrogens Fulvestrant Tamoxifen Toremifene	Hot flashes, nausea and vomiting, altered menses
Aromatase Inhibitors Aminoglutethimide Anastrozole Exemestane Letrozole	Rash, electrolytes disturbance, drowsiness, nausea, anorexia
Androgens Testosterone Methyltestosterone Fluoxymesterone	Masculinization, amenorrhea, gynecomastia, nausea, water retention, changes in libido, skin hypersensitivity, hepatotoxicity
Antiandrogens Bicalutamide Flutamide Nilutamide	Hot flashes, decreased libido, impotence, diarrhea, nausea and vomiting, gynecomastia, hepatotoxicity
LHRH Analogs Leuprolide Goserelin	Hot flashes, menstrual irregularity, sexual dysfunction, edema
LHRH antagonist Abarelix	Hypersensitivity reactions, hypotension, syncope, hot flashes, breast enlargement, prolongation of QT interval

APL, acute promyelocytic leukemia; *ATRA*, all-*trans*-retinoic acid; *CNS*, central nervous system; *LHRH*, luteinizing hormone-releasing hormone; *SIADH*, syndrome of inappropriate antidiuretic hormone.

selective inhibitor of epidermal growth factor receptor (EGFR) tyrosine kinase. EGFR is a cell surface receptor that is overexpressed in certain solid tumors. The binding of the EGFR receptor to its ligand activates tyrosine kinase, which then stimulates cell proliferation and growth of the tumor. Erlotinib blocks the tyrosine kinase signaling cascade and inhibits cancer cell growth. These agents are also known as targeted agents because they affect specific receptors to induce cancer cell death.

H. Other **miscellaneous** agents are listed in Table 57-2.

1. **Tretinoin (all-*trans* retinoic acid; ATRA)** is a retinoid derived from vitamin A, used for a specific form of acute leukemia, known as acute promyelocytic leukemia (APL), to help cells differentiate into functionally mature cells.

2. **Arsenic trioxide** is an antineoplastic arsenic compound used for APL that may induce selective apoptosis of APL cells.

3. **Bexarotene** is a selective retinoid X receptor (RXR) ligand used for cutaneous T cell lymphoma. Activation of the retinoid receptors leads to regulation of gene expression and apoptosis.

4. **Bortezomib** is a proteosome inhibitor used in patients with multiple myeloma.
   a. Proteosomes are enzyme complexes that are responsible for degrading proteins that control the cell cycle.
   b. Bortezomib is specific in that it interferes with the degradation of nuclear factor κβ (NF-κβ). NF-κβ is released from its inhibitory partner protein and moves to the nucleus. When the inhibitory partner does not degrade because of the action of bortezomib, NF-κβ is prevented from transcribing the genes that promote cancer growth.

5. **Thalidomide** is an immunomodulatory agent with a variety of mechanisms of action. It works as an angiogenesis inhibitor by interfering with the growth of new blood vessels needed for tumor growth and survival. It inhibits the production of tumor necrosis factor α (TNF-α) production, causes oxidative damage to DNA, and helps stimulate human T cells. It can be used as treatment for multiple myeloma in combination with dexamethasone.

I. **Hormones** are a class of heterogeneous compounds that have a variety of effects on cells. Table 57-2 lists some of the most commonly used hormonal agents in cancer therapy.

J. **Biological response modifiers** alter or enhance the patient's immune system to fight cancer or to lessen the side effects of the cancer treatment. Examples are given in Table 57-3.

1. **Cytokines** are soluble factors secreted or released by cells that affect the activity of other cells and/or the secreting cell itself. These agents generally act as regulatory or hematopoietic growth factors.

2. **Monoclonal antibodies** are recombinant antibodies designed to identify cancer-specific antigens, bind to the antigens on the patient's cancer cells, and allow the patient's immune system to eliminate those cells.
   a. Some monoclonal antibodies are being conjugated to antitumor agents or radioisotopes (e.g., gemtuzumab ozogamicin, ibritumomab tiuxetan) to help target cytotoxic therapy to the tumor cells.
   b. Another example of a monoclonal antibody is bevacizumab, which targets and inhibits vascular endothelial growth factor (VEGF). VEGF is an important regulator of the growth and survival of blood vessels known as angiogenesis. Bevacizumab works by inhibiting angiogenesis and, therefore, inhibiting the blood supply to the tumor.
   c. Other monoclonal antibodies are listed in Table 57-3.

3. **Immunotoxins.** Denileukin diftitox is a fusion protein composed of diphtheria toxin and interleukin 2 (IL-2). It is designed to direct the cytocidal action of diphtheria toxin to cells with the IL-2 receptor on their surface. This form of therapy is able to bypass the need for a functioning immune system, which may be defective in many cancer patients.

V. TOXICITIES OF CHEMOTHERAPY AGENTS.
Chemotherapeutic agents are most toxic to rapidly proliferating cells. The tissues most commonly affected are those of the mucous membranes, skin, hair, gastrointestinal (GI) tract, and bone marrow. Of these, bone marrow toxicity can be the most life-threatening.

Table 57-3. Biological Agents Used in Oncology

Agent	Indications	Toxicity
Cytokine		
Interferon-α -2a, -2b (Roferon-AR, Intron A)	Malignant melanoma, chronic myelogenous leukemia, hairy-cell leukemia, Kaposi sarcoma, chronic hepatitis B and C, follicular lymphoma	Flulike syndrome, anorexia, depression, fatigue
Interleukin 2 (aldesleukin, Proleukin)	Renal cell carcinoma, malignant melanoma	Chills, fever, dyspnea, pulmonary congestion, edema, nephrotoxicity, hypotension, mental status changes, anemia, thrombocytopenia, diarrhea, nausea and vomiting
Interleukin 11 (oprelvekin, Neumega)	Thrombocytopenia	Fluid retention, peripheral edema, dyspnea, tachycardia, atrial arrhythmias, dizziness, blurred vision
Filgrastim (G-CSF, Neupogen)	Decrease incidence/duration of neutropenia, hematopoietic stem-cell mobilization	Bone pain, fever, malaise
Pegfilgrastim (Neulasta)	Decrease incidence/duration of neutropenia	Bone pain, fever, malaise
Sargramostim (GM-CSF, Leukine)	Acceleration of myeloid recovery, BMT failure or engraftment delay, induction for acute myelogenous leukemia, hematopoietic stem cell mobilization, myeloid reconstitution after BMT	Bone pain, arthralgia/myalgia, chills, fever, rash, first-dose reaction (hypotension, tachycardia, dyspnea)
Epoetin α (erythropoietin, Epogen, Procrit)	Anemia associated with chronic renal failure, cancer chemotherapy or HIV treatments, reduction of blood transfusions in surgery patients	Hypertension, headache, arthralgias
Darbepoetin α (Aranesp)	Anemia associated with chronic renal failure, chronic renal insufficiency, cancer- and chemotherapy-associated anemia	Hypertension, myalgia, headache, fever, tachycardia, nausea
Monoclonal antibody		
Alemtuzumab (Campath R)	B cell chronic lymphocytic leukemia	Infusion-related fevers, chills, rash, hypotension, shortness of breath, nausea and vomiting, opportunistic infections, neutropenia, thrombocytopenia
Bevacizumab (Avastin R)	Metastatic colorectal cancer, non-small cell lung cancer (nonsquamous)	Hypertension, proteinuria, GI perforation, thrombotic events, impaired wound healing
Cetuximab (Erbitux R)	Metastatic colorectal cancer	Acneiform rash, infusion related reactions, fatigue, nausea and vomiting, diarrhea
Gemtuzumab ozogamicin (Mylotarg R)	Acute myeloid leukemia	Infusion-related fever, chills, nausea and vomiting, headache, hypotension, myelosuppression, hepatotoxicity, hypersensitivity

(Continued on next page)

Table 57-3. Continued.

Agent	Indications	Toxicity
Ibritumomab tiuxetan (Zevalin R)	Non-Hodgkin lymphoma	Infusion-related fevers, chills, rigors, hypersensitivity, hypotension, myelosuppression
Rituximab (Rituxan R)	Non-Hodgkin lymphoma	Hypersensitivity, infusion-related fevers, chills, rigors, hypotension
Tositumomab (Bexxar R)	Non-Hodgkin lymphoma	Hypersensitivity reactions, fever, chills, myelosuppression, especially thrombocytopenia, rash, nausea and vomiting, diarrhea
Trastuzumab (Herceptin R)	Breast cancer	Infusion-related fevers, chills, cardiac dysfunction including dyspnea, cough, peripheral edema, nausea and vomiting, hypersensitivity, hypotension, diarrhea
Immunotoxin		
Denileukin diftitox (Ontak R)	Cutaneous T cell lymphoma	Acute hypersensitivity, including hypotension, dyspnea, rash, chest pain, tachycardia, vascular leak syndrome, dizziness, nausea and vomiting, diarrhea

BMT, bone marrow transplant; *G-CSF,* granulocyte colony-stimulating factor; *GI,* gastrointestinal; *GM-CSF,* granulocyte-macrophage colony-stimulating factor.

A. **Bone marrow suppression** is the **most common** dose-limiting **side effect** of cancer therapy.

 1. **Complications**
    a. **Infections.** White blood cells are most affected owing to their short life span (6–12 hr).
       (1) A significant decrease in the white blood cell count, particularly a neutrophil count < 500/mm^3 (**neutropenia**), predisposes the patient to development of serious infections.
       (2) The usual signs and symptoms of infection may be absent, and fever may be the only indicator (**febrile neutropenia**).
       (3) **Colony-stimulating factors**—for example, **granulocyte colony-stimulating factor (G-CSF) and granulocyte-macrophage colony-stimulating factor (GM-CSF)**—may be used to stimulate neutrophil production and lessen the degree and duration of neutropenia.
    b. **Bleeding.** Platelets have an intermediate life span of 5–10 days. Decreased platelets (**thrombocytopenia**) can also occur from chemotherapy, which can lead to bleeding and may require platelet transfusions.
    c. **Anemia** and **fatigue** secondary to cancer chemotherapy may also occur. It generally does not occur as quickly as other bone marrow toxicities because of the long life span of red blood cells (about 120 days). **Human recombinant erythropoietin** (e.g., epoetin α, darbepoetin α) may be used to increase hemoglobin, decrease transfusion requirements, and decrease fatigue.

 2. The **time course** of myelosuppression varies with the chemotherapy regimen. In general, the onset of myelosuppression is 7–10 days after the chemotherapy has been administered. The lowest point of the counts, called the **nadir,** is usually reached in 10–14 days. Recovery of counts usually occurs in 2–3 weeks.

 3. A patient's counts must be sufficiently **recovered** before receiving subsequent chemotherapy cycles. Generally, the neutrophil count must be > 1,500/mm^3 and the platelet count > 100,000/mm^3 before the patient receives additional chemotherapy.

 4. The extent of myelosuppression is related to the **chemotherapy agents** used and **doses** given. Drugs that can cause severe myelosuppression include carmustine, cytarabine, daunorubicin, doxorubicin, and paclitaxel.

5. Some chemotherapy agents cause little or no myelosuppression. These include asparaginase, bleomycin, and vincristine.

B. **Dermatological toxicity**

1. **Alopecia** is the loss of hair associated with chemotherapy. Not all agents cause alopecia, and hair loss may be partial or complete. Chemotherapy agents that commonly cause alopecia include cyclophosphamide, doxorubicin, mechlorethamine, and paclitaxel.

2. Drugs associated with necrosis of tissue are called **vesicants. Local necrosis** may result from **extravasation** of vesicant chemotherapy drugs outside the vein during their administration. Vesicant agents include dactinomycin, daunorubicin, doxorubicin, idarubicin, mechlorethamine, mitomycin, vinblastine, vincristine, and vinorelbine.

   a. Most vesicant extravasations produce **immediate pain** or **burning.** However, a delayed reaction may occur hours or weeks later. Significant tissue injury, including ulceration or necrosis, may require plastic surgery intervention.

   b. The **treatment** of extravasations varies, depending on the vesicant. Heat or cold packs and chemicals such as hyaluronidase or dimethyl sulfoxide (DMSO) may be used.

3. Cancer chemotherapy can also cause **skin changes** such as dryness and sensitivity to sunlight. Examples are fluorouracil and methotrexate.

C. **GI toxicities** are frequently experienced by patients receiving chemotherapy.

1. **Nausea** and **vomiting** are often the most distressing toxicities from the patient's perspective. However, this side effect can generally be prevented, or better controlled, with the use of currently available antiemetics.

   a. Severe vomiting can result in dehydration, electrolyte imbalances, and esophageal tears and may cause the patient to discontinue therapy.

   b. Nausea and vomiting may be **acute, delayed,** or **anticipatory** in nature. Antiemetics should be used prophylactically to prevent the occurrence of nausea and vomiting, particularly with chemotherapeutic agents that have a high emetogenic risk.

   c. Table 57-4 lists **commonly used chemotherapeutic agents** and their emetogenic potential on a scale of 1–5.

Table 57-4. Emetogenic Potential of Cancer Chemotherapeutic Agents

Level 5: Very Highly Emetogenic	Level 4: Highly Emetogenic	Level 3: Moderately Emetogenic	Level 2: Low Emetic Risk	Level 1: Very Low Emetic Risk
Carmustine > 250 mg/m^2	Carmustine ≤ 250 mg/m^2	Carboplatin	Docetaxel	Asparaginase
Cisplatin ≥ 50 mg/m^2	Cisplatin < 50 mg/m^2	Cyclophosphamide ≤ 750 mg/m^2	Etoposide	Bleomycin
Cyclophosphamide ≥ 1500 mg/m^2	Cyclophosphamide 750–1500 mg/m^2	Cytarabine < 1000 mg/m^2	Fluorouracil	Capecitabine
Dacarbazine	Cytarabine $>$ 1000 mg/m^2	Daunorubicin	Gemcitabine	Chlorambucil
Mechlorethamine	Dactinomycin	Doxorubicin ≤ 60 mg/m^2	Irinotecan	Fludarabine
Streptozocin	Doxorubicin > 60 mg/m^2	Idarubicin	Methotrexate 50–250 mg/m^2	Hydroxyurea
	Lomustine	Ifosfamide	Mitomycin	Methotrexate ≤ 50 mg/m^2
	Methotrexate $>$ 1000 mg/m^2	Methotrexate 250–1000 mg/m^2	Paclitaxel	Melphalan
	Procarbazine	Mitoxantrone	Thiotepa $<$ 15 mg/m^2	Rituximab
	Temozolomide		Topotecan	Thioguanine
	Thiotepa ≥ 15 mg/m^2			Trastuzumab
				Vinblastine
				Vincristine
				Vinorelbine

(1) The emetogenic potential of combinations of chemotherapy agents can be estimated by identifying the most emetogenic agent in the combination.

(2) The contribution of the other agents can then be evaluated by using the following guidelines:

    (a) Level 1 agents do not contribute to the emetogenicity of the regimen.

    (b) Adding one or more level 2 agents increases the emetogenicity to one level higher than the most emetogenic agent in the combination.

    (b) Adding level 3 or 4 agents increases the level of emetogenicity by one level per agent.

  d. The occurrence of nausea and vomiting is influenced by the emetogenicity of the chemotherapeutic agent or combination of agents, the chemotherapeutic dose, the method of administration, and individual patient characteristics.

2. Stomatitis is a generalized inflammation of the oral mucosa or other areas of the GI tract. Because of the rapid turnover of epithelial cells in the GI tract, this is a common site of toxicity.

  a. Signs and **symptoms** include erythema, pain, dryness of the mouth, burning or tingling of the lips, ulcerations, and bleeding.

  b. Chemotherapy agents associated with stomatitis include capecitabine, fluorouracil, and methotrexate.

  c. Time course. Stomatitis usually appears within a week after the offending agent is administered, and resolves in 10–14 days.

  d. Consequences of stomatitis include infection of the ulcerated areas, inability to eat, pain requiring opioid analgesics, and subsequent decreases in chemotherapy doses.

  e. Topical and local analgesics in the form of mouthrinses are commonly used and can help with mouth and throat pain.

3. Other GI toxicities include **diarrhea** (e.g., irinotecan, fluorouracil), **constipation** (e.g., vincristine), **anorexia,** and **taste changes.**

D. Tumor lysis syndrome (TLS) may occur in hematological malignancies such as leukemia and lymphoma, in which there is a high tumor cell burden or rapidly growing tumors. Owing to the spontaneous lysis of cells from treatment with chemotherapy, cell lysis causes release of intracellular products, including uric acid, potassium, and phosphate, which can lead to renal failure and cardiac arrhythmias. This may be prevented by giving intravenous hydration, by alkalinizing the urine, and by giving agents such as **allopurinol** or **rasburicase** (Elitek) to decrease uric acid.

E. Hypercalcemia may occur in patients with solid or hematologic malignancies and can often be the presenting sign of malignancy. The major cause of hypercalcemia is increased osteoclastic bone resorption, which is generally caused by the release of parathyroid hormone-related protein (PTHrP) by the tumor cells. Common presenting symptoms include mental status changes, fatigue and muscle weakness, polyuria, polydipsia, nausea and vomiting. Treatment includes aggressive hydration with normal saline, calciuric therapy which consists of calcitonin, and bisphosphonates such as pamidronate (Aredia) or zoledronic acid (Zometa).

F. Chills and **fever** may occur after the administration of some chemotherapy and biological agents. This fever generally can be differentiated from fever owing to infection because of its temporal relationship to chemotherapy administration. This reaction is commonly associated with bleomycin, cytarabine monoclonal antibodies, and IL-2.

G. Pulmonary toxicity is generally irreversible and may be fatal.

1. Signs and **symptoms** are shortness of breath, nonproductive cough, and low-grade fever. In some cases, the risk of pulmonary toxicity increases as the cumulative dose of the drug increases (e.g., bleomycin).

2. Chemotherapeutic agents associated with pulmonary toxicity include bleomycin, busulfan, carmustine, and mitomycin.

H. **Cardiac toxicity** may manifest as an acute or chronic problem.

    1. **Acute changes** are generally transient electrocardiograph abnormalities that may not be clinically significant.

    2. **Chronic cardiac toxicity** is irreversible congestive heart failure. **Risk factors** include chest irradiation and high cumulative doses of cardiotoxic chemotherapy.

    3. Chemotherapy agents that are associated with chronic cardiotoxicity include daunorubicin, doxorubicin, epirubicin, idarubicin, and mitoxantrone. **Dexrazoxane** is a cardioprotective agent that may be used with doxorubicin to help prevent or lessen its toxic effects to the heart.

I. **Hypersensitivity reactions** may occur with any chemotherapy agent. Life-threatening reactions, including anaphylaxis, appear to be more common with asparaginase, carboplatin, cisplatin, etoposide, paclitaxel, and teniposide.

J. **Neurotoxicity** may occur with systemic or intrathecal chemotherapy.

    1. Vincristine is associated with **autonomic** and **peripheral** neuropathies. Patients may experience gait disturbances, numbness and tingling of hands and feet, and loss of deep-tendon reflexes. Intrathecal administration of vincristine results in fatal neurotoxicity.

    2. **Peripheral neuropathy** and **ototoxicity** are common dose-limiting toxicities of cisplatin. **Sensory** neuropathies, causing tingling or numbing of the hands and feet, may be associated with capecitabine, oxaliplatin, and paclitaxel.

    3. High doses of cytarabine may produce **cerebellar toxicity** that manifests initially as loss of eye–hand coordination and may progress to coma.

    4. **Arachnoiditis** has been associated with intrathecal administration of cytarabine and methotrexate.

K. **Hemorrhagic cystitis** is a bladder toxicity that is seen most commonly after administration of cyclophosphamide and ifosfamide. **Acrolein,** a metabolite of these agents, is thought to cause a chemical irritation of the bladder mucosa, resulting in bleeding. Preventive measures include aggressive hydration with subsequent frequent urination, and the administration of the uroprotectant mesna. **Mesna** acts by binding to acrolein and preventing it from contacting the bladder mucosa.

L. **Renal toxicity** may manifest by elevations in serum creatinine and blood urea nitrogen (BUN) as well as electrolyte abnormalities. Nephrotoxicity is associated with cisplatin, ifosfamide, methotrexate, and streptozocin. Intravenous hydration is used to protect the kidneys from the nephrotoxic effects of cisplatin. Osmotic diuresis with mannitol may also help reduce the incidence of cisplatin nephrotoxicity.

M. **Hepatotoxicity** may manifest as elevated liver function tests, jaundice, or hepatitis. Asparaginase, cytarabine, mercaptopurine, and methotrexate are known to cause hepatic toxicity.

N. **Secondary malignancies,** such as solid tumors, lymphomas, and leukemias, may occur many years after chemotherapy or radiation. Antineoplastic agents known to possess a high carcinogenic risk include cyclophosphamide, etoposide, melphalan, and mechlorethamine.

O. Chemotherapy may cause **infertility,** which may be temporary or permanent. Cyclophosphamide, chlorambucil, mechlorethamine, melphalan, and procarbazine are associated with a significant incidence of infertility in males and females.

VI. OTHER THERAPEUTIC MODALITIES

A. **Surgery** may be diagnostic (biopsy, exploratory laparotomy, second-look) or therapeutic (tumor debulking or removal). Surgery is often combined with chemotherapy and/or radiation.

B. Radiation therapy involves high doses of ionizing radiation directed at the cancerous tissue. Radiation may be combined with surgery and/or chemotherapy. Depending on the area of the body being irradiated, **adverse reactions** may include stomatitis, nausea and vomiting, diarrhea, and myelosuppression.

C. Hematopoietic stem-cell transplantation involves intravenous infusion of stem cells from a compatible donor to a recipient following high-dose chemotherapy. It is used for treatment of diseases involving the bone marrow or immune system and to allow for administration of high-dose chemotherapy or radiation for tumors resistant to standard doses. Stem cells can be obtained from bone marrow or peripheral blood.

1. In **autologous** transplants, stem cells are obtained from the patient, preserved, and later reinfused into the same patient. **Allogeneic** transplants involve two separate individuals. Cells are obtained from a matched donor and then infused into a separate patient.

2. Transplant-related complications include hepatic venoocclusive disease (VOD), acute and chronic graft versus host disease (GVHD), infection, and pulmonary complications.

STUDY QUESTIONS

Directions for questions 1–14: Each of the questions, statements, or incomplete statements in this section can be correctly answered or completed by **one** of the suggested answers or phrases. Choose the **best** answer.

1. The top four most commonly diagnosed cancers include all of the following *except*

(A) lung.
(B) prostate.
(C) colon and rectum.
(D) thyroid.
(E) breast.

2. Which statement regarding phase-specific chemotherapeutic agents is correct? They

(A) are most effective in one phase of the cell cycle.
(B) are effective in all phases of the cell cycle.
(C) are only effective in G_0 phase.
(D) include the alkylating agents.
(E) include the antitumor antibiotics.

3. Body surface area (BSA) is used in calculating chemotherapy doses because

(A) BSA is an indicator of tumor cell mass.
(B) BSA correlates with cardiac output.
(C) BSA correlates with gastrointestinal transit time.
(D) the National Cancer Institute requires that BSA be used.
(E) the U.S. Food and Drug Administration (FDA) requires that BSA be used.

4. The rationale for combination chemotherapy includes all of the following *except*

(A) biochemical enhancement of effect.
(B) rescue of normal cells.
(C) overcoming or preventing resistance.
(D) biochemical nullification of effect.
(E) cytotoxic to both resting and dividing cells.

5. All of the following chemotherapy agents can be administered intrathecally *except*

(A) methotrexate.
(B) cytarabine.
(C) hydrocortisone.
(D) thiotepa.
(E) vincristine.

6. Which of the following chemotherapeutic agents is classified as an alkylating agent?

(A) cyclophosphamide
(B) etoposide
(C) mechlorethamine
(D) paclitaxel
(E) cyclophosphamide and mechlorethamine

7. Which of the following chemotherapy agents acts by intercalation?

(A) vincristine
(B) paclitaxel
(C) doxorubicin
(D) vincristine and paclitaxel
(E) topotecan

8. How do antimetabolites exert their cytotoxic effect?

(A) inhibiting DNA synthesis by sliding between DNA base pairs
(B) inhibiting RNA synthesis by sliding between RNA base pairs
(C) acting as false metabolites in the microtubules
(D) acting as false substitutions in the production of nucleic acids
(E) promoting microtubule assembly and stabilization

9. All of the following chemotherapy agents work through affecting microtubule function *except*

(A) docetaxel.
(B) vinblastine.
(C) mitoxantrone.
(D) vincristine.
(E) vinorelbine.

10. Hormonal agents that are useful in the treatment of cancer include

(A) tamoxifen.
(B) prednisone.
(C) flutamide.
(D) tamoxifen and flutamide.
(E) tamoxifen, prednisone, and flutamide.

11. When does the neutrophil nadir associated with chemotherapy agents generally occur?

(A) during administration of the chemotherapy
(B) 1–2 days after therapy
(C) 10–14 days after therapy
(D) 1 month after therapy
(E) when the platelet count begins to rise

12. Stomatitis is characterized by all of the following signs and symptoms *except*

(A) headache.
(B) erythema.
(C) bleeding.
(D) ulcerations.
(E) dryness of mouth.

13. Which of the following statements describes hemorrhagic cystitis? It

(A) is caused by excretion of tumor cell breakdown products.
(B) is associated with ifosfamide or cyclophosphamide administration.
(C) is caused by the administration of mesna.
(D) can be prevented or treated with acrolein.
(E) can be treated with granulocyte colony-stimulating factor (G-CSF).

14. All of the following chemotherapy agents are vesicants *except*

(A) doxorubicin.
(B) mechlorethamine.
(C) vincristine.
(D) methotrexate.
(E) idarubicin.

Directions for questions 15–19: Each agent in this section is most closely associated with **one** of the following adverse effects. Each effect is used only **once**. Choose the **best** answer, **A–E.**

A cardiotoxicity
B hypersensitivity
C diarrhea
D pulmonary toxicity
E constipation

15. Vincristine

16. Irinotecan

17. Doxorubicin

18. Paclitaxel

19. Bleomycin

Directions for questions 20–22: Each of the questions, statements, or incomplete statements in this section can be correctly answered or completed by **one** of the suggested answers or phrases. Choose the **best** answer.

For questions 20–22: P.A. is a 60-year-old man who has recently been diagnosed with stage IIB lung cancer. After his case was evaluated, it was decided that he would undergo surgical resection of the primary tumor and then receive chemotherapy with carboplatin and docetaxel.

20. What type of chemotherapy is P.A. receiving?

(A) adjuvant
(B) salvage
(C) neoadjuvant

21. What side effects would you counsel P.A. about?

(A) nausea and vomiting
(B) peripheral neuropathy
(C) hemorrhagic cystitis
(D) A and B
(E) All of the above

22. If P.A. has recurrence of his lung cancer after therapy with carboplatin and docetaxel, which targeted agent may be considered for second-line therapy?

(A) doxorubicin
(B) busulfan
(C) cyclophosphamide
(D) erlotinib
(E) bleomycin

ANSWERS AND EXPLANATIONS

1. The answer is D   *[see I.B].*
Prostate cancer is the most common cancer in men, breast cancer is the most common cancer in women, followed by lung, then colon and rectum for both men and women.

2. The answer is A   *[see II.D.1–3].*
Phase-specific agents are most active in one specific phase of the cell cycle. These agents have no activity against cells in G_0, the resting phase. Examples of phase-specific agents include the mitotic inhibitors, asparaginase, the antimetabolites, and etoposide.

3. The answer is B   *[see III.B].*
BSA correlates with cardiac output, which determines renal and hepatic blood flow and thus affects drug elimination.

4. The answer is D   *[see III.D.2].*
Combination chemotherapy has been developed to have maximal cytotoxicity to tumor cells and minimal toxicity to normal cells. The drugs are dosed and scheduled such that maximal cell kill occurs, while sparing normal cells as much as possible. Combination regimens often contain agents with different spectrums of toxicity.

5. The answer is E   *[see III.E.3].*
Intrathecally administered vincristine is fatal. All syringes of vincristine must be labeled "Fatal if given intrathecally. For intravenous use only."

6. The answer is E   *[see IV.A.1].*
Cyclophosphamide and mechlorethamine are nitrogen mustards, a subgroup of the alkylating agents. Etoposide is a topoisomerase II inhibitor, and paclitaxel is a mitotic inhibitor.

7. The answer is C   *[see IV.B.1].*
Doxorubicin is an antitumor antibiotic that inhibits DNA synthesis by intercalation. Vincristine and paclitaxel are mitotic inhibitors that act on microtubule assembly. Topotecan inhibits topoisomerase I.

8. The answer is D   *[see IV.C].*
Antimetabolites are structural analogs of naturally occurring substrates for biochemical reactions. They inhibit DNA synthesis by acting as false substitutions in the production of DNA.

9. The answer is C   *[see IV.D].*
Docetaxel is a taxane, which works by promoting microtubule assembly and stabilization, resulting in inhibition of cell division. Vincristine, vinblastine, and vinorelbine are vinca alkaloids, which work by preventing microtubule formation. Mitoxantrone is an antitumor antibiotic, which works by DNA intercalation.

10. The answer is E   *[see VI; Table 57-2].*
Tamoxifen is an antiestrogen used in the treatment of breast cancer. Prednisone is used for its antilymphocytic properties in the treatment of non-Hodgkin lymphoma. Flutamide is an antiandrogen used in the treatment of prostate cancer.

11. The answer is C   *[see V.A.2].*
Bone marrow suppression, particularly of the neutrophils, usually is the most profound 10–14 days after chemotherapy.

12. The answer is A   *[see V.C.2].*
Stomatitis, or mucositis, is an inflammation of the mucous membranes, particularly the oral mucosa. Although the symptoms generally are limited to the mouth and throat, stomatitis may affect any part of the gastrointestinal tract, potentially causing diarrhea and anal fissures.

13. The answer is B *[see V.J].*
Hemorrhagic cystitis results from irritation of the lining of the bladder by acrolein, a metabolite of ifosfamide and cyclophosphamide. Mesna may be used to inactivate the acrolein, thus preventing hemorrhagic cystitis.

14. The answer is D *[see V.B.2].*
Vesicant chemotherapy agents may cause local necrosis if extravasated outside the vein. Doxorubicin, idarubicin, mechlorethamine, and vincristine are all classified as vesicants.

15. The answer is E *[see V.C.3; V.E–G].*

16. The answer is C *[see V.C.3; V.E–G].*

17. The answer is A *[see V.C.3; V.E–G].*

18. The answer is B *[see V.C.3; V.E–G].*

19. The answer is D *[see V.C.3; V.E–G].*
Cardiotoxicity is associated with cumulative doses of doxorubicin and other antitumor antibiotics. Hypersensitivity from paclitaxel may be the result of its Cremophor diluent. Severe diarrhea, requiring treatment with atropine, is associated with irinotecan. Pulmonary toxicity is associated with cumulative doses of bleomycin. Severe constipation and paralytic ileus is associated with the use of vincristine.

20. The answer is A *[see III.A.3].*
Receiving chemotherapy after potentially curative surgery is known as adjuvant chemotherapy.

21. The answer is D *[see Table 57-2].*
Nausea and vomiting are common side effects of carboplatin and docetaxel. Premedications with anti-nausea medications are given before these chemotherapy agents are given. Peripheral neuropathy can commonly be seen with docetaxel. Patients need to be counseled about this and followed up on this adverse event on routine clinic visits. If left untreated severe, disabling neuropathy can result. Hemorrhagic cystitis is an adverse event of some of the alkylating agents including ifosfamide and cyclophosphamide, but not carboplatin.

22. The answer is D *[see IV.G].*
Erlotinib is an agent targeted for the epidermal growth factor receptor tyrosine kinase. Busulfan and cyclophosphamide are alkylating agents that are non cell cycle specific. Bleomycin and doxorubicin are antitumor antibiotics that intercalate with DNA and are phase non-specific agents.

58
Pain Management
Alan F. Kaul

I. INTRODUCTION

A. Definitions

1. **Pain** is an unpleasant sensory and emotional experience that is associated with actual or potential tissue damage or described in terms of such damage. It is a subjective, individual experience that has physical, psychological, and social determinants. There is no objective measurement of pain. In the United States alone, recurrent or persistent pain is experienced by more than 75 million individuals.

2. **Acute pain** lasts > 30 days and occurs after muscle strains and tissue injury, such as trauma or surgery. The pain is usually self-limiting, decreasing with time as the injury heals. It is described as a linear process, with a beginning and an end. Increased autonomic nervous system activity often accompanies acute pain, causing tachycardia, tachypnea, hypertension, diaphoresis, and mydriasis. Increased anxiety also may occur.

3. **Chronic pain** is persistent or episodic pain of a duration or intensity that adversely affects the function or well-being of the patient and can persist after the resolution of an injury. Some define it as lasting more than 6 months.
   a. **Chronic nonmalignant pain** may be a complication of acute injury in which the healing process does not occur as expected or may be caused by a disease such as a rheumatological disorder (e.g., osteoarthritis, rheumatoid arthritis, fibromyalgia).
   b. The elderly are more likely to experience chronic pain because of the increased prevalence of degenerative disorders in this age group.
   c. The pain is constant, does not improve with time, and is described as a cyclic process (vicious circle).
   d. Compared to acute pain, there is no longer autonomic nervous system stimulation so the patient may not appear to be in pain. Instead, the patient may be depressed; suffer insomnia, weight loss, and sexual dysfunction; and may not be able to cope with the normal activities of daily living, including family and job-related activities.

4. **Chronic cancer pain** occurs in 60%–90% of patients with cancer. Its characteristics are similar to those of chronic nonmalignant pain. In addition to depression, prominent characteristics are fear, anger, and agony. The cause of chronic cancer pain can be related to the tumor or cancer therapy or can be idiosyncratic. Tumor causes of pain include bone metastasis, compression of nerve structures, occlusion of blood vessels, obstruction of bowel, or infiltration of soft tissue.

5. **Breakthrough pain** is the intermittent, transitory increase in pain that occurs at a greater intensity over baseline chronic pain. It may have temporal characteristics, precipitating factors, and predictability.

6. **Neuropathic pain** is a result of an injury or malfunction of the nervous system. Excluding patients with a progressive peripheral neuropathy or neuropathic pain associated with a cancer lesion, tissue damage is not ongoing. Neuropathic pain is described as aching, throbbing, burning, shooting, stinging and tenderness or sensitivity of the skin.

B. Principles of management

1. **Comprehensive pain assessment** should determine the characteristics of the patient's pain complaint, clinical status, and pain management history.
   a. Assessment of the pain complaint should include chronology and symptomatology of the presenting complaint such as information about onset, location, intensity, duration, quality, distribution, provocative factors, temporal qualities, severity, and pain history.
   b. Assessment of clinical status should include the extent of underlying trauma or disease. Also, the patient's physical, psychological, and social conditions should be determined.

   c. Assessment of pain management history includes drug allergies, analgesic response, onset, duration, and side effects.

2. **Appropriate pain management targets** should be established.
   a. The primary pain management goal is to improve patient comfort.
   b. For acute pain management, improved comfort can aid the healing and rehabilitation process.
   c. For chronic pain, the specific objectives are to break the pain cycle (i.e., erase pain memory) and minimize breakthrough pain.
   d. Other targets for chronic pain management include improvement of general well-being, sleep, outlook, self-esteem, activities of daily living, support, and mobility.

3. **Individualized pain management regimens** should be determined and initiated promptly.
   a. The optimal analgesic regimen, including dose, dosing interval, and mode of administration, should be selected.
   b. Additional pharmacological adjuncts and nonpharmacological therapies should be added if needed.
   c. The most common regimens for acute pain include intermittent (as needed) dosing, patient-controlled analgesia (PCA), or epidural infusions with narcotic or nonnarcotic agents.
   d. Although the practice is controversial and often not in the best interests of patients, narcotic use is often minimized or avoided for chronic nonmalignant pain. Pain management specialists are changing this suboptimal practice. Nonnarcotic analgesics and nonpharmacological management usually are maximized.
   e. For chronic cancer pain, an individualized around-the-clock analgesic regimen is established, using a long-acting analgesic. An intermittent, as-needed regimen for breakthrough pain, using a short-acting analgesic, is also determined.

4. **Monitoring** the pain management regimen and **reassessment** of the patient's pain should occur on a continuous, timely basis. Any changes in analgesic, dose, dosing interval, or method of administration should be noted in the patient's medical record and carried out in a timely fashion.

II. ANALGESICS

A. **Nonnarcotic analgesics** include aspirin; other salicylates; acetaminophen; nonsteroidal anti-inflammatory drugs (NSAIDs); selective, cyclooxygenase 2 (COX-2) inhibitors; disease-modifying antirheumatic drugs (DMARDs); and tumor-necrosis factor α (TNF-α) inhibitors (Table 58-1). Aspirin products, acetaminophen, and some low-dose NSAIDs such as ibuprofen, ketoprofen, and naproxen sodium are available as over-the-counter (OTC) products.

1. **Mechanism of action.** Salicylates and NSAIDs are prostaglandin inhibitors and prevent peripheral nociception by vasoactive substances such as prostaglandins and bradykinins. Most NSAIDs inhibit both COX-1, which produces prostaglandins that are believed to be cytoprotective of the stomach lining, and COX-2, which produces prostaglandins responsible for pain and inflammation. Selective COX-2 inhibitors like celecoxib do not inhibit COX-1. Adalimumab, etanercept, and infliximab act by binding or capturing excess TNF-α, one of the dominant cytokines, or proteins, that play an important role in the inflammatory response. The exact mechanism of action of leflunomide, a novel drug used to treat rheumatoid arthritis, is not completely known but it is thought to inhibit pyrimidine synthesis.

2. **Therapeutic effects**
   a. The peripherally acting, nonnarcotic analgesics have several effects in common. These effects distinguish these agents from narcotic analgesics.
      (1) They are antipyretic.
      (2) They are anti-inflammatory (except acetaminophen).
      (3) There is a ceiling effect to the analgesia.
      (4) They do not cause tolerance.
      (5) They do not cause physical or psychological dependence.
   b. The efficacy of nonnarcotics is compared to aspirin. Most drugs are comparable to aspirin; however, several NSAIDs have shown a superior effect to 650 mg of aspirin.

Table 58-1. Nonnarcotic Oral Analgesics and Nonsteroidal Anti-Inflammatory Drugs (NSAIDs)

Drug	Adult Dose Range (mg)	Dosing Interval (hr)	Maximum Dose/ Day (mg)
Para-aminophenol derivatives			
Acetaminophen (Tylenol)	325–1000	4–6	4000
Salicylates			
Aspirin	325–1000	4–6	4000
Choline magnesium trisalicylate			3000
(Trilisate)	1000–1500	12	
Diflunisal (Dolobid)	250–1000	8–12	1500
Salsalate (Disalcid)	500–1000	8	3000
Arylpropionic acid derivatives			
Fenoprofen (Nalfon)	200	4–6	3200
Flurbiprofen (Ansaid)	50–100	6–12	300
Ibuprofen (Motrin)	300–800	6–8	3200
Ketoprofen (Orudis)	12.5–75	6–8	300
Naproxen (Naprosyn)	200–500	12	1250
Naproxen sodium (Anaprox)	275–550	12	1375
Oxaprozin (Daypro)	600–1200	12	1200
Heteroaryl acetic acid derivatives			
Diclofenac (Voltaren)	25–75	6–12	200
Ketorolac (intramuscular)			120
(Toradol)	15–60	6	
Ketorolac (oral)	10	4–6	40
Tolmetin (Tolectin)	200–600	6–8	1800
Indole and indene acetic acid derivatives			
Etodolac (Lodine)	200–400	6–12	1200
Indomethacin (Indocin)	25–50	8–12	200
Sulindac (Clinoril)	150–200	12	400
Anthranilic acid derivatives (fenamates)			
Meclofenamate	50–100	4–6	400
Mefenamic acid (Ponstel)	250	6	1000
Alkanone derivatives			
Nabumetone (Relafen)	1000	12–24	2000
Enolic acid derivatives (oxicams)			
Piroxicam (Feldene)	20	24	20
Cyclooxygenase 2 (COX-2)			
selective inhibitors			
Celecoxib (Celebrex)	100–200	12–24	400
Disease-modifying antirheumatic drugs (DMARDs)			
Leflunomide (Arava)	20	24	20[a]
Biological response modifiers (tumor necrosis factor α inhibitors)			
Adalimumab (Humira)	40 SC injection	Every other week	TBD
Etanercept (Enbrel)	25 SC injection	Once weekly	50 SC injection
Infliximab (Remicade)	3/kg IV. infusion	Every 4-6 weeks	10/kg

[a] Excludes loading dose of 100 mg/day for 3 days.
IV, intravenous; *SC,* subcutaneous; *TBD,* to be determined.

    (1) Diflunisal (500 mg)
    (2) Ibuprofen (200–400 mg)
    (3) Naproxen sodium (550 mg)
    (4) Ketoprofen (25–50 mg)
  c. The newer classes of drugs, in general, have not been compared to aspirin.

3. **Clinical use**
   a. Generally, the nonnarcotic analgesics are used orally to manage mild to moderate pain.
      (1) They are particularly suited for acute pain of skeletal muscle (orthopedic) or oral (dental) origin.
      (2) They are used to treat pain and inflammation associated with osteoarthritis and rheumatoid arthritis.
      (3) They are used in chronic pain and can have an additive effect with narcotic analgesics.
      (4) They also may be effective in managing pain owing to bone metastases.
   b. The NSAID ketorolac is administered intramuscularly and is useful in moderate to severe pain, particularly in cases in which narcotics are undesirable (e.g., with drug addicts, excessive narcotic sedation, respiratory depression).
   c. Patients may vary in their response and tolerance to nonnarcotic analgesics. If a patient does not respond to the maximum therapeutic dose, then an alternate NSAID should be tried. Likewise, if a patient experiences side effects with one drug, then another agent should be tried.
   d. Several drugs (e.g., diflunisal, choline magnesium trisalicylate, naproxen, celecoxib, leflunomide, etanercept, infliximab, and adalimumab) have long half-lives and, therefore, may be administered less frequently.
   e. The cost of nonnarcotic analgesics is highly variable and should be considered when an agent is selected. Pharmacotherapy with the COX-2 inhibitor celecoxib, the newer DMARDs like leflunomide or TNF-α inhibitors is significantly more expensive than older agents.

4. **Adverse effects**
   a. **Gastrointestinal (GI) effects.** Most nonnarcotic analgesics cause GI symptoms secondary to prostaglandin inhibition. At normal doses, acetaminophen and choline magnesium trisalicylate produce minimal GI upset. Because of their mechanism of action, the COX-2 inhibitors have a GI toxicity similar to placebo. Adalimumab, etanercept, infliximab, and leflunomide have been associated with GI side effects including nausea, abdominal pain, dyspepsia, constipation, vomiting, hematochezia, intestinal obduction, intestinal perforation, pancreatitis, peritonitis, peptic ulcer, and diarrhea.
      (1) The most common GI symptom is dyspepsia, but ulceration, bleeding, or perforation can occur.
      (2) Patients most predisposed to severe GI effects include the elderly, patients with a history of ulcers or chronic disease, and those who smoke or use alcohol.
      (3) To minimize GI effects, the lowest possible analgesic dose should be used. Aspirin, available as enteric-coated products, may minimize GI upset. Combination therapy with a GI "protectant" (e.g., antacid, H_2-antagonist, sucralfate, misoprostol) may be needed.
   b. **Hematological effects.** Most nonnarcotic analgesics inhibit platelet aggregation. The effect is produced by reversible inhibition of prostaglandin synthetase. Aspirin is an irreversible inhibitor. Acetaminophen and choline magnesium trisalicylate lack antiplatelet effects. TNF-α inhibitors have been associated with anemia, aplastic anemia, leukopenia, neutropenia, pancytopenia, and thrombocytopenia. Leflunomide has been associated with anemia and ecchymosis.
      (1) The effect of the NSAIDs correlates to the presence of an effective serum concentration.
      (2) Use of anticoagulants (e.g., heparin, warfarin [Coumadin] is relatively contraindicated in combination with aspirin or NSAIDs.
   c. **Renal effects.** NSAIDs can produce renal dysfunction. Etanercept has not been shown to affect renal function.
      (1) The mechanism of NSAID-induced renal dysfunction includes prostaglandin inhibition, interstitial nephritis, impaired renin secretion, and enhanced tubular water/sodium reabsorption.
      (2) Many risk factors have been implicated, including congestive heart failure (CHF), chronic renal failure (CRF), cirrhosis, dehydration, diuretic use, and atherosclerotic disease in elderly patients.
      (3) Renal dysfunction is commonly manifested as abrupt onset oliguria with sodium/water retention. The effect reverses after discontinuation of the NSAID.

d. Malignancies and lymphoproliferative disorders

Agents that block TNF may affect host defenses against malignancies because TNF mediates inflammation and modulates cellular immune response. Lymphomas have occurred more frequently in patients receiving TNF-blocking agents than in controls.

e. Infections. Opportunistic and serious infections leading to sepsis and death have been associated with leflunomide and the TNF-blocking agents.

f. Miscellaneous effects

(1) Even in normal doses, acetaminophen can cause hepatotoxicity in patients with liver disease or chronic alcoholism. Hepatotoxicity has also been reported with the use of all NSAIDs including the COX-2 selective inhibitors. Leflunomide and infliximab have also been shown to cause transient elevations in liver function tests such as aspartate aminotransferase (AST)—serum glutamic-oxaloacetic transaminase (SGOT)—and alanine aminotransferase (ALT)—serum glutamic-pyruvic transaminase (SGPT)

(2) Some patients exhibit acute hypersensitivity reactions to aspirin. Manifestations include either a rhinitis or asthma presentation or a true allergic reaction (e.g., urticaria, wheals, hypotension, shock, syncope). A cross-sensitivity to other NSAIDs may develop.

(3) Some NSAIDs produce central nervous system (CNS) effects, including impaired mentation, headaches, and attention deficit disorder.

(4) Leflunomide has received a **black box warning** because of its Category X pregnancy warning. It has also been associated with weight loss, alopecia, rash, and anemia.

(5) TNF-blocking agents have been associated with reactions at the injection site and autoantibody production.

(6) As of April 2005, the U.S. Food and Drug Administration (FDA) issued a **black box warning** for celecoxib, a selective COX-2 inhibitor, because if its link to an increased risk for cardiovascular events (heart attack and stroke) This increased risk has been demonstrated to be a drug class effect for all NSAIDs, excluding aspirin. Celecoxib is also contraindicated in patients with sulfonamide allergy.

5. Drug interactions. Salicylates have two clinically significant drug interactions.

a. Oral anticoagulants. Aspirin should be carefully monitored, if used, in anticoagulated patients because it inhibits platelet function and can cause gastric mucosal damage. This can significantly increases the risk of bleeding in anticoagulated patients. Also, doses of > 3 g/day of aspirin produces hypoprothrombinemia. Choline magnesium trisalicylate or acetaminophen can be used if a nonnarcotic is needed in an anticoagulated patient.

b. Methotrexate. Salicylates may enhance the toxicity of methotrexate. The primary mechanism is blockage of methotrexate renal tubular secretion by salicylates. The resultant methotrexate toxicity has been reported as pancytopenia or hepatotoxicity. Salicylates should be avoided in patients receiving methotrexate.

c. TNF-blocking agents. Anakinra (Kineret), a recombinant interleukin 1 (IL-1) receptor antagonist, has been observed to cause an increased risk of serious infections an neutropenia when used concomitantly with etanercept in patients with rheumatoid arthritis. Consequently, its use is not recommended concomitantly with any TNF-blocking agent.

B. Narcotic analgesics include the opioid drugs (Table 58-2). Because of their abuse potential, opioids are classified as controlled drugs. Special regulations control their prescribing.

1. Mechanism of action

a. Endogenous opiates afford the body self–pain-relieving mechanisms. These endogenous peptides include the endorphins, enkephalins, and dynorphins.

b. Exogenous opiates are classified as agonists (stimulate opiate receptors), antagonists (displace agonists from opiate receptors), and mixed opiates (agonist–antagonist or partial agonist actions).

c. Opiate receptors are located in the brain and spinal cord. Several types of opiate receptors have been identified, including μ, κ, δ, σ, and ϵ.

d. Stimulation of μ receptors produces the characteristic narcotic (morphine-like) effects.

(1) Analgesia

(2) Miosis

(3) Euphoria

(4) Respiratory depression

(5) Sedation

(6) Physical dependence

(7) Bradycardia

Table 58-2. Some Commonly Used Opioid Analgesics

Drug	Parenteral Dose (mg)[a]	Oral Dose (mg)[a]	Duration (hr)
Morphine	10	60	4–7
Morphine (CR) (MS Contin)	n/a	n/a	12–24
Hydromorphone (Dilaudid)	1.3	7.5	4–6
Oxymorphone (Numorphan)	1	—	4–6
Levorphanol (Levo-Dromoran)	2	4	4–7
Methadone (Dolophine)	10	20	4–6
Meperidine (Demerol)	75	300	3–6
Fentanyl (Sublimaze)	0.1	—	1–2
Fentanyl transdermal (Duragesic)	n/a	n/a	48–72
Codeine	130	200	4–6
Hydrocodone[b]	—	5–10	4–5
Dihydrocodeine[b]	—	32	4–5
Oxycodone[b]	—	5–10	4–5
Oxycodone (CR) (OxyContin)		n/a	12–24
Propoxyphene (Darvon)	—	65–100	4–6
Nalbuphine (Nubain)	10	—	4–6
Butorphanol (Stadol)	2	—	4–6
Dezocine (Dalgan)	10	—	4–7

[a]Doses equivalent to 10 mg intramuscular or subcutaneous morphine
[b]Doses for moderate pain not necessarily equivalent to 10 mg morphine.
CR, controlled release; *n/a,* not applicable.

e. The specific mechanism (central and spinal) of opiate agonist is alteration of the effects of nociceptive neurotransmitters, possibly norepinephrine or serotonin.

2. **Clinical use**
   a. Opioid analgesics are used for the management of moderate to severe pain (acute or chronic pain) of somatic or visceral origin.
   b. The use of narcotics should be individualized for each patient. The optimal analgesic dose varies from patient to patient. Each analgesic regimen should be titrated by increasing the dose up to the appearance of limiting adverse effects. Changing to another analgesic should occur only after an adequate therapeutic trial.
   c. The appropriate route of administration should be selected for each patient.
      (1) **Oral administration** is the preferred route, particularly for patients with chronic, stable pain. Controlled-release morphine and oxycodone tablets are available for convenience in controlling continuous pain, particularly in those patients with cancer.
      (2) **Intramuscular and subcutaneous administration** are very commonly used in the postoperative period. Fluctuations in absorption may occur, particularly in elderly or cachectic patients.
      (3) **Intravenous (IV) bolus administration** has the most rapid, predictable onset of effect.
      (4) **IV infusion** is used to titrate pain relief rapidly, particularly in patients with unstable chronic pain. Morphine is most commonly used, often with supplemental IV bolus doses for breakthrough pain. A mechanical infusion device is necessary.
      (5) **IV PCA** is most often used for acute postoperative pain. It produces prompt analgesia with minimal side effects because small doses (e.g., 1–2 mg morphine) are delivered at frequent intervals (e.g., every 10 min). It allows patient control of pain management. Morphine and meperidine are the most commonly used agents. A mechanical infusion device and properly trained patient and staff are necessary.
      (6) **Epidural** and **intrathecal administration** are used for acute postoperative pain and early management of chronic cancer pain. All drugs used epidurally or intrathecally must be preservative free because of the neurotoxicity of parabens and benzyl alcohol when administered via these routes. Intrathecal doses are generally 1/10 of the corresponding drug's epidural dose.
         (a) Low opiate doses stimulate spinal opiate receptors and reduce the amount of narcotic reaching the brain. This results in delayed or minimal effects such as sedation, nausea, and respiratory depression. The opiate distribution that causes

Table 58-3. Epidurally Administered Preservative-Free Opioids: Intermittent Dosing

Drug	Dose (mg)	Onset of Action (min)	Time to Peak Effect (min)	Duration of Action (hr)
Morphine	5–10	25	60	12–24
Fentanyl	0.1	5–10	20	6
Meperidine	50–100	5–10	15–30	7
Hydromorphone	1	10–15	20	12
Buprenorphine (Subutex)	0.3	30	40–60	8–9

such effects depends on the site of spinal injection, water solubility of the opiate, and volume infused. For example, after lumbar administration of a more water-soluble opiate (morphine), severe respiratory depression can be observed 12–24 hr after initial dosing.

  (b) Local side effects of intrathecal opiate administration are itching and urinary retention. Depending on the opiate used and the type of pain being treated, intermittent doses or continuous infusions (via a mechanical infusion device) can be used (Tables 58-3 and 58-4).

  (7) Rectal administration is an alternative for patients unable to take oral narcotics. Generally, poor absorption results in an unreliable analgesic response. It is an unacceptable route of administration for many patients.

  (8) Transdermal administration is an alternative for patients with chronic pain who are unable to take oral narcotics. A controlled-release patch is available for fentanyl. Slow onset requires additional analgesia when starting treatment. The duration of analgesia is 48–72 hr per patch. A slow reduction of effect follows removal of the patch and requires 24–36 hr of monitoring.

d. Patients who have chronic pain or acute pain that is constant throughout the day should receive regularly scheduled (around-the-clock) doses of narcotics.

  (1) Long-acting opiates (e.g., controlled-release morphine and oxycodone) are preferable.

  (2) A supplement given as needed may be necessary to manage breakthrough pain, for which short-acting opiates (e.g., immediate-release morphine, hydromorphone) are preferable. If frequent supplements are required, then the around-the-clock regimen should be adjusted based on morphine equivalents (Table 58-2).

e. Although the analgesia and side effects of opiates are qualitatively similar, individual patients may respond differently. Analgesic selection is based on:

  (1) Patient's past analgesia experience

  (2) Need for a rapid onset of effect

  (3) Preference for a long (or short) duration of action

  (4) Preference for a particular mode of delivery

  (5) Preference for a particular dosage form

  (a) Controlled-release morphine or oxycodone for a long duration of action (8–12 hr) may be preferable to opiates with long half-lives (e.g., methadone, levorphanol), which can accumulate and cause overdose symptoms (e.g., respiratory depression).

  (b) Transdermal fentanyl can be used for patients who are unable to swallow.

  (c) Rectal suppositories can be used for patients who are unable to swallow. They are available for morphine, hydromorphone, and oxymorphone.

Table 58-4. Epidurally Administered Preservative-Free Opioids: Continuous Infusion

Drug	Initial Bolus Dose (mg)	Infusion Concentration (mg/mL)	Rate (mg/hr)
Morphine	2	0.05–0.25	0.2–1.5
Fentanyl	0.05–0.1	0.005–0.025	0.02–0.15
Meperidine	50–100	10–20	5–20
Hydromorphone	0.5–1	0.02–0.05	0.15–0.3

(d) Concentrated hydromorphone injection (10 mg/mL) can be used for cachectic patients who require subcutaneous injections and in patients whose injection volumes must be minimized.

(6) Individual sensitivity to side effects, which includes nausea, euphoria, sedation, and respiratory depression

(a) Partial agonists or mixed agonist–antagonists may be preferable for acute pain management in patients at risk for respiratory depression secondary to opiate agonists. These agents should not be used in patients who have received chronic doses of opiates because withdrawal symptoms will occur.

(b) Epidural administration may be preferable for critically ill patients at risk for respiratory depression secondary to systemic narcotic administration.

3. **Adverse effects.** All narcotics can produce a variety of side effects that range from bothersome to life-threatening.

   a. **Constipation** occurs as a result of decreased intestinal tone and peristalsis. There is a patient variability, but generally most patients experience constipation after several days of therapy. Constipation may be more bothersome with certain types of opiates (e.g., codeine). It may occur sooner and be more problematic in hospitalized or bedridden patients or in patients who have received anesthesia or drugs with anticholinergic effects. Prophylaxis with a laxative/stool softener combination (e.g., bisacodyl/docusate (Gentlax-S) and dietary counseling are warranted for patients who need chronic opiate therapy.

   b. **Nausea** and **vomiting** occur owing to central stimulation of the chemoreceptor trigger zone. It is more problematic with one-time or intermittent parenteral dosing for acute pain. Occasionally, patients require concomitant therapy with an antiemetic (e.g., hydroxyzine, prochlorperazine; however, these agents may add to the sedative effects of opiates.

   c. **Sedation** is a dose-related effect but sometimes is enhanced by concomitant use of other drugs with sedating effects (e.g., benzodiazepines, antiemetics). Most chronic pain patients become tolerant to this effect, but occasionally the addition of a CNS stimulant, such as dextroamphetamine or methylphenidate, is needed.

      (1) Patients starting therapy with narcotics should be warned about driving or operating machinery.

      (2) Sedation may be a sign of excessive dosing or accumulation. However, sedation should not be confused with physiological sleep in patients who have pain-control difficulties. Patients in pain often develop insomnia. When pain is brought under control by appropriate narcotic titration, the patient initially may sleep for several hours.

   d. **Respiratory depression** is the most serious adverse effect accompanying narcotic overdose. Respiratory depression may be a sign of an excessive dose, accumulation of long half-lived opiates (e.g., methadone, levorphanol), or accumulation of active morphine metabolites in renal failure patients.

      (1) Respiratory rate should be carefully monitored in patients receiving IV or epidural opiates, in neonates, in elderly patients, and in patients receiving other drugs that cause respiratory depression.

      (2) The opiate antagonists, naloxone and nalmefene are administered intravenously to reverse life-threatening respiratory depression. Use of naloxone or nalmefene (Revex) in an opiate-dependent patient (e.g., a chronic cancer pain patient) can precipitate opiate withdrawal.

   e. **Anticholinergic effects,** such as dry mouth and urinary retention, can be bothersome for some patients.

   f. **Hypersensitivity** reactions, such as itching owing to histamine release, can occur secondary to opiate use, particularly with epidural or intrathecal administration. Wheals sometimes occur at the site of morphine injection. These reactions do not represent true allergy.

   g. **CNS excitation,** such as myoclonus and other seizure-like activity, can be produced with the use of meperidine in renal failure. These symptoms have also been observed in patients with normal renal functions who receive high doses of meperidine (e.g., < 800 mg/day of intramuscular meperidine). The accumulation of the metabolite normeperidine is the cause.

4. **Drug interactions**

   a. Narcotics have additive CNS depressant effects when used in combination with other drugs that also are CNS depressants (e.g., alcohol, anesthetics, antidepressants, antihistamines, barbiturates, benzodiazepines, phenothiazines).

   b. Narcotics, particularly meperidine, can cause severe reactions such as excitation, sweating, rigidity, and hypertension in patients receiving monoamine oxidase (MAO) inhibitors. Meperidine should be avoided and other narcotics started at lower doses in patients being treated with MAO inhibitors.

5. Tolerance means that increasing doses of opiate are needed to maintain analgesia. Tolerance usually develops to the analgesic, sedative, and euphoric effects of opioids, but not to the pupillary-constricting and constipating effects. This is usually observed as a decreasing duration of analgesia in chronic pain patients. The addition of an NSAID may help delay or provide adequate analgesia in tolerant patients.

6. Dependence. The use of opiates for chronic pain may result in physical dependence, such that the abrupt discontinuation of the opiate results in the development of withdrawal symptoms.

   a. Withdrawal symptoms include anxiety, irritability, insomnia, chills, salivation, rhinorrhea, diaphoresis, nausea, vomiting, GI cramping and diarrhea, and piloerection.

   (1) The appearance and intensity of withdrawal symptoms vary according to the half-life of the opiate. For example, the withdrawal symptoms after discontinuation of chronic methadone may take several days to develop and may be less intense than those of withdrawal from morphine owing to its shorter half-life.

   (2) The development of tolerance may be associated with withdrawal symptoms.

   (3) The use of naloxone or a partial agonist–antagonist such as pentazocine in a patient receiving chronic opiate therapy produces acute withdrawal.

   b. The development of physical dependence seen in chronic pain patients is not the same as psychological dependence or addiction. Also, the drug-seeking behavior observed in many acute pain patients (i.e., from postoperative pain) is not a sign of addiction, but rather a need for adequate pain relief. Studies suggest that the addictive rates for long-term treatment of noncancer pain are low in patients without a prior history of addiction. The analgesic needs of this type of patient should be reassessed and usually necessitates increasing the dose of opiate, changing to a longer duration drug, changing to a PCA, or adding an analgesic adjunct.

C. Tramadol (Ultram) is an oral, centrally acting analgesic with weak opiate activity. It has not been placed in a controlled drug schedule.

1. Mechanism of action

   a. Tramadol is a synthetic aminocyclohexanol that binds to opiate receptors, inhibiting norepinephrine and serotonin.

   b. The analgesic effects are partially antagonized by naloxone.

2. Clinical use

   a. Tramadol is used for moderate to moderately severe pain.

   b. The recommended dosage is 50–100 mg every 4–6 hr, up to a maximum of 400 mg/day.

   c. At maximum dosage, tramadol appears no more effective than acetaminophen–codeine combinations.

3. Adverse effects

   a. GI effects include nausea, constipation, and dry mouth.

   b. CNS effects include dizziness, headache, sedation, and seizures (overdose).

   c. Diaphoresis

4. Drug interactions

   a. Tramadol can increase the sedative effect of alcohol and hypnotics.

   b. Tramadol inhibits monoamine uptake and should not be used with MAO inhibitors.

   c. Tramadol used with selective serotonin reuptake inhibitors (SSRIs) and other agents that increase serotonergic activity can cause "serotonin syndrome," which is characterized by irritability, anxiety, CNS excitation, and myoclonus.

D. Adjuvant analgesics

Adjuvant analgesics are drugs whose initial FDA approved indication was for a condition other than pain. Other classes of drugs affect nonopiate pain pathways and may be useful in certain types of pain (e.g., neuropathic pain). These drugs often are used with other analgesics and some may help manage narcotic side effects (Table 58-5).

Table 58-5. Analgesic Adjuncts

Class	Drugs	Indications
Tricyclic antidepressants	Amitriptyline (Elavil), desipramine (Norpramin), doxepin (Sinequan), imipramine (Tofranil)	Neurogenic pain; chronic pain complicated by depression or insomnia
Anticonvulsants	Gabapentin (Neurontin), pregabalin (Lyrica), carbamazepine (Tegretol), clonazepam (Klonopin), phenytoin (Dilantin), valproate (Depakote),	Lancinating neurogenic pain (e.g., trigeminal neuralgia, phantom limb pain, post-trauma neurogenic pain)
Neuroleptics	Fluphenazine (Prolixin), haloperidol (Haldol), prochlorperazine (Compazine)	Refractory neurogenic pain; pain complicated by delirium or nausea (prochlorperazine)
Corticosteroid	Dexamethasone (Decadron)	Pain from neural infiltration; pain associated with bony metastases
Antihistamine	Hydroxyzine (Atarax, Vistaril)	Pain complicated by anxiety or nausea
Benzodiazepines	Alprazolam (Xanax), lorazepam (Ativan)	Pain complicated by anxiety or muscle spasm
Amphetamines	Dextroamphetamine (Dexedrine), methylphenidate (Ritalin)	For excessive opiate-induced sedation in chronic pain patients

1. **Neuropathic pain agents** include anticonvulsants (e.g., gabapentin, pregabalin, lamotrigine, carbamazepine), systemic local anesthetic agents—for example,, 5% lidocaine (Lidoderm) patch)—and tricyclic antidepressants—such as, amitriptyline, nortriptyline, and desipramine. Gabapentin and systemic local anesthetic agents are considered first-line therapy in treating polyneuropathies.
   a. **Mechanism of action.**
      (1) Gabapentin and pregabalin may relieve neuropathic pain by the presynaptic binding of the α-2-δ subunit of voltage-sensitive calcium channels.
      (2) Pregabalin may also modulate the release of the sensory neuropeptide substance P.
      (3) Lamotrigine and carbamazepine are believed to block sodium channels at the site of ectopic discharge of damaged nerves.
      (4) The use of local anesthetics allows for local pain relief without systemic toxicity, specifically by binding to the sodium channels in the damaged nerves.
      (1) It is hypothesized that TCAs obtain their analgesic effects as a result of sodium channel blockade at the site of ectopic discharge in the peripheral nerves.
      (6) All of these agents are recommended to aid in the reduction of neuronal hyperexcitability, whether it is peripherally or centrally.
   b. **Clinical use**
      (1) Data are available to give guidance on which agents to use to treat neuropathic pain, but they do not predict which agent will provide relief for each individual patient's pain.
      (2) Typically, a **treatment algorithm** may recommend:
         (a) **First line**
            (i) Gabapentin
            (ii) Pregabalin
            (iii) 5% lidocaine patches
            (iv) TCAs
         (b) **Second line**
            (i) Other anticonvulsants (lamotrigine or carbamazepine)
            (ii) Other antidepressants (bupropion, citalopram, paroxetine, venlafaxine, imipramine)
         (c) **Other**
            (i) Capsaicin, clonidine

c. **Adverse effects.** the most common adverse events associated with anticonvulsants are dizziness, headaches, and drowsiness. Lamotrigine has been associated with the development of Stevens-Johnson syndrome (SJS). It is recommended that lamotrigine be titrated up every 2 weeks to minimize the occurrence of SJS.

E. **Miscellaneous agents**

1. **Capsaicin,** a component of red peppers, causes the release of substance P from sensory nerve fibers, resulting in prolonged cutaneous pain transmission, histamine release, and erythema because of reflex vasodilation. Repeated local application depletes the peripheral sensory C-nerve fiber of substance P, resulting in pain inhibition. Topical capsaicin cream 0.025% or 0.075% has been shown to be useful in treating joint pain and tenderness in patients with arthritis. Other uses may include treating diabetic neuralgia, reflex sympathetic dystrophy, trigeminal neuralgia, notalgia paresthetica, psoriasis and psoralen (P), and long-wave ultraviolet radiation (UVA) induced skin pain, and postherpetic neuralgia. Local toxicity may include burning, stinging, erythema, pruritus, and superficial skin ulcers.

2. **Glucosamine sulfate and chondroitin sulfate** have been used with increasing frequency in the treatment of degenerative joint disease. Glucosamine sulfate appears to act as a substrate for and stimulant to the biosynthesis of glucosaminoglycans and hyaluronic acid for forming proteoglycans found in the structural matrix of joints. Chondroitin sulfate provides additional substrates for the formation of healthy joint matrix. Short-term side effects associated with glucosamine include GI problems, drowsiness, skin reactions, and headache. Further research is needed to validate their roles.

F. **Nonpharmacological pain management.** Other therapeutic modalities for pain management include cognitive behavioral interventions and physical methods. These modalities are appropriate for interested patients, patients experiencing anxiety with their pain, patients who have incomplete relief from analgesic therapy, and patients who need to avoid or reduce analgesic use (e.g., those with chronic nonmalignant pain).

1. **Cognitive behavioral interventions** include education and instruction, simple relaxation, biofeedback, and hypnosis.

2. **Physical methods** include acupuncture, physical therapy, compression gloves, orthotic devices, heat and cold applications, massage, exercise, rest, immobilization, and transcutaneous electrical nerve stimulation (TENS).

STUDY QUESTIONS

Directions for questions 1–7: Each of the questions, statements, or incomplete statements in this section can be correctly answered or completed by **one** of the suggested answers or phrases. Choose the **best** answer.

1. An emaciated 69-year-old man with advanced inoperable throat cancer is hospitalized for pain management. He is receiving a morphine solution (40 mg orally) every 3 hr for pain. He complains of dysphagia and the frequency with which he must take morphine. An appropriate analgesic alternative for this patient would be

(A) changing to a controlled-release oral morphine.
(B) increasing the dose of the oral morphine solution.
(C) changing to intramuscular methadone.
(D) changing to transdermal fentanyl.
(E) decreasing the frequency of oral morphine administration.

For questions 2–3: A 52-year-old woman with a diagnosis of ovarian cancer presents with complaints of pain. Her pain was reasonably well controlled with two capsules of oxycodone every 4 hr until 2 weeks ago, at which point she was hospitalized for pain control. She was placed on meperidine (75 mg) every 3 hr but still complained about pain. Her meperidine dosage was increased to 100 mg every 2 hr.

2. At this dosage of meperidine, the patient is likely to experience

(A) excellent pain relief.
(B) respiratory depression.
(C) worsening renal function.
(D) myoclonic seizures.
(E) excessive sedation.

3. An appropriate next step in this patient's therapy would be to

(A) add a nonsteroidal anti-inflammatory drug (NSAID).
(B) discontinue the meperidine and convert her to a controlled-release oral morphine or oxycodone.
(C) continue the present meperidine dosage because she will eventually get relief.
(D) decrease the meperidine dose to avoid side effects.
(E) consider hypnosis or relaxation techniques.

4. A 20-year-old victim of a motor vehicle accident is 3 days postsurgery for orthopedic and internal injuries. He has been in severe pain and was placed on a regimen of intramuscular morphine (5–10 mg) every 4 hr as needed for pain. A pain consultant starts the patient with a 20-mg intravenous morphine loading dose and then begins a continuous intravenous morphine infusion with as-needed morphine boosters. About 2 hr after this regimen is started, the patient is asleep. The nurse is concerned and calls the physician. The physician should

(A) call for a psychiatric consult.
(B) administer naloxone.
(C) examine the patient and reconfirm the dosage and monitoring parameters.
(D) add an injectable nonsteroidal anti-inflammatory drug (NSAID).
(E) add an amphetamine.

5. Potential adverse effects associated with aspirin include all of the following *except*

(A) gastrointestinal ulceration.
(B) renal dysfunction.
(C) enhanced methotrexate toxicity.
(D) cardiac arrhythmias.
(E) hypersensitivity asthma.

6. All of the following facts are true about non-steroidal anti-inflammatory drugs (NSAIDs) *except* which one?

(A) They are antipyretic.
(B) There is a ceiling effect to their analgesia.
(C) They can cause tolerance.
(D) They do not cause dependence.
(E) They are anti-inflammatory.

7. Which of the following narcotics has the longest duration of effect?

(A) methadone
(B) controlled-release morphine
(C) levorphanol
(D) transdermal fentanyl
(E) dihydromorphone

Directions for questions 8–10: The questions and incomplete statements in this section can be correctly answered or completed by **one or more** of the suggested answers. Choose the answer, **A–E.**

A	if **I only** is correct
B	if **III only** is correct
C	if **I and II** are correct
D	if **II and III** are correct
E	if **I, II, and III** are correct

8. Agents that are safe to use in a patient with bleeding problems include

(I) choline magnesium trisalicylate
(II) acetaminophen
(III) ketorolac

9. Which of the following drugs bind or capture excess TNF-α?

(I) adalimumab
(II) etanercept
(III) leflunomide

10. Leflunomide has been associated with

(I) diarrhea.
(II) alopecia.
(III) anemia.

ANSWERS AND EXPLANATIONS

1. The answer is D *[see II.B.2.c.(8)].*
Patients with throat cancer often cannot take oral analgesics. The patient described in the question is also having pain difficulties with an every 3-hr regimen. Transdermal fentanyl is a good alternative because, after titration, excellent analgesia can be produced without using oral or parenteral agents. Also, the frequency of analgesic use may be decreased when titration has occurred.

2. The answer is D *[see II.B.3.g].*

3. The answer is B *[see II.B.2.c.(1); II.B.2.d.(1)].*
Myoclonic seizures can occur after frequent, high-dose meperidine owing to the accumulation of the metabolite, normeperidine. Both oxycodone and meperidine have short durations of effect. In the chronic pain patient, an around-the-clock regimen, using a controlled-released oral morphine, would be an appropriate alternative. With titration, the patient should have good pain relief with an every 8- to 12-hr regimen.

4. The answer is C *[see II.B.3.c].*
A patient suffering from pain cannot sleep properly. When the pain is adequately controlled, the patient may sleep initially for many hours. This usually is not oversedation owing to the narcotic. These patients should be monitored closely (e.g., respiratory rate), and other sedating drugs should be eliminated. Usually, no other intervention is needed.

5. The answer is D *[see II.A.4].*
Aspirin has several adverse effects and drug interactions. However, cardiac arrhythmias are not induced by aspirin.

6. The answer is C *[see II.A.2].*
Unlike the opiates, NSAID use is not associated with the development of tolerance.

7. The answer is D *[see Table 58-2].*
Transdermal fentanyl is a controlled-release dosage form that is effective for up to a 72-hr period. All of the other drugs listed in the question are effective for periods of 1–8 hr.

8. The answer is C *(I, II) [see II.A.4.b].*
Unlike aspirin and NSAIDs, acetaminophen and choline magnesium trisalicylate lack antiplatelet effects. Therefore, they are safe to use for patients with bleeding problems.

9. The answer is C *(I, II) [see II.A.1].*
Adalimumab, etanercept, and infliximab act by binding or capturing excess TNF-α, one of the dominant cytokines or proteins that play an important role in the inflammatory response. The exact mechanism of action of leflunomide, a novel drug used to treat rheumatoid arthritis, is not completely known but it is thought to inhibit pyrimidine synthesis.

10. The answer is E *(I, II, III) [see II.A.4.a; II.A.4.d.(4)].*
Leflunomide has been associated with weight loss, diarrhea, nausea, alopecia, rash, anemia, and transient elevations in liver function tests.

59
Nutrition and the Hospitalized Patient

Robert A. Quercia

Kevin P. Keating

Maria Evasovich

I. NUTRITIONAL PROBLEMS IN HOSPITALIZED PATIENTS

A. Incidence. It has been estimated that 30%–50% of patients admitted to hospitals have some degree of malnutrition. As many as 75% of patients undergo a deterioration of nutritional status while hospitalized.

B. Definitions

1. **Malnutrition** is a pathological state, resulting from a relative or absolute deficiency or excess of one or more essential nutrients.

2. **Marasmus** is a chronic disease that develops over months or years as a result of a deficiency in total caloric intake. Depletion of fat stores and skeletal protein occurs to meet metabolic needs. Marasmic patients are generally not hypermetabolic and are able to preserve their visceral protein compartment as determined by measurements of serum albumin, prealbumin, and transferrin.
   a. Marasmus is a well-adapted form of malnutrition, and despite a cachectic appearance, immunocompetence, wound healing, and the ability to handle short-term stress are generally well preserved.
   b. Nutritional support in these patients should be initiated cautiously because aggressive repletion can result in severe metabolic disturbances, such as hypokalemia and hypophosphatemia.

3. **Kwashiorkor** is an acute process that can develop within weeks and is associated with visceral protein depletion and impaired immune function. It is the result of poor protein intake with adequate to slightly inadequate caloric intake; thus patients usually appear well nourished. A hypermetabolic state (e.g., trauma, infection) combined with protein deprivation can rapidly develop into a severe kwashiorkor malnutrition characterized by hypoalbuminemia, edema, and impaired cellular immune function.
   a. In hospitalized patients, the development of kwashiorkor has been implicated in poor wound healing, gastrointestinal (GI) bleeding, and sepsis.
   b. Aggressive nutritional support to replete protein stores and decrease morbidity and mortality is indicated when the diagnosis of kwashiorkor is made.

4. **Mixed marasmic kwashiorkor** is a severe form of protein–calorie malnutrition that usually develops when a marasmic patient is subjected to an acute hypermetabolic stress, such as trauma, surgery, or infection.
   a. This condition results in depletion of fat stores, skeletal muscle protein, and visceral protein.
   b. Because of the marked immune dysfunction that develops in this state, vigorous nutritional support is indicated.

II. NUTRITIONAL ASSESSMENT AND METABOLIC REQUIREMENTS

A. Nutritional assessment. The most commonly used tools for nutritional assessment are as follows:

1. **Subjective global assessment (SGA)** relies heavily on the patient's history.
   a. SGA takes into account:
      (1) Recent weight change
      (2) Diet history
      (3) Type and length of symptoms affecting nutritional status (e.g., nausea, vomiting, diarrhea)
      (4) Functional status
      (5) Metabolic demands of the current disease process
      (6) Gross physical signs
          (a) Status of subcutaneous fat
          (b) Evidence of muscle wasting
          (c) Presence or absence of edema and ascites
   b. Patients are then classified as being well nourished or moderately or severely malnourished.

2. **Prognostic nutritional index (PNI)** is derived from a formula that attempts to quantify a patient's risk of developing operative complications based on a variety of markers of nutritional status.

   $$\text{PNI (\%)} = 158 - 16.6 \, (\text{ALB}) - 0.78 \, (\text{TSF}) - 0.20 \, (\text{TFN}) - 5.8 \, (\text{DH})$$

   where ALB is the serum albumin (g/dL); TSF is the triceps skin-fold thickness (mm); TFN is the serum transferrin (mg/dL); and DH is the delayed hypersensitivity skin-test reactivity graded 0 (nonreactive), 1 (< 5 mm induration), or 2 (≥ 5 mm induration).

   a. **Predicted risk of complications**
      (1) Low risk: PNI $< 40\%$
      (2) Intermediate risk: PNI $= 40\%$–49%
      (3) High risk: PNI $\geq 50\%$
   b. **Serum markers** (i.e., albumin, transferrin) are indicators of visceral protein status.
   c. **Delayed hypersensitivity reaction** is an indicator of immune competence.
   d. **PNI** is of value in predicting the potential for complications in stable patients scheduled to undergo elective surgery.

3. **Body composition analysis** assesses nutritional status by measuring and comparing the ratios of various body compartments.
   a. **Bioelectrical impedance.** The resistance to an electrical current is used to calculate lean body mass. The equipment is relatively inexpensive and easy to use. The results are inaccurate in critically ill patients and patients with fluid and electrolyte abnormalities.
   b. **Dual-energy x-ray absorptiometry (DEXA).** The differential attenuation of x-rays is used to measure fat and lean body mass. The equipment is expensive, and results are affected by hydration status.
   c. **Total body potassium** estimates lean body mass by using a whole body counter to measure a potassium isotope concentrated in lean tissue. This method of body composition analysis is impractical and available at only a few centers.
   d. **Total body water** estimates lean body mass from deuterium total body water measurements. This technique is clinically impractical.
   e. **In vivo neutron activation analysis.** Unlike other techniques, this analysis divides the body into several compartments. This technique requires a significant dose of radiation and is available at only a few research centers.

4. **Tests of physiological function** attempt to quantitate malnutrition based on the decrease in muscle strength caused by amino acid mobilization.
   a. **Maximum voluntary grip strength** is measured with isokinetic dynamometry. The results correlate well to total body protein. This test requires patient cooperation.
   b. **Electrical stimulation of the ulnar nerve** measures contractile function of the adductor pollicis muscle. This technique does not require voluntary patient effort and is inexpensive and easy to do. Its prognostic reliability is still under evaluation.

B. **Metabolic requirements**

1. **Energy requirements** are determined as **nonprotein calories (NPCs).** It is important to avoid excess calories to minimize complications of nutrient delivery and to optimize nutrient metabolism. Energy requirements can be determined by the following three methods.
   a. **Indirect calorimetry or measured energy expenditure (MEE)** is the most accurate method of determining caloric requirements.

(1) Oxygen (O_2) consumption and carbon dioxide (CO_2) production are measured directly.

(2) Energy expenditure is related directly to oxygen consumption and is calculated from these measurements.

(3) A respiratory quotient (RQ) can also be obtained from an MEE and is defined as the ratio of the amount of CO_2 produced to that of O_2 consumed during the course of oxidation of body fuels. The oxidation of carbohydrate results in an RQ of 1.0—that is, as much CO_2 is produced as O_2 is consumed. The oxidation of fat produces significantly less CO_2 and results in an RQ of 0.7. Normal mixed substrate oxidation results in an RQ of 0.8–0.9.

(4) The provision of excess carbohydrate calories causes their conversion to fat (lipogenesis). Lipogenesis produces significantly more carbon dioxide than oxidation does. This can result in an RQ > 1.0, which is consistent with overfeeding. The determination of RQ can, therefore, indicate patterns of substrate use.

b. **Estimated energy expenditure (EEE)** first requires the calculation of the **basal energy expenditure (BEE)** from the **Harris-Benedict equation;** the BEE is then multiplied by appropriate stress and activity factors.

(1) **Men:** BEE = 66.5 + [13.8 × weight (kg)] + [5 × height (cm)] − [6.8 × age (years)]

(2) **Women:** BEE = 655 + [9.6 × weight (kg)] + [1.8 × height (cm)] − [4.7 × age (years)]

(3) **Stress factors:** uncomplicated surgery 1.00–1.05, peritonitis 1.05–1.25, and sepsis or multiple trauma 1.25–1.5

(4) **Activity factors:** bedrest 0.95–1.10 and ambulation 1.10–1.30

c. **Simple nomogram.** The least accurate method of estimating caloric requirements, this technique is based on the patient's weight in kilograms. It is useful when the other methods cannot be used. Patients with mild to moderate degrees of stress require approximately 25–30 kcal/kg/day, whereas the severely stressed patient (e.g., a patient with major burns) may require 35 kcal/kg/day or more.

2. **Protein (nitrogen) requirements** can be determined by a number of techniques, but nitrogen balance determinations and nomograms appear to be the most practical.

a. **Nitrogen balance techniques.** The practitioner determines the patient's nitrogen output and develops a nutritional support program in which the protein administered results in a nitrogen input that exceeds losses.

(1) Nitrogen balance = 24-hr nitrogen intake − 24-hr nitrogen output.

(2) A 24-hr nitrogen intake = 24-hr total protein intake, ÷ 6.25 (approximately 16% of protein is composed of nitrogen).

(3) A 24-hr nitrogen output = [24-hr urine urea nitrogen (UUN) × 1.25 + 2, where 1.25 accounts for non-UUN losses (e.g., ammonia, creatinine) and 2 accounts for non-urine nitrogen losses (e.g., skin, feces). Total urinary nitrogen (TUN) determinations are currently available in some centers. Because TUN is a more accurate method of assessing urinary nitrogen losses, it should be used when available in place of a 24-hr UUN × 1.25 when calculating a nitrogen balance.

(4) A positive nitrogen balance of 3–6 g is the goal.

(5) This method cannot be used in renally impaired patients.

b. **Nomogram method.** This method estimates protein needs based on lean body weight. Protein requirements are 1.5–2.0 g protein/kg/day for hospitalized patients.

c. **Nonprotein calorie to nitrogen (NPC:N) ratio.** An NPC:N ratio of 125–150:1 generally has been recommended for the mildly to moderately stressed patient to achieve optimal nitrogen retention and protein synthesis. In the severely stressed patient, some studies indicate that ratios as low as 85:1 may be effective.

3. **Essential fatty acids (EFAs)** are those polyunsaturated fatty acids that cannot be synthesized by humans. EFAs affect immune responses by influencing energy production, eicosanoid synthesis, and cell membrane fluidity. They also affect levels of arachidonic acid in lymphocytes—especially monocytes, macrophages, and polymorphonuclear neutrophils (PMNs). Linoleic acid, an omega-6 polyunsaturated fatty acid (PUFA), is the principal EFA for humans. α-Linolenic acid, an omega-3 PUFA, also cannot be synthesized in vivo; its metabolic significance in humans continues to be investigated. It might be a conditionally essential fatty acid.

a. Deficiency states of **linoleic acid** are characterized by diarrhea, dermatitis, and hair loss.

   b. The currently available lipid emulsions have a high linoleic acid content.
   c. Providing 4%–7% of a patient's caloric requirements as linoleic acid from lipid emulsion prevents the development of essential fatty acid deficiency.

4. **Vitamins** are essential for proper substrate metabolism. Accepted daily allowances for oral administration have been established. **The FDA recently approved a new multivitamin preparation for adults receiving parenteral nutrition (PN).**
   a. Vitamin A (fat soluble). Normal stores can last up to 1 year but are rapidly depleted by stress. Vitamin A has essential functions in vision, growth, and reproduction. Recommended oral intake is 2500–5000 IU/day. **The recommended requirement is 3300 IU/ day in PN formulations.**
   b. Vitamin D (fat soluble). In conjunction with parathormone and calcitonin, vitamin D helps regulate calcium and phosphorous homeostasis. Recommended oral intake is 100–400 IU/day. **The PN requirement is 200 IU/day.**
   c. Vitamin E (fat soluble) appears to function as an antioxidant, inhibiting the oxidation of free unsaturated fatty acids. Recommended daily oral allowances are 12–15 IU/day. **The requirement in PN formulations is 10 IU/day.** The presence of polyunsaturated fatty acids increases the requirement for vitamin E, which needs to be considered with the use of lipid system PN.
   d. Vitamin K (fat soluble) plays an essential role in the synthesis of clotting factors. The suggested oral intake is 0.7–2.0 mg/day. **The recommended PN requirement is 150 μg/day.**
   e. Vitamin B_1 (thiamine; water soluble) functions as a coenzyme in the phosphogluconate pathway and as a structural component of nervous system membranes. The development of its deficiency state (i.e., acute pernicious beriberi with high output cardiac failure) is well described in patients on PN receiving inadequate thiamine replacement. A prolonged deficiency state can cause Wernicke encephalopathy. Recommended doses are 0.5 mg/1000 oral calories/day and **6 mg/day in PN formulations.**
   f. Vitamin B_2 (riboflavin; water soluble) functions as a coenzyme in oxidative phosphorylation. Essentially, no intracellular stores are maintained. Oral requirements are 1.3–1.7 mg/day. **The requirement in PN formulations is 3.6 mg/day.**
   g. Vitamin B_3 (niacin; water soluble) functions as a coenzyme in oxidative phosphorylation and biosynthetic pathways. Pellagra is the well-described deficiency state. Oral requirements are 14.5–19.8 mg/day. **The recommended PN requirement is 40 mg/ day.**
   h. Vitamin B_5 (pantothenic acid; water soluble). The functional form of vitamin B_5 is coenzyme A, which is essential to all acylation reactions. Oral requirements are 5–10 mg/day. Intravenous (IV) requirements are 10–29 mg/day.
   i. Vitamin B_6 (pyridoxine; water soluble) functions as a coenzyme in a variety of enzymatic pathways. Deficiency states are accentuated by some medications, including isoniazid, penicillamine, and cycloserine. Oral requirements are 1.5–2.0 mg/day. **The recommended PN requirement is 6.0 mg/day.**
   j. Vitamin B_7 (biotin; water soluble) functions in carboxylation reactions. It is synthesized by intestinal flora; therefore, deficiency states are rare. **The requirement in PN formulations is 60 μg/day.**
   k. Vitamin B_9 (folic acid; water soluble) is involved in a variety of biosynthetic reactions and amino acid conversions. Folate cofactors are necessary for purine and pyrimidine (DNA) synthesis. Stores usually last 3–6 months; however, rapid depletion is seen with metabolic stress. Deficiency of vitamin B_{12} causes deficiency in folate. A megaloblastic anemia is classic in the deficiency state. Deficiency of folic acid in a pregnant mother can cause neural tube defects in the fetus. Oral requirements are 200–400 μg/day. **The recommended requirement in PN formulations is 600 μg/day.**
   l. Vitamin B_{12} (cyanocobalamin; water soluble) has a variety of metabolic and biosynthetic functions. Because of large stores, deficiency states can take years to develop. Megaloblastic (pernicious) anemia is one manifestation of deficiency. Another manifestation of deficiency is peripheral neuropathy because B_{12} is responsible for biosynthesis of the insulation sheet on nerves called myelin. Oral requirements are 2 μg/day. **The requirement in PN formulations is 5.0 μg/day.**

5. **Trace mineral deficiency** may develop during PN because of reduced intake, increased use, decreased plasma binding, or increased excretion.

   a. **Iron** is necessary for hemoglobin and myoglobin production and is a necessary cofactor in a variety of enzymatic reactions. Deficiency is classically demonstrated by a hypochromic, microcytic anemia as well as by the development of immune deficiency. Oral requirements are 16–18 mg/day. IV requirements are 0.5–1.0 mg/day.
   b. **Zinc** is necessary for DNA and RNA synthesis and is a necessary cofactor in a variety of enzymatic reactions. Zinc deficiency results in impaired wound healing, growth retardation, hair loss, dermatitis, diarrhea, anorexia, and glucose intolerance. Patients at high risk for developing zinc deficiency are those with long-term steroid therapy, malabsorption syndromes, fistulas, sepsis, and major surgery. Oral requirements are 10–15 mg/day. IV requirements are **3.0-5.0 mg/day.**
   c. **Copper** is necessary for heme synthesis, electron transport, and wound healing. Deficiency that develops during PN usually manifests as anemia, leukopenia, and neutropenia. Oral requirements are 30 μg/kg/day. **Intravenous requirements are 0.5–1.5 mg/day.**
   d. **Manganese** is involved in protein synthesis and possibly glucose use. Oral requirements are 0.7–22 mg/day. **Intravenous requirements are 150–300 μg/day.**
   e. **Selenium** is important in antioxidant reactions. Deficiency during PN has been associated with muscle pain and cardiomyopathy. **Intravenous** requirements are **40–60 μg/day.**
   f. **Iodine** is a component of the thyroid hormones. Deficiency manifests as a goiter. Recommended intake is 1 μg/kg/day.
   g. **Chromium** is important in glucose use and potentiates the effect of insulin. Signs of deficiency include hyperglycemia and abnormal glucose tolerance. Oral requirements are 70–80 μg/day. Intravenous (IV) maintenance requirements are 0.14–0.2 μg/kg/day (10–15 μg/day). **Suggested IV requirements for deficiency and severe glucose intolerance are 150–200 μg/day.**
   h. **Molybdenum** is essential to xanthine oxidase. Oral requirements are 2.0 μg/kg/day.

III. METHODS OF SUPPORT

A. PN is also called **total parenteral nutrition (TPN)** and **hyperalimentation.** It is used to meet the patient's nutritional requirements when the enteral route cannot accomplish this.

   1. **Indications.** When the enteral route cannot be used because of dysfunction or disease states (e.g., acute pancreatitis, inflammatory bowel disease, complete bowel obstruction), PN is instituted.

   2. **Initiation** of PN should be undertaken within 1–3 days in moderately to severely malnourished patients when the inadequacy of enteral support is anticipated for more than 5–7 days. In healthy or mildly malnourished patients, PN should be initiated within 5–7 days if enteral support has not been initiated.

   3. **Routes of administration**
      a. **A central venous route** is used with hypertonic PN formulations (i.e., dextrose concentrations > 10%). Most commonly, dextrose concentrations of 25% are used centrally, and the osmolarity exceeds 2000 mOsm/L. Such highly osmolar solutions must be infused into a large-diameter central vein (e.g., superior vena cava), where they are rapidly diluted by high flow rates.
      b. **A peripheral venous route** can be used when the dextrose concentration is 10% or less.
         (1) Solutions with 10% dextrose, amino acids, electrolytes, and trace minerals have a resulting osmolarity of 900–1000 mOsm/L. Higher osmolarity is associated with a higher incidence of thrombophlebitis.
         (2) The major reason for use of the central venous PN rather than the peripheral route is the development of thrombophlebitis. Maintaining the osmolality of the peripheral PN solution < 900 mOsm/kg and preferably between 600 and 800 mOsm/kg with intravenous lipid emulsion administered concurrently over 24 hr minimizes the incidence of thrombophlebitis. Also, the development of new peripheral fine-bore catheters made from polyurethane or silicone has been shown to be significantly less thrombogenic. In addition, the use of low-dose heparin (1 unit/mL) and

hydrocortisone (5 mg/L) delivered in the PN solutions has been shown to protect against thrombophlebitis.

(3) **Glyceryl trinitrate** patches (5 mg), when applied over the area where the tip of the catheter is expected to lie, have been shown to significantly reduce peripheral PN infusion failure caused by phlebitis. With the use of this new catheter technology and new techniques for infusion, it is now feasible to administer peripheral PN in selected patients for short-term therapy (7–10 days) with a low incidence of peripheral vein thrombophlebitis.

4. **NPC sources**
   a. **Dextrose monohydrate** is the form of dextrose used for parenteral administration. It yields 3.4 kcal/g. It is the component in PN formulas that contributes the most to osmolarity. It is available commercially in concentrations up to 70%.
   b. **Intravenous lipids** are commercially available as 10% or 20% emulsions derived from soybean oil (Intralipid) or a combination of soybean oil and safflower oil (Liposyn II).
      (1) Both the 10% and 20% emulsions are isotonic (280 and 340 mOsm/L, respectively) and can be administered via the peripheral vein with a low incidence of phlebitis; these emulsions provide 1.1 and 2.0 kcal/mL, respectively. They contain 1.2% egg yolk phospholipids as the emulsifying agent and 2.25%–2.5% glycerol to make the emulsions isosmotic.
      (2) Lipid emulsions can be given as part of the daily NPC requirement or 2–3 times per week to prevent essential fatty acid deficiency. Both types of lipid emulsion contain particles of 0.4–0.5 μm, which prevents the use of 0.22 μm bacterial retention filters.

5. **Protein (nitrogen) source. Synthetic crystalline amino acids** are currently used as the nitrogen source in PN formulations.
   a. **These formulations are available commercially without electrolytes and dextrose in concentrations of 5.5% (Travasol), 8.5% (Travasol), 10% (Aminosyn II, Travasol), 15%. (Aminosyn II, Clinisol) and 20% (Prosol).**
   b. These formulations yield 4 kcal/g.
   c. These solutions generally contain a mixture of free essential and nonessential L-amino acids.
   d. Specialized amino acid formulations are available for specific disease states.

6. **Systems of PN**
   a. **Glucose system PN**
      (1) **Definition.** The glucose system PN is a parenteral formulation in which dextrose is used exclusively as the NPC source. Nitrogen is provided as crystalline amino acids. Electrolytes, vitamins, and trace minerals are added to the formulation as needed.
      (2) **Administration.** The glucose system PN formulations usually have dextrose concentrations of 25% or greater and must be administered by the central venous route. These formulations are also referred to as two-in-one formulations because the dextrose and amino acids are usually mixed in one container with electrolytes, vitamins, and trace minerals.
         (a) Because of the high dextrose concentration, initial administration should be at low hourly rates (e.g., 50 mL/hr) and increased gradually over 24 hr to avoid hyperglycemia (> 200 mg/dL).
         (b) To avoid reactive hypoglycemia (< 70 mg/dL), discontinuation should be gradual over several hours.
         (c) Lipid emulsions should be administered for **essential fatty acid replacement** in a dose that provides 4%–7% of required calories as linoleic acid. This can be accomplished by the administration of 250 mL of 20% or 500 mL of 10% emulsion, two to three times weekly.
   b. **Lipid system PN**
      (1) **Definition.** The lipid system PN is a parenteral formulation in which lipid is administered daily to provide a substantial proportion of the NPC. Nitrogen is provided as crystalline amino acids. Electrolytes, vitamins, and trace minerals are added to the formulation as needed.
      (2) **Administration.** The lipid system PN is administered peripherally when the dextrose concentration is less than or equal to 10% and centrally when the dextrose concentration is more than 10%.

(a) **Piggyback method.** The solution with amino acids, dextrose, electrolytes, trace minerals, and vitamins is infused concurrently with a separate bottle of lipid emulsion through a Y site on the intravenous administration set.

(b) **Total nutrient admixture** (TNA) **method**—three-in-one, all-in-one. Lipids, amino acids, dextrose, electrolytes, trace minerals, and vitamins are mixed in one container and administered by the central or peripheral route, depending on dextrose concentration.

   (i) **Advantages** include simplification of administration and decreased training time for home PN patients.

   (ii) **Disadvantages** include the inability to inspect for particulate matter in the opaque admixture, the inability to use 0.22-μm bacterial retention filters, and stability problems.

   (iii) Because the presence of lipid emulsion in TNAs obscure the presence of a precipitate and may present a life-threatening hazard to patients, the U.S. Food and Drug Administration (FDA) suggests that the piggyback method be used to administer lipid emulsion. If a TNA is deemed medically necessary, then specific admixture guidelines recommended by the FDA should be followed. Also, a particle filter (i.e., 1.2 μ) should be used with TNA administration.

(c) **Lipid dosage**

   (i) Lipid calories should not exceed 60% of total daily calories, including protein calories.

   (ii) Maximum dosage of lipids for adults is 2.5 g/kg/day.

   (iii) Baseline and weekly serum triglycerides must be monitored in patients on lipid system PN.

(3) **Adverse effects** of lipids are uncommon. The most frequent adverse effects include fever, chills, sensation of warmth, chest pain, back pain, vomiting, and urticaria (overall incidence < 1%). Severe hypoxemia has been reported with rapid infusion of lipid emulsion.

7. **Additives**

   a. **Electrolytes.** PN formulations must include adequate amounts of sodium, magnesium, calcium, chloride, potassium, phosphorus, and acetate. The intracellular "anabolic" electrolytes—potassium, magnesium, and phosphate—are essential for protein synthesis. Requirements vary widely, depending on a patient's fluid and electrolyte losses; renal, hepatic, and endocrine status; acid–base balance; metabolic rate; and type of PN formula used. The electrolyte composition of the PN formula must be adjusted to meet the needs of the individual patient.

   b. **Vitamins and trace minerals.** Vitamins are usually added to PN solutions in the form of commercially available multivitamin preparations. Currently, there is a new adult multiple vitamin infusion formula available (Infuvite Adult, MVI-Adult) that meets the recently amended requirements of the FDA for adult parenteral multivitamins.

   (1) The new FDA requirements are based on the prior multivitamin formulation recommended by the Nutrition Advisory Group of the Department of Foods and Nutrition of the American Medical Association (NAG-AMA) but with increased dosages of vitamins B_1, B_6, C, and folic acid and the addition of vitamin K.

   (2) The FDA also approved the same multivitamin formulation without vitamin K (MVI-12; multivitamin infusion without vitamin K) for those patients who receive warfarin-type anticoagulant therapy. Because of stability problems, one vial of Infuvite Adult and MVI-Adult contains vitamins A, D, E, B_1, B_2, B_3, B_5, B_6, and K. MVI-12 contains the same vitamins in one vial without vitamin K. The second vial for both preparations contains vitamins B_{12}, biotin, and folic acid.

   (3) Trace minerals may be added individually or as a commercially available multielement preparation. Precise requirements for trace minerals have yet to be determined.

   c. **Insulin** may be required for patients receiving PN formulations (especially glucose system PN) to maintain blood glucose levels < 200 mg/dL. If insulin is required, it is best provided by the addition of an appropriate amount of regular insulin to the PN formulation at the time of admixture. Although a small amount of insulin (5–10 U per bag) may be adsorbed to the container and tubing, such losses can be overcome by appropriate titration of the dose. The addition of insulin to the PN formulation has the advantage of changes in the rate of PN infusion being automatically accompanied by appropriate changes in the rate of insulin infusion.

  d. **Miscellaneous drugs.** A number of medications have been successfully admixed with PN formulations for continuous infusion. The H_2-receptor antagonists are the most common drugs used in this way. The routine addition of medications to PN formulations remains controversial because of:

  (1) **Questions of stability** over the wide range of PN component concentrations

  (2) Possible **therapeutic inadequacy** or toxicity secondary to PN rate changes and loss of peak and trough levels

  (3) Increased **potential for waste** with dose changes

8. **Complications** with the use of PN can be serious and potentially life-threatening but can be avoided by careful management. Complications can be divided into mechanical, infectious, and metabolic.

  a. **Mechanical** complications generally relate to the central venous catheter or its placement and include pneumothorax, catheter occlusion, and venous thrombosis.

  b. **Infectious** complications usually are related to the central venous catheter. This line-related sepsis is secondary to multiple catheter manipulations, contamination during insertion, or contamination during routine maintenance. Hyperglycemia and IV lipids also have been implicated. Maintaining blood sugars < 200 mg/dL has been shown to significantly reduce septic complications in certain subsets of patients.

  c. **Metabolic** complications are the most common. These include hyperglycemia, hypoglycemia, hypokalemia, hypomagnesemia, hypophosphatemia, metabolic acidosis, respiratory acidosis, prerenal azotemia, and zinc deficiency. A transient self-limited hepatic dysfunction is also seen with long-term PN.

B. **Enteral nutrition (EN).** Use of the GI tract to achieve total nutritional support or partial support in combination with the parenteral route should be attempted whenever possible in the face of inadequate oral intake. Theoretical advantages include maintenance of normal digestion, absorption, and gut mucosal barrier function.

  1. **Contraindications** to EN include complete intestinal obstruction, high-output intestinal fistulas, severe acute pancreatitis, severe acute inflammatory bowel disease, and severe diarrhea.

  2. **Routes of administration.** Tube feedings can be administered via nasogastric, nasoduodenal, nasojejunal, gastrostomy, and jejunostomy tubes.

  3. **EN formulations** can be classified as being standard (complete) or modular.

  a. **Standard formulas** generally contain carbohydrates, fats, vitamins, trace minerals, and a nitrogen source. They are further classified according to their nitrogen source.

  (1) **Monomeric** formulas contain crystalline amino acids as their nitrogen source. These formulas are usually marketed commercially for specific indications (e.g., ileus, pancreatitis, hepatic coma).

  (2) **Short-chain peptide** formulas contain dipeptides and tripeptides from hydrolyzed protein or de novo synthesis as their nitrogen source. They are currently marketed for the metabolically stressed patient.

  (3) **Polymeric** formulas contain either intact proteins or protein hydrolysates as their nitrogen source. Most patients can be managed with these formulas.

  b. **Modular formulas** consist of separate modules of specific nutrients that can be combined or administered separately. They are used for supplemental use or to custom design an EN formula to meet a specific clinical situation.

  (1) **Carbohydrate** modules differ in the type of carbohydrate present (e.g., polysaccharides, disaccharides, monosaccharides).

  (2) **Protein** modules contain either intact protein, hydrolyzed protein, or crystalline amino acids.

  (3) **Fat** modules contain either long-chain triglycerides (LCTs) prepared from vegetable oils or medium-chain triglycerides (MCTs) prepared from coconut oil. MCTs are more water soluble and more easily absorbed than LCTs. (Bypassing the intestinal lacteal and lymphatic system, MCTs are transported directly to the portal system.) MCTs are, however, relatively expensive and contain no essential fatty acids.

4. **Complications.** The two **most common** complications of EN are diarrhea and improper tube placement.
   a. **Diarrhea** in patients receiving EN is usually secondary to concomitant administration of medication (e.g., antibiotics and sorbitol-containing liquids). Infectious causes should be eliminated (e.g., *Clostridium difficile*), after which antidiarrheal medications may be beneficial. Reducing the rate or concentration may also be effective.
   b. A **feeding tube improperly placed** into the tracheobronchial tree can have disastrous consequences. Tube feedings should never be initiated without radiological verification of tube position.
   c. **Aspiration**

IV. MONITORING SUPPORT

A. **PN.** In addition to appropriate general medical and nursing care, patients receiving PN initially require daily and weekly laboratory monitoring to assess nutritional progress and metabolic status.

1. **Electrolytes**
   a. Initially, **potassium, sodium,** and **chloride** should be determined daily. Potassium is used intracellularly; thus hypokalemia is not an uncommon finding.
   b. **Calcium, magnesium,** and **phosphate** are primarily intracellular electrolytes, serum levels of which become depleted during protein synthesis. Serum levels generally do not fall as rapidly as potassium; therefore, monitoring two to three times a week is recommended initially until the patient is stabilized, then weekly thereafter.
   c. **Bicarbonate** should be monitored to assess acid–base balance. Hyperchloremic metabolic acidosis may develop in patients on PN. This imbalance can be corrected by providing the potassium and sodium as acetate (converted to bicarbonate in the serum) rather than as the chloride salt. After initial correction, provision of one half the sodium and potassium requirements as the acetate salt and one half as the chloride salt may be beneficial.

2. **Serum glucose** should be monitored daily, particularly in central glucose systems. Maintaining a blood glucose concentration between 100–200 mg/dL is generally recommended.

3. **Weights** obtained on a daily or every other day basis track optimum lean body weight gain of 0.25–0.50 lb/day. Weight gain in excess of 0.5 lb/day generally indicates fluid overload or fat deposition.

4. **Visceral proteins** (e.g., albumin, prealbumin, transferrin) are important indicators of the adequacy of nutritional support.
   a. **Albumin** is useful in the initial assessment of nutritional status, but its long half-life (18–21 days) limits its utility as a short-term marker of nutritional repletion.
   b. **Prealbumin** has a short half-life (2–3 days) and is a more sensitive and early indicator of the adequacy of nutritional support. Its serum value is falsely elevated in renal failure.
   c. **Transferrin** has an intermediate half-life (7–10 days), which makes weekly monitoring useful. Transferrin may be falsely elevated in iron-deficiency states.

5. **Serum creatinine** and **blood urea nitrogen (BUN)** should be obtained at least weekly. Evidence of renal impairment may require modification of the PN formula. Elevation of the BUN in the absence of renal impairment may be secondary to the PN formula (e.g., excess nitrogen, low NPC:N ratio) and appropriate adjustments need to be made.

6. **Liver function tests**—aspartate aminotransferase (AST), alanine aminotransferase (ALT), alkaline phosphatase, lactate dehydrogenase (LDH), and bilirubin—require baseline and periodic monitoring because of potential toxicity from the PN formulation (i.e., fatty infiltration of the liver). Abnormal liver function studies may necessitate changes in the PN formulation.

7. **Serum triglycerides** should be measured for a baseline and weekly thereafter for patients on lipid system PN. It is not necessary to monitor triglycerides on a weekly basis for patients receiving lipids two to three times per week for essential fatty acid replacement.

8. A **24-hr UUN** should be obtained weekly to determine nitrogen balance for patients in whom nitrogen requirements are uncertain. These are usually highly stressed, severely ill, or injured patients in an intensive care unit (ICU) setting.

9. **Serum iron** levels should be obtained weekly to determine deficiency and to allow appropriate interpretation of serum transferrin levels.

B. **EN** generally requires less intense laboratory monitoring. Specific laboratory guidelines for monitoring EN support vary from institution to institution.

V. SUPPORT OF SPECIFIC STATES

A. **Conditionally essential nutrients**

1. **Glutamine.** Because of its instability, glutamine is currently not a component of commercially available standard PN amino acid solutions and is found in free form in relatively few EN formulas. It is known to be used as a primary fuel source by enterocytes and may exert a trophic effect on the gut mucosa. It is most widely used as a PN component for bone marrow transplant patients and short gut syndrome. Glutamine-containing dipeptides that are stable and highly soluble are being investigated as a source of glutamine in PN. At present, glutamine must be added to the PN solution at the time of compounding. Optimum PN dose, contraindications, and EN necessity in free form are controversial and require further investigation.

2. **Arginine** has been shown experimentally and clinically to enhance immune function. EN formulas enriched with arginine are available commercially. Optimum dose has yet to be determined.

3. **Antioxidant formulations.** Oxidant production occurs as part of the normal inflammatory response and has been implicated in reperfusion injury. The body also produces antioxidant defenses to limit oxidant damage to healthy tissue. These defenses rely on adequate intake of dietary nutrients, such as the sulfur-containing amino acids, vitamin E, vitamin C, selenium, and zinc. Several investigators believe provision of these nutrients should be an early priority in critically ill patients. Optimum doses remain controversial.

4. **Tyrosine, cysteine,** and **taurine** are either absent or present in low concentrations in commercially available PN formulas. They are believed to be conditionally essential amino acids by some investigators.

5. **Omega-3 polyunsaturated fatty acids** are derived from fish oils and are currently found in some EN formulations. These fatty acids have been shown experimentally to enhance immune response, protect against tumor growth, and inhibit some of the proinflammatory effects of omega-6 fatty acids. In addition, they have been shown to lower cardiovascular risk factors by decreasing platelet activation, lowering blood pressure, and reducing triglycerides. However, well-controlled clinical trials in humans are needed to confirm the beneficial effects of immunomodulation seen in animal models.

B. **Nutritional support for renal failure.** The goal of nutritional support in acute renal failure (ARF) is to meet the patient's NPC requirements while minimizing volume, protein load, and potential electrolyte imbalance.

1. **PN formulations** used in ARF are low-nitrogen, high-caloric density formulas (e.g., 2% amino acid/47% dextrose), resulting in NPC:N ratios of approximately 500:1.

2. **Commercial renal failure formulations** (e.g., NephrAmine, RenAmin, Aminosyn RF), containing primarily essential amino acids, have shown no clinical advantage over less expensive, low-concentration standard amino acid formulations.

3. **Standard glucose system formulations** (4.25% amino acid/25% dextrose) can generally be used in renal failure patients who are being dialyzed on a regular basis. This formulation is particularly useful in severely malnourished patients because it can provide adequate protein to attain positive nitrogen balance, which is not possible with renal failure PN.

4. **Monitoring transferrin** is a more sensitive and accurate visceral protein marker compared to albumin and prealbumin for assessing nutritional progress in these patients.

5. **Enteral formulations** that are low in nitrogen and calorie dense (1.7–2.0 NPC/mL) are available for patients with renal failure.

C. **Nutritional support for hepatic failure.** Patients with hepatic failure have altered protein metabolism, resulting in decreased serum levels of branched-chain amino acids (i.e., leucine, isoleucine, valine) and increased levels of aromatic amino acids (i.e., phenylalanine, tyrosine, tryptophan), methionine, and glutamine. A similar amino acid profile can exist in the cerebrospinal fluid (CSF) and is thought to contribute to hepatic encephalopathy. Fluid and electrolyte disturbances are frequently associated with hepatic failure as well.

1. **PN formulations** enriched in branched-chain amino acids (36%) and low in aromatic amino acids (e.g., HepatAmine) improve mental status in patients with altered serum amino acid profiles and hepatic encephalopathy. However, studies have not demonstrated definitive clinical differences in morbidity and mortality with these expensive formulations compared to standard formulas.

2. **Adequate NPC** with a 20–40 g/day protein load (e.g., 2% amino acid/25% dextrose) is an alternative approach to the use of hepatic failure amino acid formulations. Protein load can be liberalized slowly as long as mental status does not deteriorate.

3. **EN formulations** (e.g., Hepatic-Aid II) enriched with branched-chain amino acids and low in aromatic amino acids are commercially available for patients with hepatic failure.

D. **Nutritional support for respiratory failure.** The type and amount of substrate administered as NPC can have an effect on a patient's ventilatory status. Overfeeding with resultant lipogenesis and increased carbon dioxide production can be a cause of respiratory acidosis and/or increased minute ventilation and, therefore, should be avoided. Even in the presence of appropriate amounts of NPC administered as carbohydrate, the normal carbon dioxide load generated by glycolysis may be excessive for the patient with underlying pulmonary dysfunction—for example, chronic obstructive pulmonary disease (COPD).

1. **PN lipid system formulations** (e.g., 4.25% amino acid/15% dextrose with daily lipid emulsion), where the lipid component constitutes 40%–50% of the total NPC, may be beneficial in reducing the ventilatory demands in respiratory failure patients because lipolysis generates less carbon dioxide than glycolysis.

2. **EN formulations** containing similar amounts of fat can be prepared from standard EN formulas with the use of lipid modules (i.e., MCT oil, corn oil). More expensive commercial pulmonary formulas are also available.

3. **Oxepa,** a low-carbohydrate enteral formula containing antioxidants, eicosapentaenoic acid, and γ-linolenic acid, is currently available for adult respiratory distress syndrome (ARDS). It modulates the phospholipid fatty acid composition of inflammatory cell membranes, decreases the synthesis of the proinflammatory eicosanoids of lung injury, and attenuates endotoxin-induced increases in pulmonary microvascular protein permeability. Limited studies have shown some improvement in cardiopulmonary hemodynamics and respiratory gas exchange in ARDS.

E. **Nutritional support for cardiac failure.** The goal in these patients is to meet metabolic needs while restricting fluid and sodium intake.

1. **PN formulations** that provide protein and calories in as high a concentration as possible is the goal of nutritional therapy. This can be accomplished with both central glucose or lipid system PN formulations (e.g., 5% amino acid/35% dextrose; 7% amino acid/21% dextrose/ 20% lipid emulsion).

2. **Serum electrolyte monitoring** and **adjustment** are imperative in cardiac failure patients receiving PN, particularly when potent diuretics are used concurrently.

3. **EN formulations** with high nutrient density are available for oral supplementation or tube feedings. Infusion of enteral tube feedings should begin at one third to one half the strength, with a gradual increase in concentration, while maintaining a slow infusion rate (30–50 mL/hr) to avoid rapid increases in fluid load, cardiac output, heart rate, and myocardial oxygen consumption.

F. **Nutritional support in pancreatitis.** Severe acute pancreatitis is a hypercatabolic state that without nutritional support renders the patient a poor surgical candidate and at increased risk of infection. The goal of nutritional support in severe acute pancreatitis is to rest the pancreas by limiting exocrine stimulation while providing adequate nutrition.

1. **PN** is generally favored over EN to achieve this goal in the early phases of pancreatitis. Lipid system PN has been shown to be safe and effective when administered to these patients, provided there is no concurrent hyperlipidemia; in fact, it may be valuable in the patient with recalcitrant hyperglycemia.

2. **EN,** using chemically defined (elemental), low-fat formulas administered into the jejunum, results in minimal pancreatic stimulation and has been used safely in these patients.

G. **Nutritional support in stress/critical care.** In hypermetabolic critically ill patients, alterations in substrate use, the development of conditional nutrient deficiencies, and modulation of the immune response provide the rationale for specific nutritional formulations.

1. In critical illness, branched-chain amino acids (i.e., isoleucine, leucine, valine) are released from skeletal muscle for protein synthesis and as an energy substrate. PN formulations enriched in branched-chain amino acids (45%)—for example, FreAmine HBC, BranchA-min, Aminosyn-HBC—have been made available with the rationale that, being the preferred fuel source in this patient population, it would enhance protein synthesis, decrease protein catabolism, and improve the patient's clinical outcome. However, these more expensive branched-chain amino acid formulations have not been shown to favorably influence clinical outcomes in critically ill patients.

2. Enteral formulations are currently being produced (e.g., Impact, Perative) with various amounts of the conditionally essential nutrients of critical illness and immunomodulatory substrates (e.g., omega-3 polyunsaturated fatty acids, arginine, glutamine). Clinical studies of the ability of these formulas to improve outcomes in critical illness have been mixed.

3. **Hyperglycemia** and **insulin resistance** are common occurrences in critically ill patients. Recent data involving mechanically ventilated patients in the surgical intensive care unit who received intensive insulin therapy to maintain blood glucose levels between 80 and 110 mg/dL showed a significant reduction in mortality when compared to more conventional therapy of maintaining blood glucose levels between 180 and 200 mg/dL. The greatest reduction in mortality was associated with deaths caused by multiple organ failure with a proven septic focus. These data point out the importance of striving for a tight glucose control in critically ill patients on PN while avoiding the complications of hypoglycemia.

4. Thermal injury is one of the most hypermetabolic conditions observed in the critical care setting.
   a. Methods for estimating the calorie requirements in this patient population are conflicting owing to differences in bias and precision. One of the more accurate unbiased methods reported for estimating energy requirements in thermal injury is

$$Kcal = (1000 \text{ kcal} \times BSA) + (25 \times \%BSAB)$$

   where BSA is body surface area and BSAB is body surface area burned.

   b. Protein requirements in thermally injured patients are high at 2–2.5 g/kg/day because of the significant degree of catabolism associated with this injury.
   c. The increased dermal losses of nitrogen from their burn wounds renders the use of the conventional nitrogen balance formulas less accurate in assessing nitrogen requirements especially with thermal injuries > 40% of BSA. The UUN plus the insensible loss factor can differ significantly from total nitrogen losses in this patient population.

H. **Nutritional support in pregnancy.** Nutritional support in pregnancy can have a significant affect on fetal outcome. Weight gain throughout pregnancy is the primary indicator of the adequacy of the nutritional state of mother and child. A weight gain of 11.5–16.0 kg should be the desired goal in women with normal prepregnancy body mass index. PN and EN have both been used successfully during pregnancy, with both modalities demonstrating adequate maternal weight gain, appropriate fetal growth, and term delivery. The calories required to achieve appropriate weight gain throughout the entire pregnancy per the World Health Organization recommendations are an additional 300 kcal/day above the estimated basal energy expenditure (based on the pregravid weight) during all trimesters. The recommended daily protein intake during a normal pregnancy is approximately 1 g/kg/day. This amount represents the normal recommended daily allowance for females plus an additional 10 g/day. In pregnant patients with moderate to severe stress, both calories and protein requirements need to be adjusted in the same manner as for other hypermetabolic nonpregnant patients.

1. PN glucose system and lipid system formulations can both be used successfully to meet the nutrient requirements of pregnant patients. PN is most commonly used during pregnancy in patients with severe hyperemesis gravidarum.

2. Essential fatty acids (EFAs) are required by both mother and fetus. They are necessary for prostaglandin synthesis and normal fetal lipid development. The provision of at least 4.5–7.0% of calorie requirements as EFAs has been estimated to meet the minimum requirements during pregnancy.

3. The **daily vitamin requirements** in a normal pregnancy based on the 1999 dietary reference intakes (DRI) can be met with the parenteral vitamin infusion Infuvite Adult and MVI-Adult. If MVI-12 is used as the parenteral vitamin preparation, an additional 65 ug of vitamin K needs to be added to the daily PN formulation to meet the daily DRI requirements.

4. Prealbumin appears to be the preferred biochemical marker to assess protein status in pregnancy because albumin is falsely depressed and transferrin is falsely elevated in pregnant patients.

5. EN may be useful during pregnancy for patients with less severe hyperemesis gravidarum. The composition of polymeric formulas should be adequate for meeting the nutritional requirements of most pregnant patients.

6. Blood glucose levels should be kept at approximately 100 mg/dL during prolonged continuous PN or EN infusion because chronically elevated maternal glucose levels can result in fetal anomalies, increased risk of miscarriages, and stillbirth.

VI. TECHNICAL ASPECTS OF PN PREPARATIONS

A. PN formula preparation is performed **aseptically** in the pharmacy under a laminar flow hood that filters the air, removing airborne particles and microorganisms.

B. **Compatibility** of the various components of PN formulations is determined by several factors, including their concentration, solution pH, temperature, and the order of admixture. The **most common** compatibility concern is in regard to the addition of calcium and phosphate salts to PN solutions.

C. After admixture of the various components, the PN solution should be **visually inspected** for precipitate or particulate matter. After labeling and final checking, the PN solution should be refrigerated until delivery to the nursing unit.

D. A statistically valid, continuous **sterility testing program** should be an essential component of quality control in preparing PN solutions.

VII. HOME PARENTERAL NUTRITION (HPN) has become a widely accepted and useful technique for provision of complete nutritional requirements in the home setting. When used appropriately, this modality benefits the patient medically and psychologically, with a decreased cost to the healthcare system.

A. **Indications** for HPN include short bowel syndrome, severe inflammatory bowel disease, radiation enteritis, enterocutaneous fistulae, and selected malignancies.

B. **Candidate selection** requires a multidisciplinary approach to determine if the patient and family can assume the responsibility and training needed for safe and successful HPN.

C. **Administration.** HPN is infused through a central venous Silastic catheter (e.g., Hickman, Broviac), which allows for prolonged PN with low clotting and infection rates. The PN solution is generally infused over a 12- to 15-hr period at night. This type of cycling program allows the patient to be free from the infusion pump during the day, allowing for a more normal lifestyle.

D. **Clinical monitoring** and follow-up are done periodically, depending on the needs of the individual patient. Long-term HPN patients generally are seen by the physician on a monthly basis after initial stabilization.

VIII. MISCELLANEOUS

A. **Soluble fiber** is present in some commercially available EN formulas. This fiber is fermented by normal large intestinal flora to short-chain fatty acids that are used by colonocytes as a fuel source. These short-chain fatty acids also seem to have a trophic effect on the large intestinal mucosa.

B. **Growth factors.** The use of recombinant human growth hormone, insulin-like growth factor, and anabolic steroids, in combination with nutritional support to improve nitrogen balance and reduce hospital length of stay in select patient populations, is currently under investigation. To date, recombinant growth hormone (Humatrope) is available for nutritional support in children with cystic fibrosis, sickle cell anemia, and thalassemia and in adults with AIDS-related cachexia.

STUDY QUESTIONS

Directions: Each of the questions, statements, or incomplete statements in this section can be correctly answered or completed by **one** of the suggested answers or phrases. Choose the **best** answer.

1. A 32-year-old well-nourished man involved in a motor vehicle accident was admitted to the surgical intensive care unit with multiple long bone fractures and abdominal injuries with no nutritional support for 4 days. This patient is most likely

(A) suffering from moderate to severe kwashiorkor malnutrition.
(B) at low risk for hospital-acquired infection and other complications.
(C) not suffering from protein or calorie malnutrition.
(D) suffering from severe marasmus malnutrition.
(E) not a candidate for aggressive nutritional support.

2. A patient in the intensive care unit on a ventilator was placed on a glucose system parenteral nutrition (PN) formulation providing 2040 kcal/day and 98 g protein/day. A measured energy expenditure (MEE) of 2038 kcal and a respiratory quotient (RQ) of 1.1 were subsequently obtained. Which of the following is correct based on this information?

(A) The patient is receiving adequate glucose calories, and an adjustment in the program is not necessary.
(B) The daily protein intake has to be decreased to reduce the patient's RQ.
(C) The PN formulation should be switched to a lipid system formulation to reduce the carbon dioxide load.
(D) The patient is retaining oxygen from the glucose calories in the PN formulation.
(E) Lipid emulsion should be added to the current PN formulation to enhance lipogenesis.

3. Total nutrient admixture (TNA)

(A) is more complicated to administer for home parenteral nutrition (PN) patients.
(B) should be filtered with a 1.2-μ filter.
(C) consists of glucose, amino acids, electrolytes, and trace minerals mixed in one container.
(D) is the method recommended by the U.S. Food and Drug Administration (FDA) to administer lipid system PN.
(E) can be visualized for particulate matter.

4. The calorie requirements of a moderately hypermetabolic hospitalized patient are best estimated by uisng the

(A) nomogram method.
(B) nitrogen balance method.
(C) estimated energy expenditure (EEE) method.
(D) prognostic nutritional index (PNI).
(E) subjective global assessment method.

5. Lipid system parenteral nutrition (PN)

(A) can be administered by peripheral vein if the glucose concentration is less than 15%.
(B) requires daily serum triglyceride monitoring.
(C) is contraindicated in patients with elevated carbon dioxide levels.
(D) requires daily lipid administration to provide a portion of the patient's nonprotein calorie requirements.
(E) can be administered with a maximum lipid dosage of 4.5 g/kg/day.

6. Commercial parenteral nutrition (PN) formulations for hypermetabolic critically ill patients

(A) are enriched in branched-chain amino acids and contain low concentrations of aromatic amino acids.
(B) contain primarily essential amino acids.
(C) have not demonstrated a positive clinical outcome benefit in this patient population.
(D) are the preferred PN formulation used in this clinical setting.
(E) are enriched with arginine to enhance immune function.

7. Which of the following methods of parenteral nutritional support would be most appropriate in a severely protein calorie malnourished patient with acute renal failure?

(A) 2% amino acid/47% dextrose.
(B) 4.25% amino acid/25% dextrose.
(C) 4% essential amino acid/47% dextrose.
(D) 4.25% amino acid/25% dextrose with dialysis on a regular basis.
(E) 2% amino acid/47% dextrose/20% lipid emulsion.

8. Which of the following statements regarding the monitoring of nutritional support is true?

   (A) Prealbumin is not the optimal marker to follow for short-term nutritional progress.
   (B) Transferrin is falsely depressed in patients with iron deficiency.
   (C) Albumin is falsely elevated in renal failure.
   (D) A positive nitrogen balance of 3–6 g of nitrogen daily is optimal.
   (E) A weight gain of 1.5–2 lb/day indicates optimal lean body weight gain.

9. Patients with end-stage liver disease

   (A) generally have increased levels of branched-chain amino acids and decreased levels of aromatic amino acids.
   (B) should be placed on a low-branched chain, high aromatic amino acids parenteral nutrition (PN) solution.
   (C) can tolerate 20–40 g protein/day with a 2% standard amino acid PN solution.
   (D) require glutamine-enriched amino acid solutions.
   (E) can tolerate standard glucose system formulations 4.25% amino acid/25% dextrose with regular dialysis.

For questions 10–12: A 67-year-old white female presented to the attending physician with a 3-month history of progressive difficulty swallowing and a 10-kg weight loss. She is currently 160 cm tall and weighs 50 kg. She has just undergone a distal esophagectomy and proximal gastrectomy for distal esophageal cancer. At the time of surgery, she had a feeding jejunostomy tube inserted.

10. The dieticians who are adept at using the Harris-Benedict equation have gone home for the day, and the surgeon calls you for your best guess at what the hourly goal rate for this patient should be using isotonic enteral formula, which provides 0.85 nonprotein calories (NPCs)/mL. Your answer should be

    (A) 65 mL/hr.
    (B) 75 mL/hr.
    (C) 85 mL/hr.
    (D) 95 mL/hr.
    (E) 50 mL/hr.

11. The enteral formulation the surgeon has selected is enriched with fish oils. He is hoping this additive will

    (A) prevent diarrhea.
    (B) prevent dermatitis.
    (C) prevent hyperglycemia.
    (D) improve immune function.
    (E) improve neurological function.

12. On the 5th postoperative day, the feeding jejunostomy tube becomes clogged and unusable. The patient will be NPO an additional 5 days to ensure the integrity of her surgical anastomosis. The most appropriate course at this time is

    (A) start the patient on a lipid-based peripheral parenteral nutrition program.
    (B) keep the patient NPO and without parenteral nutritional support.
    (C) have a central venous catheter inserted, and initiate a lipid-based parenteral nutrition program.
    (D) start the patient on a glucose-based peripheral parenteral nutritional program.
    (E) have a central venous catheter inserted, and start the patient on a high branched-chain amino acid parenteral program.

For questions 13–14: RJ is a 28-year-old pregnant woman. She is in the 9th week of her pregnancy and is diagnosed with hyperemesis gravidarum. Her pregravid weight was 57 kg, and her height is 5 ft., 5 in. She has lost 7 kg (12.3%) during her pregnancy. She was placed on a central glucose PN program.

13. Which one of the following represents the best estimate of her daily caloric requirements?

    (A) 1675 kcal
    (B) 1790 kcal
    (C) 2261 kcal
    (D) 2062 kcal
    (E) 1925 kcal

14. MVI-12 is used as the parenteral vitamin preparation in the PN formulation. Which of the following vitamin(s) need to be supplemented in the daily PN formulation to meet the daily requirements during pregnancy?

    (A) vitamin K
    (B) thiamine (B_1)
    (C) folic acid
    (D) A and C
    (E) pyridoxine (B_6)

1270 *Chapter 59*

For questions 15–17: A 55-year old male with multiple traumatic injuries and type II diabetes was admitted to the surgical ICU. He was placed on mechanical ventilation and initiated on glucose system PN. After 3 days of PN therapy his blood glucose levels have ranged from 250 to 285 mg/dL over the past 24 hr with 80 U of insulin/L in his PN formulation. He is on no other insulin supplementation at this time.

15. The nutritional support service recommends an insulin drip with the goal of achieving a blood glucose level of

(A) 180-225 mg/dL.
(B) 200-215 mg/dL.
(C) 80-110 mg/dL.
(D) 65-100 mg/dL.
(E) 70-105 mg/dL.

16. What parenteral trace mineral therapy may be an effective adjunct if the insulin drip fails to achieve the glucose level goal?

(A) 20–40 mg zinc/day
(B) 150–200 μg chromium/day
(C) 0.5–1.5mg copper/day
(D) 150–400mcg manganese/day
(E) 40–60 μg selenium/day

17. Appropriate insulin control in this patient setting has been shown to provide which of the following clinical outcomes?

(A) decreased length of time on the ventilator
(B) significant reduction in mortality
(C) decreased duration of PN therapy
(D) a decrease in multiple organ failure with a proven septic focus
(E) B and D

ANSWERS AND EXPLANATIONS

1. The answer is A *[see I.B.3].*
A hypermetabolic state (e.g., trauma, infection) combined with protein deprivation can rapidly develop into a severe kwashiorkor malnutrition characterized by hypoalbuminemia, edema, and impaired cellular immune function.

2. The answer is *C [see V.D.1].*
Even in the presence of appropriate amounts of NPCs administered as carbohydrate, the normal carbon dioxide load generated by glycolysis may be excessive for the patient with underlying pulmonary dysfunction. PN lipid system formulations, in which the lipid component constitutes 40%–50% of the total NPCs, may be beneficial in reducing the ventilatory demands in respiratory failure patients because lipolysis generates less carbon dioxide than glycolysis.

3. The answer is B *[see III.A.6.b.(2)(b).(iii)].*
A particle filter (i.e., 1.2 μ) should be used with TNA administration.

4. The answer is C *[see II.B.1].*
Energy requirements are determined as nonprotein calories by indirect calorimetry, estimated energy expenditure, and the simple nomogram method. The nomogram method is the least accurate method of estimating caloric requirements.

5. The answer is D *[see III.A.6.b.(1)].*
The lipid system PN is a formulation in which lipid is administered daily to provide a substantial portion of the NPCs.

6. The answer is C *[see V.G.1].*
PN formulations enriched in branched-chain amino acids have been made available with the rationale that, being the preferred fuel source in this patient population, it would enhance protein synthesis, decrease protein catabolism, and improve the patient's clinical outcome. However, these more expensive branched-chain amino acid formulations have not been shown to favorably influence clinical outcomes in critically ill patients.

7. The answer is D *[see V.B.3].*
Standard glucose system formulations (4.25% amino acid/25% dextrose) can generally be used in renal failure patients who are being dialyzed on a regular basis. This formulation is particularly useful in severely malnourished patients because it can provide adequate protein to attain positive nitrogen balance, which is not possible with renal failure PN.

8. The answer is D *[see II.B.2.a.(4)].*
A positive nitrogen balance of 3–6 g is the goal.

9. The answer is C *[see V.C.2].*
Adequate NPCs with a 20–40 g/day protein load (e.g., 2% amino acid/25% dextrose) is an alternative approach to the use of hepatic failure amino acid formulations.

10. The answer is B *[see II.B.1.c].*
Use the nomogram of 30 kcal/kg to determine the NPCs/day, and divide that by the NPCs/mL of the enteral formula to determine the volume of formula per day, which is divided by 24 hr to yield the hourly goal rate.

11. The answer is D *[see V.A.5].*
Omega-3 polyunsaturated fatty acids are derived from fish oils and are currently found in some enteral formulations. These fatty acids have been shown experimentally to enhance immune response.

12. The answer is A *[see III.A.3.b].*
With the use of new catheter technology and new techniques for infusion, it is now feasible to administer peripheral PN in selected patients for short-term therapy (7–10 days) with a low incidence of peripheral vein thrombophlebitis. This method of PN administration avoids the potential of more serious complications associated with central venous route administration.

13. The answer is A   *[see V.H].*
The estimated basal energy expenditure is calculated using the pregravid weight in the Harris-Benedict equation. An additional 300 kcal/day is added to the basal energy expenditure to provide the required calories per day during pregnancy.

14. The answer is A   *[see V.H.3].*
An additional 65 μg of vitamin K needs to be added to the daily PN formulation when MVI-12 is used as the parenteral vitamin preparation to meet the daily requirements during pregnancy.

15. The answer is C   *[see V.G.3].*
Recent data involving critically ill, mechanically ventilated patients in the surgical intensive care unit indicate intensive insulin therapy to maintain blood glucose levels between 80 and 110 mg/dL.

16. The answer is B   *[see II.B.5.g]*
Suggested IV requirements of chromium for deficiency and severe glucose intolerance are 150–200 μg/day.

17. The answer is E   *[see V.G.3]*
The greatest reduction in mortality in patients maintained on tight insulin control was associated deaths owing to multiple organ failure with a proven septic focus.

60

Immunosuppressive Agents in Organ Transplantation

David I. Min

I. ORGAN TRANSPLANTATION

A. **Definition.** Replacement of a diseased vital organ with a viable organ from a living or cadaver donor. Solid organ transplantation has become the therapy of choice for many patients with end-organ failure (i.e., heart, liver, lung, and kidney disease). However, it generally requires immunosuppression to overcome the immunological barrier between donor and recipient, except in syngenic (i.e., twins) or autologous transplantation.

B. **Classification**

1. **Solid organ transplantation**
   a. **Life-saving transplantation** (e.g., heart, heart–lung, lung, and liver transplantation). There is no alternative life-sustaining method available.
   b. **Non-life-saving transplantation** (i.e., kidney, pancreas, and cornea transplantation). There are alternative life-sustaining methods available, such as dialysis or external insulin injection. In these cases, transplantation will improve the patient's quality of life or long-term survival significantly.

2. **Bone marrow transplantation** is used mainly for hematological malignancy or aplastic anemia.

II. GRAFT REJECTION

A. **Transplant immunology** (see Chapter 8)

1. **Graft rejection.** The body's immune system recognizes the allograft (transplanted organ) as a foreign antigen, and it initiates the immune response to remove or destroy the transplanted graft. This reaction is called *rejection.* The degree of the reaction depends on the genetic similarities or differences between the organ of the donor and the immune system of the recipient.

2. **Histocompatibility.** The antigen determining the compatibility between the donor and the recipient is called a **histocompatibility antigen,** the gene being located on chromosome 6. In many transplants (e.g., bone marrow or kidney transplant), this histocompatibility matching is an important factor for determining the long-term survival of the graft. However, more selective, potent immunosuppression may alleviate the importance of tissue matching between donor and recipient (*exception:* in bone marrow, the tissue matching is still important).

3. **Other factors.** Another group of substances that also plays an important role is the **ABO blood group system** of red blood cells. The donor and recipient must be ABO-compatible; otherwise, immediate graft destruction occurs. Some patients may have preformed antibody for unspecified donors because of multiple blood transfusions or other reason. In this case, patients may destroy the transplanted organ immediately. To detect the preformed antibody, the recipient's serum will be tested immediately before the transplantation (cross-match).

B. **Types of graft rejection**

1. **Types of graft rejection according to the time course**
   a. **Hyperacute rejection.** Immediate destruction (within minutes or hours) of the transplant organ by a preformed antibody or complement system. Today, this is extremely rare. It occurs only in an ABO-mismatched organ or a cross-match positive (preformed antibody) organ. There is no adequate treatment available.

   b. **Acute rejection** occurs within a few days to several months after transplantation. It is mediated by T lymphocyte (cell-mediated immunity), and this rejection can be reversible by steroids or antibody therapy such as muromonab/CD3 or antithymocyte globulin.
   c. **Chronic rejection** occurs several months to several years after transplantation. This reaction is mediated by B lymphocyte (antibody), and there is no adequate treatment available.

2. **Graft versus host, host versus graft.** In most solid organ transplants, rejection occurs as the host immune system rejects or attacks the transplant organ (host versus graft). However, in bone marrow transplant, the host is generally immune deficient and the transplanted graft is immune competent, which attracts host tissues (graft versus host).

III. PROPHYLAXIS AND TREATMENT OF GRAFT REJECTION (TABLE 60-1)

A. CALCINEURIN INHIBITORS

1. **Cyclosporine (Neoral, Sandimmune, Gengraf)**
   a. **Mechanism of action.** Cyclosporine binds an intracellular receptor, cyclophilin. This complex inhibits calcineurin, an intracellular phosphatase, which involves activation of the promoter region for the gene-encoding cytokine, such as interleukin 2. This results in inhibiting T cell activation in the early stage of immune response to a foreign antigen such as a graft.
   b. **Dosing and monitoring.** Cyclosporine pharmacokinetics is unpredictable, and many factors such as age, time after transplant, different oral formulation (Neoral or Sandimmune), or drugs affect it. Oral bioavailability is about 30%. Generally, 8 mg/kg/day of oral cyclosporine as two divided doses is used in solid organ transplantation and adjusted according to the blood levels. Serum creatinine should be monitored with the blood levels of cyclosporine. The blood levels are useful in the clinical monitoring.
   c. **Side effects. Nephrotoxicity** is the major side effect. Neurotoxicity and hepatotoxicity are also common. Hirsutism and gingival hyperplasia are also cumbersome side effects. Numerous drug interactions have been reported (Table 60-2).

2. **Tacrolimus (Prograf)**
   a. **Mechanism of action.** It is very similar to cyclosporine (see III.A.1.a).
   b. **Dosing and monitoring.** Tacrolimus pharmacokinetics is also variable, and oral bioavailability is about 25%. Blood levels are useful in clinical monitoring.
   c. **Side effects. Nephrotoxicity** is the major side effect. Neurotoxicity and gastrointestinal (GI) toxicity are more common than with cyclosporine.

B. Antimetabolites

1. **Azathioprine (Imuran)**
   a. **Mechanism of action.** It is converted to 6-mercaptopurine in the body and is a nonspecific purine synthesis inhibitor. It interferes with DNA and RNA synthesis so that it may reduce both cell-mediated and humoral immune responses.
   b. **Dosage and monitoring.** An initial dose of 3–5 mg/kg/day is administered preoperatively. Immediately after transplantation, the dose is usually tapered to a maintenance dose of 1–3 mg/kg/day or titrated to the patient's white blood cell (WBC) count. The WBC count is generally maintained > 3000/mm^3.
   c. **Side effects. Bone marrow suppression** (leukopenia, thrombocytopenia) is the major side effect. In addition, xanthine oxidase inhibitor allopurinol inhibits azathioprine metabolism. When these drugs are used concurrently, the azathioprine dose should be reduced by 80%. Otherwise, the patient may develop severe leukopenia owing to azathioprine overdose.

2. **Mycophenolic acid (CellCept, Myfortic)**
   a. **Mechanism of action.** Two forms are available. Mycophenolate mofetil (CellCept) is a prodrug, which is converted to mycophenolic acid in the body, which is the active form. In the body, mycophenolic acid (Myfortic) inhibits de novo purine synthesis pathway by inhibiting inosine dehydrogenase. As a result, it inhibits DNA and RNA synthesis in the immune cells.

Table 60-1. Current Immunosuppressive Agents Used in Organ Transplantation

Classification	Drug	Usual Initial Dose	Major Side Effects	Monitoring
Calcineurin inhibitors	Cyclosporine (Neoral, Sandimmune)	8 mg/kg/day	Nephrotoxicity	Blood concentrations and serum creatinine concentrations
	Tacrolimus (Prograf)	0.1–0.3 mg/kg/day	Neurotoxicity	
Antimetabolites	Azathioprine (Imuran)	1.5–3 mg/kg/day	Bone marrow suppression	WBC count
	Mycophenolate mofetil (CellCept)	1 g twice daily		
	Mycophenolic acid sodium (Myfortic)	720 mg twice daily		
	Methotrexate (Rheumatrex)	15 mg/m² on day 1, 10 mg/m²/day on days 3, 6, and 11		
mTOR inhibitor	Sirolimus (Rapamune)	6–15 mg loading dose and 2–5 mg once daily	Hyperlipidemia, leukopenia and thrombocytopenia	Blood concentrations and WBC, platelet, and lipid profile
Antibody products	Muromonab/CD3 (Orthoclone OKT3)	5 mg daily for 7–14 days	Cytokine release syndromes (flulike syndrome)	Signs and symptoms, CD+ cell count
	Antithymocyte globulin (Atgam, Thymoglobulin)	15–20 mg/kg/day for 7–14 days (Atgam) or 1.5 mg/kg/day for 7–14 days (Thymoglobulin)	Leukopenia and thrombocytopenia	T cell count
	Daclizumab (Zenapax)	1 mg/kg (max. 100 mg), on day 0, and every 2 weeks for a total of 5 doses	No significant side effects reported	No special monitoring required
	Basiliximab (Simulect)	For adults, 2 doses of 20 mg each (day 0 and day 4)		
Corticosteroids	Prednisone (Deltasone) or methylprednisolone (Solu-Medrol)	500 mg IV on the day of surgery and rapidly tapering to 10 mg daily at 1 month	Fluid retention, psychosis, cataracts, osteonecrosis	Signs and symptoms

IV, intravenous; *mTOR*, mammalian target of rapamycin; *WBC*, white blood cell.

Table 60-2. Major Drug Interactions of Cyclosporine and Tacrolimus with Other Drugs and Their Management

Drugs	Mechanism	Effects	Management
Antiepileptic drugs Phenytoin Phenobarbital Carbamazepine Rifampin or isoniazid	Increased metabolism by inducing cytochrome P450 enzyme	Cyclosporine or tacrolimus trough levels drop within 48 hr after initiation of these drugs	Increase cyclosporine dose or tacrolimus with frequent monitoring of blood levels. Valproic acid does not interfere with cyclosporin or tacrolimus levels
Azole antifungal agents Ketoconazole Fluconazole Itraconazole	Inhibition of liver cytochrome P450 enzyme by these drugs	Significant increase of cyclosporine or tacrolimus levels	Reduce cyclosporine or tacrolimus dose with frequent monitoring of levels
Macrolide antibiotics Erythromycin Josamycin	Inhibition of liver and GI cytochrome P450 enzyme	Increase AUC ($\times$ 2) and cyclosporine or tacrolimus trough levels ($\times$ 2–3)	Same as above
Calcium-channel blockers Verapamil Diltiazem Nicardipine			Reduce cyclosporine or tacrolimus dose, or use nifedipine or isradipine
Grapefruit juice	Inhibition of GI cytochrome P450 enzyme	Increase AUC and peak concentrations of cyclosporine and possibly tacrolimus, and increase variability of blood levels	Avoid grapefruit juice

AUC, area under the curve; *GI,* gastrointestinal.

   b. **Dosing and monitoring.** A dose of 2 g/day (CellCept) or 1440 mg/day (Myfortic) is administered as two divided doses. The WBC and GI symptoms should be monitored.
   c. **Side effects. Bone marrow suppression** (leukopenia, thrombocytopenia) is the major side effect, as in azathioprine. In addition, GI side effects are more common than with azathioprine.

  3. **Methotrexate.** This agent is used mainly in autoimmune disease and preventing graft versus host disease in bone marrow transplant (BMT) patients.
   a. **Mechanism of action.** It prevents dihydrofolic acid from converting to tetrahydrofolic acid by inhibiting the enzyme dihydrofolate reductase. As a result, DNA and protein synthesis are inhibited.
   b. **Dosing and monitoring.** Dosage regimens in BMT patients usually consist of 15 mg/m^2/day on day 1 after transplant and 10 mg/m^2/day on days 3, 6, and 11 with other agents such as cyclosporine.
   c. **Side effects. Bone marrow suppression** (leukopenia, thrombocytopenia) is the major side effect as in azathioprine. In addition, diarrhea and mucositis are common.

 C. **Mammalian target of rapamycin (mTOR) inhibitor** is the alkylating agent mainly used for BMT patients. Rarely is it used as a substitute agent for azathioprine in solid organ transplantation.

1. Sirolimus (Rapamune)

    a. Mechanism of action. Sirolimus binds the intracellular receptor FK binding protein-12 (FKBP-12). This complex inhibits the mTOR, which is a key regulatory kinase. This results in inhibiting T cell activation in a later stage of immune response to foreign antigen such as a graft.

    b. Dosing and monitoring. A dose of 2–10 mg/day is administered as a once-daily dose. Usually, a loading dose of 6–15 mg with a maintenance dose of 2–5 mg once daily is used. Blood levels are useful in clinical monitoring. The serum lipid profile, WBC count, and GI symptoms should be monitored.

    c. Side effects. Hyperlipidemia is the major side effect. In addition, leukopenia, thrombocytopenia, and GI side effects are common.

D. Alkylating agent. Cyclophosphamide is the alkylating agent mainly used for BMT patients. Rarely, it is used as a substitute agent for azathioprine in solid organ transplantation.

    1. Mechanism of action. It is converted to the active metabolite phosphoramide mustard in the liver, which inhibits the cross-linking of DNA, leading to cell death.

    2. Dosing and monitoring. Doses of cyclophosphamide up to 3–4 mg/kg/day for 4 days followed by a reduction to 1 mg/kg/day to treat graft rejection. The dosage should be titrated to maintain a WBC count greater than 4000/mm^3.

    3. Side effects. Hemorrhagic cystitis and **bone marrow suppression** (leukopenia, thrombocytopenia). In addition, nausea, vomiting, and diarrhea are common.

E. Antibody products

    1. Muromonab CD3 (Orthoclone; OKT3) is the first therapeutic mouse monoclonal antibody produced for use in humans.

        a. Mechanism of action. OKT3 is a mouse IgG2α immunoglobulin that binds to the CD3 structure on T lymphocytes. Once OKT3 is bound to the CD3 region of T cells, they lose the antigen recognition function and cannot initiate the rejection process.

        b. Dosing and monitoring. The dosage is 5 mg/day intravenously for 7–14 days for prevention or treatment of rejection. The CD3 + lymphocyte counts are monitored, and it is desirable that CD + cell be maintained at < 30/mm^3.

        c. Side effects. With the first few doses, the patient will develop severe flulike symptoms such as fever, chills, nausea, vomiting, and headache. The OKT3 stimulates T cells, and these symptoms are caused by abrupt release of cytokines such as interleukin 1, tumor necrosis factor α, and interleukin 6 from opsonized T cells (cytokine release syndrome). It requires premedications such as acetaminophen, diphenhydramine, and corticosteroids to reduce these side effects before OKT3 injection.

    2. Antithymocyte globulin (Thymoglobulin, Atgam)

        a. Mechanism of action. It is a purified polyclonal immunoglobulin from rabbits (Thymoglobulin) or horses (Atgam), which binds to the human T cells. However, it may have cross-reactivity against the red blood cells, platelets, and granulocytes.

        b. Dosing and monitoring. The dosage is 1.5 mg/kg (Thymoglobulin) or 15–20 mg/kg (Atgam) infusion daily through a central line for 7–14 days for prevention or treatment of rejection. The T-lymphocyte counts are monitored and maintained < 100/mm^3.

        c. Side effects. Antithymocyte globulin may cause fever, chills, erythema, leukopenia, thrombocytopenia, and anaphylactic reaction or serum sickness.

    3. Daclizumab (Zenapax)

        a. Mechanism of action. It is a molecularly engineered humanized immunoglobulin active against interleukin 2 receptor (CD25, or Tac), which binds to block the interleukin 2 receptor on the surface of activated T lymphocytes, thus preventing T cell activation and proliferation.

        b. Dosing and monitoring. It is indicated only for the prevention of acute rejection. The usual recommended dosage is 1 mg/kg (maximum of 100 mg) within 24 hr post-transplantation and every 2 weeks up to 8 weeks (a total of five doses).

        c. Side effects. Based on results of clinical trials, no specific safety monitoring is required with daclizumab.

4. **Basiliximab (Simulect)**
   a. **Mechanism of action.** It is a chimeric (murine/human) monoclonal antibody (IgG1κ), produced by recombinant DNA technology, that binds to block the interleukin 2 receptor on the surface of activated T lymphocytes; as a result, it prevents T lymphocyte activation, thus preventing acute rejections.
   b. **Dosing and monitoring.** It is indicated only for the prevention of acute rejection. The usual recommended dosage for the adult patient is two doses of 20 mg each at day 0 and day 4 after kidney transplantation. No special monitoring is required.
   c. **Side effects.** Based on results of clinical trials, no cytokine release syndromes have been noticed.

F. **Corticosteroids. Prednisone (Deltasone)** and **methylprednisolone (Solu-Medrol)** are the major corticosteroid products used for transplant patients.

1. **Mechanisms of action.** Corticosteroids have multiple pharmacological effects in various cells. Corticosteroids bind with intracellular glucocorticoid receptors, which results in altering DNA and RNA translation. As a result, corticosteroids cause a rapid and profound drop in circulating T lymphocytes. They have potent anti-inflammatory effects by inhibiting arachidonic acid release and macrophage phagocytosis.

2. **Dosing and monitoring.** They are used in both preventing and treating graft rejection and acute graft versus host disease. In general, prophylactic doses in solid organ transplantation are in the range of 1–2 mg/kg/day and tapered over months to 0.1–0.3 mg/kg/day. In the case of treatment, the dosage is 500 mg of methylprednisolone IV for 3–5 days or 1–2 mg/kg/day of oral prednisone, which should be tapered rapidly.

3. **Side effects.** In the long-term, corticosteroids cause more troubling side effects. They include psychological disturbances (i.e., euphoria, depression), adrenal axis suppression, hypertension, sodium and water retention, myopathy, impaired wound healing, increased appetite, osteoporosis, hyperglycemia, and cataracts.

IV. COMPLICATIONS OF IMMUNOSUPPRESSION

A. **Infections**

1. **Risk.** Transplant patients have a high risk of acquiring an infection owing to patient factors such as diabetes mellitus, hepatitis, or uremia. In addition, immunosuppressive agents can cause various effects, such as leukopenia, lymphopenia, or T cell dysfunction, which inhibit adequate immune response to the infection.

2. **Time course.** The risk of infection is greatest during the first 3 months after transplantation, when higher doses of immunosuppression are used, and again after a rejection episode is treated. This risk correlates with the overall level of immunosuppression.

3. **Types of infections** include bacterial, fungal, viral, and protozoan.

4. **Prevention**
   a. **Trimethoprim-sulfamethoxazole (Bactrim).** One single- or double-strength tablet daily for 6 months significantly reduces *Pneumocystis carinii* pneumonia and bacterial urinary tract infection. After 6 months, three times a week is effective.
   b. **Herpes and cytomegalovirus (CMV) infection.** Oral acyclovir (200 mg twice a day for normal renal function, with doses adjusted according to renal function) for herpes prophylaxis. For CMV prophylaxis, various prophylaxis can be used. High doses of acyclovir (800 mg four times a day for normal renal function, with doses adjusted according to renal function), oral ganciclovir (1 g three times a day for normal renal function, with doses adjusted according to renal function), valganciclovir (Valcyte) 900 mg daily, or high-titer CMV immunoglobulin are effective in reducing the incidence of CMV infection and invasive CMV disease.
   c. **Nystatin solution or clotrimazole troche** reduce oral candidiasis (thrush).

B. **Increased risk of malignancy**

1. **Cause.** Continuous immunosuppression interferes with normal immune surveillance and function for malignancy. In addition, some of the immunosuppressive drugs may be directly carcinogenic or activate oncogenic virus, such as Epstein-Barr virus (EBV).

2. **Characteristics.** Cancers that occur most frequently in the general population (e.g., lung, breast, colon) are not increased among transplant patients. However, various cancers uncommon in the general population are often more prevalent in transplant patients: lymphomas, squamous cell carcinomas of the lip and skin, Kaposi sarcoma, other sarcoma.

3. **Post-transplant lymphoproliferative diseases (PTLDs).** The incidence of lymphoma appears to correlate with the intensity of immunosuppression. It is especially well documented that T cell specific agents, including OKT3, cyclosporine, and tacrolimus, increase the incidence of lymphoproliferative diseases.

4. **Treatment.** In case of nonvital organ transplant, immunosuppression should be reduced or stopped. If EBV-related lymphoma occurs, acyclovir or ganciclovir therapy appears to be effective; the B cell–specific monoclonal antibody rituximab (Rituxan), is also used.

C. **Hypertension.** Many immunosuppressive agents cause hypertension. Cyclosporine and tacrolimus clearly increase arterial blood pressure, and steroids may exacerbate hypertension after transplantation from fluid and sodium retention. Treatment usually requires the use of multiple agents, including diuretics and calcium-channel blockers.

STUDY QUESTIONS

Directions for question 1: The question in this section can be correctly answered or completed by **one or more** of the suggested answers. Choose the answer, **A–E.**

A	if **I only** is correct
B	if **III only** is correct
C	if **I and II** are correct
D	if **II and III** are correct
E	if **I, II, and III** are correct

1. S.T., a 48-year-old, received her living related kidney transplant 2 months ago. At her clinic visit today, she complains of tiredness, shortness of breath, and pedal edema. The following lab results were obtained: serum creatinine is 2.1 mg/dL (1.3 mg/dL 3 weeks ago), BUN is 43 mg/dL (24 mg/dL 3 weeks ago), and cyclosporine levels 40 ng/mL (therapeutic range 150–300 ng/mL). She was diagnosed as having acute graft rejection. She was admitted to the hospital and was treated by Thymoglobulin. Which of the following regarding Thymoglobulin is true?

    I.   It is a horse serum against human B cells.
    II. It is an interleukin 2 receptor antagonist against human T cells.
    III. It is a rabbit immunoglobulin against human T cells.

Directions for question 2: The question in this section can be correctly answered or completed by **one** of the suggested answers or phrases. Choose the **best** answer.

2. After 7-day course of Thymoglobulin therapy, S.T's renal function improved by Thymoglobulin treatment. Her Thymoglobulin was completed and her blood cyclosporine level was 250 ng/mL. She was discharged to her home. Several days later, she developed diabetic coma and seizures. Her seizures were controlled by intravenous diazepam, and the local physician wanted to start phenytoin 200 mg daily as a maintenance therapy. What is appropriate advice for this prescription?

    (A) Phenytoin will reduce cyclosporine metabolism, so please reduce the cyclosporine dose by 100% and check cyclosporine level twice a week.
    (B) Phenytoin will increase cyclosporine metabolism, so please switch cyclosporine to tacrolimus.
    (C) Phenytoin will increase cyclosporine metabolism, so please switch phenytoin to valproic acid.
    (D) Phenytoin will not affect cyclosporine metabolism, so continue same dose of cyclosporine.
    (E) Phenytoin will reduce cyclosporine metabolism, so please monitor cyclosporine level more frequently.

Directions for question 3: The question in this section can be correctly answered or completed by **one or more** of the suggested answers. Choose the answer, **A–E.**

A	if **I only** is correct
B	if **III only** is correct
C	if **I and II** are correct
D	if **II and III** are correct
E	if **I, II, and III** are correct

3. On examination 6 months later, her renal function was good: creatinine 1.6 mg/dL and BUN 28 mg/dL. Today her blood pressure is 160/105. Which of the following medications contributes her hypertension?

   I. Neoral
   II. Deltasone
   III. CellCept

Directions for questions 4–6: Each of the questions, statements, or incomplete statements in this section can be correctly answered or completed by **one** of the suggested answers or phrases. Choose the **best** answer.

4. The physician asked you whether the immunosuppressant, basiliximab (Simulect) is useful in treating this patient's acute rejection.

(A) It is a humanized immunoglobulin G (IgG) product against interleukin 2 (IL-2) receptor and it is useful only in preventing acute rejection.

(B) It is a useful agent to treat rejection, but chest x-ray and monitoring of patient's fluid status are required before this therapy.

(C) It is useful, but patient's weight gain should be > 3% from the dry weight before therapy

(D) It is a chimeral IgG with specificity against IL-2 receptor and is useful only for prevention of rejection.

(E) It is a humanized horse serum against T cells and is a new agent useful for prevention and treatment of rejection.

5. All of the following are correct regarding infection prophylaxis in an organ transplant patient *except* which one?

(A) trimethoprim-sulfamethoxazole for *Pneumocystis carinii* pneumonia prophylaxis
(B) nystatin for fungal infection
(C) oral acyclovir for herpes simplex
(D) clotrimazole troche for oral thrush
(E) cefaclor for urinary tract infection

6. A 16-year-old girl who had received her transplant 2 years ago complained of hair growth on her face and did not want to take her medications any more. Which of the following is the likely cause of her problem?

(A) cyclosporine
(B) tacrolimus
(C) prednisone
(D) azathioprine
(E) mycophenolic acid

ANSWERS AND EXPLANATIONS

1. The answer is B *(III) [see III.E.2].*
Thymoglobulin is a antibody from rabbit against the human thymocytes. This drug can be used as a rejection prevention agent or a treatment agent for ongoing rejection. The dose for rejection treatment is 1.5 mg/kg daily for 7–10 days. Atgam is a horse antibody against the human thymocytes. Daclizumab (Zenapax) or basiliximab (Simulect) is an monoclonal antibody against an IL-2 receptor.

2. The answer is C *[see Table 60-2].*
Phenytoin is a potent cytochrome P450 enzyme inducer, which increases cyclosporine metabolism. When cyclosporine is used concurrently with phenytoin, it is necessary to increase cyclosporine dose by 500% to maintain the therapeutic levels, which is costly. Valproic acid is another antiepileptic agent, which does not interact with cyclosporine. So it is a good alternative for phenytoin in this case.

3. The answer is C *(II, III) [see III.A.1; III.F]*
Neoral (cyclosporine) and prednisone increase the blood pressure. Cyclosporine promotes the vasoconstriction and causes renal dysfunction, which contributes to hypertension. Deltasone (prednisone) increases fluid and sodium retention, which contributes to hypertension. CellCept (mycophenolate mofetil) is an antimetabolite inhibiting DNA synthesis and cell proliferation. Its side effects include leukopenia and thrombocytopenia and does not cause hypertension.

4. The answer is D *[see III.E.4.c].*
Basiliximab (Simulect) is a chimeric monoclonal antibody to the IL-2 receptor on the T cells. The chimeric antibody contains two parts from different origins in the one body (chimeric). The binding site of this antibody is originated from mouse, but the other part is humanized IgG. Interleukin 2 is T cell growth factor, initiating T cell proliferation. The basiliximab opsonizes this IL-2 receptor, which prevents T cell growth and proliferation, which are essential for the graft rejection process. Unlike OKT3 or antithymocyte globulin, it does not show any serious side effects, so it does not require premedications such as acetaminophen, diphenhydramine, and corticosteroids before its administration.

5. The answer is E *[see IV.A].*
All except for cefaclor are correct. Cefaclor is a broad-spectrum oral cephalosporin, which is not appropriate for prophylactic regimen.

6. The answer is A *[see III.A.1].*
Facial hair growth (hirsutism) is one of the cumbersome side effects of cyclosporine, which may discourage a patient's compliance.

61
Outcomes Research and Pharmacoeconomics

Peter K. Wong

Alan H. Mutnick

I. GENERAL CONCEPTS

A. Outcomes research (OR) is the study of healthcare interventions (treatment modalities such as drug therapies, surgery, and palliative therapy), care delivery processes, and healthcare quality that are evaluated to measure the extent to which optimal and desirable outcomes can be reached. Normally, the purpose of OR is to assess the value of a program or therapy in question.

1. The **Economic, Clinical, Humanistic Outcome (ECHO) model** provides a framework for comprehensive evaluation of outcomes. Three areas of outcomes identified by Kozma and Reeder (1998) are economic outcomes, clinical outcomes, and humanistic outcomes.

2. **Outcomes research methodologies** include retrospective chart review, prospective clinical trials, observational studies, and computer modeling studies.

3. **Examples of outcomes measures**
   a. Economic outcomes include acquisition costs associated with care, labor costs associated with care, costs to treat adverse drug reactions, costs of treatment failure, costs of hospital readmission, and costs of emergency room and clinic visits.
   b. Clinical outcomes include length of hospital stay, adverse drug reactions, hospital readmission, and death.
   c. Humanistic outcomes include patient satisfaction, functional status as measured by a validated instrument, and quality-of-life assessment.

B. Pharmacoeconomics (PE), a division of health economics, is designed to provide decision makers with information about the value of the different pharmacotherapies. According to Bootman, Townsend, McGhan (2006), PE research identifies, measures, and compares the costs (resources consumed) and consequences (clinical, economic, and humanistic) of pharmaceutical products and services.

II. COST

A. Definitions

1. **Total cost.** All expenses that are directly and indirectly necessary to provide a product or service

2. **Average cost.** The average cost per unit of output (total cost divided by quantity)

3. **Fixed cost.** Costs that do not vary with the quantity of output for a short-run production (e.g., rent, fixtures, fixed salary, depreciation, administrative costs)

4. **Variable cost.** Costs that vary with the level of output (e.g., wages, supplies)

5. **Marginal cost.** The extra cost of producing *one extra* unit of output

6. **Incremental cost.** Additional costs when comparing one alternative to another

7. **Direct cost.** Costs directly related to producing/providing a specific quantity of services or output (e.g., salary, drug cost and supply cost for the provision of pharmacy services)

8. **Indirect cost.** Costs that are allocated to the area(s) that produce/provide a specific quantity of services or output (e.g., overhead cost)

9. **Allowable cost.** A cost that is eligible to claim for purposes of reimbursement as necessary and relevant to the delivery of a unit of output

10. **Opportunity cost.** The cost of the benefit of pursuing an alternative course of action

11. **Operating cost.** Any cost that supports the operations to provide the output

B. **Cost and charge**

1. The meaning of the term *cost* depends on the perspective for the analysis. The following examples show differing perspectives.

2. Providers may include hospitals, physician offices, or ambulatory surgery centers, and the term *cost* means the total costs for providing the specific service(s).

3. Payors may include insurance companies, Medicare, or Medicaid, and the term *cost* means the price that they have to pay to obtain the service (i.e., charges by providers).

4. Charges do not equal the payment to providers. Depending on the contractual terms, many providers receive only a percentage of the charges for payment. These are called discounted charges. Many provides today receive a lump sum amount of dollars for each episode of care, e.g., diagnosis-related groups (DRGs) or case rate payment. This may also apply to both inpatient and outpatient treatments.

5. Contractual terms are rarely reviewed and vary with different insurance carriers. This creates additional confusion as to the costs associated for various services or therapies.

6. A recognizable way to resolve these hurdles is to use the cost to charge (RCC) ratio for the cost estimation. Multiply the RCC by the patient's charge to yield the estimated cost. RCC can be obtained from the individual hospital's Centers for Medicare and Medicaid Services (CMS) yearly cost report.

C. **Basic steps in assessing cost**

1. Define the units of service or output

2. Determine the number of service or output units provided

3. Determine cost drivers of these units of service or output

4. Calculate total costs, direct or indirect, related to the provision of this output or service

5. Calculate the average cost and incremental cost

III. ELEMENTS OF A GOOD STUDY

A. **Sound objective(s).** The study has well-defined objective(s) and answerable question(s).

B. **Perspective(s).** There is a defined perspective for analysis (e.g., patient, payor, provider, society). In many cases, study perspective determines the cost-effectiveness of an intervention. Most of the published PE guidelines suggest that societal perspective be considered as an additional perspective for analysis.

C. **Patient population** chosen must be within the scope of analysis. Patient selection criteria that are too stringent pose a threat to external validity. Patient selection criteria that are too liberal are a threat to internal validity. Consideration is also given to comorbidity and multiple treatment modalities.

D. **Possible comparators and their effectiveness.** All relevant alternatives for comparison are identified. Chosen comparator(s) should be reasonable and is the current preferred standard treatment. In some instances no treatment (placebo) is considered as an alternative.

E. Metrics for costs and consequences. Measures chosen for costs and consequences can affect the results of the analysis. Biases can be introduced into the analysis if units of measures are not clearly defined. This may pose a problem with a multicountry study in the aggregation of the final costs and consequences because currency exchange rates may fluctuate from time to time.

F. Inclusion of relevant costs and consequences in the analysis are based on the perspective chosen. The computation of costs and consequences should be transparent to readers. The key is reproducibility. Readers should be able to use the published computation methods with the local data to validate the findings.

G. A valid data source. Depending on the design of the study, data can come from clinical trials, observational studies, healthcare claim databases, chart reviews, and epidemiological data. Each of the sources of these data were designed for some other purpose than economic analysis. Limitations are listed in VIII.

H. Discounting for costs and consequences. Much discussion has been devoted to the appropriateness of discounting costs and consequences as well as the discount rate. The consensus at this time is to discount both costs and consequences. The discount rate normally is the opportunity cost of using resources. Many researchers have used the government bond rate. Regardless, the researcher must offer the justification for the chosen discount rate(s).

I. Incremental analysis provides an insight on the comparison for cost generated from one alternative to another alternative, and the additional benefit yielded from the increased cost.

J. Sensitivity analysis should include all the plausible values and their justification for the key parameters.

K. Time horizon of the analysis covers the full duration of treatment for the disease process. For example, the time horizon for the cholesterol-lowering agent's treatment should be the life span from the start day of treatment to the end of life.

L. Appropriateness and comprehensiveness of presentation and discussion of the study results. Similar to the clinical studies, the presentation of study results should not be biased. Interventional alternatives and study limitations must be addressed. Generalizability and applicability are also discussed.

IV. PHARMACOECONOMIC METHODOLOGIES

A. Cost of illness (COI) is the evaluation and assessment of the resources used in treating an illness. This technique is used to obtain the baseline cost information before the introduction of a new intervention. Costs are measured in terms of dollars. Like any PE analysis, the evaluator needs to define the analysis perspective. A different perspective will change the cost structure. For example, from a patient's perspective, the cost of illness will include the transportation to and from the treatment site. Time duration of the disease can be critical in determining the cost and may be a source of bias. No comparison is made in this type of analysis.

B. Cost–benefit analysis (CBA) is a tool used to determine priority for the resource allocation. The technique can be applied to the comparison of healthcare programs and with non-healthcare programs, such as social welfare programs. For example, one can compare the costs and benefits of a coronary risk factor reduction program and the childhood immunization program and the domestic violence prevention program. This technique consists of identifying all of the benefits that accrue from the program and converting them into dollars in the year that they occur. The stream of costs and benefits are then discounted to present value at the selected discount rate. Net benefit is computed for each program and can then be compared with other programs.

C. Cost-minimization analysis (CMA). The underlying assumption for this type of analysis assumes that consequences are equivalent. Therefore, only cost is compared. The cheapest intervention will be chosen for implementation. Equivalent outcomes may not necessarily be equal. One needs to determine the key outcome of each comparator. For example, two drugs may have the equivalent therapeutic value but different side effect profiles. In such cases, consequences may not be equivalent, and this technique is not appropriate. CEA should be used instead.

D. **Cost-effectiveness analysis (CEA)** is a technique to assist the decision maker in identifying a preferred choice among possible alternatives within similar consequences (e.g., same therapeutic category) in terms of health improvement created (e.g., life year gained, clinical cures). It is not to be used to compare different consequences for each alternative, such as blood pressure reduction to degree of cholesterol lowering. Consequences can be intermediate outcomes or surrogate outcomes such as the reperfusion time of the vessel after thrombolytic therapy. Generally, the incremental cost of a program or an intervention from a specified perspective is compared to the incremental health effects. An example is the cost per unit of blood pressure reduction with each antihypertensive agent compared. The results of the analysis normally are stated in terms of cost per unit of effectiveness.

E. **Cost-utility analysis (CUA).** Unlike CEA, CUA measures the consequences in terms of the quality-adjusted life year (QALY) gained. The results of the analysis are normally expressed as a cost per QALY. The metric of QALY incorporates both the improvement in quantity of life, quality of life, and the preference (utility value) of the health state. There are three sources of obtaining utility values for health states in CUA: judgment to estimate the utility values, values from the literature, or values elicited from a sample of subjects. Common techniques for eliciting utility values are rating scale (visual analog scale), standard gamble, and time trade-off. Five circumstances have been summarized that detail when CUA may be the appropriate technique to apply.

1. When quality of life is the only outcome

2. When quality and quantity of life are health outcomes

3. When the intervention affects both mortality and morbidity and a combined unit of outcome is desired

4. When the intervention being compared has a wide range of potential outcomes and a common unit of outcome is needed

5. When the objective is to compare a gold standard intervention that already has the cost per QALY. QALY is calculated by multiplying the utility values obtained for the specific health state with the quantity of life years spent in that specific health state. Comparison can then be made for the program and intervention.

F. **Multiattribute utility theory (MAUT) or analysis (MAUA)** is another technique frequently used in assessing utilities. In this situation, several attributes can be included, such as clinical effect and financial effect as well as quality of life. It is possible to preferentially weigh the decision based on what the priorities are for the decision maker and then apply the weights to identify the most preferable therapy, service, and so on. As evidenced from the following three examples, the individual's perspective will have a major effect on the final decision made, based on the levels of priority chosen for evaluation.

1. A physician may view clinical outcome to represent 70% of the decision, followed by patient's quality of life (20%), and last the costs (10%).

2. A hospital administrator may view the financial outcomes (70%) as a major priority, followed by the clinical outcome (20%), and last the quality of life (10%).

3. A patient with health insurance might view the clinical outcome (45%) and quality of life (45%) as the top priorities and have minimal concern for the financial outcomes (10%) of such a decision.

G. **Willingness to pay (WTP)** technique is used to assess the perceived value or benefit of a product and service. The WTP values can be obtained through two approaches:

1. Indirect measurement, which examines in actual payments previous real-world decisions that involve trade-offs between money and expected outcomes

2. Direct measurement, which uses survey methods to elicit stated dollar on the perceived benefits. In this second approach, researchers are seeking to provide sufficient background information to create within the respondent's mind a hypothetical market in which the person provides a judgment of the value of the proposed service.

3. The challenge of using contingent valuation is to present within the questionnaire sufficient, clearly organized information to allow this judgment to occur. Basic facts need to be given at the appropriate time. Unlike CBA, WTP takes into consideration the psychological aspects of the illness as well as the physical deterioration. The use of WTP as an outcome measure is theoretically consistent with welfare economics. It also provides a means to assign dollar values to health outcomes.

V. DECISION ANALYSIS is a systematic approach to decision making under conditions of uncertainty. It is a tool for helping the decision makers identify options that are available, predict the consequences and value of each option based on the probabilities assigned to each option, and choose the option that has the best payoff. Decision analysis can be incorporated into the pharmacoeconomics evaluation. Steps in performing a decision analysis are as follows:

A. Identify and bound the decision. All the ground rules such as analysis perspective, comparators selection, time span, and decision rules are identified and clarified.

B. Develop a decision tree (Figure 61-1). The decision maker will structure the decision in the form of a tree with branches from left to right. Each branch is a segment of a path that leads to an outcome. The process of setting up the tree helps the decision maker put thoughts on paper and provides an evaluation for each option that occurs.

C. Assess and assign probabilities. Probability related to each branch is assessed and assigned. Probabilities can be obtained from the published literature, an expert panel, or clinical trials.

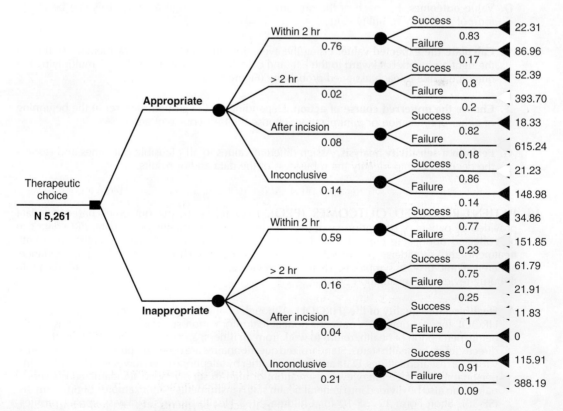

Figure 61-1. Decision tree with probabilities included.

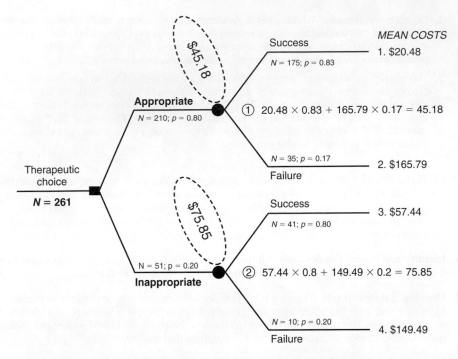

Figure 61-2. Completed decision tree after averaging out and folding back.

D. Value outcomes. For each of the outcome possibilities, assign a value. This can be in the form of monetary or utility values.

E. Calculate the expected value. Using the averaging-out and folding-back method, start from the right and work backward to the left, and calculate the expected value by multiplying the outcome value to each assigned probability (Figure 61-2).

F. Choose the preferred course of action. Depending on the ground rules set in the beginning of either optimization or minimization, choose the best course of action.

G. Perform a sensitivity analysis. Assign different values to all plausible outcomes and resolve the decision tree to identify the robustness of the data and/or results.

VI. PATIENT-REPORTED OUTCOMES (PRO). PRO refers to any outcomes based on data provided by patient or patient proxy. It includes health-related quality of life data. PRO data can be collected during the clinical trial. Examples of PRO data include patient satisfaction with treatment and providers, functional status, psychosocial well-being, treatment compliance/adherence, and disease symptoms. There is a growing amount of interest in adding PRO data into the drug-review and evaluation process.

A. Health-related quality of life (HRQOL). Although quality of life focuses on all aspects of life, HRQOL focuses only on a patient's nonclinical information such as functional status, well-being, perception of health, return to work from an illness, and other health outcomes that are directly affect by health status. Standardized questionnaires are used to capture HRQOL data in a variety of research settings. Data are obtained either by telephone interview, self-administration, personal face-to-face interview, observation, or mail-in survey. Such standardized questionnaires can also be divided into general health status instruments—for example,, Short-Form 36 (SF-36), Short-Form 12, SF-10 for Children, SF-8 Health Surveys, sickness impact profiles (SIP)—or disease-specific instrument (e.g., McGill Pain Inventory, Beck Depression Scale, Functional Living Index—Cancer). The general health status instruments measure the global health status, whereas the disease-specific instruments target the disease-specific issues.

B. **Short form surveys** are the most frequently used general health status instruments. There are a variety of dimensions available, depending on the chosen short form instrument. The original SF-36 includes physical functions, social functions, emotional role, physical role, bodily pain, mental health, general health, and vitality. Other survey instruments may contain only some of these dimensions. Interested readers can explore the the following Web site: www.quality-metric.com for more information.

C. **Psychometric properties.** Before using any instrument, the researcher must understand the psychometric properties of the chosen instrument. The psychometric properties consist of the reliability and validity information of the instrument. In addition, the sensitivity and specificity of the instrument are also important.

   1. **Reliability** is a measure of consistency. Can we reproduce the same score under the same conditions with the same individual? Statistical methods of measuring reliability are Cronbach's α, Pearson's r coefficient, and the κ statistic.

   2. **Validity** is a measure of accuracy. Is the instrument measuring what it is supposed to measure? Types of validity are content validity, construct validity, criterion validity, and convergent/divergent validity.

   3. **Use of the instrument.** The psychometric properties preclude "mixing and matching" sections of established questionnaires or selection of a section of an established questionnaire for administration without recalibrating the instrument's psychometric properties.

VII. MODELING STUDIES.
Mathematical modeling is widely used today in the economic evaluation of medications and healthcare technologies.

A. The goal for modeling is to assemble evidence of costs and outcomes in a form that can project long-term consequences. Model-based evaluations are great tools for healthcare decision makers.

B. Mathematical models provide the cost–consequence estimates that cannot be revealed by randomized control trials or epidemiological studies because of the duration required for long-term studies (10–20 years).

C. Results derived from modeling assist decision makers in making informed decisions. However, the quality of the decision is based completely on the truthfulness of the projected results, which in turn depends on the input information and assumptions imposed for each model.

D. The International Society of Pharmacoeconomics and Outcomes Research (ISPOR) recommends the following criteria for assessing the quality of models: model structure, data used as inputs for the model, and model validation.[1]

VIII. 1997 FDA MODERNIZATION ACT, SECTION 114, HEALTH CARE ECONOMIC INFORMATION

A. "Health care economic information provided to a formulary committee, or other similar entity, in the course of the committee or entity carrying out its responsibilities for the selection of drugs for managed care or other similar organizations, shall not be considered to be false or misleading under this paragraph if the health care economic information directly relates to an indication approved . . . for such drug and is based on competent and reliable scientific evidence." (From the FDA's Modernization Act of 1997, http://www.fda.gov/cder/guidance/s830enr.txt)

---

[1]Weinstein MC, O'Brien B, Hornberger J, et al. ISPOR Task Force on Good Research Practices. Principles of good practice for decision analytic modeling in health-care evaluation. Value in Health 2003;6:9–17.

B. Health economic information means any analysis that identifies, measures, or compares the economic consequences including the costs of the represented health outcomes, or the use of a drug to the use of another drug, or to another healthcare intervention, or to no intervention.

C. Key concepts of the act

1. A venue for the pharmaceutical industry to provide OR and/or PE research studies to decision makers

2. Economic information can be provided in the form of CMA, CBA, CUA, COI, and cost-quality of life.

3. Competent and reliable scientific information pertaining to an approved indication

4. Standard of competent and reliable scientific information has not been addressed.

IX. PRACTICAL ISSUES IN INTERPRETING OUTCOMES RESEARCH AND PHARMACOECONOMIC STUDIES

A. Comparisons between economic study and randomized clinical trials (RCTs)

1. Economic studies are carried out in an observational environment, whereas RCTs depend on rigorous experimental design with strict inclusion/exclusion criteria.

2. RCTs rely on highly controlled and artificial clinical settings to demonstrate clinical efficacy. Clinical and economic end points of the study may not be the same. In addition, RCTs tend to have additional protocol costs (e.g., extra tests) and inflated benefits (e.g., medication compliance, appropriateness of utilization).

3. Economic studies have large sample sizes, whereas RCTs are limited to a relatively small sample size.

4. Economic studies are generalizable to the broader patient population, whereas RCTs are limited to those included within the stringent entry criteria, which might not represent the typical patient receiving the tested therapy.

B. Multiple countries' OR and PE studies

1. There are significant differences in physician practice patterns and care-delivery systems among different countries.

2. Different methods of funding healthcare and allocating health expenditures make it almost impossible to calculate costs.

3. Patients' concerns and beliefs are different.

C. Budgetary constraints. Decision making should not be solely based on the information from the PE analysis because most published PE studies do not impose budgetary constraint as part of the analysis. *Cost-effective* does not equal *affordable*. In addition, one should also consider the implementation costs of the program. In many instances, implementation costs may exceed the benefits or effectiveness of the program.

D. Reproducibility

1. Often, owing to journal space limitation, lengthy cost computations are eliminated from the published article. Such practice creates an impossible auditing mechanism for the derivation and computation of costs. Critical assessment of this section of the published article is necessary to ensure the validity and reliability of the results.

2. Modeling is an appropriate method when the disease and treatment in question has a lengthy time span and ethical dilemma of withdrawing treatment. However, assumptions and input values to these models are not transparent to readers.

3. Both issues make it almost impossible to reproduce the study results using the local data.

E. **Limitations of claim data studies.** Claim data are designed for billing purposes. There is no differentiation between comorbid conditions and complications in coding data. This can pose a problem in quality benchmark studies. In addition, coding practice may be different from one institution to another, a threat to reliability.

STUDY QUESTIONS

Directions: Each of the questions, statements, or incomplete statements in this section can be correctly answered or completed by **one** of the suggested answers or phrases. Choose the **best** answer.

1. The underlying assumption of cost-minimization analysis (CMA) is

(A) calculation of cost minimization ratio.
(B) consequences are equivalent.
(C) costs are equivalent.
(D) no more than two comparators in any analysis.

2. Which one of these statements is *not* true for the differences between economic studies and randomized clinical trials (RCTs)?

(A) Generalizability and applicability of the results differ between economic studies and RCTs.
(B) Clinical end point and economic end point are identical.
(C) RCTs tend to have inflated benefits and additional protocol-driven costs.
(D) Sample size of the economic study is normally larger than in the RCT.

3. In choosing an instrument to measure the health-related quality of life (HRQOL), attention should be paid to

(A) reliability and validity of the instrument.
(B) sensitivity and specificity of the instrument.
(C) length of the instrument.
(D) All of the above

4. In choosing a study perspective, the current pharmacoeconomic (PE) guidelines have suggested which one of the following perspectives to be included?

(A) society
(B) payors
(C) patients
(D) providers

5. When interpreting a multination economic clinical trial, what issue needs special attention?

(A) cost computations
(B) healthcare funding and cost-allocating mechanisms?
(C) patients' variations and beliefs
(D) All of the above

6. Which one of these pharmacoeconomic (PE) techniques does not address both cost and consequences?

(A) cost-benefit analysis
(B) cost-effectiveness analysis
(C) cost-utility analysis
(D) cost of illness

7. Which of the following is an example of a clinical outcome indicator?

(A) dollars spent treating acute myocardial infarction
(B) resources used in diagnosing the presence of medical errors
(C) duration of hospitalization and mortality versus discharge rate for ventricular fibrillation patients treated with amiodarone
(D) functional capacity of patients treated with ramipril in the presence of cardiovascular risk factors

ANSWERS AND EXPLANATIONS

1. The answer is B *[see IV.C].*
CMA assumes all consequences compared are equivalent. For this reason, only the cost of each alternative is compared. The least expensive alternative will be chosen.

2. The answer is B *[see IX.A].*
Clinical and economic end points are generally not equal. In the sequence of the study events, efficacy should come before effectiveness.

3. The answer is D *[see VI.C.1–3].*
All of the characteristics listed require attention.

4. The answer is A *[see III.B].*
The societal perspective must be included. It is critical in the healthcare environment to identify the perspective from which a decision is being made because that perspective directly affects the final decision. The decision to add a high-cost, moderately effective therapy for the treatment of hospitalized septic patients might be different if viewed from a hospital formulary committee (in-house budgetary concerns) than from the local community (saving lives at whatever expense).

5. The answer is D *[see IX.B.1–3].*
All of the issues stated need special attention and play a major role in developing multination economic evaluations to avoid carrying out a study, which when completed cannot be generalized to the broad patient population.

6. The answer is D *[see IV.A].*
The cost of illness methodology is carried out as an assessment of the necessary resources, which will be used to treat a designated illness. Resources are measured in terms of dollars, and there are no comparator groups in the evaluation.

7. The answer is C *[see I.A.3.].*
Clinical outcomes include the following: length of hospital stay, adverse drug reactions, hospital readmission, and death. These are definable measures of a patient's response to a given treatment, such as amiodarone used for the treatment of ventricular fibrillation.

PRESCRIPTION DISPENSING INFORMATION AND METROLOGY

Prescriptions

PARTS OF THE PRESCRIPTION

A prescription is an order for medication for use by a patient that is issued by a physician, dentist, veterinarian, or other licensed practitioner who is authorized to prescribe medication or by their agent via a collaborative practice agreement. A prescription is usually written on a single sheet of paper that is commonly imprinted with the prescriber's name, address, and telephone number. A medication order is similar to a prescription, but it is written on the patient chart and intended for use by a patient in an institutional setting.

All prescriptions should contain accurate and appropriate information about the patient and the medication that is being prescribed. In addition, a prescription order for a **controlled substance** must contain the following information:

1. Date of issue
2. Full name and address of the patient
3. Drug name, strength, dosage form, and quantity prescribed
4. Directions for use
5. Name, address, and Drug Enforcement Agency (DEA) number of the prescriber
6. Signature of the prescriber

A written prescription order is required for substances listed in **Schedule II.** Prescriptions for controlled substances listed in **Schedule II** are **never** refillable. Any other prescription that has no indication of refills is not refillable.

Prescriptions for medications that are listed in Schedules III, IV, and V may be issued either in writing or orally to the pharmacist. If authorized by the prescriber, these prescriptions may be refilled up to five times within 6 months of the date of issue. If the prescriber wishes the patient to continue to take the medication after 6 months or five refills, a new prescription order is required.

THE PRESCRIPTION LABEL

In addition to the name of the patient, the pharmacy, and the prescriber, the prescription label should accurately identify the medication and provide directions for its use.

The label for a prescription order for a controlled substance must contain the following information:

1. Name and address of the pharmacy
2. Serial number assigned to the prescription by the pharmacy
3. Date of the initial filling
4. Name of the patient
5. Name of the prescriber
6. Directions for use
7. Cautionary statements as required by law*

AUXILIARY LABELS

Auxiliary, or cautionary, labels provide additional important information about the proper use of the medication. Examples include "Shake Well" for suspensions or emulsions; "For External Use Only" for

---

*The label of any drug that is listed as a controlled substance in Schedule II, III, or IV of the Controlled Substances Act must contain the following warning: **CAUTION: Federal law prohibits the transfer of this drug to any person other than the patient for whom it was prescribed.**

topical lotions, solutions, or creams; and "May Cause Drowsiness" for medications that depress the central nervous system. The information contained on auxiliary labels should be brought to the attention of the patient when the medication is dispensed. The pharmacist should place only appropriate auxiliary labels on the prescription container because too many labels may confuse the patient.

BEFORE DISPENSING THE PRESCRIPTION

Double-check the accuracy of the prescription.
Provide undivided attention when filling the prescription.

1. Check the patient information (e.g., name, address, date of birth, telephone number).
2. Check the patient profile (e.g., allergies, medical conditions, other drugs, including over-the-counter medications).
3. Check the drug (e.g., correct drug name, correct spelling, appropriate drug for the patient's condition), and verify that there are no known drug interactions. **Always verify the name of the drug. Beware of drug names that look alike (see table).**
4. Check the dosage, including the drug strength, the dosage form (e.g., capsule, liquid, modified release), the individual dose, the total daily dose, the duration of treatment, and the units (e.g., mg, mL, tsp, tbsp).
5. Check the label. Compare the drug dispensed with the prescription. Verify the National Drug Code (NDC) number. Ensure that the information is accurate, that the patient directions are accurate and easily understood, and that the auxiliary labels are appropriate.
6. **Provide patient counseling. Be sure that the patient fully understands the drug treatment as well as any precautions.**

Examples of Drugs with Similar Names

Brand name	Celebrex	Cerebyx	Celexa
Generic name	Celecoxib capsules	Fosphenytoin sodium injection	Citalopram HCl
Manufacturer	Searle	Parke-Davis	Forest
Indication	Osteoarthritis and rheumatoid arthritis	Prevention and treatment of seizures	Major depression

Dangerous or Confusing Abbreviations

Numerous common abbreviations and symbols have been associated with errors. Detailed lists of these can be found at the websites of the Institute for Safe Medication Practices (ISMP) and Joint Commission for the Accreditation of Healthcare Organizations (JCAHO) at :

http://www.ismp.org/Tools/abbreviationslist.pdf.
http://www.jcaho.org/accredited + organizations/patient + safety/06_dnu_list.pdf.

The JCAHO has created a "Do Not Use" list of abbreviations that its accredited organizations should not allow to be used.

➤**"U" or "IU" for units**: the "U" has been misinterpreted as various numbers such as zero, four; serious harm has occurred with insulin and heparin as a result of confusion. For example, a patient received 66 units of insulin instead of 6 units. The order was written for "6u" of regular insulin but was misinterpreted. The word "units" should be written out in full.
➤**"QD, Q.D, qd, q.d."**: common abbreviations for daily have been misinterpreted as "QID" or "qid" and overdoses have occurred. "Daily" should be written out in full.
➤**"Q.O.D, QOD, qod"**: common abbreviations for every other day have been misinterpreted as QID (four times daily). This should be written out completely as "every other day."

➤**Trailing zero**: when a dose is ordered and followed with a decimal point and a zero, such as 2.0 mg. or 25.0 mg., errors can occur. The decimal point may be missed and an overdose can occur. For example, Warfarin 2.0 mg may be misinterpreted as 20 mg. Trailing zeros should be avoided and the dose written without the additional zero, for example Warfarin 2 mg. rather than 2.0 mg.

➤**Lack of leading zero**: a drug's dose may be less than 1 mg., such as Digoxin. Often the dose may be written without a leading zero, such as Digoxin .25 mg., rather than as Digoxin 0.25 mg. Errors have occurred because the decimal point is missed. For example, Warfarin .5 mg may be interpreted as Warfarin 5 mg. Leading zeroes should be included, so the dose is written as "Digoxin 0.25 mg. or Warfarin 0.5 mg."

➤**MS, MSO4, MgSO$_4$: Abbreviations for morphine sulfate (MS, MSO4) have been confused with Magnesium sulfate (MgSO4). It is recommend to write out each name in full rather than using abbreviations: morphine sulfate or magnesium sulfate.**

In addition to the above abbreviations, there are numerous other hazardous symbols and abbreviations which should be reviewed with caution when used on prescriptions. Examples include:

➤**"cc"** : Often used instead of "ml." this has been misinterpreted as a "0" (zero). Use "ml."

➤**"µg"**: Used for "micrograms," for example, Levothyroxine 250 µg. daily. The symbol has been mistaken for "mg." and overdoses have occurred. Best to use "mcg." Or write out "micrograms."

➤**"<" or " >"** : Symbols for " less than" (<) or "greater than" (>) have been mistaken for each other or misinterpreted as numbers. Best to write out as "less than" or "greater than."

➤**"HCT"** : An abbreviation for "hydrocortisone" has been misinterpreted as "hydrochlorothiazide. " Best to write name out completely.

➤**"HCl"**: An abbreviation for "hydrochloric acid" has been misinterpreted as "KCl" (potassium chloride). Best to write out name completely.

Common Abbreviations

Considerable variation occurs in the use of capitalization, italicization, and punctuation in abbreviations. The following list shows the abbreviations that are most often encountered by pharmacists.

A, aa., or aa	of each	mcg, mcg., or μg	microgram
a.c.	before meals	mEq	milliequivalent
ad	to, up to	mg or mg.	milligram
a.d.	right ear	ml or mL	milliliter
ad lib.	at pleasure, freely	μl or μL	microliter
a.m.	morning	ℳ	minim
amp.	ampule	N&V	nausea and vomiting
ante	before	Na	sodium
aq.	water	N.F.	National Formulary
a.s.	left ear	No.	number
asa	aspirin	noct.	night, in the night
a.u.	each ear, both ears	non rep.	do not repeat
b.i.d.	twice a day	NPO	nothing by mouth
BP	British Pharmacopoeia	N.S., NS, or N/S	normal saline
BSA	body surface area	1/2 NS	half-strength normal saline
c. or c	with	O	pint
cap. or caps.	capsule	o.d.	right eye, every day
cp	chest pain	o.l. or o.s.	left eye
D.A.W.	dispense as written	OTC	over the counter
cc or cc.	cubic centimeter	o.u.	each eye, both eyes
comp.	compound, compounded	oz.	ounce
dil.	dilute	p.c.	after meals
D.C., dc, or disc.	discontinue	PDR	*Physicians' Desk Reference*
disp.	dispense	p.m.	afternoon, evening
div.	divide, to be divided	p.o.	by mouth
dl or dL	deciliter	Ppt	precipitated
d.t.d.	give of such doses	pr	for the rectum
DW	distilled water	prn or p.r.n.	as needed
D5W	dextrose 5% in water	pt.	pint
elix.	elixir	pulv.	powder
e.m.p.	as directed	pv	for vaginal use
et	and	q.	every
ex aq.	in water	q.d.	every day
fl or fld	fluid	q.h.	every hour
fl oz	fluid ounce	q. 4 hr.	every four hours
ft.	make	q.i.d.	four times a day
g or Gm	gram	q.o.d.	every other day
gal.	gallon	q.s.	a sufficient quantity
GI	gastrointestinal	q.s. ad	a sufficient quantity to make
gr or gr.	grain	R	rectal
gtt or gtt.	drop, drops	R.L. or R/L	Ringer's lactate
H	hypodermic	℞	prescription
h. or hr.	hour	s. or s	without
h.s.	at bedtime	Sig.	write on label
IM	intramuscular	sol.	solution
inj.	injection	S.O.B.	shortness of breath
IV	intravenous	s.o.s.	if there is need (once only)
IVP	intravenous push	ss. or ss	one-half
IVPB	intravenous piggyback	stat.	immediately
K	potassium	subc, subq, or s.c.	subcutaneously
l or L	liter	sup. or supp	suppository
lb.	pound	susp.	suspension
μ	Greek mu	syr.	syrup
M	mix	tab.	tablet
m² or M²	square meter	tal.	such, such a one

tal. dos.	such doses	**U or u.**	unit
tbsp. or T	tablespoonful	**u.d. or ut dict.**	as directed
t.i.d.	three times a day	**ung.**	ointment
tr. or tinct.	tincture	**U.S.P. or USP**	United States Pharmacopoeia
tsp. or t.	teaspoonful	**w/v**	weight/volume
TT	tablet triturates		

Metrology

THE METRIC, APOTHECARY, AND AVOIRDUPOIS SYSTEMS

Metric system

1. Basic units

Mass = g or gram
Length = m or meter
Volume = L or liter
1 cc (cubic centimeter) of water is approximately equal to 1 mL and weighs 1 g.

2. Prefixes

kilo- 10^3, or 1000 times the basic unit
hekto- 10^2, or 100 times the basic unit
deka- 10^1, or 10 times the basic unit
deci- 10^{-1}, or 0.1 times the basic unit
centi- 10^{-2}, or 0.01 times the basic unit
milli- 10^{-3}, or 0.001 times the basic unit
micro- 10^{-6}, or one-millionth of the basic unit
nano- 10^{-9}, or one-billionth of the basic unit
pico- 10^{-12}, or one-trillionth of the basic unit

Examples of these prefixes include milligram (mg), which equals one-thousandth of a gram, and deciliter (dL), which equals 100 mL, or 0.1 L.

Apothecary system

1. Volume (fluids or liquid)

60 minims (℥) = 1 fluidrachm or fluidram (f℥) or (℥)
8 fluidrachms (480 minims) = 1 fluidounce (f℥ or ℥)
16 fluidounces = 1 pint (pt or 0)
2 pints (32 fluidounces) = 1 quart (qt)
4 quarts (8 pints) = 1 gallon (gal or C)

2. Mass (weight)

20 grains (gr) = 1 scruple (℈)
3 scruples (60 grains) = 1 drachm or dram (℥)
8 drachms (480 grains) = 1 ounce (℥)
12 ounces (5760 grains) = 1 pound (lb)

Avoirdupois system

1. Volume

1 fluidrachm = 60 min.
1 fluid ounce = 8 fl. dr.
= 480 min.
1 pint = 16 fl. oz.
= 7680 min.

```
1 quart  = 2 pt.
         = 32 fl. oz.
1 gallon = 4 qt.
         = 128 fl. oz.
```

2. Mass (weight)

The grain is common to both the apothecary and the avoirdupois systems.

437.5 grains (gr) = 1 ounce (oz)
16 ounces (7000 grains) = 1 pound (lb)

CONVERSION

Exact equivalents

Exact equivalents are used for the conversion of specific quantities in pharmaceutical formulas and prescription compounding.

1. Length

1 meter (m) = 39.37 in.
1 inch (in) = 2.54 cm.

2. Volume

```
       1 ml = 16.23 minims (♏)
       1 ♏ = 0.06 mL
      1 f℥ = 3.69 mL
      1 f℥ = 29.57 mL
       1 pt = 473 mL
1 gal (U.S.) = 3785 mL
```

3. Mass

```
        1 g = 15.432 gr
       1 kg = 2.20 lb (avoir.)
       1 gr = 0.065 g or 65 mg
1 oz (avoir.) = 28.35 g
  1 ℥ (apoth.) = 31.1 g
1 lb (avoir.) = 454 g
1 lb (apoth.) = 373.2 g
```

4. Other equivalents

```
 1 oz (avoir.) = 437.5 gr
  1 ℥ (apoth.) = 480 gr
  1 gal (U.S.) = 128 fl ℥
1 fl ℥ (water) = 455 gr
 1 gr (apoth.) = 1 gr (avoir.)
```

Approximate equivalents

Physicians may use approximate equivalents to prescribe the dose quantities using the metric and apothecary systems of weights and measures, respectively. Household units are often used to inform the patient of the size of the dose. In view of the almost universal practice of using an ordinary household teaspoon to administer medication, a teaspoon may be considered 5 mL. However, when accurate measurement of a liquid dose is required, the USP recommends the use of a calibrated oral syringe or dropper.

```
 1 fluid dram = 1 teaspoonful
              = 5 mL
4 fluidounces = 120 mL
8 fluidounces = 1 cup
              = 240 mL
      1 grain = 65 mg
        1 kg = 2.2 pounds (lb)
```

APPENDIX **B**

COMMON PRESCRIPTION DRUGS AND OVER-THE-COUNTER PRODUCTS

The FDA Approved Drug Products With Therapeutic Equivalence Evaluation: The *Orange Book*

The United States Food and Drug Administration (FDA) publishes the book, *Approved Drug Products With Therapeutic Equivalence Evaluation,* often known as the *Orange Book.* An electronic version of the *Orange Book* is available on the Internet at http://www.fda.gov/cder/ob/. This book is also reproduced by the United States Pharmacopeial Convention, Inc., in the publication, USP DI, Volume III, *Approved Drug Products and Legal Requirements.*

The texts, which are published annually, identify the prescription and nonprescription products that are formally approved by the FDA on the basis of safety and effectiveness. They also provide the FDA's therapeutic equivalence evaluations for approved multiple-source prescription drug products.

The *Orange Book* is a drug product selection guide for pharmacists to use when dispensing a generic drug product as a substitute for the brand-name equivalent. A few drug products that were on the market before 1938 received a "grandfathered" FDA approval. These products are assumed to be safe and effective because of their long usage (e.g., digoxin tablets, phenobarbital tablets). These older products do not have therapeutic equivalence ratings at this time.

The *Orange Book* uses various codes to indicate therapeutic equivalence. The first letter "A" designates drug products that the FDA considers therapeutically equivalent to a pharmaceutically equivalent drug product. These products can be safely substituted. The first letter "B" designates drug products that, for various reasons, the FDA does not consider bioequivalent to the pharmaceutically equivalent drug product.

Therapeutic Equivalence Evaluation Codes

A Codes

Drug products that the FDA considers therapeutically equivalent to other pharmaceutically equivalent products

AA Products in conventional dosage forms that do not present bioequivalence problems
AB Products that meet necessary bioequivalence requirements
AN Solutions and powders for aerosolization
AO Injectable oil solutions
AO Injectable aqueous solutions, and in certain instances, intravenous nonaqueous solutions
AT Topical products

B Codes

Drug products that the FDA does not consider therapeutically equivalent to other pharmaceutically equivalent products at this time

B* Drug products that require further FDA investigation and review to determine therapeutic equivalence
BC Extended-release dosage forms (capsules, injectables, and tablets)
BD Active ingredients and dosage forms that have documented problems with bioequivalence
BE Delayed-release oral dosage forms
BN Products in aerosol-nebulizer drug-delivery systems

1300

BP Active ingredients and dosage forms that have potential problems with bioequivalence
BR Suppositories or enemas that deliver drugs for systemic absorption
BS Drug products that have drug standard deficiencies
BT Topical products that have bioequivalence issues
BX Drug products for which the data are sufficient to determine therapeutic equivalence

Top 200 Prescription Drugs by Trade Name and Generic Name[a]

Rank	Trade Name	Generic Name
1	Lipitor	Atorvastatin
2	Synthroid	Levothyroxine
3	Lortab	Hydrocodone/acetaminophen
4	Toprol-XL™	Metoprolol succinate
5	Hydrochlorothiazide	Hydrochlorothiazide
6	Norvasc	Amlodipine
7	Zithromax	Azithromycin
8	Proventil	Albuterol
9	Tenormin	Atenolol
10	Zoloft	Sertraline
11	Lasix	Furosemide
12	Lexapro	Escitalopram
13	Amoxil	Amoxicillin
14	Coumadin	Warfarin
15	Singulair	Montelukast
16	Fosamax	Alendronate
17	Zestril	Lisinopril
18	Prevacid	Lansoprazole
19	Potassium Chloride	Potassium chloride
20	Allegra	Fexofenadine
21	Advair	Fluticasone/salmeterol
22	Effexor (XR)	Venlafaxine
23	Zyrtec	Cetirizine
23	Nexium	Esomeprazole
25	Ambien	Zolpidem
26	Wellbutrin (SR, XL)	Bupropion
27	Maxzide™	Triamterene/hydrochlorothiazide
28	Premarin	Conjugated estrogens
29	Flonase™	Fluticasone
30	Plavix	Clopidogrel
31	Levaquin	Levofloxacin
32	Keflex & Keflet	Cephalexin
33	Lanoxin	Digoxin
34	Celebrex	Celecoxib
35	Xanax	Alprazolam
36	Protonix	Pantoprazole
37	Glucophage (XR)	Metformin ER
38	Darvocet–N	Propoxyphene/acetaminophen
39	Diovan	Valsartan
40	Lotrel	Amlodipine/benazepril
41	Zetia	Ezetimibe
42	Prilosec	Omeprazole
43	Lopressor	metoprolol tartrate
44	Ortho-Novum 7/7/7	Ethinyl estradiol/norethindrone
45	Avandia	Rosiglitazone
46	Zocor	Simvastatin
47	Actos	Pioglitazone
48	Motrin	Ibuprofen
49	Tylenol with Codeine	Acetaminophen/codeine
50	Zantac	Ranitidine

(*Continued on next page*)

Continued.

Rank	Trade Name	Generic Name
51	Lantus	Insulin Glargine
52	Actonel	Risedronate
53	Altace	Ramipril
54	Ortho Tri-Cyclen	Ethinyl estradiol/norgestimate
55	Seroquel	Quetiapine
56	Amitriptyline	Amitriptyline
57	Diovan-HCT	Valsartan/hydrochlorothiazide
58	Adderall (XR)	Dextroamphetamine/amphetamine
59	TriCor	Fenofibrate
60	Ativan	Lorazepam
61	Paxil (CR)	Paroxetine
62	Viagra	Sildenafil
63	Pravachol	Pravastatin
64	Coreg	Carvedilol
65	Flomax	Tamsulosin
66	Humulin	Insulin
67	Augmentin (XR)	Amoxicillin/clavulanate
68	Crestor	Rosuvastatin
69	Nasonex	Mometasone
70	Concerta	Methylphenidate
71	Glucotrol (XL)	Glipizide ER
72	Yasmin	Ethinyl estradiol/drospirenone
73	Ortho Evra	Ethinyl estradiol/norelgestromin
74	Allegra-D	Fexofenadine/pseudoephedrine
75	Depakote (ER)	Divalproex
76	Amaryl	Glimepiride
77	Folic Acid	Folic Acid
78	Isoptin (SR)	Verapamil SR
79	Percocet	Oxycodone/acetaminophen
80	Combivent	Ipratropium/albuterol
81	Risperdal	Risperidone
82	Xalatan™	Latanoprost
83	Prozac	Fluoxetine
84	Zyloprim	Allopurinol
85	Flexeril	Cyclobenzaprine
86	Neurontin	Gabapentin
87	AcipHex	Rabeprazole
88	Vytorin	Simvastatin/ezetimibe
89	Detrol (LA)	Tolterodine
90	Mobic	Meloxicam
91	Evista	Raloxifene
92	Deltasone	Prednisone
93	Dyazide	Triamterene/hydrochlorothiazide
94	Celexa	Citalopram
95	Humalog	Insulin Lispro
96	Catapres	Clonidine
97	Ultram	Tramadol
98	Dilantin	Phenytoin
99	Imdur	Isosorbide mononitrate
100	Inderal (LA)	Propranolol LA
101	Aricept™	Donepezil
102	Desyrel	Trazodone
103	Omnicef	Cefdinir
104	Anaprox (DS)	Naproxen sodium
105	Veetids	Penicillin V K
106	Bactrim™ (DS)	Sulfamethoxazole/trimethoprim
107	Klonopin	Clonazepam

Continued.

Rank	Trade Name	Generic Name
108	Valtrex	Valacyclovir
109	Zyprexa	Olanzapine
110	Topamax	Topiramate
111	OxyContin	Oxycodone ER
112	Strattera	Atomoxetine
113	Cozaar	Losartan
114	Hyzaar	Losartan/hydrochlorothiazide
115	Valium	Diazepam
116	Niaspan	Niacin SR
117	Biaxin (XL)	Clarithromycin ER
118	Benicar	Olmesartan
119	Cymbalta	Duloxetine
120	Patanol	Olopatadine
121	Relafen	Nabumetone
122	MiraLax™	Polyethylene glycol
123	Avapro	Irbesartan
124	Cardizem (CD)	Diltiazem
125	Ultracet	Tramadol/acetaminophen
126	Flovent	Fluticasone
127	Clarinex	Desloratadine
128	Imitrex™	Sumatriptan
129	Accupril	Quinapril
130	Avalide	Irbesartan/hydrochlorothiazide
131	Lopid	Gemfibrozil
132	Lamictal	Lamotrigine
133	Antivert	Meclizine
134	Zyrtec-D	Cetirizine
135	Ditropan(XL)	Oxybutynin
136	Mytussin AC	Guaifenesin/codeine
137	Mircette	Ethinyl estradiol/desogestrel
138	Micronase	Glyburide
139	Hytrin	Terazosin
140	Rhinocort AQ	Budesonide
141	Nitrostat	Nitroglycerin
142	Prempro™	Estrogens: conjugated/equine, medroxyprogesterone
143	Benicar-HCT	Olmesartan/hydrochlorothiazide
144	Cipro (XR)	Ciprofloxacin
145	Lescol (XL)	Fluvastatin
146	Alesse™	Ethinyl estradiol/levonorgestrel
147	Vasotec	Enalapril
148	Lotrisone	Betamethasone/clotrimazole
149	Ortho-Cept	Ethinyl estradiol/desogestrel
150	Pulmicort	Budesonide
151	Skelaxin	Metaxalone
152	Remeron	Mirtazapine
153	Ketek	Telithromycin
154	Methotrexate	Methotrexate
155	Cosopt	Dorzolamide/timolol
156	Abilify™	Aripiprazole
157	Zestoretic	Lisinopril/hydrochlorothiazide
158	Spiriva	Tiotropium
159	Procardia (XL)	Nifedipine
160	Kenalog	Triamcinolone
161	Miacalcin	Calcitonin
162	Namenda	Memantine
163	Tessalon	Benzonatate

(*Continued on next page*)

Continued.

Rank	Trade Name	Generic Name
164	Estrace	Estradiol
165	Vigamox	Moxifloxacin
166	Cialis	Tadalafil
167	Phenergan with Codeine	Promethazine/codeine
168	Reglan	Metoclopramide
169	Ortho-Cyclen	Ethinyl estradiol/norgestimate
170	Medrol	Methylprednisolone
171	Alphagan P	Brimonidine
172	Ceftin	Cefuroxime
173	Lumigan	Bimatoprost
174	Macrodantin & Macrobid	Nitrofurantoin
175	Histinex HC	Phenylephrine/hydrocodone/chlorpheniramine
176	Feldene	Piroxicam
177	Sinemet	Carbidopa/levodopa
178	Lo/Ovral	Ethinyl estradiol/norgestrel
179	Restoril	Temazepam
180	Sumycin	Tetracycline
181	Ritalin	Methylphenidate
182	Travatan	Travoprost
183	Naprosyn & EC-Naprosyn™	Naproxen
184	Lamisil	Terbinafine
185	Necon 1/35	Ethinyl estradiol/norethindrone
186	Cardura	Doxazosin
187	Atacand	Candesartan
188	Voltaren	Diclofenac
189	Mirapex	Pramipexole
190	Prometrium	Progesterone
191	Pamelor	Nortriptyline
192	Triphasil	Ethinyl estradiol/levonorgestrel
193	Xopenex Inhalation Solution	Levalbuterol
194	Serevent	Salmeterol
195	Timoptic	Timolol
196	DuoNeb	Albuterol/ipratropium
197	BenzaClin	Clindamycin/benzoyl peroxide
198	Ciprodex	Ciprofloxacin/dexamethasone
199	Vibramycin & Vibra-Tabs	Doxycycline
200	Mevacor	Lovastatin

[a]This table contains the top 200 prescription drugs dispensed through independent, chain, food store, mass merchandiser, and deep discount pharmacies. All forms of the same generic equivalent drug are grouped together and listed under the brand name when appropriate. Rankings are based on total number of prescriptions for August 2004 to August 2005, as measured by SFI's Prescription Drug Audit. Insulin products are included in the tally.
Adapted with permission from Prescription Drug Cards, 21st ed. SFI Medical Publishing, 2005.

Top Over-the-Counter (OTC) Drugs[a]

Trade Name	Drug Use
Abreva	Cold sore medication
Actifed	Allergy and cold relief
Advil	Analgesic
Afrin	Nasal decongestant
Aleve	Analgesic
ALternaGEL	Antacid
Anbesol	Oral cavity analgesic
Anusol	Hemorrhoidal agent
Azo Standard	UTI analgesic
Bayer Aspirin	Analgesic
Benadryl Oral	Allergy and cold relief
BEN-GAY	Topical analgesic
Betadine	Antiseptic
Bonine	Motion sickness medication
Bufferin	Analgesic
Caladryl	Topical antipruritic
Campho-Phenique	Topical antiseptic/antibiotic
Capastat	Oral cavity analgesic
Chlor-Trimeton	Allergy and cold relief
Chloraseptic	Oral cavity analgesic
Citrucel	Laxative
Claritin	Allergy and cold relief
Claritin-D	Allergy and cold relief
Colace	Stool softener
COLD-EEZE	Cold relief
Compound W	Keratolytic
Comtrex	Cough and cold relief
Cortaid	Topical antipruritic
Debrox	Ear wax removal aid
Delsym	Cough suppressant
Dramamine & Dramamine II	Motion sickness medication
Dulcolax	Laxative
Duofilm	Keratolytic
Emetrol	Antiemetic
Estroven	Menopause support
Excedrin	Analgesic
FiberCon	Laxative
Fungi-Nail	Topical antifungal
Gas-X	Antiflatulent
Gyne-Lotrimin	Vaginal antifungal
Imodium A-D	Antidiarrheal
Kank-A	Oral cavity analgesic
Kaopectate	Antidiarrheal
Lactaid	Digestive aid
Lactinex	Antidiarrheal
Lamisil AT	Antifungal
Listerine	Oral cavity antiseptic
Lotrimin AF	Topical antifungal
Maalox & Maalox Plus	Antacid
Metamucil	Laxative
Midol & Midol PMS	Analgesic
Monistat Vaginal	Vaginal antifungal
Motrin IB	Analgesic
Mucinex	Expectorant
Mylanta	Antacid
Mylicon Drops	Antiflatulence
Myoflex	Topical analgesic

(Continued on next page)

Continued.

Trade Name	Drug Use
Naphcon A	Ophthalmic anti-allergy
NasalCrom	Allergy and cold relief
Neo-Synephrine	Nasal decongestant
Neosporin	Topical anti-infective
NicoDerm CQ	Smoking cessation aid
Nicorette	Smoking cessation aid
Nix	Pediculicide
Nizoral Shampoo	Topical antifungal
NoDoz	Analeptic
NyQuil	Cough and cold relief
Ocean	Nasal decongestant
Opcon-A	Ophthalmic anti-allergy
Orabase	Oral cavity analgesic
OralBalance	Oral moisturizer
Os-Cal	Essential mineral
Pamprin	Analgesic
PediaCare	Cough and cold relief
Pepcid Complete	Acid reducer
Pepcid-AC	Acid reducer
Pepto Bismol	Antidiarrheal
Peri-Colace	Stool softener plus laxative
Phillips' MOM	Laxative / antacid
Pin-X	Anthelmintic
Preparation H	Hemorrhoidal agent
Prilosec OTC	Acid reducer
RID	Pediculicide
Robitussin (Adult)	Cough relief
Rogaine	Hair growth stimulant
Salivart	Saliva substitute
Senokot	Laxative
Similasan Earache Relief	Earache relief
Slow-Mag	Essential mineral
Sominex	Sleeping aid
Sudafed	Allergy and cold relief
Tagamet HB 200	Acid reducer
Tavist	Allergy and cold relief
Tears Naturale	Artificial tears
Triaminic Oral	Cough and cold relief
Tums	Antacid
Tylenol	Analgesic
Tylenol Allergy & Sinus	Allergy and cold relief
Tylenol Cold & Flu (Adult)	Allergy and cold relief
Tylenol PM	Analgesic
Unisom	Sleeping aid
Zantac 75	Acid reducer
Zicam Cold Remedy	Cold relief
Zostrix	Topical analgesic

[a]This table contains the top OTC drugs by pharmacist recommendation in specific therapeutic classes.
Adapted with permission from Nonprescription Drug Cards, 4th ed. SFI Medical Publishing, 2003.

REFERENCE CHARTS FOR PATIENT COUNSELING

Drugs That Should Not Be Crushed

Listed below are various slow-release as well as enteric-coated products that should not be crushed or chewed. Slow-release (sr) represents products that are controlled-release, extended-release, long-acting, or timed-release. Enteric-coated (ec) represents products that are delayed-release.

In general, capsules containing slow-release or enteric-coated particles may be opened and their contents administered on a spoonful of soft food. Instruct patients not to chew the particles, though. (Patients should, in fact, be discouraged from chewing any medication unless it is specifically formulated for that purpose.)

This list should not be considered all-inclusive. Generic and alternate brands of some products may exist. Tablets intended for sublingual or buccal administration (not included in this list) should also be administered only as intended, in an intact form.

Drug	Manufacturer	Form
Aciphex	Eisai	ec
Adalat CC	Schering Plough	sr
Adderall XR	Shire US	sr
Advicor	KOS	sr
Aerohist	Aero	sr
Aerohist Plus	Aero	sr
Afeditab CR	Watson	sr
Aggrenox	Boehr, Ingelheim	sr
Aldex	Zyber	sr
Aldex-G	Zyber	sr
Aleve Cold & Sinus	Bayer Healthcare	sr
Aleve Sinus & Headache	Bayer Healthcare	sr
Allegra-D 12 Hour	Senofi-Aventis	sr
Allegra-D 24 Hour	Senofi-Aventis	sr
Allerx	Cornerstone	sr
Allerx-D	Cornerstone	sr
Allfen	MCR American	sr
Allfen-DM	MCR American	sr
Alophen	Numark	ec
Altex-PSE	Alphagen	sr
Altoprev	First Horizon	sr
Ambi 1000/55	Ambi	sr
Ambi 45/800	Ambi	sr
Ambi 45/800/30	Ambi	sr
Ambi 60/580	Ambi	sr
Ambi 60/580/30	Ambi	sr
Ambi 80/700	Ambi	sr
Ambi 80/700/40	Ambi	sr
Ambifed-G	Ambi	sr
Ambifed-G DM	Ambi	sr
Amdry-C	Prasco	sr
Amdry-D	Parsco	sr
Amibid DM	Amide	sr
Amibid LA	Amide	sr

(*Continued on next page*)

Drug	Manufacturer	Form
Amidal	Amide	sr
Aminoxin	Tyson Neutraceuticals	ec
Ami-Tex PSE	Amide	sr
Anextuss	Cypress	sr
Aquabid-DM	Alphagen	sr
Aquatab C	Adams	sr
Aquatab D	Adams	sr
Aquatab DM	Adams	sr
Arithrotec	Pharmacia	ec
Asacol	Procter & Gamble	ec
Ascocid-1000	Key	sr
Ascocid-500-D	Key	sr
Ascriptin Enteric	Novartis Consumer	ec
ATP	Tyson Neutraceuticals	ec
Atrohist Pediatric	Celltech	sr
Augmentin XR	GlaxoSmithKline	sr
Avinza	Ligand	sr
Azulfidine Entabs	Pharmacia	ec
Bayer Aspirin Regimen	Bayer Healthcare	ec
Bellahist-D LA	Cypress	sr
Bellatal ER	Qualitest	sr
Biaxin XL	Abbott	sr
Bidex-DM	Stewart-Jackson	sr
Bidhist	Cypress	sr
Bidhist-D	Cypress	sr
Biohist LA	Ivax	sr
Bisac-Evac	G & W	ec
Biscolax	Global Source	ec
Blanex-A	Blansett	sr
Bontril Slow-Release	Valeant	sr
Bromfed	Victory	sr
Bromfed-PD	Victory	sr
Bromfenex	Ethex	sr
Bromfenex PD	Ethex	sr
Bromfenex PE	Ethex	sr
Bromfenex PE Pediatric	Ethex	sr
Budeprion SR	Teva	sr
Buproban	Teva	sr
Calan SR	Pharmacia	sr
Campral	Forest	ec
Carbatrol	Shire US	sr
Cardene SR	Roche	sr
Cardizem CD	Biovall	sr
Cardizem LA	KOS	sr
Carox Plus	Seneca	sr
Cartia XT	Andrx	sr
Catemine	Tyson Neutraceuticals	ec
Cemill 1000	Miller	sr
Cemill 500	Miller	sr
Certuss-D	Capellon	sr
Cevi-Bid	Lee	sr
Chlorex-A	Cypress	sr
Chlor-Phen	Truxton	sr
Chlor-Trimeton Allergy	Schering Plough	sr
Chlor-Trimeton Allergy Decongestant	Schering Plough	sr
Cipro XR	Schering Plough	sr
Clarinex-D 24 Hour	Schering Plough	sr
Coldamine	Breckenridge	sr
Coldec D	Breckenridge	sr
Coldec TR	Breckenridge	sr

Drug	Manufacturer	Form
Coldex-A	United Research	sr
ColdMist DM	Breckenridge	sr
ColdMist Jr	Breckenridge	sr
ColdMist LA	Breckenridge	sr
Colfed-A	Breckenridge	sr
Concerta	McNeil Consumer	sr
Contac 12-Hour	GlaxoSmithKline	sr
Correctol	Schering Plough	ec
Cotazym-S	Organon	ec
Covera-HS	Pharmacia	sr
CPM 8/PE 20/MSC 1.25	Cypress	sr
Crantex ER	Breckenridge	sr
Crantex LA	Breckenridge	sr
Crantex Lac	Breckenridge	sr
Creon 10	Solvay	ec
Creon 20	Solvay	ec
Creon 5	Solvay	ec
Cymbalta	Eli Lilly	ec
Cypex-LA	Cypress	sr
Dacex-PE	Cypress	sr
Dairycare	Plainview	ec
Dallergy	Laser	sr
Dallergy-Jr	Laser	sr
D-Amine-SR	Alphagen	sr
Deconamine SR	Kenwood Therapeutics	sr
Deconex	Poly	sr
Decongest II	Qualitest	sr
De-Congestine	Qualitest	sr
Deconsal II	Cornerstone	sr
Depakote	Abbott	ec
Depakote ER	Abbott	sr
Depakote Sprinkles	Abbott	ec
Despec SR	Int'l Ethical	sr
Detrol LA	Pharmacia	sr
Dexaphen SA	Major	sr
Dexcon-PE	Cypress	sr
Dexedrine Spansules	GlaxoSmithKline	sr
D-Feda II	WE Pharm.	sr
Diabetes Trio	Mason Vitamins	sr
Diamox Sequels	Duramed	sr
Dilacor XR	Watson	sr
Dilantin Kapseals	Pfizer	sr
Dilatrate-SR	Schwarz Pharma	sr
Diltia XT	Andrx	sr
Dilt-XR	Apotex	sr
Dimetane Extentabs	Wyeth	sr
Disophrol Chronotab	Schering Plough	sr
Ditropan XL	Ortho-McNeil	sr
Donnatal Extentabs	PBM	sr
Doryx	Warner Chilcott	ec
Drexophed SR	Qualitest	sr
Drihist SR	Prasco	sr
Drixomed	Iopharm	sr
Drixoral	Schering Plough	sr
Drixoral Plus	Schering Plough	sr
Drixoral sinus	Schering Plough	sr
Drize-R	Monarch	sr
Drysec	A. G. Marin	sr
Dulcolax	Boehr. Ingelheim	ec

(*Continued on next page*)

Drug	Manufacturer	Form
Duomax	Capellon	sr
Duradex	Proethic	sr
Duradryl Jr	Breckenridge	sr
Durahist	Proethic	sr
Durahist D	Proethic	sr
Durahist PE	Proethic	sr
Duraphen DM	Proethic	sr
Duraphen Forte	Proethic	sr
Duraphen II	Proethic	sr
Duraphen II DM	Proethic	sr
Duratuss	Victory	sr
Duratuss GP	Victory	sr
Dynabac	Muro	ec
Dynabac D5-Pak	Muro	ec
Dynacirc CR	Reliant	sr
Dynahist-ER Pediatric	Breckenridge	sr
Dynex	Athlon	sr
Dytan-CS	Hawthorn	sr
Easprin	Harvest	ec
EC Naprosyn	Roche	ec
Ecotrin	GlaxoSmithKline	ec
Ecotrin Adult Low Strength	GlaxoSmithKline	ec
Ecotrin Maximum Strength	GlaxoSmithKline	ec
Ecpirin	Prime Marketing	ec
Ed A-Hist	Edwards	sr
Ed-Chlor-Tan	Edwards	sr
Effexor-XR	Wyeth	sr
Efidac 24 Chlorpheniramine	Novartis Consumer	sr
Efidac 24 Pseudoephedrine	Novartis Consumer	sr
Enablex	Novartis	sr
Endal	Pediamed	sr
Entab-DM	Rising	sr
Entercote	Global Source	ec
Entex ER	Andrx	sr
Entex LA	Andrx	sr
Entex PSE	Andrx	sr
Entocort EC	Prometheus	ec
Equetro	Shire US	sr
ERYC	Warner Chilcott	ec
Ery-Tab	Abbott	ec
Eskalith-CR	GlaxoSmithKline	sr
Exefen-DM	Larken	sr
Exefen-PD	Larken	sr
Extendryl Jr	Fleming	sr
Extendryl SR	Fleming	sr
Extress-30	Key	sr
Extuss LA	Cypress	sr
Feen-A-Mint	Schering Plough	ec
Femilax	G & W	ec
Fero-Folic-500	Abbott	sr
Fero-Grad-500	Abbott	sr
Ferro-Sequels	Inverness Medical	sr
Ferro-Time	Time-Cap	sr
Ferrous Fumarate DS	Vita-Rx	sr
Fetrin	Lunsco	sr
Flagyl ER	Pharmacia	sr
Fleet Bisacodyl	Fleet, C. B.	ec
Focalin XR	Novartis	sr
Folitab 500	Rising	sr
Fortamet	First Horizon	sr

Drug	Manufacturer	Form
Fumatinic	Laser	sr
G/P 1200/75	Cypress	sr
Genacote	Ivax	ec
GFN 1000/DM 50	Cypress	sr
GFN 1200/DM 20/PE 40	Cypress	sr
GFN 1200/DM 60/PSE 60	Cypress	sr
GFN 1200/Phenylephrine 40	Cypress	sr
GFN 1200/PSE 50	Cypress	sr
GFN 500/DM 30	Cypress	sr
GFN 550/PSE 60	Cypress	sr
GFN 550/PSE 60/DM 30	Cypress	sr
GFN 595/PSE 48	Cypress	sr
GFN 595/PSE 48/DM 32	Cypress	sr
GFN 795/PSE 85	Cypress	sr
GFN 800/DM 30	Cypress	sr
GFN 800/PE 25	Cypress	sr
GFN 800/PSE 60	Cypress	sr
Gilphex TR	Gil	sr
Giltuss TR	Gil	sr
Glucophage XR	Bristol-Myers Squibb	sr
Glucotrol XL	Pfizer	sr
GP-1200	Iopharm	sr
Guaifed	Victory	sr
Guaifed-PD	Victory	sr
Guaifenex DM	Ethex	sr
Guaifenex GP	Ethex	sr
Guaifenex PSE 120	Ethex	sr
Guaifenex PSE 60	Ethex	sr
Guaifenex PSE 80	Ethex	sr
Gualmax-D	Schwarz Pharma	sr
Gua-SR	Seatrace	sr
Guia-D	Breckenridge	sr
Guiadex D	Breckenridge	sr
Guiadex PD	Breckenridge	sr
Guiadrine DM	Breckenridge	sr
Guiadrine G-1200	Breckenridge	sr
Guiadrine GP	Breckenridge	sr
Guiadrine PSE	Breckenridge	sr
H 9600 SR	Hawthorn	sr
Halfprin	Kramer	ec
Hemax	Pronova	sr
Histacol LA	Breckenridge	sr
Histade	Breckenridge	sr
Histade MX	Breckenridge	sr
Hista-Vent DA	Ethex	sr
Hista-Vent PSE	Ethex	sr
Histex CT	Teamm	sr
Histex I/E	Teamm	sr
Histex SR	Teamm	sr
Humavent LA	WE Pharm.	sr
Humibid DM	Carolina	sr
Humibid L.A.	Carolina	sr
Hydro Pro DM SR	Breckenridge	sr
Hyoscyamine TR	Breckenridge	sr
Iberet-500	Abbott	sr
Iberet-Folic-500	Abbott	sr
Icar-C Plus SR	Hawthorn	sr
Imdur	Schering Plough	sr
Inderal LA	Wyeth	sr

(*Continued on next page*)

Drug	Manufacturer	Form
Indocin SR	Forte Pharma	sr
Innopran XL	Reliant	sr
Iobid DM	Iopharm	sr
Ionamin	Celltech	sr
Iosal II	Iopharm	sr
Iotex PSE	Iopharm	sr
Isochron	Forest	sr
Isoptin SR	FSC	sr
Kadian	Alphagen	sr
Kaon-Cl 10	Savage	sr
K-Dur 10	Schering Plough	sr
K-Dur 20	Schering Plough	sr
Klor-Con 10	Upsher-Smith	sr
Klor-Con 8	Upsher-Smith	sr
Klor-Con M10	Upsher-Smith	sr
Klor-Con M15	Upsher-Smith	sr
Klor-Con M20	Upsher-Smith	sr
Klotrix	Bristol-Myers Squibb	sr
Kronofed-A	Ferndale	sr
Kronofed-A-Jr	Ferndale	sr
K-Tab	Abbott	sr
K-Tan	Prasco	sr
Lescol XL	Novartis	sr
Levall G	Athlon	sr
Levbid	Schwarz Pharma	sr
Levsinex	Schwarz Pharma	sr
Lexxel	Astra Zeneca	sr
Lipram 4500	Global	ec
Lipram-CR10	Global	ec
Lipram-CR20	Global	ec
Lipram-CR5	Global	ec
Lipram-PN10	Global	ec
Lipram-PN16	Global	ec
Lipram-PN20	Global	ec
Lipram-UL12	Global	ec
Lipram-UL18	Global	ec
Lipram-UL20	Global	ec
Liquibid-D	Capellon	sr
Liquibid-D 1200	Capellon	sr
Liquibid-PD	Capellon	sr
Lithobid	JDS Pharm.	sr
Lodine XL	Wyeth	sr
Lodrane 12 Hour	ECR	sr
Lodrane 12D	ECR	sr
Lodrane 24	ECR	sr
Lohist-12	Larken	sr
Lohist-12D	Larken	sr
Lusonex	Wraser	sr
Mag Delay	Major	ec
Mag64	Rising	ec
Mag-SR	Cypress	sr
Mag-SR Plus Calcium	Cypress	sr
Mag-Tab SR	Niche	sr
Maxifed	MCR American	sr
Maxifed DM	MCR American	sr
Maxifed DMX	MCR American	sr
Maxifed-G	MCR American	sr
Maxiphen DM	Ambi	sr
Maxovite	Tyson Neutraceuticals	sr
Medent DM	Stewart-Jackson	sr

Drug	Manufacturer	Form
Medent LD	Stewart-Jackson	sr
Mega-C	Merit	sr
Melfiat	Numark	sr
Menopause Trio	Mason Vitamins	sr
Mestinon Timespan	Valeant	sr
Metadate CD	Celltech	sr
Metadate ER	Celltech	sr
Methylin ER	Mallinckrodt	sr
Micro-K	Ther-Rx	sr
Micro-K 10	Ther-Rx	sr
Mild-C	Carison, J. R.	sr
Mindal	Breckenridge	sr
Mindal DM	Breckenridge	sr
Mintab C	Breckenridge	sr
Mintab D	Breckenridge	sr
Mintab DM	Breckenridge	sr
Miraphen PSE	Caraco	sr
Modane	Savage	ec
MS Contin	Purdue	sr
MSP-BLU	Cypress	ec
Mucinex	Adams	sr
Muco-Fen DM	Ivax	sr
Multi-Ferrous Folic	United Research	sr
Multiret Folic-500	Amide	sr
Myfortic	Novartis	ec
Nacon	Cypress	sr
Nalex-A	Blansett	sr
Nasatab LA	ECR	sr
Nasex	Cypress	sr
Nd Clear	Seatrace	sr
Nescon-PD	Cypress	sr
New Ami-Tex LA	Amide	sr
Nexium	Astra Zeneca	ec
Niaspan	KOS	sr
Nicomide	Sirius	sr
Nifediac CC	Teva	sr
Nifedical XL	Teva	sr
Nitrocot	Truxton	sr
Nitro-Time	Time-Cap	sr
Nohist	Larken	sr
Norel SR	U.S. Pharm. Corp.	sr
Norpace CR	Pharmacia	sr
Obstetrix EC	Seyer Pharmatec	ec
Omnihist L.A.	WE Pharm.	sr
Oramorph SR	AAI Pharma	sr
Oruvail	Wyeth	sr
Oxycontin	Purdue	sr
Palcaps 10	Breckenridge	ec
Palcaps 20	Breckenridge	ec
Palgic-D	Pamlab	sr
Pancrease	McNeil Consumer	ec
Pancrease MT 10	McNeil Consumer	ec
Pancrease MT 16	McNeil Consumer	ec
Pancrease MT 20	McNeil Consumer	ec
Pancrecarb MS-16	Digestive Care	ec
Pancrecarb MS-4	Digestive Care	ec
Pancrecarb MS-8	Digestive Care	ec
Pangestyme CN-10	Ethex	ec
Pangestyme CN-20	Ethex	ec

(*Continued on next page*)

Drug	Manufacturer	Form
Pangestyme EC	Ethex	ec
Pangestyme MT16	Ethex	ec
Pangestyme UL12	Ethex	ec
Pangestyme UL18	Ethex	ec
Pangestyme UL20	Ethex	ec
Panmist DM	Pamlab	sr
Panmist Jr	Pamlab	sr
Panmist LA	Pamlab	sr
Pannaz	Pamlab	sr
Panocaps	Breckenridge	ec
Panocaps MT 16	Breckenridge	ec
Panocaps MT 20	Breckenridge	ec
Papacon	Consolidated Midland	sr
Para-Time SR	Time-Cap	sr
Paser	Jacobus	sr
Pavacot	Truxton	sr
Paxil CR	GlaxoSmithKline	sr
PCE Dispertab	Abbott	sr
PCM LA	Cypress	sr
Pendex	Cypress	sr
Pentasa	Shire US	sr
Pentopak	Zoetica	sr
Pentoxil	Upsher-Smith	sr
Pharmadrine	Breckenridge	sr
Phenabid	Gil	sr
Phenabid DM	Gil	sr
Phenavent	Ethex	sr
Phenavent D	Ethex	sr
Phenavent LA	Ethex	sr
Phenavent PED	Ethex	sr
Phendiet-105	Truxton	sr
Phenytek	Mylan Bertek	sr
Plendil	Astra Zeneca	sr
Poly Hist Forte	Poly	sr
Poly-Vent	Poly	sr
Poly-Vent Jr	Poly	sr
Prehist D	Marnel	sr
Prelu-2	Roxane	sr
Prevacid	Tap	ec
Prilosec	Astra Zeneca	ec
Prilosec OTC	Procter & Gamble	sr
Procanbid	Monarch	sr
Procardia XL	Pfizer	sr
Profen Forte	Ivax	sr
Profen Forte DM	Ivax	sr
Profen II	Ivax	sr
Profen II DM	Ivax	sr
Prolex PD	Blansett	sr
Prolex-D	Blansett	sr
Pronestyl-SR	Bristol-Myers Squibb	sr
Prosed EC	Star	ec
Proset-D	Blansett	sr
Protid	Lunsco	sr
Protonix	Wyeth	ec
Prozac Weekly	Eli Lilly	ec
Pseubrom	Alphagen	sr
Pseubrom-PD	Alphagen	sr
Pseudatex	Breckenridge	sr
Pseudocot-C	Truxton	sr
Pseudocot-G	Truxton	sr

Drug	Manufacturer	Form
Pseudovent	Ethex	sr
Pseudovent 400	Ethex	sr
Pseudovent DM	Ethex	sr
Pseudovent PED	Ethex	sr
P-Tuss DM	Prasco	sr
Qdall	Atley	sr
Quibron-T/SR	Monarch	sr
Quindal	Qualitest	sr
Ralix	Cypress	sr
Razadyne ER	Ortho-McNeil	sr
Reliable Gentle Laxative	Ivax	ec
Rescon-Jr	Capellon	sr
Rescon-MX	Capellon	sr
Respa-1ST	Respa	sr
Respa-AR	Respa	sr
Respa-DM	Respa	sr
Respahist	Respa	sr
Respaire-120 SR	Laser	sr
Respaire-60 SR	Laser	sr
Respa-PE	Respa	sr
Rhinabid	Breckenridge	sr
Rhinabid PD	Breckenridge	sr
Rhinacon A	Breckenridge	sr
Ribo-2	Tyson Neutraceuticals	ec
Risperdal Consta	Janssen	sr
Ritalin LA	Novartis	sr
Ritalin-SR	Novartis	sr
Rodex Forte	Legere	sr
Rondec-TR	Biovail	sr
Ru-Tuss 800	Sage	sr
Ru-Tuss 800 DM	Sage	sr
Ru-Tuss Jr	Sage	sr
Ryneze	Stewart-Jackson	sr
Rythmol SR	Reliant	sr
Sam-E	Pharmavite	ec
Sinemet CR	Bristol-Myers Squibb	sr
Sinutuss DM	WE Pharm.	sr
Sinuvent PE	WE Pharm.	sr
Sitrex	Vindex	sr
Sio-Niacin	Upsher-Smith	sr
Slow Fe	Novartis Consumer	sr
Slow Fe With Folic Acid	Novartis Consumer	sr
Slow-Mag	Purdue	ec
Spacol T/S	Dayton	sr
St. Joseph Pain Reliever	McNeil Consumer	ec
Sta-D	Magna	sr
Stahist	Magna	sr
Stamoist E	Magna	sr
Sudafed 12 Hour	Pfizer	sr
Sudafed 24 Hour	Pfizer	sr
Sudal DM	Atley	sr
Sudal SR	Atley	sr
Sular	First Horizon	sr
Sulfazine EC	Qualitest	ec
Symax Duotab	Capellon	sr
Symax-SR	Capellon	sr
Tarka	Abbott	sr
Taztia XT	Andrx	sr
Tegretol-XR	Novartis	sr

(*Continued on next page*)

Drug	Manufacturer	Form
Tenuate Dospan	Sanofi-Aventis	sr
Theo-24	UCB	sr
Theocap	Forest	sr
Theochron	Forest	sr
Theo-Time	Major	sr
Thiamilate	Tyson Neutraceuticals	ec
Tiazac	Forest	sr
Time-Hist	MCR American	sr
Toprol XL	Astra Zeneca	sr
TotalDay	Nat'l Vitamin Co.	sr
Touro Allergy	Dartmouth	sr
Touro CC	Dartmouth	sr
Touro CC-LD	Dartmouth	sr
Touro DM	Dartmouth	sr
Touro HC	Dartmouth	sr
Touro LA	Dartmouth	sr
Touro LA-LD	Dartmouth	sr
Tranxene-SD	Ovation	sr
Trental	Sanofi-Aventis	sr
Trikof-D	Respa	sr
Trinalin Repetabs	Schering Plough	sr
Trituss-ER	Everett	sr
Tussafed-LA	Everett	sr
Tussall-ER	Everett	sr
Tussbid	Breckenridge	sr
Tussi-Bid	Capellon	sr
Tussitab	Iopharm	sr
Tylenol Arthritis	McNeil Consumer	sr
Ultrabrom	WE Pharm.	sr
Ultrabrom PD	WE Pharm.	sr
Ultracaps MT 20	Breckenridge	ec
Ultrase	Axcan Scandipharm	ec
Ultrase MT12	Axcan Scandipharm	ec
Ultrase MT18	Axcan Scandipharm	ec
Ultrase MT20	Axcan Scandipharm	ec
Uniphyl	Purdue	sr
Uni-Tex	United Research	sr
Urimax	Xanodyne	ec
Urocit-K 10	Mission	sr
Urocit-K 5	Mission	sr
Uroxatral	Sanofi-Aventis	sr
Ultra	Hawthron	sr
V-Dec-M	Seatrace	sr
Veracolate	Numark	ec
Verelan	Schwarz Pharma	sr
Verelan PM	Schwarz Pharma	sr
Versacaps	Seatrace	sr
Videx EC	Bristol-Myers Squibb	ec
Vivotif Berna	Berna Products	ec
Voltaren	Novartis	ec
Voltaren-XR	Novartis	sr
Vospire ER	Odyssey	sr
We Mist II LA	WE Pharm.	sr
We Mist LA	WE Pharm.	sr
Wellbid-D	Prasco	sr
Wellbid-D 1200	Prasco	sr
Wellbutrin SR	GlaxoSmithKline	sr
Wellbutrin XL	GlaxoSmithKline	sr
Wobenzym N	Marlyn	ec
Xanax XR	Pharmacia	sr

Drug	Manufacturer	Form
Xiral	Hawthorn	sr
XpeCT-At	Hawthorn	sr
XpeCT-HC	Hawthorn	sr
Z-Cof LA	Zyber	sr
Z-Cof LAX	Zyber	sr
Zephrex LA	Sanofi-Aventis	sr
Zorprin	Par	sr
Zyban	GlaxoSmithKline	sr
Zymase	Organon	ec
Zyrtec-D	Pfizer	sr

Reprinted with permission from *The Drug Topics Red Book.* Montvale NJ: Thomson Medical Economics, 2006.

Sugar-Free Products

Listed below, by therapeutic category, is a selection of drug products that contain no sugar. When recommending these products to diabetic patients, keep in mind that many may contain sorbitol, alcohol, or other sources of carbohydrates. This list should not be considered all-inclusive. Generics and alternate brands of some products may be available. Check product labeling for a current listing of inactive ingredients.

Analgesics

Actamin Maximum Strength Liquid	Cypress
Addaprin Tablet	Dover
Aminofen Tablet	Dover
Aminofen Max Tablet	Dover
Aspirtab Tablet	Dover
Back Pain-Off Tablet	Textilease Medique
Backprin Tablet	Hart Health and Safety
Buffasal Tablet	Dover
Dyspel Tablet	Dover
Febrol Liquid	Scot-Tussin
I-Prin Tablet	Textilease Medique
Medi-Seltzer Effervescent Tablet	Textilease Medique
Ms.-Aid Tablet	Textilease Medique
PMS Relief Tablet	Textilease Medique
Silapap Children's Elixir	Silarx

Antacids/Antiflatulents

Almag Chewable Tablet	Textilease Medique
Alcalak Chewable Tablet	Textilease Medique
Aldroxicon I Suspension	Textilease Medique
Aldroxicon II Suspension	Textilease Medique
Baby Gasz Drops	Lee
Dimacid Chewable Tablet	Otis Clapp & Son
Diotame Chewable Tablet	Textilease Medique
Diotame Suspension	Textilease Medique
Gas-Ban Chewable	Textilease Medique
Mallamint Chewable	Textilease Medique
Mylanta Gelcaplet	Johnson & Johnson/Merck
Neutralin Tablet	Dover
Tums E-X Chewable Tablet	GlaxoSmithKline Consumer

(*Continued on next page*)

Antiasthmatic/Respiratory Agents

Jay-Phyl Syrup	Pharmakon

Antidiarrheals

Diarrest Tablet	Dover
Di-Gon II Tablet	Textilease Medique
Imogen Liquid	Pharmaceutical Generic

Blood Modifiers/Iron Preparations

I.L.X. B-12 Elixir	Kenwood
Irofel Liquid	Dayton
Nephro-Fer Tablet	R & D

Corticosteroids

Pediapred Solution	Celltech

Cough/Cold/Allergy Preparations

Accuhist DM, Pediatric Drops	Pediamed
Accuhist Pediatric Drops	Pediamed
Alacol DM Syrup	Ballay
Amerifed DM Liquid	MCR American
Amerifed Liquid	Ambi
Amerituss AD Solution	Ambi
Anaplex DM Syrup	ECR
Anaplex DMX Syrup	ECR
Anaplex HD Syrup	ECR
Andehist DM Liquid	Cypress
Andehist DM NR Liquid	Cypress
Andehist DM NR Syrup	Cypress
Andehist DM Syrup	Cypress
Andehist Liquid	Cypress
Andehist NR Liquid	Cypress
Andehist NR Syrup	Cypress
Andehist Syrup	Cypress
Atuss EX Liquid	Atley
Atuss NX Solution	Atley
Baltussin Solution	Ballay
Bellahist-D LA Tablet	Cypress
Benadryl Allergy/Sinus Children's Solution	Warner-Lambert Consumer
Boidec DM Drops	Bio-Pharm
Bromaxefed DM RF Syrup	Morton Grove
Bromaxefed RF Syrup	Morton Grove
Bromdec Solution	Scientific Laboratories
Bromdec DM Solution	Scientific Laboratories
Bromhist-DM Solution	Cypress
Bromhist Pediatric Solution	Cypress
Bromophed DX Syrup	Qualitest
Bromphenex DM Solution	Breckendridge
Bromphenex HD Solution	Breckenridge
Bromplex DM Solution	Prasco
Bromplex HD Solution	Prasco
Broncotron Liquid	Seyer Pharmatec
Broncotron-D Suspension	Seyer Pharmatec
Brovex HC Solution	Athlon
B-Tuss Liquid	Blansett
Carbaphen 12 Ped Suspension	Gil
Carbaphen 12 Suspension	Gil
Carbatuss-CL Solution	GM
Carbetaplex Solution	Breckenridge
Carbihist Solution	Boca Pharmacal
Carbinoxamine PSE Solution	Boca Pharmacal

Carbofed DM Liquid	Hi-Tech
Carbofed DM Syrup	Hi-Tech
Carbofed DM Drops	Hi-Tech
Carboxine Solution	Cypress
Carboxine-PSE Solution	Cypress
Cardec DM Syrup	Qualitest
Cetafen Cold Tablet	Hart Health and Safety
Cheratussin DAC Liquid	Qualitest
Chlordex GP Syrup	Cypress
Codal-DM Syrup	Cypress
Colace Solution	Purdue Pharma
ColdCough EXP Solution	Breckenridge
ColdCough HC Solution	Breckenridge
ColdCough PD Solution	Breckenridge
ColdCough Solution	Breckenridge
ColdCough XP Solution	Breckenridge
Coldec DS Solution	Breckenridge
ColdMist DM Syrup	Breckenridge
Coldonyl Tablet	Dover
Colidrops Pediatric Liquid	A.G. Marin
Cordron-D Solution	Cypress
Cordron-DM Solution	Cypress
Cordron-HC Solution	Cypress
Corfen DM Solution	Cypress
Co-Tussin Liquid	American Generics
Cotuss-V Syrup	Alphagen
Coughtuss Solution	Breckenridge
Crantex HC Syrup	Breckenridge
Crantex Syrup	Breckenridge
Cypex-LA Tablet	Cypress
Cytuss HC Syrup	Cypress
Dacex-A Solution	Cypress
Dacex-DM Solution	Cypress
Dacex-PE Solution	Cypress
Decahist-DM Solution	Cypress
De-Chlor DM Solution	Cypress
De-Chlor DR Solution	Cypress
De-Chlor G Solution	Cypress
De-Chlor HC Solution	Cypress
De-Chlor HD Solution	Cypress
De-Chlor MR Solution	Cypress
De-Chlor NX Solution	Cypress
Decorel Forte Tablet	Textilease Medique
Denaze Solution	Cypress
Despec Liquid	International Ethical
Despec-SF Liquid	International Ethical
Dexcon-DM Solution	Cypress
Diabetic Tussin Allergy Relief Liquid	Health Care Products
Diabetic Tussin Allergy Relief Gelcaplet	Health Care Products
Diabetic Tussin C Expectorant Liquid	Health Care Products
Diabetic Tussin Cold & Flu Gelcaplet	Health Care Products
Diabetic Tussin DM Liquid	Health Care Products
Diabetic Tussin EX Liquid	Health Care Products
Dimetapp Allergy Children's Elixir	Wyeth Consumer
Diphen Capsule	Textilease Medique
Double-Tussin DM Liquid	Reese
Drocon-CS Solution	Cypress
Duratuss DM Solution	Victory
Dynatuss Syrup	Breckenridge
Dynatuss HC Solution	Breckenridge

(Continued on next page)

Dynatus HCG Solution	Breckenridge
Dytan-CS Tablet	Hawthorn
Emagrin Forte Tablet	Otis Clapp & Son
Endacof DM Solution	Larken Laboratories
Endacof HC Solution	Larken Laboratories
Endacof XP Solution	Larken Laboratories
Endacof-PD Solution	Larken Laboratories
Endal HD Liquid	Pediamed
Endal HD Plus Liquid	Pediamed
Endotuss-HD Syrup	American Generics
Enplus-HD Syrup	Alphagen
Entex Syrup	Andrx
Entex HC Syrup	Andrx
Exo-Tuss Syrup	American Generics
Ganidin NR Liquid	Cypress
Gani-Tuss NR Liquid	Cypress
Gani-Tuss-DM NR Liquid	Cypress
Genebronco-D Liquid	Pharm Generic Developers
Genecof-HC Liquid	Pharmaceutical Generic
Genecof-XP Liquid	Pharmaceutical Generic
Genedel Syrup	Pharmaceutical Generic
Genedotuss-DM Liquid	Pharmaceutical Generic
Genelan Liquid	Pharm Generic Developers
Genetuss-2 Liquid	Pharm Generic Developers
Genexpect DM Liquid	Pharmaceutical Generic
Genexpect-PE Liquid	Pharmaceutical Generic
Genexpect-SF Liquid	Pharmaceutical Generic
Gilphex TR Tablet	Gil
Giltuss Liquid	Gil
Giltuss HC Syrup	Gil
Giltuss Pediatric Liquid	Gil
Giltuss TR Tablet	Gil
Guai-Co Liquid	Alphagen
Gualcon DMS Liquid	Textilease Medique
Guai-DEX Liquid	Alphagen
Guaitussin AC Solution	Scientific Laboratories
Guaitussin DAC Solution	Scientific Laboratories
Guapetex HC Solution	Scientific Laboratories
Guapetex Syrup	Scientific Laboratories
Guiatuss AC Syrup	Alpharma
Guiatuss AC Syrup	Ivax
Halotussin AC Liquid	Watson
Hayfebrol Liquid	Scot-Tussin
Histacol DM Pediatric Solution	Breckenridge
Histex PD Liquid	TEAMM
Histex PD 12 Suspension	Teamm
Histinex HC Syrup	Ethex
Histinex PV Syrup	Ethex
Histuss HC Solution	Scientific Laboratories
Histuss PD Solution	Scientific Laboratories
Hydex-PD Solution	Cypress
Hydone Liquid	Hyrex
Hydro-DP Solution	Cypress
Hydro-GP Syrup	Cypress
Hydro PC Syrup	Cypress
Hydro PC II Plus Solution	Cypress
Hydro Pro Solution	Breckenridge
Hydrocof-HC Solution	Morton Grove
Hydron CP Syrup	Cypress
Hydron EX Syrup	Cypress
Hydron KGS Liquid	Cypress

Hydron PSC Liquid	Cypress
Hydro-Tussin CBX Solution	Ethex
Hydro-Tussin DM Elixir	Ethex
Hydro-Tussin HC Syrup	Ethex
Hydro-Tussin HD Liquid	Ethex
Hydro-Tussin XP Syrup	Ethex
Hytuss Tablet	Hyrex
Hytuss 2X Capsule	Hyrex
Jaycof Expectorant Syrup	Pharmakon
Jaycof-HC Liquid	Pharmakon
Jaycof-XP Liquid	Pharmakon
Kita LA Tos Liquid	R.I.D.
Lodrane Liquid	ECR
Lodrane D Suspension	ECR
Lodrane XR Suspension	ECR
Lohist-LQ Solution	Larken
Lortuss DM Solution	Proethic Laboratories
Lortuss HC Solution	Proethic Laboratories
Marcof Expectorant Syrup	Marnel
Maxi-Tuss HCX Solution	MCR American
M-Clear Syrup	McNeil, R.A.
M-Clear Jr Solution	McNeil, R.A.
Metanx Tablet	Pamlab
Mintex PD Liquid	Breckenridge
Mintuss NX Solution Syrup	Breckenridge
Mytussin DAC Syrup	Morton Grove
Nalex DH Liquid	Blansett
Nalex-A Liquid	Blansett
Nasop Suspension	Hawthorn
Neotuss S/F Liquid	A.G. Marin
Nescon-PD Tablet	Cypress
Niferex Elixir	Ther-Rx
Norel DM Liquid	U.S. Corp
Nycoff Tablet	Dover
Onset Forte Tablet	Textilease Medique
Orgadin Liquid	American Generics
Orgadin-Tuss Liquid	American Generics
Orgadin-Tuss DM Liquid	American Generics
Organidin NR Liquid	Wallace
Organidin NR Tablet	Wallace
Palgic-DS Syrup	Pamlab
Pancof Syrup	Pamlab
Pancof EXP Syrup	Pamlab
Pancof HC Solution	Pamlab
Pancof XP Liquid	Pamlab
Pancof XP Solution	Pamlab
Panmist DM Syrup	Pamlab
Pediatex Solution	Zyber
Pediatex D	Zyber
Pediatex DM Liquid	Zyber
Pediatex DM Solution	Zyber
Pediatex HC Solution	Zyber
Phanasin Syrup	Pharmakon
Phanasin Diabetic Choice Syrup	Pharmakon
Phanatuss Syrup	Pharmakon
Phanatuss DM Diabetic Choice Syrup	Pharmakon
Phanatuss-HC Diabetic Choice Solution	Pharmakon
Phena-HC Solution	GM
Phenabid DM Tablet	Gil
Phenydryl Solution	Scientific Laboratories

(*Continued on next page*)

Pneumotussin 2.5 Syrup	ECR
Poly Hist DM Solution	Poly
Poly Hist PD Solution	Poly
Poly-Tussin Syrup	Poly
Poly-Tussin DM Syrup	Poly
Poly-Tussin HD Syrup	Poly
Poly-Tussin XP Syrup	Poly
Pro-Clear Solution	Pro-Pharma
Pro-Cof D Liquid	Qualitest
Pro-Red Solution	Pro-Pharma
Prolex DH Liquid	Blansett
Prolex DM Liquid	Blansett
Protex Solution	Scientific Laboratories
Protex D Solution	Scientific Laboratories
Protuss Liquid	First Horizon
Quintex Syrup	Qualitest
Quintex HC Syrup	Qualitest
Relacon-DM Solution	Cypress
Relacon-HC Solution	Cypress
Rescon-DM Liquid	Capellon
Rhinacon A Solution	Breckenridge
Rhinacon DH Solution	Breckenridge
Rindal HD Liquid	Breckenridge
Rindal HD Plus Solution	Breckenridge
Rindal HPD Solution	Breckenridge
Romilar AC Liquid	Scot-Tussin
Romilar DM Liquid	Scot-Tussin
Rondamine DM Liquid	Major
Rondec Syrup	Biovail
Rondec DM Syrup	Biovail
Rondec DM Drops	Biovail
Ru-Tuss A Syrup	Sage
Ru-Tuss DM Syrup	Sage
Scot-Tussin Allergy Relief Formula Liquid	Scot Tussin
Scot-Tussin DM Cough Chasers Lozenge	Scot-Tussin
Scot-Tussin Original Liquid	Scot Tussin
Siladryl Allergy Liquid	Silarx
Siladryl DAS Liquid	Silarx
Sildec Syrup	Silarx
Sildec Drops	Silarx
Sildec-DM Syrup	Silarx
Silexin Syrup	Otis Clapp & Son
Silexin Tablet	Otis Clapp & Son
Sil-Tex Liquid Liquid	Silarx
Siltussin DM DAS Cough Formula Syrup	Silarx
S-T Forte 2 Liquid	Scot-Tussin
Statuss Green Liquid	Magna
Sudodrin Tablet	Textilease Medique
Sudafed Children's Cold & Cough Solution	Pfizer
Sudafed Children's Solution	Pfizer
Sudafed Children's Tablet	Pfizer
Sudanyl Tablet	Dover
Sudatuss-SF Liquid	Pharm Generic Developers
Sudodrin Tablet	Textilease Medique
Supress DX Pediatric Drops	Kramer-Novis
Suttar-SF Syrup	Gil
Triant-HC Solution	Hawthorn
Tricodene Syrup	Pfeiffer
Trispec-PE Liquid	Deliz
Trituss DM Solution	Breckenridge
Trituss Solution	Everett

Tri-Vent DM Solution	Ethex
Tusdec-DM Solution	Cypress
Tusdec-HC Solution	Cypress
Tusnel Solution	Llorens
Tussafed Syrup	Everett
Tussafed-EX Pediatric Drops	Everett
Tussafed-HC Syrup	Everett
Tussafed-HCG Solution	Everett
Tussall Solution	Everett
Tuss-DM Liquid	Seatrace
Tuss-ES Syrup	Seatrace
Tussi-Organidin DM NR Liquid	Wallace
Tussi-Organidin NR Liquid	Wallace
Tussi-Organidin-S NR Liquid	Wallace
Tussi-Pres Liquid	Kramer-Novis
Tussirex Liquid	Scot-Tussin
Uni Cof EXP Solution	United Research Labs
Uni Cof Solution	United Research Labs
Uni-Lev 5.0 Solution	United Research Labs
Vazol Solution	Wraser
Vi-Q-Tuss Syrup	Qualitest
Vitussin Expectorant Syrup	Cypress
Welltuss EXP Solution	Prasco
Welltuss HC Solution	Prasco
Z-Cof HC Solution	Zyber
Z-Cof HC Syrup	Zyber
Ztuss Expectorant Solution	Magna
Zyrtec Syrup	Pfizer

Fluoride Preparations

Ethedent Chewable Tablet	Ethex
Fluor-A-Day Tablet	Pharmascience
Fluor-A-Day Lozenge	Pharmascience
Flura-Loz Tablet	Kirkman
Lozi-Flur Lozenge	Dreir
Sensodyne w/Fluoride Gel	GlaxoSmithKline Consumer
Sensodyne w/Fluoride Tartar Control Toothpaste	GlaxoSmithKline Consumer
Sensodyne w/Fluoride Toothpaste	GlaxoSmithKline Consumer

Laxatives

Citrucel Powder	GlaxoSmithKline Consumer
Colace Solution	Purdue Pharma
Fiber Ease Liquid	Plainview
Fibro-XL Capsule	Key
Genfiber Powder	Ivax
Konsyl Easy Mix Formula Powder	Konsyl
Konsyl-Orange Powder	Konsyl
Metamucil Smooth Texture Powder	Procter & Gamble
Reguloid Powder	Rugby
Senokot Wheat Bran	Purdue Products

Miscellaneous

Acidoll Capsule	Key
Alka-Gest Tablet	Key
Bicitra Solution	Ortho-McNeil
Colidrops Pediatric Drops	A.G. Manin
Cytra-2 Solution	Cypress
Cytra-K Solution	Cypress
Cytra-K Crystals	Cypress

(*Continued on next page*)

Melatin Tablet	Mason Vitamins
Methadose Solution	Mallinckrodt
Neutra-Phos Powder	Ortho-McNeil
Neutra-Phos-K Powder	Ortho-McNeil
Polycitra-K Solution	Ortho-McNeil
Polycitra-LC Solution	Ortho-McNeil
Questran Light Powder	Par

Mouth/Throat Preparations

Aquafresh Triple Protection Gum	GlaxoSmithKline Consumer
Cepacol Maximum Strength Spray	J.B. Williams
Cepacol Sore Throat Lozenges	J.B. Williams
Cheracol Sore Throat Spray	Lee
Cylex Lozenges	Pharmakon
Fisherman's Friend Lozenges	Mentholatum
Fresh N Free Liquid	Geritrex
Isodettes Sore Throat Spray	GlaxoSmithKline Consumer
Larynex Lozenges	Dover
Listerine Pocketpaks Film	Pfizer Consumer
Medikoff Drops	Textilease Medique
Oragesic Solution	Parnell
Orasept Mouthwash/Gargle Liquid	Pharmakon
Robitussin Lozenges	Wyeth Consumer
Sepasoothe Lozenges	Textilease Medique
Thorets Maximum Strength Lozenges	Otis Clapp & Son
Throto-Ceptic Spray	S.S.S.
Vademecum Mouthwash & Gargle Concentrate	Dermatone

Potassium Supplements

Cena K Liquid	Century
Kaon Elixir	Savage
Kaon-Cl 20% Liquid	Savage
Rum-K Liquid	Fleming

Vitamins/Minerals/Supplements

Action-Tabs Made For Men	Action Labs
Adaptosode For Stress Liquid	HVS
Adaptosode R + R for Acute Stress Liquid	HVS
Alamag Tablet	Textilease Medique
Alcalak Tablet	Textilease Medique
Aldroxicon I Suspension	Textilease Medique
Aldroxicon II Suspension	Textilease Medique
Aminoplex Powder	Tyson
Aminostasis Powder	Tyson
Aminotate Powder	Tyson
Apetigen Elixir	Kramer-Novis
Apptrim Capsule	Physician Therapeutics
Apptrim-D Capsule	Physician Therapeutics
B-C-Bid Caplet	Lee
Bevitamel Tablet	Westlake
Biosode Liquid	HVS
Biotect Plus Caplet	Gil
C & M Caps-375 Capsule	Key
Calbon Tablet	Emrex/Economed
Cal-Cee Tablet	Key
Calcet Plus Tablet	Mission Pharmacal
Calcimin-300 Tablet	Key
Cal-Mint Chewable Tablet	Freeda Vitamins
Cena K Solution	Century
Cerefolin Tablet	Pamlab

Cevi-Bid Tablet	Lee
Choice DM Liquid	Bristol-Myers Squibb
Cholestratin Tablet	Key
Chromacaps Tablet	Key
Chromium K6 Tablet	Rexall Consumer
Citrimax 500 Plus Tablet	Mason Vitamins
Combi-Cart Tablet	Atrium Bio-Tech
Delta D3 Tablet	Freeda Vitamins
Detoxosode Liquids	HVS
Dexfol Tablet	Rising
DHEA Capsule	ADH Health Products
Diabeze Tablet	Key
Diatx Tablet	Pamlab
Diatx ZN Tablet	Pamlab
Diet System 6 Gum	Applied Nutrition
Dimacid Tablet	Otis Clapp & Son
Diucaps Capsule	Legere
Di-Phen-500 Capsule	Key
Electrolab Tablet	Hart Health And Safety
Endorphenyl Capsule	Tyson
Ensure Nutra Shake Pudding	Ross Products
Enterex Diabetic Liquid	Victus
Essential Nutrients Plus Silica Tablet	Actions Labs
Evening Primrose Oil Capsule	National Vitamin
Evolve Softgel	Bionutrics Health Products
Ex-L Tablet	Key
Extress Tablet	Key
Eyetamins Tablet	Rexall Consumer
Fem-Cal Tablet	Freeda Vitamins
Fem-Cal Plus Tablet	Freeda Vitamins
Ferrocite F Tablet	Breckenridge
Folacin-800 Tablet	Key
Folbee Plus Tablet	Breckenridge
Folplex 2.2 Tablet	Breckenridge
Foltx Tablet	Pamlab
Gabadone Capsule	Physician Therapeutics
Gram-O-Leci Tablet	Freeda Vitamins
Hemovit Tablet	Dayton
Herbal Slim Complex Capsule	ADH Health Products
Irofol Liquid	Dayton
Lynae Calcium/Vitamin C Chewable Tablet	Boscogen
Lynae Chondroitin/Glucosamine Capsule	Boscogen
Lynae Ginse-Cool Chewable Tablet	Boscogen
Mag-Caps Capsule	Rising
Mag-Ox 400 Tablet	Blaine
Mag-SR Tablet	Cypress
Magimin Tablet	Key Company
Magnacaps Capsule	Key Company
Mangimin Capsule	Key Company
Mangimin Tablet	Key Company
Medi-Lyte Tablet	Textilease Medique
Metanx Tablet	Pamlab
Multi-Delyn w/Iron Liquid	Silarx
Nephro-Fer Tablet	Watson
Neutra-Phos Powder	Ortho-Mcneil
Neutra-Phos-K Powder	Ortho-Mcneil
New Life Hair Tablet	Rexall Consumer
Niferex Elixir	Ther-Rx
Nutrisure OTC Tablet	Westlake
O-Cal Fa Tablet	Pharmics

(Continued on next page)

Plenamins Plus Tablet	Rexall Consumer
Powervites Tablet	Green Turtle Bay Vitamin
Prostaplex Herbal Complex Capsule	ADH Health Products
Prostatonin Capsule	Pharmaton Natural Health
Protect Plus Liquid	Gil
Protect Plus NR Softgel	Gil
Pulmona Capsule	Physician T
Quintabs-M Tablet	Freeda Vitamins
Re/Neph Liquid	Ross Products
Replace Capsule	Key
Replace w/o Iron Capsule	Key
Resource Arginaid Powder	Novartis Nutrition
Ribo-100 T.D. Capsule	Key
Samolinic Softgel	Key
Sea Omega 30 Softgel	Rugby
Sea Omega 50 Softgel	Rugby
Sentra Am Capsule	Physician Therapeutics
Sentra PM Capsule	Physician Therapeutics
Soy Care for Bone Health Tablet	Inverness Medical
Soy Care for Menopause Capsule	Inverness Medical
Span C Tablet	Freeda Vitamins
Strovite Forte Syrup	Everett
Sunnie Tablet	Green Turtle Bay Vitamin
Sunvite Tablet	Rexall Consumer
Super Dec B100 Tablet	Freeda Vitamins
Super Quints-50 Tablet	Freeda Vitamins
Supervite Liquid	Seyer Pharmatec
Suplevit Liquid	Gil
Theramine Capsule	Physician Therapeutics
Triamin Tablet	Key
Triamino Tablet	Freeda Vitamins
Ultramino Tablet	Freeda Vitamins
Uro-Mag Capsule	Blaine
Vinatal 600 Kit	Breckenridge
Vitalize Liquid	Scot-Tussin
Vitamin C/Rose Hips Tablet	ADH Health Products
Vitrum Jr Chewable Tablet	Mason Vitamins
Xtramins Tablet	Key
Yohimbe Power Max 1500 For Women Tablet	Action Labs
Yohimbized 1000 Capsule	Action Labs
Ze-Plus Softgel	Everett

Alcohol-Free Products

The following is a selection of alcohol-free products by therapeutic category. The list is not comprehensive. Generic and alternate brands may exist. Always check product labeling for definitive information on specific ingredients.

Analgesics

Acetaminophen Infants Drops	Ivax
Actamin Maximum Strength Liquid	Cypress
Addaprin Tablet	Dover
Advil Children's Suspension	Wyeth Consumer
Aminofen Tablet	Dover
Aminofen Max Tablet	Dover
APAP Elixir	Bio-Pharm
Aspirtab Tablet	Dover

Buffasal Tablet	Dover
Demerol Hydrochloride Syrup	Sanofi-Synthelabo
Dolono Elixir	R.I.D.
Dyspel Tablet	Dover
Genapap Children Elixir	Ivax
Genapap Infant's Drop	Ivax
Motrin Children's Suspension	McNeil Consumer
Motrin Infant's Suspension	McNeil Consumer
Silapap Children's Elixir	Silarx
Silapap Infant's Drops	Silarx
Tylenol Children's Suspension	McNeil Consumer
Tylenol Extra Strength Solution	McNeil Consumer
Tylenol Infant's Drops	McNeil Consumer
Tylenol Infant's Suspension	McNeil Consumer

Antiasthmatic Agents

Dilor-G Liquid	Savage
Dy-G Liquid	Cypress
Elixophyllin-GG Liquid	Forest

Anticonvulsants

Zarontin Syrup	Pfizer

Antiviral Agents

Epivir Oral Solution	GlaxoSmithKline

Cough/Cold/Allergy Preparations

Accuhist Pediatric Drops	Propst
Alacol DM Syrup	Ballay
Allergy Relief Medicine Children's Elixir	Hi-Tech Pharmacal
Altarussin Syrup	Altaire
Amerifed DM Liquid	MCR American
Amerifed Liquid	Ambi
Anaplex DM Syrup	ECR
Anaplex DMX Suspension	ECR
Anaplex HD Syrup	ECR
Andehist DM Drops	Cypress
Andehist DM Syrup	Cypress
Andehist DM NR Liquid	Cypress
Andehist DM NR Syrup	Cypress
Andehist NR Syrup	Cypress
Andehist Syrup	Cypress
Aquatab DM Syrup	Adams
Atuss DR Syrup	Atley
Atuss EX Liquid	Atley
Atuss G Liquid	Atley
Atuss HC Syrup	Atley
Atuss MS Syrup	Atley
Baltussin Solution	Ballay Pharm
Benadryl Allergy Solution	Pfizer Consumer
Benadryl Allergy/Sinus Children's Solution	Pfizer
Biodec DM Drops	Bio-Pharm
Bromaline Solution	Rugby
Bromaline DM Elixir	Rugby
Bromanate Elixir	Alpharma USPD
Bromatan-DM Suspension	Cypress
Bromaxefed DM RF Syrup	Morton Grove
Bromaxefed RF Syrup	Morton Grove
Broncotron Liquid	Seyer Pharmatec

(*Continued on next page*)

Bromdec Solution	Scientific Laboratories
Bromdec DM Solution	Scientific Laboratories
Bromhist Pediatric Solution	Cypress
Bromhist-DM Pediatric Syrup	Cypress
Bromhist-DM Solution	Cypress
Bromphenex HD Solution	Breckenridge
Bromplex DM Solution	Prasco Laboratories
Broncotron-D Suspension	Seyer Pharmatec
Bron-Tuss Liquid	American Generics
Brovex HC Solution	Athlon
B-Tuss Liquid	Blansett
Carbaphen 12 Ped Suspension	Gil
Carbaphen 12 Suspension	Gil
Carbatuss Liquid	GM
Carbatuss-CL Solution	GM
Carbaxefed DM RF Liquid	Morton Grove
Carbetaplex Solution	Breckenridge
Carbihist Solution	Boca Pharmacal
Carbofed DM Drops	Hi-Tech Pharmacal
Carbofed DM Syrup	Hi-Tech Pharmacal
Carboxine Solution	Cypress
Carboxine-PSE Solution	Cypress
Cardec Syrup	Qualitest
Cardec DM Syrup	Qualitest
Cepacol Sore Throat Liquid	J. B. Williams
Chlordex GP Syrup	Cypress
Chlor-Mes D Solution	Cypress
Chlor-Trimeton Allergy Syrup	Schering Plough
Codal-DH Syrup	Cypress
Codal-DM Syrup	Cypress
Codotuss Liquid	Major
Coldec DS Solution	Breckenridge
Coldec-DM Syrup	United Research Labs
Coldmist DM Solution	Breckenridge
Coldmist DM Syrup	Breckenridge
Coldmist S Syrup	Breckenridge
Coldonyl Tablet	Dover
Coldtuss DR Syrup	United Research Labs
Colidrops Pediatric Liquid	A. G. Marin
Complete Allergy Elixir	Cardinal Health
Cordron-D Solution	Cypress
Cordron-DM Solution	Cypress
Cordron-HC Solution	Cypress
Corfen DM Solution	Cypress
Co-Tussin Liquid	American Generics
Cotuss-V Syrup	Alphagen
Crantex HC Syrup	Breckenridge
Crantex Syrup	Breckenridge
Creomulsion Complete Syrup	Summit Industries
Creomulsion Cough Syrup	Summit Industries
Creomulsion For Children Syrup	Summit Industries
Creomulsion Pediatric Syrup	Summit Industries
Cytuss HC Syrup	Cypress
Dacex-A Solution	Cypress
Dacex-DM Solution	Cypress
Decahist-DM Solution	Cypress
De-Chlor DM Solution	Cypress
De-Chlor DR Solution	Cypress
Dehistine Syrup	Cypress
Deka Liquid	Dayton
Deka Pediatric Drops Solution	Dayton

Deltuss Liquid	Deliz
Denaze Solution	Cypress
Despec Liquid Labs	International Ethical
Dex PC Syrup	Boca Pharmacal
Dexcon-DM Solution	Cypress
Diabetic Tussin Allergy Relief Liquid	Healthcare Products
Diabetic Tussin C Expectorant Liquid	Healthcare Products
Diabetic Tussin Cold & Flu Tablet	Healthcare Products
Diabetic Tussin DM Liquid	Healthcare Products
Diabetic Tussin DM Maximum Strength Liquid	Healthcare Products
Diabetic Tussin DM Maximum Strength Capsule	Healthcare Products
Diabetic Tussin EX Liquid	Healthcare Products
Dimetapp Allergy Children's Elixir	Whitehall-Robins
Dimetapp Cold & Fever Children's Suspension	Wyeth Consumer
Dimetapp Decongestant Pediatric Drops	Wyeth Consumer
Double-Tussin DM Liquid	Reese
Drocon-CS Solution	Cypress
Duradal HD Plus Syrup	Prasco Laboratories
Duratan DM Suspension	Proethic Laboratories
Duratuss DM Solution	Victory
Dynatuss Syrup	Breckenridge
Dynatuss EX Syrup	Breckenridge
Dynatuss HC Solution	Breckenridge
Dynatuss HCG Solution	Breckenridge
Endacof DM Solution	Larken Laboratories
Endacof HC Solution	Larken Laboratories
Endacof XP Solution	Larken Laboratories
Endagen-HD Syrup	Monarch
Endal HD Solution	Pediamed
Endal HD Syrup	Propst
Endal HD Plus Syrup	Propst
Endotuss-HD Syrup	American Generics
Enplus-HD Syrup	Alphagen
Entex Syrup	Andrx
Entex HC Syrup	Andrx
Exo-Tuss	American Generics
Father John's Medicine Plus Drops	Oakhurst
Friallergia DM Liquid	R.I.D.
Friallergia Liquid	R.I.D.
Ganidin NR Liquid	Cypress
Gani-Tuss NR Liquid	Cypress
Gani-Tuss-DM NR Liquid	Cypress
Genahist Elixir	Ivax
Genebronco-D Liquid	Pharm Generic
Genecof-HC Liquid	Pharm Generic
Genecof-XP Liquid	Pharm Generic
Genecof-XP Syrup	Pharm Generic
Genedel Syrup	Pharm Generic
Genedotuss-DM Liquid	Pharm Generic
Genepatuss Liquid	Pharm Generic
Genetuss-2 Liquid	Pharm Generic
Genexpect-DM Liquid	Pharm Generic
Genexpect-PE Liquid	Pharm Generic
Genexpect-SF Liquid	Pharm Generic
Giltuss HC Syrup	Gil
Giltuss Liquid	Gil
Giltuss Pediatric Liquid	Gil
Guai-Co Liquid	Alphagen
Guaicon DMS Liquid	Textilease Medique
Guai-Dex Liquid	Alphagen

(*Continued on next page*)

Guaifed Syrup	Muro
Guaitussin AC Solution	Scientific Laboratories
Guaitussin DAC Solution	Scientific Laboratories
Guapetex HC Solution	Scientific Laboratories
Guapetex Syrup	Scientific Laboratories
Halotussin AC Liquid	Watson Pharma
Hayfebrol Liquid	Scot-Tussin
H-C Tussive Syrup	Vintage
Histacol DM Pediatric Solution	Breckenridge
Histacol DM Pediatric Syrup	Breckenridge
Histex HC Syrup	TEAMM
Histex Liquid	TEAMM
Histex PD Drops	TEAMM
Histex PD Liquid	TEAMM
Histinex HC Syrup	Ethex
Histinex PV Syrup	Ethex
Histuss HC Solution	Scientific Laboratories
Hi-Tuss Syrup	Hi-Tech Pharmacal
Hycomal DH Liquid	Alphagen
Hydex-PD Solution	Cypress
Hydone Liquid	Hyrex
Hydramine Elixir	Ivax
Hydro PC Syrup	Cypress
Hydro PC II Plus Solution	Cypress
Hydro Pro Solution	Breckenridge
Hydrocol-HC Solution	Morton Grove
Hydro-DP Solution	Cypress
Hydron CF Syrup	Cypress
Hydron EX Syrup	Cypress
Hydron KGS Liquid	Cypress
Hydron PSC Liquid	Cypress
Hydro-Tussin DM Elixir	Ethex
Hydro-Tussin HC Syrup	Ethex
Hydro-Tussin HD Liquid	Ethex
Hydro-Tussin XP Syrup	Ethex
Hyphen-HD Syrup	Alphagen
Jaycof Expectorant Syrup	Pharmakon
Jaycof-HC Liquid	Pharmakon
Jaycof-XP Liquid	Pharmakon
Kita La Tos Liquid	R.I.D.
Levall Liquid	Andrx
Levall 5.0 Liquid	Andrx
Lodrane Liquid	ECR
Lodrane D Suspension	ECR
Lodrane XR Suspension	ECR
Lohist D Syrup	Larken Laboratories
Lohist-LQ Solution	Larken
Lortuss DM Solution	Proethic
Lortuss HC Solution	Proethic
Marcof Expectorant Syrup	Marnel
Maxi-Tuss HCX Solution	MCR American
M-Clear Jr Solution	McNeil, R.A.
M-Clear Syrup	McNeil, R.A.
Medi-Brom Elixir	Medicine Shoppe
Mintex Liquid	Breckenridge
Mintex PD Liquid	Breckenridge
Mintuss DM Syrup	Breckenridge
Mintuss EX Syrup	Breckenridge
Mintuss G Syrup	Breckenridge
Mintuss HD Syrup	Breckenridge
Mintuss MR Syrup	Breckenridge

Mintuss MS Syrup	Breckenridge
Mintuss NX Solution	Breckenridge
Motrin Cold Children's Suspension	McNeil Consumer
Mytussin-PE Liquid	Morton Grove
Nalex DH Liquid	Blansett Pharmacal
Nalex-A Liquid	Blansett Pharmacal
Nalspan Senior DX Liquid	Morton Grove
Nasop Suspension	Hawthorn
Neotuss S/F Liquid	A.G. Marin
Neotuss-D Liquid	A.G. Marin
Norel DM Liquid	U.S. Pharmaceutical
Nucofed Syrup	Monarch
Nycoff Tablet	Dover
Orgadin Liquid	American Generics
Orgadin-Tuss Liquid	American Generics
Orgadin-Tuss DM Liquid	American Generics
Organidin NR Liquid	Wallace
Palgic-DS Syrup	Pamlab
Pancof Syrup	Pamlab
Pancof EXP Syrup	Pamlab
Pancof HC Liquid	Pamlab
Pancof HC Solution	Pamlab
Pancof XP Liquid	Pamlab
Pancof XP Solutuion	Pamlab
Panmist DM Syrup	Pamlab
Panmist-S Syrup	Pamlab
PediaCare Cold + Allergy Children's Liquid	Pharmacia
PediaCare Cough + Cold Children's Liquid	Pharmacia
PediaCare Decongestant Infants Drops	Pharmacia
PediaCare Decongestant Plus Cough Drops	Pharmacia
PediaCare Multi-Symptom Liquid	Pharmacia
PediaCare Nightrest Liquid	Pharmacia
Pediahist DM Syrup	Boca
Pedia-Relief Liquid	Major
Pediatex Liquid	Zyber
Pediatex Solution	Zyber
Pediatex-D Liquid	Zyber
Pediatex D Solution	Zyber
Pediatex DM Solution	Zyber
Pediox Liquid	Atley
Phanasin Syrup	Pharmakon
Phanatuss Syrup	Pharmakon
Phanatuss-HC Diabetic Choice Solution	Pharmakon Labs
Phena-HC Solution	GM
Phena-S Liquid	GM
Pneumotussin 2.5 Syrup	ECR
Poly Hist DM Solution	Poly
Poly Hist PD Solution	Poly
Poly-Tussin Syrup	Poly
Poly-Tussin DM Syrup	Poly
Poly-Tussin HD Syrup	Poly
Poly-Tussin XP Syrup	Poly
Primsol Solution	Medicis
Pro-Clear Solution	Pro-Pharma
Pro-Cof Liquid	Qualitest
Pro-Cof D Liquid	Qualitest
Prolex DH Liquid	Blansett Pharmacal
Prolex DM Liquid	Blansett Pharmacal
Pro-Red Solution	Pro-Pharma

(*Continued on next page*)

Protex Solution	Scientific Laboratories
Protex D Solution	Scientific Laboratories
Protuss Liquid	First Horizon
Protuss-D Liquid	First Horizon
Pyrroxate Extra Strength Tablet	Lee
Q-Tussin PE Liquid	Qualitest
Qual-Tussin DC Syrup	Pharm. Associates
Quintex Syrup	Qualitest
Quintex HC Syrup	Qualitest
Relacon-DM Solution	Cypress
Relacon-HC Solution	Cypress
Rescon-DM Liquid	Capellon
Rescon-GG Liquid	Capellon
Rhinacon A Solution	Breckenridge
Rhinacon DH Solution	Breckenridge
Rindal HD Liquid	Breckenridge
Rindal HD Plus Solution	Breckenridge
Rindal HPD Solution	Breckenridge
Robitussin Cough & Congestion Liquid	Wyeth Consumer
Robitussin DM Syrup	Wyeth Consumer
Robitussin PE Syrup	Wyeth Consumer
Robitussin Pediatric Drops	Wyeth Consumer
Robitussin Pediatric Cough Syrup	Wyeth Consumer
Robitussin Pediatric Night Relief Liquid	Wyeth Consumer
Romilar AC Liquid	Scot-Tussin
Romilar DM Liquid	Scot-Tussin
Rondamine DM Liquid	Major
Rondec Syrup	Biovail
Rondec DM Drops	Biovail
Rondec DM Syrup	Biovail
Ru-Tuss A Syrup	Sage
Ru-Tuss DM Syrup	Sage
Scot-Tussin Allergy Relief Formula Liquid	Scot-Tussin
Scot-Tussin DM Liquid	Scot-Tussin
Scot-Tussin Expectorant Liquid	Scot-Tussin
Scot-Tussin Original Syrup	Scot-Tussin
Scot-Tussin Senior Liquid	Scot-Tussin
Siladryl Allergy Liquid	Silarx
Siladryl DAS Liquid	Silarx
Sildec Liquid	Silarx
Sildec Syrup	Silarx
Sildec-DM Drops	Silarx
Sildec-DM Syrup	Silarx
Sil-Tex Liquiduid Liquid	Silarx
Siltussin DAS Liquid	Silarx
Siltussin DM Syrup	Silarx
Siltussin DM DAS Cough Formula Syrup	Silarx
Siltussin SA Syrup	Silarx
Simply Cough Liquid	McNeil Consumer
Simply Stuffy Liquid	McNeil Consumer
S-T Forte 2 Liquid	Scot-Tussin
Statuss DM Syrup	Magna
Sudafed Children's Cold & Cough Solution	Pfizer
Sudafed Children's Solution	Pfizer
Sudafed Children's Tablet	Pfizer
Sudanyl Tablet	Dover
Sudatuss DM Syrup	Pharmaceutical Generic
Sudatuss-2 Liquid	Pharmaceutical Generic
Sudatuss-SF Liquid	Pharmaceutical Generic
Triaminic Infant Decongestant Drops	Novartis Consumer
Triant-HC Solution	Hawthorn

Trispec-PE Liquid	Deliz
Trituss DM Solution	Breckenridge
Trituss Solution	Everett
Tri-Vent DM Solution	Ethex
Tri-Vent DPC Syrup	Ethex
Tusdec-DM Solution	Cypress
Tusdec-HC Solution	Cypress
Tusnel Pediatric Solution	Llorens Pharma
Tusnel Solution	Llorens Pharma
Tussafed Syrup	Everett
Tussafed-EX Syrup	Everett
Tussafed-EX Pediatric Liquid	Everett
Tussafed HC Syrup	Everett
Tussafed-HCG Solution	Everett
Tussall Solution	Everett
Tussbid Capsule	Breckenridge
Tuss-DM Liquid	Seatrace
Tuss-ES Syrup	Seatrace
Tussex Syrup	H. L. Moore
Tussinate Syrup	Pediamed
Tussi-Organidin DM NR Liquid	Wallace
Tussi-Organidin NR Liquid	Wallace
Tussi-Pres Liquid	Kramer-Novis
Tussirex Liquid	Scot-Tussin
Tussirex Syrup	Scot-Tussin
Tylenol Allergy-D Children's Liquid	McNeil Consumer
Tylenol Cold Children's Liquid	McNeil Consumer
Tylenol Cold Children's Suspension	McNeil Consumer
Tylenol Cold Infants' Drops	McNeil Consumer
Tylenol Cold Plus Cough Children's Liquid	McNeil Consumer
Tylenol Cold Plus Cough Infants' Suspension	McNeil Consumer
Tylenol Flu Children's Suspension	McNeil Consumer
Tylenol Flu Night Time Max Strength Liquid	McNeil Consumer
Tylenol Sinus Children's Liquid	McNeil Consumer
Uni-Lev 5.0 Solution	United Research
Vanex-HD Syrup	Monarch
Vazol Solution	Wraser Pharm
Vicks 44E Pediatric Liquid	Procter & Gamble
Vicks 44M Pediatric Liquid	Procter & Gamble
Vicks Dayquil Multi-Symptom Liquicap	Procter & Gamble
Vicks Dayquil Multi-Symptom Liquid	Procter & Gamble
Vicks 44 Liquid Capsules Cold, Flu, Cough	Procter & Gamble
Vicks Nyquil Children's Liquid	Procter & Gamble
Vicks Sinex 12 Hour Spray	Procter & Gamble
Vicks Sinex Spray	Procter & Gamble
Vi-Q-Tuss Syrup	Vintage
V-Tann Suspension	Breckenridge
Vitussin Expectorant Syrup	Cypress
Vortex Syrup	Superior
Welltuss EXP Solution	Prasco Laboratories
Welltuss HC Solution	Prasco Laboratorues
Z-Cof DM Syrup	Zyber
Z-Cof DMX Solution	Zyber
Z-Cof HC Syrup	Zyber
Ztuss Expectorant Solution	Magna

Ear/Nose/Throat Products

4-Way Saline Moisturizing Mist Spray	Bristol-Myers
Ayr Baby Saline Spray	B.F. Ascher

(*Continued on next page*)

Bucalcide Solution	Seyer Pharmatec
Bucalcide Spray	Seyer Pharmatec
Bucalsep Solution	Gil
Bucalsep Spray	Gil
Cepacol Sore Throat Liquid	Combe
Cheracol Sore Throat Spray	Lee
Fresh N Free Liquid	Geritrex
Gly-Oxide Liquid	GlaxoSmithKline
Isodettes Sore Throat Spray	GlaxoSmithKline
Lacrosse Mouthwash Liquid	Aplicare
Larynex Lozenges	Dover
Listermint Liquid	Pfizer Consumer
Nasal Moist Gel	Blairex
Orajel Baby Liquid	Del
Orajel Baby Nighttime Gel	Del
Oramagic Oral Wound Rinse Powder for Suspension	MPM Medical
Orasept Mouthwash/Gargle Liquid	Pharmakon Labs
Tanac Liquid	Del
Tech 2000 Dental Rinse Liquid	Care-Tech
Throto-Ceptic Spray	S.S.S.
Zilactin Baby Extra Strength Gel	Zila Consumer

Gastrointestinal Agents

Axid	Pediamed Pharm
Axid Solution	Reliant
Baby Gasz Drops	Lee
Colidrops Pediatric Drops	A.G. Marin
Colace Solution	Purdue Pharma
Diarrest Tablet	Dover
Imogen Liquid	Pharmaceutical
Kaodene NN Suspension	Pfeiffer
Liqui-Doss Liquid	Ferndale
Mylicon Infants' Suspension	J&J-Merck
Neoloid Liquid	Kenwood
Neutralin Tablet	Dover
Senokot Children's Syrup	Purdue Frederick

Hematinics

Irofol Liquid	Dayton

Miscellaneous

Cytra-2 Solution	Cypress
Cytra-K Solution	Cypress
Emetrol Solution	Pharmacia
Fluorinse Solution	Oral B
Primsol Solution	FSC
Rum-K Liquid	Fleming

Psychotropics

Thorazine Syrup	

Topical Products

Aloe Vesta 2-N-1 Antifungal Ointment	Convatec
Blistex Complete Moisture Stick	Blistex
Blistex Fruit Smoothies Stick	Blistex
Blistex Herbal Answer Gel	Blistex
Blistex Herbal Answer Stick	Blistex
Dermatone Lips N Face Protector Ointment	Dermatone
Dermatone Moisturizing Sunblock Cream	Dermatone
Dermatone Outdoor Skin Protection Cream	Dermatone

Dermatone Skin Protector Cream	Dermatone
Eucapsulein Facial Lotion	Beiersdorf, Inc.
Evoclin Foam	Connetics
Fleet Pain Relief Pads	Fleet
Fresh & Pure Douche Solution	Unico
Handclens Solution	Woodward
Joint-Ritis Maximum Strength Ointment	Naturopathic Laboratories
Neutrogena Acne Wash Liquid	Neutrogena
Neutrogena Antiseptic Liquid	Neutrogena
Neutrogena Clear Pore Gel	Neutrogena
Neutrogena T/Derm Liquid	Neutrogena
Neutrogena Toner Liquid	Neutrogena
Podiciens Spray	Woodward
Propa pH Foaming Face Wash Liquid	Del
Sea Breeze Foaming Face Wash Gel	Clairol
Shade Uvaguard Lotion	Schering Plough
Sportz Bloc Cream	Med-Derm
Stri-Dex Maximum Strength Pad	Blistex
Stri-Dex Sensitive Skin Pad	Blistex
Stri-Dex Super Scrub Pad	Blistex
Therasoft Anti-Acne Cream	SFC/Solvent Free
Therasoft Skin Protectant Cream	SFC/Solvent Free
Tiger Balm Arthritis Rub Lotion	Prince of Peace Enterprises

Vitamins/Minerals/Supplements

Adaptosode For Stress Liquid	HVS
Adaptosode R+R For Acute Stress Liquid	HVS
Apetigen Elixir	Kramer-Novis
Biosode Liquid	HVS
Detoxosode Products Liquid	HVS
Folbic Tablet	Breckenridge
Folplex 2.2 Gel	Breckenridge
Genesupp-500 Liquid	Pharmaceutical
Genetect Plus Liquid	Pharmaceutical
Multi-Delyn w/Iron Liquid	Silarx
Poly-Vi Sol Drops	Mead Johnson
Poly-Vi Sol w/Iron Drops	Mead Johnson
Poly-Vi Solution Liquid	Mead Johnson
Poly-Vi Solution w/Iron Liquid	Mead Johnson
Protect Plus Liquid	Gil
Soluvite-F Drops	Pharmics
Strovite Forte Syrup	Everett
Supervite Liquid	Seyer Pharmatec
Suplevit Liquid	Gil
Tri-Vi-Sol Drops	Mead Johnson
Tri-Vi-Sol w/Iron Drops	Mead Johnson
Vitafol Syrup	Everett
Vitalize Liquid	Scot-Tussin
Vitamin C/Rose Hips Tablet, Extended Release	ADH Health Products

Drugs That May Cause Photosensitivity

The drugs in this table are known to cause photosensitivity in some individuals. Effects can range from itching, scaling, rash, and swelling to skin cancer, premature skin aging, skin and eye burns, cataracts, reduced immunity, blood vessel damage, and allergic reactions.

The list is not all-inclusive, and shows only representative brands of each generic. When in doubt, always check specific product labeling. Individuals should be advised to wear protective clothing and to apply sunscreens while taking the medications listed below.

Generic	Brand
Acamprosate	Campral
Acetazolamide	Diamox
Acitretin	Soriatane
Acyclovir	Zovirax
Alendronate	Fosamax
Alitretinoin	Panretin
Almotriptan	Axert
Amilloride/hydrochlorothiazide	Moduretic
Aminolevulinic acid	Levulan Kerastick
Amiodarone	Cordarone, Pacerone
Amitriptyline	Elavil
Amitriptyline/chlordiazepoxide	Limbitrol
Amitriptyline/perphenazine	Triavil
Amlodipine/atorvastatin	Caduet
Amoxapine	
Anagrelide	Agrylin
Apripiprazole	Abilify
Atazanavir	Reyataz
Atenolol/chlorthalidone	Tenoretic
Atorvastasin	Lipitor
Atovaquone/proguanil	Malarone
Azatadine/pseudoephedrine	Ryanatan, Trinalin
Azithromycin	Zithromax
Benazepril	Lotensin
Benazepril/hydrochlorothiazide	Lotensin HCT
Bendroflumethiazide/nadolot	Corzide
Bexarotene	Targretin
Bismuth/metronidazole/tetracycline	Helidac
Bisoprolol/hydrochlorothiazide	Ziac
Brompheniramine/dextromethorphan/phenylephrine	Alacol DM
Brompheniramine/dextromethorphan/pseudoephedrine	Bromfed-DM
Buffered aspirin/pravastatin	Pravigard PAC
Bupropion	Wellbutrin, Zyban
Candesartan/hydrochlorothiazide	Atacand HCT
Capecitabine	Xeloda
Captopril	Capoten
Captopril/hyrdrochlorothiazide	Capozide
Carbamazepine	Carbatrol, Tegretol, Tegretol-XR
Carbinoxamine/pseudoephedrine	Palgic-D, Palgic-DS, Pediatex-D
Carvedilol	Coreg
Celecoxib	Celebrex
Cetirizine	Zyrtec
Cetirizine/pseudoephedrine	Zyrtec-D
Cevimeline	Evoxac
Chlorhexidine gluconate	Hibistat
Chloroquine	Aralen
Chlorothiazide	Diuril
Chlorpheniramine/hydrocodone/pseudoephedrine	Tussend
Chlorpheniramine/phenylephrine/pyrilamine	Rynatan
Chlorpromazine	Thorazine
Chlorpropamide	Diabinese
Chlorthalidone	Thalitone
Chlorthalidone/clonidine	Clorpres
Cidofovir	Vistide
Ciprofloxacin	Cipro
Citalopram	Celexa
Clemastine	Tavist

Generic	Brand
Clonidine/chlorthalidone	Clorpres
Clozapine	Clozaril, Fazaclo
Cromolyn sodium	Gastrocrom
Cyclobenzaprine	Flexeril
Cyproheptadine	Cyproheptadine
Dacarbazine	DTIC-Dome
Dantrolene	Dantrium
Demeclocycline	Declomycin
Desipramine	Norpramin
Diclofenac potassium	Cataflam
Diclofenac sodium	Voltaren
Diclofenac sodium/misoprostol	Arthrotec
Diflunisal	Dolobid
Dihydroergotamine	D.H.E. 45
Diltiazem	Cardizem, Tiazac
Diphenhydramine	Benadryl
Divalproex	Depakote
Doxepin	Sinequan
Doxycycline hyclate	Doryx, Periostat, Vibra-Tabs,Vibramycin
Doxycycline monohydrate	Monodox
Duloxetine	Cymbalta
Enalapril	Vasotec
Enalapril/felodipine	Lexxel
Enalapril/hydrochlorothiazide	Vaseretic
Enalaprilat	Vasotec I.V.
Epirubicin	Ellence
Eprosartan mesylate/hydrochlorothiazide	Teveten HCT
Erythromycin/sulfisoxazole	Pediazole
Estazolam	ProSom
Estradiol	Gynodiol, Estrogel
Eszopiclone	Lunesta
Ethionamide	Trecator-SC
Etodolac	Lodine
Felbamate	Felbatol
Fenofibrate	Tricor, Lofibra
Floxuridine	Sterile FUDR
Flucytosine	Ancobon
Fluorouracil	Efudex
Fluoxetine	Prozac, Sarafem
Fluphenazine	Prolixin
Flutamide	Eulexin
Fluvastatin	Lescol
Fluvoxamine	Luvox
Fosinopril	Monopril
Fosphenytoin	Cerebyx
Furosemide	Lasix
Gabapentin	Neurontin
Gatifloxacin	Tequin
Gemfibrozil	Lopid
Gemifloxacin mesylate	Factive
Gentamicin	Garamycin
Glatiramer	Copaxone
Glimepiride	Amaryl
Glipizide	Glucotrol
Glyburide	DiaBeta, Glynase, Micronase
Glyburide/metformin HCI	Glucovance
Griseofulvin	Fulvicin P/G, Grifulvin, Gris-PEG

(Continued on next page)

Generic	Brand
Haloperidol	Haldol
Hexachlorophene	pHisoHex
Hydralazine/hydrochlothiazide	Hydra-zide
Hydrochlorothiazide	HydroDIURIl, Microzide, Oretic
Hydrochlorothiazide/fosinopril	Monopril HCT
Hydrochlorothiazide/irbesartan	Avalide
Hydrochlorothiazide/lisinopril	Prinzide, Zestoretic
Hydrochlorothiazide/losartan potassium	Hyzaar
Hydrochlorothiazide/methyldopa	Aldoril
Hydrochlorothiazide/moexipril	Uniretic
Hydrochlorothiazide/propanolol	Inderide
Hydrochlorothiazide/quinapril	Accuretic
Hydrochlorothiazide/spironolactone	Aldactazide
Hydrochlorothiazide/telmisartan	Micardis HCT
Hydrochlorothiazide/timolol	Timolide
Hydrochlorothiazide/triamterene	Dyazide, Maxzide
Hydrochlorothiazide/valsartan	Diovan HCT
Hydroflumethiazide	Hydroflumethiazide
Hydroxychloroquine	Plaquenil
Hypericum	Kira, St. John's Wort
Hypericum/vitamin B_1/vitamin C/kava-kava	One-A-Day Tension & Mood
Ibuprofen	Motrin
Imatinib Mesylate	Gleevec
Imipramine	Tofranil
Imiquimod	Aldara
Indapamide	Lozol
Interferon alfa-2b, recombinant	Intron A
Interferon alfa-n3 (human leukocyte derived)	Alferon-N
Interferon beta-1a	Avonex
Interferon beta-1b	Betaseron
Irbesartan/hydrochlorothiazide	Avalide
Isoniazid/pyrazinamide/rifampin	Rifater
Isotrentinoin	Accutane, Amnesteem
Itraconazole	Sporanox
Ketoprofen	Orudis, Oruvail
Lamotrigine	Lamictal
Leuprolide	Lupron
Levamisole	Levamisole
Lisinopril	Prinivil, Zestril
Lisinorpil/hydrochlorothiazide	Prinivil, Zestoretic
Lomefloxacin	Maxaquin
Loratadine	Claritin
Loratadine/pseudoephedrine	Claritin-D
Losartan	Cozaar
Losartan/hydrochlorothiazide	Hyzaar
Lovastatin	Altoprev, Mevacor
Lovastatin/niacin	Advicor
Maprotiline	Maprotiline
Mefenamic acid	Ponstel
Meloxicam	Mobic
Mesalamine	Pentasa
Methazolamide	
Methotrexate	Trexall
Methoxsalen	Uvadex, Oxsoralen 8-MOP
Methyclothiazide	Enduron
Methyldopa/hydrochlorothiazide	Aldoril
Metolazone	Mykrox, Zaroxolyn
Minocycline	Dynacin, Minocin
Mirtazapine	Remeron

Generic	Brand
Moexipril	Univasc
Moexipril/hydrochlorothiazide	Uniretic
Moxilfloxacin	Avelox
Nabumetone	Relafen
Nadolol/bendroflumethiazide	Corzide
Nalidixic acid	Nalidixic acid
Naproxen	Naprosyn, EC-Naprosyn
Naproxen sodium	Anaprox, Naprelan
Naratriptan	Amerge
Nefazodone	Serzone
Nifedipine	Adalat CC, Procardia
Nisoldipine	Sular
Norfloxacin	Noroxin
Nortriptyline	Pamelor
Ofloxacin	Floxin
Olanzapine	Zyprexa
Olanzapine/fluoxetine	Symbyax
Olmesartan medoxomil/hydrochlorothiazide	Benicar HCT
Olsalazine	Dipentum
Oxaprozin	Daypro
Oxcarbazepine	Trileptal
Oxycodone	Roxicodone
Oxytetracycline	Terramycin
Pantoprazole	Protonix
Paroxetine	Paxil
Pastinaca sativa	Parsnip
Pentosan polysulfate	Elmiron
Pentostatin	Perphenazine
Pilocarpine	Salagen
Piroxicam	Feldene
Polythiazide	Renese
Polythiazide/prazosin	Minizide
Porfimer sodium	Photofrin
Pravastatin	Pravachol
Prochlorperazine	Compazine, Compro
Promethazine	Phenergan
Protriptyline	Vivactil
Pyrazinamide	Pyrazanamide
Quetiapine	Seroquel
Quinapril	Accupril
Quinapril/hydrochlorothiazide	Accuretic
Quinidine gluconate	Quinidine
Quinidine sulfate	Quinidex
Raberprazole sodium	Aciphex
Ramipril	Altace
Riluzole	Rilutek
Risperidone	Risperdal, Risperdal Consta
Ritonavir	Norvir
Rizatriptan	Maxalt
Ropinirole	Requip
Rosuvastatin	Crestor
Ruta graveolens	Rue
Saquinavir	Fortovase
Saquinavir mesylate	Invirase
Selegiline	Eldepryl
Sertraline	Zoloft
Sibutramine	Meridia
Sildenafil	Viagra
Simvastatin	Zocor
Simvastatin/ezetimibe	Vytorin

(*Continued on next page*)

Generic	Brand
Somatropin	Serostim
Solatol	Betapace, Betapace AF
Sulfamethoxazole/trimethoprim	Bactrim, Septra
Sulfasalazine	Azulfidine
Sulindac	Clinoril
Sumatriptan	Imitrex
Tacrolimus	Prograf, Protopic
Tazarotene	Tazorac
Telmisartan/hydrochlorothiazide	Micardis HCT
Tetracycline	Sumycin
Thalidomide	Thalomid
Thioridazine hydrochloride	Mellaril
Thiothixene	Navane
Tiagabine	Gabitril
Tolazamide	Tolazamide
Tolbutamide	Tolbutamide
Topiramate	Topamax
Tretinoin	Retin-A
Triamcinolone	Azmacort
Triamterene	Dyrenium
Triamterene/hydrochlorothiazide	Dyazide, Maxzide
Trifluoperazine	Trifluoperazine
Trimipramine	Surmontil
Trovafloxacin	Trovan
Valacyclovir	Valtrex
Valdecoxib	Bextra
Valproate	Depacon
Valproic acid	Depakene
Valsartan/hydrochlorothiazide	Diovan HCT
Vardenafil	Levitra
Venlafaxine	Effexor
Verteporfin	Visudyne
Vinblastine	Vinblastine
Voriconazole	Vfend
Zalcitabine	Hivid
Zaleplon	Sonata
Ziprasidone	Geodon
Zolmitriptan	Zomig
Zolpidem	Ambien

Drug/Alcohol Interactions

Product	Interaction	Onset	Severity
ACETAMINOPHEN	ETHANOL Concurrent use of ACETAMINOPHEN and ETHANOL may result in an increased risk of hepatotoxicity	2	2
ACETOPHENAZINE	ETHANOL Concurrent use of ACETOPHENAZINE and ETHANOL may result in increased CNS depression and an increased risk of extrapyramidal reactions.	1	2

Product	Interaction	Onset	Severity
ACITRETIN	ETHANOL Concurrent use of ACITRETIN and ETHANOL may result in a prolonged risk of teratogenicity.	2	1
ALFENTANIL	ETHANOL Concurrent use of ALFENTANIL and ETHANOL may result in decreased therapeutic effects for alfentanil.	2	2
ALPRAZOLAM	ETHANOL Concurrent use of ALPRAZOLAM and ETHANOL may result in increased sedation.	1	2
AMITRIPITYLINE	ETHANOL Concurrent use of AMITRIPTYLINE and ETHANOL may result in enhanced CNS depression and impairment of motor skills.	1	2
AMOBARBITAL	ETHANOL Concurrent use of AMOBARBITAL and ETHANOL may result in excessive CNS depression	1	2
AMOXAPINE	ETHANOL Concurrent use of AMOXAPINE and ETHANOL may result in enhanced drowsiness and impairment of motor skills.	1	2
AMPRENAVIR	ETHANOL Concurrent use of AMPRENAVIR and ETHANOL may result in an increased risk of propylene glycol toxicity (seizures, tachycardia, lactic acidosis, renal toxicity, and hemolysis).	2	1
APROBARBITAL	ETHANOL Concurrent use of APROBARBITAL and ETHANOL may result in excessive CNS depression.	1	2
ASPIRIN	ETHANOL Concurrent use of ASPIRIN and ETHANOL may result in increased gastrointestinal blood loss.	1	2
BUPROPION	ETHANOL Concurrent use of BUPROPION and ETHANOL may result in an increased risk of seizures.	2	1
BUTABARBITAL	ETHANOL Concurrent use of BUTABARBITAL and ETHANOL may result in excessive CNS depression.	1	2
BUTALBITAL	ETHANOL Concurrent use of BUTALBITAL and ETHANOL may result in excessive CNS depression.	1	2
CALAMUS	ETHANOL Concurrent use of CALAMUS and ETHANOL may result in increased sedation.	1	2

(*Continued on next page*)

Product	Interaction	Onset	Severity
CANNABIS	ETHANOL Concurrent use of CANNABIS and ETHANOL may result in increased intoxication.	1	2
CEFAMANDOLE	ETHANOL Concurrent use of CEFAMANDOLE and ETHANOL may result in disulfiram-like reactions.	2	1
CEFMENOXIME	ETHANOL Concurrent use of CEFMENOXIME and ETHANOL may result in disulfiram-like reactions.	1	1
CEFOPERAZONE	ETHANOL Concurrent use of CEFOPERAZONE and ETHANOL may result in disulfiram-like reactions.	2	1
CEFOTETAN	ETHANOL Concurrent use of CEFOTETAN and ETHANOL may result in disulfiram-like reactions.	2	1
CHAPARRAL	ETHANOL Concurrent use of CHAPARRAL and ETHANOL may result in elevated liver transaminases with or without concomitant hepatic damage.	1	2
CHLORAL HYDRATE	ETHANOL Concurrent use of CHLORAL HYDRATE and ETHANOL may result in increased sedation.	1	3
CHLORDIAZEPOXIDE	ETHANOL Concurrent use of CHLORDIAZEPOXIDE and ETHANOL may result in increased sedation.	1	2
CHLORPROMAZINE	ETHANOL Concurrent use of CHLORPROMAZINE and ETHANOL may result in increased sedation.	1	2
CHLORPROPAMIDE	ETHANOL Concurrent use of CHLORPROPAMIDE and ETHANOL may result in disulfiram-like reactions.	1	1
CIMETIDINE	ETHANOL Concurrent use of CIMETIDINE and ETHANOL may result in increased ethanol concentrations.	1	3
CISAPRIDE	ETHANOL Concurrent use of CISAPRIDE and ETHANOL may result in increased blood levels of ethanol.	1	2
CITALOPRAM	ETHANOL Concurrent use of CITALOPRAM and ETHANOL may result in potentiation of the cognitive and motor effects of alcohol.	0	2
CLOMIPRAMINE	ETHANOL Concurrent use of CLOMIPRAMINE and ETHANOL may result in enhanced drowsiness and impairment of motor skills.	1	2

Product	Interaction	Onset	Severity
CLORAZEPATE	ETHANOL Concurrent use of CLORAZEPATE and ETHANOL may result in increased sedation.	1	2
COCAINE	ETHANOL Concurrent use of COCAINE and ETHANOL may result in increased heart rate and blood pressure.	1	2
CODEINE	ETHANOL Concurrent use of CODEINE and ETHANOL may result in increased sedation.	1	2
COMFREY	ETHANOL Concurrent use of COMFREY and ETHANOL may result in elevated liver transaminases with or without concomitant hepatic damage.	1	1
CYCLOSERINE	ETHANOL Concurrent use of CYCLOSERINE and ETHANOL may result in an increased risk of seizures.	1	1
DESIPRAMINE	ETHANOL Concurrent use of DESIPRAMINE and ETHANOL may result in enhanced drowsiness and impairment of motor skills.	1	2
DIAZEPAM	ETHANOL Concurrent use of DIAZEPAM and ETHANOL may result in increased sedation.	1	2
DIMETHINDENE	ETHANOL Concurrent use of DIMETHINDENE and ETHANOL may result in inceased sedation.	1	2
DIPHENHYDRAMINE	ETHANOL Concurrent use of DIPHENHYDRAMINE and ETHANOL may result in increased sedation.	1	2
DISULFIRAM	ETHANOL Concurrent use of DISULFIRAM and ETHANOL may result in ethanol intolerance.	1	1
DOTHIEPIN	ETHANOL Concurrent use of ETHANOL and DOTHIERIN may result in enhanced drowsiness and impairment of motor skills.	1	2
DOXEPIN	ETHANOL Concurrent use of DOXEPIN and ETHANOL may result in enhanced drowsiness and impairment of motor skills.	1	2
ESCITALOPRAM	ETHANOL Concurrent use of ESCITALOPRAM and ETHANOL may result in potentiation of the cognitive and motor effects of alcohol.	0	2

(*Continued on next page*)

Product	Interaction	Onset	Severity
ESZOPICLONE	ETHANOL Concurrent use of ESZOPICLONE and ETHANOL may result in impaired psychomotor functions and risk of increased sedation.	1	2
ETEROBARB	ETHANOL Concurrent use of ETEROBARB and ETHANOL may result in excessive CNS depression.	1	2
ETHOPROPAZINE	ETHANOL Concurrent use of ETHOPROPAZINE and ETHANOL may result in increased CNS depression and an increased risk of extrapyramidal reactions.	1	2
FLUNITRAZEPAM	ETHANOL Concurrent use of FLUNITRAZEPAM and ETHANOL may result in excessive sedation and psychomotor impairment.	1	2
FLUPHENAZINE	ETHANOL Concurrent use of FLUPHENAZINE and ETHANOL may result in increased CNS depression and an increased risk of extrapyramidal reactions.	1	2
FOMEPIZOLE	ETHANOL Concurrent use of FOMEPIZOLE and ETHANOL may result in the reduced elimination of both drugs.	2	2
FOSPHENYTOIN	ETHANOL Concurrent use of FOSPHENYTOIN and ETHANOL may result in decreased phenyloin serum concentrations, increased seizure potential, and additive CNS depressant effects.	1	2
FURAZOLIDONE	ETHANOL Concurrent use of FURAZOLIDONE and ETHANOL may result in disulfiram-like reactions.	1	1
GERMANDER	ETHANOL Concurrent use of GERMANDER and ETHANOL may result in elevated liver transaminases with or without concomitant hepatic damage.	2	1
GLIPIZIDE	ETHANOL Concurrent use of GLIPIZIDE and ETHANOL may result in prolonged hypoglycemia and disulfiram-like reactions.	1	1
GLICLAZIDE	ETHANOL Concurrent use of ETHANOL and GLICLAZIDE may result in prolonged hypoglycemia and disulfiram-like reactions.	1	1
GLUTETHIMIDE	ETHANOL Concurrent use of GLUTETHIMIDE and ETHANOL may result in increased sedation.	1	2

Product	Interaction	Onset	Severity
GLYBURIDE	ETHANOL Concurrent use of GLYBURIDE and ETHANOL may result in prolonged hypoglycemia and disulfirma-like reactions.	1	1
GOSSYPOL	ETHANOL Concurrent use of GOSSYPOL and ETHANOL may result in delayed effects of gossypol and/or increased toxic effects of ethanol.	1	2
GRISEOFULVIN	ETHANOL Concurrent use of GRISEOFULVIN and ETHANOL may result in disulfiram-like reactions.	1	1
GUAR GUM	ETHANOL Concurrent use of GUAR GUM and ETHANOL may result in increased intoxication effects of ethanol.	2	2
GUARANA	ETHANOL Concurrent use of GUARANA and ETHANOL may result in increased risk of ethanol intoxication.	1	3
HYDROCODONE	ETHANOL Concurrent use of HYDROCODONE and ETHANOL may result in increased sedation.	1	2
HYDROMORPHONE	ETHANOL Concurrent use of HYDROMORPHONE and ETHANOL may result in increased sedation.	1	2
IMIPRAMINE	ETHANOL Concurrent use of IMIPRAMINE and ETHANOL may result in enhanced drowsiness and impairment of motor skills.	1	2
INSULIN	ETHANOL Concurrent use of INSULIN and ETHANOL may result in increased hypoglycemia.	1	2
INSULIN LISPRO, HUMAN	ETHANOL Concurrent use of INSULIN LISPRO, HUMAN and ETHANOL and may result in increased hypoglycemia	1	2
ISONIAZID	ETHANOL Concurrent use of ISONIAZID and ETHANOL may result in decreased isoniazid concentrations and disulfiram-like reactions.	2	1
ISOTRETINOIN	ETHANOL Concurrent use of ISOTRETINOIN and ETHANOL may result in disulfiram-like reactions.	1	1
KAVA	ETHANOL Concurrent use of KAVA and ETHANOL may result in increased CNS depression and/or increased risk of hepatotoxicity.	1	2

(*Continued on next page*)

Product	Interaction	Onset	Severity
KETOCONAZOLE	ETHANOL Concurrent use of KETOCONAZOLE and ETHANOL may result in disulfiram-like reactions (Flushing, vomiting, increased respiratory rate tachycardia).	1	1
LOFEPRAMINE	ETHANOL Concurrent use of LOFEPRAMINE and ETHANOL may result in enhanced drowsiness and impairment of motor skills.	1	2
LORAZEPAM	ETHANOL Concurrent use of LORAZEPAM and ETHANOL may result in increased sedation.	1	2
MA HUANG	ETHANOL Concurrent use of MA HUANG and ETHANOL may result in effects on mental status.	1	1
MATE	ETHANOL Concurrent use of MATE and ETHANOL may result in increased risk of ethanol intoxication.	1	3
MEPERIDINE	ETHANOL Concurrent use of MEPERIDINE and ETHANOL may result in increased sedation.	1	2
MEPHOBARBITAL	ETHANOL Concurrent use of MEPHOBARBITAL and ETHANOL may result in excessive CNS depression.	1	2
MEPROBAMATE	ETHANOL Concurrent use of MEPROBAMATE and ETHANOL may result in increased sedation.	1	2
MESORIDAZINE	ETHANOL Concurrent use of MESORIDAZINE and ETHANOL may result in increased CNS depression and an increased risk of extrapyramidal reactions.	1	2
METFORMIN	ETHANOL Concurrent use of METFORMIN and ETHANOL may result in an increased risk of lactic acidosis.	2	2
METHADONE	ETHANOL Concurrent use of METHADONE and ETHANOL may result in increased sedation.	1	2
METHOHEXITAL	ETHANOL Concurrent use of METHOHEXITAL and ETHANOL may result in excessive CNS depression.	1	2
METHOTREXATE	ETHANOL Concurrent use of METHOTREXATE and ETHANOL may result in increased hepatotoxicity.	2	2

Product	Interaction	Onset	Severity
METHOTRIMEPRAZINE	ETHANOL Concurrent use of METHOTRIMEPRAZINE and ETHANOL may result in increased CNS depression and an increased risk of extrapyramidal reactions.	1	2
METRONIDAZOLE	ETHANOL Concurrent use of METRONIDAZOLE and ETHANOL may result in disulfiram-like reactions (Flushing, increased respiratory rate, tachycardia) or sudden death.	1	1
MIRTAZAPINE	ETHANOL Concurrent use of MIRTAZAPINE and ETHANOL may result in psychomotor impairment.	1	2
MORPHINE	ETHANOL Concurrent use of MORPHINE and ETHANOL may result in increased risk of respiratory depression, hypotension, profound sedation, or coma.	1	2
MORPHINE SULFATE LIPOSOME	ETHANOL Concurrent use of MORPHINE SULFATE LIPOSOME and ETHANOL may result in increased risk of respiratory depression, hypotension, profound sedation, or coma.	1	1
MOXALACTAM	ETHANOL Concurrent use of ETHANOL and MOXALACTAM may result in disulfiram-like reactions.	2	1
NEFAZODONE	ETHANOL Concurrent use of NEFAZODONE and ETHANOL may result in an increased risk of CNS side effects.	1	3
NIACIN	ETHANOL Concurrent use of NIACIN and ETHANOL may result in increased side effects of flushing and pruritus.	0	2
NILUTAMIDE	ETHANOL Concurrent use of NILUTAMIDE and ETHANOL may result in an increased risk of ethanol intolerance (facial flushing, malaise, and hypotension).	1	3
NITROGLYCERIN	ETHANOL Concurrent use of NITROGLYCERIN and ETHANOL may result in hypotension.	1	2
NORTRIPTYLINE	ETHANOL Concurrent use of NORTRIPTYLINE and ETHANOL may result in enhanced drowsiness and impalment of motor skills.	1	2
OLANZAPINE	ETHANOL Concurrent use of OLANZAPINE and ETHANOL may result in excessive CNS depression.	1	2

(*Continued on next page*)

Product	Interaction	Onset	Severity
OXYCODONE	ETHANOL Concurrent use of OXYCODONE and ETHANOL may result in increased sedation.	1	2
PARALDEHYDE	ETHANOL Concurrent use of PARALDEHYDE and ETHANOL may result in metabolic acidosis.	2	2
PAROXETINE	ETHANOL Concurrent use of PAROXETINE and ETHANOL may increase the risk of mental and motor-skill impairment.	1	3
PENNYROYAL	ETHANOL Concurrent use of PENNYROYAL and ETHANOL may result in elevated liver transaminases with or without concomitant hepatic damage.	1	1
PENTAZOCINE	ETHANOL Concurrent use of PENTAZOCINE and ETHANOL may result in increased sedation.	1	2
PERPHENAZINE	ETHANOL Concurrent use of PERPHENAZINE and ETHANOL may result in increased CNS depression and an increased risk of extrapyramidal reactions.	1	2
PHENELZINE	ETHANOL Concurrent use of PHENELZINE and ETHANOL may result in hypertensive urgency or emergency.	1	2
PHENOBARBITAL	ETHANOL Concurrent use of PHENOBARBITAL and ETHANOL may result in excessive CNS depression.	1	2
PHENYTOIN	ETHANOL Concurrent use of PHENYTOIN and ETHANOL may result in decreased phenytoin serum concentrations, increased seizure potential, and additive CNS depressant effects.	1	2
PIPOTIAZINE	ETHANOL Concurrent use of PIPOTIAZINE and ETHANOL may result in increased CNS depression and an increased risk of extrapyramidal reactions.	1	2
PRIMIDONE	ETHANOL Concurrent use of PRIMIDONE and ETHANOL may result in excessive CNS depression.	1	2
PROCARBAZINE	ETHANOL Concurrent use of PROCARBAZINE and ETHANOL may result in disulfiram-like reactions and increased sedation.	1	1
PROCHLORPERAZINE	ETHANOL Concurrent use of PROCHLORPERAZINE and ETHANOL may result in increased CNS depression and an increased risk of extrapyramidal reactions.	1	2

Product	Interaction	Onset	Severity
PROMAZINE	ETHANOL Concurrent use of PROMAZINE and ETHANOL may result in increased CNS depression and an increased risk of extrapyramidal reactions.	1	2
PROPIOMAZINE	ETHANOL Concurrent use of PROPIOMAZINE and ETHANOL may result in increased CNS depression and an increased risk of extrapyramidal reactions.	1	2
PROTRIPTYLINE	ETHANOL Concurrent use of PROTRIPTYLINE and ETHANOL may result in enhanced drowsiness and impairment of motor skills.	1	2
QUETIAPINE	ETHANOL Concurrent use of QUETIAPINE and ETHANOL may result in potentiation of the cognitive and motor effects of alcohol.	1	2
SECOBARBITAL	ETHANOL Concurrent use of SECOBARBITAL and ETHANOL may result in excessive CNS depression.	1	2
SERTRALINE	ETHANOL Concurrent use of SERTRALINE and FTHANOL may increase the risk of mental and motor-skill impairment.	1	2
SULFAMETHOXAZOLE	ETHANOL Concurrent use of SULFAMETHOXAZOLE and ETHANOL may result in disulfiram-like reactions (flushing, sweating, palpitations, drowsiness).	1	1
TADALAFIL	ETHANOL Concurrent use of TADALAFIL and ETHANOL may result in an increased risk of hypotension and orthosiatic signs and symptoms.	1	2
TEMAZEPAM	ETHANOL Concurrent use of TEMAZEPAM and ETHANOL may result in impaired psychomotor functions.	1	2
THIETHYLPERAZINE	ETHANOL Concurrent use of THIETHYLPERAZINE and ETHANOL may result in increased CNS depression and an increased risk of extrapyramidal reactions.	1	2
THIOPENTAL	ETHANOL Concurrent use of THIOPENTAL and ETHANOL may result in excessive CNS depression.	1	2
THIORIDAZINE	ETHANOL Concurrent use of THIORIDAZINE and ETHANOL may result in increased CNS depression and an increased risk of extrapyramidal reactions.	1	2

(*Continued on next page*)

Product	Interaction	Onset	Severity
TIZANIDINE	ETHANOL Concurrent use of TIZANIDINE and ETHANOL may increase the risk of tizanidine adverse effects (excessive CNS depression).	1	2
TOLAZAMIDE	ETHANOL Concurrent use of TOLAZAMIDE and ETHANOL may result in prolonged hypoglycemia and disulfiram-like reactions.	1	1
TOLAZOLINE	ETHANOL Concurrent use of TOLAZOLINE and ETHANOL may result in disulfiram-like reactions.	2	1
TOLBUTAMIDE	ETHANOL Concurrent use of TOLBUTAMIDE and ETHANOL may result in prolonged hypoglycemia and disulfiram-like reactions.	1	1
TRAMADOL	ETHANOL Concurrent use of TRAMADOL and ETHANOL may increase the risk of excessive CNS depression.	1	2
TRANYLCYPROMINE	ETHANOL Concurrent use of TRANYLCYPROMINE and ETHANOL may result in hypertensive urgency or emergency.	1	2
TRIAZOLAM	ETHANOL Concurrent use of TRIAZOLAM and ETHANOL may result in increased sedation	1	2
TRIFLUOPERAZINE	ETHANOL Concurrent use of TRIFLUOPERAZINE and ETHANOL may result in increased CNS depression and an increased risk of extrapyramidal reactions.	1	2
TRIFLUPROMAZINE	ETHANOL Concurrent use of TRIFLUPROMAZINE and ETHANOL may result in increased CNS depression and an increased risk of extrapyramidal reactions.	1	2
TRIMETHOPRIM	ETHANOL Concurrent use of ETHANOL and COTRIMOXAZOLE may result in disulfiram-like reactions.	1	1
TRIMIPRAMINE	ETHANOL Concurrent use of TRIMIPRAMINE and ETHANOL may result in enhanced drowsiness and impairment of motor skills.	1	2
VALERIAN	ETHANOL Concurrent use of VALERIAN and ETHANOL may result in increased sedation.	1	2
VENLAFAXINE	ETHANOL Concurrent use of VENLAFAXINE and ETHANOL may result in an increased risk of CNS effects.	1	3

Product	Interaction	Onset	Severity
VERAPAMIL	ETHANOL Concurrent use of VERAPAMIL and ETHANOL may result in enhanced ethanol intoxication (impaired psychomotor functioning).	1	2
WARFARIN	ETHANOL Concurrent use of WARFARIN and ETHANOL may result in increased or decreased international normalized ratio (INR) or prothrombin time.	2	2
YOHIMBINE	ETHANOL Concurrent use of YOHIMBINE and ETHANOL may result in increased ethanol intoxication and increased anxiety and blood pressure.	1	2
ZALEPLON	ETHANOL Concurrent use of ZALEPLON and ETHANOL may result in impaired psychomotor functions.	1	2
ZOLPIDEM	ETHANOL Concurrent use of ZOLPIDEM and ETHANOL may result in increased sedation.	1	2

ONSET: 0 = Unspecified
          1 = Rapid (within 24 hours)
          2 = Delayed (after 24 hours)
SEVERITY: 1 = Major (possibly life threatening or potential permanent damage)
             2 = Moderate (may exacerbate patient's condition)
             3 = Minor (little if any clinical effect)
Note: Disulfiram-like reactions include nausea, vomiting, diarrhea, flushing, tachycardia, and hypotension.
Reprinted with permission from *The Drug Topics Red Book*. Montvale, NJ: Thomson Medical Economics, 2006.

Drug/Tobacco Interactions

Product	Interaction	Onset	Severity
ALPRAZOLAM	TOBACCO Concurrent use of ALPRAZOLAM and TOBACCO may result in decreased alprazolam plasma concentrations and efficacy.	0	2
CONTRACEPTIVES, COMBINATION	TOBACCO Concurrent use of CONTRACEPTIVES, COMBINATION and TOBACCO may result in an increased risk of cardiovascular disease.	2	3
ERLOTINIB	TOBACCO Concurrent use of ERLOTINIB and TOBACCO may result in increased erlotinib clearance and reduced serum concentrations.	0	2

(*Continued on next page*)

Product	Interaction	Onset	Severity
FLUVOXAMINE	TOBACCO Concurrent use of FLUVOXAMINE and TOBACCO may result in increased fluvoxamine metabolism.	2	3
IMIPRAMINE	TOBACCO Concurrent use of IMIPRAMINE and TOBACCO may result in decreased imipramine concentrations.	2	2
PENTAZOCINE	TOBACCO Concurrent use of PENTAZOCINE and TOBACCO may result in decreased pentazocine concentrations.	2	2
PROPOXYPHENE	TOBACCO Concurrent use of PROPOXYPHENE and TOBACCO may result in decreased propoxyphene concentrations.	2	2
ROPINIROLE	TOBACCO Concurrent use of ROPINIROLE and TOBACCO may result in decreased ropinirole plasma concentrations and efficacy.	0	2
THEOPHYLLINE	TOBACCO Concurrent use of THEOPHYLLINE and TOBACCO may result in decreased theophylline concentrations.	2	2
TOLBUTAMIDE	TOBACCO Concurrent use of TOLBUTAMIDE and TOBACCO may result in decreased tolbutamide concentrations.	2	2
WARFARIN	TOBACCO Concurrent use of WARFARIN and TOBACCO may result in increased or decreased international normalized ratio (INR) or prothrombin time.	2	2

ONSET: 0 = Unspecified
             1 = Rapid (within 24 hours)
             2 = Delayed (after 24 hours)
SEVERITY: 1 = Major (possibly life threatening or potential permanent damage)
             2 = Moderate (may exacerbate patient's condition)
             3 = Minor (little if any clinical effect)
Note: Disulfiram-like reactions include nausea, vomiting, diarrhea, flushing, tachycardia, and hypotension.
Reprinted with permission from *The Drug Topics Red Book*. Montvale, NJ: Thomson Medical Economics, 2006.

Use-In-Pregnancy Ratings

The U.S. Food and Drug Administration's Use-in-Pregnancy rating system weighs the degree to which available information has ruled out risk to the fetus against the drug's potential benefit to the patient. Below is a listing of drugs (by generic name) for which ratings are available.

X

CONTRAINDICATED IN PREGNANCY

Studies in animals or humans, or investigational or post-marketing reports, have demonstrated fetal risk which clearly outweighs any possible benefit to the patient.

Acitretin
Amlodipine Besylate/
    Atorvastatin Calcium
Amprenavir

Anisindione
Atorvastatin Calcium
Bexarotene
Bicalutamide
Bosentan
Cetrorelix Acetate
Choriogonadotropin Alfa
Chorionic Gonadotropin

Clomiphene Citrate
Desogestrel/Ethinyl Estradiol
Diclofenac Sodium/
　Misoprostol
Dihydroergotamine Mesylate
Dutasteride
Estazolam
Estradiol
Estradiol Acetate
Estradiol Cypionate/
　Medroxyprogesterone
　Acetate
Estradiol Valerate
Estradiol/Levonorgestrel
Estradiol/Norethindrone
　Acetate
Estrogens, Conjugated
Estrogens, Conjugated,
　Synthetic A
Estrogens, Conjugated/
　Medroxyprogesterone
　Acetate
Estrogens, Esterified
Estrogens, Esterified/
　Methyltestoterone
Estropipate
Ethinyl Estradiol/Drospirenone
Ethinyl Estradiol/Ethynodiol
　Diacetate
Ethinyl Estradiol/Etonogestrel
Ethinyl Estradiol/Ferrous
　Fumarate/Norethindrone
　Acetate
Ethinyl Estradiol/
　Levonorgestrel
Ethinyl Estradiol/
　Norelgestromin
Ethinyl Estradiol/
　Norethindrone
Ethinyl Estradiol/
　Norethindrone Acetate
Ethinyl Estradiol/Norgestimate
Ethinyl Estradiol/Norgestrel
Ezetimibe/Simvastatin
Finasteride
Fluorouracil
Flurazepam Hydrochloride
Fluvastatin Sodium
Follitropin Alfa
Follitropin Beta
Ganirelix Acetate
Goserelin Acetate
Histrelin Acetate
Hyrdromorphone
　Hydrochloride
Interferon Alfa-2B,
　Recombinant/Ribavirin
Iodine I 131 Tositumomab/
　Tositumomab

Isotretinoin
Leflunomide
Leuprolide Acetate
Levonorgestrel
Lovastatin
Lovastatin/Niacin
Medroxyprogesterone Acetate
Megestrol Acetate
Menotropins
Mequinol/Tretinoin
Mestranol/Norethindrone
Methotrexate Soduim
Methyltestosterone
Miglustat
Misoprostol
Nafarelin Acetate
Norethindrone
Norethindrone Acetate
Norgestrel
Oxandrolone
Oxymetholone
Plicamycin
Pravastatin Sodium
Pravastatin Sodium/Aspirin
　Buffered
Raloxifene Hydrochloride
Ribavirin
Rosuvastatin Calcium
Simvastatin
Tazarotene
Testosterone
Testosterone Enanthate
Thalidomide
Triptorelin Pamoate
Urofollitropin
Warfarin Sodium

D

POSITIVE EVIDENCE OF RISK

Investigational or postmarketing data show risk to the fetus. Nevertheless, potential benefits may outweigh the potential risk.

Alitretinoin
Alprazolam
Altretamine
Amiodarone Hydrochloride
Amlodipine Besylate/
　Benazepril Hydrochloride
Anastrozole
Arsenic Trioxide
Aspirin Buffered/Pravastatin
　Sodium
Aspirin/Dipryridamole
Atenolol

Azathioprine
Azathioprine Sodium
Benazepril Hydrochloride*
Benazepril Hydrochloride/
　Hydrochlorothiazide*
Bortezomib
Busulfan
Candesartan Cilexetil*
Candesartan Cilexetil/
　Hydrochlorothiazide*
Capecitabine
Captopril*
Carbamazepine
Carboplatin
Carmustine (Benu)
Chlorambucil
Cladribine
Clofarabine
Clonazepam
Cytarabine Liposome
Dactinomycin
Daunorubicin Citrate
　Liposome
Daunorubicin Hydrochloride
Demeclocycline
　Hydrochloride
Diazepam
Divalproex Sodium
Docetaxel
Doxorubicin Hydrochloride
Doxorubicin Hydrochloride
　Liposome
Doxycycline Calcium
Doxycycline Hyclate
Doxycycline Monohydrate
Efavirenz
Enalapril Maleate*
Enalapril Maleate/
　Hydrochlorothiazide*
Epirubicin Hydrochloride
Eprosartan Mesylate
Eriotinib
Exemestane
Felodipine/Enalapril Maleate
Floxuridine
Fludarabine Phosphate
Flutamide
Fosinopril Sodium*
Fosinopril Sodium/
　Hydrochlorothiazide*
Fosphenytoin Sodium
Fulvestrant
Gefitinib
Gemcitabine Hydrochloride
Gemtuzumab Ozogamicin
Goserelin Acetate
Ibritumomab Tiuxetan
Idarubicin Hydrochloride
Ifosfamide

(Continued on next page)

Imatinib Mesylate
Irbesartan*
Irbesartan/
    Hydrochlorothiazide*
Irinotecan Hydrochloride
Letrozole
Lisinopril*
Lisinopril/
    Hydrochlorothiazide*
Lithium Carbonate
Losartan Potassium*
Losartan Potassium/
    Hydrochlorothiazide*
Mechlorethamine
    Hydrochloride
Melphalan
Melphalan Hydrochloride
Mephobarbital
Mercaptopurine
Methimazole
Midazolam Hydrochloride
Minocycline Hydrochloride
Mitoxantrone Hydrochloride
Moexipril Hydrochloride*
Moexipril Hydrochloride/
    Hydrochlorothiazide*
Neomycin Sulfate/Polymyxin
    B Sulfate
Nicotine
Olmesartan Medoxomil
Oxaliplatin
Pamidronate Disodium
Pemetrexed
Penicillamine
Pentobarbital Sodium
Pentostatin
Perindropil Erbumine*
Phenytoin
Procarbazine Hydrochloride
Quinapril Hydrochloride*
Quinapril Hydrochloride/
    Hydrochlorothiazide*
Ramipril
Streptomycin Sulfate
Tamoxifen Citrate
Telmisartan
Telmisartan/
    Hydrochlorothiazide
Temozolomide
Thioguanine
Tigecycline
Tobramycin
Topotecan Hydrochloride
Toremifene Citrate
Trandolapril*
Trandolaprill/Verapamil
    Hydrochloride*
Tretinoin
Valproate Sodium
Valproic Acid
Valsartan*

Valsartan/
    Hydrochlorothiazide*
Vinorelbine Tartrate
Voriconazole
Zoledronic Acid

C

RISK CANNOT BE RULED OUT

Human studies are lacking, and animal studies are either positive for risk or are lacking as well. However, potential benefits may outweigh the potential risk.

Abacavir Sulfate
Abacavir Sulfate/Lamivudine
Abacavir Sulfate/Lamivudine/
    Zidovudine
Abciximab
Acamprosate Calcium
Acetaminophen
Acetaminophen/Butalbital/
    Caffeine
Acetaminophen/Caffeine/
    Chlorpheniramine Maleate/
    Hydrocodone Bitartrate/
    Phenylephrine
    Hydrochloride
Acetazolamide
Acetazolamide Sodium
Acyclovir
Adapalene
Adefovir Dipivoxil
Adenosine
Alatroflaxacin Mesylate
Albendazole
Albumin (Human)
Albuterol
Albuterol Sulfate
Albuterol Sulfate/Ipratropium
    Bromide
Alclometasone Dipropionate
Aldesleukin
Alemtuzumab
Alendronate Sodium
Alendronate Sodium/
    Cholecalciferol
Altopurinol Sodium
Almotriptan Malate
Alpha1-Proteinase Inhibitor
    (Human)
Alprostadil
Alteplase
Amantadine Hydrochloride
Amifostine

Aminocaproic Acid
Aminohippurate Sodium
Aminolevulinic Acid
    Hydrochloride
Aminosalicylic Acid
Amlodipine Besylate
Amlodipine Besylate/
    Benazepril Hydrochloride
Amoxicillin/Clarithromycin/
    Lansoprazole
Amphetamine Aspartate/
    Amphetamine Sulfate/
    Dextroamphetamine
    Saccharate/
    Dextroamphetamine Sulfate
Amprenavir
Anagrelide Hydrochloride
Anthralin
Antihemophilic Factor
    (Human)
Antihemophilic Factor
    (Recombinant)
Anti-inhibitor Coagulant
    Complex
Anti-Thymocyte Globulin
Apomorphine Hydrochloride
Aripiprazole
Arnica Montana/Herbals,
    Multiple/Sulfur
Asparaginase
Atomoxetine Hydrochloride
Atovaquone
Atovaquone/Proguanil
    Hydrochloride
Atropine Sulfate/Benzoic Acid/
    Hyoscyamine Sulfate/
    Methenamine/Methylene
    Blue/Phenyl Salicylate
Atropine Sulfate/Hyoscyamine
    Sulfate/Scopolamine
    Hydrobromide
Azelastine Hydrochloride
Bacitracin Zinc/Neomycin
    Sulfate/Polymyxin B Sulfate
Baclofen
Bcg. Live (Intravesical)
Becaplermin
Beclomethasone Dipropionate
Beclomethasone Dipropionate
    Monohydrate
Benzepril Hydrochloride*
Benazepril Hydrochloride/
    Hydrochlorothiazide*
Bendroflumethiazide
Benzocaine
Benzonatate
Benzoyl Peroxide
Benzoyl Peroxide/Clindamycin
Benzoyl Peroxide/
    Erythromycin
Betamethasone Dipropionate

Betamethasone Dipropionate/
    Chlotrimazole
Betamethasone Valerate
Betaxolol Hydrochloride
Bethanechol Chloride
Bevacizumab
Bimatoprost
Bisacodyl/Polyethylene
    Glycol/Potassium Chloride/
    Sodium Bicarbonate/
    Sodium Chloride
Bisoprolol Fumarate
Bisoprolol Fumarate/
    Hydrochlorothiazide
Bitolterol Mesylate
Black Widow Spider
    Antivenin (Equine)
Botulinum Toxin Type A
Botulinum Toxin Type B
Brinzolamide
Brompheniramine Maleate/
    Dextromethorphan
    Hydrobromide/
    Phenylephrine
    Hydrochloride
Budesonide
Bupivacaine Hydrochloride
Bupivacaine Hydrochloride/
    Epinephrine Bitartrate
Buprenorphine Hydrochloride
Buprenorphine Hydrochloride/
    Naloxone Hydrochloride
Butabarbital/Hyoscyamine
    Hydrobromide/
    Phenazopyridine
    Hydrochloride
Butalbital/Acetaminophen
Butenafine Hydrochloride
Butoconazole Nitrate
Butorphanol Tartrate
Caffeine Citrate
Calcipotriene
Calcitonin-Salmon
Calcitriol
Calcium Acetate
Candesarta Cilexetil*
Candesartan Cilexetil/
    Hydrochlorothiazide*
Capreomycin Sulfate
Captropil*
Carbetapentane Tannate/
    Chlorpheniramine Tannate
Carbetapentane Tannate/
    Chlorpheniramine Tannate/
    Ephedrine Tannate/
    Phenylephrine Tannate
Carbidopa/Entacapone/
    Levodopa
Carbidopa/Levodopa

Carbinoxamine Maleate/
    Dextromethorphan
    Hydrobromide/
    Pseudoephedrine
    Hydrochloride
Carteolol Hydrochloride
Carvedilol
Caspofungin Acetate
Celecoxib
Cetirizine Hydrochloride
Cetuximab
Cevimeline Hydrochloride
Chloramphenicol
Chloroprocaine
    Hydrochloride
Chlorothiazide
Chlorothiazide Sodium
Chlorpheniramine Maleate/
    Methscopolamine Nitrate/
    Phenylephrine
    Hydrochloride
Chlorpheniramine Maleate/
    Pseudoephedine
    Hydrochloride
Chlorpheniramine Polistirex/
    Hydrocodone Polistirex
Chlorpheniramine Tannate/
    Phenylephrine Tannate
Chlorpropamide
Chlorthalidone/Clonidine
    Hydrochloride
Choline Magnesium
    Trisalicylate
Cidofovir
Cilostazol
Cinacalcet Hydrochloride
Ciprofloxacin Hydrochloride
Ciprofloxacin Hydrochloride/
    Hydrocortisone
Ciprofloxacin/
    Dexamethasone
Citalopram Hydrobromide
Clarithromycin
Clobetasol Propionate
Clonidine
Clonidine Hydrochloride
Codeine Phosphate/
    Acetaminophen
Colistimethate Sodium
Colistin Sulfate/
    Hydrocortisone/Acetate/
    Neomycin Sulfate/
    Thonzonium Bromide
Corticorelin Ovine Triflutate
Cycloserine
Cyclosporine
Cytomegalovirus Immune
    Globulin
Dacarbazine

Daclizumab
Dantrolene Sodium
Dapsone
Darbepoetin Alia
Darifenacin
Deferoxamine Mesylate
Delavirdine Mesylate
Denileukin Diftitox
Desloratadine
Desloratadine/
    Pseudoephedrine Sulfate
Desoximetasone
Dexamethasone
Dexamethasone Sodium
    Phosphate
Dexmethylphenidate
    Hydrochloride
Dexrazoxane
Dextroamphetamine Sufate
Diazoxide
Dichlorphenamide
Diclofenac Potassium
Diclofenac Sodium
Diflorasone Diacetate
Diflunisal
Digoxin
Digoxin Immune Fab (Ovine)
Diltiazem Hydrochloride
Dimethyl Sulfoxide
Dinoprostone
Diphtheria & Tetanus Toxoids
    and Acellular Pertussis
    Vaccine Adsorbed
Diphtheria & Tetanus Toxoids
    and Acellular Pertussis
    Vaccine Adsorbed/Hepatitis
    B Vaccine, Recombinant/
    Poliovirus Vaccine
    Inactivated
Dirithromycin
Dofetilide
Donepezil Hydrochloride
Dorzolamide Hydrochloride
Dorzolamide Hydrochloride/
    Timolol Maleate
Doxazosin Mesylate
Dronabinol
Drotrecogin Alfa (Activated)
Duloxetine Hydrochloride
Echothiophate Iodide
Econazole Nitrate
Efalizumab
Eflornithine Hydrochloride
Eletriptan Hydrobromide
Enalapril Maleate*
Enalapril Maleate/Felodipine*
Enalapril Maleate/
    Hydrochlorothiazide*
Entacapone
                (Continued on next page)

Entecavir
Epinastine Hydrochloride
Epinephrine
Epoetin Alfa
Eprosartan Mesylate
Erythromycin Ethylsuccinate/
   Sulfisoxazole Acetyl
Escitalopram Oxalate
Esmolol Hydrochloride
Eszopiclone
Ethionamide
Ethotoin
Etidronate Disodium
Exenatide
Ezetimibe
Factor Ix Complex
Felodipine
Fenofibrate
Fentanyl
Fentanyl Citrate
Ferrous Fumarate/Folic
   Acid/Intrinsic Factor
   Concentrate/Liver
   Preparations/Vitamin B12/
   Vitamin C/Vitamins with
   Iron
Fexofenadine Hydrochloride
Fexofenadine Hydrochloride/
   Pseudoephedrine
   Hydrochloride
Filgrastim
Flecainide Acetate
Fluconazole
Flucytosine
Fludrocortisone Acetate
Flumazenil
Flunisolide
Fluocinolone Acetonide
Fluocinolone Acetonide/
   Hydroquinone/Tretinoin
Fluocinonide
Fluorometholone
Fluorometholone/
   Sulfacetamide Sodium
Fluoxetine Hydrochloride
Fluoxetine Hydrochloride/
   Olanzapine
Flurandrenolide
Flurbiprofen Sodium
Fluticasone Propionate
Fluticasone Propionate Hfa
Fluticasone Propionate/
   Salmeterol Xinafoate
Fomivirsen Sodium
Formoterol Fumarate
Fosamprenavir Calcium
Foscarnet Sodium*
Fosinopril Sodium*
Fosinopril Sodium/
   Hydrochlorothiazide*
Frovatriptan Succinate

Furosemide
Gabapentin
Gallium Nitrate
Ganciclovir
Ganciclovir Sodium
Gatifloxacin
Gemfibrozil
Gemifloxacin Mesylate
Gentamicin Sulfate
Gentamicin Sulfate/
   Prednisolone Acetate
Glimepiride
Glipizide
Glipizide/Metformin
   Hydrochloride
Globulin, Immune (Human)
Globulin, Immune (Human)/
   Rho (D) Immune Globulin
   (Human)
Glyburide
Gramicidin/Neomycin Sulfate/
   Polymyxin B Sulfate
Guaifenesin/Hydrocodone
   Bitartrate
Haemophilus B Conjugate
   Vaccine
Haemophilus B Conjugate
   Vaccine/Hepatitis B Vaccine,
   Recombinant
Halobetasol Propionate
Haloperidol Decanoate
Hemin
Heparin Sodium
Hepatitis A Vaccine, Inactivated
Hepatitis A Vaccine,
   Inactivated/Hepatitis B
   Vaccine, Recombinant
Hepatitis B Immune Globulin
   (Human)
Hepatitis B Vaccine,
   Recombinant
Homatropine Methylbromide/
   Hydrocodone Bitartrate
Homeophatic Formulations
Hydralazine Hydrochloride/
   Isosorbide Dinitrate
Hydrochlorothiazide
Hydrocodone Bitartrate
Hydrocodone Bitartrate/
   Acetaminophen
Hydrocodone Bitartrate/
   Ibuprofen
Hydrocortisone
Hydrocortisone Acetate
Hydrocortisone Acetate/
   Neomycin Sulfate/Polymyxin
   B Sulfate
Hydrocortisone Acetate/
   Pramoxine Hydrochloride
Hydrocortisone Butyrate
Hydrocortisone Probutate

Hydrocortisone/Neomycin
   Sulfate/Polymyxin B Sulfate
Hydromorphone
   Hydrochloride
Hydroquinone
Hyoscyamine Sulfate
Ibandronate Sodium
Ibutilide Fumarate
Iloprost
Imiglucerase
Imipenem/Cilastatin
Imiquimod
Immune Globulin Intravenous
   (Human)
Indinavir Sulfate
Indocyanine Green
Influenza Virus Vaccine
Insulin Aspart
Insulin Aspart Protamine,
   Human/Insulin Aspart,
   Human
Insulin Glargine
Insulin Glulisine
Interferon Alfa-2A,
   Recombinant
Interferon Alfa-2B,
   Recombinant
Interferon Alfacon-1
Interferon Alfa-N3 (Human
   Leukocyte Derived)
Interferon Beta-1A
Interferon Beta-1B
Interferon Gamma-1B
Iodoquinol/Hydrocortisone
Irbesartan*
Irbesartan/
   Hydrochlorothiazide*
Iron Dextran
Isoniazid/Pyrazinamide/
   Rifampin
Isosorbide Mononitrate
Isradipine
Itraconazole
Ivermectin
Ketoconazole
Ketorolac Tromethamine
Ketotifen Fumarate
Labetalol Hydrochloride
Lamivudine
Lamivudine/Zidovudine
Lamotrigine
Lanthanum Carbonate
Latanoprost
Levalbuterol Hydrochloride
Levalbuterol Tartrate
Levamisole Hydrochloride
Levetiracetam
Levobunolol Hydrochloride
Levofloxacin
Linezolid
Lisinopril*

Lisinopril/
  Hydrochlorothiazide*
Lopinavir/Ritonavir
Losartan Potassium*
Losartan Potassium/
  Hydrochlorothiazide*
Loteprednol Etabonate
Mafenide Acetate
Magnesium Salicylate
  Tetrahydrate
Measles Virus Vaccine, Live
Measles, Mumps & Rubella
  Virus Vaccine, Live
Mebendazole
Mecamylamine Hydrochloride
Mecasermin [Rdna Origin]
Medrysone
Mefenamic Acid
Mefloquine Hydrochloride
Meloxicam
Meningoccal Polysaccharide
  Diphtheria Toxoid
  Conjugate Vaccine
Meningococcal
  Polysaccharide Vaccine
Meperidine Hydrochloride
Mepivacaine Hydrochloride
Metaproterenol Sulfate
Metaraminol Bitartrate
Metformin Hydrochloride/
  Pioglitazone Hydrochloride
Metformin Hydrochloride/
  Rosiglitazone Maleate
Methamphetamine
  Hydrochloride
Methazolamide
Methenamine Mandelate/
  Sodium Acid Phosphate
Methocarbamol
Methoxsafen
Methscopolamine Nitrate/
  Pseudoephedrine
  Hydrochloride
Methyldopa Chlorothiazide
Methyldopa/
  Hydrochlorothiazide
Methylphenidate
  Hydrochloride
Metipranolol
Metoprolol Succinate
Metoprolol Tartrate
Metoprolol Tartrate/
  Hydrochlorothiazide
Metyrosine
Mexiletine Hydrochloride
Micafungin Sodium
Mododrine Hydrochloride
Mivacurium Chloride
Modafinil
Moexipril Hydrochloride*

Moexipril Hydrochloride/
  Hydrochlorothiazide*
Mometasone Furoate
Mometasone Furoate
  Monohydrate
Morphine Sulfate
Morphine Sulfate, Liposomal
Moxifloxacin Hydrochloride
Mumps Virus Vaccine, Live
Muromonab-Cd3
Mycophenolate Mofetil
Mycophenolate Mofetil
  Hydrochloride
Mycophenolic Acid
Nabumetone
Nadolol
Nadolol/Bendroflumethiazide
Naloxone Hydrochloride/
  Pentazocine Hydrochloride
Naltrexone Hydrochloride
Naphazoline Hydrochloride
Naproxen
Naproxen Sodium
Naratriptan Hydrochloride
Natamycin
Nateglinide
Nefazodone Hydrochloride
Neomycin Sulfate/
  Dexamethasone Sodium
  Phosphate
Neomycin Sulfate/Polymyxin
  B Sulfate/Prednisolone
  Acetate
Nesiritide
Nevirapine
Niacin
Nicardipine Hydrochloride
Nifedipine
Nilutamide
Nimodipine
Nisoldipine
Nitroglycerin
Norfloxacin
Ofloxacin
Olanzapine
Olmesartan Medoxomil/
  Hydrochlorothiazide
Olopatadine Hydrochloride
Olsalazine Sodium
Omega-3-Acid Ethyl Esters
Omeprazole
Oprelvekin
Orphenadrine Citrate
Oseltamivir Phosphate
Oxcarbazepine
Oxycodone Hydrochloride/
  Acetaminophen
Oxycodone Hydrochloride/
  Ibuprofen
Oxymorphone Hydrochloride

Palifermin
Palivizumab
Pancrelipase
Paricalcitol
Paroxetine Hydrochloride
Paroxetine Mesylate
Peg-3350/Potassium Chloride/
  Sodium Bicarbonate/Sodium
  Chloride
Pegademase Bovine
Pegaspargase
Pegfilgrastim
Peginterferon Alfa-2A
Peginterferon Alfa-2B
Pemirolast Potassium
Pentazocine Hydrochloride/
  Acetaminophen
Pentoxifylline
Perindopril Erbumine*
Phenoxybenzamine
  Hydrochloride
Phentermine Hydrochloride
Pilocarpine Hydrochloride
Pimercrolimus
Pimozide
Pioglitazone Hydrochloride
Pirbuterol Acetate
Piroxicam
Plasma Fractions, Human/
  Rabies Immune Globulin
  (Human)
Plasma Protein Fraction
  (Human)
Pneumococcal Vaccine,
  Diphtheria Conjugate
Pneumococcal Vaccine,
  Polyvalent
Podofilox
Polyethylene Glycol
Polyethylene Glycol/
  Potassium Chloride/
  Sodium Bicarbonate/
  Sodium Chloride
Polyethylene Glycol/
  Potassium Chloride/Sodium
  Bicarbonate/Sodium
  Chloride/Sodium Sulfate
Polymyxin B Sulfate/
  Trimethoprim Sulfate
Polythiazide/Prazosin
  Hydrochloride
Porfimer Sodium
Potassium Acid Phosphate
Potassium Chloride
Potassium Citrate
Potassium Phosphate/Sodium
  Phosphate
Pralidoxime Chloride
Pramipexole Dihydrochloride
Pramlintide Acetate
(*Continued on next page*)

Pramoxine Hydrochloride/
  Hydrocortisone Acetate
Prazosin Hydrochloride
Prednisolone Acetate
Prednisolone Acetate/
  Sulfacetamide Sodium
Prednisolone Sodium
  Phosphate
Pregabalin
Proclainamide Hydrochloride
Promethazine Hydrochloride
Propafenone Hydrochloride
Proparacaine Hydrochloride
Propranolol Hydrochloride
Pseudoephedrine
  Hydrochloride
Pyrimethamine
Quetiapine Fumerate
Quinapril Hydrochloride*
Quinidine Sulfate
Rabies Vaccine
Ramelteon
Ramipril*
Rasburicase
Remifentanil Hydrochloride
Repaglinide
Reteplase
Rho (D) Immune Globulin
  (Human)
Rifampin
Rifapentine
Rifamixin
Riluzole
Rimantadine Hydrochloride
Risedronate Sodium
Risedronate Sodium/Calcium
  Carbonate
Risperidone
Ritumixab
Rizatriptan Benzoate
Rocuronium Bromide
Rofecoxib
Ropinirole Hydrochloride
Rosiglitazone Maleate
Rubella Virus Vaccine, Live
Salmeterol Xinafoate
Sargamostim
Scopolamine
Selegiline Hydrochloride
Sertaconazole Nitrate
Sertraline Hydrochloride
Sevelamer Hydrochloride/
  Monohydrate
Sirolimus
Sodium Benzoate/Sodium
  Phenylacelate
Sodium Phenylbutyrate
Sodium Sulfacetamide/Sulfur
Solifenacin Succinate
Somatropin
Somatropin (rDNA Origin)

Stavudine
Streptokinase
Succimer
Sulfacetamide Sodium
Sulfamethoxazole Trimethoprim
Sulfanilamide
Sumatriptan
Sumatriptan Succinate
Tacrine Hydrochloride
Tacrolimus
Telithromycin
Telmisartan
Telmisartan/
  Hydrochlorothiazide*
Tenecteplase
Terazosin Hydrochloride
Teriparatide
Tetanus & Diphtheria Toxoids
  Adsorbed
Tetanus Immunde Globulin
  (Human)
Theophylline
Theophylline Anhydrous
Thiabendazole
Thrombin
Thyrotropin Alfa
Tiagabine Hydrochloride
Tiludronate Disodium
Timolol Hemihydrate
Timolol Maleate
Timolol Maleate
  Hydrochlorothiazide
Tinidazole
Tiotropium Bromide
Tipranavir
Tizanidine Hydrochloride
Tobramycin/Dexamethasone
Tobramycin/Loteprednol
  Etabonate
Tolcapone
Tolterodine Tartrate
Topiramate
Tramadol Hydrochloride
Tramodol Hydrochloride/
  Acetaminophen
Trandolapril*
Trandolapril/Verapamil
  Hydrochloride*
Travoprost
Tretinoin
Triamcinolone Acetonide
Triamterene
Triamterene/
  Hydrochlorothiazide
Trientine Hydrochloride
Triethanolamine Polypeptide
  Oleate-Condensate
Trifluridine
Trimethoprim Hydrochloride
Trimipramine Maleate
Tropicamide/

Hydroxyamphetamine
  Hydrobromide
Trospium Chloride
Trovafloxacin Mesylate
Tuberculin Purified Protein
  Derivative, Diluted
Typhoid Vaccine Live Oral
  Ty21A
Unprostone Isopropyl
Urea
Valdecoxib
Valganciclovir Hydrochloride
Valsartan*
Valsartan/
  Hydrochlorothiazide*
Varicella Virus Vaccine, Live
Venlafaxine Hydrochloride
Verapamil Hydrochloride
Verteporfin
Vitamin K1
Yellow Fever Vaccine
Zalcitabine
Zaleplon
Zavamivir
Zidovudine
Zileuton
Ziprasidone Mesylate
Zolmitriptan
Zonisamide

B

NO EVIDENCE OF RISK IN HUMANS

Either animal findings show risk while human findings do not, or, if no adequate human studies have been done, animal findings are negative.
Acarbose
Acrivastine
Acyclovir
Acyclovir Sodium
Adalimumab
Agalsidase Beta
Alefacept
Alfuzosin Hydrochloride
Alosetron Hydrochloride
Amiloride Hydrochloride
Amiloride Hydrochloride/
  Hydrochlorthiazide
Amoxicillin
Amoxicillin/Clavulanate
  Potassium
Amphotericin B
Amphotericin B Lipid
  Complex
Amphotericin B, Liposomal

Amphotericin B/Cholesteryl
  Sulfate Complex
Ampicillin Sodium/Sulbactam
  Sodium
Anakinra
Anithrombin III
Aprepitant
Aprotinin
Argatroban
Arginine Hydrochloride
Atazanavir Sulfate
Azalaic Acid
Azithromycin
Azithromycin Dihydrate
Aztreonam
Balsalazide Disodium
Basiliximab
Bivalirudin
Brimonidine Tartrate
Budesonide
Bupropion Hydrochloride
Cabergoline
Carbenicillin Indanyl Sodium
Cefaclor
Cefazolin Sodium
Cefdinir
Cefditoren Pivoxil
Cefepime Hydrochloride
Cefixime
Cefoperazone Sodium
Cefotaxime Sodium
Cefotetan Disodium
Cefoxitin Sodium
Cefpodoxime Proxetil
Cefprozil
Ceftazidime Sodium
Ceftibuten Dihydrate
Ceftizoxime Sodium
Ceftriaxone Sodium
Cefuroxime
Cefuroxime Axetil
Cephalexin
Cetirizine Hdyrochloride
Ciclopirox
Ciclopirox Olamine
Cimetidine
Cimetidine Hydrochloride
Cisatracurium Besylate
Clindamycin Hydrochloride/
  Clindamycin Phosphate
Clindamycin Palmitate/
  Hydrochloride
Climdamycin Phosphate
Clopidogrel Bisulfate
Clotrimazole
Clozapine
Colesevelam Hydrochloride
Cromolyn Sodium
Cyclobenzaprine
  Hydrochloride

Cyproheptadine
  Hydrochloride
Dalfopristin/Quinupristin
Dalteparin Sodium
Dapiprazole Hydrochloride
Daptomycin
Desflurane
Desmopressin Acetate
Dicyclomine Hydrochloride
Didanosine
Diphenhydramine
  Hydrochloride
Dipivefrin Hydrochloride
Dipyridamole
Dolasetron Mesylate
Dornase Alfa
Doxapram Hydrochloride
Doxepin Hydrochloride
Doxercalciferol
Edetate Calcium Disodium
Emtricitabine
Emtricitabine/Tenofovir
  Disoproxil Fumarate
Enfuvirtide
Enoxaparin Sodium
Eplerenone
Epoprostenol Sodium
Ertapenem
Erythromycin
Erythromycin Ethylsuccinate
Erythromycin Stearate
Esomeprazole Magnesium
Esomeprazole Sodium
Etanercept
Ethacrynate Sodium
Ethacrynic Acid
Famciclovir
Famotidine
Fenoldopam Mesylate
Fondaparinux Sodium
Galantamine Hydrobromide
Glatiramer Acetate
Glucagon
Glyburide/Metformin
  Hydrochloride
Granisetron Hydrochloride
Hydrochlorothiazide
Ibuprofen
Indapamide
Infliximab
Insulin Lispro Protamine,
  Human/Insulin Lispro,
  Human
Insulin Lispro, Human
Ipratropium Bromide
Iron Sucrose
Isosorbide Mononitrate
Lactulose
Lansoprazole
Lansoprazole/Naproxen

Laronidase
Lepirudin
Levocarnitine
Lidocaine
Lidocaine Hydrochloride
Lidocaine/Prilocaine
Lindane
Loperamide Hydrochloride
Loracarbef
Loratadine
Malathion
Meclizine Hydrochloride
Memantine Hydrochloride
Meropenem
Mesalamine
Metformin Hydrochloride
Methohexital Sodium
Methyldopa
Metolazone
Metronidazole
Miglitol
Montelukast Sodium
Mupirocin
Mupirocin Calcium
Naftifine Hydrochloride
Nalbuphine Hydrochloride
Nalmefene Hydrochloride
Naloxone Hydrochloride
Naproxen Sodium
Nedocromil Sodium
Nevlfinavir Mesylate
Nitazoxanide
Nitrofurantoin Macrocrystals
Nitrofurantoin Macrocrystals/
  Nitrofurantoin
  Monohydrate
Nizatidine
Ocreotide Acetate
Omalizumab
Ondansetron
Ondansetron Hydrochloride
Orlistat
Oxiconazole Nitrate
Oxybutynin
Oxybutynin Chloride
Oxycodone Hydrochloride
Palonosetron Hydrochloride
Pancrelipase
Pantoprazole Sodium
Pegvisomant
Pemoline
Penciclovir
Penicillin G Benzathine
Penicillin G Benzathine/
  Peniciillin G Procaine
Penicillin G Potassium
Pentosan Polysulfate Sodium
Pergolide Mesylate
Permethrin
Piperacillin Sodium
(*Continued on next page*)

Piperacillin Sodium/
  Tazabactam Sodium
Praziquantel
Progesterone
Propofol
Pseudoephedrine
  Hydrochloride
Pseudoephedrine Sulfate
Psyllium Preparations
Rabeprazole Sodium
Ranitidine Hydrochloride
Rifabutin
Ritonavir
Rivastigmine Tartrate
Ropivacaine Hydrochloride
Saquinvair
Saquinvair Mesylate
Sevoflurane
Sildenafil Citrate
Silver Sulfadiazine

Sodium Ferric Gluconate
Somatropin
Sotalol Hydrochloride
Sucralfate
Sulfasalazine
Tadalafil
Tamsulosin Hydrochloride
Tegaserod Maleate
Tenofovir Disoproxil Fumarate
Terbinafine Hydrochloride
Ticarcillin Disodium/
    Clavulanate Potassium
Ticlopidine Hydrochloride
Tirofiban Hydrochloride
Torsemide
Trastuzumab
Treprostinil Sodium
Urokinase
Ursodiol
Valacyclovir Hydrochloride

Vancomycin Hydrochloride
Vardefanil Hydrochloride
Zafirlukast
Zolpidem Tartrate

A

**CONTROLLED STUDIES
SHOW NO RISK**
*Adequate, well-controlled
studies in pregnant women
have failed to demonstrate
risk to the fetus.*
Levothyroxine Sodium
Liothyronine Sodium
Liotrix
Nystatin

Reprinted with permission from *The Drug Topics Red Book.* Montvale NJ: Thomson Medical Economics, 2006.

Drugs Excreted in Breast Milk

The following list is not comprehensive; generic forms and alternate brands of some products may be available. When recommending drugs to pregnant or nursing patients, always check product labeling for specific precautions.

Accolate
Accuretic
Aciphex
Actiq
Activella
Actonel with Calcium
ActoPlus Met
Actos
Adalat
Adderall
Advicor
Aggrenox
Aldactazide
Aldactone
Aldomet
Aldoril
Alesse
Allegra-D
Alfenta
Aloprim
Altace
Ambien
Anaprox
Ancef
Androderm
Antara
Apresoline
Aralen
Arthrotec
Asacol
Ativan

Augmentin
Avalide
Avandia
Avetox
Axid
Axocet
Azactam
Azasari
Azathloprine
Azulfidine
Bactrim
Baraclude
Benadryl
Bentyl
Betapace
Bextra
Bexxar
Bicllin
Biocadren
Boniva
Brethine
Brevicone
Brontex
Byetta
Caduet
Cafergot
Calan
Campral
Capoten
Capozide
Captopril

Carbatrol
Cardizem
Cataflam
Catapres
Ceclor
Cefizox
Cefobid
Cefotan
Ceftin
Celebrex
Celexa
Ceptaz
Cerebyx
Ceredase
Cipro
Ciprodex
Claforan
Clarinex
Claritin
Claritin-D
Cleocin
Climara
Clozaril
Codeine
CombiPatch
Combipres
Combivir
Combunox
Compazine
Cordarone
Corgard

Cortisporin	Enduron	Lamprene
Corzide	Epzicom	Lanoxicaps
Cosopt	Equetro	Lanoxin
Coumadin	ERYC	Lariam
Covera-HS	EryPed	Lescol
Cozaar	Ery-Tab	Levbid
Crestor	Erythrocin	Levitra
Crinone	Erythromycin	Levlen
Cyclessa	Esgic-plus	Levlite
Cymbalta	Eskalith	Levora
Cystospaz	Estrogel	Levothroid
Cytomel	Estrostep	Levoxyl
Cytotec	Ethmozine	Levsin
Cytoxan	Evista	Levsinex
Dapsone	FazaClo	Lexapro
Daraprim	Felbatol	Lexiva
Darvon	Feldene	Lexxel
Darvon-N	femhrt	Lindane
Decadron	Florinal	Lioresal
Deconsal II	Flagyl	Lipitor
Demerol	Florinef	Lithium
Demulen	Floxin	Lithobid
Depacon	Foradil	Lo/Ovral
Depakene	Fortamet	Loestrin
Depakote	Fortaz	Lomotil
DepoDur	Fosamax Plus D	Loniten
Depo-Provera	Furosemide	Lopressor
Desogen	Gabitril	Lortab
Desoxyn	Galzin	Lostensin
Desyrel	Garamycin	Lotrel
Dexedrine	Glucophage	Luminal
DextroStat	Glyset	Luvox
D.H.E.45	Guaifed	Lyrica
Diabinese	Halcion	Macrobid
Diastat	Haldol	Macrodantin
Diflucan	Helidac	Marinol
Digitek	Hydrocet	Maxipime
Dilacor	Hydrocortone	Maxzide
Dilantin	HydroDIURIL	Mefoxin
Dilaudid	Iberet-Folic	Menostar
Diovan	Ifex	Methergine
Diprivan	Imitrex	Methotrexate
Diuril	Imuran	MetroCream/
Dolobid	Inderal	Gel/Lotion
Dolophine	Ideride	Mexitil
Doral	Indocin	Micronor
Doryx	INFed	Microzide
Droxia	Inspra	Midamor
Duracion	Invanz	Migranal
Duragesic	Inversine	Miltown
Duramorph	Isoptin	Minizide
Duratuss	Kadlan	Minocin
Duricef	Keflex	Mirapex
Dyazide	Keppra	Mircette
Dyrenium	Kerlone	M-M-R II
E.E.S.	Ketek	Mobic
EC-Naprosyn	Klonopin	Modicon
Ecotrin	Kronofed-A	Moduretic
Effexor	Kutrase	Monodox
Elestat	Lamictal	Monopril
EMLA	Lamisil	Morphine

(*Continued on next page*)

MS Contin
MSIR
Myambutol
Mycamine
Mysoline
Namenda
Naprelan
Naprosyn
Nascobal
Necon
NegGram
Nembutal
Neoral
Niaspan
Nicotrol
Niravam
Nizoral
Norco
Nor-QD
Nordette
Norinyl
Noritate
Normodyne
Norpace
Norplant
Novantrone
Nubain
Nucofed
Nydrazid
Oramorph
Oretic
Ortho-Cept
Ortho-Cyclen
Ortho-Novum
Ortho Tri-Cyclen
Orudis
Ovcon
Oxistat
OxyContin
OxyFast
OxyIR
Pacerone
Pamelor
Pancrease
Paxil
PCE
Pediapred
Pediazole
Pediotic
Pentasa
Pepcid
Periostat
Persantine
Pfizerpen
Phenergan
Phenobarbital
Phrenilin
Pipracil
Plan B
Ponstel
Pravachol

Premphase
Prempro
Prevacid
Prevacid NapraPAC
PREVPAC
Prinzide
Procanbid
Prograf
Proloprim
Prometrium
Pronestyl
Propofol
Prosed/DS
Protonix
Provera
Prozac
Pseudoephedrine
Pulmicort
Pyrazinamide
Quinidex
Quinine
Raptiva
Reglan
Relpax
Renese
Requip
Reserpine
Restoril
Retrovir
Rifadin
Rifamate
Rifater
Rimactane
Risperdal
Rocaltrol
Rocephin
Roferon A
Roxanol
Rozerem
Sanctura
Sandimmune
Sarafem
Seconal
Sectral
Semprex-D
Septra
Seroquel
Sinequan
Slo-bid
Soma
Sonata
Spiriva
Sporanox
Stadol
Streptomycin
Stromectol
Symbyax
Symmetrel
Synthroid
Tagamet
Tambocor

Tapazole
Tarka
Tavist
Tazicef
Tazidime
Tegretol
Tenoretic
Tenormin
Tenuate
Tequin
Testoderm
Thalitone
Theo-24
The-Dur
Thorazine
Tiazac
Timolide
Timoptic
Tindamax
Tobi
Tofranil
Tolectin
Toprol-XL
Toradol
Trandate
Tranxene
Trental
Tricor
Triglide
Trilafon
Trileptal
Tri-Levlen
Trilisate
Tri-Norinyl
Triostat
Triphasil
Trivora
Trizivir
Trovan
Truvada
Tygacil
Tylenol
Tylenol with Codeine
Ultane
Ultram
Unasyn
Uniphyl
Uniretic
Unithroid
Urimax
Valium
Valtrex
Vanceril
Vancocin
Vantin
Vascor
Vaseretic
Vasotec
Ventavis
Verelan
Vermox

Versed	Zantac	Zomig
Vibramycin	Zarontin	Zonalon
Vibra-Tabs	Zaroxolyn	Zonegran
Vicodin	Zegerid	Zosyn
Vigamox	Zemplar	Zovia
Viramune	Zestoretic	Zovirax
Voltaren	Zetia	Zyban
Vytorin	Ziac	Zydone
Wellbutrin	Zinacef	Zyloprim
Xanax	Zithromax	Zyprexa
Xolair	Zocor	Zyrtec

Reprinted with permission from *The Drug Products Red Book.* Montvale NJ: Thomson Medical Economics, 2006.

Low Potassium Diet

Potassium is a mineral found in most foods except sugar and lard. It plays a role in maintaining normal muscle activity and helps keep body fluids in balance. Too much potassium in the blood can lead to changes in the heartbeat and can lead to muscle weakness. The kidneys normally help keep blood potassium controlled, but in kidney disease or when certain drugs are taken, dietary potassium must be limited to maintain a normal level of potassium in the blood.

The following guidelines include 2–3 g of potassium per day.

- **Milk group.** Limit to 1 cup serving of milk or milk product (yogurt, cottage cheese, ice cream, pudding).
- **Fruit group.** Limit to two servings daily from the low potassium choices. Watch serving sizes. Avoid the high potassium choices.
- **Low potassium**

Apple, 1 small
Apple juice, applesauce $^1/_2$ cup
Apricot, 1 medium or $^1/_2$ cup canned in syrup
Blueberries, $^1/_2$ cup
Cherries, canned in syrup $^1/_3$ cup
Cranberries, cranberry juice $^1/_2$ cup
Fruit cocktail, canned in syrup $^1/_2$ cup
Grapes, 10 fresh
Lemon, lime 1 fresh
Mandarin orange, canned in syrup $^1/_2$ cup
Nectar: apricot, pear, peach $^1/_2$ cup
Peach, 1 small or $^1/_2$ cup canned with syrup
Pear, 1 small or $^1/_2$ cup canned with syrup
Pineapple, $^1/_2$ cup raw or canned with syrup
Plums, 1 small or $^1/_2$ cup canned with syrup
Tangerine, 1 small
Watermelon, $^1/_2$ cup

- **High potassium**

Avocado
Banana
Cantaloupe
Cherries, fresh
Dried fruits
Grapefruit, fresh and juice
Honeydew melon
Kiwi
Mango
Nectarine
Orange, fresh and juice
Papaya
Prunes, prune juice
Raisins

- **Avoid.** Avoid using the following salt substitutes owing to their high potassium content: Adolph's, Lawry's Season Salt Substitute, No Salt, Morton Season Salt Free, Nu Salt, Papa Dash, and Morton Lite Salt.

Tyramine Content of Foods

Food	Allowed	Minimize Intake	Not Allowed
Beverages	Milk, decaffeinated coffee, tea, soda	Chocolate beverage, caffeine-containing drinks, clear spirits	Acidophilus milk, beer, ale, wine, malted beverages
Breads/cereals	All except those containing cheese	None	Cheese bread and crackers
Dairy products	Cottage cheese, farmers or pot cheese, cream cheese, ricotta cheese, all milk, eggs, ice cream, pudding (except chocolate)	Yogurt (limit to 4 oz. per day)	All other cheeses (aged cheese, American, Camembert, Cheddar, Gouda, Gruyère, mozzarella, parmesan, provolone, Romano, Roquefort, stilton)
Meat, fish, and poultry	All fresh or frozen	Aged meats, hot dogs, canned fish and meat	Chicken and beef liver, dried and pickled fish, summer or dry sausage, pepperoni, dried meats, meat extracts, bologna, liverwurst
Starches— potatoes/rice	All	None	Soybean (including paste)
Vegetables	All fresh, frozen, canned, or dried vegetable juices except those not allowed	Chili peppers, Chinese pea pods	Fava beans, sauerkraut, pickles, olives, Italian broad beans
Fruit	Fresh, frozen, or canned fruits and fruit juices	Avocado, banana, raspberries, figs	Banana peel extract
Soups	All soups not listed to limit or avoid	Commercially canned soups	Soups which contain broad beans, fava beans, cheese, beer, wine, any made with flavor cubes or meat extract, miso soup
Fats	All except fermented	Sour cream	Packaged gravy
Sweets	Sugar, hard candy, honey, molasses, syrups	Chocolate candies	None
Desserts	Cakes, cookies, gelatin, pastries, sherbets, sorbets	Chocolate desserts	Cheese-filled desserts
Miscellaneous	Salt, nuts, spices, herbs, flavorings, Worcestershire sauce	Soy sauce, peanuts	Brewer's yeast, yeast concentrates, all aged and fermented products, monosodium glutamate, vitamins with brewer's yeast

NATIONAL AND STATE BOARDS OF PHARMACY CONTACT INFORMATION

This appendix contains the most recent contact information for the national and state boards of pharmacy. A current listing of contact information for state boards of pharmacy is maintained at the National Association of Boards of Pharmacy website, www.napb.com. In addition, contact information for all the pharmacy schools in the United States can be found at the American Association of Colleges of Pharmacy Web site, www.aacp.org.

National Association of Boards of Pharmacy
Carmen A. Catizone
Executive Director
1600 Feehanville Drive
Mount Prospect, IL 60056
Phone: 847/391-4406
Fax: 847/391-4502
Web site: www.nabp.net

State Boards of Pharmacy
Alabama State Board of Pharmacy
Louise Foster Jones
Executive Secretary
10 Inverness Center, Suite 110
Birmingham, AL 35242
Phone: 205/981-2280
Fax: 205/981-2330
Web site: www.albop.com
E-mail: ljones@albop.com

Alaska Board of Pharmacy
Sher Zinn
Licensing Examiner
PO Box 110806
Juneau, AK 99811-0806
Phone: 907/465-2589
Fax: 907/465-2974
Web site: www.commerce.state.ak.us/occ/ppha.htm
E-mail: sher_zinn@commerce.state.ak.us
(through the Division of Occupational Licensing)

Arizona State Board of Pharmacy
Harlan Wand
Executive Director
4425 West Olive Avenue, Suite 140
Glendale, AZ 85302-3844
Phone: 623/463-2727
Fax: 623/934-0583
Web site: www.pharmacy.state.az.us
E-mail: hwand@azsbp.com

Arkansas State Board of Pharmacy
Charles S. Campbell
Executive Director
101 East Capitol, Suite 218
Little Rock, AR 72201
Phone: 501/682-0190
Fax: 501/682-0195
Web site: www.arkansas.gov/asbp
E-mail: charlie.campbell@arkansas.gov

California State Board of Pharmacy
Patricia F. Harris
Executive Officer
1625 North Market Boulevard, N219
Sacramento, CA 95834
Phone: 916/574-7900
Fax: 916/574-8618
Web site: www.pharmacy.ca.gov/
E-mail: patricia_harris@dca.ca.gov

Colorado State Board of Pharmacy
Susan L. Warren
Program Director
1560 Broadway, Suite 1310
Denver, CO 80202-5143
Phone: 303/894-7800
Fax: 303/894-7764
Web site: www.dora.state.co.us/pharmacy
E-mail: susan.warren@dora.state.co.us

Connecticut Commission of Pharmacy
Michelle Sylvestre
Drug Control Agent and Board Administrator
State Office Building, 165 Capitol Avenue Room 147
Hartford, CT 06106
Phone: 860/713-6070
Fax: 860/713-7242
Web site: www.ct.gov/dcp/site/default.asp
E-mail: michelle.sylvestre@ct.gov

Delaware State Board of Pharmacy
David W. Dryden
Executive Secretary
Division of Professional Regulation
Cannon Bulding
861 Silver Lake Boulevard, Suite 203
Dover, DE 19904
Phone: 302/744-4526
Fax: 302/739-2711
Web site: www.dpr.delaware.gov
E-mail: debop@state.de.us

District of Columbia Board of Pharmacy
Bonnie Rampersaud
Executive Director
717 Fourteenth Street NW, Suite 600
Washington, DC 20005
Phone: 202/724-4900
Fax: 202/727-8471
Web site: www.dchealth.dc.gov
E-mail: graphelia.ramseur@dc.gov

Florida Board of Pharmacy
Rebecca Poston
Executive Director
4052 Bald Cypress Way, Bin #C04
Tallahassee, FL 32399-3254
Phone: 850/245-4292
Fax: 850/413-6982
Web site: www.doh.state.fl.us/mga
E-mail: rebecca_poston@doh.state.fl.us

Georgia State Board of Pharmacy
Sylvia L. "Sandy" Bond
Executive Director
Professional Licensing Boards
237 Coliseum Drive
Macon, GA 31217-3858
Phone: 478/207-1640
Fax: 478/207-1660
Web site: www.sos.state.ga.us/plb/pharmacy
E-mail: sibond@sos.state.ga.us

Guam Board of Examiners for Pharmacy
Jane M. Diego
Secretary for the Board
PO Box 2816
Hagatna, GU 96932
Phone: 671/735-7406 ext 11
Fax: 671/735-7413
E-mail: jmdiego@dphss.govguam.net

Hawaii State Board of Pharmacy
Lee Ann Teshima
Executive Officer
PO Box 3469
Honolulu, HI 96801
Phone: 808/586-2694
Fax: 808/586-2874
Web site: www.hawaii.gov/dcca/areas/pvl/
  boards/pharmacy
E-mail: pharmacy@dcca.hawaii.gov

Idaho Board of Pharmacy
Richard Markuson
Executive Director
3380 Americana Terrace, Suite 320
Boise, ID 83706
Phone: 208/334-2356
Fax: 208/334-3536
Web site: www.accessidaho.org/bop/
E-mail: rmarkuson@bop.state.id.us

Illinois Department of Financial and Professional
  Regulation, Division of Professional
  Regulation-State Board of Pharmacy
Kim Scott
Pharmacy Board Liaison
320 West Washington, 3rd Floor
Springfield, IL 62786
Phone: 217/782-8556
Fax: 217/782-7645
Web site: www.idfpr.com
E-mail: PRFGROUP10@idfpr.com
(through Department of Professional
  Regulation)

Indiana Board of Pharmacy
Marty Allain, Director
Director
402 West Washington Street, Room W072
Indianapolis, IN 46204-2739
Phone: 317/234-2067
Fax: 317/233-4236
Web site: http://www.in.gov/pla/bandc/isbp/
E-mail: pla4@pla.IN.gov

Iowa Board of Pharmacy Examiners
Lloyd K. Jessen
Executive Director/Secretary
400 Southwest Eighth Street, Suite E
Des Moines, IA 50309-4688
Phone: 515/281-5944
Fax: 515/281-4609
Web site: www.state.ia.us/ibpe
E-mail: Lloyd.jessen@ibpe.state.ia.us

Kansas State Board of Pharmacy
Debra L. Billingsley
Executive Secretary/Director
Landon State Office Building, 900 Jackson,
  Room 560
Topeka, KS 66612-1231
Phone: 785/296-4056 Fax: 785/296-8420
Web site: http://www.kansas.gov/pharmacy
E-mail: pharmacy@pharmacy.state.ks.us

Kentucky Board of Pharmacy
Michael A. Burleson
Executive Director
Spindletop Administration Building, Suite 302,
2624 Research Park Drive,
Lexington, KY 40511
Phone: 859/246-2820
Fax: 859/246-2823
Web site: http://pharmacy.ky.gov/
E-mail: mike.burleson@ky.gov

Louisiana Board of Pharmacy
Malcolm J. Broussard
Executive Director
5615 Corporate Boulevard, Suite 8E
Baton Rouge, LA 70808-2537
Phone: 225/925-6496
Fax: 225/925-6499
Web site: www.labp.com
E-mail: mbroussard@labp.com

Maine Board of Pharmacy
Geraldine Betts
Board Administrator
Department of Professional/Financial Regulation
35 State House Station
Augusta, ME 04333
Phone: 207/624-8689
Fax: 207/624-8637
Hearing Impaired: 207/624-8563
PFR/OLR Web site:
  www.maineprofessionalreg.org
E-mail: for all Licensing and Board Meeting
  Information/Inquires and for Application
  packets: kelly.l.mclaughlin@maine.gov
Enforcement inquiries:
  gregory.w.cameron@maine.gov
Administration and all other Inquiries:
  geraldine.l.betts@maine.gov

Maryland Board of Pharmacy
La Verne George Naesea
Executive Director
4201 Patterson Avenue
Baltimore, MD 21215-2299
Phone: 410/764-4755
Fax: 410/358-6207
Web site: http://www.dhmh.state.md.us/
  pharmacyboard/
E-mail: lnaesea@dhmh.state.md.us

Massachusetts Board of Registration in
  Pharmacy
Charles R. Young
Executive Director
239 Causeway Street, 2nd Floor
Boston, MA 02114
Phone: 617/973-0800
Fax: 617/973-0983
Web site: www.mass.gov/dpl/boards/ph/
  index.htm
E-mail: charles.young@state.ma.us

Michigan Board of Pharmacy
Rae Ramsdell
Director, Licensing Division
611 West Ottawa, 1st Floor
PO Box 30670
Lansing, MI 48909-8170
Phone: 517/335-0918
Fax: 517/373-2179
Web site: http://www.michigan.gov/healthlicense
Email: rhramsd@michigan.gov

Minnesota Board of Pharmacy
Cody C. Wiberg
Executive Director
2829 University Avenue SE, Suite 530
Minneapolis, MN 55414-3251
Phone: 612/617-2201
Fax: 612/617-2212
Web site: http://www.phcybrd.state.mn.us
E-mail: Cody.Wiberg@state.mn.us

Mississippi State Board of Pharmacy
Leland McDivitt
Executive Director
204 Key Drive, Suite C
Madison, MS 39110
Phone: 601/605-5388 Fax: 601/605-9546
Web site: www.mbp.state.ms.us
E-mail: lmcdivitt@mbp.state.ms.us

Missouri Board of Pharmacy
Kevin E. Kinkade
Executive Director
PO Box 625
Jefferson City, MO 65102
Phone: 573/751-0091
Fax: 573/526-3464
Web site: http://www.pr.mo.gov/pharmacists.asp
E-mail: kevin.kinkade@pr.mo.gov

Montana Board of Pharmacy
Executive Director
PO Box 200513
301 South Park Avenue, 4th Floor
Helena, MT 59620-0513
Phone: 406/841-2355
Fax: 406/841-2305
Web site: http://mt.gov/dli/bsd/license/
  bsd_boards/pha_board/board_page.asp
E-mail: dlibsdpha@state.mt.us

Nebraska Board of Pharmacy
Becky Wisell
Executive Secretary
PO Box 94986
Lincoln, NE 68509-4986
Phone: 402/471-2118
Fax: 402/471-3577
Web site: www.hhs.state.ne.us
E-mail: becky.wisell@hhss.ne.gov

Nevada State Board of Pharmacy
Larry L. Pinson
Executive Secretary
555 Double Eagle Circuit, Suite 1100
Reno, NV 89521
Phone: 775/850-1440
Fax: 775/850-1444
Web site: http://state.nv.us/pharmacy
E-mail: pharmacy@govmail.state.nv.us

New Hampshire Board of Pharmacy
Paul G. Boisseau
Executive Secretary
57 Regional Drive
Concord, NH 03301-8518
Phone: 603/271-2350
Fax: 603/271-2856
Web site: www.nh.gov/pharmacy
E-mail: pharmacy.board@nh.gov

New Jersey Board of Pharmacy
Joanne Boyer
Executive Director
124 Halsey Street
Newark, NJ 07101
Phone: 973/504-6450
Fax: 973/648-3355
Web site: http://www.state.nj.us/lps/ca/
  boards.htm
E-mail: boyerj@dca.lps.state.nj.us

New Mexico Board of Pharmacy
William Harvey
Executive Director/Chief Durg Inspector
5200 Oakland NE, Suite A
Albuquerque, NM 87113
Phone: 505/222-9830
Fax: 505/222-9845
Web site: www.state.nm.us/pharmacy
E-mail: William.Harvey@state.nm.us

New York Board of Pharmacy
Lawrence H. Mokhiber
Executive Secretary
89 Washington Avenue, 2nd Floor W
Albany, NY 12234-1000
Phone: 518/474-3817 ext. 130
Fax: 518/473-6995
Web site: www.op.nysed.gov
E-mail: pharmbd@mail.nysed.gov

North Carolina Board of Pharmacy
Jack W. Campbell IV
Executive Director
PO Box 4560
Chapel Hill, NC 27515-4560
Phone: 919/942-4454
Fax: 919/967-5757
Web site: www.ncbop.org
E-mail: jcampbell@ncbop.org

North Dakota State Board of Pharmacy
Howard C. Anderson Jr
Executive Director
PO Box 1354
Bismarck, ND 58502-1354
Phone: 701/328-9535
Fax: 701/328-9536
Web site: www.nodakpharmacy.com
E-mail: ndboph@btinet.net

Ohio State Board of Pharmacy
William T. Winsley
Executive Director
77 South High Street Room 1702
Columbus, OH 43215-6126
Phone: 614/466-4143
Fax: 614/752-4836
Web site: www.pharmacy.ohio.gov
E-mail: exec@bop.state.oh.us

Oklahoma State Board of Pharmacy
Bryan H. Potter
Executive Director
4545 Lincoln Boulevard, Suite 112
Oklahoma City, OK 73105-3488
Phone: 405/521-3815
Fax: 405/521-3758
Web site: www.pharmacy.ok.gov
E-mail: pharmacy@pharmacy.ok.gov

Oregon State Board of Pharmacy
Gary A. Schnabel
Executive Director
800 Northeast Oregon Street, Suite 150
Portland, OR 97232
Phone: 971/673-0001
Fax: 971/673-0002
Web site: www.pharmacy.state.or.us
E-mail: pharmacy.board@state.or.us

Pennsylvania State Board of Pharmacy
Melanie Zimmerman
Executive Secretary
PO Box 2649
Harrisburg, PA 17105-2649
Phone: 717/783-7156
Fax: 717/787-7769
Web site: www.dos.state.pa.us/pharm
E-mail: st-pharmacy@state.pa.us

Puerto Rico Board of Pharmacy
Madga Bouet
Executive Director, Department of Health, Board
  of Pharmacy
Call Box 10200, Santurce, PR 00908
Phone: 787/724-7282
Fax: 787-725-7903
E-mail: mbouet@salud.gov.pr

Rhode Island Board of Pharmacy
Catherine A. Cordy
Executive Director
3 Capitol Hill, Room 205
Providence, RI 02908-5097
Phone: 401/222-2837
Fax: 401/222-2158
Web site: http://www.health.ri.gov/hsr/
  professions/pharmacy.php
E-mail: cathyc@doh.state.ri.us

South Carolina Department of Labor, Licensing, and Regulation-Board of Pharmacy
LeeAnn Bundrick
Administrator
Kingstree Building
110 Centerview Drive, Suite 306
Columbia, SC 29210
Phone: 803/896-4700
Fax: 803/896-4596
Web site: www.llronline.com/POL/pharmacy
E-mail: bundrici@llr.sc.gov

South Dakota State Board of Pharmacy
Dennis M. Jones
Executive Secretary
4305 South Louise Avenue, Suite 104
Sioux Falls, SD 57106
Phone: 605/362-2737
Fax: 605/362-2738
Web site: www.state.sd.us/doh/pharmacy
E-mail: dennis.jones@state.sd.us

Tennessee Board of Pharmacy
Terry Webb Grinder
Interim Executive Director
Tennessee Department of Commerce and
    Insurance,
Board of Pharmacy
Davy Crockett Tower, 2nd Floor
500 James Robertson Pkwy
Nashville, TN 37243-1149
Phone: 615/741-2718
Fax: 615/741-2722
Web site: www.state.tn.us/commerce/boards/
    pharmacy
E-mail: terry.grinder@state.tn.us

Texas State Board of Pharmacy
Gay Dodson
Executive Director
333 Guadalupe, Tower 3, Suite 600
Austin, TX 78701-3942
Phone: 512/305-8000
Fax: 512/305-8082
Web site: www.tsbp.state.tx.us
E-mail: gay.dodson@tsbp.state.tx.us

Utah Board of Pharmacy
Diana L. Baker
Bureau Manager
PO Box 146741
Salt Lake City, UT 84114-6741
Phone: 801/530-6179
Fax: 801/530-6511
Web site: http://www.dopl.utah.gov/
E-mail: dbaker@utah.gov
(through Division of Occupational and
    Professional Licensing)

Vermont Board of Pharmacy
Peggy Atkins
Board Administrator
Office of Professional Regulation
26 Terrace Street
Montpelier, VT 05609-1106
Phone: 802/828-2373
Fax: 802/828-2465
Web site: www.vtprofessionals.org
E-mail: patkins@sec.state.vt.us

Virgin Islands Board of Pharmacy
Lydia T. Scott
Executive Assistant
Department of Health
Schneider Regional Center
48 Sugar Estate
St. Thomas, VI 00802
Phone. 340/774-0117
Fax: 340/777-4001
E-mail:lydia.scott@usvi-doh.org

Virginia Board of Pharmacy
Elizabeth Scott Russell
Executive Director
6603 West Broad Street, 5th Floor
Richmond, VA 23230-1712
Phone: 804/662-9911
Fax: 804/662-9313
Web site: www.dhp.state.va.us/pharmacy/
    deafault.htm
(or through Department of Health Professions at
    www.dhp.state.va.us)
E-mail: scotti.russell@dhp.virginia.gov

Washington State Board of Pharmacy
Steven M. Saxe
Executive Director
PO Box 47863
Olympia, WA 98504-7863
Phone: 360/236-4825
Fax: 360/586-4359
Web site: https://fortress.wa.gov/doh/hpqa1/hps4/
    pharmacy/default.htm
E-mail: Steven.Saxe@doh.wa.gov

West Virginia Board of Pharmacy
William T. Douglass Jr
Executive Director and General Counsel
232 Capitol Street
Charleston, WV 25301
Phone: 304/558-0558
Fax: 304/558-0572
Web site: http://www.wvbop.com/
E-mail: wdouglass@wvbop.com

Wisconsin Pharmacy Examining Board
Tom Ryan
Bureau Director
1400 East Washington
PO Box 8935
Madison, WI 53708-8935
Phone: 608/266-2112
Fax: 608/267-0644
Web site: http://www.drl.state.wi.us/
E-mail: thomas.ryan@drl.state.wi.us

Wyoming State Board of Pharmacy
James T. Carder
Executive Director
632 South David Street
Casper, WY 82601
Phone: 307/234-0294
Fax: 307/234-7226
Web site: http://pharmacyboard.state.wy.us/
E-mail: wybop@state.wy.us

Reprinted with permission from National Association of Boards of Pharmacy, Mount Prospect, IL.

APPENDIX E

BUDGETING FOR DRUG INFORMATION RESOURCES

Basic Library

References	Cost[a]
American Hospital Formulary Service (AHFS) Drug Information	$ 209.00
Drug Facts and Comparisons	$ 205.00
Handbook on Injectable Drugs	$ 219.00
Handbook of Non-Prescription Drugs: An Interactive Approach to Self-Care	$ 145.00
Martindale: The Complete Drug Reference	$ 470.00
Nonprescription Product Therapeutics	$ 90.00
Physicians' Desk Reference	$ 95.00
Remington's Pharmaceutical Sciences	$ 125.00
USP DI (three-volume set)	$ 412.00

Additional Resources

References	Cost[a]
Drug–drug interaction	
Drug Interactions Analysis and Management	$ 195.00
Drug Interaction Facts	$ 217.00
Evaluations of Drug Interactions	$ 230.00
Herbal	
PDR for Herbal Medicines	$ 60.00
The Review of Natural Products	$ 173.00
Internal medicine	
Cecil Textbook of Medicine	$ 149.00
Harrison's Principles of Internal Medicine	$ 135.00
Pediatrics	
Pediatric Dosage Handbook	$ 47.00
The Harriet Lane Handbook	$ 40.00
Pharmacokinetics	
Applied Biopharmaceutics and Pharmacokinetics	$ 60.00
Clinical Pharmacokinetics	$ 69.00
Concepts in Clinical Pharmacokinetics	$ 100.00
Applied Pharmacokinetics and Pharmacodynamics: Principles of Therapeutic Drug Monitoring	$ 73.00
Pharmacology	
Goodman and Gilman's The Pharmacological Basis of Therapeutics	$ 139.00
Pregnancy/breast-feeding	
Drugs in Pregnancy and Lactation	$ 99.00
Therapeutics	
Applied Therapeutics: The Clinical Use of Drugs	$ 206.00
Pharmacotherapy: A Pathophysiologic Approach	$ 200.00
Textbook of Therapeutics: Drug and Disease Management	$ 157.00

(Continued on next page)

Continued.

References	Cost[a]
CD ROM computer systems/programs	
AHFS first WEB	$ 3,500.00
Clinical Pharmacology (online)	$ 495.00
Lexi–Comp online	$ 2,550.00
CliniTrend software	$ 722.00
DataKinetics software	$ 719.00
Facts and Comparisons 4.0 online (individual subscription)	$ 496.00
Iowa Drug Information System (online)	$ 9,600.00
IPA	$ 900.00
MD Consult (core collection, individual)	$ 220.00
Medline (primary component of PubMed)	0
MedTeach software	$ 565.00
Micromedex > 200 licensed bed facility	
Diseasedex	$16,000.00
Drugdex System	$16,500.00
Poisindex System	$16,900.00
Other Micromedex databases	
CareNotes System	$12,123.00
Drug–Reax	$ 2,081.00
Kinetidex	$ 4,126.00
Martindale: The Complete Drug Reference	$ 2,081.00
PDR	$ 6,954.00
P&T Quik	$ 1,669.00
Reprorisk	$ 3,164.00
UpToDate (stand-alone)	$1,495.00
Major online vendors	
Dialog	
EBSCOInformation Services	
Gale Group	
National Library of Medicine	
Ovid	
OCLC First Search	
Thomson Scientific	

[a]Costs are approximate and are based on 2005 figures. Costs depend on selection of format, site versus individual license fees, and concurrent users. Institutional subscriptions cost more than individual subscriptions.

Index

Pages in *italics* denote figures; those followed by a t denote tables.